Martino Ruggieri
Ignacio Pascual-Castroviejo
Concezio Di Rocco
(Eds.)

Neurocutaneous Disorders
Phakomatoses and Hamartoneoplastic Syndromes

SpringerWienNewYork

Martino Ruggieri
Institute of Neurological Science, National Research Council, Catania, Italy

Ignacio Pascual-Castroviejo
University Hospital La Paz, Madrid, Spain

Concezio Di Rocco
Institute of Neurosurgery, Catholic University of the Sacred Heart, Rome, Italy

© 2008 Springer-Verlag/Wien
Printed in Germany

SpringerWienNewYork is part of Springer Science + Business Media
springer.com

Typesetting: Thomson Press Ltd., Chennai, India
Printing: Strauss GmbH, 69509 Mörlenbach, Deutschland

Printed on acid-free and chlorine-free bleached paper
SPIN: 10997437

With numerous figures, some of them in colour

Library of Congress Control Number: 2006937726

ISBN 978-3-211-21396-4 SpringerWienNewYork

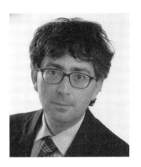

**Martino Ruggieri** is First Researcher in Paediatrics at the Institute of Neurological Science of the Italian National Research Council and at the Department of Paediatrics of the University of Catania, Italy and Associate Professor of Paediatrics (board certified, 2006). He graduated at the University of Catania and completed his postgraduate training at the Departments of Medical Genetics and Paediatrics, Churchill and John Radcliffe Hospitals, University of Oxford, UK and of Neurology and Neurogenetics, Massachusetts General Hospital, Harvard Medical School, Boston, USA. He trained on neurocutaneous disorders along with professors Lorenzo Pavone in Catania, Italy and Susan M. Huson in Oxford, UK. His postgraduate thesis was on the neurological manifestations of hypomelanosis of Ito and his PhD thesis on the different forms of neurofibromatosis. He is the International Deputy Editor of the *Journal of Brachial Plexus and Peripheral Nerve Injury* and the International Associate Editor (Paediatric Neurology) of *Child's Nervous System*. He is editor of a textbook of general paediatric neurology (in Italian). He currently runs in Catania, Italy a clinical and research programme devoted to neurocutaneous diseases. Research interests include the clinical manifestations of the different forms of neurofibromatosis in childhood, mosaic neurocutaneous phenotypes and paediatric multiple sclerosis.

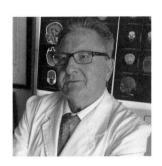

**Ignacio Pascual-Castroviejo** has been associate Professor of Paediatrics (Paediatric Neurology) at the University of Madrid and Chairman of Paediatric Neurology at the University Hospital "La Paz", Madrid, Spain from 1965 to 2004. He graduated at the Complutensis University of Madrid in 1962. He completed his postgraduate training in Madrid, in Würzbourg (Germany) and in Strasbourg (France). He obtained the board in Neurology in 1965 and the board in Paediatrics in 1971. He got his PhD in 1968 with a thesis on "Cerebral malformations and the Classification of corpus callosum and septum pellucidum malformations by pneumoencephalography". He has been one of the founding members of the International Child Neurology Association (ICNA) (1973) and the European Society of Neuroradiology (ESNR) (1969) and the President of the Spanish Society of Neurology and Spanish National Commission of Neurology. He is honorary member of several International Scientific Societies of Neurology, Neuroradiology, Paediatric Neurology and Paediatrics. He is member of the board of several international journals of Paediatric Neurology. He is editor of many textbooks (in Spanish and English) on general paediatric neurology, spinal tumours in infancy, attention-deficit hyperactivity disorder (ADHD), neurocutaneous disorders and contributed with chapters in the most acclaimed books on Neurocutaneous Disorders. Research interests include general paediatric neurology, neurocutaneous disorders, ADHD, vascular pathology, and neuroradiology.

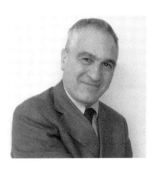

**Concezio Di Rocco** is Professor and Chairman of Paediatric Neurosurgery at the Catholic University of the Sacred Heart in Rome and Director of the Training Programme in Neurosurgery at the "Gemelli" University Hospital, Rome, Italy. He graduated at the Catholic University in Rome and completed his postgraduate trainings in Neurosurgery, Paediatric Neurosurgery and Paediatrics at the University of Genoa and at the North-western University Medical School, Children's Memorial Hospital of Chicago, USA. He has been President of the International Society for Paediatric Neurosurgery, European Society for Paediatric Neurosurgery and Vice- President of the European Association of Neurosurgical Societies. Currently, he is Chairman of the Paediatric Committee of the World Federation of Neurosurgical Societies and member of the teaching faculty at INI-China in Beijing. Professor Di Rocco is the Editor-in Chief of *Child's Nervous System* and member of board of several international journals of Neurosurgery and Neurosciences. Research interests include brain malformations, hydrocephalus, tumours, craniosynostoses, and neurocutaneous disorders.

To our wonderful Wives
Agata, Alicia and Paola

# NEUROCUTANEOUS DISORDERS

M. Ruggieri, I. Pascual-Castroviejo, and C. Di Rocco

## Phakomatoses and hamartoneoplastic diseases

The striking association of some neurological diseases with cutaneous abnormalities has long attracted the attention of physicians. Many such associations have been recognized; many are relatively rare conditions but, collectively, they account for a significant proportion of the neurological disorders especially in children. Their clinical manifestations are polymorphous, they may involve many others organs or systems in addition to skin and nervous system and they may be difficult to diagnose. Their clinical interest, their causes and mechanisms are closely related to several major basic biological problems and their study has contributed to shed light on such basic biological issues as the growth regulation and differentiation of tissues, opening new perspectives and leading to the introduction of new ideas and revision of others. Thus, the concepts that skin and CNS are entirely derived from the ectoderm had to be modified as mesoderm and endoderm are also involved. Likewise, the view that each of the three-germ layers is committed to generate specific derivatives had to be qualified as no developmental function appears to be restricted to a single layer and developmental genes appear to exert their specifying and signalling functions also on other layers. The essential role of the neural crest whose cells are of single origin as the major source of many neurocutaneous disorders is being now generally accepted. In the past few decades, molecular genetic studies have permitted considerable progresses in understanding the causes, mechanisms and classification, and new discoveries continue to challenge time-honoured concepts and generate new ones for example that of somatic mosaicism.

The neurocutaneous diseases have also proved to be of broad biological and clinical importance as their study may help unravel some of the causes and mechanisms of tumour formation and understand many aspects of oncogenesis, clearly a major theme of current and future investigation with major implications for public health and medical practice.

The amount of recent acquisitions, both on the clinical and basic aspects of the neurocutaneous diseases, has grown tremendously especially as a result of the recent development in neuroimaging and molecular genetics and it is now difficult to find an overall synthetic view of the complexities of this group of conditions. This difficulty makes the present work that brings together up to date data both timely and of considerable value for the many different categories of physicians and scientists that may become involved with these disorders.

Indeed, the general panorama of the neurocutaneous diseases is rapidly changing. New conditions have been recognized and the respective frequencies of the various types have changed with recent studies: for example the relatively recently described PHACE syndrome is now considered the commonest of all the neurocutaneous disorders.

There is no universal agreement on a definition of the neurocutaneous diseases. Early work mainly concerned the pakomatoses, especially tuberous sclerosis and the neurofibromatosis. The domain has considerably grown to include many other conditions in which variable amounts of cutaneous and neurological abnormalities tend to occur in persons with one same condition but not necessarily in the same person and most often with relatively independent involvement of various systems or organs. As a result, the clinical presentation of these conditions is extremely variable. Even major features may be missing in many accepted cases. In addition, extra-neurological and extra-cutaneous anomalies have been increasingly recognized and in some cases can represent the dominant clinical abnormalities. The causes and mechanisms are clearly multiple. Such heterogeneity further complicates the issues of classification and diagnosis. Indeed, if criteria for several specific entities have been established, no definite criteria have been adopted for the group as a whole, so the limits of the group of neurocutaneous syndromes can vary to some extent with the authors.

The editors of this book have opted for a broad definition of the neurocutaneous disorders, encompassing diseases in which the clinical association of the cutaneous and the neurological manifestations is not fortuitous, regardless of the mode of transmission, genetic or otherwise, of the mechanisms of disease, of the relative involvement of tissues or systems and of the possible involvement of tissues other than skin or the nervous system, provided that the cutaneous and neurological features are present.

This definition is not stringent and, in some cases, the decision as to whether minor dermatological of neurological features are sufficient to satisfy the requirement for dual tissue or organ involvement association may be somewhat arbitrary. However, it is eminently practical from the point of view of diagnosis as no clear borderline exists between the various causes and categories of neurocutaneous disorders and indeed the conditions included in the group have varied widely with authors. It does not attempt to give any cue about aetiology and classification and is admittedly imperfect and temporary.

However, such a simple approach permits to give a comprehensive description of all major neurocutaneous diseases on one simple clinical basis without having to justify their inclusion on the basis of dubious and not universally accepted criteria even though some conditions included may be regarded by some as disputable.

The comprehensive text is written by distinguished clinicians and investigators who have contributed significantly to their study, several of them having indeed given the first or early descriptions of the disease described, covers in great detail the clinical presentations and brings about complementary up to date biological data which will be of help in selecting the best investigations for confirmation of the diagnosis. Over seventy erudite chapters together with profuse and excellent illustrations and explanatory schemes and diagrams will guide the reader in the interpretation of the highly polymorphous clinical features and the significance of the necessary diagnostic investigations for these conditions many of which are rare or uncommon. The rarity and complexity of the neurocutaneous diseases point to the difficulties to master the topic in full, none the less, and this is a dilemma familiar to physicians, whether common or rare, these diseases exist, therefore the persons affected deserve to receive correct diagnosis and management.

Contrary to an unfortunately too common opinion, making a correct diagnosis is by no means an 'insect collection' exercise but is indeed of vital importance. For example, recognizing the minimal signs of neurofibromatosis I will radically alter the therapeutic approach to a brainstem tumour that may not necessitate irradiation when part of this disorder as opposed to isolated tumours, thus avoiding the tragic irradiation brain damage that was all too often observed in the past. Likewise, the diagnosis of many genetic conditions often rests critically on cutaneous, morphological or others non-obvious clinical or imaging details, essential to avoid incorrect genetic counselling which currently may have practical consequences including legal ones.

Given the complexity and the rarity of some of the neurocutaneous disorders, the necessity of imaging and connections with specialized laboratory facilities and the multiple skills necessary for their management, no single physician can cover both the diagnosis and management requirements of all patients. As a result, many centres are now offering a team approach to difficult cases, with multidisciplinary units or specialized clinics for the neurocutaneous diseases which can help doctors in their task to alleviate the burden that these conditions represent for the patients and society at large.

This work will go a long way to help clinicians face the complex challenges posed by the neurocutaneous disorders. It responds to the need for an up to date text about a group of conditions still largely unexplained and imperfectly diagnosed. I firmly believe it will become the standard text in the field for many years. It will obviously be a 'must' for neurologists and dermatologists especially those working with children, given the early age of clinical manifestations in most cases. Moreover, because the manifestations of the diseases studied can affect so many different tissues or organs, few clinicians will not need to use it for some cases and will like to find it at least in the hospital library as an essential reference work.

This book will also be helpful for the more biologically oriented physicians and biologists who want to keep abreast of many general biological problems such as carcinogenesis and molecular genetics and hopefully improve the condition of persons affected by the neurocutaneous diseases.

*Jean Aicardi MD, FRCP, Hon FRCPCH*

# PREFACE

This book sees the light of day after more than 5-year "gestation". The idea behind it originated in the early 2000' and was originally inspired by the superb manual (published in 1987) by the late professor Manuel Rodriguez Gomez (*Neurocutaneous Disorders. A Practical Approach*. Boston: Butterworths). The manual was a practical and comprehensive guide to compile the diagnosis and management of nearly all the common and rare neurocutaneous disorders recognised at that time. It was an exhaustive and authoritative source of clinical information coupled with the pathological and pathogenetic knowledge of the time, enriched by historical pearls on the "men behind the syndromes".

Since the publication of that edition, there have been significant advances in many aspects of this field, especially in molecular genetics and cellular biology. As a consequence of that the general panorama of the neurocutaneous disorders has changed. New entities have been delineated expanding the nosology of the whole group. The old concepts on the natural history and treatment of the various syndromes have been largely modified by the most recent large, population-based, clinical and genotype studies. In addition, it has become clearer that the most appropriate approach for the management of these disorders is multidisciplinary. At the same time, further important works on this and related topic(s) have been published delineating and establishing the present accepted definition(s) of the whole group of these disorders.

As all of the present editors have been running special clinics devoted to the diagnosis and management of children and adults with neurocutaneous disorders and have research interests in this field, we set out to create a new text, which could reflect all these recent acquisitions coupling the practical clinical and bedside diagnostic approaches with the current management issues and the modern basic science. To this purpose, we congregated an internationally renowned group of contributors, many of them the very same experts who first explored a particular disorder or established its present accepted definition.

Different from what was done in prior publications, in the present text we have included disorders, which had been only seldom reported or reported under such a variety of names that it was not clear they were distinct entities. By doing that we have opted in the end for a broad definition of the neurocutaneous disorders. This definition is not stringent and, in some cases, the decision as to whether minor skin or nervous system features were sufficient to satisfy the requirement for dual tissue or organ involvement association was on the basis of our personal clinical and research experience. In some cases, the inclusion of a certain condition among the spectrum of neurocutaneous disorders was dictated, besides its clinical phenotype, by a common pathogenic mechanism or a shared metabolic/cellular pathway. In a rapidly changing panorama of proteins, effectors, metabolites and receptors acting in common "cascades" (see for example Fig. 16, Chapter 5; Fig. 9, Chapter 19; or Fig. 8, Chapter 66) we opted for unifying rather than splitting groups of disorders. For these and other reasons (e.g., historical) we have also maintained in this book the handling of some conditions even when an overt skin (e.g., von Hippel-Lindau disease) or a frequent nervous system involvement (e.g., ILVEN syndrome) was lacking. In other cases the frequent similarities and/or overlaps between some disorders (e.g., Sturge-Weber vs Klippel-Trenaunay vs Parkes Weber syndromes; or CHILD syndrome vs CDP Conradi-Hunermann-Happle type/CDPX2 syndrome) prompted us to treat the whole spectrum of disorders. To this purpose we also chose to subtitle the book "*Phakomatoses and Hamartoneoplastic syndromes*" [borrowing the latter term from the classical (4th edition; published in 2001) of the text by Robert J. Gorlin, Michael M. Cohen Jr and Raoul C.M. Hennekam (*Syndromes of the Head and Neck*. Oxford: Oxford University Press)] – i.e., to emphasise that one of the aims of the present book was to encompass the whole spectrum of the classic neurocutaneous disorders and the less known conditions with "*phakomas*" and "*hamartomas*".

The book is deliberately in the format of a textbook rather than a manual and is conceived to address neurocutaneous disorders in a different way from other existing publications in the field. Its main philosophy consists in the discussion and wide illustration of neurocutaneous disorders, as it is much easier to recognise a disorder by seeing images rather than by only reading about clinical phenotypes. In line with such philosophy we also included many sections not only to detail historical and biographical aspects for the readers with a "historical turn of mind" but also to credit all the "women and men behind the eponyms" who attained their place in history not by accident, but by virtue of great gifts and consistent hard work of the highest quality in many fields besides medical field.

The 72 chapters were authored and co-authored by leading, world-renowned authorities in the various fields many times co-authored by one or more of us. We also undertook an enormous editorial revision of all contributions to give the book a homogeneous structure. This entailed editing the text and sometimes adding our own case material where we considered it useful to enrich or complete the various presentations. We would like to thank all contributors for their patience in accepting these frequent "intrusions" in their work. We also drew most of the line drawings ourselves, and included pathologic illustrations and anatomic preparations. Because the work on this book spanned several years, we also undertook a review, sometimes painful but hopefully thorough, of the more recent literature throughout the text.

Last but not least, we wish to thank all the people at Springer in Vienna, Austria, and especially our first contact person Mr Raimund Petri-Wieder and the current medical editor Mrs. Mag. Franziska Brugger; the production editors Mag. Judith Martiska and Ing. Mag. (FH) Karim Ernst Karman; the selling editor Mrs. Petra Kern; and the typesetter Thomson Digital, A Division of Thomson Press (India) Ltd., for the enduring kindness, patience, and trust that they bestowed in us, graciously accepting our too often controversial requests, believing that we would eventually succeed, and especially in pursuing a common goal. Their efforts coupled with the Springer's superb quality of printing and laying out made our initial aims concrete facts.

*Catania, Madrid and Rome,* July 2008

*Martino Ruggieri, MD, PhD*
*Ignacio Pascual-Castroviejo, MD, PhD*
*Concezio Di Rocco, MD*

# Contents

Subject index

Acknowledgements for figures or else

**Jean Aicardi MD, MRCP, Hon MRCPCH**
Institute of Child Health
30 Guilford Street
London WC1N 1EH
*Foreword*
jean.aicardi@free.fr

**Carmelo Amato, MD**
Unit of Neuroradiology
I.R.C.C.S. Oasi M. Santissima
Via Conte Ruggero, 73
940128 – Troina
Italy

**Enrico Bertini, MD**
Unit of Molecular Medicine
Department of Laboratory Medicine
Bambino Gesù Children's Research Hospital
Piazza S. Onofrio, 4
00165 – Rome
*Corresponding author: chapter 71*
ebertini@tin.it

**Maria del Carmen Boente, MD**
Department of Dermatology
Hospital del Niño Jesús
Pasaje Felipe, Bertrés 224
4000 – San Miguel de Tucumán,
Tucumán
Argentina
*Corresponding author: chapter 22*
mboente@arnet.com.ar

**Julita Borkowska, MD**
Department of Neurology and Epileptology
Children's Memorial Health Institute
Aleja Dzieci Polskich 20
04-730 – Warsaw
Poland

**Judith V.M.C. Bovée, MD**
Department of Pathology
Leiden University Medical Center
Albinusdreef 2, 2333 ZA
Leiden
The Netherlands

**Claudio Bruno, MD, PhD**
Muscular and Neurodegenerative Diseases Unit
Department of Pediatrics
University of Genoa
Giannina Gaslini Institute
Largo Gerolamo Gaslini, 5
16147 – Genoa
Italy
*Corresponding author: chapter 69*
claudiobruno@ospedale-gaslini.ge.it

**Luciana Chessa, MD, PhD**
Department of Experimental Medicine
2nd Faculty of Medicine
University "La Sapienza"
Via di Grottarossa, 1035
00160 - Rome
*Corresponding author: chapter 49*
Luciana.chessa@uniroma1.it

**Jill Clayton-Smith, MBChB, FRCP, FRCPCH, MD**
Academic Department of Medical Genetics
St Mary Hospital
St Mary's Hospital for Women & Children
Oxford Road
Manchester M13 9WL
United Kingdom

**Maria Rosa Cordisco, MD**
Department of Dermatology
Hospital de Pediatria "Prof. Dr. Juan P. Garrahan"
Combate de los Pozos 1881, 1245
Buenos Aires
Argentina
*Corresponding author: chapters 13*
cordisco@netizen.com.ar

**Concezio Di Rocco, MD**
Section of Pediatric Neurosurgery
Department of Pediatrics
Catholic University of Sacred Heart
Policlinico Gemelli
Largo Gemelli, 8
00168 – Rome
Italy
*Co-editor*
cdirocco@rm.unicatt.it

**Carlo Dionisi-Vici, MD**
Division of Metabolic Disorders
Department of Neuroscience
Bambino Gesù Children's Research Hospital
Piazza S. Onofrio, 4
00165 – Rome

**Maria Teresa Dotti, MD**
Department of Neurological and Behavioral Science
Medical School
University of Siena
Policlinico "Le Scotte"
Viale Bracci
53100 – Siena

**Carola Duràn-McKinster, MD**
Department of Dermatology
National Institute of Pediatrics
Insurgente Sur 3700-C
Mexico City 04530
Mexico

**May El Hachen, MD**
Division of Dermatology
Department of Pediatric Medicine
Department of Laboratory Medicine
Bambino Gesù Children's Research Hospital
Piazza S. Onofrio, 4
00165 – Rome

**Nancy Esterly, MD**
Department of Dermatology
Medical College of Wisconsin
Milwaukee
Wisconsin
101 Calle Contenta
Corrales, NM 87048
USA

**Raffaele Falsaperla, MD**
Unit of Pediatrics
University Hospital "Vittorio Emanuele"
via Plebiscito, 628
95100 – Catania
Italy
*Corresponding author: chapter 72*
raffaelefalsaperla@hotmail.com

**Antonio Federico, MD**
Department of Neurological and Behavioral Science
Medical School
University of Siena
Policlinico "Le Scotte"
Viale Bracci, 2
53100 – Siena
*Corresponding author: chapter 68*
federico@unisi.it

**Laura Flores-Sarnat, MD**
Division of Pediatric Neurology
Alberta Children's Hospital
2888 Shaganappi Trail NW
Calgary, AB T3B 6A8
Canada
*Corresponding author: chapter 1*
laura.flores-sarnat@calgaryhealthregion.ca

**Annalia Gabriele, MD**
Molecular Genetics Unit
Institute of Neurological Science
Italian National Research Council
Località Burga
87050 – Piano Lago Mangone
Italy

**Gian Nicola Gallus, MD**
Department of Neurological and Behavioral Science
Medical School
University of Siena
Policlinico "Le Scotte"
Viale Bracci
53100 – Siena

**Simone Gangarossa, MD**
Pediatric Unit
ASL 7
Via Risorgimento, 66
Ragusa
Italy

**Robert J. Gorlin, MD** [* *the late professor R.J. Gorlin*]
Department of Oral Pathology and Genetics
University of Minnesota
School of Dentistry
Twin Cities Campus

16-127 Moos Tower
515 Delaware Street S.E.
Minneapolis MN 55455
USA

**Jessica E. Gosnell, MD**
Department of Surgery and UCSF Comprehensive
   Cancer Center
1600 Divisadero, Room C348
University of California San Francisco/Mount Zion
   Medical Center
San Francisco
USA

**Takahiro Hamada, MD**
Department of Dermatology
Kurume University School of Medicine
67 Asahimachi
Kurume
Fukuoka
830-011
Japan
*Corresponding author: chapter 57*
hamataka@kurume-u.ac.jp

**Rudolf Happle, MD**
Department of Dermatology
Philipp University of Marburg
Deutschhausstr. 9
35037 Marburg
Germany

**Anna-Christine Hauser, MD**
Department of Medicine III
Division of Nephrology and Dialysis
Medical University of Vienna
Wahringergurtel 18-20
1090 Vienna
Austria
*Corresponding author: chapter 67*
anna-christine.hauser@meduniwien.ac.at

**Pancras C. W. Hogendoorn, MD, PhD**
Department of Pathology
Leiden University Medical Center
Albinusdreef 2, 2333 ZA
(Postbus 9600, 2300 RC)

Leiden
The Netherlands
*Corresponding author: chapter 15*
p.c.w.hogendoorn@lumc.nl

**Karl Hormann, MD**
Department of Otorhinolaryngology, Head and
   Neck Surgery
University Hospital Mannheim
Theodor-Kutzer-Ufer 1-3
D-68167 Mannheim
Germany

**Paola Iannetti, MD**
2nd Chair of Pediatrics
Division of Pediatric Neurology
Department of Pediatrics
University "La Sapienza"
Viale R. Elena 324
00186 – Rome
Italy

**S. Taylor Jarrell, MD**
Surgical Neurology Branch
National Institute of Neurological Disorders
   and Stroke
National Institutes of Health
10 Center Drive
Building 10, Room 5D37
Bethesda, MD 20892-1414
USA

**Sergiusz Jòzwiak, MD, PhD**
Department of Neurology and Epileptology
Children's Memorial Health Institute
Aleja Dzieci Polskich 20
04-730 – Warsaw
Poland
*Corresponding author: chapters 5, 20, 26 and 30*
s.jozwiak@czd.pl

**Electron Kebebew, MD, FACS**
Department of Surgery and UCSF Comprehensive
   Cancer Center
1600 Divisadero, Room C348
University of California San Francisco/Mount Zion
   Medical Center

San Francisco
USA
*Corresponding author: chapter 46*
kebebew@surgery.ucsf.edu

**Ingo Kennerknecht, MD**
Institute of Human Genetics
Westfalische Wilhelms
University of Munster
Schlossplatz 2
Munster D – 48149
Germany

**Orhan Konez, MD**
Department of Radiology, Vascular and
    Interventional Radiology
St. John West Shore Hospital
University Hospitals Case Medical Center
29000 Center Ridge Road
Westlake, Ohio 44145
USA
*Corresponding author: chapter 9*
konez@ccf.org

**Kenneth H. Kraemer, MD, PhD**
Basic Research Laboratory
Center for Cancer Research
National Cancer Institute
National Institute of Health
Bethesda, MD 20892
USA

**Pablo Lapunzina, MD**
Department of Medical Genetics
University Hospital La Paz
University of Madrid
Paseo de la Castellana, 261
28046 – Madrid
Spain
*Corresponding author: chapter 12*
plapunzina.hulp@salud.madrid.org

**Russell R. Lonser, MD**
Surgical Neurology Branch
National Institute of Neurological Disorders
    and Stroke
National Institutes of Health

10 Center Drive
Building 10, Room 5D37
Bethesda, MD 20892-1414
USA
*Corresponding author: chapter 6*
lonser@ninds.nih.gov

**Nicola Migone, MD, PhD**
Department of Genetics, Biology and Biochemistry
Medical Genetics Unit
University of Turin
S. Giovanni Battista Hospital
Corso Bramante, 88-90
10126 – Turin
Italy

**Pietro Milone, MD**
Institute of Radiology
University of Catania
Via S. Sofia, 78
95123 – Catania
Italy

**Carlo Minetti, MD, PhD**
Muscular and Neurodegenerative Diseases Unit
Department of Pediatrics
University of Genoa
Giannina Gaslini Institute
Largo Gerolamo Gaslini, 5
16147 – Genoa
Italy

**Dennis A. Nowak, MD**
Department of Neurology
University of Cologne
Department of Neurology
50924 Cologne
Germany
*Corresponding author: chapter 28*
dennis.nowak@uk-koeln.de

**Edward H. Oldfield, MD**
Surgical Neurology Branch
National Institute of Neurological Disorders
    and Stroke
National Institutes of Health

10 Center Drive
Building 10, Room 5D37
Bethesda, MD 20892-1414
USA

**Luz Orozco-Covarrubias, MD**
Department of Dermatology
National Institute of Pediatrics
Insurgente Sur 3700-C
Mexico City 04530
Mexico

**Laura Papi, MD, PhD**
Department of Physiopathology
Medical Genetics Unit
University of Florence
Viale Pieraccini, 6
50139 – Florence
Italy
*Corresponding author: chapter 47*
l.papi@dfc.unifi.it

**Ignacio Pascual-Castroviejo, MD**
Pediatric Neurology Service
University Hospital La Paz
Madrid
Paseo de la Castellana, 261
28046 – Madrid
Spain
*Co-editor*
*Corresponding author: chapters 2, 10, 18, 21, 38, 54, 55, 58,59,60,61,62,66 and 70*
p.castroviejo@telefonica.net

**Scott Randall Plotkin, MD, PhD**
Department of Neurology
Massachusetts General Hospital
Harvard Medical School
55 Fruit Street
02114 – Boston
USA
*Corresponding author: chapter 4*
splotkin@partners.org

**Agata Polizzi, MD, PhD**
Department of Experimental Medicine

University "La Sapienza"
Via di Grottarossa, 1035
00160 – Rome

**Emily Reiff, MD**
Department of Surgery and UCSF Comprehensive
  Cancer Center
1600 Divisadero, Room C348
University of California San Francisco/Mount Zion
  Medical Center
San Francisco
USA

**Domenico A. Restivo, MD**
Neurology Unit
Garibaldi Hospital
Via Palermo, 636
95121 – Catania
Italy

**Mario Roggini, MD**
Pediatric Radiology Unit
Department of Pediatrics
University "La Sapienza"
Viale R. Elena 324
00186 – Rome
Italy

**Corrado Romano, MD**
Unit of Pediatrics and Medical Genetics
I.R.C.S.S. Oasi M. Santissima
Via Conte Ruggero, 73
940128 – Troina
Italy
*Corresponding author: chapters 27 and 29*
cromano@oasi.en.it

**Leida B. Rozeman, PhD**
Department of Pathology
Leiden University Medical Center
Albinusdreef 2, 2333 ZA
Leiden
The Netherlands

**Ramòn Ruiz-Maldonado, MD**
Department of Dermatology
National Institute of Pediatrics

Insurgente Sur 3700-C
Mexico City 04530
Mexico
*Corresponding author: chapters 19, 23, 37, 40, 42, 43,
44 and 63*
rrm@servidor.unam.mx

**Martino Ruggieri, MD, PhD**
Institute of Neurological Science
Italian National Research Council
Viale R. Margherita, 6
95125 – Catania
Italy
*Co-editor*
*Corresponding author: chapters 3, 7, 8, 14, 16, 24, 25,
31, 33, 34, 36, 39 and 65*
m.ruggieri@isn.cnr.it

**Haneen Sadick, MD, PhD**
Department of Otorhinolaryngology, Head
and Neck Surgery
University Hospital Mannheim
Theodor-Kutzer-Ufer 1-3
D-68167 Mannheim
Germany
*Corresponding author: chapter 11*
haneen.sadick@hno.ma.uni-heidelberg.de

**Maliha Sadick, MD**
Department of Clinical Radiology
University Hospital Mannheim
Theodor-Kutzer-Ufer 1-3
D-68167 Mannheim
Germany

**Marimar Saez-De-Ocariz, MD**
Department of Dermatology
National Institute of Pediatrics
Insurgente Sur 3700-C
Mexico City 04530
Mexico

**Harvey B Sarnat, MD, FRCPC**
Division of Pediatric Neurology
Alberta Children's Hospital

2888 Shaganappi Trail NW
Calgary, AB T3B 6A8
Canada

**Salvatore Savasta, MD**
Department of Pediatrics
I.R.C.S.S. Hospital S. Matteo
University of Pavia
Piazzale Golgi, 2
27100 – Pavia
Italy
*Corresponding author: chapter 56*
s.savasta@smatteo.pv.it

**Carmelo Schepis, MD**
Unit of Dermatology
I.R.C.S.S. Oasi M. Santissima
Via Conte Ruggero, 73
940128 – Troina
Italy
*Corresponding author: chapters 17 and 48*
cschepis@oasi.en.it

**Yvonne M. Schrage, MD**
Department of Pathology
Leiden University Medical Center
Albinusdreef 2, 2333 ZA
Leiden
The Netherlands

**Maddalena Siragusa, MD**
Unit of Dermatology
I.R.C.S.S. Oasi M. Santissima
Via Conte Ruggero, 73
940128 – Troina
Italy

**Miria Stefanini, MD, PhD**
Institute of Molecular Genetics
Italian National Research Council
Via Abbiategrasso, 207
27100 – Pavia
Italy
*Corresponding author: chapters 51,52 and 53*
stefanini@igm.cnr.it

**Jeffrey L. Sugarman, MD, PhD**
Departments of Dermatology and Community
  and Family Medicine
University of California San Francisco
CA 95404
San Francisco
USA
*Corresponding author: chapters 32 and 35*
pediderm@yahoo.com

**Christer Ullbro, MD**
Department of Pedodontics
Institute of Postgraduate Education
5511 Jönköping
Sweden
*Corresponding author: chapter 41*
cullbro@hotmail.com

**Meena Upadhyaya, PhD, FRCP**<sup>ath</sup>
Institute of Medical Genetics
University of Wales College of Medicine
Heath Park
Cardiff CF14 4XN
United Kingdom

**Maurizia Valli, MD**
Department of Biochemistry
Section of Medicine and Pharmacy
University of Pavia
Piazzale Golgi, 2
27100 – Pavia
Italy

**Corry Weemaes, MD, PhD**
Department of Pediatrics
Radboud University Nijmegen Medical Centre
Geert Grooteplein 20
P.O. Box 9101
6500 Nijmegen
The Netherlands
*Corresponding author: chapter 50*
C.Weemaes@cukz.umcn.nl

**Janice Zunich, MD**
Department of Medical Genetics
Indiana University School of Medicine
Northwest
3400 Broadway
Gary, IN 46408
USA
*Corresponding author: chapter 64*
jzunich@iun.edu

# Chapter 1

# EMBRYOLOGY OF NEUROCUTANEOUS SYNDROMES

Laura Flores-Sarnat and Harvey B. Sarnat

Alberta Children's Hospital (LFS) (HBS), and University of Calgary Faculty of Medicine (HBS), Calgary, Alberta, Canada

## Introduction

The neurocutaneous diseases and neurocutaneous syndromes are a broad group of congenital disorders with diverse genetic, clinical and pathological features that share in common developmental lesions of the skin and of the central and peripheral nervous systems. Subcutaneous and systemic involvement is common. In many of these conditions another feature is a tendency to develop tumors in multiple sites of the body. Many of these disorders are hamartomatous in nature, and produce benign tumors, but patients also may develop malignant tumors. The etiology has been identified in several conditions: such cases are properly referred to as *neurocutaneous diseases*. In the case of neurofibromatosis and tuberous sclerosis complex, neoplasias can be explained because the genes responsible for the disease also are tumor-suppressor genes. Many neurocutaneous syndromes manifest overgrowth in one area, region or one side of the body, usually progressive (Cohen et al. 2001). Asymmetry and hemimegalencephaly are common features in several neurocutaneous syndromes (Flores-Sarnat 2002). The clinical features may be present at birth or become manifest later.

One of the constant and intrinsic features of the neurocutaneous syndromes, the skin lesions (mainly in the form of flat spots), occur in a big variety of shapes (round, oval, ash leaf, lines, whorls, etc.), sizes and number. There is little variation in color: they are hypo- or hyperpigmented, or red if vascular lesions. These spots may appear in any site on the body. In particular cases the hair, iris and meninges also may be affected. Abnormalities in vascular and adipose tissue, in the form of angiomas or lipomas, are a common feature.

Initially this group of disorders was named "phakomatosis" and consisted of only three entities: tuberous sclerosis, neurofibromatosis, and von Hippel-Lindau disease. Over time, more than 50 disorders have been added to this category, some without a developmental basis; the list continues to grow. It is, therefore, important to distinguish two categories of neurocutaneous syndromes as *primary* and *secondary* because of their different origins and prognoses.

Traditionally, it was considered that the common origin of skin and central nervous system from ectoderm explained the pathogenesis of the neurocutaneous syndromes. However, it was soon noted that mesodermal and endodermal tissues also were involved. Furthermore, with the advent of molecular genetics, the traditional concept of three germ layers has been challenged because the expression of many developmental genes is not restricted to one germinal layer. At present, there are many clues, both clinical and molecular, that support the new concept that an abnormality in the formation, migration or differentiation of neural crest cells is the common pathogenesis for most, if not all, *primary* neurocutaneous syndromes.

Many derivatives of the neural crest are involved in the neurocutaneous syndromes, particularly melanocytes that explain most of the skin lesions. Another clue is the abnormal pattern of migration of the melanocytes in several neurocutaneous syndromes that follow the lines of Blaschko, as observed in hypomelanosis of Ito and incontinentia pigmenti.

Neural crest cells are first recognized shortly after gastrulation, though they are not committed to their diverse lineages until later. After dorsal closure of the neural tube, neural crest cells separate and migrate throughout the embryo to form many structures of ectodermal origin (e.g. dorsal root and autonomic ganglia, peripheral nerve sheaths) and mesodermal origin (e.g. blood vessels, melanocytes, adipose tissue, membranous bone, connective tissue, most of ocular globe). Terminal differentiation occurs after migration is complete. Three regions of the neural tube generate neural crest: rhombencephalon, mesencephalon and prosencephalon, each with a different migratory pattern. Some of the most important genes promoting neural crest differentiation and migration are those with a dorsalizing influence in the vertical axis of the neural tube (e.g. *PAX3*, *BMP4*, *ZIC2*), some segmentation genes (e.g. *WNT1*), genes that inhibit neural crest (e.g. *EGR2*) and neural crest-specific differentiating genes (e.g. *SLUG*, *SOX10*). In the neurocutaneous syndromes, diverse features may result from abnormal neural crest differentiation, providing a more encompassing embryological basis for these disorders than the traditional view that these syndromes are somehow related to skin and brain because both are ectodermal derivatives. Abnormal angiogenesis, regions of abnormal pigmentation, nerve sheath proliferations, lipomas and disorders of chromaffin tissue are frequent features. Interactions between genes associated with these disorders and others essential to neural crest formation, migration and differentiation, are a likely molecular genetic basis for these diseases. The craniofacial abnormalities associated with many neurocutaneous syndromes and the characteristic skin lesions emphasize an important inductive role of the neural tube upon the development of non-neural tissues, mediated through neural crest.

The classification of neurocristopathies can now be expanded to include many neurocutaneous syndromes. On the other hand, known neurocristopathies such as multiple endocrine neoplasia type II and familial medullary thyroid carcinoma are now included in the group of neurocutaneous syndromes. Waardenburg syndrome, recognized as a typical neurocristopathy, also can be considered a neurocutaneous syndrome.

## Historical perspective and terminology

Though many diseases we now identify as neurocutaneous syndromes were described in the 19th cen-

tury, the association of brain and skin developmental abnormalities was first made in 1920 by Van der Hoeve, a Dutch ophthalmologist, who observed similar retinal lesions between tuberous sclerosis, neurofibromatosis and von Hippel-Lindau disease. He coined the term *phakoma* and the concept of *phakomatosis* (*phakos* Greek = lentil, spot; lens-shaped), to describe the disseminated lentiform retinal lesions observed in that group of hereditary disorders (Van der Hoeve 1920, 1932). The term became inappropriate when Van der Hoeve included Sturge-Weber syndrome, which is not associated with phakomas or hamartomas. Etymologically it also is inadequate because it does not include the nervous system. It continues to be used by some contemporary authors, in a less broad context. In any case, its use should be reserved to those conditions which manifest retinal hamartomas ("phakomas"), corresponding to the original description.

The term *neurocutaneous syndromes* was introduced by Yakovlev and Guthrie in 1931 to describe "congenital malformations affecting more or less electively the ectodermal structures, i.e., the nervous system, the skin, the retina, the eyeball and its contents; sometimes visceral organs are also involved" (Yakovlev and Guthrie 1931). In their review they cited neurofibromatosis 1, tuberous sclerosis and Sturge-Weber syndrome. At that time the neurocutaneous syndromes were considered to originate from ectoderm, even though they recognized that the vascular anomalies in Sturge-Weber syndrome were mesodermal derivatives. However, the term "neurocutaneous" also is technically incorrect because *cutaneous* denotes only the epidermis and dermis, but subcutaneous lesions such as lipomas and subcutaneous neurofibromas also frequently appear in neurocutaneous syndromes. Moreover, it is now known that these syndromes involve not only ectodermal derivatives, but many structures other than brain and skin. Another problem is that *neurocutaneous* is a nonspecific term which might include any condition that affects the skin and nervous system, without being developmental in nature. It has the merit of linking the two most obvious manifestations of this group of disorders. Because of its long established and widespread usage, the introduction of another nomenclature at this time would impede, rather than enhance, scientific communication.

*Hamartoma* refers to any abnormal growth that is made up of tissue composed of disorganized cells with dysplastic cytoarchitecture and situated within its organ of origin. A hamartoma occurs when a tissue does not develop completely or has ambiguous or mixed cellular lineage. Hamartomas can occur throughout the body, in any tissue.

It is important to make a distinction between *primary* and *secondary* neurocutaneous syndromes because, as mentioned previously, they have different pathogeneses and prognosis and the approach to management also is different. Primary neurocutaneous syndromes are developmental, dysgenetic conditions. Secondary neurocutaneous syndromes are not developmental disorders; they are the result of, or complications of, previous conditions, usually metabolic diseases. Examples include: Fabry disease, a lysosomal storage disease caused by deficiency of a-galactosidase; Lesch-Nyhan disease, due to a disorder in purine metabolism, exhibits cutaneous lesions secondary to accidental or self-inflicted injuries; Menkes disease is secondary to abnormal copper transport and metabolism; the cutaneous and central nervous system lesions are secondary to the metabolic defect.

Many neurocutaneous syndromes are now really diseases. A *syndrome* is a constellation of symptoms and signs, of unknown etiology, shared by a group of patients. When the etiology is discovered, whether it be infectious, metabolic or genetic, the syndrome is promoted in status to a *disease*.

## Pathogenesis and molecular genetics

Throughout most of the 20th century, clinicians and pathologists tried to discover a common pathogenetic theme in the group of neurocutaneous syndromes, but this approach has been difficult because each disease varies greatly from the others in clinical presentation, genetics, pathological findings and imaging characteristics. Despite the traditional view is that they are diseases of ectoderm, even early 20th century investigators were troubled by the fact that many, if not all primary neurocutaneous syndromes, also involved tissues of mesodermal or endodermal origin. Tuberous sclerosis complex was the prototype of multisystemic involvement most frequently cited, with hamartomas not only of the brain and skin (ectoderm), but also of the heart and kidneys (mesoderm) and of endocrine glands and liver (endoderm) (Gómez et al. 1999, Curatolo 2003). Even some cutaneous lesions, such as the facial angiofibromas (inappropriately named "adenoma sebaceum" because they are neither adenomatous nor sebaceous), are of mesodermal origin. Angiomas are features common to many neurocutaneous syndromes, and also are mesodermal (Roach and Miller 2004, Santos et al. 2004). In our attempt to understand the embryology of neurocutaneous syndromes, we found the traditional theory of three germ layers unsatisfactory. The search for a common pathogenesis led us to conclude that the neural crest was the common thread in all of these syndromes.

With the advent of molecular genetics in the late 1980s, it soon became apparent that genetic expression does not restrict itself to the artificially assigned boundaries of the classical, time-honored "germ layers" and that the same gene families and individual genes contribute to developmental programming in multiple tissues. The entire traditional concept of germ layers is now under scrutiny and revision by contemporary embryologists. It may, in the future, become a concept cited only as an historical footnote. With it, the explanation that the neurocutaneous syndromes have a common link because brain and skin are both ectodermal derivatives no longer is tenuous as a rational basis.

## Embryology of neural crest tissue

The first description of the neural crest was done by the Swiss/German anatomist-embryologist His (1868); however, it took almost a century for this structure to attract the attention of clinical investigators (Pages 1955, Small 1955).

Neural crest cells are first recognized at the lateral margin of the neural placode shortly after gastrulation, though they are not committed to their diverse fates until later. The neural crest is a transient population of embryonic cells derived from ectoderm and defined by their migratory behavior and ability to form numerous derivatives (Basch et al. 2000). As neurulation proceeds, the curling of the neural placode results in these cells becoming dorsomedial in the neural groove. With closure of the dorsal midline to form the neural tube, the neural crest cells separate and begin migrating along prescribed routes throughout the embryo rather than remaining confined to the neural tube, initiating the formation of the peripheral nervous system, including dorsal root and autonomic ganglia, Schwann cells of peripheral nerves and chromaffin tissue in the adrenal medulla, carotid body and other sites. Neural crest also differentiates as cells traditionally regarded as mesodermal in origin, including melanocytes, endothelial cells, smooth muscle of blood vessels, interstitial connective tissue, the cranial meninges, the sclera of the eye, cartilage and membranous (but not endochondral) bone, especially the craniofacial skeleton (Tan and Morriss-Kay 1985, Le Douarin and Kalcheim 1999, Basch et al. 2000). When neural crest meets an epithelium, cartilage forms; when it meets mesodermal tissue, membranous bone forms. This explains why we have cartilage in our ears and bone in our orbits. Neural crest cells terminally differentiate into their diverse lineages only after reaching their final destination.

Neural crest is so pervasive that some authors have suggested its status be promoted as a fourth germ layer (Le Douarin and Kalcheim 1999, Hall 1999) but we disagree. Though incipient neural crest cells first appear at the lateral margins of the neuroepithelial placode on the day of gastrulation, these cells are not irreversible "committed" to a specific fate. Lineage analyses demonstrate that individual neural fold cells can form epidermis or neural crest cells, hence they are not truly neural crest until after gastrulation. Moreover, to create a fourth germ layer, other germ layers would have to yield tissues previously classified as derived from ectoderm and mesoderm in particular. But since the whole concept of embryonic germ layers may, in future, be regarded as an obsolete concept from the pre-molecular genetic era, this point is of little importance.

The development of neural crest derivatives can be divided into stages: a) specification of cells at the lateral borders of the neural plate as potential neural crest precursors; b) commitment of these cells at the time of closure of the neural tube as neural crest precursors, situated adjacent to the midline in the dorsomedial part of the closed neural tube; c) delamination or separation of these cells from the neural tube; d) migration into the periphery of the body, but not crossing the midline except in unpaired structures such as the heart and intestine; e) terminal differentiation as specific types of cells, or cellular lineage and diversification, after reaching the final position in the body. All of these stages are genetically programmed or influenced by genetic factors in surrounding tissues (Baker 2005). A cell is not formally regarded as neural crest until after it "delaminates" or separates from the neural tube; failure to delaminate and migrate results in further differentiation of neural crest precursor cells within the neural tube (Borchers et al. 2001).

Neural crest arises segmentally in all three primitive cerebral vesicles: rhombencephalon, mesencephalon and prosencephalon. Neural crest cells migrate in a somewhat different manner from each part of the embryonic neural tube after segmentation and the formation of neuromeres at 4–8 weeks gestation. The neural crest may be divided into three groups on this basis. The prosencephalic neural crest migrates rostrally into the head as a midline *vertical sheet* of cells (Puelles and Rubinstein 2003). The mesencephalic neural crest, which arises not only from the mesencephalic neuromere (i.e. r0, future midbrain), but also from the first two hindbrain rhombomeres (neuromeres r1 and the rostral half of r2), migrates as *streams* of cells (Fig. 1). The rhombencephalic neural crest, arising from the hindbrain (caudal half of r2 through r7 and also r8, which forms the spinal cord), migrates as *segmental blocks* of cells (Bronner-Fraser 1994, Carstens 2004).

Lists of structures derived from the neural crest are traditionally arranged according to anatomical zones and histological categories (Jambart et al. 1979; Jones 1990; Bolande 1974, 1997). We are modifing these lists to provide an embryological approach, with the current terminology (Table 1). The next stage awaits the discovery of specific genes involved in the development of each of these structures.

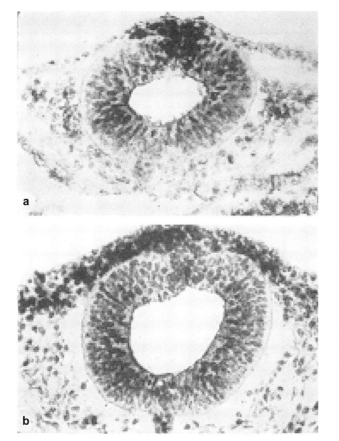

**Fig. 1.** Transverse sections of mesencephalic rhombomere (midbrain) in chick embryo. (**a**) Immediately after neural tube closure at the midbrain, neural crest cells (marked in black) are seen dorsomedially next to the midline. (**b**) A few hours later, these same cells are seen migrating away from the neural tube into the periphery as a stream, where they will proceed rostrally to form many structures of the face and cranium. A defect in the dorsal part of the neural tube at this level can interfere with mesencephalic neural crest formation and/or migration, resulting in midfacial hypoplasia. Reproduced with permission from: Le Douarin N and Kalcheim C (1999) The Neural Crest, 2nd ed. Cambridge: Cambridge University Press.

Neural crest is responsible for much of craniofacial development, including membranous bones of the face and cranial vault, though not the cranial base. In the face, mesencephalic neural crest forms not only structures of the peripheral nervous system, such as the ciliary ganglion and Schwann cells of nerves, but also many non-neural tissues of mesodermal origin: melanocytes of the skin and iris, stria vascularis of the cochlea, most of the globe of the eye including the sclera and cornea; connective tissues and vascular structures (Bronner-Fraser 1994, Le Douarin and Kalcheim 1999, Hall 1999).

Though patterns of genetic expression in the hindbrain contribute to the segmental arrangement of neural crest cells, cellular migratory pathways also are guided by attractant and repulsant paracrine molecules secreted by surrounding tissues such as the otic capsule, the somites, and the vertebral neural arches. In addition, neural crest cells possess *integrin* receptors for interacting with extracellular matrix molecules (Bronner-Fraser 1994). Changes in the distribution of *extracellular matrix* components during neural crest migration impose migratory guidance limits as well (Sadaghiani et al. 1994). The extracellular matrix glycoprotein *tenascin* is required for proper cranial neural crest migration and its absence in the chick embryo leads to neural tube defects and aggregates of ectopic neural crest cells (Bronner-Fraser 1988). Other extracellular matrix molecules that promote neural crest migration include fibronectin, laminin and collagen types I, IV and VI (Perris and Perissinotto 2000). Ephrins, by contrast, repulse neural crest divert caudally (Kalcheim 2000, Krull 2001, Baker 2005).

Protein kinase C is an inhibitory factor on neural crest at various stages. If this protein is inhibited in mouse embryos at the neural tube stage and in cell cultures, neural crest precursor cells precociously delaminate and migrate away from the neural tube before their programmed time (Newgreen and Minichiello 1995, Rathjen et al. 2002). *Sox10*, associated with later differentiation of neural crest cells (see below), also is upregulated by protein kinase C inhibition (Rathjen et al. 2002). The phase of the mitotic cell cycle, in particular the transition from G1 to S-phase, is another important determinant of delamination; blocking this transition also impedes delamination of the neural crest (Burstyn-Cohen and Kalcheim 2002, Baker 2005).

The neural crest consists of a series of overlapping cell populations that thus differ in their migratory pathways and fates. Why neural crest precursors are so heterogeneous, why neural crest stem cells exist with multiple potentials, and even whether stem cells arising from the neural tube are joined by surrounding cells from the mesodermal germ layer are not as well understood as are their migratory pathways outside the neural tube (Selleck et al. 1993). As with other parts of the neural tube, neural crest tissue has a rostrocaudal gradient of differentiation. The fate of neural crest cells is not entirely predetermined; environmental factors may induce differentiation as other cells than were originally intended. For example, although early-migrating neural crest cells generally form dorsal root ganglion cells, when these early-migrating cells are ablated, the late-migrating neural crest cells that ordinarily form mesodermal structures change their fate to become

**Table 1.** Embryonic distribution of neural crest derivatives

**Prosencephalic Neural Crest**
Paramedian frontal bones around metopic suture
Melanocytes of skin at frontal midline, extending onto midline of nose
Melanocytes of hair follicles of rostral frontal midline scalp ("forelock")
Subcutaneous connective tissue, including adipocytes, microvasculature of frontal
   midline and Schwann cells of small cutaneous nerves

**Mesencephalic Neural Crest**
Membranous bones of face including orbit, otic capsule, sphenoid
Membranous bones of cranial vault including rostral 2/3 of parietal bone
Cartilage of face, including nasal root and ears
Hard and soft palate
Trigeminal neurovascular bundles (including ganglia, Schwann cells and vessels)
Stria vascularis of cochlea
Ciliary ganglion
Parasympathetic nerves (except axons) to face and iris
Connective tissue, including adipocytes, and vasculature of face and cranium, including
   smooth muscle of arterioles and venules, part of dermis
Connective tissue of adenohypophysis (anterior pituitary)
Cranial leptomeninges and dura mater (not spinal meninges or tentorium cerebelli)
Most of ocular globe (except retina, choroid, cornea)
Odontoblasts
Melanocytes of iris, skin of face and most of scalp hair

**Rhombencephalic Neural Crest (includes spinal cord)**
Facial neurovascular bundle
Glossopharyngeal neurovascular bundle
Vagal neurovascular bundles
Spinal nerve roots and dorsal root ganglia (except neurons and axons)
Sympathetic nerves and ganglia (except axons), including those of face, paravertebral sympathetic
   chain, superior cervical ganglion, periaortic complexes, celiac ganglion, mesenteric nerves
Adrenal medulla
Carotid body and other chemoreceptors
Parasympathetic nerves and ganglia (except axons) including submucosal and intramuscular
   plexus of intestine and to lungs, dermal and endocrine glands, pelvic plexus
Melanocytes of skin and hair of posterior 1/3 of scalp, neck and body (trunk and extremities)
Cartilage of pharyngeal arches and part of chondrocranium (not cranial base or basioccipital,
   exoccipital or supraoccipital bones)
Connective tissue of lingual, salivary buccal, parathyroid glands and thymus; adipocytes
Thyroid C-cells

neurons. Nevertheless, transplantation of early-migrating neural crest cells does not result in production of neurons under all conditions (Raible and Eisen 1996).

Neurotrophic factors, such as neurotrophin-3 (NT-3), also influence the fate of neural crest cells and are essential for survival of sympathetic neuroblasts and innervation of specific organs (El Shamy et al. 1996). NT3 is the principal and perhaps the only neurotrophin needed by neurons of the myenteric plexus (Gershon 1999; Chalazonitis 1996, 2004), but other neural crest derivatives require other factors. Gene products of *bone morphogenic proteins* (*BMP2* and *BMP4*) regulate the onset of NT3 during fetal gut development, and *BMP4* and NT3 (with its receptor TrkC) are needed to preserve the integrity of the submucosal and myenteric plexuses. Nerve growth factor (NGF), the first neurotrophin identified, was first demonstrated in dorsal root ganglia. Brain-derived neurotrophic factor (BDNF), ciliary neurotrophic factor (CNTF) and glial-derived neurotrophic factor (GNTF) all are associated with neural crest migration or differentiation (Sieber-Blum 1999).

The origin of neural crest is topographically unequal in the neuraxis. The streams of cells arising in the midbrain contribute to craniofacial structure. In the hindbrain, migratory mesencephalic neural crest cells from r1 and r2 populate the trigeminal ganglion and streams of rhombencephalic neural crest form the mandibular arch; cells from r4 form the hyoid arch, the geniculate and vestibular and cochlear ganglia; those from r6 populate the third and fourth pharyngeal arches and associated peripheral ganglia (Bronner-Fraser 1994, 1995). Rhombomeres 3 and 5 do not appear to have neural crest cells, but actually neural crest cells are generated in r3 and r5 but they fuse rostrally and caudally with neural crest cells of adjacent rhombomeres to migrate together, because of the EGR2 gene expressed only in r3 and r5 as discussed below (Bronner-Fraser 1994). This also explains the fusion of the proximal maxillary and mandibular branches of the trigeminal nerve.

In phylogenetic evolution, neural crest tissue is unique in vertebrates and absent in invertebrates. Some protochordates, such as amphioxus, express some genes that also are expressed in vertebrate neural crest, but these are not detected either in the lateral border of the neural plate during development or in the dorsal "neural tube" in the adult (Meulemans et al. 2003). The central nervous system of the mature amphioxus remains in a stage resembling the neural groove of vertebrates, however, because the dorsal midline does not fuse to form a complete neural tube and this is the region where neural crest originates in vertebrates; the central canal in amphioxus is a vertical slit lined by ependyma but without a roof plate and open at the dorsal surface (Sarnat and Netsky 1981).

## Genetic programming of neural crest

Many genes are involved in the formation and migration of neural crest and, finally, the terminal differentiation into the various types of cells it forms. Neural crest cells do not differentiate until they arrive in their target zone. The recent explosion of molecular genetic data diminishes the importance of embryonic germ layers, long believed to be fundamental in cellular lineage, because it is now recognized that the same organizer and regulator genes program development and cytological differentiation in various tissues, and that genes do not restrict their expression to individual embryonic germ layers. Examples are the *HOX* and *PAX* families, both primordial in the embryonic segmentation of the neural tube, but also in the ontogenesis of bone, kidney, gut and many other tissues. Even single gene deletions or mutations may downregulate other downstream genes in a cascade, permit the overexpression of antagonistic genes or otherwise alter complex multigenetic interactions. Trophic factors important in neural crest migration and maturation also might be defective in some of these syndromes. Neural crest induction occurs continuously over a long period starting at gastrulation and persisting well past the time of neural tube closure [4]. Neural crest can be induced to form in early neuroectoderm by the proximity of non-neural surface ectoderm (Lumsden et al. 1991, García-Castro and Bronner-Fraser 1999). Exposure of the most rostral neuroectoderm at its boundary with epidermis in *Xenopus*, to *BMP* plus bFGF, *Wnt8* or retinoic acid, transforms this tissue into neural crest (Villanueva et al. 2002). The lateral border of the primitive neural plate, where neural crest precursors first develop, is specified by the activity of *BMP* and *Dlx* transcription products, but these molecules do not specify neural crest cells (Villanueva et al. 2002, McLarren et al. 2003, Woda et al. 2003).

Many genes are essential to the formation of neural crest, but the most important are those having a strong dorsalizing effect in the vertical axis of the neural tube: *ZIC2, BMP4, BMP7, PAX3*. The transforming growth factor-beta (TGFβ) superfamily, and in particular *BMP4* and *BMP7*, promote neural crest differentiation at the time of neural tube closure; these two genes can even substitute for non-neural ectoderm in inducing neural crest cells (Liem et al. 1995). Ventralizing genes of the vertical axis, such as *SHH*, produced by both notochord and floor plate cells of the neural tube, inhibit neural crest formation (Bronner-Fraser 1995). Experimentally, either notochordal tissue or *Shh*-expressing cells grafted adjacent to the neural folds prevent neural crest formation (Selleck et al. 1998). The gene *Noggin*, a strong antagonist of *BMP* genes, also inhibits neural crest formation (Dickinson et al. 1995).

Delamination of neural crest precursor cells from the dorsal neural tube to the periphery is mediated or regulated by several genes, that include *FoxD2, RhoB* (activated by *BMP4*), and *Slug* in particular (Nieto et al. 1994, Cano et al. 2000, Dottori et al. 2001, Baker 2005).

At a later stage in neural tube development, the segmentation genes that program the formation of neuromeres also can promote neural crest, especially those with a dorsalizing effect in the vertical axis. The segmentation homebox *Wingless* family, particularly *Wnt1* and *Wnt3a*, not only are important for the formation of neuromeric compartments and their boundaries in the hindbrain, but also promote neural crest formation (Dickinson et al. 1995, LaBonne 2002). The human gene *EGR2* (known as *Krox-20* in the mouse) is another segmentation homeobox gene, but expressed only in rhombomeres r3 and r5. *EGR2* inhibits neural crest formation, but the incipient neural crest cells of these two rhombomeres shift to adjacent rhombomeres where

*EGR2* is not expressed, and mix with the neural crest being generated in those rhombomeres, so that neural crest cells that migrate caudally around the otic vesicle are from both r5 and r6 (Bronner-Fraser 1994). *Hox-1.5* and *Hox-2.9* regulate the premigratory and migratory neural crest cells from r4 (Chisaka and Capecchi 1991, Hunt et al. 1991). *Hox* family genes encode the posterior part of the brain, rhombencephalic neural crest and the pharyngeal arches, whereas this programming function in the rostral brain, including the mesencephalic and prosencephalic neural crest and viscerocranium (cranial vault) is correspondingly regulated by the gene *Otx2* (Kuratani et al. 1997). Expression of *Otx2* is regulated by two "enhancers" with their caudal limit at the isthmus or mesencephalic-metancephalic boundary (Kurokawa et al. 2004). At least part of the migratory patterning is not as rigidly preprogrammed as previously thought, however, and the cranial neural crest may partly be a passive transfer of positional information from the brain to the periphery by not inhibiting, rather than actively promoting, cellular migration (Trainor and Krumlauf 2000).

The gene *SLUG* (*Snail* in invertebrates) seems to be essential for later stages of neural crest differentiation. Though it also is detected in early stages of the neural placode prior to neural crest migration and in early migratory cells to the periphery, its transcript is later is downregulated in later migration and also in vitro in the absence of tissue interactions (Basch et al. 2000, LaBonne and Bronner-Fraser 2000). *SLUG* then is later re-expressed in stronger form. *SLUG* is a "zinc-finger", defined as DNA-binding, gene-specific transcription factors consisting of 28 amino acid repeats with pairs of cysteine and histadine residues, each sequence folded around an ion of zinc (Nieto et al. 1994). In the amphibian embryo, *Slug* expression does not itself induce neural crest, but in the presence of *Wnt* signals. It yields a robust neural crest (LaBonne and Bronner-Fraser 2000). *BMP4* is upregulated in the isolated neural folds just prior to the expression of *Slug* (LaBonne and Bronner-Fraser 1998). *SOX10* is another gene involved in terminal neural crest differentiation, particularly in the rhombencephalic neural crest migration to the gut and differentiation of ganglion cells for the submucosal and myenteric plexuses (Honore et al. 2003, Paratore et al. 2001).

Other genes implicated in neural crest development include *OTX* (*EMX1,2*), *PHOX*, *DLX*, *MASH1* and *TWIST*. The *PAX* and *MSX* families are of particular importance in craniofacial development associated with prosencephalic and mesencephalic neural crest migration (Bei et al. 2002). The proto-oncogene *c-myc* is another essential regulator of neural crest formation (Bellmeyer et al. 2003). Mutations of the RET proto-oncogene resulting in overexpression is associated with several neurocristopathies including multiple endocrine neoplasias type 2 and medullary carcinoma of the thyroid (Donis-Keller et al. 1993, Hofstra et al. 1994), neuroblastoma (Ikeda et al. 1990) and Hirschprung disease (Edery et al. 1994, Romeo et al. 1994).

Terminal differentiation of neural crest cells also is genetically regulated. The choice between differentiating as sensory (i.e. dorsal root ganglionic) neurons or autonomic ganglionic neurons depends upon exposure to *BMP2* expression in peripheral tissues, that probably emanates from the dorsal aorta; *BMP2* initiates *MASH1* expression, which leads to autonomic differentiation (Anderson 1997). Sensory neurons form in the absence of *BMP2*.

## The concept of "neurocristopathies"

The term *neurocristopathy* was first introduced by Bolande in 1974 to denote a group of diverse diseases having a common origin in neural crest maldevelopment (Bolande 1974), with later updates (Bolande 1981, 1997). He divided the neural crest disorders into *simple* and *complex*; *dysgenetic* and *neoplastic*. A simple neurocristopathy is exemplified by aganglionic megacolon (Hirschsprung disease), in which segments of intestine lack submucosal and myenteric plexi of parasympathetic ganglion cells. Neurofibromatosis and neurocutaneous melanosis were cited by Bolande as examples of complex neurocristopathies, but he did not extend the concept to encompass all neurocutaneous syndromes. Bolande also noted that the complex diseases tended to follow Mendelian inheritance, and that simple neurocristopathies were usually sporadic.

In recent years, and particularly with the fountainhead of new molecular genetic data that continues to emerge, the importance of neural crest as an inducer not only of peripheral neural structures such as ganglia but of many tissues in craniofacial development and other peripheral mesodermal structures is becoming more and more evident.

We submit that many manifestations of the category traditionally been regarded as "primary neurocutaneous syndromes" may be attributed in large part to abnormal neural crest migration and differentiation as well, thus expanding Bolande's original concept of neurocristopathies to an entire category of abnormal neural tube induction of non-neural peripheral structures of the body that represent neural crest derivatives. Bolande's original and updated division of the neurocristopathies into "simple" and "complex" (Bolande 1974, 1997) has merit for convenience in clinical classification, but the two categories may blend when the genetic basis of all become known.

## Relation between neural crest and neurocutaneous disorders

For the past three decades, neurofibromatosis and neurocutaneous melanosis were the only neurocutaneous syndromes consistently considered to be related to abnormal neural crest. A few authors have speculated on a possible role of neural crest in the pathogenesis of other neurocutaneous syndromes in isolated cases, but until now we have not found publications with the proposal that the embryological basis for the entire group of "primary" neurocutaneous diseases is defective neural crest tissue due to genetic mutations that impede or alter the formation, migration or terminal differentiation of neural crest cells. In the case of encephalocraniocutaneous lipomatosis or Haberland syndrome, a link with cephalic neural crest was suggested in 1989 (Bamforth et al. 1989), but only rarely cited in further publications (Jozwiak and Janniger 2005)

The primary neurocutaneous syndromes are here reexamined in this context, with a premise that they are embryological disorders of neural crest tissue, hence can be considered neurocristopathies (Sarnat and Flores-Sarnat 2005).

A common theme amongst the various neurocutaneous syndromes, despite their diverse genetics and clinical presentation, is that all include many features explicable as defects in neural crest. Examples include the circumscribed cutaneous lesions with deficient or excessive melanin pigment, frequent vascular malformations in skin and in other organs and involvement of peripheral nerve sheaths. Even many lipomas associated with several neurocutaneous syndromes are terminal overgrowths due to dysregulation of neural crest. Some examples of proliferation of adipose tissue are: epidermal nevus syndromes, Proteus syndrome, Klippel-Trenaunay syndrome, encephalocraniocutaneous lipomatosis, Cowden syndrome, Bannayan-Riley-Ruvalcaba syndrome, Delleman syndrome.

Another characteristic feature in several neurocutaneous syndromes is the pattern of skin lesions that follow Blaschko lines, described in detail by this author a century ago, who noted this pattern assumed by many different naevoid and acquired skin and mucosae diseases does not follow nerves, vessels, or lymphatics (Blaschko 1901). He observed that these lines not only did not correspond to any known anatomical basis, but were remarkably consistent both from patient to patient and even from one disease to another. He proposed an embryonic origin for these lines, but did not suggest a mechanism. Their cause remained unknown, but we now can attribute this unique abnormal pattern of linear cutaneous pigmentation to abnormal migration of neural crest cells in the skin.

The following are examples of well known neurocutaneous syndromes in the context of derivation from neural crest tissue. We include Waardenburg syndrome, because it easily fulfills the criteria of a primary neurocutaneous syndrome:

*Neurofibromatosis 1*: This autosomal dominant disease is the most frequent and clinically well described of the neurocutaneous syndromes (Pascual-Castroviejo 2001, Roach and Miller 2004, Santos et al. 2004)). Many features support the concept

that its pathogenesis is indeed a result of defective neural crest: a) Café-au-lait and depigmented spots involve abnormal melanocyte differentiation, excessive or deficient, from rhombencephalic neural crest in particular. b) Neurofibromas (and also Schwannomas) of peripheral nerves, including small cutaneous and subcutaneous nerves, are benign nerve sheath growth disorders of neural crest origin. c) A high incidence of pheochromocytoma in the adrenal medulla is of neural crest origin. d) An increased incidence of hypertelorism is found in patients with neurofibromatosis 1, a minor dysmorphism indicating involvement of prosencephalic neural crest with incomplete formation of the intercanthal ligament, as described below. e) Nerve sheath tumors may be directly attributed to defective neural crest, but the *NF1* gene also is a tumor-suppressor gene and its impairment predisposes to neoplasia. It should be noted that the cranial meninges are of neural crest origin, but that the spinal meninges are derived from paraxial mesoderm (Table 1).

Optic nerve gliomas are common in this disease, but are not of neural crest origin; the defective tumor-suppressor function of the *NF1* gene is more likely the basis, because this effect is not limited to neural crest.

*Tuberous sclerosis complex*: This is the most complicated of the neurocutaneous syndromes and involves the largest number of tissues arising from all three germ layers of classical embryology (Gómez et al. 1999, Curatolo 2003). Some, but not all, lesions can be attributed to neural crest defects: a) Cutaneous lesions, particularly hypomelanotic macules, b) Shagreen patches, are due in part to abnormal segmental melanocytic distribution. c) The characteristic facial angiofibromas are derived from mesencephalic neural crest. d) Poliosis or hypopigmented scalp hair is another neural crest defect of melanocyte differentiation.

Hamartomas in the periventricular region and in the cerebral cortex ("tubers") are not neural crest derivatives. The two tuberous sclerosis genes also function as tumor-suppressor genes and this may promote the tumoural transformation of hamartomas in the periventricular region. One report has suggested that a link between a primitive neuroectodermal tumor of bone and tuberous sclerosis may be a "maldevelopment of the neural crest or neurocristopathy" (Hindman et al. 1997).

*Epidermal nevus syndromes*: This umbrella term includes several disorders with different types of epidermal nevi and diverse systemic involvement. One of the best known epidermal lesions, the *linear sebaceous nevus of Jadasshohn*, is the prototype that initially drew our attention to the neural crest because of its characteristic features: a) This midline vertical linear pigmented, or occasionally depigmented, lesion of the forehead is a clear marker of prosencephalic neural crest distribution: the prosencephalic neural crest migrates as a vertical sheet in the midline of the head. b) The subcutaneous lipoma that affects the face asymmetrically (Egan et al. 2001, Flores-Sarnat 2002) is of neural crest origin. This lesion is often referred as "facial hemihypertrophy" or "facial hypertrophy" (Pavone et al. 1991, Zhang et al. 2003). Some patients develop a more severe, infiltrative lesion, called "congenital infiltrating lipomatosis of the face" (Slavin et al. 1983, Unal et al. 2000, Aydingöz 2002). c) The inflamatory linear verrocous epidermal nevus (ILVEN) has a particular pattern following lines of Blaschko that we consider of neural crest origin. d) Ocular (but not retinal) dysplasia is a common complication that may arise from neural crest.

*Incontinentia pigmenti (Bloch-Sulzberger syndrome)*: a) The linear pigmented lesions on the trunk and extremities in this X-linked dominant disease are often said to correspond to "cleavage lines in the skin" (lines of Blaschko), but they are better explained as rhombencephalic neural crest migratory pathways to the dermis. b) Verrucous plaques and epidermal hyperplasia with hyperpigmentation, already observed at birth, indicate epidermal as well as dermal involvement of the same origin. c) Neovascularity and microangiomas in the eye and brain cause microinfarcts, the predisposing vascular lesions probably being of neural crest origin.

*Hypomelanosis of Ito*: a) The hypopigmented macules arranged over the body surface in sharply demarcated whorls, streaks and patches are present from birth (Pascual-Castroviejo et al. 1998), also following the lines of Blaschko that represent deficient melanocyte differentiation in rhombencephalic neural crest dermal territories. b) Dysfunction in sweating in some patients, with anhidrosis in the hypomelanotic areas, suggest abnormal eccrine gland cells, which derive from the neural crest (Steijlen et al. 2000). c) Neuroblastoma, a neoplasm derived from neural crest, has been reported in this syndrome (Oguma et al. 1996). Mental retardation, epilepsy and muscular hypotonia are present as evidence of CNS involvement.

*Neurocutaneous melanosis*: This rare syndrome was described in 1861 by Rokitansky and is characterized by the presence of giant or multiple congenital pigmented nevi, associated with benign or malignant melanocytic tumors of the CNS, particularly of the leptomeninges (Rokitansky 1861). The nevi are usually localized in the head, neck and dorsal spine, suggesting a rhombomeric distribution. Both melanocytes and cranial leptomeninges are neural crest derivatives. Neurocutaneous melanosis is frequently reported in association with the Dandy-Walker malformation (Cramer 1988, Chaloupka et al. 1996, Berker et al. 2000), but the common pathogenesis is not evident. Since Bolande first included this disorder as a neurocristopathy, other authors also have accepted the premise that neurocutaneous melanosis is a disorder of neural crest (Bolande 1974, 1981, 1997).

*Sturge-Weber disease*: The remarkable concordance of the cutaneous vascular lesions with branches of the trigeminal nerve has been observed for many years, with the inference that somehow the nerves are involved with the formation of capillary malformations of the face and scalp (Roach and Millar 2004). Fetal sensory nerves secrete a neurotrophic factor that serves as a potent stimulant of angiogenesis, accounting for arterial differentiation and the "neurovascular bundles" in the fetus (Mokouyama et al. 2002). An alternative explanation is that rather than the nerves causing the vascular malformation, both are in territories corresponding to neural crest migrations that form both nerve sheaths and small blood vessels. Many cases of Sturge-Weber disease are more extensive, beyond the territories of the trigeminal nerve, with microcapillary malformations involving the neck, chest and back, but still within the distribution of rhombencephalic neural crest. Cutaneous lesions may be unilateral or bilateral. Epilepsy in this disease may result from microvascular malformations in the meninges, of neural crest origin, or in the brain. Gómez pointed out that Sturge-Weber syndrome is neither phakomatosis nor hamarmatosis (Gómez et al. 1999).

*Klippel–Trenaunay syndrome, Klippel–Trenaunay-Weber syndrome*: These terms are sometimes used interchangeably; however, Cohen et al. (2001) distinguishes between the syndrome described by Klippel and Trenaunay (1900) and that described by Parkes Weber (1907). Even when they are similar conditions, usually sporadic and characterized by developmental vascular abnormalities, there are some important clinical differences. The classical triad of Klippel–Trenaunay syndrome consists of: a) vascular malformations of the capillary, venous and lymphatic vessels; b) varicosities of unusual distribution, particularly the lateral venous anomaly; and c) unilateral limb enlargement, usually the lower extremity. In Parkes Weber syndrome, the arteriovenous fistulas, are the predominating feature. The cutaneous vascular lesions that characterize these syndromes derive from cells of neural crest origin.

*Waardenburg syndrome (WS)*: This condition was first reported by Van der Hoeve in 1916 in 3 patients (Van der Hoeve 1916). Waardenburg added more cases and defined the main features of this condition (Waardenburg 1948, 1951). Waardenburg syndrome was amongst the first genetic diseases to be associated with neural crest (Ommen and McKusick 1979). Waardenburg syndrome is classified into four types: WS type I (WS1), WS type II (WS2), WS type III (WS3), and WS type IV (WS4). Though not previously cited as neurocutaneous syndromes, both cutaneous (hair, skin) and neurological deficits (neurosensory hearing loss) are constant features, hence can be grouped under this rubric. WS types I and III are caused by mutations of *PAX3* gene. Waardenburg syndrome type III (*Klein-Waardenburg*) includes variable musculoskeletal anomalies, and

occasionally meningomyelocele and mental retardation. All of the characteristic facial features observed in Waardenburg type I that together present a pleasant feline facies (Flores-Sarnat 2007) can be explained by neural crest defects: a) The hypopigmentation of hair (typical white forelock of hair adjacent to the midline in the scalp) is due to lack of hair follicle melanocytes in the distribution of prosencephalic neural crest. b) Hypopigmented irides, sometimes asymmetrical (heterochromia), are due to a paucity of melanocytes in the iris. The reason for the asymmetry in some cases is uncertain, but may involve interactions with genes of bilateral symmetry. c) Lateral displacement of the medial canthi of the eyes (dystopia canthorum). d) The tubular nose due to hypoplasia of the alae nasi with a hyperplastic,

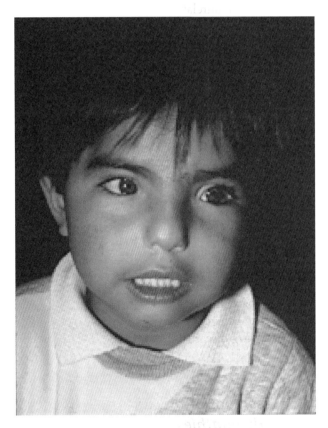

**Fig. 2.** Five-year-old boy with Waardenburg syndrome (WS) type I, showing typical features: sapphire blue eyes with dystopia canthi, hypertelorism, high nasal root with tubular nose and a small white forelock. He also has profound bilateral neurosensory deafness. His mother also has WS type I.

broad and high nasal bridge, suggests a defect of prosencephalic neural crest, probably with defective formation of the intercanthal ligament. e) A square jaw is explained by the derivation of membranous bone of the lower jaw from neural crest (Fig. 2). The neurosensory hearing loss is also the result of involvement of the cochlear *stria vascularis*, another neural crest derivative, secondarily causing degeneration of the cochlear hair cells and the auditory nerve.

WS type II was recognized by Arias and distinguished from WS1 for the lack of dystopia canthorum (Arias 1971). This is a melanocyte-specific disorder also characterized by deafness and hypopigmentation because of lack of melanocytes in the inner ear and skin, but without a distinctive face as in WS type I. It is due to a mutation in the *MITF* gene, essential for melanocyte differentiation. Recently, in two unrelated patients with WS2, homozygous deletions in SLUG were demonstrated (Sánchez-Martín et al. 2002).

Waardenburg type IV (*Shah-Waardenburg*) includes aganglionic megacolon (Hirschsprung disease) (Ommen and McKusick 1979), a defect of rhombencephalic neural crest; many of these patients have defective expression of *SOX10* during fetal development (Touraine et al. 2000, Chan et al. 2003), an essential gene for neural crest migration to the gut (Paratore et al. 2001). Mutations of the *SOX10* gene also are involved in some patients with Waardenburg type IV who additionally have congenital hypomyelinating neuropathy (Inoue et al. 2002), incorporating a defect in Schwann cell function, yet another cell of neural crest origin.

Because the genetic bases of the four forms are known, Waardenburg syndrome is ready to be elevated to the category of a disease and can be called "Waardenburg disease".

## Reassessment of the classification of *neurocristopathies*

The classification of "neurocristopathies" can be expanded to include many primary neurocutaneous syndromes, in addition to neurofibromatosis and neurocutaneous melanosis. Waardenburg syndrome, on the other hand, is a recognized neurocristopathy, but not previously considered a neurocutaneous syndrome, though it easily fulfills the criteria. A better understanding of the primordial role of neural crest in the pathogenesis of the neurocutaneous syndromes may enable further subclassification of these diseases, based upon a common pathogenesis of abnormal neural crest induction of non-neural tissues. This category would supplement the scheme we previously proposed as an integrated morphological and molecular genetic classification of nervous system malformations (Sarnat 2000, Sarnat and Flores-Sarnat 2004). We also include Waardenburg syndrome as a neurocutaneous syndrome for the same reason that unifies the other diseases in this category.

This new concept of the embryology of neurocutaneous syndromes deriving from disturbances of neural crest formation or migration may lead to a reclassification of *primary* neurocutaneous syndromes as a category of neurocristopathies. Ultimately, the classification of the neurocristopathies and of the neurocutaneous syndromes will rest upon the identification of genetic mutations and interrelations with embryonic neural crest. How defective genes in the neurocutaneous syndromes interact with the many genes, including some that program symmetry, with transcription factors and with neurotrophic factors during normal neural crest development is largely unknown, but offers the promise of insight into the pathogenesis of these diseases.

## References

Anderson DJ (1997) Cellular and molecular biology of neural crest cell lineage determination. Trends Genet 13: 276–280.

Arias S (1971) Genetic heterogeneity in the Waardenburg syndrome. Birth Defects 7: 87–101.

Aydingöz U, Emir S, Karh-Oguz K, Kose G, Buyukpamukcu M (2002) Congenital infiltrating lipomatosis of the face with ipsilateral hemimegalencephaly. Pediatr Radiol 32: 106–109.

Baker C (2005) Neural crest and cranial ectodermal placodes. In: Developmental Neurobiology (Rao MS, Jacobson M, eds.), 4th ed., pp. 67–127. New York: Kluwer Academic/Plenum Publishers.

Bamforth JS, Riccardi VM, Thisen P, Chitayat D, Friedman JM, Caruthers J, Hall BK (1989) Encephalocraniocutaneous lipomatosis. Report of two cases and a review of the literature. Neurofibromatosis 2: 166–173.

Basch ML, Selleck MAJ, Bronner-Fraser M (2000) Timing and competence of neural crest formation. Devel Neurosci 22: 217–227.

Bei M, Peters H, Maas RL (2002) The role of *PAX* and *MSX* genes in craniofacial development. In: Craniofacial Surgery (Lin KY, Ogle RC, Jane JA, eds.), pp. 101–112. Philadelphia: WB Saunders.

Bellmeyer A, Krase J, Lindgren J, LaBonne C (2003) The protooncogene *c-myc* is an essential regulator of neural crest formation in *Xenopus*. Devel Cell 4: 827–839.

Berker M, Oruckaptan HH, Oge HK, Benli K (2000) Neurocutaneous melanosis associated with Dandy-Walker malformation. Pediatr Neurosurg 33: 270–273.

Blaschko (1901) Die Neven-verteilung in der Haut in ihrer Beziehung zu den Erkrankungen der Haut. Beilage zu den Verhandlungen der Deutschen Dermatologischen Gesellschaft VII Congress, Breslau.

Bolande RP (1974) The neurocristopathies. A unifying concept of disease arising in neural crest maldevelopment. Hum Pathol 5: 409–429.

Bolande RP (1981) Neurofibromatosis – the quintessential neurocristopathy: pathogenetic concepts and relationships. Adv Neurol 29: 67–75.

Bolande RP (1997) Neurocristopathy: its growth and development in 20 years. Pediatr Pathol Lab Med 17: 1–25.

Borchers A, David R, Wedlich D (2001) *Xenopus* cadherin-11 restrains cranial neural crest migration and influences neural crest specification. Development 128: 3049–3060.

Bronner-Fraser M (1988) Distribution and function of tenascin during cranial neural crest development in the chick. J Neurosci Res 21: 135–147.

Bronner-Fraser M (1994) Neural crest formation and migration in the developing embryo. FASEB J 8: 699–706.

Bronner-Fraser M (1995) Origins and developmental potential of the neural crest. Exp Cell Res 218: 405–417.

Burstyn-Cohen T, Kalcheim C (2002) Association between the cell cycle and neural crest delamination through specific regulation of G1/S transition. Dev Cell 3: 383–395.

Cano A, Pérez-Moreno MA, Rodrigo I et al. (2000) The transcription factor snail controls epithelial-mesenchymal transitions by repressing E-cadherin expression. Nat Cell Biol 2: 76–83.

Carstens MH (2004) Neural tube programming and craniofacial cleft formation. I. The neuromeric organization of the head and neck. Eur J Paediatr Neurol 8: 181–210.

Chalazonitis A (1996) Neurotrophin-3 as an essential signal for the developing nervous system. Mol Neurobiol 12: 39–53.

Chalazonitis A (2004) Neurotrophin-3 in the development of the enteric nervous system. Progr Brain Res 146: 243–263.

Chaloupka JC, Wolf RJ, Varma PK (1996) Neurocutaneous melanosis with the Dandy-Walker malformation: a possible rare pathoetiologic association. Neuroradiology 38: 486–489.

Chan KK, Wong CK, Lui VC et al. (2003) Analysis of *SOX10* mutations identified in Waardenburg-Hirschsprung patients: differential effects on target gene regulation. J Cell Biochem 90: 573–583.

Chisaka O, Capecchi MR (1991) Regionally restricted developmental defects resulting from targeted disruption of the mouse homeobox gene *Hox 1.5*. Nature 350: 473–479.

Cohen MM Jr, Neri G, Weksberg R (2001) Overgrowth Syndromes. Oxford University Press, New York.

Cramer SF (1988) The melanocytic differentiation pathway in congenital melanocytic nevi: theoretical considerations. Pediatr Pathol 8: 253–265.

Curatolo P (ed.) (2003) Tuberous Sclerosis Complex: From Basic Science to Clinical Phenotypes. International Child Neurology Association and MacKeith Press, London, UK.

Dickinson M, Selleck M, McMahon A, Bronner-Fraser M (1995) Dorsalization of the neural tube by the non-neural ectoderm. Development 121: 2099–2106.

Donis-Keller H, Dou S, Chi D, Carlson KM, Toshima K, Lairmore TC, Howe JR, Moley JF, Goodfellow P, Wells SA Jr (1993) Mutations in the RET proto-oncogene are associated with MEN 2A and FMTC. Hum Mol Genet 2: 851–856.

Dottori M, Gross MK, Labosky P, Goulding M (2001) The winged helix transcription factor *Foxd3* suppresses interneuron differentiation and promotes neural crest cell fate. Development 128: 4127–4138.

Edery P, Lyonnet S, Mulligan LM, Pelet A, Dow E, Abel L, Holder S, Nihoul-Fekete C, Ponder BA, Munnich A (1994) Mutations of the RET proto-oncogene in Hirschsprung's disease. Nature 367(6461): 378–380.

Egan CA, Meadows KP, Van Orman CB, Vanderhoof SL (2001) Neurologic variant of epidermal nevus syndrome with a facial lipoma. Int J Dermatol 40: 189–190.

El Shamy WM, Linnarsson S, Lee K-F et al. (1996) Prenatal and postnatal requirements of NT-3 for sympathetic neuroblast survival and innervation of specific targets. Development 122: 491–500.

Flores-Sarnat L (2002) Hemimegalencephaly. Part 1. Genetic, clinical and imaging aspects. J Child Neurol 17: 373–384.

Flores-Sarnat L (2007) Waardenburg syndrome. MedLink (internet medical data system), San Diego.

García-Castro M, Bronner-Fraser M (1999) Induction and differentiation of the neural crest. Curr Opin Cell Biol 11: 695–698.

Gershon MD (1999) Neurotrophins in enteric nervous system development. In: Neurotrophins and the Neural Crest (Sieber-Blum M, ed.), pp. 173–202. CRC Press: Boca Raton, Florida.

Gómez M, Sampson JR, Whittemore VH (eds.) (1999) Tuberous Sclerosis Complex, 3rd ed. New York: Oxford University Press.

Hall BK (1999) The Neural Crest in Development and Evolution. New York Berlin: Springer.

Hall BK (2000) The neural crest as a fourth germ layer and vertebrates as quadroblastic not triploblastic. Evol Devel 2: 3–5.

Hindman BW, Gill HK, Zuppan CW (1997) Primitive neuroectodermal tumor in a child with tuberous sclerosis. Skel Radiol 26: 184–187.

His W (1868) Untersuchungen über die erste Anlage der Wirtbeltierleibes die erste Entwickelung des Hunchens im Ei. Vogel, Leipzig.

Hofstra RM, Landsvater RM, Ceccherini I, Stulp RP, Stelwagen T, Luo Y, Pasini B, Hoppener JW, van Amstel HK, Romeo G et al. (1994) A mutation in the RET proto-oncogene associated with multiple endocrine neoplasia type 2B and sporadic medullary thyroid carcinoma. Nature 367(6461): 375–376.

Honore SM, Aybar MJ, Mayor R (2003) *Sox10* is required for the early development of the prospective neural crest in Xenopus embryos. Devel Biol 260: 79–96.

Hunt P, Wilkinson DG, Krumlauf R (1991) Patterning of the vertebrate head: murine *Hox-2* genes mark distinct subpopulations of premigratory and migrating neural crest. Development 112: 43–51.

Ikeda I, Ishizaka Y, Tahira T, Suzuki T, Onda M, Sugimura T, Nagao M (1990) Specific expression of the ret proto-oncogene in human neuroblastoma cell lines. Oncogene 5: 1291–1296.

Inoue K, Shilo K, Boerkoel CF et al. (2002) Congenital hypomyelinating neuropathy, central demyelination and Waardenburg-Hirschsprung disease: phenotypes linked by *SOX10* mutation. Ann Neurol 52: 836–842.

Jambart S, Turpin G, de Gennes JL (1979) Neurocristopathies: embryology, physiology, and pathology of the neural crest derivatives. Semaine des Hopitaux 55: 1679–1688.

Jones MC (1990) The neurocristopathies: reinterpretation based upon the mechanism of abnormal morphogenesis. Cleft Palate J 27: 136–140.

Jozwiak S, Janniger CK (2005) Haberland syndrome. eMedicine, 3 May.

Kadonaga JN, Frieden IJU (1991) Neurocutaneous melanosis: definition and review of the literature. J Am Acad Dermatol 24: 747–755.

Kalcheim C (2000) Mechanisms of early neural crest development: from cell specification to migration. Int Rev Cytol 200: 143–196.

Klippel M, Trenaunay P (1900) Du naevus variqueux ostëohypertrophique. Arch Génét Méd (Paris) 3: 611–672.

Krull CE (2001) Segmental organization of neural crest migration. Mech Devel 105: 37–45.

Kuratani S, Matsuo I, Aizawa S (1997) Developmental patterning and evolution of the mammalian viscerocranium: genetic insights into comparative morphology. Devel Dynam 209: 139–155.

Kurokawa D, Kiyonari H, Nakayama R et al. (2004) Regulation of *Otx2* expression and its functions in mouse forebrain and midbrain. Development 131: 3319–3331.

LaBonne C (2002) Vertebrate development: *wnt* signals at the crest. Curr Biol 12: R743–R744.

LaBonne C, Bronner-Fraser M (1998) Neural crest induction in *Xenopus*: evidence for a two-signal model. Development 125: 2403–2414.

LaBonne C, Bronner-Fraser M (2000) *Snail*-related transcriptional repressors are required in *Xenopus* for both the induction of the neural crest and its subsequent migration. Devel Biol 221: 195–205.

Le Douarin N, Kalcheim C (1999) The Neural Crest. 2nd ed. Cambridge University Press, Cambridge, UK.

Liem KF Jr, Tremmi G, Roelink H, Jessell TM (1995) Dorsal differentiation of neural plate cells induced by *BMP*-mediated signals from epidermal ectoderm. Cell 82: 969–979.

Lumsden A, Sprawson N, Graham A (1991) Segmental origin and migration of neural crest cells in the hindbrain region of the chick embryo. Development 113: 1281–1291.

McLarren KW, Litsiou A, Streit A (2003) *DLX5* positions the neural crest and preplacode region at the border of the neural plate. Dev Biol 259: 34–47.

Meulemans D, McCauley D, Bronner-Fraser M (2003) *Id* expression in amphioxus and lamprey highlights the role of gene cooption during neural crest evolution. Devel Biol 264: 430–442.

Mokouyama M, Shin D, Britsch S, Taniguichi M, Anderson DJ (2002) Sensory nerves determine the pattern of arterial differentiation and blood vessel branching in the skin. Cell 109: 693–705.

Newgreen DF, Minichiello J (1995) Control of epitheliomesenchymal transformation. I. Events in the onset of neural crest cell migration are separable and inducible by protein kinase inhibitors. Dev Biol 170: 91–101.

Nieto MA, Sargent MG, Wilkinson DG, Cooke J (1994) Control of cell behaviour during vertebrate development by *Slug*, a zinc finger gene. Science 264: 835–839.

Oguma E, Aihara T, Shimanuki Y et al. (1996) Hypomelanosis of Ito associated with neuroblastoma. Pediatr Radiol 26: 273–275.

Ommen GS, McKusick VA (1979) The association of Waardenburg syndrome and Hirschsprung megacolon. Am J Med Genet 3: 217–223.

Pages A (1955) Essai sur le systeme des "cellules claires" de Feyrter. P. Dehan Edt., Montpellier.

Parkes-Weber F (1907) Haemangiectatic hypertrophies of the foot and lower extremity. Med Press, London, UK, pp. 136–261.

Pascual-Castroviejo I (ed.) (2001) Neurofibromatosis. Escuela Libre Editorial, Madrid.

Pascual-Castroviejo I, Roche E, Martínez-Bermejo A et al. (1998) Hypomelanosis of Ito. A study of 76 infantile cases. Brain Dev 20: 36–43.

Pavone L, Curatolo P, Rizzo R et al. (1991) Epidermal nevus syndrome: a neurologic variant with hemimegalencephaly, gyral malformation, mental retardation, seizures and facial hemihypertrophy. Neurology 41: 266–71.

Perris R, Perissinotto D (2000) Role of the extracellular matrix during neural crest cell migration. Mech Devel 95: 3–21.

Puelles L, Rubinstein JL (2003) Forebrain gene expression domains and the evolving prosomeric model. Trends Neurosci 26: 469–476.

Raible DW, Eisen JS (1996) Regulative interactions in zebrafish neural crest. Development 122: 501–507.

Rathjen J, Haines BP, Hudson KM et al. (2002) Directed differentiation of pluripotent cells to neural lineages: homogeneous formation and differentiation of a neurectoderm population. Development 129: 2649–2661.

Roach ES, Miller VS (eds.) (2004) Neurocutaneous Disorders. Cambridge University Press, Cambridge, UK.

Rokitansky J (1861) Ein ausgezeichneter Fall von Pigment-Mal mit ausgrebreiteter Pigmentierung der inneren Hirn-und Rückenmarkshäute. Allg Wien Med 1: 113–116.

Romeo G, Ronchetto P, Luo Y, Barone V, Seri M, Ceccherini I, Pasini B, Bocciardi R, Lerone M, Kääriäinen H et al. (1994) Point mutations affecting the tyrosine kinase domain of the RET proto-oncogene in Hirschsprung's disease. Nature 367(6461): 377–378.

Sadaghiani B, Crawford BJ, Vielkind JR (1994) Changes in the distribution of extracellular matrix components during neural crest development in *Xiphophorus* spp. embryos. Can J Zool 72: 1340–1353.

Sánchez-Martín M, Rodríguez-García A, Pérez-Losada J, Sagrera A, Read AP, Sánchez-García I (2002) *SLUG*

(*SNAIL2*) deletions in patients with Waardenburg disease. Hum Mol Genet 11: 3231–3236.

Santos CC, Miller VS, Roach ES (2004) Neurocutaneous syndromes. In: Neurology in Clinical Practice (Bradley WG, Daroff RB, Fenichel GM, Jankovic J, eds.) 4th ed., pp. 1867–1900. Philadelphia: Butterworth-Heinemann (Elsevier).

Sarnat HB (2000) Molecular genetic classification of central nervous system malformations. J Child Neurol 15: 675–687.

Sarnat HB, Netsky MG (1981) Evolution of the Nervous System. 2nd ed. Oxford University Press, NY, London.

Sarnat HB, Flores-Sarnat L (2004) Integrative classification of morphology and molecular genetics in central nervous system malformations. Am J Med Genet 126A: 386–392.

Sarnat HB, Flores-Sarnat L (2005) Embryology of the neural crest: its inductive role in the neurocutaneous syndromes. J Child Neurol 20: 637–643.

Selleck MAJ, Scherson TY, Bronner-Fraser M (1993) Origins of neural crest cell diversity. Dev Biol 159: 1–11.

Selleck MAJ, García-Castro M, Artinger KB, Bronner-Fraser M (1995) Dorsalization of the neural tube by the non-neural ectoderm. Development 121: 2099–2106.

Selleck MAJ, García-Castro M, Artinger KB, Bronner-Fraser M (1998) Effects of *Shh* and *noggin* on neural crest formation demonstrate that *BMP* is required in the neural tube but not ectoderm. Development 125: 4919–4930.

Sieber-Blum M (ed.) (1999) Neurotrophins and the Neural Crest CRC Press, Boca Raton, Florida.

Slavin SA, Baker DC, McCarthy JG, Mufarrij A (1983) Congenital infiltrating lipomatosis of the face: clinicopathologic evaluation and treatment. Plast Reconstr Surg 72: 158–164.

Small JM (1955) Some disturbances of the neural crest affecting the nervous system. Proc Roy Soc Med 48: 597–601.

Steijlen PM, Vietor HE, Steensel MV, Happle R (2000) Sweat testing in Hypomelanosis of Ito: divergent results reflecting genetic heterogeneity. Eur J Dermatol 10: 217–219.

Tan SS, Morriss-Kay GM (1985) The development and distribution of the cranial neural crest in the rat embryo. Cell Tiss Res 240: 403–416.

Touraine RL, Attie-Bitach T, Manceau E et al. (2000) Neurological phenotype in Waardenburg syndrome type 4 correlates with novel *SOX10* truncating mutations and expression in developing brain. Am J Hum Genet 66: 1496–1503; *erratum* 2000; 66: 2020.

Trainor P, Krumlauf R (2000) Plasticity in mouse neural crest cells reveals a new patterning role for cranial mesoderm. Nature Cell Biol 2: 96–102.

Unal O, Cirak B, Bekerecioglu M, Kutluhan A, Ugras S, Tali T (2000) Congenital infiltrating lipomatosis of the face with cerebral abnormalities. Eur Radiol 10: 1610–1613.

Van der Hoeve J (1916) Abnorme Länge der Tränen-röhrchen mit Ankyloblepharon. Klin Mbl Augenheilk 56: 232–238.

Van der Hoeve J (1920) Eye symptoms in tuberous sclerosis of the brain. Trans Ophthalmol Soc UK 20: 329–334.

Van der Hoeve J (1921) Augengeschwulst bei der tuberosen Hirnskleose (Bourneville). Albrecht Graefes Arch Klin Ophthalmol 105: 880–898.

Van der Hoeve J (1932) Eye symptoms in phakomatoses (The Doyle Memorial Lecture). Tr Ophthalmol Soc UK 52: 380–401.

Villanueva S, Glavic A, Ruiz P, Mayor R (2002) Posterior-ization by *FGF*, *Wnt* and retinoic acid is required for neural crest induction. Dev Biol 241: 289–301.

Waardenburg PJ (1948) Dystopia punctorum lachri-marum, blepharophimosis en partiele irisatrophie bij een doofstomme. Ned Tschr Geneeskd 92: 3463–3465.

Waardenburg PJ (1951) A new syndrome combining devel-opmental anomalies of the eyelids, eyebrows and nose root with pigmentary defects of the iris and head hair and with congenital deafness. Am J Hum Genet 3: 195–253.

Woda JM, Pastagia J, Mercola M, Artinger KB (2003) *Dlx* proteins position the neural plate border and etermine adjacent cell fates. Development 130: 331–342.

Yakovlev PO, Guthrie RH (1931) Congenital ectodermoses (neurocutaneous syndromes) in epileptic patients. Arch Neurol Psychiat 26: 1145.

Zhang W, Simos PG, Isibashi H (2003) Neuroimaging fea-tures of epidermal nevus syndrome. Am J Neuroradiol 24: 1468–1470.

# Chapter 2

# VASCULAR BIRTHMARKS OF INFANCY: PHACE ASSOCIATION (PASCUAL-CASTROVIEJO TYPE II SYNDROME) AND COBB SYNDROME

Ignacio Pascual-Castroviejo

Paediatric Neurology Service, University Hospital La Paz, University of Madrid, Madrid, Spain

## Introduction, historical perspective and terminology

Cutaneous hemangiomas and associated pathology (PHACE association) (OMIM 606519), first described by Pascual-Castroviejo in 1978, is the most frequent neurocutaneous syndrome (Pascual-Castroviejo et al. 1996, Pascual-Castroviejo 2004).

The terminology used to describe *congenital vascular birthmarks* has been a source of confusion in the medical literature (Hand and Frieden 2002) until Mulliken and Glowacki (1982) described a biologic classification system, simplifying and clarifying concepts: this has become the most widely accepted framework for classifying vascular birthmarks and is currently regarded as the official classification schema by the International Society for the Study of Vascular Anomalies (ISSVA). The relationship of the two main groups of cutaneous vascular anomalies, *hemangiomas* and *vascular malformations*, with intracranial and/or extracranial vascular and non-vascular abnormalities was established by the papers of Pascual-Castroviejo (1978, 1985) and Pascual-Castroviejo et al. (1995, 1996). These vascular lesions are now well-known to be present anywhere in the body, to be associated with internal lesions in subjacent or in distant structures (Pascual-Castroviejo et al. 1996, Drolet et al. 1999, Metry et al. 2001, Hand and Frieden 2002, Pascual-Castroviejo 2004), and to depict the most frequent neurocutaneous disorder (Pascual-Castroviejo et al. 1996, Pascual-Castroviejo 2004).

**Hemangiomas** are the most common benign tumors in infancy, occurring in up to 10% of children less than 1 year of age (Frieden et al. 1996). They are between likely more than five fold more common in girls than boys (Watson and McCarthy 1940; Pascual-Castroviejo 1978, 1985; Persky 1986; Enjolras et al. 1990; Byard et al. 1991; Gorlin et al. 1994; Pascual-Castroviejo et al. 1996). In 60 percent of cases, they occur on the head and neck (Esterly 1995). Hemangiomas are usually not present at birth, and most develop during the first few weeks of life. After growing over months or more rarely over years because of rapid endothelial cell proliferation, they spontaneously involute (Mulliken and Glowacki 1982). In some cases, hemangiomas can proliferate in utero and manifest as fully developed tumors at birth (Boon et al. 1996). Their presence was observed in 23% of premature infants with weigh less than 1000 g (Amir et al. 1986). The risk of hemangioma is 10 times higher in children born to women who underwent chorionic-villus sampling compared to children of women who did not undergo this procedure (Burton et al. 1995, Metry et al. 2006).

Hemangioma is not the only vascular anomaly that appears as a birthmark during infancy (Mulliken and Glowacki 1982; Cohen 2006, 2007). **Vascular malformations** can also be found on the skin in a distribution similar to hemangiomas, although without having the appearance of a tumor. Vascular malformations are composed of dysplastic vessels without cellular proliferation and never regress. They are subcategorized depending on the flow (high- or slow-flow malformations) and on the predominant anomalous channels (arteriovenous and lymphatic malformations) (see also chapter on "Kippel-

Trenaunay, Parkes Weber and Sturge-Weber syndromes") (Mulliken 1992; Dubois and Garel 1999; Cohen 2006, 2007).

The first serious problems, apart from the esthetic and psychological factors linked to the facial hemangioma, were those associated with central nervous system malformations and extracranial and intracranial arterial anomalies as well as congenital cyanotic cardiopathies and anomalies of the aortic arch (Pascual-Castroviejo 1978). The presence of cutaneous hemangioma not only in the head, face and/or neck, but also in other parts of the body, such as the genitalia, associated with vascular, cardiac and aortic arch anomalies, was also emphasized in the papers by Pascual-Castroviejo (1985) and Pascual-Castroviejo et al. (1996).

Hemangiomas have been also associated with skeletal changes (Boyd et al. 1984), sternal malformations (Hersh et al. 1985), constitutional deformities (Burns et al. 1991, Baker et al. 1993), coarctation of the aorta (Schneeweiss et al. 1982, Vaillant et al. 1988, Pascual-Castroviejo et al. 1996), midabdominal raphè (Igarashi et al. 1985) or sacral and genitourinary defects (Goldberg et al. 1986). Hemangiomas may involve not only the face, but also the pharynx, larynx, arms, shoulders, chest, back, mediastinum, limbs, trunk, genitalia, liver, gastrointestinal tract and/or other anatomical locations (Pascual-Castroviejo 1985, 2004; Enjolras et al. 1990; Geller et al. 1991; Reese et al. 1993; Pascual-Castroviejo et al. 1996; Capin et al. 1997; Metry et al. 2001). Visceral hemangiomas are associated with bulky cervicocephalic hemangiomas or with small hemangiomas scattered over the body (Enjolras et al. 1990, Pascual-Castroviejo et al. 2002). Spinal arteriovenous malformations are associated with cutaneous vascular malformations in the Cobb's syndrome (Cobb 1915, Pascual-Castroviejo et al. 2002). Cutaneous hemangiomas or vascular malformation may be associated with one, two or several lesions as described in the first papers on the syndrome (Pascual-Castroviejo 1978, 1985; Pascual-Castroviejo et al. 1995, 1996) and this association corresponds to a true syndrome and not to an incomplete phenotypic expression (Rossi et al. 2001).

It was suggested that cutaneous hemangiomas associated with vascular and/or nonvascular abnormalities of surrounding structures in the body could constitute well defined syndromes. We could, therefore, identify a syndrome associating cutaneous hemangioma of the gluteal and sacrococcygeal regions and spinal dysraphism (recently named SACRAL syndrome achromin for Spinal dysraphism, Amogenital, Cutaneous, Renal and Urologic anomalies associated with on angioma of lumbosacral localization) (Stockman et al. 2007); another associating sternal malformation or aplasia associated with hemangioma in the face, neck and chest (Hersh et al. 1985); another associating facial cavernous hemangioma, cerebellar hypoplasia and coarctation of the aorta (that was named the *3C syndrome*) (Goh and Lo 1993) (all these three signs added to several others had been included as part of the pathological findings in the syndrome already described by Pascual-Castroviejo in 1978); and another associating midabdominal raphe with facial cavernous hemangioma (Igarashi et al. 1985). Later on Pascual-Castroviejo et al. (1996) described the associated pathology of any type with hemangiomas of the head, neck and chest in 17 cases, some of them with a follow-up of more than twenty years. They found cerebral and cerebellar malformations, intracranial and extracranial arterial anomalies, mainly consisting of persistent embryonic arteries, absence or hypoplasia of the carotid and/or vertebral arteries, anomalies of the aortic arch, congenital cardiac malformations, as well as intra-abdominal hemangioma affecting an extensive segment of the intestine. In this paper, the authors presented a case with regression of intracranial and extracranial vascular anomalies and extreme narrowing of the intracranial arteries. They suggested that this complex malformation syndrome could show as many complications as other systemic classical neurocutaneous diseases, such as neurofibromatosis type 1, tuberous sclerosis, and hypomelanosis of Ito, and concluded that **cutaneous hemangioma-vascular complex syndrome** (a name that did not satisfy the authors, but at least included the term complex that means "wide" and/or "large" as they wished to imply) could be one of the most frequent neurocutaneous diseases.

A type of hemangioma, called "*disseminated*" or "*diffuse*" *neonatal hemangiomatosis* (Burke et al. 1964,

Holden and Alexander 1970, Enjolras et al. 1990) shows a rapid growth and extension of the hemangiomas during the neonatal period and is associated with visceral hemangiomas in which any organ can be affected. Holden and Alexander (1970) included as diffuse neonatal hemangiomas only cases with: 1). Recognized visceral hemangiomas in neonatal period; 2). Three or more organ systems affected by the hemangiomas; 3). Not malignant hemangiomas. The prognosis is not always linked to the size of the hemangioma, and lethal visceral hemangiomas associated with small cutaneous hemangiomas have been reported (Enjolras et al. 1990). The systemic involvement cannot be predicted by the number and/or size of cutaneous hemangiomas (Enjolras et al. 1990). Diffuse neonatal hemangiomatosis is thus a differentiated type of hemangioma, but it does not seem to correspond to a different entity.

The eponym "**PHACE**" is used by some authors (Frieden et al. 1996) to denote the major features described by Pascual-Castroviejo (1978 and 1985), and Pascual-Castoviejo et al. (1996). P derives from Posterior fossa malformations, H from Hemangioma, A from Arterial anomalies, C from Coarctation of the aorta and other cardiac defects, and E from Eye abnormalities (mostly secondary to eye closure by the facial hemangioma). The term **PHACES** syndrome is used when sternal clefting or a supraumbilical abdominal raphe is present. The eponymic *Pascual-Castroviejo type II* has also been applied (Torres-Mohedas et al. 2001, Bèlanger-Quintana et al. 2002). Pascual-Castroviejo et al. had described in 1975 another entity, the **Pascual-Castroviejo type 1** or "cerebro-facio-thoracic dysplasia" (Rufo-Campos et al. 2004). Distribution patterns of the hemangiomas or vascular malformations suggest dermatological involvement in some cases, but not in all, which is typical of the well described trigeminal patterns V1, V2, and V3 (Pascual-Castroviejo 1978; Frieden et al. 1996; Guian-Almeida et al. 1996; Pascual-Castroviejo et al. 1996, 2002a; Mohammadi et al. 2004).

PHACE syndrome or Pascual-Castroviejo type II is a widespread disease with possibility of clinical and pathological expression in any region of the body (Pascual-Castroviejo et al. 1996, Drolet et al. 1999, Pascual-Castroviejo 2004). The lesions most commonly involve the skin, but any organ can be affected, including CNS (intracranial and intraspinal areas), gastrointestinal tract, liver, lungs, spleen, kidneys, oral cavity, genito-urinary system, lumbosacral or any region of the spine (possibly, it may include the Cobb syndrome as well). Such systemic involvement cannot be predicted based of the number or size of the cutaneous hemangiomas. The frequency of this syndrome largely surpasses that of the other neurocutaneous disorders. Its prevalence is about 10% in infancy, although the clinical meaning and phenotype expression are variable. This syndrome is not only the most frequent vascular neurocutaneous disorder, but also the most frequent neurocutaneous disease and perhaps the most frequent general or systemic congenital defect.

## PHACE(S) association/Pascual-Castroviejo II syndrome

### Clinical manifestations

This systemic syndrome can show clinical manifestations localized anywhere in the body.

The main clinical manifestations include: a) cutaneous hemangiomas, b) ocular alterations, c) mental and psychological problems, d) intracranial and extracranial abnormalities, e) cerebellar malformations, f) congenital cardiovascular disease with coarctation of the aortic arch and congenital cardiopathy, g) thoracic and abdominal malformations, h) hepatic and/or intestinal hemangiomas, i) sacral and ano-genitourinary malformations, j) spinal anomalies.

In one of the earliest important series of hemangiomas in 210 children (Margileth and Museles 1965), lesions were located in any area of the body: the head and neck, 38%; and the trunk, 29%. The majority were: strawberry lesions in 81%; cavernous type in 7%; and mixed in 9%.

Not only is the size of the cutaneous hemangioma important, but also its localization. The latter can determine many of the associated complications, particularly involvement of the face, nose, orbits, neck and ears, followed by the genitalia, hands, feet and anal region. These locations can complicate the life of a patient with cutaneous hemangiomas as much as the size of the lesion. However, small size hemangiomas may be associated with severe internal malformations that can also lead to death (Pascual-Castroviejo et al. 2005).

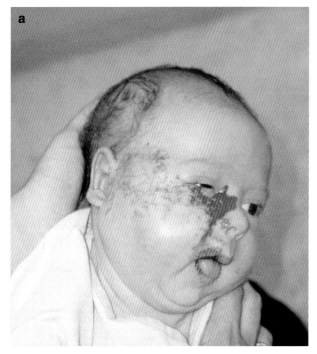

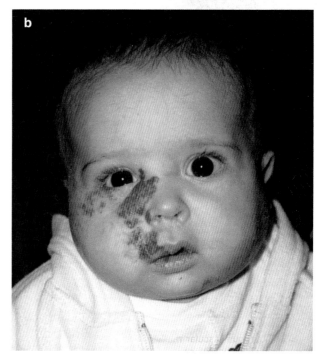

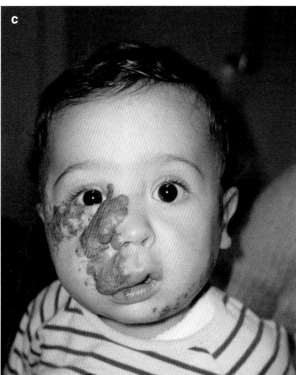

**Fig. 1.** Cutaneous hemangioma extending to the right facial area innervated by the second branch of the right trigeminal and by the third branch of the left trigeminal nerve at the age of: (**a**) 1 month, (**b**) 6 months, and (**c**) 12 months.

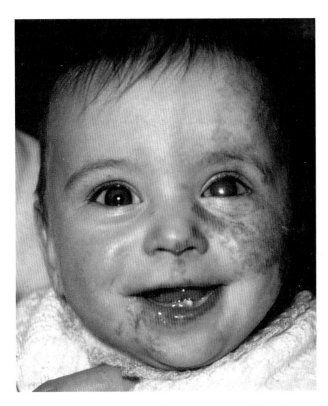

**Fig. 2.** Cutaneous vascular malformation of the left facial area innervated by the first and the second sensory division of the trigeminal nerve and of the right lower lip and neighboring area.

## Hemangioma and other external malformations

Cutaneous vascular anomalies can be distributed anywhere in the body. These vascular anomalies are of two types according to the classification of Mulliken and Glowacki (1982): a) hemangiomas (Fig. 1) (benign vascular tumors) and b) vascular malformations (Fig. 2). Both anomalies may be located in the same regions of the body and are associated with many common complications. These appear more frequently in the head, face, neck, shoulders and chest but any area of the skin may show one or more hemangiomas (Fig. 3) (Pascual-Castroviejo et al. 1996, Frieden et al. 1996, Metry et al. 2001). A few malformations appear to be in tight connection with the hemangioma in many cases, including ventral sternal clefting and supraumbilical abdominal raphe, sacral and/or genitourinary defects and coarctation of the aortic arch (Burns et al. 1991). Small bowel (Fig. 4) and pancreatic involvement were described by Hersh et al. (1985). Facial and neck hemangiomas and vascular malformations are best known, and their association with cerebellar and arterial malformations and, less frequently, with aortic arch anomalies and cardiac congenital malformations constitute a recognized entity (Pascual-Castroviejo 1978, Pascual-Castroviejo et al. 1996).

Sternal defects and/or supraumbilical midline raphe have been described in isolated reports in which these malformations appear to be associated with cutaneous facial hemangiomas as well as with internal angiomas (Haque 1984, Hersh et al. 1985).

The presence of a hemangioma or other type of lesions in internal subjacent zones to those of the cutaneous hemangiomas or vascular malformations must be always suspected and investigated. Internal lesions, however, may be found distantly from the cutaneous hemangioma (Chateil et al. 2000). We found a hepatic hemangioma and another hemangioma in the mediastinum in a case that had an ipsilateral cutaneous strawberry hemangioma in the upper part of the right abdomen. Both, cutaneous and hepatic hemangiomas showed increased size at the same time during the first year of age and later involuted concomitantly (Pascual-Castroviejo et al. 2002). Another patient who showed cutaneous vascular malformations in the middle zone of the back had an intramedullary arteriovenous malformation at the thoracic level. This association was given the name of Cobb syndrome (Cobb 1915). We believe that this phenotype can be a localized form of the same disease.

Periorbital hemangiomas are associated with ophthalmic complications (Coats et al. 1999). The occlusion of the eye as a result of the size of the hemangioma can be prolonged over a long period and therefore the eye is subject to stimulus deprivation. Amblyopia (defined as reduced visual acuity of 20/30 or more) was found closely correlated with the duration of eyelid closure (Stigmar et al. 1978).

Many patients with cervicofacial hemangioma, especially those associated with intracranial arterial abnormalities, frequently have developmental delay

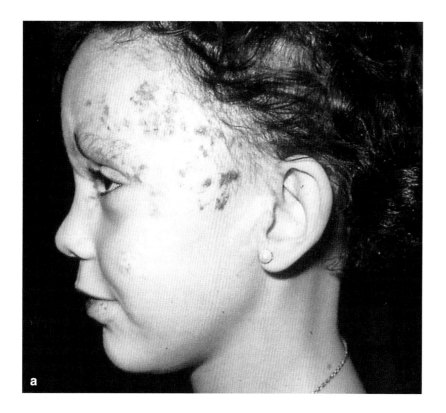

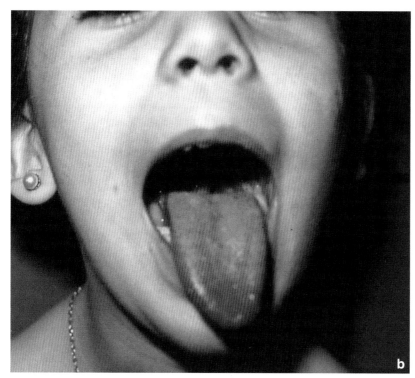

**Fig. 3.** A patient shows cutaneous hemangiomas located in different areas of the body: (**a**) face; (**b**) tongue; (**c**) scarococcigeal and genitalia regions; and (**d**) left foot.

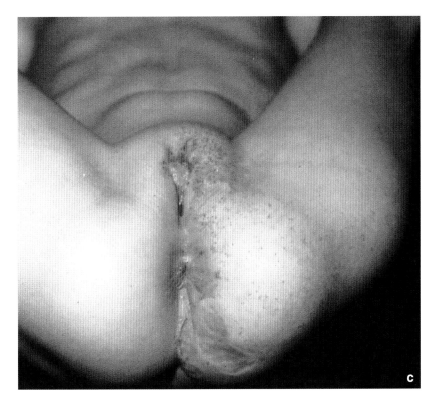

**Fig. 3.** (Continued)

and borderline mental levels (Pascual-Castroviejo et al. 1996).

Facial hemangioma has a significant impact on the patients and their families. Although the condition may be temporary, they must confront not only their own emotional reactions, but also the strangers who repeatedly reinforce the stigmatising nature of the condition (Tanner et al. 1998) and most parents wish to have the hemangioma removed before the child enters school (Dieterich-Miller and Safford 1992).

Another possible location of cutaneous vascular anomalies is the sacral hemangioma and/or vascular malformation (Fig. 5). It can extend to the lumbar, perineal, buttock and genital regions, and most are associated with genitourinary, neurological and skeletal anomalies, such as imperforate anus, tethered spinal cord, occult spinal cord dysraphism, lipomeningocele, diastematomyelia, renal anomalies, abnormal genitalia, abnormal intergluteal sulcus trajectory, lower extremity deformities, and sphincter malformations. Motor paralysis and sensory deficits are not uncommon.

Bony abnormalities occur in association with hemangiomas (Fig. 6) in only 1 per cent of patients, in contrast with 34 percent of patients with vascular malformations (Boyd et al. 1984).

## Cerebellar malformation

Dandy-Walker malformation and hemispheric hypoplasia are the two most frequent central nervous system anomalies. Dandy-Walker malformation and other cerebellar anomalies are present in 50% (Pascual-Castroviejo et al. 1996) to 90% (Poetke et al. 2002) of cases. They usually do not cause neurological signs of cerebellar disturbances and the presence of the cerebellar defects is a neuroradiological finding that should be routinely looked for in all cases with cutaneous facial and/or neck hemangiomas and vascular malformations after the first description of the syndrome by Pascual-Castroviejo in 1978.

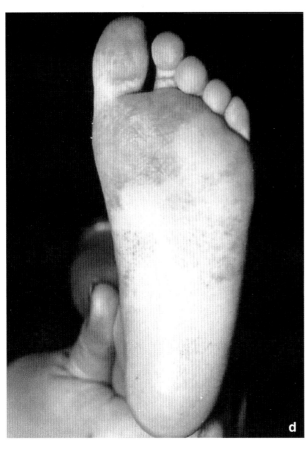

**Fig. 3.** (Continued)

## Coarctation of the aortic arch and congenital cardiopathy

Anomalous aortic arch and congenital cardiopathy are often associated with the cutaneous hemangiomas or the vascular malformations. Both anomalies were reported in the first complete description of this syndrome (Pascual-Castroviejo 1978). Although rare, the presence of cardiopathy in some patients with cutaneous hemangiomas had been previously reported (Cooper and Bolande 1965) along with coarctation of the aorta (Fig. 7) and of right aortic arch (Honey et al. 1975). Further reports associating coarctation of the aorta with mild congenital cardiopathy, hemangioma of the face (Schneeweiss et al. 1982) and cerebellar hypoplasia (Goh and Lo 1993) suggested a new syndrome. More complete information on the previously reported cases (Pascual-Castroviejo 1993) prompted same authors to assume that the syndrome was broader and that the facial hemangioma, the coarctation of the aorta and the cerebellar hypoplasia, besides the previous description, were only some features of the problem, but not the problem itself, which presented many more alterations (Pascual-Castroviejo 1996). At that time, some authors considered the possibility of a single causal entity in the association

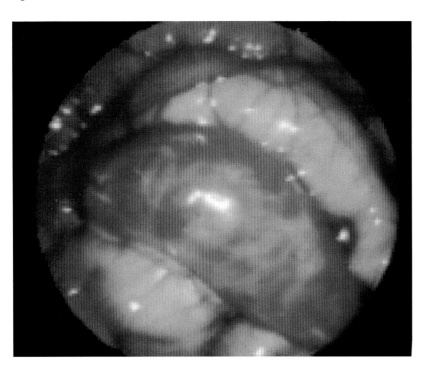

**Fig. 4.** Small bowel involvement (see text for explanation).

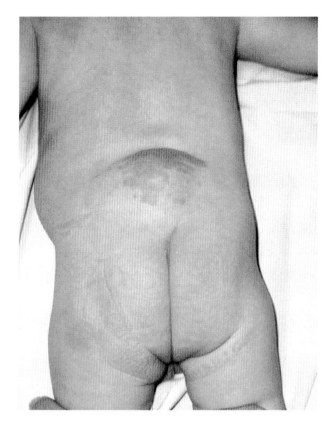

**Fig. 5.** Cutaneous hemangioma extends to the sacrogluteal areas. Note the deformity of the intergluteal sulcus.

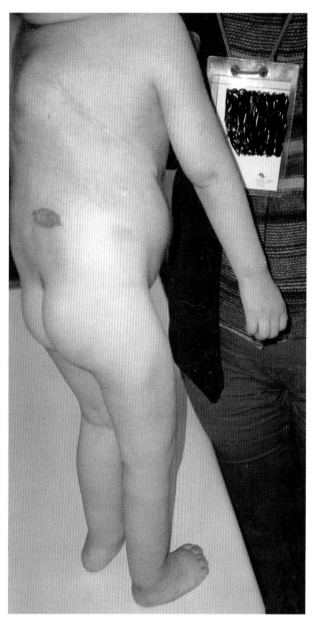

**Fig. 6.** Strawberry-shaped lumbar hemangioma associated with severe spinal malformations.

of hemangioma, supraumbilical midline raphè and coarctation of the aorta (Kishnani et al. 1995).

Aortic arch anomalies may be of several different types: anomalous aortic arch (Pascual-Castroviejo 1978), later identified as aortic arch coarctation (Pascual-Castroiejo et al. 1996); coarctation of the aorta with right aortic arch (Vaillant et al. 1988, Kishnani et al. 1995); double aortic arch and double aortic coarctation (Gorlin et al. 1994). Congenital aneurysm with cutaneous hemangioma, cleft sternum and supraumbilical raphè (Schieken et al. 1987, Raas-Rothschild et al. 2000, Slavotinek et al. 2002) have been reported less frequently.

Congenital cardiopathy can be associated equally with cutaneous cavernous hemangioma and with vascular malformations located in regions of the face, neck, chest or shoulder. The types of congenital cardiopathies are multiple: ductus arteriosus, tricuspid atresia, ventricular septal defect, tetralogy of Fallot, and others.

## Natural history of the skin lesions

Cutaneous hemangiomas in any location of the body are known to regress spontaneously in the majority of cases, although corticosteroids, interferon, thalidomide, and perhaps other therapies may shorten the time of involution. Also intracranial arterial anomalies show diminution of the thickness and tortuos-

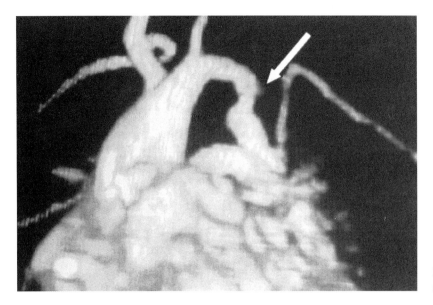

**Fig. 7.** Cardiac MR study shows marked coarctation of the aortic arch (white arrow).

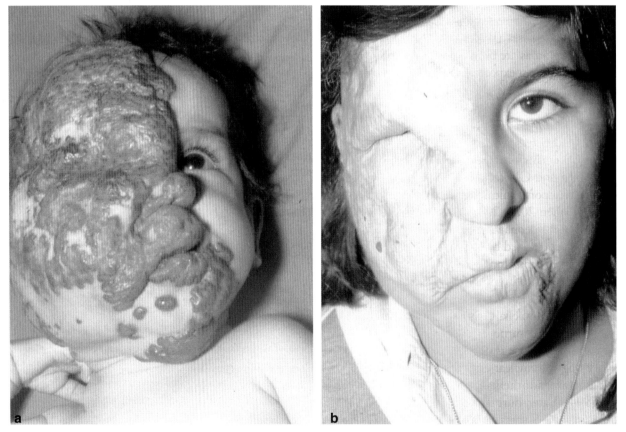

**Fig. 8.** Facial aspect of a patient: (**a**) at few months of age, during the evolution of the hemangioma; (**b**) during adult age, after regression of the hemangioma.

ity in many cases (Pascual-Castroviejo et al. 1996, 2003; Burows et al. 1998). Only minor skin changes remain after regression of the majority of lesions. However, large hemangiomas severely affecting the involved area of skin even after regression may result in excessively slack skin (Fig. 8), pigmentary changes, and a fibrofatty residues (Enjolras et al. 1990).

It is possible, however, to demonstrate atypical cases in which an hemangioma with onset in childhood which was apparently cured redeveloped in adult life (Murotani and Hiramoto 1985).

Cutaneous hemangiomas regress in months or years in the majority of cases. In the series of Margileth and Museles (1965), spontaneous regression between 2 and 6 years was recorded in the strawberry (81%), cavernous (79%), and mixed (83%) types. However, spontaneous regression is not rapid. In the series of Margileth and Museles (1965), regression occurred : at the age 3 years in 30% and by age 7 years in 76%. However, congenital hemangiomas can regress rapidly in some cases (Boon et al. 1996). In general, most hemangiomas are best left untreated, particularly the small ones on unexposed areas (Esterly 1995).

## Pathology

Vascular birthmarks were differentiated into vascular tumors or hemangiomas and vascular malformations by Mulliken and Glowacki in 1982. They based their classification upon clinical, histological and cytological features (Cohen 2006, 2007). 1) *Hemangiomas* have a history of rapid neonatal growth and slow involution. They are characterized by endothelial cell proliferation followed by diminishing hyperplasia and progressive fibrosis. Histologically, in the early proliferating phase, the hemangiomas are made of plump, proliferative, hyperplastic, endothelial cells forming syncytial masses with an increased turnover and increased number of mast cells. This phase is defined by high expression of proliferating cell nuclear antigen, type IV collagenase, and vascular endothelial growth factor (Takahashi et al. 1994). Later, during the involuting phase which starts by age 1–5 years, and continues improvement until 6–12 years of age, there is progressive perivascular deposition of fibrofatty tissue and thinning of the endothelial lining. Increased expression of the tissue inhibitor of metalloproteinase, TIMP 1, an inhibitor of new blood vessel formation, is observed exclusively in the involuting phase (Takahashi et al. 1994). Clinically, hemangiomas appear as subcutaneous bluish-red masses that resemble the surface of a strawberry. They are seen three to four times more frequently in females than in males. 2) *Vascular malformations* are present at birth, grow commensurately with the child, and are characterized histologically by a normal rate of endothelial cell turnover, flat endothelium, thin (normal) basal membrane and normal mast cells (Mulliken and Glowacki 1982). Vascular malformations can be: a) simple or b) combined. Vascular malformations of type simple include: capillary, venous, arterial and lymphatic malformations. The combined type includes arteriovenous, capillary-venous, and lymphatic-venous malformations (Dubois and Garel 1999). Vascular malformations are present at birth, though not always visible. They grow commensurately with the child, and do not regress spontaneously. Boys and girls are equally affected.

## Embryologic development and vascular abnormalities of the brain

In placing these vascular anomalies into an ontogenetic perspective it is necessary to make a chronological summary of the embryonic development of the cerebral arteries, including both their origin from the aortic arch and their intracranial trajectories (Mall 1912, Streeter 1918, Congdon 1922, Padget 1948). Carotid and vertebral arteries begin their development in the aortic arch. Two stages of this development are recognized: the *primary* or *brachial stage* appears at about 22 days and involves the appearance of a vascular apparatus destined to become the precursor of the posterior arteries; in the *second* or *postbrachial stage* the vascular apparatus mentioned is replaced by the adult arterial system during a period lasting about 28 days. The brachial stage starts with the formation of the first aortic arch and terminates somewhat arbitrarily with the interruption of the sixth arch. The sequence reflects the appearance of the different structures: first aortic arch in the embryo of

1.5 mm (3 weeks) and formation of angioblastic nests and preexisting capillaries; second aortic arch in the embryo of 3 mm ($3^1/2$ weeks); third aortic arch in the embryo of 4 mm ($3^1/2$ weeks); fourth aortic arch in the embryo of 4.6 mm (4 weeks); fifth aortic arch immediately after the sixth; sixth aortic arch in the embryo of 5 mm ($4^1/2$ weeks). Each arch is formed from three elements, an outpouching from the aortic sac, a similar outpouching from the wall of the aorta and an intermediate endothelial capillary plexus in the corresponding visceral arch. The formative process is sequential, the first and the second arches disappearing with the formation of the third and fourth. The fifth appears after the sixth and is very transitory, disappearing almost as soon as it is formed. The fourth left arch takes part in the development of the aortic arch, the fourth right arch in that of the subclavian artery and the third arch of each side in the development of the common and internal carotid arteries.

There is disagreement with respect to the development of the external carotid arteries. Congdon (1922) concluded that they originate as an external growth from the aortic sac after the first and second aortic arches have disappeared. Their subsequent origin displaces the third aortic arch, becoming separated into a proximal part that forms the primitive carotid artery and a distal portion that gives origin to the proximal part of the internal carotid artery. Consequently, the common carotid arteries are formed after the involution of the wall of the aorta between the third and fourth arches in the embryo of 12–14 mm (35–36 days). The internal carotid artery appears in the embryo of 3 mm, and as soon as it reaches 4 mm this vessel begins to present an anterior division, that is the outline of the future anterior cerebral, middle cerebral, and anterior choroidal arteries. The posterior division gives origin to the posterior communicating and posterior cerebral arteries in the embryo of 5.3 mm; at this time the anterior cerebral artery is well defined and extends from the third aortic arch. The caudal division of the carotid artery has now formed a secondary anastamosis with the extreme cranial branch of the neural longitudinal artery in the mesencephalon, an embryonic vessel that will soon constitute the definitive posterior communicating artery and be totally substituted for the trigeminal artery.

When the embryo is in the third and last phase of the brachial stage, with a length of approximately 7–12 mm (32–35 days) the internal carotid artery already shows filling with blood in its intracerebral course, in contrast with its small trunk in the third aortic arch. The first important cerebral vessel in this location is the primitive dorsal ophthalmic artery. Subsequently, the primitive anterior carotid artery appears and the first evidence of what will constitute the trunk of the middle cerebral arteries. In the transitional epochs of the brachial and postbrachial development, when the embryo is 12–14 mm (35–38 days), the common carotid artery may be identified and for the first time the cerebral ramification of the internal carotid artery and of its collateral vessels may be described as the earliest adult configuration.

The trigeminal artery begins to be recognized in the embryo of 3 mm (<3 weeks) as the second of the three vascular arms that are derived from the first aortic arch, passes dorsally arching next to the medial zone of the Gasserian ganglion. It constitutes the first source of blood supply to the posterior part of the primordial brain. When the embryo reaches 4 mm (28 days) the trigeminal artery communicates with fragments of the walls of the neural longitudinal arteries, from which the basilar artery forms completely when the embryo has reached 7–12 mm ($4^1/2$–5 weeks) by consolidation of the wall of the longitudinal neural arteries, although there are still discontinuous stretches. The formation of the basilar artery is accompanied by the involution of the trigeminal artery or its annexation by the internal carotid, becoming complete in the embryo of 14 mm (5–$5^1/2$ weeks). If the trigeminal artery is present after birth it constitutes an important vascular malformation anastomosing the internal carotid system with the basilar artery, a function normally substituted by the posterior communicating artery. The superior cerebellar arteries appear during the 7–10 mm stage ($4^1/2$ weeks), supplying part of the anterior zone formerly provided by the trigeminal artery.

The embryo of 9–11 mm (32 days) with a completely formed basilar artery is in an intermediate phase of anastomosis with the carotid system (still across the trigeminal arteries) and with the vertebral system. If the vascular development is arrested or is occluded between 32 and 36 days, the basilar artery could exist without the vertebral artery having formed. The vertebral arteries begin to form when the embryo is 9 mm (32 days) by longitudinal anastomoses between the superior longitudinal segmental arms of the dorsal aorta with subsequent obliteration of all aortic connection except those of the seventh cervical segmental arches, which remain as the subclavian trunk. By the time the embryo measures 12.5 mm (35 days) the vertebral arteries complete their formation but still originate from the wall of the aorta. The vertebral arteries finish their maturation when the embryo reaches 14–16 mm (between 36 and 40 days), with their origin having been displaced at the level of the ductus arteriosus.

The mechanism for normal and abnormal external and internal vascular development is related with the causative genes, that probably are the same in familial and in sporadic cases (see below) (Breugem et al. 2002).

## Abnormalities in the vasculature and brain

From our findings, we deduce that the embryo should be affected in the zone of development of the Gasserian ganglion in earlier periods when the teratogenic possibilities are pluripotential, although related to one another. The type of cutaneous vascular lesion depends on the state of embryonic development, but the possibilities to develop hemangioma or vascular malformation could depend on the regulatory genes which are involved in shaping the specific structures. The association of facial hemangiomas and vascular malformations with alterations in the formation of the embryonic cerebral arteries of more precocious appearance is beyond doubt. For genetically uncertain reasons there is a failure of formation of some definitive arteries that were intended to ascend to the cerebral hemisphere, mostly ipsilateral to that of the hemangioma, which obliges the arteries of first appearance to persist, including the development of contralateral connections and great embryologic com-

plication. Intracranial and extracranial abnormalities including persistence of the trigeminal artery, absence of the carotid or vertebral arteries, angiomatous malformations near the siphon coarctation of the aortic arch and/or congenital cardiac malformations, are associated equally with facial and neck cutaneous hemangioma and vascular malformations.

## Imaging findings

### Vascular abnormalities

Vascular anomalies, particularly of the arterial system, are the most frequent malformations associated with the cutaneous hemangioma and the vascular malformations. Absence of the internal carotid and/or vertebral arteries (Fig. 9) and persistence of the trigeminal artery (Fig. 10) are the most frequent malformations. The largest series analysing data on conventional and/or magnetic resonance angiography (MRA) (Pascual-Castroviejo 1978, 1985; Pascual-Castroviejo et al. 1996; Drolet et al. 2006) showed absence of the vertebral artery in 35% of patients, persistence of the trigeminal artery in about 30%, absence of the internal carotid artery in about 25%, hypoplasia of the internal carotid artery in a 10%, intracranial angiomatous malformations in 10% and isolated cases with other less common malformations, such as arterial angiomatous malformation in the extracranial or intracranial proximal zones to the siphon, intracavernous anterior cerebral artery origin, segmental intervertebral anastomosis, carotid bifurcation of both sides located at different level in the neck (Fig. 11), persistence of the proatlantal artery, persistence of embryonic vascularization (Fig. 12), absence of an external carotid artery (this anomaly was associated with agenesis of the ear of the same side). All the three anomalies (facial hemangioma, absence of external carotid artery and agenesis of the ear) seem to be related. The association of several malformations is common in this syndrome (Fig. 13).

Absence of the internal carotid artery and persistence of the trigeminal artery were seen ipsilateral to the external hemangioma in all cases of our series.

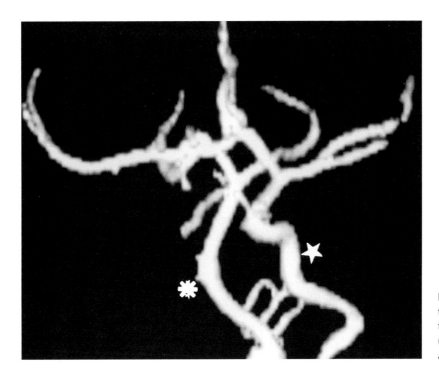

**Fig. 9.** MR arteriography shows absence of the left vertebral and right internal carotid arteries and presence of an enlarged left carotid (white star) and right vertebral (white asterisk) arteries.

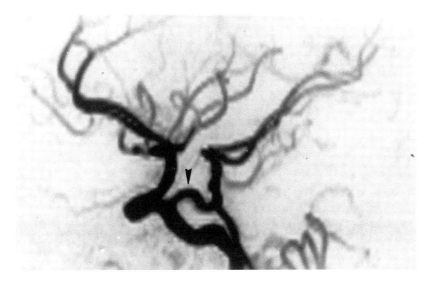

**Fig. 10.** MR arteriography shows the presence of a persistent right trigeminal artery (arrowhead).

Absence of the vertebral artery also was ipsilateral to the external hemangioma in most cases, but not in all. Some patients showed absence of the vertebral artery on the contralateral side to the facial hemangioma.

The cerebral hemisphere ipsilateral to the absence of the internal carotid artery is moderately smaller than the contralateral hemisphere, and cerebral cortical dysplasia can be found in the hypoplas-

tic hemisphere (Pascual-Castroviejo et al. 1995), but alterations of the cortical organization are also seen in other cases with different types of intracranial vascular anomalies related to cutaneous hemangioma or to vascular malformations.

When the hemangioma is located in the orbital zone, the vascular filling is derived from branches of the superficial anterior temporal artery. In the ma-

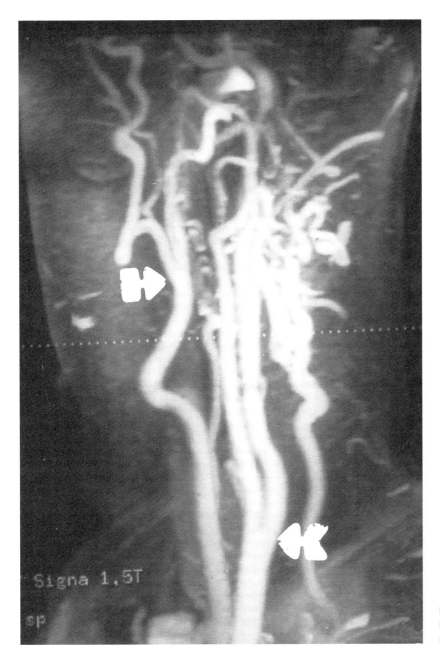

**Fig. 11.** MR arteriography shows the carotid bifurcation of both sides located at different levels (white arrows) in the neck.

jority of cases some blood also is provided via the ophthalmic artery. While this vessel usually arises from the internal carotid and the anterior part of the carotid siphon, in some of these cases we have also seen the ophthalmic artery originate anomalously from a branch of the external carotid artery. In the cases with intraorbital angiomas, vascularization from both sides may be identified.

All types of vascular anomalies, as well as cerebellar defects, coarctation of the aortic arch and/or congenital cardiac malformations, are equally associated with cutaneous hemangiomas on with capillary-telangiectatic or capillary-venous malformations (Pascual-Castroviejo et al. 1996). In our series a girl with capillary-telangiectatic malformation on both sides of her face showed a very rare vascular malfor-

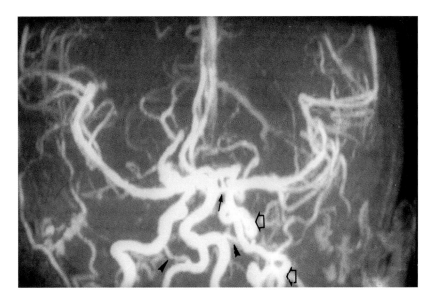

**Fig. 12.** Magnetic resonance angiography (MRA). The coronal view shows the presence of bilateral proatlantal artery (small arrowheads), left trigeminal artery (arrow), kinking of left internal carotid in two zones (empty arrows) and asymmetry of the posterior cerebral arteries, thinner in the left side (shown on right in the figure).

mation that consisted of absence of the left internal cerebral artery and the left vertebral artery; intracranial vascularization, however, was supplied through the right vertebral artery, which connected with the trigeminal artery on the left side after crossing at the level of the clivus. She also had left hemispheric cerebellar hypoplasia, aortic arch coarctation and tricuspid atresia (patient 3 in Pascual-Castroviejo et al. 1996).

Apart from our previous reports (Pascual-Castroviejo 1978, 1985; Pascual-Castroviejo et al. 1995, 1996) angiographic studies of this syndrome have been sparse and mostly incomplete (Prensky and Gado 1973, Mizuno et al. 1982, Murotami and Hiramoto 1985, Matsui et al. 1997, Burrows et al. 1998, Tortori-Donati et al. 1999) including isolated cases of absent carotid or vertebral arteries, persistence of the trigeminal artery, intracranial arterial angiomatous malformation near the siphon and sinus pericranii (Drosou et al. 2006).

Conventional arteriography is not the most suitable study to have a complete view of the vascular malformations. It is necessary to visualize all cerebral arteries (both carotids and both vertebrals) from their origin in the aortic arch and to follow the route of

each vessel extra-and intracranially with images in axial, coronal and sagittal views. The only study that makes this possible is magnetic resonance angiography (MRA) that permits us to find the embryonic arteries, the absence or hypoplasia of some cerebral arteries, and the evolution of extracranial and intracranial hemangiomas or vascular angiomatous anomalies. Venous malformations are not visible on MRA (Pascual-Castroviejo et al. 1995, 1996; Ziyeh et al. 2003).

## Cerebellar malformations

The Dandy-Walker syndrome has been associated with facial hemangiomas since the initial description (Pascual-Castroviejo 1978). Later, it has been considered as one of the most frequent alterations related to angiomas located on the face or anywhere on the trunk or extremities (Pascual-Castroviejo 1985; Pascual-Castroviejo et al. 1991, 1996; Reese et al. 1993). However, the presence of any type of cutaneous hemangioma or vascular malformation in patients with Dandy-Walker malformation was

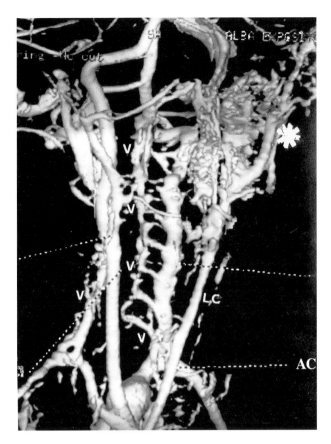

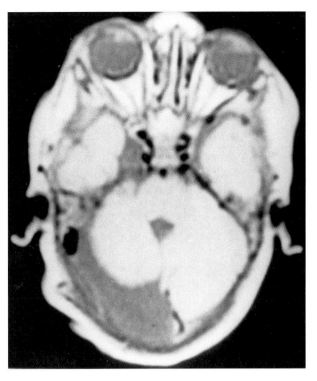

Fig. 14. Axial MRI study of the brain shows a complex cerebellar malformation consisting in a Dandy-Walker malformation and hypoplasia of the right cerebellar hemisphere.

Fig. 13. Magnetic resonance angiography (MRA) in coronal view shows a voluminous hemangioma in the left neck and parotid (asterisk), a thin left common carotid artery that ends in the hemangioma, right common and internal carotids and a hypoplastic external carotid artery. Both vertebral arteries show embryonic state with persistance of cervical segmental arteries.

observed by Dandy and Blackfan (1914) and later were reported by some authors (Pascual-Castroviejo et al. 1991). Less severe cerebellar defects, mostly of the type of unilateral hypoplasia (Fig. 14) located on the same side as the facial hemangioma, have been reported frequently (Pascual-Castroviejo 1978, 1995; Mizuno et al. 1982; Reese et al. 1993; Goh and Lo 1993; Pascual-Castroviejo et al. 1996; Matsui et al. 1997; Burrows et al. 1998). Between 50% (Pascual-Castroviejo et al. 1996) and 90% (Poetke et al. 2002) of patients with facial and/or neck hemangiomas also have some type of cerebellar defects. Neither the presence of Dandy-Walker syndrome nor the less severe cerebellar defects usually cause clinical cerebellar symp-

tomatology as expected. Hemispheric cerebellar hypoplasia commonly appears ipsilaterally to the external vascular abnormalities.

## Cerebral malformations

Cerebral hemispheric malformations were first described by Pascual-Castroviejo et al. (1995). They reported a girl who presented with a facial hemangioma, associated with homolateral internal carotid agenesis, hypoplasia of the cerebral hemisphere and dysplasia of the cerebral cortex (Fig. 15). Cases of facial hemangioma, intracranial vascular abnormalities and malformations of cortical development have been later reported by Aeby et al. (2003) and Grosso et al. (2004). Seizures and/or low mental level of different degrees may be associated with the brain abnormality. Cerebral hemispheric dysplasia and hypoplasia can be severe (Fig. 16). A statistical significant difference was found for structural brain abnormalities in males vs females in one study (Metry et al. 2008).

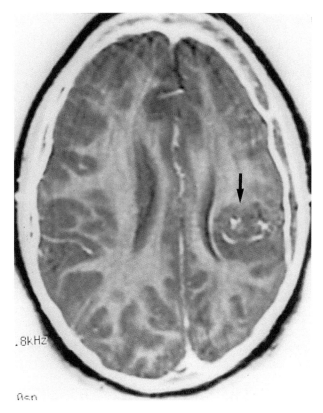

**Fig. 15.** Axial MR image of the brain shows a left hemispheric hypoplasia with cerebral cortical dysplasia (arrow).

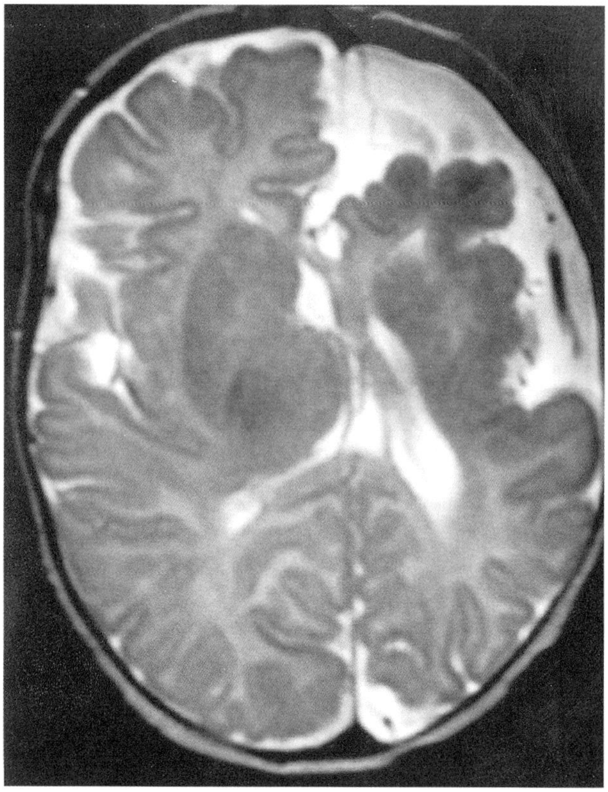

**Fig. 16.** Axial MR image of the brain shows a left cortical dysplasia with hemispheric hypoplasia.

## Evolution of vascular anomalies

Regression in parallel of the internal and external hemangiomas has been demonstrated (Fig. 17) (Pascual-Castroviejo et al. 1996, 2003, 2003a). Spontaneous regression of cutaneous hemangiomas has been known for many years. Only a few cases of progressive occlusion of the intracranial arteries or the hemangiomas without treatment have been described (Pascual-Castroviejo et al. 1996, 2003, 2003a). This regression causes progressive occlusive cerebrovascular disease and increases the occurrence of acute cerebral infarction (Burrows et al. 1998, Drolet et al. 2006, Heyer et al. 2007), although chronic cerebral infarction may be seen as well. Vascular regression has been attributed to the medication given to treat the cutaneous hemangioma (Burrows et al. 1998). However, progressive regression of intracranial and extracranial arteries and occlusive cerebrovascular disease has been equally re-

ported in untreated (Pascual-Castroviejo et al. 1996) and in treated patients (Burrows et al. 1998). There are cases in the literature described more than twenty or thirty years ago whose facial hemangiomas were treated by radiation therapy which was customary at that time (Taveras 1969, Wright and Bresnan 1976). Some years later, an angiographic study performed because of the presence of neurological symptoms discovered the occlusion of both internal carotid and basilar arteries, with filling of the intracranial branches by way of transdural external-internal anastomoses (Fig. 18). In both cases, the lack of filling of some cerebral arteries or perhaps occlusion (Taveras 1969) and the occlusion of intracranial arteries (Wright and Bresnan 1976) were attributed to the radiotherapy, but at that time it was not yet known that there is an association of facial hemangioma with the absence of internal carotid and/or vertebral arteries, first described in 1978 (Pascual-Castroviejo 1978) and a spontaneous

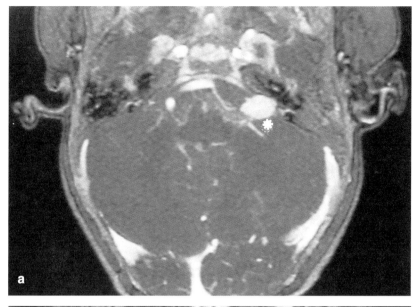

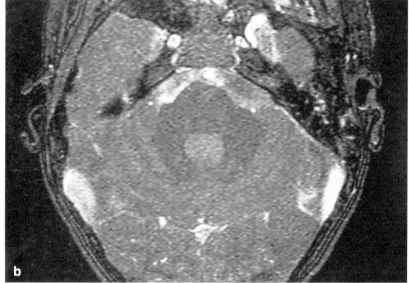

**Fig. 17.** MRI study of the brain after gadolinium administration in a girl with left facial hemangioma: (**a**) the axial scan obtained at age 7 months shows an ovoid-shaped hemangioma (asterisk) in the left pontocerebellar region; (**b**) same study at age 4 years, shows absence of the ponto-cerebellar hemangioma.

regression and occlusion of intracranial and extracranial hemangiomas (Pascual-Castroviejo et al. 1996, 2003, 2003a; Burrows et al. 1998). There are many cases of spontaneous regression and occlusion of intracranial vascular malformation in the literature that make us to believe that perhaps these are patients with this syndrome. However, the reports do not mention the presence of a facial hemangioma and, therefore, these patients must be excluded from this syndrome.

Spontaneous regression in parallel with cutaneous and internal hemangiomas can occur in any region of the body: that is to say, intracranially and/or in any organ of the body (liver, intestines, gluteal, perineal or any other zone) (Pascual-Castroviejo et al. 2002, 2005). Regression of the lesions has also been seen after treatment with corticosteroids (Prensky and Gado 1973) and/or interferon (Capin et al. 1997). The process of regression and occlusion of the pathologic vessels is unclear. Cutaneous and internal

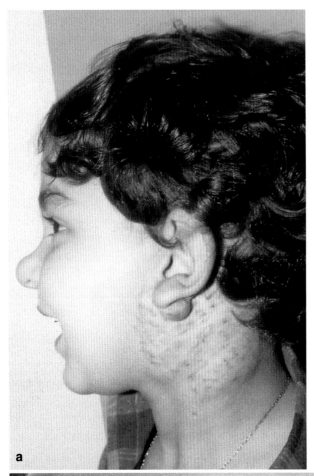

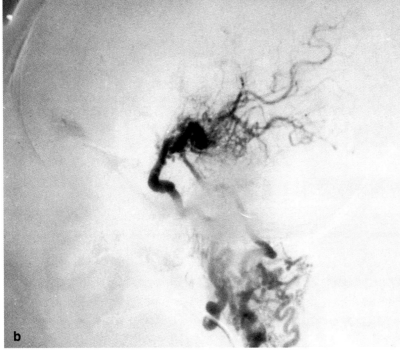

Fig. 18. (a–b): a patient with an hemangioma of the left neck (a) at age 17 months; conventional arteriography of the left carotid and vertebral system at the same age (b) shows a tortuous and angiomatous aspect of both arteries and an intracranial angioma vascularized through the carotid and vertebral arteries; (c) The same hemangioma of the neck after regression in the same patient at 19 years of age; (d) MRI arteriography at 19 years of age shows in lateral view that the intracranial vascular malformation appeared at age 17 months has disappeared while still are present the persistence of the basilar artery (arrow) along with some overdeveloped branches of the externals carotids (arrow heads); (e) Axial view of the same study (at 19 years of age) shows left carotid (open arrow) and trigeminal (large arrow) arteries without presence of intracranial vascular malformation or angioma. Absence of carotid and vertebral arteries on the right side; presence of several overdeveloped arterial branches of the external carotid arteries (arrowheads) for a collateral vascularization.

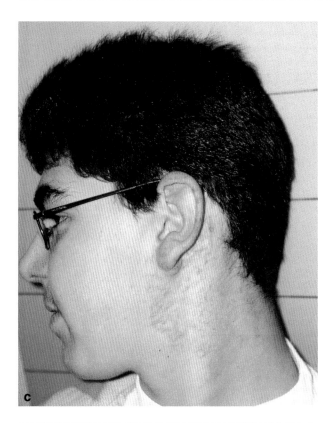

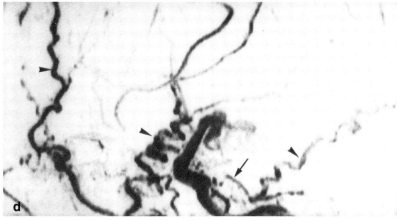

**Fig. 18.** (Continued)

hemangiomas may increase in size during the first months or years and then spontaneously regress. Anatomical changes in the internal and external vessels would mainly occur in cases with the hemangioma, in accordance with the histologic difference between the two types of vascular anomalies (Mulliken and Glowacki 1982). Clinical and histologic features suggest that mitochondrial cytochrome b plays a role in both spontaneous and steroid-induced/accelerated regression of hemangioma by increasing apoptosis (Hasan et al. 2001).

Neither cutaneous vascular malformations nor associated arterial anomalies located intracranially, in the neck and/or in the aortic arch show a regressive process or any change after time or after any treatment.

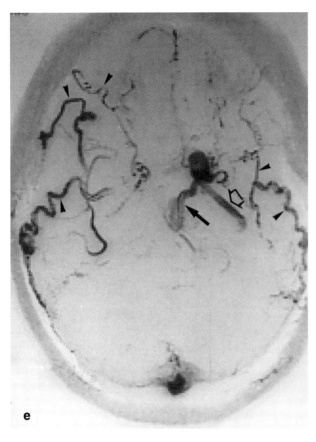

**e**

**Fig. 18.** (Continued)

## Molecular genetics

Hemangiomas almost always are sporadic (Breugem et al. 2002, 2002a). Familial forms may represent a small minority of the total cases (Blei et al. 1998, Walter et al. 1999). A marked female predilection is seen in this syndrome, especially in cases with facial hemangioma (Pascual-Castroviejo 1978, 1985; Mulliken 1992; Gorlin et al. 1994; Pascual-Castroviejo et al. 1996).

Gorlin et al. (1994) reported 29 females and 2 males in a series in which facial hemangioma was associated only with partial or complete sternal agenesis and/or supraumbilical raphè, while in other series there was not sex predilection (Tasnadi 1993).

Evidence for linkage to 5q and for locus heterogeneity was seen in all reported genetic studies on familial cases with cutaneous hemangioma or vascular malformation. Walter et al. (1999) found three candidate genes involved with the growth of blood vessels mapping to the region of chromosome 5q31–33 which corresponds to the interval spans 38cM between markers D5S1469 and D5S211. The three genes are: fibroblast growth factor receptor-4 (FGFR4), platelet-derived growth factor receptor-β (PDGFRB), and fm1-related tyrosine kinase-4 (FLT4). Further investigations mapped a locus for an autosomal dominant disorder in a three-generation family that manifested multiple cutaneous capillary malformations to chromosome 5q13–22 (Breugem et al. 2002). This locus spans 48cM between the markers D5S647 and D5S659 and harbours several candidate genes. Eerola et al. (2002) identified a susceptibility locus for capillary malformation – arteriovenous malformation (CMAVM) (OMIM 608354) on chromosome 5q14–21 (CMC1) with a minimally linked region of 23cM between markers D5S1962 and D5S652. Eerola et al. (2003) detected heterozygous inactivating RASA 1 mutations in six families manifesting multiple, small, round to oval in shape, and pinkish red in color cutaneous hemangiomas. The phenotypic variability can be explained by the involvement of p120-Ras GAP in signaling for various growth factor receptors that control proliferation, migration, and survival of several cell types, including vascular endothelial cells (Eerola et al. 2003). Brancati et al. (2003) also mapped a locus for *hereditary benign telangiectasia* (HBT) (OMIM 187260) a benign type of Rendu-Osler-Weber disease on chromosome 5q14 in a large kindred from northern Italy. Notably, the locus for CMC1 was assigned to a 19Mb region on 5q13–15 (Breugem et al. 2002, Eerola et al. 2002), while the linked interval in the HBT spans 7Mb on chromosome 5q14 physical map and coincides to CMC1 (Brancati et al. 2003). CMAVM and HBT (and possibly other vascular cutaneous conditions as well) share not only similar cutaneous characteristics, but also similar histopathologic changes and association with vascular or nonvascular alterations. These observations suggest that HBT and CMAVM may represent variable clinical presentations of the same disorder. Linkage of HBT to CMC1 corroborates this hypothesis (Brancati et al. 2003). The linked region contains 15 genes, some of which represent suitable candidates for cutaneous vascular anomalies. It is likely that genes implicated in familial cases may be also involved in sporadic cases (Berg et al. 2001, Breugem et al. 2002a). On the contrary, in Sturge-Weber syndrome, another disorder of the group of vascular birthmarks, somatic mosaicism was seen in chromosomes 10 and 4 (Huq et al. 2002). Hemangiomas and vascular malformations are linked to several causative genes that have been identified during the last 10 years (Brouillard and Vikkula 2003), some of which have already mentioned.

The vascular system is developed by a process through which this complex network is developed. It is divided into vasculogenesis, angiogenesis and lymphangiogenesis. During vasculogenesis the formation of blood vessels in the embryo, is based on "in situ" differentiation of precursor cells, the hemangioblasts, to form the primary capillary plexus. Many factors that play a role in this process are already known (Brouillard and Vikkula 2003). Angiogenesis denotes the growth and remodeling of this primary capillary plexus into a complex network of vessels composed of capillaries, arteries and veins (Risau 1997). Small blood vessels consist only of endothelial cells (ECs), whereas larger vessels are surrounded by mural cells (pericytes in medium-sized and smooth muscle cells (SMC$_s$) in large vessels). Several congenital or inherited diseases are caused by abnormal vascular remodeling. Vessels can grow in several ways. Endothelial progenitors differentiate to mature EC$_s$, but not all EC$_s$ are alike. Dysregulation of the vasculogenesis and angiogenesis development contributes to numerous disorders (Carmeliet 2000, 2003). In the "cutaneous hemangioma and associated pathology", vascular disorders affect almost exclusively arteries. From an embryological point of view, little is known about the various pathways specifying the identity of arterial and venous SMC$_s$, but genetic studies offer insight into the signals controlling arterial and venous identities of Ec$_s$ (Wang et al. 1998, Zhong et al. 2001, Lawson et al. 2001). Wang et al. (1998) described the arterial, but not venous expression of Ephrin-B$_2$ (Efnb2), an Eph family transmembrane ligand. In contrast, Eph-B4 (Efnb4), a receptor tyrosine kinase that bins Efnb2, is found at much higher levels in veins than in arteries.

The Notch pathway, with its ligands (Delta-like-4, Jagged-1 and Jagged-2) and receptors (Notch-1, Notch-3 and Notch-4), promotes arterial fate of Ecs by repressing venous differentiation (Zhong et al. 2001, Lawson et al. 2001). Sonic Hedgehog and vascular endothelial growth factor (VEGF) act upstream, whereas Gridlock probably acts downstream of Notch to determine arterial fate, even before the onset of flow (Zhong et al. 2001; Lawson et al. 2000, 2002). VEGF is a key regulator of physiological angiogenesis during embryogenesis and is also implicated in pathological angiogenesis associated with a lot of conditions. The biological effects of VEGF are mediated by two receptor tyrosine kinases (RTKs), VEGF-1 and VEGF-2, which differ considerably in signaling properties (Ferrara et al. 2003). Some other genes, such as homeobox (HOX) and Eph genes and ephrin proteins, have been linked to capillary (Boudreau et al. 1997, Myers et al. 2000), and neural (Studer et al. 1998, Holder and Klein 1999) development.

In 1 of 15 infantile capillary hemangiomas (also known as *hemangioma capillary infantile* or HCI, OMIM 602089) specimens, Walter et al. (2002) identified mutations in the FLT4 gene, whilst mutations in the VEGFRZ gene were identified in another of 15 specimens, suggesting that alteration of the FTL4 signalling pathway in endothelial and/or pericytic cells may be a mechanisms involved in hemangioma formation.

For a more thorough analysis the readers is referred to the reviews of Cohen (2006, 2007).

## Management

Most cutaneous hemangiomas regress spontaneously over months or years. Small solitary hemangiomas do not need any treatment. On the contrary, some types of hemangiomas, especially those considered to be alarming, cause serious problems, especially periorbital hemangiomas that are associated with ophthalmic complications and voluminous facial hemangiomas that have a significant impact on the family and on society. These lesions have to be treated as soon as possible. Most parents prefer to have the hemangioma removed before the child enters school and not to wait for sporadic regression (Dieterich-Miller and Safford 1992).

Corticosteroids, interferon alfa -2a or -2b, embolization and/or surgery and/or intralesional photocoagulation are the most used therapies. Radiation therapy was the only available treatment more than twenty years ago. However, at present has not indication despite the fact that it was not the cause of further arterial occlusion, as it was previously believed (Taveras 1969, Wright and Bresnan 1975), because of the natural evolution to spontaneous regression of cutaneous hemangiomas and intracranial and/or extracranial aneurysmal dilatation of the arteries. The substances employed are angiogenesis inhibitors used to treat endangering hemangiomas. They appear to accelerate the regression of this tumors with response rates ranging between 30% to 90% although realistic good results are nearer the 30% (Bartoshesky et al. 1978, Enjolras et al. 1990). Bad responses to corticosteroids are also seen in a 30%, and doubtful response in a 40% (Enjolras et al. 1990). No factors are found to predict a response or nonresponse to steroids treatments (Enjolras et al. 1990).

## Corticosteroids

A sufficient daily starting dose should be prednisone or prednisolone, 2 or 3 mg/kg of body weight per day, given at a full dose for 1 month and then slowly tapered to discontinue the administration of the drug by the time the infant is 10–12 months of age (Enjolras et al. 1990, Boon et al. 1999). If there is no evidence of regression or stabilization of the hemangioma after 2 weeks with prednisone or predisolone at a dose of 2–3 mg/kg/day possibly the hemangioma will not respond to therapy and children should be treated with interferon (Boon et al. 1999) or perhaps with other methods. Higher initial doses do not provide more successful response than an initial dose of 2 mg/kg/day (Boon et al. 1999).

The treatment should not be stopped early because of the risk of recrudescence (Enjolras et al. 1990). Malocclusion and skin sequelae but also ocular sequelae in cases of periorbital hemangiomas, are commonly seen with and/or without steroids treatment. Live vaccines must be withheld during corticosteroids therapy.

Side effects of corticosteroids are several and well documented (Boon et al. 1999).

## Interferon

Interferon – alfa (-2a or -2b) appears to accelerate the regression of the hemangiomas due to its angiogenesis inhibitory action (White 1990, Ezekowitz et al. 1992) Urinary levels of basic fibroblast growth factor topically decrease in parallel with clinical signs of response of hemangiomas to corticosteroids or interpheron (Burrows et al. 1998). Interferon is generally used when steroid therapy fails. Subcutaneous daily injections of interferon alfa -2a or -2b in continued treatment over 6–9 months is recommended.

Neurotoxicity (spastic diplegia), however, has been occasionally reported using interferon alfa -2a (Barlow et al. 1998) or alfa -2b (Dubois and Garel 1999). In the series of Barlow et al. (1998), five infants from a group of 26 children treated with interferon alfa -2a displayed diplegia that persisted in three infants, and in the remaining two was followed by significant recovery after medication was discontinued.

## Intralesional photocoagulation

Periorbital hemangiomas can be reduced quickly and effectively by the use of intralesional photocoagulation (Achauer et al. 1999). Low power laser type Nd: YAG has been recommended for its versatility in the treatment of capillary hemangiomas. Alternatively, the laser can be used to produce an incision with hemostatic action in surgical resection. Intralesional photocoagulation has been described in recent years. The Nd: YAG or KTP wavelength with a bare fiber or fiberoptic is inserted directly into the hemangioma (Achauer et al. 1998). This method reduces the size of large hemangiomas and minimizes damage to the overlying skin.

## Thalidomide

Oral administration of thalidomide has been shown to inhibit angiogenesis via an unknown mechanism.

However, thalidomide has no effect on proliferation of endothelial cells in culture (D'Amato et al. 1994), and it is unlikely that the drug will have effects on cavernous hemangiomas and/or vascular malformations in vivo.

## Cobb syndrome

Berenbruch first described the disorder in 1890, but it was not widely known until Cobb's report (1915) who described a syndrome that associated port-wine stains on the posterior thorax with underlying venous or arteriovenous malformation of the spinal cord, potentially causing cord compression in an 8-year-old boy (Morwood and Kriyda 2007). It is also known as cutaneous meningospinal angiomatosis and consists of a capillary malformation that has a high-flow nature on the posterior thorax in association with on arteriovenous malformations of the spine. The association of cutaneous vascular malformations with spinal arteriovenous malformations is much higher than usually reported (Doppman et al. 1969). Six of 28 patients with spinal cord arteriovenous malformations had cutaneous vascular anomalies in an important series, which also reviewed 10 cases previously described by others (Doppman et al. 1969). However, close scrutiny of the back is required in some cases to obtain a true visualization of the cutaneous lesions. In some cases, this can be made more evident by the Valsalva maneuver (Doppman et al. 1969); in others, stroking the skin makes the lesion remarkably obvious (Fig. 19) (Pascual-Castroviejo et al. 2002, 2002b). Internal vascular and/or other types of alterations, however, are not different in patients showing cutaneous hemangiomas or vascular malformations (Pascual-Castroviejo 1978, Pascual-Castroviejo et al. 1996). Spinal cord arteriovenous malformations are frequently associated with metameric vascular malformations involving the skin and deep soft tissues (Cobb 1915; Pascual-Castroviejo 1978; Pascual-Castroviejo et al. 1996, 2002).

The genetic framework of Cobb syndrome is unclear, although the presence of cutaneous vascular malformations in persons of the same family has been reported (Mercer et al. 1978, Maramattom et al. 2005), hinting at an inherited predisposition (Mercer et al. 1978).

Contrast media myelography usually reveals numerous serpentine vessels (Chateil et al. 2000). These images, however, are not demonstrated by transfemoral angiography in all cases. Magnetic resonance arteriography (Fig. 20) combined with selective intercostal arteriography is the diagnostic procedure of choice. Both studies complement each other. Selective intercostal arteriography is more specific than magnetic resonance

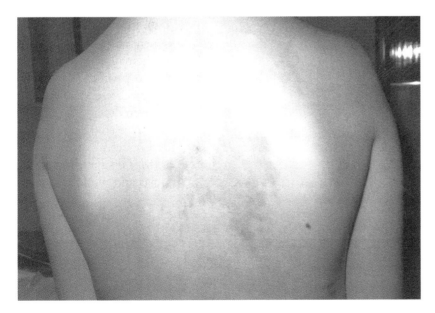

**Fig. 19.** Area of cutaneous vascular malformation on the middle-right region of the back that is remarkably obvious after stroking.

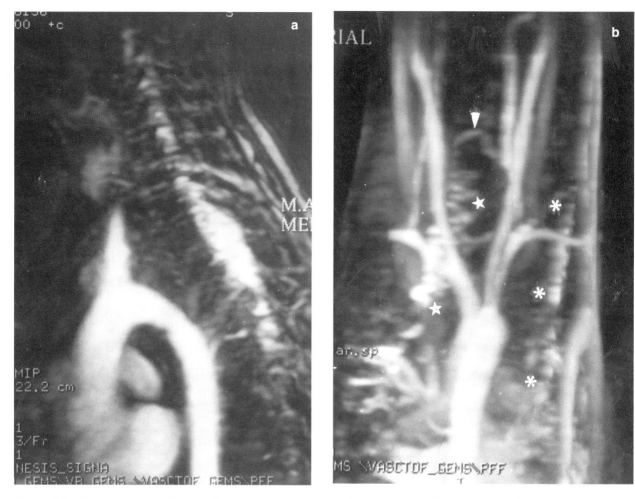

**Fig. 20.** Spinal MR arteriography. (**a**) The sagittal view shows an intraspinal arteriovenous malformation extending between the seventh cervical and the fourth dorsal metamere. (**b**) The coronal view shows two arteriovenous malformations: one intraspinal, extending between the seventh cervical and the fourth dorsal metamere (asterisks), and the other extraspinal, located in the right paraspinal region (stars) and ascending to the azygos-caval system (arrowhead).

arteriography in demonstrating the precise feeding vessels and the draining veins of the arteriovenous malformation (Fig. 21). Magnetic resonance arteriography can show the local extension and the presence of one or more arteriovenous malformations. Specific maneuvers to bring out port-wine stains are indicated in patients with deep arteriovenous malformations.

Cutaneous vascular lesions are rarely reported in association with intraspinal vascular anomalies. Spinal arteriovenous malformations, however, have occasionally been associated with hereditary cutaneous hemangiomas (Kaplan et al. 1976).

We suggest that Cobb syndrome, which is limited to the spinal region, as well as other syndromes with larger clinical and anatomic alterations (Frieden et al. 1996, Torres-Mohedas et al. 2001, Holtzman et al. 1999) may be localized manifestations of the same disease (Pascual-Castroviejo 1978, 2004; Pascual-Castroviejo et al. 1996) on counterparts of PHACE association (Stockman et al. 2007).

Management of intraspinal arteriovenous malformations is very difficult and most often not advisable neither by surgical nor by interventional neuroradiology because of the risk of irreversible medullary injury.

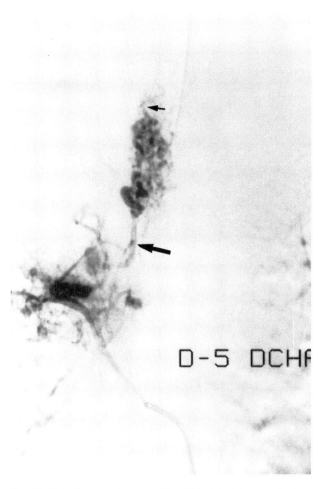

**Fig. 21.** Selective arteriogram of the fifth right intercostal artery showing an intraspinal arteriovenous malformation with the feeder branch (long arrow) and the draining veins (small arrow).

Endovascular embolization, however, has been made (Miyatake et al. 1996, Soeda et al. 2003, Maramattom et al. 2005), with questionable results to date.

Extramedullary vascular malformations may be treated by surgical resection, or by intravascular occlusion, or by a combination of both.

## References

Achauer BM, Celikoz B, Vanderkam VM (1998) Intralesional bare fiber laser treatment of hemangioma of infancy. Plast Reconstr Surg 101: 1212–1217.

Achauer BM, Chang CJ, Vanderkam VM, Boyko A (1999) Intralesional photocoagulation of periorbital hemangiomas. Plas Reconstr Surg 103: 11–16.

Aeby A, Guerrini R, David P, Rodesch G, Raybaud C, Van Bogaert P (2003) Facial hemangioma and cerebral corticovascular dysplasia. A syndrome associated with epilepsy. Neurology 60: 1030–1032.

Amir J, Knikler A, Reisner SH (1986) Strawberry hemangioma in preterm infants. Pediatr Dermatol 3: 131–132.

Baker LL, Dillon WP, Hieshima GB, Dowd CF, Frieden I (1993) Hemangiomas and vascular malformations of the head and neck: MR characterization. Am J Neuroradiol 14: 307–314.

Barlow CF, Priebe CJ, Mulliken JB, Barnes PD, McDonald D, Folkman J, Ezekowith RAB (1998) Spastic diplegia as a complication of interferon alfa -2a treatment of hemangiomas of infancy. J Pediatr 132: 527–530.

Bartoshesky LE, Bull M, Feingold M (1978) Corticosteroid treatment of cutaneous hemangiomas: how effective? Clin Pediatr 17: 625–638.

Belánger Quintana A, Aparicio Meix JM, Quintana Castilla A (2002) Sìndrome de Pascual-Castroviejo II: asociación de hemangioma facial, alteración de la fosa posterior y cardiopatìa congènita. An Esp Pediatr 57: 588–589.

Berg JN, Walter JW, Thisanagayam M, Evans M, Blei F, Waner M, Diamond AG, Marchuk DA, Porteous ME (2001) Evidence for loss of heterozygosity of 5q in sporadic haemangiomas: are somatic mutations involved in haemangioma formation? J Clin Patol 54: 249–252.

Blei F, Walter J, Orlow SJ, Marchuk DA (1998) Familial segregation of hemangiomas and vascular malformations as an autosomal dominant trait. Arch Dermatol 134: 718–722

Boon LM, Enjolras O, Mulliken JB (1996) Congenital hemangioma: evidence of accelerated involution. J Pediatr 128: 329–335.

Boon LM, McDonald DM, Mulliken JB (1999) Complications of systemic corticosteroid therapy for problematic hemangioma. Plast Reconstr Surg 104: 1616–1623.

Boudreau N, Andrews C, Srebrow A, Ravanpay A, Cheresh DA (1997) Hox D3 induces an angiogenic phenotype in endothelial cells. J Cell Biol 139: 257–264.

Boyd JB, Mulliken JB, Kaban LB, Upton J, Murray JE (1984) Skeletal changes associated with vascular malformations. Plast Reconstr Surg 74: 789–795.

Brancati F, Valente EM, Tadini G, Caputo V, Di Benedetto A, Gelmetti C, Dallapiccola B (2003) Autosomal dominant hereditary benign telangiectasia maps to the CMC1 locus for capillary malformation on chromosome 5q14. J Med Genet 40: 849–853.

Breugem CC, Alders M, Salieb-Beugelaar GB, Mannens MMAM, Van dr Horst CM, Hennekam RCM (2002) A locus for hereditary capillary malformations mapped on chromosome 5q. Hum Genet 110: 343–347.

Breugem CC, van der Horst CMAM, Hennekam RCM (2002a) Progress toward understanding vascular malformations. Plast Reconstr Surg 107: 1509–1523.

Brouillard P, Vikkula M (2003) Vascular malformations: localized defects in vascular morphogenesis. Clin Genet 63: 340–351.

Burke EC, Winkelman RK, Strickland MK (1964) Disseminated hemangiomatosis: The newborn with central nervous system involvement. Am J Dis Child 108: 418–424.

Burns AJ, Kaplan LC, Mulliken JB (1991) Is there an association between hemangioma and syndromes with dysmorphic features? Pediatrics 88: 1257–1267.

Burrows PE, Robertson RL, Mulliken JB, Beardsley DS, Chaloupka JC, Ezekowitz RA (1998) Cerebral vasculopathy and neurologic sequelae in infants with cervicofacial hemangioma: Report of eight patients. Radiology 207: 601–607.

Burton BK, Schulz CJ, Angle B, Burd LI (1995) An increased incidence of haemangiomas in infants born following chorionic villus sampling (CVS). Prenat Diagn 15: 209–214.

Byard RW, Burrows PE, Izakawa T, Silver MM (1991) Diffuse infantile hemangiomatosis: clinicopathological features and management problems in five fatal cases. Eur J Pediatr 150: 224–227.

Capin DM, Gottlieb S, Rosman NP (1997) Central nervous system hemangiomatosis in early childhood. Pediatr Neurol 17: 365–370.

Carmeliet P (2000) Developmental biology. One cell, two fates. Nature 408: 43–45.

Carmeliet P (2003) Angiogenesis in health and disease. Nat Med 9: 653–660.

Chateil JF, Saragne-Feuga C, Pèrel Y, Brun M, Neuenschwander S, Vergnes P, Diard F (2000) Capillary haemangioma of the greater omentum in a 5-month-old female infant: a case report. Pediatr Radiol 30: 837–839.

Coats DK, Paysse EA, Levy ML (1999) PHACE: a neurocutaneous syndrome with important ophthalmology implication. Case report and literature review. Ophthalmology 106: 1739–1741.

Cobb S (1915) Haemangioma of the spinal cord associated with skin naevi of the same metamere. Ann Surg 62: 641–649.

Cohen MM Jr (2006) Vascular update: morphogenesis, tumors, malformations, and molecular dimensions. Am J Med Genet A 140: 2013–2038.

Cohen MM Jr (2007) Hemangiomas: their uses and abuses. Am J Med Genet A 143: 235–240.

Congdon ED (1922) Transformation of aortic arch system during the development of the human embryo. Contrib Embryol 14: 47–110.

Cooper AG, Bolande RP (1965) Multiple hemangiomas in an infant with cardiac hypertrophy. Post-mortem angiographic demostration of the arteriovenous fistulae. Pediatrics 35: 27–35.

D'Amato RJD, Loughnan MS, Flynn E, Folkman J (1994) Thalidomide is an inhibitor of angiogenesis. Proc Natl Acad Sci 91: 4082–4085.

Dandy WE, Blackfan KD (1914) Intenal hydrocephalus: an experimental, clinical and pathological study. Am J Dis Child 8: 406–482.

Dieterich-Miller CA, Safford PL (1992) Psychosocial development of children with hemangiomas: home school, health care collaboration. Children's Health Care 21: 84–89.

Doppman JL, Wirth FP Jr, Di Chiro G, Ommaya AK (1969) Value of cutaneous angiomas in the arteriographic localization of spinal cord arteriovenous malformations. N Engl J Med 281: 1440–1444.

Drolet BA, Esterly NB, Frieden IJ (1999) Hemangiomas in children. N Engl J Med 341: 173–181.

Drolet BA, Dohil M, Golomb MR, Wells R, Murowski L, Tamburro J, Sty J, Friedlander SF (2006) Early stroke and cerebral vasculopathy in children with facial hemangiomas and PHACE association. Pediatrics 117: 959–964.

Drosou A, Benjamin L, Linfante I, Mallin K, Trowers A, Wakhloo AK, Thaller SR, Schachner LA (2006) Infantile midline facial hemangioma with agenesis of the corpus callosum and sinus pericranii: another face of the PHACE syndrome. J Am Acad Dermatol 54: 348–352.

Dubois J, Garel L (1999) Imaging and therapeutic approach of hemangiomas and vascular malformations in the pediatric age group. Pediatr Radiol 29: 879–893.

Eerola I, Boom LM, Watanabe S, Grynberg H, Mulliken JB, Vikkula M (2002) Locus for susceptibility for familial capillary malformation ("port-wine staine") maps to 5q. Eur J Hum Genet 10: 375–380.

Eerola I, Boon LM, Mulliken JB, Burrows PE, Dompmartin A, Watanabe S, Vanwijck R, Vikkula M (2003) Capillary malformation-arteriovenous malformation, a new clinical and genetic disorder caused by RASA1 mutations. Am J Hum Genet 73: 1240–1249.

Enjolras O, Riche MC, Merland JJ, Escaude JP (1990) Management of alarming hemangiomas in infancy: a review of 25 cases. Pediatrics 85: 491–498.

Esterly N (1995) Cutaneous hemangiomas, vascular stains and malformations and associated syndromes. Current Prob Dermatol 7: 65–108.

Ezekowitz RAB, Mulliken JB, Folkman J (1992) Interferon-alfa -2a therapy for life – threatening hemangiomas of infancy. N Engl J Med 326: 1456–1463.

Ferrara N, Gerber HP, Le Couter J (2003) The biology of VEGF and its receptors. Nat Med 9: 669–676.

Frieden IJ, Reese V, Cohen D (1996) PHACE syndrome. The association of posterior fossa brain malformations, hemangiomas, arterial anomalies, coarctation of the aorta and cardiac defects, and eye abnormalities. Arch Dermatol 132: 307–311.

Geller JD, Topper SF, Hashimoto K (1991) Diffuse neonatal hemangiomatosis: a new constellation of findings. J Am Acad Dermatol 24: 816–818.

Goh WHS, Lo R (1993) A new 3C syndrome: cerebellar hypoplasia, cavernous hemangioma and coarctation of the aorta. Develop Med Child Neurol 35: 637–641.

Goldberg NS, Hevert AA, Sterly NB (1986) Sacral hemangiomas and multiple congenital abnormalities. Arch Dermatol 122: 684–687.

Gorlin RJ, Kantaputra P, Aughton DJ Mulliken JB (1994) Marked female predilection in some syndromes associated with facial hemangiomas. Am J Med Genet 52: 130–135.

Grosso S, De Cosmo L, Bonifazi E, Galluzzi P, Farnetani MA, Loffredo P, Anichini C, Berardi R, Morgese G, Balestri P (2004) Facial hemangioma and malformation of the cortical development: a bradening of the PHACE spectrum or a new entity? Am J Med Genet 124A: 192–195.

Guian-Almeida ML, Richieri-Costa A, Saavedra D, Cohen Jr MM (1996) Cerebro-facio-thoracic syndrome. Am J Med Genet 61: 152–153.

Hand JL, Frieden IJ (2002) Vascular birthmarks in infancy: resolving neurologic confusion. Am J Med Genet 108: 257–264.

Haque KN (1984) Isolated asternia: an idependent entity. Clin Genet 25: 362–365.

Hasan Q, Tan ST, Gush J, Davis PF (2001) Altered mitochondrial cytochrome b gene expression during the regression of hemangioma. Plast Reconstr Surg 108: 1477–1478.

Hersh JH, Waterfill D, Rutledge J, Harrod MJE, O'Sheal SF, Verdi G, Martinez S, Weisskopf B (1985) Sternal malformation/vascular dysplasia association. Am J Med Genet 21: 177–186.

Heyer GL, Millar WS, Ghatan S, Gorzon MC (2006) The neurologic aspects of PHACE: case report and review of the literature. Pediatr Neural 35: 419–424

Holden KR, Alexander F (1970) Diffuse neonatal hemangiomatosis. Pediatrics 46: 411–421.

Holder N, Klein R (1999) Eph receptors and ephrins: effectors of morphogenesis. Development 126: 2034–2044.

Honey M, Lincoln JCR, Osborne MP, de Bono DP (1975) Coarctation of aorta with right aortic arch. (Case 2) Brit Heart J 37: 937–945.

Holtzman RN, Brisson PM, Pearl RE, Gruber ML (1999) Lobular capillary hemangioma of the cauda equina. Case report. J Neurosurg 90 (Suppl Spine 2): 239–241.

Huq AHMM, Chugani DC, Hukku B, Serajee FJ (2002) Evidence of somatic mosaicism in Sturge-Weber syndrome. Neurology 59: 780–782.

Igarashi M, Uchida H, Kajaii T (1985) Supraumbilical mid-abdominal raphè and facial cavernous hemangiomas. Clin Genet 27: 196–198.

Kaplan P, Hollenberg RD, Fraser FC (1976) A spinal arteri-ovenous malformation with hereditary cutaneous hemangiomas. Am J Dis Child 130: 1329–1333.

Kishnani P, Lafolla AK, McConkie-Rossell A, Van Hove JLK, Kanter RJ, Kahler SG (1995) Hemangioma, supraumbilical midline raphè, and coarctation of the aorta with a right aortic arch. Single causal entity. Am J Med Genet 59: 44–48.

Lawson ND, Scheer N, Phan VN, Kim CH, Chitnis AB, Campos-Ortega JA, Weinstein BM (2001) Notch signalling is required for arterial-venous differentiation during embryonic vascular development. Development 128: 3675–3683.

Lawson ND, Vogel AM, Weinstein BM (2002) Sonic hedgehog and vascular endothelial growth factor act upstream of the Notch pathway during arterial endothelial differentiation. Dev Cell 3: 127–136.

Mall FP (1912) Determination of the age of embryos and fetuses. In: Kebel VI, Mall FP (eds.) Manual of Human Embryology. Philadelphia, pp. 180–201.

Maramattom BV, Cohen-Gadol AA, Vijdicks EFM, Kallmes D (2005) Segmental cutaneous hemangioma and spinal arteriovenous malformation (Cobb syndrome). Case report and historical perspective. J Neurosurg Spine 3: 249–252.

Margileth AM, Museles M (1965) Cutaneous hemangiomas in children. Diagnosis and conservative management. JAMA 194: 135–138.

Matsui T, Ono T, Kito M, Yoshioka S, Ikeda T (1997) Extensive facial strawberry mark associated with cerebellar hypoplasia and vascular abnormalities. J Dermatol 24: 113–116.

Mercer RD, Rothner AD, Cook SA (1978) The Cobb syndrome: association with hereditary cutaneous hemangiomas. Cleve Clin Q 45: 237–240.

Metry DW, Dowd CF, Barkovich AJ, Frieden IJ (2001) The many faces of PHACE syndrome. J Pediatr 139: 117–123.

Metry DW, Haggstrom AN, Drolet BA, Baselga E, Chamlin S, Garzon M, Horii K, Lucky A, Mancini AJ, Newell B, Heyer G, Frieden IJ (2006) A prospective study of PHACE syndrome in infantile hemangiomas : demographic features, clinical findings, and complications. Am J Med Genet A 140: 975–986.

Metry DW, Siegel DH, Cordisco MR, Pope E, Prendiville J, Drolet BA, Horii KA, Stein SL, Frieden IJ (2008) A comparison of disease severity among affected male versus female patients with PHACE syndrome. J Am Acad Dermatol 58: 81–87.

Miyatake S, Kikuchi H, Yamagata S, Nagata I, Minami S, Asato R (1996) Cobb's syndrome and its treatment with embolization. Neurosurgery 38: 558–562.

Mizuno Y, Kurokawa T, Numaguchi Y, Goya M (1982) Facial hemangioma with cerebro-vascular anomalies and cerebellar hypoplasia. Brain Dev 4: 373–378.

Mohammadi M, Mohebbi MR, Holden KR (2004) Facial hemangioma and associated malformations: a case report. Neuropediatrics 35: 194–197.

Mulliken JB (1992) A biologic approach to cutaneous vascular anomalies. Pediatr Dermatol 9: 356–357.

Mulliken JB, Glowacki J (1982) Hemangiomas and vascular malformations in infants and children: a classification based on endothelial characteristics. Plastic Reconstr Surg 69: 412–422.

Murotani K, Hiramoto M (1985) Agenesis of the internal carotid artery with a large hemangioma of the tongue. Neuroradiology 27: 357–359.

Myers C, Charboneau A, Boudreau N (2000) Homeobox B3 promotes capillary morphogenesis and angiogenesis. J Cell Biol 148: 343–351.

Morwood C, Kriyda S (2007) Cobb Syndrome. e-medicine from the web. http://www.emedicine.com/derm/topic769.html

Padget DH (1948) The development of the cranial arteries in the human embryo. Contrib Embryol 32: 205–262.

Pascual-Castroviejo I (1978) Vascular and nonvascular intracranial malformations associated with external capillary hemangiomas. Neuroradiology 16: 82–84.

Pascual-Castroviejo I (1985) The association of extracranial and intracranial vascular malformations in children. Can J Neurol Sci 12: 139–148.

Pascual-Castroviejo I (1993) New 3C syndrome (letter) Dev Med Child Neurol 35: 1026.

Pascual-Castroviejo I (2004) Cutaneous hemangiomas: vascular anomaly complex. In: Roach ES, Miller VS (eds.) Neurocutaneous Disorders. Cambridge: Cambridge University Press, pp. 172–178.

Pascual-Castroviejo I, Santolaya JM, Lopez Martìn V, Rodriguez-Costa T, Tendero A, Mulas F (1975) Cerebro-facio-thoracic dysplasia: report of three cases. Dev Med Child Neurol 17: 343–351.

Pascual-Castroviejo I, Velez A, Pascual-Pascual SI, Roche MC, Villarejo F (1991) Dandy-Walker malformation: analysis of 38 cases. Childs Nerv Syst 7: 88–97.

Pascual-Castroviejo I, Viaño J, Pascual-Pascual SI, Martinez V (1995) Facial hemangioma, agenesis of internal carotid artery and cerebral cortex dysplasia: case report. Neuroradiology 37: 693–695.

Pascual-Castroviejo I, Viaño J, Moreno F, Palencia R, Martinez-Fernandez V, Pascual-Pascual SI (1996) Hemangiomas of the head, neck, and chest with associated vascular and brain anomalies: A complex neurocutaneous syndrome. Am J Neuroradiol 17: 461–471.

Pascual-Castroviejo I, Fernández-Cuadrado J, Cortès P, De la Flor-Crespo M, Pascual-Pascual SI (2002) Hemangioma cutáneo asociado a hemangioma hepático y a neurofibromatosis tipo 1 (NF1). Rev Neurol 34: 652–654.

Pascual-Castroviejo I, Pascual-Pascual SI, Rafia S, Viaño J (2002a) Hemangiomas y malformaciones vasculares cutaneas e intracraneales (Sìndrome de Pascual-Castroviejo tipo II). Presentación de un caso. Rev Neurol 35: 1034–1036.

Pascual-Castroviejo I, Frutos R, Viaño J, Pascual-Pascual SI, Gonzalez P (2002b) Cobb sìndrome: case report. J Child Neurol 17: 847–849.

Pascual-Castroviejo I, Viaño J, Pascual-Pascual SI, Martinez V (2003) Do cutaneous hemangiomas and internal vascular anomalies follow the same evolution? Neurology 61: 140–141.

Pascual-Castroviejo I, Pascual-Pascual SI, Moreno F, Viaño J, Martinez V (2003a) Anomalias vasculares extracraneales e intracraneales y nevus de Ota en la misma familia. Neurologìa 18: 102–106.

Pascual-Castroviejo I, Pascual-Pascual SI, Garcìa-Guereta L, Goded F (2005) Cutaneous hemangioma in chest and internal vascular anomalies. J Pediatr Neurol 3: 103–106.

Persky MS (1986) Congenital vascular lesions of the head and neck. Laryngoscope 96: 1002–1015.

Philip N, Guala A, Moncla A, Monlouis M, Aymè S, Giraud F (1992) Cerebro-facio-thoracic dysplasia: a new family. J Med Genet 29: 497–499.

Poetke M, Frommeld T, Berlien HP (2002) PHACES syndrome: new views on diagnostic criteria. Eur J Pediatr Surg 13: 366–374.

Prensky AL, Gado M (1973) Angiographic resolution of a neonatal intracranial cavernous hemangioma coincident with steroid therapy. Case report. J Neurosurg 39: 99–103.

Raas-Rothschild A, Nir A, Gillis R, Rein AJJ (2000) Giant congenital aortic aneurysm with cleft sternum, supraumbilical raphè, and hemangiomatosis: report and review. Am J Med Genet 90: 243–245.

Reese V, Frieden IJ, Paller AS, Esterly NB, Ferriero D, Levy ML, Lucky AW, Gellis SE, Siegfried EC (1993) Associaton of facial hemangiomas with Dandy-Walker and other posterior fossa malformations. J Pediatr 122: 379–384.

Risau W (1997) Mechanisms of angiogenesis. Nature 386: 671–674.

Rossi A, Bava GL, Biancheri R, Tortori-Donati P (2001) Posterior fossa and arterial abnormalities in patients with capillary haemangioma: presumed incomplete phenotypic expression of PHACES syndrome. Neuroradiology 43: 934–940.

Rufo-Campos M, Riveros-Huckstadt P, Rodriguez-Criado G, Hernandez-Soto R (2004) Another case of cerebrofacio-thoracic dysplasia (Pascual-Castroviejo syndrome). Brain Dev 26: 209–212.

Schieken LS, Brenner JI, Baker KR, Ringel RE, Pacìfico A (1987) Aneurysm of the ascending aorta associated with sternal cleft, cutaneous hemangioma and occlusion of the right innominate artery in a neonate. Am Heart J 113: 202–204.

Schneeweis A, Blieden LC, Shem-Tov A, Motro M, Feigel A, Neufeld HN (1982) Coarctation of the aorta with congenital hemangioma of the face and neck and aneurysm or dilatation of subclavian or innominate artery: a new syndrome? Chest 82: 186–187.

Slavotinek AM, Dubovsky E, Dietz HC, Lacbawan F (2002) Report of a child with aortic aneurysm, orofacial clefting, hemangioma, upper sternal defect, and marfanoid features: possible PHACE syndrome. Am J Med Genet 110: 283–288.

Soeda A, Sakai N, Iihara K, Nagata I (2003) Cobb syndrome in an infant: treatment with endovascular embolization and corticosteroid therapy: case report. Neurosurgery 52: 711–715.

Stigmar G, Crawford JS, Ward CM, Thomson HG (1978) Ophthalmic sequelae of infantile hemangiomas of the eyelids and orbit. Am J Ophthalmol 85: 806–813.

Stockman A, Boralevi F, Taieb A, Leaute-Labreze C (2007) SACRAL syndrome: spinal dysraphism, anogenital, cutaneous, renal and urologic anomalies, associated with an angioma of lumbosacral localization. Dermatology 214: 40–45.

Streeter GL (1918) The development alterations in the vascular system of the brain of human embryo. Contrib Embryol 8: 5–38.

Studer M, Gavalas A, Marshall H, Ariza-McNaughton L, Rijili FM, Chambon P, Krumlauf R (1998) Genetic interactions between Hox A1 and Hox B1 reveal new roles in regulation of early hindbrain patterning. Development 125: 1025–1036.

Takahashi K, Mulliken JB, Kozakewich HPW, Rogers RA, Folkman J, Ezekowitz RAB (1994) Cellular markes that distinguish the phases of hemangioma during infancy and childhood. J Clin Invest 93: 2357–2364.

Tanner JL, Dechert MP, Frieden IJ (1998) Growing up with a facial hemangioma: parent and child coping and adaptation. Pediatrics 101: 446–452.

Tasnadi G (1993) Epidemiology and etiology of congenital vascular malformations. Sem Vascul Surg 6: 200–203.

Taveras JM (1969) Multiple progressive intracranial arterial occlusions: a syndrome of children and young adults. Am J Roentgenol Rad Ther Nucl Med 106: 235–268.

Torres-Mohedas J, Verdú A, Vidal B, Jadraque R (2001) Presentación conjunta de hemangioma facial, malformación de fosa posterior e hipoplasia carótido-vertebral (sìndrome de Pascual-Castroviejo II): aportación de dos nuevos casos. Rev Neurol 32: 50–54.

Tortori-Donati P, Fondelli MP, Rossi A, Bava GL (1999) Intracranial contrast enhancing masses in infants with capillary hemangioma of the head and neck: intracranial capillary haemangioma? Neuroradiology 41: 369–375.

Vaillant L, Lorette G, Chantepie A, Marchand M, Alison D, Vaillant MC et al. (1988) Multiple cutaneous hemangiomas and coarctation of the aorta with right aortic arch. Pediatrics 81: 707–710.

Walter JW, Blei F, Anderson JL, Orlow SJ, Speer MC, Marchuk DA (1999) Genetic mapping of a novel familial form of infantile hemangioma. Am J Med Genet 82: 77–83.

Walter JW, Morth PE, Werner M, Mizonacki A, Blei F, Walker JWT, Reinisch JF, Marchuk DA (2002) Somatic mutation of Vascular endothelial growth factor receptors in furverile hemangioma. Genes Chromosomes Cancer 33: 295–303.

Wang HU, Chen ZF, Anderson DJ (1998) Molecular distinction and angiogenic interaction between embryonic arteries and veins revealed by ephrin-B2 and its receptor eph-B4. Cell 93: 741–753.

Watson WL, McCarthy WD (1940) Blood and lymph vessel tumors. A report of 1056 cases. Surg Gynecol Obstet 71: 569–588.

White CW (1990) Treatment of hemangiomatosis with recombinant interferon alfa-2a. Sem Hematol 27: 15–22.

Wright TL, Bresnan MJ (1976) Radiation-induced cerebrovascular disease in children. Neurology 26: 540–543.

Zhong TP, Childs S, Leu JP, Fishman MC (2001) Gridlock signalling pathway fashions the first embryonic artery. Nature 414: 216–220.

Ziyeh S, Shumacher M, Strecker R, Rössler J, Hochmuth A, Klisch J (2003) Head and neck vascular malformations: time-resolved MR proyection angiography. Neuroradiology 45: 681–686.

# Chapter 3

# NEUROFIBROMATOSIS TYPE 1 & RELATED DISORDERS

**Martino Ruggieri, Meena Upadhyaya, Concezio Di Rocco, Annalia Gabriele, and Ignacio Pascual-Castroviejo**

Institute of Neurological Science, National Research Council, Catania, and Department of Paediatrics, University of Catania, Italy (MR); Institute of Medical Genetics, University of Wales College of Medicine, Cardiff, United Kingdom (MU); Section of Paediatric Neurosurgery, Department of Paediatrics, Catholic University of Sacred Heart, Rome, Italy (CDR); Molecular Genetics Unit, Institute of Neurological Science, National Research Council, Cosenza, Italy (AG); Paediatric Neurology Service, University Hospital La Paz, Madrid, Spain (IPC)

## Introduction

The last decades have seen major developments in our knowledge of the different forms of neurofibromatosis (Ferner 2007a, b; Ferner et al. 2007; Friedman et al. 1999; Huson and Hughes 1994; Korf and Rubenstein 2005; North 1997; Ruggieri 2007; Upadhyaya and Cooper 1998a). Evidence based clinical diagnostic criteria and management guidelines have been developed (Baser et al. 2002; Ferner et al. 2007; Gutman et al. 1997; Listernick et al. 1997; Listernick and Charrow 2004a, b; North et al. 1997; Maria 2002; Ruggieri 1999; Wolkenstein et al. 1996). The genes for the two major forms, neurofibromatosis type 1 (NF1) and type 2 (NF2), have been cloned and the gene products, *neurofibromin* and *merlin* (also called *Schwannomin*), respectively, fully characterised (reviewed in Baser et al. 2003, Ferner 2007a, Friedman et al. 1999, Korf and Rubenstein 2005, Upadhyaya and Cooper 1998b).

Until the late '70s, however, many clinicians did not distinguish between the different forms of neurofibromatosis and used the terms *von Recklinghausen disease* or *multiple neurofibromatosis* to describe all patients with variable combinations of café-au-lait spots and tumours of the peripheral and/or central nervous system (CNS) (Gorlin et al. 2005, Hecht 1989, Huson and Hughes 1994). As systematic clinical research began it became clearer that within this umbrella term there were several distinct diseases (Ferner et al. 2007, Huson and Hughes 1994, Ruggieri 1999). The differentiation of these disorders is not simply an academic exercise – the natural history and management of the various forms of neurofibromatosis is very different (Friedman et al. 1999, Gutman et al. 1997, Huson and Ruggieri 2006, Ruggieri 1999).

## Classification of the different types of neurofibromatosis

The definition of the different forms of neurofibromatosis depends on the occurrence, number and distribution of café-au-lait spots, tumours of the nervous system (neurofibromas and schwannomas) and ophthalmologic findings (which are frequently asymptomatic) (Gorlin et al. 2005, Huson and Hughes 1994). *Riccardi* in 1982 (also reviewed in Friedman et al. 1999, Huson and Hughes 1994) proposed a classification of neurofibromatosis, which included seven different types and an eight category for cases "not otherwise specified". This classification has not come into general use partly because type III "mixed", type IV "variant", type VI "multiple, café-au-lait spots only" and type VII "late onset" forms were not defined sufficiently to permit their general use (Ruggieri 1999). *Gorlin et al.* (reviewed in 2005) later added two further categories of type VIII "gastrointestinal" and type IX "Neurofibromatosis/Noonan" forms. *Viskochil and Carey* (1992) proposed in the 90s an alternative classification, which lays the basis for differentiation combining clinical and molecular knowledge. They divided the different forms of neurofibromatosis into two broad categories: 1) *alternate* forms (having some of the respective clinical features of either NF1 or NF2 yet not demonstrating the "typical" presentation); these included mixed type, localised types (segmental and gastrointestinal neurofibromatosis, and multiple café-au-lait spots only) and Schwannomatosis; 2) *related* forms (having classical clinical features of neurofibromatosis in addition to distinctive clinical features not typically seen in either NF1 or NF2), including Noonan/neurofibromatosis, Watson syndrome, Duodenal/carcinoid/phaechromocytoma/NF1 and juvenile xanthogranuloma/NF1.

However, at present, the most widely used classification continues to be that recommended in 1987 by the ***NIH Consensus Conference on neurofibromatosis*** (National Institute of Health Consensus Development Conference Statement 1988) and updated by Gutman et al. (1997). This is a numerical rather than descriptive or eponymous nomenclature, with *NF1* replacing the classic term von Recklinghausen or peripheral neurofibromatosis or multiple neurofibromatosis, and *NF2* replacing bilateral acoustic or central neurofibromatosis (Gutman et al. 1997). The Consensus statement acknowledges that there are other types (and subtypes), which, at that time were not defined well enough to be part of the formal classification (Gutman et al. 1997). Apart from *mosaic/segmental NF1 and NF2* (Ruggieri and Huson 2001) (formerly type V of Riccardi's classification) (Ruggieri 2001) and *Schwannomatosis* (most likely a true different form of neurofibromatosis, which has been proposed as NF3) (MacCollin et al. 2005) they are all extremely rare (Ferner et al. 2007, Ruggieri 1999).

# Neurofibromatosis type 1

NF1 is the most common form of neurofibromatosis and one of the commonest autosomal dominant disorders in man, with an estimated birth incidence of 1/2,500 and disease prevalence in population-based studies of 1/4,000 (Huson et al. 1988, Huson and Hughes 1994). It is an extremely variable disease, even within families and is characterised by age-related: (1) **major features** which include pigmentary lesions (i.e., café-au-lait spots, freckling in specific areas and a mild to moderate skin hyperpigmentation which can be localised or more

diffuse) and peripheral neurofibromas in the eyes (i.e., Lisch nodules of the iris) and/or skin (cutaneous and/or nodular types); (2) **minor features** (e.g., macrocephaly, stature at low percentiles, dysmorphic features, thoracic abnormalities and hemihypertrophy); and (3) **systemic complications** mostly affecting the skeletal, nervous and vascular systems. From the patient's perspective, it is this variability, as well as the unpredictability of what will happen and when, that makes NF1 a difficult disease for families to come to terms with and for clinicians to manage.

# Historical perspective and eponyms

## Earliest descriptions and medical curiosities

### Roman Empire (ca. 200 BC)

The earliest example of a neurofibromatosis sufferer could be traced in the remnants of a Roman statue representing a man with skin nodules in his trunk and arms resembling neurofibromas (Bruno Dallapiccola, personal communication 2004).

### From 200 AD to the 12th century

There is a manuscript called *Tiberius B V* in the British Museum (Zanca and Zanca 1980) which is part of a series of texts dealing with the "Marvels of the East" originated between the 7th and 10th century. In these treatises (Wittkower 1942; Zanca and Zanca 1980), monstrous human races of oriental origin are described. At fol. 83[v] there is a specimen of the mythical race with large, long ears, represented with his snakelike ears wound round his arms which in the opinion of Zanca and Zanca (1977, 1980) might be "an individual with two enormous plexiform neurofibromas hanging from his cheeks". In the text is maintained the description of creatures with enormous fanlike ears that at night lie down on one ear and fold the other on themselves.

## Year 1200 AD

Code 507, is a collection of drawings from the abbey of Reun in Styria dating from about the year 1200 (Zanca and Zanca 1980). The code, now in Vienna, was published by Baltrusaitis (1960) and contains a miniature showing in the lower part of the illustration a human figure with three large nodules hanging from the face in front of the neck and from the left mandibular region plus two additional long sack-like tumours hanging from under the armpits down to the waist labelled as plexiform neurofibromas by Zanca and Zanca (1980).

## Early 1300 AD

An early 13th century illustration, probably composed by the Cistercian scribe a monk named Heiricus from the abbey near Graz, Austria, has been suggested to depict a patient with NF1 (Hermann 1926, Morse 1999, Mulvhill 1988). The image represents a man with skin nodules resembling cutaneous neurofibromas and was later added to the original diagram portraying the different species of amphibian.

## Conrad von Magenberg (1309–1374) and the "Buch der Natur"

This Bavarian philosopher, historian and naturalist freely translated the "De natura rerum" of Thomas of Cantimpré publishing it as the *Buch der Natur*. In the 12th Tome of the Ausgburg edition, printed in 1475, one can observe various types of monsters with as the sciapod with webbed foot, the headless monster with six arms, the cinocephalus and the Cyclops, among the others. In the lower row of the xylograph, near the bearded woman can be seen another woman who, according to Choulant (1963), has a large goiter whereas according to other authors had either "full blown" NF1 (Zanca and Zanca 1980) or mosaic/segmental NF1) (Ruggieri and Polizzi 2003).

## The 16th century: Ambroise Paré and José de Ribera (the "Spagnoletto")

Among the various figures published in "*Des monstres et prodiges*" by the famous French surgeon Ambroise Paré (1510–1590) (author of many books on anatomy, surgery and medicine) (Céard 1971, Deux livres de chirurgie 1573, Les oeuvres d'Ambroise Paré 1585) is that of a monster born on January 17th 1578, in Piedmont, at Chicri, near Turin, Italy (Fig. 3) (Zanca and Zanca 1980). The face, writes Paré "… was well-proportioned in every way, but there were five horn-like growths on the head and a long, fleshy mass hanging down from the head along the back" "en maniere d'un chaperon de damoyselle" ("like a woman's hat"); "… another double fleshy mass like a shirt collar was visible around the neck". Besides the more or less fantastic deformations (horns, claw-like hands, etc.) and relying on the accuracy with which Paré himself reported this case, that fleshy mass hanging down along the back, might be diagnosed as a plexiform neurofibroma (Ruggieri and Polizzi 2003; Zanca and Zanca 1980).

Another xylograph of a "man with an enormous protuberance hanging down from the mandible" (likely a plexiform neurofibroma) may be seen in a work of José de Ribeira (1588–1656) know also as the "Spagnoletto".

## Ulisse Aldrovandi and the "homuncio" in the Monstrorum Historia

In 1592, Ulisse Aldrovandi (1522–1605), an Italian physician, philosopher, and naturalist (Caprotti 1980, Il Teatro della Natura di Ulisse Aldrovandi 2001, Tega 2002) recorded the extraordinary case of a man of low stature ("homuncio"), of Indian origin who presented enormous, flabby masses of flesh less than two inches thick, hanging from the left side of his head and trunk (Madigan and Masello 1989; Hecht 1989; Ruggieri and Polizzi 2003; Zanca and Zanca 1980). This illustration, along with a Latin text, appeared on page 587 and 585, respectively, of the Monstrorum Historia, published posthumously in 1642 under Aldrovandi's name and edited by Bartolomeo Ambrosino (Aldrovandi 1642). Zanca and Zanca (1980) inferred that this mis-shapen man would represent a full-blown NF1 case. The English translation of the original (and earlier) version (1592) of Aldrovandi's manuscript reads (Ruggieri and Polizzi 2003):

"The monster. Homunculus, as refers the Aegisthus, born in India, of six palms in stature. Between his mouth and left ear, he had a double fleshy mass hanging forward towards the chest: one [mass] was nearer the mouth, the other shorter, and adhered to the ear. Behind and under the left ear, likewise, a similar flesh rolled down dropping over the shoulder, spread with some tufts of hair as were the former two [masses] on the left side of his mouth covered with hairs such as of beard, particularly in the folds. At the beginning of the chest, under the chin and springing up around almost the entire chest, another very large and very wide [fleshy mass] extending from the left shoulder hung downward across almost the entire abdomen, enlarging from the right breast to the opposite side or rather the left armpit. Indeed that flesh and that loose substance was less than two fingers thick and with the hands it could be raised from the body, as it did not adhere [to the skin] except in the place of its own origin, up to the beginning of the chest and over the breasts. That same part of the body felt exceedingly warm, and therefore it must be believed that the red portion of the growth could be invaded by heat of some kind. This monstrous homunculus was brought to my attention by the Bolognese nobleman Bovio."

Ruggieri and Polizzi (2003) proposed that the diagnosis in this case was mosaic/segmental NF1 rather than "full-blown NF1 as inferred by other authors (Hecht 1989; Madigan and Masello 1989; Morse 1999; Zanca and Zanca 1977, 1980).

## The Waldassen (oriental) "curious fool"

During the abbacy of Eugen Schmid (1724–1764) in the Monastry of "Waldassen" (located near the forest along the central arm of the Wondreb River, in Germany) began the work of decoration of the library as planned in previous years by the Jesuit frater Johannes Hoermann. Abbot Schmid developed a unique and highly complex figural programme of large-scale carved figures (likely depictions of fooled probably influenced by Egerland carnival figures as in the "Comedy of Art") supporting the walls under the galleries and balconies of the library. Among the "angry", the "stupid and lazy", the "vain" and the "hypocritical" fools, the crank, the vain mocker, the braggart, the ignoramus and the arrogant pride in the south gallery of the window wall is the so-called oriental "curious fool", carved in lindenwood around years 1720–1730. He wears a turban set with precious stones, a long robe with buttoned-up pockets and above this a jacket with super buttons and a large pointed collar, hanging down. He holds a bottle gourd behind his back in his right hand and his left hand is raised. The object he once held in this hand is now lost but is said it was a mirror and the figure would thus have been a reference to self-knowledge. Notably, his oriental face is disfigured by wart-like prominences resembling cutaneous neurofibromas. The figure's disproportionately large right ear is conspicuous and it is usually interpreted as a symbol of curiosity. Drs. Riccardi and Krone interpreted these findings as "full-blown" NF1 (Riccardi 1987, 1992).

## The Buffon's girl and the Wart Man of Tilesius

Other portraits of NF1 sufferers can be traced in the drawings of a child by B. de Bakker which and appeared in Buffon's (1707–1788) *Histoire Naturelle* ("Natural history") (Buffon's girl) (Zanca and Zanca 1980, Ruggieri and Polizzi 2003) and the "Wart Man" of Tilesius (Tilesius von Tilenau 1793). In both cases we are confronted by reproductions of severe generalised NF1 phenotypes. The Tilesius' patient, Johan Gottfried Rheinhard, was reported under the title "Case History of Extraordinary Unsightly Skin" and described as having "countless growths [fibrous tumours] on the skin, café-au-lait spots, macrocephaly, and scoliosis".

## Initial clinical descriptions

### The first English report

The first English language, more plausible, clinical report however is that of Akenside (1768) who in 1761 observed a man about threescore years of age coming to St. Thomas Hospital … "to obtain present assistance for an uncommon disorder: he had been accustomed during the greater part of his life to a constant succession of wens (tumours) that shot our in several places of his head, trunk, arms and legs; which indisposition he inherited from his father" Akenside (1768).

### Virchow and his "pupil" von Recklinghausen

Rudolf L. Virchow perhaps deserves more credit than his student von Recklinghausen in describing clinical and neuropathological features of neurofibromatosis in a series of reports dating from 1847 to 1863.

Born in 1821 in East Prussia in modest circumstances, Virchow formed his rebellious ideas – which decades later would make him an outspoken antagonist of a leading politician authority such as Bismark – during his childhood by seeing the treatment of the poor by the great landowners of Pomerania. Thus, he became opposed at an early age to the ruling class of "Junkers", who were the mainstay of the Prussian kingdom. He had no difficulty in entering medical school at the king's institute for future army doctors, where he was a brilliant student, receiving his medical degree in 1843 at Berlin and becoming resident physician and clinical pathologist ("prosector") at the Berlin *Charité Hospital.*

He was a born fighter, and he liked to take on authorities. An excellent orator, he was elected speaker for various celebrations of the institute at which he attacked vitalism, empiricism, and humoural pathology. He preached clinical observation, animal experimentation, and necropsy, including microscopic examination. He contended that life is the sum of cellular phenomena, regulated by physical and chemical laws. Such revolutionary thoughts were not then acceptable to the leading medical journals

of Germany. So, in 1847 while becoming "Privatdozent" in Berlin, at the ripe old age of 26 he founded his own and celebrated medical journal, later known as *Virchow's Archiv fur pathologische Anatomie und Physiologie und fur klinische Medizin.*

By 1849, for his revolutionary (political) ideas was suspended from his post at the Charité and had to leave Berlin to Wurzburg in Bavaria where he was appointed as pathologist and teacher. After seven years, Virchow was called back to Berlin where a Pathological Institute was built for him. In this Institute, Recklinghausen and many other future pathologists were trained, so that about half the professors of pathology in Germany were Virchow's former pupils. Virchow's books on cellular pathology and on tumours appeared in this period (about 1858 to 1865). He entered politics again and was elected to the Prussian Parliament. While a member of Parliament, he was even challenged to a duel by Bismark, one challenge he did not accept. He was the king of German pathology and was regarded as the leading figure in medicine in the world. In 1888, Virchow was on the wrong side in the violent debate about the (malignant) laryngeal lesion of Frederick III, Emperor of Germany. Although innocent of error (he was called as consultant on a biopsy taken from the Emperor's lesion and found no sign of malignancy – having however received only benign tissue) he was actively involved in the tragedy of the Emperor's death for cancer. He died at age 81 after jumping off a moving streetcar.

Virchow's classification of neuromas and fibromas on pathological basis laid the groundwork for von Recklinghausen's landmark presentation. In a series addressing the overall classification and terminology of growths and tumours, he placed neurofibromata in the category fibroma molluscum (elephantiasis molluscum):

"I had the opportunity to pursue the exact details of an outstanding case of this type. A 47-year-old woman bore over the entire body a large number of small and large growths, some of which had grown slowly over years. Many of them were rather small, pea-to cherry-sided, round and covered with smooth skin, others were larger, walnut-sized and of the same soft consistency."

In another part of the same treatise, Virchow noted the familial nature of the fibromas:

"These presentations will even more therefore favour that cases of decidedly hereditary transmission of a fibromatosis disposition occur. I have seen a young man whose body was quite covered with lumps from pinhead-sized to pigeon egg-sized, and in such families these peculiarities have existed in an inherited manner already over three generations."

Virchow felt that fibromas involving nerves, known as neuromas, had to be classified in a different category. In 1847, he reported a case of multiple neuromas, and noted the presence of nerve elements as a part of the tumour; later (1857) he distinguished "false" and "true" neuromas based on the histological appearance.

## The eponym

### The studies of Friedrich Daniel von Recklinghausen

**Von Recklinghausen** was born in 1833 in Gutersloh, Westphalia (West Prussia), and was generally considered one of Germany's great pathologists. After a "happy childhood and routinely schooling" he began, at the age of 19 years, his medical studies in Bonn, then went to Wurzburg and to Berlin, where he received his doctor of medicine degree in 1855. He was appointed assistant to Professor Virchow at the Pathological Institute in Berlin at the rather young age of 22 years owing to his outstanding abilities. After nine years, he moved to Konisberg, where he became Professor of Pathological Anatomy at the age of 31. In 1872, he was called to the new University of Strassbourg as chairman of pathology. There he remained, an outstanding member of the faculty, for the rest of his life.

During the 55 years of his professional life, he taught, did autopsies, and investigated. He gave an enormous number of detailed case reports and wrote several excellent papers describing in great details different pathological conditions. Whether Recklinghausen was a good teacher of medical students we are not told, but his postgraduates were many and outstanding. His colleagues honoured

him by attaching his name to osteitits fibrosa generalisata (secondary to hyperparathyroidism) and to neurofibromatosis. It is doubtful that his colleagues did a favour for Recklinghausen by these eponymic honours as both conditions connected with his name had been described previously by others.

As part of a Festschrift honouring the 25th anniversary of the Berlin Pathological Institute in 1882, von Recklinghausen dedicated to Professor Virchow a report, "On Multiple Cutaneous Fibroma and their Relationship to Multiple Neuromas", in which he reviewed the existing literature and added 2 cases, with extensive description of the clinical and pathological characteristics by means of 23 figures grouped into five plates. He concluded:

"In the case presented ... it appears that these multiple neuromas and cutaneous fibromas existed simultaneously. It also appears that this was not a fortuitous combination, but rather that the tumours were related structurally... The evidence for the latter is 1) the nature of the neoplastic tissue in both types of tumour was almost identical, 2) nerve tumours penetrated the undersurface of the tumour of the skin and sometimes could be peeled out of them, and 3) the cutaneous fibromas presented an arrangement different from the usual multiple fibromatous neoplasms...".

He linked the simultaneously existence of fibromas and neuromas for the first time and used the term neurofibroma to underscore the postulated structural similarity between the two lesions. He conjectured that the skin and nerve tumours resulted from the "mingling" of neural elements and connective tissue cells. Although he was not the first to describe neurofibromatosis, and his cases exhibited only a few of its numerous features, it is on the basis of this article that the eponym "von Recklinghausen" disease was applied to NF1.

## Misconceptions

### Sir Frederick Treves and Joseph C. Merrick: the "Elephant Man" unmasked?

On 2nd December 1884, at a meeting of the Pathological Society of London, Sir Frederick Treves –

surgeon at the London Hospital – showed "a man who presented an extraordinary appearance, owing to a series of deformities … From the massive distortion of the head, and the extensive areas covered by papillomatous growth, the patient had been called "the elephant-man". The subject of these deformities was later reported in detail and illustrated by photographs at a further meeting of the Society on Tuesday 17th March 1885 and an account of this was later published in the Society's Transactions (vol. XXXVI, 1885, page 494) as "A Case of Congenital Deformity", and figured at Plate XX. A biographical sketch of this misshapen man "who earned his living at one time by exhibiting himself under the name which he still bears" (i.e., the "elephant man") was accounted in the 11th December 1886 issue of the British Medical Journal, accompanied by four drawings representing the patient's condition at that time. Even though no definitive diagnosis could be reached in that century "elephantiasis" and "dermatolysis and pachydermatocele" were raised as possibilities. In 1905 the dermatologist Dr. Henry Radcliffe Crocker, who was familiar with the monograph of von Recklinghausen, and attended the 1885's presentation of Treves examining his patient closely later on, was of the opinion that this poor man suffered from neurofibromatosis. His colleague Parkes Weber, who saw the elephant man while he was at the London Hospital, also subscribed to the same diagnosis and this was widely accepted. The reasons that led contemporary physicians and early commentators to a diagnosis of neurofibromatosis can be readily discerned. However, many of the elephant man's features are unique to him.

Joseph Carey Merrick (the so-called elephant man) was born on 5 August 1862 at 50 Lee Street, Leicester to Mary Jane Merrick, née Potterton, and Joseph Rockley Merrick, the obstetric history apparently having been normal. Both parents (in their twenties at the time of his birth) and two subsequent siblings (a brother born in 1886 and a sister in 1867) had no evidence of the disorder (notably, the sister died at age 23½ years of "myoletic convulsions). At birth he had no obvious congenital abnormalities, but a firm swelling of the right cheek became to develop at about 18 months and this ex-

tended forwards under the upper lip. The other soft-tissue swellings began to be evident at about 5 years of age and the skeletal abnormalities somewhat later. Joseph fell at age 4–5 years injuring his left hip. At age 12 years left school and took a job rolling cigars, which he had to give up at age 15 years because of increasing clumsiness of his deformed right hand. When he was 20 a large portion (20–23 cm in length and 85–115 g in weight) of his facial deformity was successfully removed. It was to 123 Whitechapel Road (now 259) that Tom Norman, a showman who exhibited freaks, brought Merrick towards the end of November 1884. There, Frederick Treves' house surgeon, Dr. Reginald Tuckett, saw him and then told Treves about the Elephant Man. Treves saw the Elephant Man and negotiated to take him, now aged 24 years, to his room at the London Hospital Medical College across road. It was on this occasion that Treves demonstrated Merrick to his London colleagues.

Other renowned "patients" could have been the Duke Federico of Montefeltro painted by Piero Della Francesca in the 15th century and Quasimodo, the "hunchback" in Notre Dame de Paris by Victor Hugo (Ruggieri and Polizzi 2003).

## Incidence and prevalence

Most studies have found a disease prevalence of around 1 in 4–5,000 (Huson et al. 1989b, Samuelson and Axelson 1981), although two studies in New Zealand and Israel (Fuller et al. 1989, Garty et al. 1994) have shown a significant higher prevalence. Crowe et al. (1956) and Huson et al. (1989b) estimated the birth incidence to be 1 in 2,500–3,300. When the prevalence studies are analysed in relation to age, there is a decreased prevalence in the older age groups (Fuller et al. 1989, Huson et al. 1989b, Samuelson and Axelson 1981).

## Clinical features

The clinical features of NF1 are diverse and can affect almost any organ system. The NIH Conference

**Table 1.** NIH Diagnostic criteria for NF1

*Two or more* of the following criteria:

1. Six or more **café-au-lait macules**
   - 5 mm in greatest diameter in pre-pubertal individuals
   - 15 mm in greatest diameter in post-pubertal individuals
2. Two or more **neurofibromas** of any type or one **plexiform neurofibroma**
3. **Freckling** in the axillary or inguinal region
4. **Optic glioma**
5. Two or more **Lisch nodules** (iris *hamartomas**)
6. A distinctive **osseous lesion** such as sphenoid wing dysplasia or thinning of the long bone cortex with or without peudarthrosis.
7. **First degree relative** (parent, sibling or offspring) with **NF1** by the above criteria.

Adapted and modified from (Gutman et al. 1997, National Institutes of Health Consensus Development Conference 1988, Ruggieri 1999).

* = Currently regarded as neurofibromas (see below and Richetta et al. 2004).

on NF1 (National Institute of Health Consensus Development Conference Statement 1988) formulated the diagnostic criteria for NF1, underlying the pivotal involvement of the skin, bone, and the nervous system in the condition (Ferner et al. 2007) (Table 1).

We find it useful to consider the NF1 features in three main groups (Huson and Hughes 1994, Huson and Ruggieri 2006, Ruggieri 1999):

*1. Major defining features*: these are café-au-lait spots, freckling in specific places, peripheral neurofibromas and Lisch nodules. They manifest with an age-dependant pattern (see Table 2) and develop in the vast majority of affected individuals forming the basis for the diagnostic criteria (see Table 1).

## Café-au-lait spots

Café-au-lait spots are macules varying in diameter from 0.5 to 50 cm having usually a typical smooth contour or, the larger ones, irregular outlines. Their colour varies with background skin pigmentation. They are not unique to NF1 patients and from 11% to 25% of individuals in the general population may

**Table 2.** Major features and most frequent age related complications in NF1

| Major features | Complications |
|---|---|
| ***Birth – 2 years of life*** | |
| Café-au-lait spots | Plexifrom neurofibroma |
| Macrocephaly | Sphenoid wing dysplasia |
| Stature at 10–20th percentie | Pseudarthrosis |
| Thoracic abnormalities | Hypertension [renal artery stenosis or phaechromocytoma] |
| Hypertelorism | Glaucoma |
| | Optic pathway glioma (unusual) |
| | Scoliosis (unusual) |
| ***Pre-school children*** | |
| Café-au-lait spots ± | Learning difficulties |
| Skinfold freckles | Optic pathway glioma |
| Macrocephaly | [peak incidence 4–6 years] |
| Stature at 10–25th percentile | Other central nervous system tumours |
| | Scoliosis (unusual) |
| | Hypertension [renal artery stenosis or phaechromocytoma] |
| | Cerebrovascular disease |
| ***Late childhood and adolescence*** | |
| Café-au-lait spots+ | Learning difficulties |
| Skinfold freckling | Optic pathway glioma |
| Lisch nodules | Other central nervous system tumours |
| Occasional neurofibromas | Scoliosis |
| Macrocephaly | Hypertension [renal artery stenosis or phaechromocytoma] |
| Short stature | Cerebrovascular disease |
| ***Adulthood*** | |
| Café-au-lait spots+ | Spinal neurofibromas |
| Skinfold freckling | Malignancy secondary to NF1 |
| Lisch nodules | Endocrine tumours |
| Neurofibromas | Hypertension [phaechromocytoma] |
| Macrocephaly | Duodenal carcinoid |
| Short stature | |

Adapted and modified from (Ferner et al. 2007, Huson and Ruggieri 2006, Ruggieri 1999)

have one to three/four such skin lesions. Clinically, there are no major differences between café-au-lait spots in NF1 patients and those in the general popu-

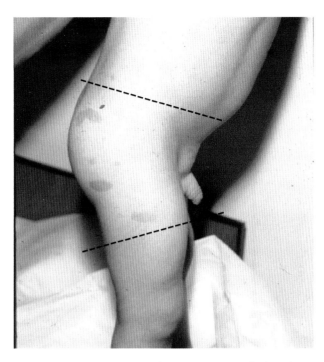

**Fig. 1.** A 1.5-year-old child with NF1 showing multiple *café-au-lait spots* prevalently distributed in the area of the "napkin".

Jeghers syndrome and Piebaldism; 2) those associated with *localised overgrowth* such as Proteus syndrome and Klippel-Trenaunay syndrome; and 3) those associated with *cutaneous or subcutaneous tumours* including lipomatosis, Banayan-Riley-Ruvalcaba syndrome, MEN type 2B and the congenital generalised/localised fibromatoses. Café-au-lait spots may be present at birth or develop within the first 1-year of life. They increase in number in early childhood, but tend to fade with age or become obscured by numerous dermal neurofibromas. Hence, in adulthood it may be difficult to recognise or count a number greater than six. They are not found on the scalp, eyebrows, palms and soles. There is no correlation between the location of café-au-lait spots and the location of other NF1-associated lesions, such as neurofibromas, nor there is a correlation of the overall number of café-au-lait spots with the severity of disorder: however, a darker background skin pigmentation associated with darker café-au-lait spots and more intense and diffuse freckling has been associated with a more severe neurocutaneous phenotype (Gabriele et al. 2007).

Hypopigmented macules may coexist with café-au-lait spots in NF1 and are found in a similar distribution (Ferner et al. 2007) or in close proximity to café-au-lait spots: the latter is interpreted as a twin-spotting phenomenon (see Happle 1997).

## Skin-fold freckling

These are hyperpigmented macules resembling café-au-lait spots, 1–3 mm in diameter, not related to sun exposure, seen in the axillae (Fig. 2A, B), groins and around the base of the neck They can also occur in the inframammary regions (Fig. 2C) or spread over the entire trunk. In their "sprinkle" pattern are unique to NF1, appearing after café-au-lait spots and usually before dermal neurofibromas develop (Huson and Hughes 1994, Listernick and Charrow 2004b).

Café-au-lait spots and skin-fold freckling do not usually cause complications, however, may be patients are distressed by the appearance of pigmentation and may be helped by skin camouflage advice. There is no evidence to support the routine use of laser treatment for café-au-lait macules (Ferner et al. 2007).

lation (even though café-au-lait spots in non-NF1 individuals have usually more irregular margins and a paler pigmentation); it is the increased number (and the time of increasing: usually, within the first months to one year of life) that is significant (Table 2). Notably, when they first appear the napkin (Fig. 1) and this is related to the stimuli to melanin provoked by the physiologic napkin erythema (S. Calvieri, personal communication 2006). Occasionally in children with very pale complexions, café-au-lait spots may be difficult to see with the naked eye and are best assessed with a Wood's lamp. Few other conditions give rise to more than six typical café-au-lait spots, and are all extremely rare (reviewed in Huson and Ruggieri 2006, Ruggieri 1999): these include ring/mosaic chromosome syndromes, DNA repair defects (see chapters 49 to 53) and Schimke osseous dysplasia. The other conditions that are confused with NF1 largely fall into three groups (see also Ferner et al. 2007): 1) those associated with *abnormal skin pigmentation* confused with café-au-lait spots, such as McCune-Albright syndrome, Leopard syndrome, Peutz-

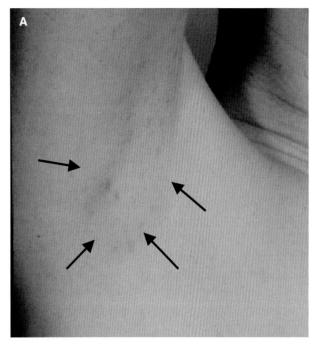

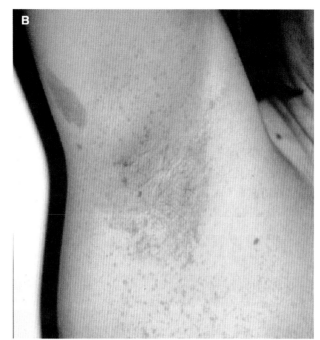

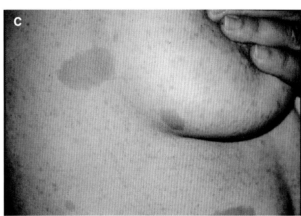

**Fig. 2.** *Skin freckling*: Note the initial appearance (**A**) of the typical NF1 freckles in a confined area of the axilla (arrows) and their later distribution (**B**) to the entire axilla, the arm and the upper chest including in females (**C**) the submammary region.

## Neurofibromas

Nearly all-adult patients have *dermal* (*cutaneous*) neurofibromas (Friedman et al. 1999, Korf and Rubinstein 2005, Listernick and Charrow 2004b). These lie within the dermis and epidermis and move passively with the skin. Most are discrete nodules, soft, almost gelatinous in consistency, violaceous in colour (Fig. 3A). In older patients they tend to increase in size and become papillomatous. Dermal neurofibromas are found mainly on the trunk, but can appear in any body part. Their number is only roughly proportional to age, severely and mildly affected individuals being seen in all age groups. At present there is no means of predicting how many neurofibromas a patient will develop: in our experience individuals with a more pigmented background (and larger number of café-au-lait spots and freckles) have an increased risk of developing larger amounts of neurofibromas. The pattern of growth is unpredictable, with periods of rapid growth followed by relative quiescence. New neurofibromas or increased growth of pre-existing lesions are often noted during pregnancy (Huson and Hughes 1994).

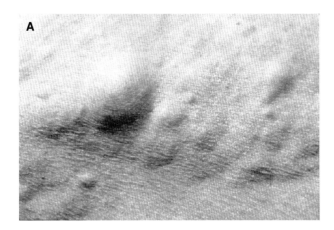

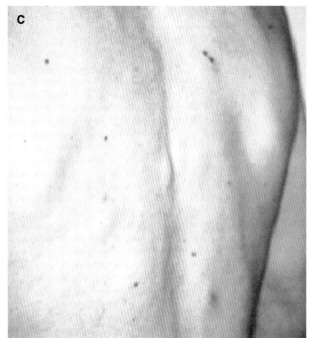

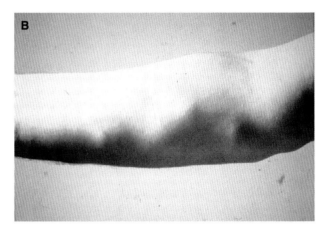

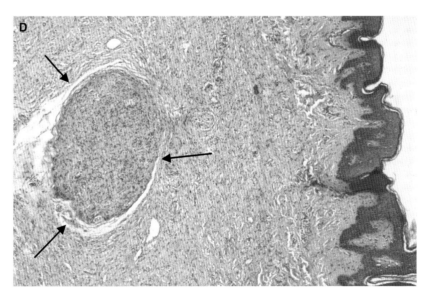

**Fig. 3.** Clinical appearance of cutaneous (**A**) and subcutaneous (**B**) *neurofibromas*: note their average distribution at older ages (**C**). Histologically (**D**), they show maldefined margins, are characteristically fusiform due to their intrinsic development, and involve multiple Schwann cells. At imaging [magnetic resonance (MR)] studies (**E–G**) show (slightly) greater signal intensity than skeletal muscle on $T_1$-weighted sequences (**E**, **F**). On $T_2$-weighted sequences, the signals tend to be of higher intensity in the peripheral areas with respect to the muscle, whereas the centre of the lesion is often of low signal intensity ("target sign") (**E**, **F** arrowheads). After gadolinium administration, neurofibromas show almost uniform enhancement with a tendency to greater signal intensity in the peripheral area (arrowhead) and lower intensity in the center (**G**).

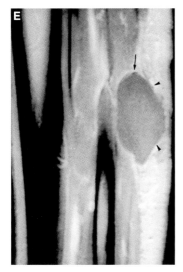 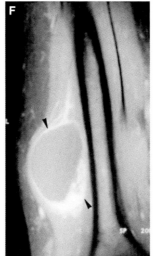 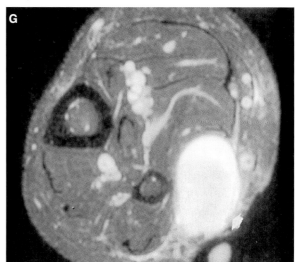

**Fig. 3.** (Continued)

A less common form of peripheral neurofibroma is the *nodular (subcutaneous)* neurofibroma, present in about 5% of NF1 patients. These develop subcutaneously on the major peripheral nerve trunks; have a much firmer consistency and more defined margins. They are palpated under the skin or found in deeper parts of the body (Fig. 3B, C).

Histopathology reveals a mixture of cell types including Schwann cells, perineural-like cells, fibroblasts, mast cells, endothelial cells, lympohocytes, and cells with intermediate features. Basically, neurofibromas are WHO grade I tumours which infiltrate the nerve, show maldefined margins, are characteristically fusiform due to their intrinsic development, are unencapsulated, and involve multiple Schwann cells (Fig. 3D). Their growth is initially along the course of nerve fibres, which become encased by tumours. Staining for S-100 protein is invariably seen (less extensively that in Schwannomas: see chapter 4, NF2) and the tumour is EMA-negative.

Dermal neurofibromas are rarely painful but often can cause itching. There have been no reports of these skin tumours undergoing sarcomatous change, but are prudent to remove rapidly enlarging or painful lesions. On the contrary, nodular neurofibromas often give rise to neurological symptoms such as sensorimotor deficit due to pressure on the peripheral nerves (tingling in the distribution of the affected nerve) and are a source of pain. Malignant changes can rarely occur (Ferner and Gutman 2002, Woodruff 1999) – in our experience more frequently from multinodular lesions. Average age of malignancy for neurofibromas in patients with NF1 is 26 years while in patients with no other stigmata of NF1 (see also mosaic/segmental NF1) is 62 years.

Solitary neurofibromas at imaging [magnetic resonance (MR)] studies show slightly greater signal intensity than skeletal muscle on $T_1$-weighted sequences. On $T_2$-weighted sequences, the lesions have variable signal intensity (Barkovich 2005). Most commonly, the signals tend to be of higher intensity in the peripheral areas with respect to the muscle, whereas the centre of the lesion is often of low signal intensity (Barkovich 2005, Suh et al. 1992); this has been referred to as the "target sign" (Fig. 3E, F). The central area of decreased intensity is probably related to the known dense central core of collagen within these lesions (collagen has a low mobile proton density and therefore is of low signal intensity on $T_2$-weighted images) (Barkovich 2005). After gadolinium administration, neurofibromas show almost uniform enhancement (Fig. 3G). Malignant transformation may appear as non-homogeneous masses with low signal intensity on $T_1$-weighted and high signal intensity on $T_2$-weighted images.

## Lisch nodules

These are harmless, asymptomatic iris nodules, which appear on slit-lamp examination as smooth dome-shaped, usually light orange/brown in colour (Fig. 4A), the colour of burnt sienna, appearing darker than blue irides but paler than brown irides. Most are round and evenly distributed on the ante-rior surface of the iris (Fig. 4C–E). Their size varies from a pinpoint to involvement of a segment of iris. They are usually bilateral and may be confluent. They develop during childhood, after the appearance of café-au-lait spots but before peripheral neurofibromas: they are present in one-third of 2.5 year olds, half of 5 year olds, three-quarters of 15-year olds and almost all adults over 30. As they are

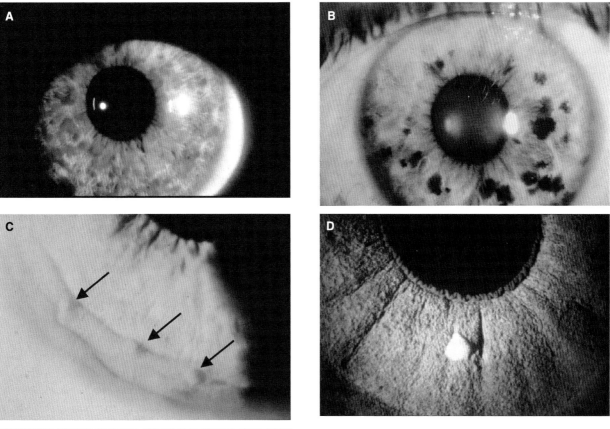

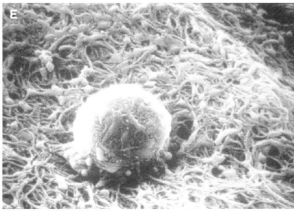

**Fig. 4.** *Lisch nodules* of the iris: note the typical appearance of the iris nodules (**A**) as seen at slip lamp examination as compared to (**B**) hyper-pigmented naevi of the iris; slit lamp magnification of the iris (**C**), scan (**D**) and electron (**E**) microscopy reveal the dome-shaped (**C**, arrows) or rounded appearance of nodules which look like neurofibromas (courtesy of Susan M. Huson, Manchester, UK).

unique to NF1 (Fig. 4B) and are present in over 90% of adults with NF1 they are useful to confirm the diagnosis (see Table 1). Several studies have reported that the Lisch nodules are melanocytic hamartomas but its pathogenesis is still debated. Richetta et al. (2004) studied the histopathological and ultrastructural features of a Lisch nodule in a 50-year-old woman and found that this was composed of three main cytotypes: pigmented cells, firboblast-like cells and mast cells, showing a pattern similar to neurofibromas.

*2. Minor features*: These are features present in a significant proportion of patients but that are not so specific that they can be used as part of the diagnostic criteria (Cnossen et al. 1997, 1998b; Huson et al. 1988, Ruggieri 1999).

## Macrocephaly

Macrocephaly (harbouring an underlying megalencephaly with altered ratio between grey/white matter) (Korf and Rubinstein 2005, Ruggieri et al. 2007) is seen in about 50% of people with NF1. A child with NF1 and macrocephaly, therefore, does not need to be investigated unless there are other symptoms or signs suggestive of intracranial pathology or serial measurements of head circumference are showing progressive enlargement.

## Stature at low percentiles

Since Crowe et al. wrote the first modern book on neurofibromatosis in 1956, stature at low percentiles has been a common feature of patients with NF1. Approximately 30% of NF1 patients are at the 10th–25th percentile and fewer below the 3rd percentile in height. The study of large series of patients with NF1 with ages between 6 and 15 years without suprasellar lesion, showed a 44.5% with centiles below 25%, and 27% with centiles below 10% (Vassilopoulou-Sellin et al. 2000). When compared with unaffected siblings or schoolmates, the NF1 patients are usually 7 to 8 centimetres shorter. Short stature persists during adult life and it is constated in all races (Szudek et al. 2000). The cause is unknown. As the clinical expression in the second generation is more pronounced, the underlying mechanism seems to be mediated by yet undefined genetic factors. However, short adult height is strongly linked with familial background of NF1 (Carmi et al. 1999). Short stature is also related with precocious puberty despite normal pituitary gland and thyroid function test in most children and adolescent with NF1.

## Additional cutaneous features

**Nevus aneamicus** and **benign cherry angiomas** (Campbell de Morgan spots), mostly on the trunk and thighs, are more common in NF1 patients than in the general population irrespective of age. Cutaneous abdominal hemangioma with subjacent hepatic hemangioma associated with NF1 has been reported (Pascual-Castroviejo et al. 2002).

Multiple juvenile **xanthogranulomas** (JXG) may develop in 1–2% of children with NF1 predominantly on the head (Fig. 5), extremities and trunk. They present as orange papules that appear transiently in early childhood and disappear with age. Occasionally they can take the form of xanthogranuloma disseminatum (XD) (Savasan et al. 2005). There was some suggestion in the literature that NF1 patients with JXG were at increased risk for developing juvenile chronic myeloid leukaemia (JCML) (Gurney et al. 1996, Zvulunov et al. 1995). However, routine haematological studies are not warranted in this group (Ferner et al. 2007, Friedman and Birch 1997) and a recent follow-up study did not reveal any features distinguishable from those of classical JXG or haematological malignancies in 14 children with NF1 and JXG (Cambiaghi et al. 2004). This was also our experience in an ongoing study (mean follow-up of 7 years; range 3–15 years) of 40 children with such association (Ruggieri et al. manuscript in preparation). Thus, JCML in NF1 patients with JXG could well be regarded as a coincidental occurrence of rare NF1 features due to report bias (Burgdorf and Zelger 2004).

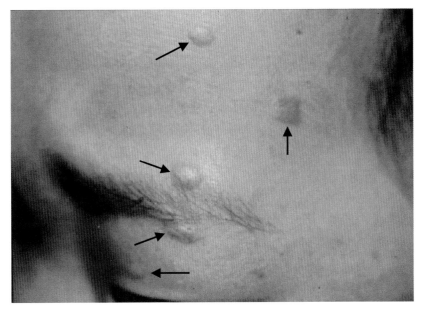

**Fig. 5.** Xanthogranulomas (arrows) of the face in a child with NF1.

## Hypertelorism

*Hypertelorism* and *thoracic abnormalities* including pectus excavatum and pectus carinatum have been documented in 63% and 37.6% of patients in one series respectively (Cnossen et al. 1997). Documentation of such features may be a helpful aid in assessing the possibility of a diagnosis of NF1 in children with only CAL spots (Ruggieri 1999).

## Hemihypertrophy

Localised or generalised hemihypertrophy or hemihyperplasia is a disease manifestation in 6% of NF1 patients (Pascual-Castroviejo 1992). Hemihyperplasia is characterised by asymmetric growth of cranium, face (Fig. 6A), tongue (Fig. 6B), trunk (Fig. 6C), limbs (Fig. 6D), and/or digits, with or without visceral involvement. It may occur in several syndromes. In patients with NF1, it may be an isolated finding, but more frequently it is associated with underlying plexiform neurofibroma.

*3. Disease complications*: We define a complication as any condition that occurs at an increased frequency in individuals with NF1 compared with the general population. Few of the complications are specific to NF1; most are also seen as isolated findings in the general population. It is the disease complications, which make NF1 a condition with significant morbidity and mortality. Their occurrence cannot be predicted, even within families (Boulanger et al. 2005). We will discuss the major NF1 complications in their order of appearance at different ages.

## Orthopaedic complications

Skeletal system is one of the most frequently involved structures (Alwan et al. 2005; Crawford and Schorry 1999, 2006). Some type of bone anomalies may affect approximately 40% of patients with NF1 irrespective of age (Friedman and Birch 1997). In children, the prevalence may be lower (Crawford and Schorry 2006). Ruggieri et al. (1999) reported 8.8% of congenital bone malformations in a series of 135 NF1 patients.

## Spine (scoliosis & kyphoscoliosis)

Osseous anomalies most often involve the spine and cause scoliosis and, in severe cases, kyphoscoliosis (Figs. 7 and 8). The prevalence of scoliosis is estimated to be between 10% and 30% (Akbarnia et al. 1992, Holt 1977). Other studies reported variable prevalence figures in individuals with NF1: 24% (Friedman and Birch 1997); 10% (Huson 1994); and 7% (in children only) (Pascual-Castroviejo 1992). The scale of severity of the scoliosis is very large and

one can see patients with very moderate spinal curvature (Fig. 7A) or scoliosis or kyphoscoliosis with narrow angles of the spine (Fig. 8A) which may prove extremely dangerous for the spinal cord, with severe

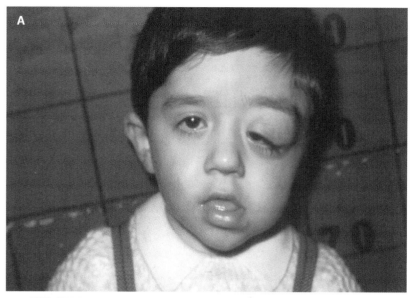

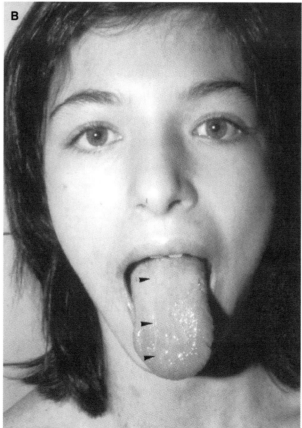

**Fig. 6.** Hemihypertrophy of the left facies (**A**) associated with ipsilateral plexiform neurofibroma; (**B**) hemihypertrophy of the left half of the tongue which displaces the normally structured right half of the tongue (arrowheads); (**C**) hemihypertrophy of the right lower limb which includes the right buttock (arrows) (this girl had a huge plexiform neurofibroma of the lower end of the spine); (**D**) hemihypertrophy of the left upper limb (black arrows) and left shoulder (white arrows) with severe hyperpigmentation of the affected area.

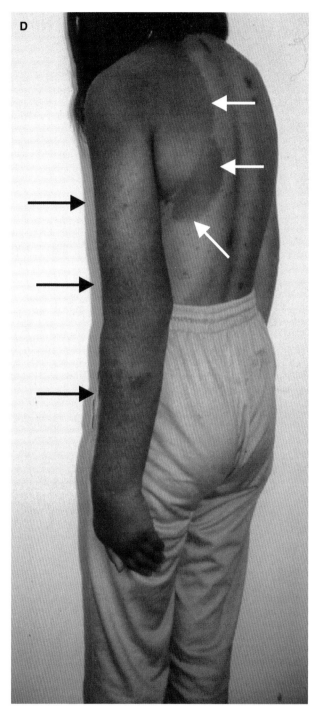

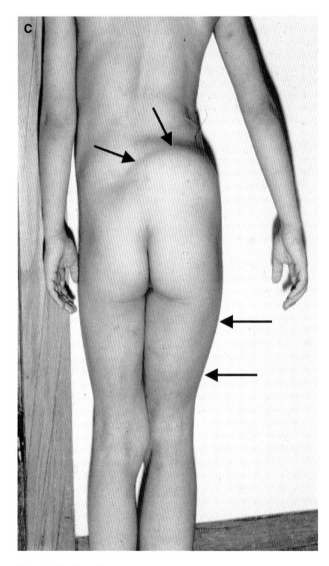

**Fig. 6.** (Continued)

motor, sensory, sphinterian and sexual problems (Chaglassian et al. 1976). The type of scoliosis, which is associated with NF1 is commonly located in the thoracic spine and mostly is of a discrete degree (Fig. 7B, C). However, in some patients may show pronouncing curvatures, involving four to six vertebrae with a progressive natural history. Cases with kyphoscoliosis that show severe kyphosis are at risk

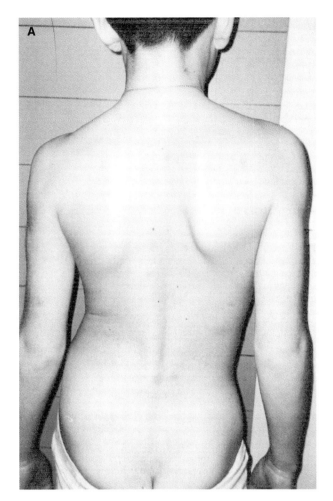

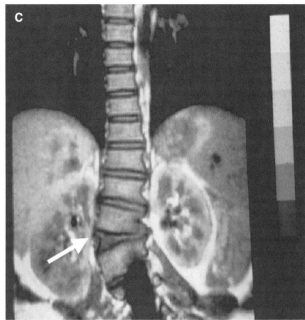

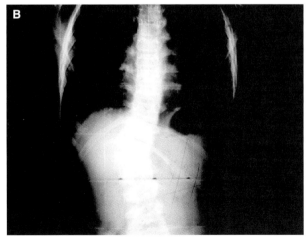

**Fig. 7.** Clinical (**A**) and radiographic (**B**) appearance of a right curved scoliosis: (**A**) this moderate scoliosis is responsible for the contracted paravertebral muscles and asymmetric shoulders and scapulae in this 12-year-old NF1 boy; (**C**) note the dysplastic vertebral body (hemivertebra).

of medullar compression and severe neurological disease (Fig. 8A). There are two recognised types of scoliosis depending on the presence or absence of lo-

calised vertebral dystrophy. The most severe type of scoliosis (*dystrophic scoliosis*) is associated with partial or total dystrophy of one (Fig. 8B) or several verte-

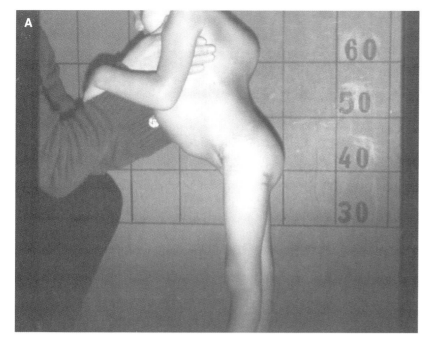

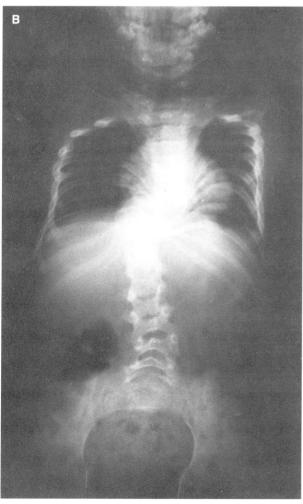

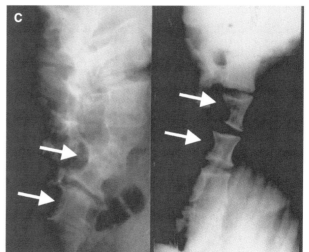

Fig. 8. (A) Severe cyphoscoliosis in a 4-year-old NF1 girl; (B) skeletal radiograph of the same patient showing severe scoliosis and dysplastic vertebrae; (C) typical radiographic appearance of the vertebral scalloping (white arrows).

brae. Vertebral dystrophy may not be present during the first years manifesting only during the maturation process of the NF1 patient (Crawford and Bagamery 1986). Dystrophic scoliosis is associated with severe and pronounced curvatures, mostly of left convexity, with severe deformity of the involved vertebrae. An enlarged vertebral canal is often observed in this zone reducing the risk of medullar lesion. Surgical treatment must be performed in cases with curvatures up or > than 20 degrees because the degree of severity of the scoliosis which follows has a progressive evolution. Surgical actitude must be very aggressive, often needing repeated interventions, aimed to get a solid arthrodesis to avoid the regression of the deformity (Perez-Grueso 2001). Orthopaedic corset is not effective in these cases.

## Long bone dysplasia/pseudoarthrosis

Pseudoarthrosis is a severe disease that involves the long bones, most often of the inferior extremities, but also of the upper limbs of patients with NF1. The orthopaedic surgeons favour the term "congenital dysplasia of long bones" rather than "pseudoarthrosis" as the latter is a consequence of the first event, i.e., the skeletal dysplasia. The bone dysplasia may not be present at birth manifesting during the first years or decade of life. Some newborns with NF1, however, may show a curvature in the inferior region of the tibia that can gradually and progressively evolve into a frank pseudoarthrosis. This complication may cause serious motor problems. Most patients show cutaneous-subcutaneous changes that presage the subjacent osseous lesion (Fig. 9A, B). The pseudoarthrosis affects between 2% and 4% of the general population irrespective of age (Friedman and Birch 1997, Huson 1994, North 2000, Pascual-Castroviejo 1992). Osseous changes involve all bones of the affected region to the same degree (radius and cubitus, tibia and fibula). Functional prognosis may be conditioned by the extension of the bone lesion (Fig. 9C) and the pseudoarthrotic lesion. Tibial pseudoarthrosis is associated with a worst prognosis than the lesions localised to the cubitus and the radius (Fig. 9E–G): this is due

to the body weight that an affected tibia has to support as compared to an affected arm. This is also one of the reasons for which the orthopaedic surgery is more successful on arms than on legs. A very important prognostic factor is the age of appearance of fracture(s) in the tibia. Fractures occurring after age 4 years have a better response to surgery and need less surgical interventions than fractures in children with less than 4 years (average of 1.5 vs. 4.2 surgical actions, respectively) (Fig. 9H, I) (Traub et al. 1999, Tudisco et al. 2000). The recent literature shows that 95% of cases requiring amputation first manifested this bobe complication before 4 years of age (Grill et al. 2000, Lehman et al. 2000, Tudisco et al. 2000, Crawford and Schorry 2006).

## Sphenoid wing dysplasia

Dysplasia of the greater sphenoid wing is a distinctive manifestation of NF1 forming one of the six clinical criteria for the diagnosis of NF1 (see Table 1). In most patients it can be identified during the first years of life. Sphenoid dysplasia has been reported to occur in 1 to 7% of patients with NF1 (Bognanno et al. 1988, Poole 1989). This manifestation, however, is not always pathognomonic of NF1 (Rasmusen and Friedman 2000): it may also be found in various diseases, including craniosinostosis (especially in plagiocephaly in which the malformation is unilateral) and any type of acrocephalo-syndactily showing bilateral malformation of the sphenoidal wings. Dysplasia of the greater sphenoid wing is associated with increased size of the temporal fossa and facial, orbitary and eyes asymmetry (Fig. 10). The condition is usually primitive, but tumours of the temporal fossa or the orbit, commonly neurofibromas, may cause this greater wing deformity. Orbital fissure enlargement is found in primitive sphenoid dysplasia and also in cases with deformity secondary to contiguous neurofibroma. Orbital changes and enlargement of the cranial foramina support the concept of secondary dysplasia. The condition may have a progressive evolution (Jacquemin et al. 2002, Mcfarlane et al. 1995). Current neuroimaging suggest that secondary dysplasia may have multifaceted and interactive pathogenesis (Jacquemin et al. 2002).

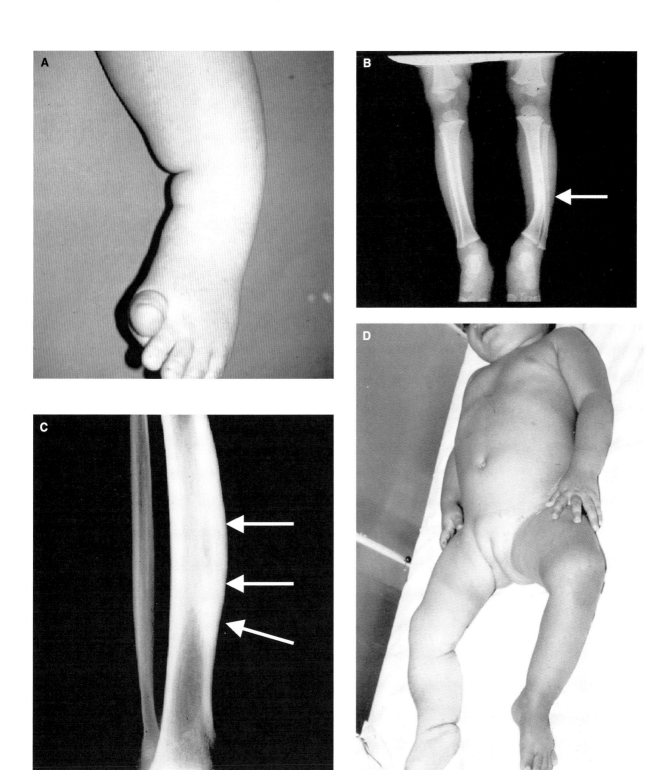

**Fig. 9.** (**A**) A 9-month-old boy showing the earliest manifestations of the long bone dysplasia (in this case localised to the left leg); (**B**) his plain radiograph shows bowing of the left tibia (white arrow); (**C**) a plain radiograph obtained few months later shows cortical hyperostosis (white arrows); (**D**) a 2-year-old girl with right lower limb pseudoarthrosis presents with the external cutaneous and motor anomalies of the disease; (**E**) plain radiograph of the same patient in (**D**) shows severe disease with pseudoarthrosis of tibia and fibula with decreased density of all bones of the limb; (**F**) plain radiograph of the right arm in a 2-year-old boy shows severe pseudoarthrosis of the cubitus; (**G**) plain radiograph of the same patient in (**F**) at 19 years of age: the cubitus shows distal pseudoarthrosis and moderate decreased length, and the radius, that was not affected, adopted a functional form in its distal portion; (**H**) fractures of the fibula secondary to long bone dysplasia and pseudoarthrosis; (**I**) post-surgery results in the fractured long bone.

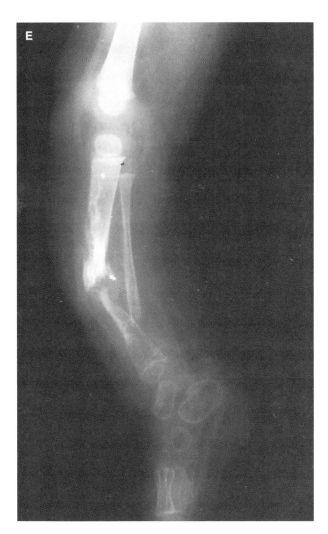

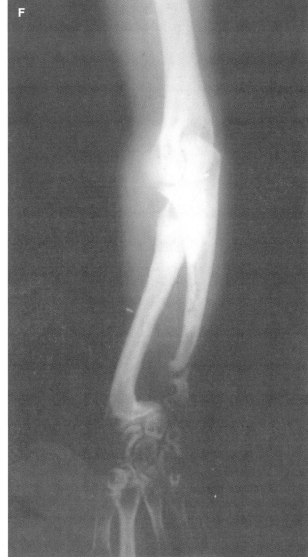

**Fig. 9.** (Continued)

Primary sphenoidal dysplasia manifests very early in life, whilst, in secondary dysplasia, contiguous tumours, arachnoid cysts or other pathological processes usually lead to the osseous deformities. Helicoidal CT and MRI studies offer the chance to see the sphenoid dysplasia, the greater wing and the contiguous structures in three dimensions-coronal, axial and saggital planes and to make the differential diagnosis between primary or secondary disease (Fig. 11).

## Other (less frequent) bone manifestations

### Bone cyst formation

Cyst-like rarefactions (Fig. 12) occur as a result of proliferation of tissue within the medullary cavity (Fig. 12D). These osteolytic lesions tend to increase in number and size over the years (compare

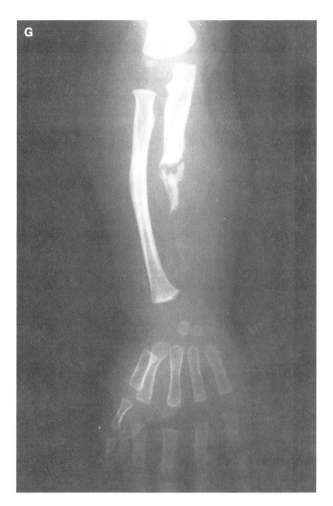

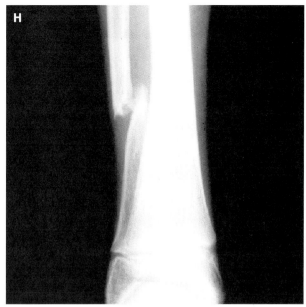

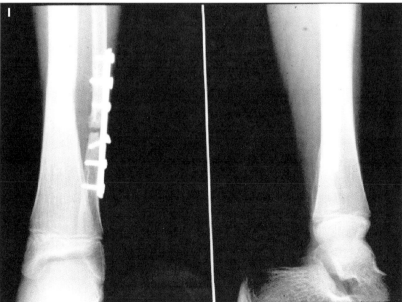

**Fig. 9.** (Continued)

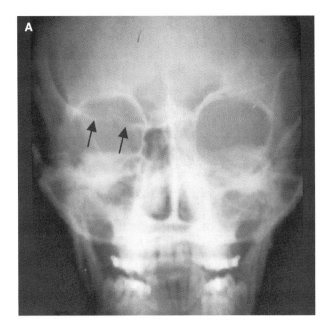

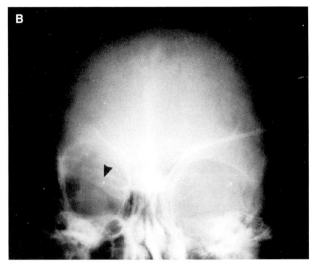

**Fig. 10.** (**A**, **B**) Sphenoid wing dysplasia: frontal radiographs of the head show absence of the right greater wing which is normal in the right side (**A**, arrows; **B**, arrowhead).

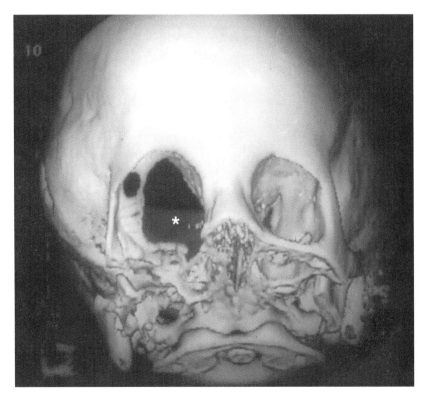

**Fig. 11.** Cranial helicoidal CT study shows secondary right sphenoid greater wing dysplasia (asterisk) due to a plexiform neurofibroma involving the first and the second sensory trigeminal nerves: note the enlargement of the right orbital fissure, supraorbital and rotundum foramina.

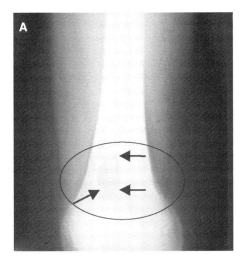
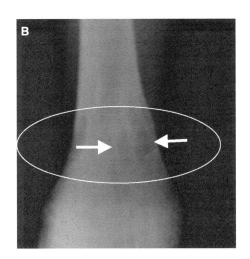
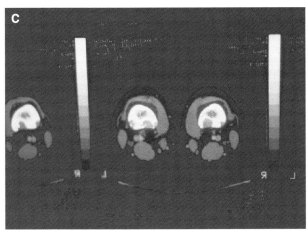
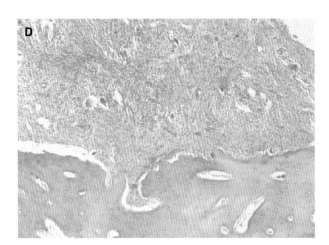

**Fig. 12.** (**A**, **B**) Radiographic and (**C**) CT scan appearance of the typical osteolytic lesions of the long bones: these lesions usually start as single cystic cavities (**A**) in the metaphysical end of the bone (black circle and arrows) and later enlarge (**B**) and increase their number (white circle and arrows); on axial CT scans (**C**) appear as erosions of the cortical and medullary parts of the bone; at histological examination (**D**) the abnormal fibrous tissue (upper part of the figure) almost entirely substitutes the bone (seen in the lower portion of the figure).

Figs. 12A and 12B) becoming stable around puberty. X-ray or CT scan (Fig. 12C) can see cortical bone defects investigation: these are usually caused by NF1 tissue irritating the periosteum.

## Bony lacunae

Besides macrocranium and macrocephaly and sphenoid wing dysplasia, other skull and facial anomalies that occur in NF1 include mandibular enlargement, osseous dysplasia of the lambdoid suture (Fig. 13)

and foraminal enlargement. In one study, these and other abnormalities were found in 92% of 38 patients with neurofibromatosis (D'Ambrosio et al. 1988). In our experience the frequency of cranial vault lacunae was around 5% (Ruggieri et al. 1999).

## Decreased bone density

NF1 patients undergoing orthopaedic surgery often have osteopenic bone (Crawford and Schorry 1999, Illes et al. 2001). Similar findings have been

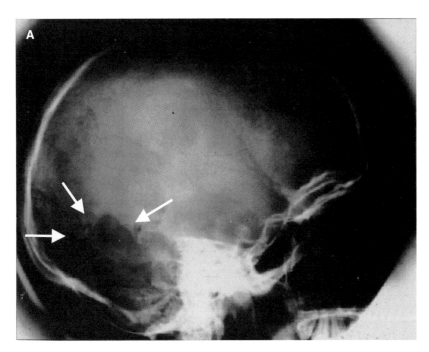

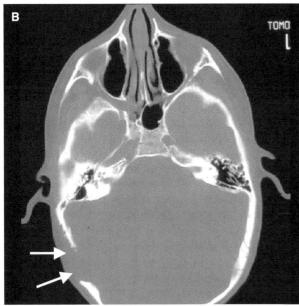

**Fig. 13.** (**A**) Lateral skull x-rays and axial (**B**) CT scan of the head revealing an interrupted bone of the cranial vault (white arrows).

recorded incidentally in children and adults undergoing x-ray investigation during follow-ups of previous orthopaedic complications (Crawford and Schorry 1999, 2006). Based on such observations some clinical research groups have recently assessed the bone mineral density in NF1 patients with and without orthopaedic defects (Dulai et al. 2007, Kuorilehto et al. 2005, Lammert et al. 2005, Stevenson et al. 2007, Yilmaz et al. 2007) recording a general tendency toward osepopenia in NF1 children with lowered bone mineral density and content irrespective to sex (Schindeler and Little 2008).

The location of the lowest local bone mineral densities was clustered in the load-carrying parts of the body (Kuorilehto et al. 2005). The decreased bone mineral density was more significant in patients with typical NF1 skeletal complications (Duman et al. 2008). Stevenson et al. (2007) postulated that individuals with NF1 have a unique generalised skeletal dysplasia predisposing to localised osseous defects.

## Tumours

### Generalities

Most tumours in patients with NF1 are neurofibromas (see above under major defining features) (Woodruff et al. 2005). NF1 can be associated however with benign or malignant tumours of the central nervous system (CNS), irrespective of age (Blatt et al. 1986). These tumours can be seen in 40% to 94% of patients with NF1 (North 1997, Friedman and Birch 1997).

Glioma (astrocytoma) is the predominat CNS tumour type in NF1 and occurs in all parts of the nervous system, with a predilection for the optic pathways, brainstem and cerebellum (Ferner et al. 2007, Rodriguez et al. 2008). In children, optic pathway gliomas are the most frequent tumours and are seen in 15% of cases (Listernick et al. 1989, Pascual-Castroviejo 1992), followed by the benign brainstem tumours. Most intracranial gliomas found in NF1 are histologically classified as benign pilocytic astrocytomas (WHO grade 1). Higher grade (malignant) gliomas (WHO II to IV), are recorded with higher frequencies in adults (Blatt et al. 1986): they are very rare in children aged less than 10 years (Riccardi 1987).

### Optic pathway gliomas

Optic pathway gliomas are the most common primary brain abnormality (and most important disease complication) seen in NF1 during childhood. Their prevalence is estimated at around 15% (Tenny et al. 1982, Hochstrasser et al. 1988, Listernick et al. 1989, 1995; Pascual-Castroviejo 1992, Pascual-Castroviejo

et al. 1994). Higher (up to 44%), but likely biased, prevalence figures have been seldom reported (Hoyt and Baghdassarian 1969, Guillamo et al. 2003). Despite the high incidence, only about half of affected patients ever develop signs or symptoms of their tumours; therefore, the incidence of symptomatic optic pathway tumours is only 5% to 7%. Optic pathway gliomas are more frequent (2:1) in girls than in boys, with lower prevalences in Afro-Americans than in people from other ethnic groups (Gutman 2002). Similar distribution in both sexes has been also reported (Czyzyk et al. 2003). Optic gliomas in monozygotic twins with NF1 have been reported in few instances (Crawford and Buckler 1983, Pascual-Castroviejo et al. 1988).

These tumours usually develop during the first 6 to 7 years of age (Listernick et al. 1999). They can be located in one (Fig. 14A, B) or both optic nerves (Fig. 14C, D) and/or in the chiasm (Fig. 15A, B) showing an independent and asymmetric growth in some cases or a symmetric extension in others. An intracerebral growth may occur in the optic tracts (Fig. 15C, D), the corpus geniculatus and seldom the optic radiations and the occipital area. Tumours that are restricted to the optic nerves may be asymptomatic or may present with mild to moderate visual impairment that rarely progress (Barkovich 2005): those patients with tumours that involve the optic chiasm and hypothalamus may develop precocious puberty (Czyzyk et al. 2003, Laue et al. 1985, Listernick et al. 1997). Clinical studies indicate a poorer prognosis for tumours that involve the optic chiasm or the optic tracts as compared to those restricted to the optic nerves.

The most important phase of growth of this tumour commonly occurs during the first 4 to 6 years of life: thereafter, most of these tumours stop and maintain the same appearance for the rest of life. Tumour progression however has been also recorded later Listernick et al. (2004). Several cases in the literature have specifically documented a neoplasm shrunk without treatment in children with NF1 irrespective of age and sex (Brzowski et al. 1992, Liu and Lessell 1992, Parazzini et al. 1995, Parsa et al. 2001). Spontaneous involution of non-optic astrocitomas in patients with NF1 has been also reported (Cakirer and

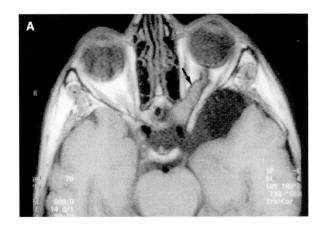
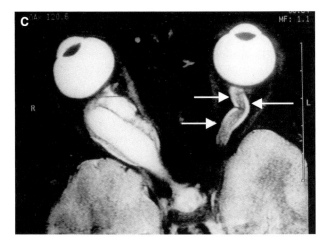
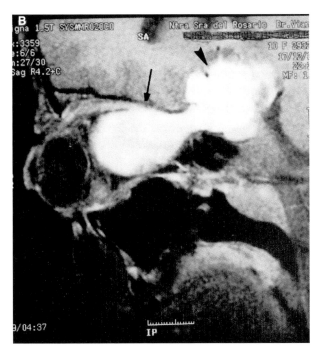
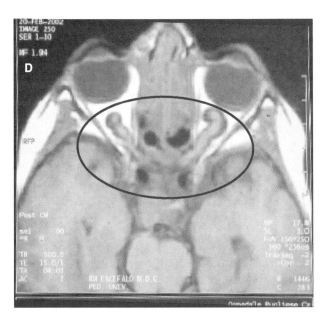

**Fig. 14.** Axial (**A, C, D**) and sagittal (**B**) $T_1$- (**A, D**) and $T_2$-weighted (**B, C**) magnetic resonance images of the head at the level of the orbitae reveal unilateral enlargement of the left optic nerve (**A**, arrow) which appears voluminous (**B**) either in its intraorbital (arrow) and intracranial (arrowhead) component showing the typical increase in signal which follows the nerve contour (**C**, white arrows); (**D**) typical enlargement of both optic nerves.

Karaaslan 2004). On the contrary, rapid development of optic glioma has been recorded in a patient with supposedly mixed NF1/tuberous sclerosis phenotypes (Erbay et al. 2004). Optic pathway gliomas are sometimes associated with homolateral palpebral neurofibroma(s), with local or hemifacial

hypertrophy, occlusion of the eye and often complete lost of vision in the involved eye.

Optic pathway gliomas are often asymptomatic and more indolent than their counterparts in the general population (Czyzyk et al. 2003). However, some tumours may produce impaired visual acuity, abnormal colour vision, visual field loss, squint, papillary abnormalities (Fig. 16), pale optic disc, proptosis (in patients with orbital location of the tumour), failure to thrive, and hypothalamic dysfunction (Fig. 17) (Ferner et al. 2007). Young children do not complain of visual impairment until it is advanced and sometimes only when they have bilateral visual loss. A 52% of patients with NF1 and optic gliomas also show other tumours that

commonly appear about 4 years after the diagnosis of the optic glioma (Kuenzle et al. 1994). Parents need to be alert to possible pointers of visual problems: for example, failure to pick up small toys and bumping into objects. Optic pathway gliomas are often associated with various benign gliomas (Pascual-Castroviejo et al. 2001) and stenosis of the aqueduct (Pascual-Castroviejo et al. 1988, 1994). Most optic pathway gliomas remain clinically silent whilst others

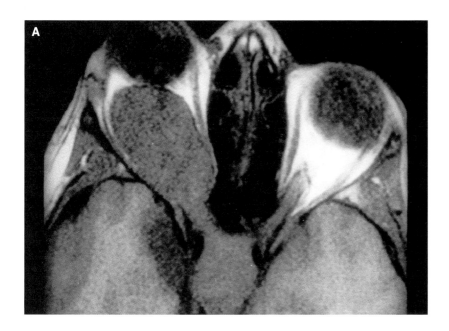

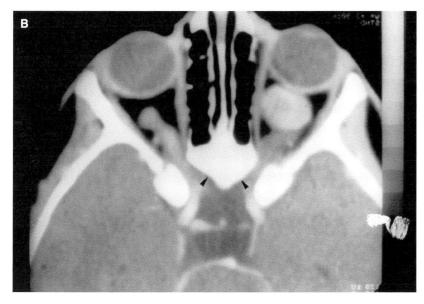

Fig. 15. Axikal computerised tomography (**A**, **B**) and T$_2$-weighted magnetic resonance (**C**, **D**) images showing large bilateral optic nerve and chisamatic glioma (more voluminous on the right side) with enlarged otpic foramina (**B**) caused by bone erosion. Axial T$_2$-weighted magnetic resonance images of the brain show retro-chiasmatic high signal lesions (**C** and **D**, arrowheads) in the optic pathways.

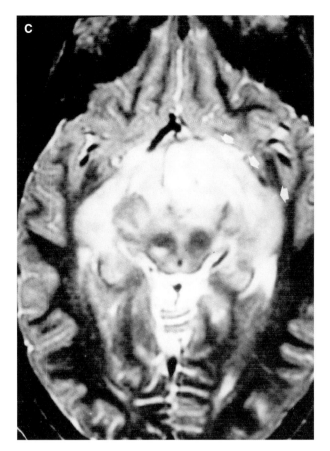

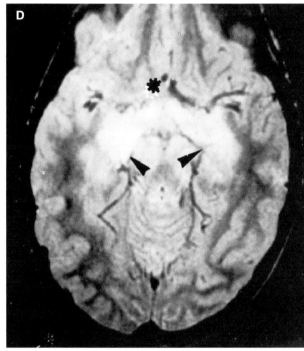

**Fig. 15.** (Continued)

experience a period of growth that may result in ophthalmologic complications or hypothalamic dysfunction. However, even symptomatic tumours may not progress to the point that requires medical intervention (Ferner et al. 2007).

Computerised tomography (CT) is a good method for evaluating tumours of the intraorbital optic nerves (Fig. 15A); enlargement of the optic canals can be seen if bone windows are used. CT however cannot distinguish the two architectural forms of optic pathway gliomas and is less sensitive in assessing intracranial involvement (Fig. 15B) (Barkovich 2005, Tortori-Donati et al. 2005).

Magnetic resonance imaging (MRI) is the preferred imaging modality for evaluating the entire CNS in NF1 (Figs. 14 and 15C, D) (Barkovich 2005). MRI beautifully demonstrates not only the anatomical extension of tumour but also its size,

trajectory, tumoural sheath involvement, involvement of the surrounding structures and destruction of (intratumoural and surrounding) tissues. In addition, the use of MRI eliminates exposure of the child's eyes to ionising radiation. $T_1$-weighted axial and coronal sequences, using slice thickness of 3 mm or less, should be obtained through the globes, optic nerves, and optic chiasm (Barkovich 2005). These are best supplemented by rapid acquisition relaxation-enhanced $T_2$-weighted volumetric images with fat suppression. A routine brain scan should follow to look for involvement of the optic tracts and other areas of the brain (Barkovich 2005). Enlargement of the optic nerves is usually fusiform (Fig. 14A, C, D), although occasionally the enlargement can be rather eccentric. Postcontrast MRI using fat saturation will distinguish the two *architectural forms* of optic pathway glioma: (1)

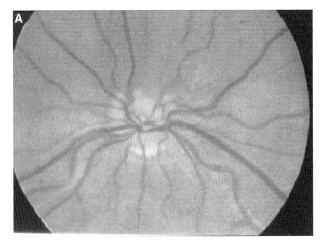

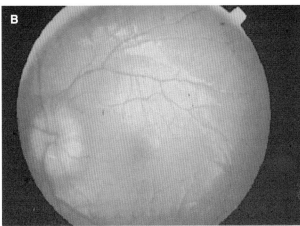

**Fig. 16.** Optic disc examination showing enlarged vessels (**A**) and elevated papillae (**B**) in two NF1 children with intraorbital optic nerve glioma.

Visual evoked potentials (VEP) show a sensitivity of 90% and a specificity of 60% for the detection of optic pathway tumours (North et al. 1994), but their sensitivity to substantiate the routine use is questionable. MR examination shows images that permit to compare the findings between patients with and those without NF1.

On pathologic examination, optic pathway gliomas appear identical to pilocytic (WHO Grade 1) astrocytomas found in other CNS locations. The tumour frequently presents abundant mucus, and histologically, is composed of microcystic regions, made of cells containing brightly eosinophilic granular bodies, alternating with compact pilocytic areas consisting of elongated, fibrillary cells (Rosser and Packer 2002). Although vascularity is prominent, mitosis and signs of malignant degeneration are rare. Some optic (pathway) tumours are not gliomas, but gangliogliomas (Bergin et al. 1988), a tumour that associates neural and glial elements, which may show a rapid growth in some cases (Sadun et al. 1996).

The *diagnostic work-up* of optic pathway gliomas is difficult as visual assessment is problematic in young children and those with cognitive deficits. Recognition of visual acuity can be assessed at a developmental age of 3 years, colour vision at 5 years, and visual fields at age 8 years. In our experience we have not yet detected an asymptomatic child on screening who later required treatment. Nonetheless, the greatest risk of developing optic pathway gliomas is in young children, and those under 7 years should have annual visual acuity and fundoscopy looking for optic disc pallor, vessels abnormalities and disc elevation. One baseline assessment of colour vision and visual fields should be undertaken when the child is mature enough to cope with the test (Ferner et al. 2007). Brain MRI screening for optic pathway gliomas is not indicated, as treatment is not required in the absence of progressive visual disturbance or proptosis.

*Management* of optic gliomas (once diagnosed) is still controversial, especially for asymptomatic patients (or patients with apparently stable lesions) as well for those with larger tumours (Hoffman et al. 1993, Kuenzle et al. 1994, Listernick and Gutmann 1999, Pascual-Castroviejo et al. 1994). The usual

when the nerve is diffusely infiltrated (the enhancing tumour will fill the optic nerve sheath) (Fig. 14B); and (2) when the tumour infiltrates the subarachnoid spaces (showing a rim of enhancing tumour around a minimally enhancing optic nerve) (Fig.14C) (Barkovih 2005). The most common site of involvement in NF1 patients is the orbital nerve (66%) followed by the chiasm (62%) vs. the chiasmatic and post-chiasmatic lesions in children with non-NF1 optic pathway gliomas. The presence of a cystic component is significantly more common in the non-NF1 group (66% vs. 9% in the NF1 group) (Barkovich 2005, Kornreich et al. 2001, Tortori-Donati et al. 2005).

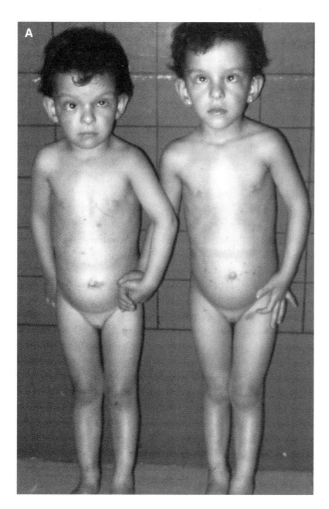 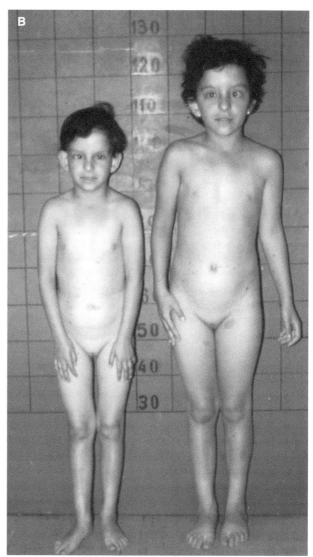

**Fig. 17.** Monozygotic NF1 twins with optic nerve glioma "in mirror" (one in the right and the other one in the left optic nerve) photographed at age 4 years (**A**) and 11 years (**B**). The girl on left who was treated with radiotherapy developed severe endocrinological sequelae.

management policy for patients with stable vision is to "wait and see" scheduling follow-up (non-invasive) work-ups (MRI and VEP). Other authors also believe that patients with anterior visual pathway gliomas associated with NF1 should not be treated unless there is a clear clinical or imaging evidence of progression (Tow et al. 2003). A full ophthalmologic screening protocol for these NF1 children with optic pathway lesions who do not have ocular symptoms may help their follow-up (Listernick et al. 1997,

Listernick and Gutmann 1999). Congenital glaucoma, non-associated with optic pathway tumours, in NF1 children has been reported (Payne et al. 2003).

## Brainstem tumours

Brainstem gliomas (Fig. 18) are the second most frequent intracranial tumours in patients with NF1. They are surpassed only by the optic pathway tumours, and represent about 8.5% of the tumours in large series (Pollack et al. 1996). Main features include paralysis of cranial nerves, gross motor incoordination, ataxia, dysphagia, disarthria, abnormal head movements, macrocephaly and hydrocephaly caused by aqueduct obstruction that is observed between 25% (Pollack et al. 1996) and 41% (Molloy et al. 1995).

Tumours are located primarily in the medulla (82% in the series of Molloy 1995) (Fig. 18C, D), in contrast to the pontine tumour location in the non-NF1 population. Shunt placement or ventriculostomy is required in many patients if ventricular enlargement is seen. Aqueductal obstruction caused by the brainstem glioma is common, but both diseases, obstruction of the aqueduct and brainstem glioma, can coexist independently in the same patient. Most brainstem gliomas are benign and well delimited and seldom invade the surrounding structures. However, some brainstem gliomas can growth to one cerebellar hemisphere, and gliomas with cerebellar origin can growth to the brainstem as well (Fig. 18). Localised brainstem gliomas commonly are benign and tumours that invade the cerebellar can show malignity, especially if they show hyposignal on $T_1$-weighted MR and hypersignal on $T_2$-weighted MR, with intratumoural zones with distinct grade of signal. The MRI characteristics of brainstem gliomas could be subdivided into four distinct groups (Pollack et al. 1996): 1) Diffuse, poorly circumscribed enlargement of a sizable portion of the brainstem with hyperintensity on $T_1$-weighted MR images. 2) Focal enhancing brainstem masses. 3) Intrinsic tectal tumours. 4) Large, sharply margined, nonenhancing area of focal hypointensity on $T_1$-weighted MR images or diffuse brainstem lesion in association with a focal area of enhancement or hypodensity. Optic pathways and brainstem gliomas are frequently associated in patients with NF1.

Brainstem gliomas can not completely seen by computed tomography (CT) (Pascual-Castroviejo et al. 1986) and they require MRI study to know the location and MR spectroscopy (MRS) if malignancy is suspected (Fig. 19). Both MRI measurements and MRS seem to be useful for distinguishing patients with NF1 and diffuse brain stem enlargement from patients without NF1 but with diffuse pontine glioma (PG). They are most helpful in differentiating symptomatic patients with NF1 from patients with PG, thereby minimizing aggressive treatment and its side effects in patients destined to have better outcomes (Broniscer et al. 1997). Most brainstem gliomas show to be biologically benign tumours (Pascual-Castroviejo et al. 1986, Raffel et al. 1989, Pollack et al. 1996).

Brainstem gliomas in patients with NF1 carry a more favourable prognosis than patients with PG with similar MRI appearances. Most patients with brainstem gliomas associated with NF1 usually exhibit spontaneous stabilisation and, in some cases, regression without therapeutic intervention. Indications for intervention on these lesions must be conservative. Only those symptomatic lesions that produce significant (and progressive) local mass effect or that exhibit clinical and radiographic progression, which together constitute a minority of brainstem lesions in patients with NF1 should be considered for treatment (Pollack et al. 1996). Those lesions that do progress have a favourable response to surgical resection, radiotherapy or chemotherapy. Brainstem tumours require clinical and MRI control at least 1 to 2 times a year.

## Tumours of cerebral hemispheres

Cerebral hemispheres are rare location for tumours in patients with NF1. In our series of more than 600 patients, only less than 2% of the tumours were located in the cerebral hemispheres. Most of the tumours are grade 1 astrocytomas, that may be located anywhere of the brain hemispheres (Fig. 20). Intracerebral schwannoma (Bruni et al. 1984), ganglioglioma (Parizel et al. 1991), eosinophilic granuloma, and intracranial neurofibroma are occasionally found. Focal seizures and motor disease, most times hemiparesis, are the main clinic features. MRI reveals all the anatomic changes of the tumours (Fig. 20). MR spectroscopy (MRS) shows the biological characteristics, with the image corresponding with benign or malignant profile. Clinical evolution of the apparently malignant tumours of patients with

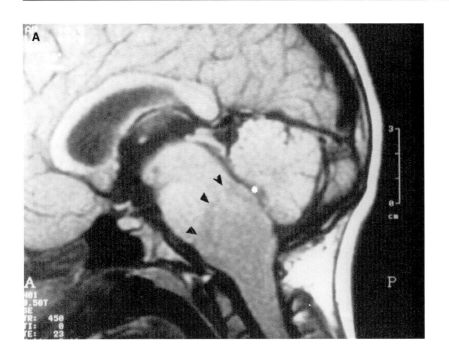

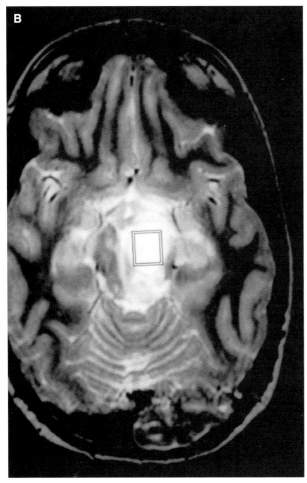

**Fig. 18.** Sagittal (**A**, **C**), axial (**B**) and coronal (**D**) T$_1$- (**A**, **C**, **D**) and T$_2$-weighted (**B**) magnetic resonance images of the brain showing astrocytomas of the ponds and medulla (**A**, arrowheads; **B**, square) and of the medulla oblongata (**C**, **D** arrows).

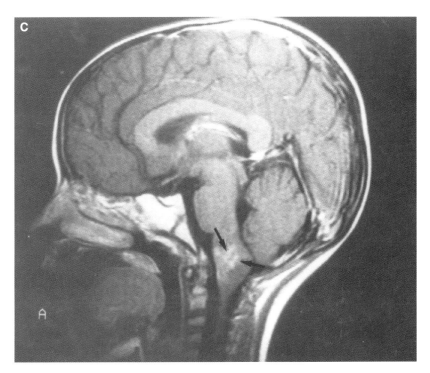

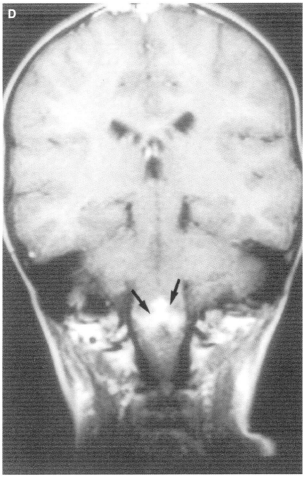

**Fig. 18.** (Continued)

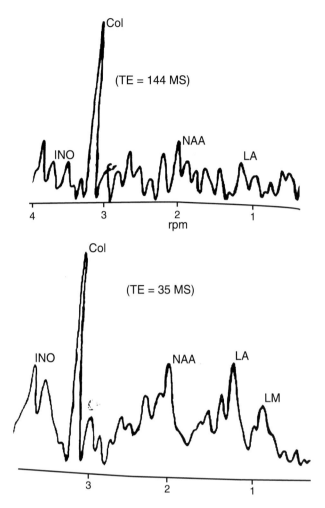

**Fig. 19.** Magnetic resonance spectroscopy (MRS) showing altered peaks in a NF1-associated brainstem tumour.

NF1, in accordance with the MRS findings, is better than that of patients without NF1 and similar MRS results.

### Tumours of the cerebellum

Most cerebellar tumours are benign astrocytomas, commonly located in the cerebellar hemispheres, with frequent extension to the lateral zones of the brainstem. Despite the cerebellar astrocitoma is a benign tumour (Fig. 21), malignancy may be occasionally found (Carella and Medicamento 1997). MRS may be necessary to distinguish the benign or malignant nature of the tumour (Castillo et al. 1995). Malignant

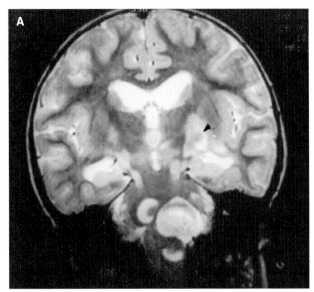

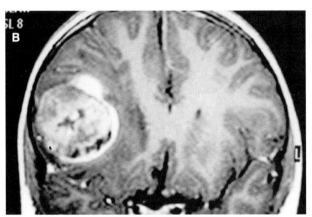

**Fig. 20.** Coronal $T_2$-weighted (**A**) and inversion recovery (**B**) magnetic resonance images of the brain show a temporal grade I (**A**, arrowheads) and a parietotemporal grade III astricytoma in two different patients with NF1.

tumours, such as medulloblastoma and sarcoma of the cerebellum are very uncommon, and there are very few cases described in the literature (Corkill and Ross 1969, Meadows et al. 1977). We have seen only one case of medulloblastoma who survived 3 years after resection and posterior chemotherapy.

### Spinal tumours

Spinal tumours are common in patients with NF1 (Fig. 22). They are most often neurofibromas (Lee et al. 1996). Incidence of these tumours is, however,

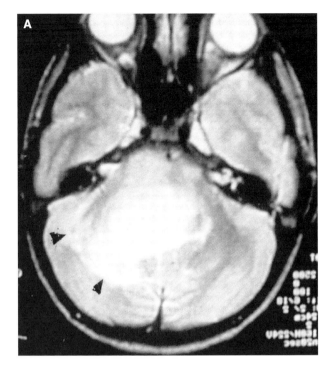

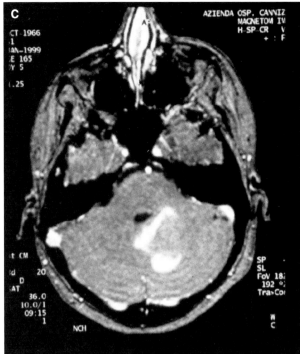

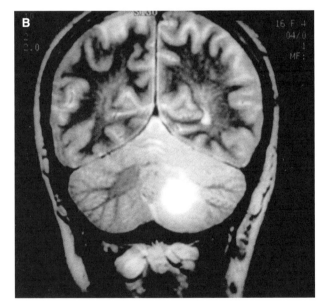

**Fig. 21.** Axial (**A**, **C**) and coronal (**B**) T$_2$-weighted magnetic resonance images of the brain showing cerebellar astrocytomas in the right (**A**, arrowheads) and left (**B**) cerebellar hemispheres; note the enhancement (**C**) in the peripheral region of the tumour after gadolinium administration.

lower than in NF2. Intramedullar location also is uncommon in NF1 as compared to NF2. Intramedullar spinal tumours are also different in NF1 in that most often are astrocytomas; conversely, in NF2 the most frequent tumour is the ependymoma (Lee et al. 1996, Ruggieri et al. 2005). Only 5% of patients with NF1 have neurological features (Huson 1989, Halliday et al. 1991, Von Deimling et al. 1995), while spinal MRI enhanced with gadolinium demonstrates spinal neurofibromas in 36% (Egelhoff et al. 1992) to 38% (Pohynen et al. 1997), and only 5 to 7% with neurological features.

## Tumours of the peripheral nervous system

The peripheral nerves may be affected by solitary/multiple **neurofibroma(s)** involving single or multiple cutaneous and/or subcutaneous nerve(s), and/or **plexiform neurofibromas**, which may affect some, several, most or all nerves of the body (Pascual-Castroviejo et al. 2000). Most neurofibromas are discrete nodules of variable consistence, more numerous and bigger in adults than in children. Dermal and nodular neurofibromas have been covered in the section on major diseases features (see above). Here below we will discuss the plexiform neurofibroma.

### Plexiform neurofibroma (PNF)

Plexiform neurofibromas are locally aggressive congenital lesions composed of tortuous cords of Schwann cells, neurons, and collagen in an unorganised intercellular matrix (Barkovich 2005). They may affect one nerve (usually small, unidentified nerves)

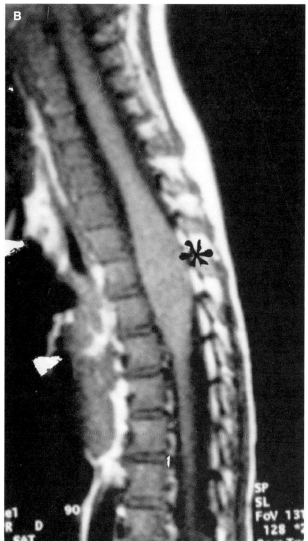

**Fig. 22.** (Continued)

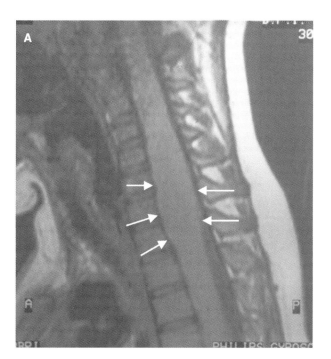

**Fig. 22.** Sagittal T$_1$-weighted magnetic resonance images of the spine showing intraspinal astrocytomas (**A**, arrows; **B**, asterisk).

but more often involve multiple nerves or multiple nerve branches (Fig. 23) growing along the length of the nerve of origin into the anatomic spaces or body cavities in close proximity to them causing significant morbidity. They may involve primarily the sensory sheath rather than the nervous fibers secondarily affecting all the structures (sensory and motor) of peripheral nerves giving rise to neurological symptoms such as sensory/motor deficits due to pressure on the irradiating peripheral nerve (or on the branches or the plexus), and/or pain or sys-

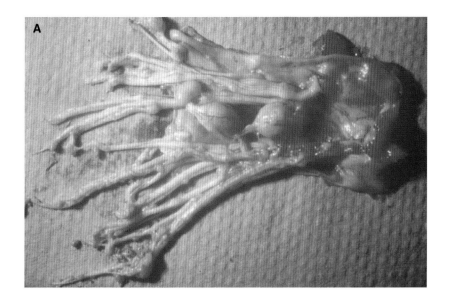

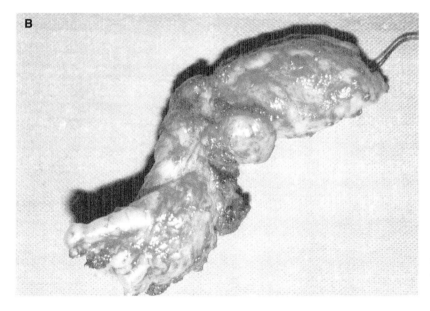

**Fig. 23.** (**A**, **B**) Gross anatomy appearance of two large plexiform neurofibromas removed from the lumbar plexus (**A**) and the sciatic nerve (**B**).

temic manifestations due to the space occupying effect of the mass. The lesions are usually nodular and multiple discrete tumours may develop along the nerve branches. They may affect all nerves of the body in some patients (Fig. 24) (Pascual-Castroviejo et al. 2000). Their prevalence has been estimated between 17.3% (Albisi et al. 1993), 18% (Cnossen et al. 1998A) and 26.7% (Huson et al. 1989B).

They commonly present as large subcutaneous swelling, soft in consistency, with ill-defined mar-gins, varying from a few centimetres in diameter to a whole area of the body. The overlying skin is often hypertrophied (Fig. 25A, B), hyperpig-mented (Fig. 25B, C), or shows excessive hair growth (Fig. 25C, D). The growth rate is unpre-dictable and there may be periods of rapid growth, particularly in early childhood and/or adolescence, followed by periods of relative inactivity, which can last all life. Neurophysiologic studies show de-creased sensory and motor velocity conduction in the zone of the nerve tumour.

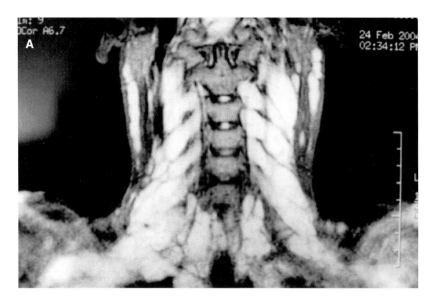

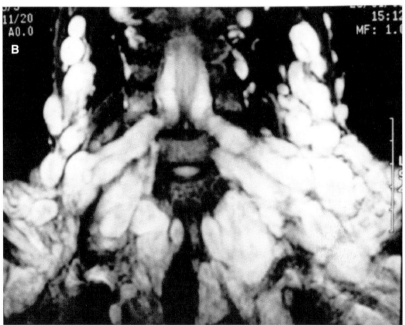

**Fig. 24.** Diffuse plexiform neurofibroma involving almost all nerve branches of the neck, spine and upper thoracic regions in a case of *hereditary spinal neurofibromas*. Coronal (**A–D**) and axial (**E**) T$_2$-weighted magnetic resonance images are taken at the cervical (**A, B**), thoraco-lumbar (**C**) and gluteal (**D**) levels; the axial scan (**E**) shows the extension of tumour along the nerve branches.

The *principal locations* of plexiform neurofibromas are the **face** (Fig. 26A) and the **neck** involving the sensory branches of the trigeminal (V), glossopharyngeal (IX) and vagus (X) nerves or, occasionally, the facial (VII) nerves. Facial unilateral hypertrophy involving the territory innervated by the 1$^{st}$ sensory branch of the trigeminal nerve may be associated with homolateral facial disfigurement (Fig. 26B) and/or hyperplasia of the cerebral hemi-sphere (Fig. 26C). In patients with plexiform neurofibromas involving the 2$^{nd}$ and 3$^{rd}$ sensory branches of the trigeminal nervea along with the neck and the thoracic regions, the hyperplasia can affect the homolateral cerebellar hemisphere as well (Fig. 26D). The etiology and the pathogenesis of the intracranial overgrowth changes, which do not correspond to hemimegalencephaly, remain controversial. Loss of heterozygosity in the entire region (affecting the

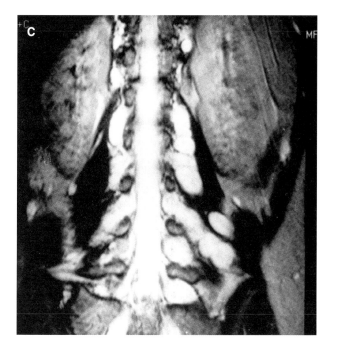
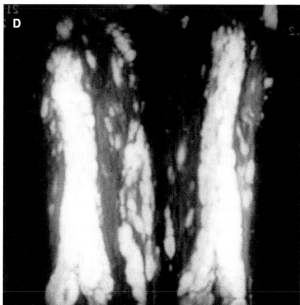
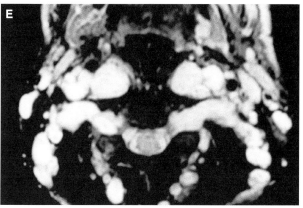

**Fig. 24.** (Continued)

soft tissues and the brain) has been postulated (see below pathogenesis/molecular genetics). Plexiform neurofibromas involving the branches of the glossopharyngeus and pneumogastricus or vagus nerves are located in the pharynx, neck and cranial base (Tortori-Donati et al. 2005, Yumoto et al. 1996). Plexiform neurofibromas affecting the branches of the vagus nerve can extend through the thoracic wall into the mediastinum, the abdominal and pelvic regions. Intrathoracic tumours derived from the vagus nerve may cause sudden death (Chow et al. 1993).

Plexiform neurofibromas usually do not cause pain unless they are located superficially or are injured. Local pain in the area of a plexiform neurofibroma without an explaining cause constitutes suspicion for a malignant transformation (into a neurofibrosarcoma). NF1 patients should seek advise from specialist neurofibromatosis clinics or soft tissue tumour units if they develop any of the following in association with a (subcutaneous) nodular or a plexiform neurofibroma: (1) persistent pain lasting for more than a month or pain that disturbs sleep; (2) new or unexplained neuro-

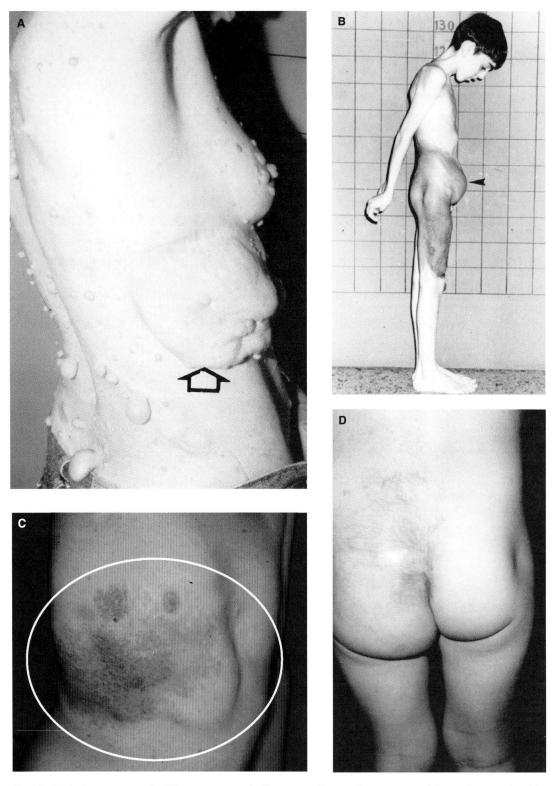

**Fig. 25.** Clinical appearance of a diffuse cutaneous plexiform neurofibroma (**A**, empty arrow); hyperpigmentation (**B**, arrowhead; **C**, circle) with tufts of hair in the affected areas (**C**, **D**).

logical deficit or sphincter disturbance; (3) alteration in the texture of a neurofibroma from soft to hard; (4) rapid increase in the size of a neurofibroma (Ferner and Gutman 2002, Ferner et al. 2007).

The risk for NF1 patients to develop *malignant peripheral nerve sheath tumours* (**MPNST**) (previously known as neurofibrosarcoma) is about 10% (Ferner et al. 2007, Mc Gaughran et al. 1999, Mautner et al. 2003). This represents the major cause of limited survival in NF1 sufferers, especially for NF1 gene carriers aged less than 40 years (Rasmusen et al. 2001). MPNST usually, but not invariably, originate from pre-existing plexiform neurofibromas (Evans et al. 2002b, Ferner and Gutman 2002, Ferner et al. 2007) (Fig. 27). Ma-

lignant transformation can produce metasthases on the adjacent structures. Radiotherapy and chemotherapy usually are not effective on MPNST, and only a complete removal before the appearance of metastases may be effective (see also below MPNST) (Ducatman et al. 1986, Ferner et al. 2007, Greager et al. 1992).

*Imaging studies* should be always considered when undertaking the diagnostic work-up of a plexiform neurofibroma to well delineate the extent of tumoural involvement and to monitor lesion progression. On both CT and MR studies, plexiform neurofibromas appear as masses that can be located anywhere in the body. They tend to be of low attenuation on CT and generally do not enhance after administration of intravenous contrast (Barkovich 2005). On MR, the

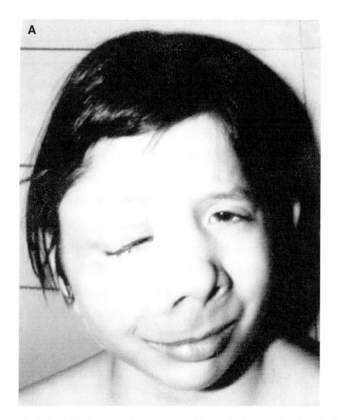
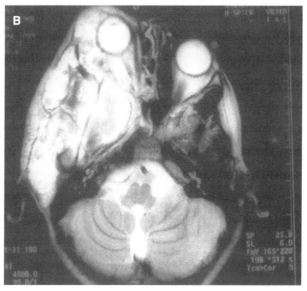

**Fig. 26. (A, B)** Facial and cerebral hemihyperplasia associated with NF1: (**A**) a girl with right palpebral and forehead plexiform neurofibroma shows right hemifacial hyperplasia; (**B**) axial T$_2$-weighted magnetic resonancer images after gadolinium administration show enhancement in the large plexiform neurofibroma associated with right proptosis of the globe; (**C**) coronal T$_2$-weighted images show right cerebral hyperplasia: the right lateral ventricle and the subarachnoid spaces are also enlarged, the subcortical white matter and cortical grey matter appear well formed and perfectly differentiated; (**D**) axial T$_2$-weighted MRI shows left cerebellar hemisphere hyperplasia associated with ipsilateral orbital, palpebral and facial plexiform neurofibroma in an adult with NF1.

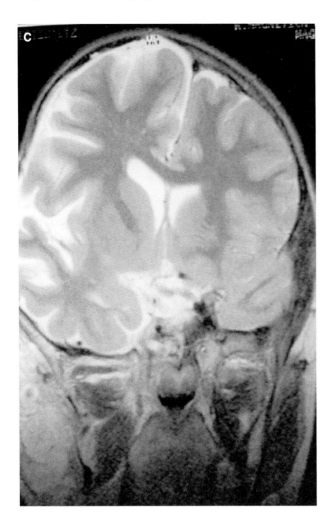

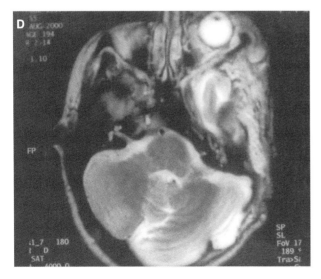

**Fig. 26.** (Continued)

masses are heterogeneous displaying mostly low signal intensity as compared to the brain on $T_1$-weighted images and high signal intensity on $T_2$-weighted images. Enhancement after administration of gadolinium is variable, although at least a portion of the tumour usually enhances. Careful evaluation of the images often reveals extension of the tumour into the adjacent anatomic spaces or invasion of the nearby cavities. [18]Fluorodeoxyglucose positron emission tomography (PET) allows the visualisation and quantification of glucose metabolism in cells and may help in differentiating benign plexiform neurofibromas from cases suspected of having malignant degeneration or at risk of malignancy (Ferner et al. 2000a, King et al. 2000).

Despite the advances in imaging studies, biopsy of a tumoural fragment may be required in some cases before a definitive treatment is undertaken (see below treatment).

## Plexiform neurofibromas at specific locations

Plexiform neurofibromas can be found anywhere in the body. Clinical features are related to the particular location and to the involved organ(s).

### • Retroperitoneal

Retroperitoneal locations are not commonly referred to as such. They, however, are frequent and often show voluminous size. They mostly appear as enlarged spinal nerves, commonly bilateral, growing along the nerve of origin in the paraspinal area towards a distant region. Enlargement of the spinal conjunction foramina is usually caused by the intra- and extra-spinal location of the mass. These tumours can affect any region of the spine (i.e., cervical, thoracic, lumbar or sacral), often extending for multiple (transitional) segments (e.g., cervicothoracic, thoraco-lumbar or lumbosacral). The lumbar and sacral locations are the most common. Patients with plexiform neurofibromas extending to pre-lumbar and pre-sacral organs may present severe disease in specific organs including kidneys (Fig. 28A), rectum (Fig. 28B), bladder (Fig. 28B), ureters and internal sexual organs or, in some cases, in all intrapelvic or-

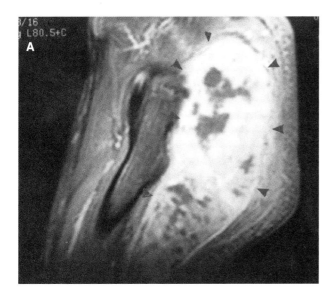

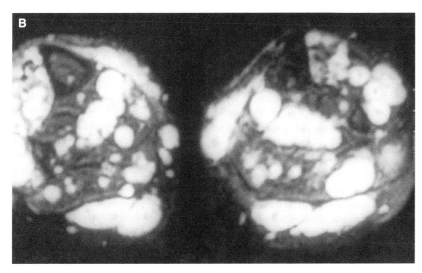

**Fig. 27.** Sagittal (**A**) and axial (**B**) T$_2$-weighted magnetic resonance images show a malignant peripheral nerve sheath tumour (MPNST) at the level of the gluteal region and the thighs. Note the distinct types of signal within the MPNST tumour (arrowheads): this patient had been operated of a benign neurofibroma one year before this scan was taken.

gans (Fig. 28C). MR imaging usually delineates the extension of the mass and, to a certain extent, its benign or malignant behaviour (Barkovich 2005, Bass et al. 1994, Tortori-Donati et al. 2005). The malignant appearance at MR usually takes the form of nerve enlargement(s) with loss of the external limits and variability of signals in the intratumoural regions (Tortori-Donati et al. 2005).

• **Genitourinary**

Plexiform neurofibromas of the genitourinary tract are relatively uncommon. Hypertrophy of the exter-

nal genitalia in NF1 can be observed either in children with precocious puberty or in individuals with plexiform neurofibromas affecting the clitoris and/or the labia majora or the penis (Fig. 29A), the prepucious (Fig. 29B) and the scrotum. The hypertrophy secondary to pubertal anomalies can be seen by age 8 to 10 years whereas plexiform neurofibromas involving the external genitalia can present at any age (even though these are more frequently recorded during childhood and adolescence). A common association is the genito-urinary tract involvement with the bladder and lower ureter being the organs

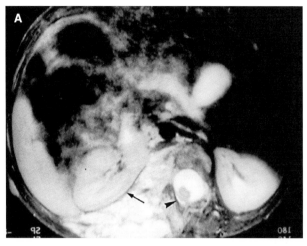

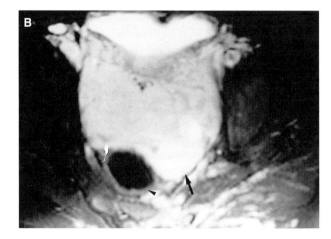

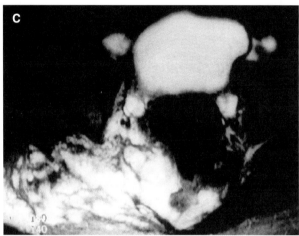

**Fig. 28.** (**A**) Plexiform neurofibroma that involves the right subcutaneous region and extends to the retroperitoneal zone displacing the right kidney (arrow) and eroding the adjacent vertebra (arrowhead); (**B**) axial $T_1$-weighted MRI enhanced with gadolinium shows a large plexiform neurofibroma that invades the posterior zone of the bladder (arrow) and displaces the rectum (arrowhead); (**C**) Coronal view of a generalised neurofibroma that involve all pelvic organs.

most often affected. Plexiform neurofibromas of the bladder have been recorded 3 times more frequently in boys than in girls (Deniz et al. 1966), whereas plexiform neurofibromas of the external genital are twice more frequent in girls. Plexiform neurofibromas of the bladder and genitalia can be found either in association or independently (Hess 1938, Mc Donnell 1936, Rink and Mitchell 1983, Sutphen et al. 1995). Solitary plexiform neurofibromas have been also reported in the external genitalia, such as the clitoris, the gland penis and penile shaft or scrotum (see mosaic segmental/NF1).

In females, clitoral hypertrophy is the most frequent presenting feature, but, neurofibromas of one or both labia majora have been described in about 25% of cases (Sutphen et al. 1995). Genitalia hyper-

trophy (with clitoral hypertrophy) is usually pathognomonic of NF1: to the best of our knowledge, only one case of NF2 and clitoral hypertrophy has been reported so far (Yüksel et al. 2003). Most patients with clitoral involvement and histological confirmation of the plexiform neurofibroma had a syndrome with abnormal hormonal stimulation that provoked intersexual problems (Labardini et al. 1968). Tumours can affect the uterus as well (Fig. 29C)

Most affected males have large tumours involving the genitourinary system (Kaefer et al. 1997, Ogawa and Watanabe 1986, Rink and Mitchell 1983). The penis affected by the plexiform neurofibroma often shows moderate overgrowth (Fig. 29A), but some cases have been described as elephantiatic, enlarged, giant or voluminous because of

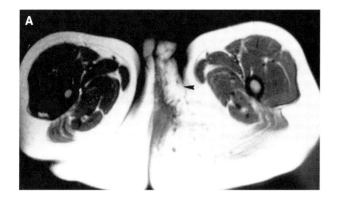

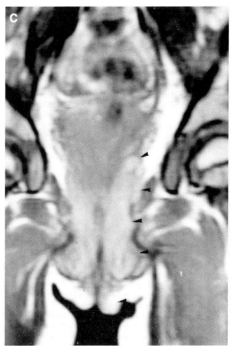

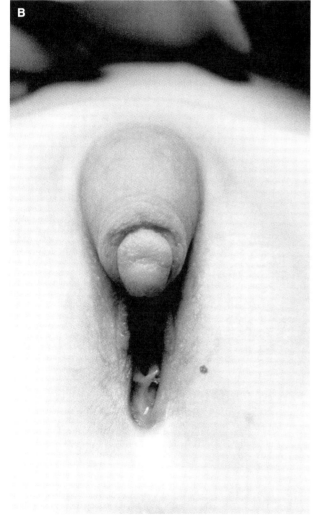

**Fig. 29.** (**A**) Axial T$_2$-weighted magnetic resonance images showing a plexiform neurofibroma of the left gluteal region that involves the perineum and the external genitals causing left half penial hypertrophy (arrowhead); (**B**) external appearance of the patent in (**B**); (**C**) coronal T$_2$-weighted MR images showing a plexiform neurofibroma in the left lower bladder wall and in the lower urinary and genital regions including the uterus (arrowheads).

the macrosomic phalon (Thomson et al. 1992). Asymmetric overgrowth with neurofibroma affecting only a half of the penis is a rare presentation (Fig. 29A).

Imaging (CT and MR) studies of the external genitalia and the pelvic region well delineate the location, size, extension, and in some cases the behaviour of the masses.

• **Tongue, mouth, larynx and pharynx**

These sites are infrequent but not so rare (Colledge 1930, Masip et al. 1996). Probably, a routine MR study of all NF1 patients would demonstrate a higher prevalence of lesions in these locations. The most frequent presenting signs (besides the chance of detecting a nodule or a mass in the tongue or the mouth at physical examination) include dyspnoea, dysphagia, and loss or change of voice. The laryngeal location is commonly supraglottal (Fig. 30A), although subglottal locations involving the trachea (Fig. 30B) have been reported as well. The tongue is usually affected on one side with initial displacement of the contralateral region; later on, if the lesion enlarges (Fig. 30C) it can occupy part of or the entire oral cavity causing (besides a cosmetic burden) dental displacement, chewing and swallowing difficulties and ultimately respiratory impairment. Imaging studies usually show well-defined masses, which displace but do not invade the soft tissues. Histologically, the tumours of this region are neurofibromas and/or plexiform neurofibromas; seldom plexiform ganglioneurofibromas (Chang-Lao 1977). Most of these tumours have a good prognosis after surgical excision (Chang-Lao 1977). Abnormal and rapid aggressive growth of the tongue needing subtotal excision and postsurgical radiotherapy has been reported in children (Chen et al. 1989).

• **Thorax**

About 3.5% of children with NF1 have tumours in the thorax, most often of the plexiform neurofibroma type (Fig. 31) (Schorry et al. 1997). Most commonly these are asymptomatic and remain undiscovered if an imaging study is not performed for other reasons. They usually originate from the chest wall, especially from the intercostal and sensory nerves and/or from the sympathetic fibers that innerve the pleura (Manoli et al. 1969). Tumours also can originate from the mediastinum, particularly in its posterior region. Malignant plexiform neurofibromas of the thorax frequently metastasise in contiguous areas.

• **Gastrointestinal**

Gastrointestinal involvement is not very common in patients with NF1, with three possible histological tumours: tumours of the stromal, neuronal hyperplasia, and ganglioneuromatosis (Hochberg et al. 1974, Artaza et al. 1999), being the stromal the most frequent (Fuller and Williams 1991). Stromal tumours include neurofibroma, malignant schwannoma, leiomyoma and leiomyosarcoma. Plexiform neurofibroma is pathognomonic of NF1 nerves (Fuller and Williams 1991). Plexiform neurofibromas of the gut have a characteristic "bag of worms" fell on palpation. They can be located anywhere between esophagus and anus. The jejunum, followed by stomach, ileon, duodene, colon and small intestine mesenterium are the most frequent location (Horcher et al. 1974). A segmental involvement of any intestinal tract may be found (Fig. 32) (Yang et al. 2002, Magro et al. 2000). Benign plexiform neurofibromas can be commonly removed. They may be voluminous (Fig. 32). Malignancy of these tumours occurs in less than 5% of cases (Allan 1985), and is clinically manifested as rapid growth of the abdominal mass with local pain. MRI studies of mesenteric plexiform neurofibromas show concentric images in $T_2$-weighted MRI (Yang et al. 2002).

## Malignant tumours

Malignant tumours occur more frequently in subjects with NF1 than in the general population (four times as often) (Ruggieri and Packer 2001). They are histological defined by a high cellular proliferation and dissemination to the rest of the body, and a high risk of recurrence after excision. In our series of NF1, approximately 10% of the tumours were malignant. Some of these tumours are common in childhood including rhabdomyosarcomas, neuroblastomas, Wilms tumours, and some types of leukaemias. In children with NF1, however, malignant transformation of plexiform neurofibromas (or MPNSTs ab initio) and other soft tissue tumours, including the rare angiosarcoma (usually associated with other types of malignancies or benign tumours in the same individual) (Lederman et al. 1987), are seen more often. Malignancies can occur some or many years after radiotherapy in the same or in a different area originally irradiated.

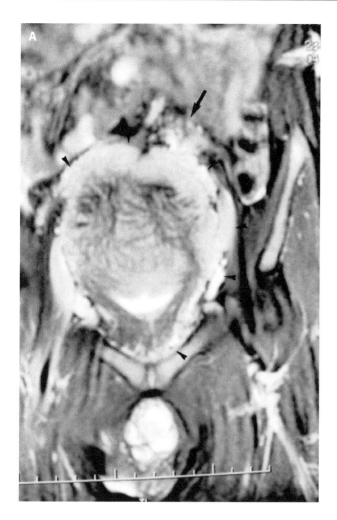

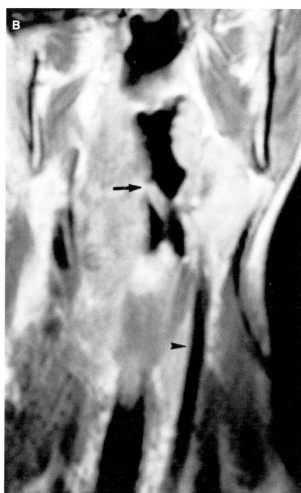

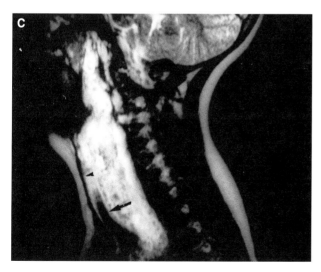

**Fig. 30.** Coronal (**A**) magnetic resonance images show a large plexiform neurofibroma involving the vocal cords; Coronal (**B**) and sagittal (**C**) magnetic resonance images show enhancement after gadolinium administration in a voluminous plexiform neurofibroma that displaces the trachea (arrow) and the esophagus (arrowhead) which is displaced to the left.

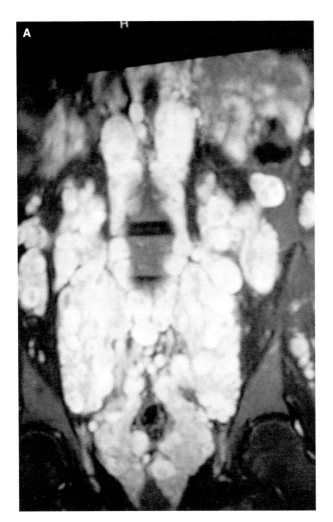

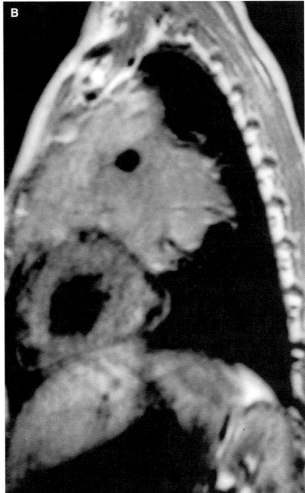

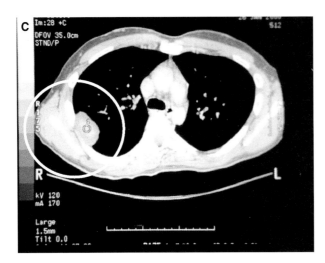

**Fig. 31.** (**A**) Coronal and (**B**) sagittal magnetic resonance images show a voluminous intrathoracic tumour; (**C**) axial CT scan study of the chest showing a plexifomr neurofibroma of the thoraci wall.

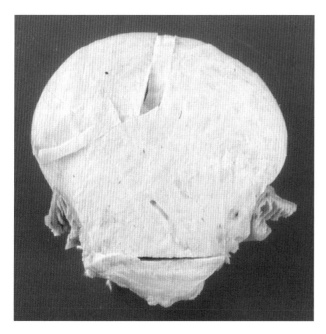

**Fig. 32.** Anatomic appearance of a large isolated neurofibroma of the peritoneum and ileal wall.

during surgery due to the frequent oscillations of blood pressure.

Children with NF1 are more predisposed to have myeloid malignant disease (particularly preleukaemic syndrome and myeloid proliferative syndromes) than the normal population (Luria et al. 1997, Shannon et al. 1994, Weiberg 1991). Approximately 10% of cases with myeloproliferative syndromes are associated with NF1 (Gadner and Hass 1992, Shannon et al. 1992). For the chance occurrence of juvenile chronic myeloyd leukaemia (JCML) and xanthogranulomas in NF1 see above (minor disease features). Most patients with JCML are associated with monosomy of chromosome 7 commonly leading to an acute myeloid leukaemia or to death caused by intercurrent complications (Gadner and Haas 1992, Shannon et al. 1992). For the pathogenic role played by the P[53] and neurofibromin proteins see below (pathogenesis and molecular genetics).

## Other tumours

Some other tumours are seldom associated to NF1 (Shorry et al. 1997) including *desmoplastic neurotropic tumours* (Gutzmer et al. 2000), malignant cutaneous or uveal *melanomas* (Duve and Rekoski 1994, Specht and Smith 1988), *adenocarcinoma of the pancreas* (Keller and Logan 1977), *tumours of the thyroid* (Anagnostouli et al. 2002) and the *parathyroid glands and penis* (Kouseff and Hoover 1999).

An association has been also reported between *glomus tumours* and NF1 (De Smet et al. 2002). The glomus tumour is usually solitary but multiple lesions have been observed in NF1 individuals: these are located most frequently under the fingernail (the glomus bodies are small, dermal, encapsulated arteriovenous anstomoses, commonest in the fingertips where they regulate peripheral blood flow and body temperature) and presents with pain, cold sensitivity and excruciating very localised tenderness. The treatment is local excision of the tumour (De Smet et al. 2002, Ferner et al. 2007).

Rhabdomyosarcomas represent 1% of tumours in NF1 patients (Mc Keen et al. 1978). These tumours may be located anywhere in the body with their higher frequency in the genitourinary tract. The presence of mesenchimal (striated muscle) tissue and epithelial glands may be seen in (benign and) malignant peripheral nerve tumours (Triton tumours) (Woodruff and Perino 1994).

Neuroblastoma has been also associated with NF1 (Witzleben and Landy 1974), running in NF1 families in some cases (Clausen et al. 1989).

Wilms tumours are associated to NF1 in approximately 1% of cases in the large series: 3/342 cases in the review of Stay and Vawter (1977).

The association pheochromocytoma/NF1 records similar figures (approximately 1%) (Hope and Mulvihill 1981). A familial presentation of pheochromocytomas in individuals with NF1 has been seldom reported (Ogawa et al. 1994): MRI studies in these families demonstrated abdominal pheochromocytomas in 100% of cases, some of them as small as 1 cm in diameter (Mc Grath et al. 1998). Treatment of this tumour is surgical, taking precautions

## Secondary malignazing tumours

The presence of a second malignant tumour in a patient with NF1 who had been treated for a primary (or simply for another) malignant tumour is often observed in adults (30% according to Sorensen et al. 1986), but it is rare in children (Maris et al. 1997). Second malignant tumours are most frequently seen in subjects who had been treated for malignant tumours with radiotherapy or chemotherapy some or many years before (Maris et al. 1997).

## Endocrinologic disorders

The most frequent endocrinologic disorders associated with NF1 are: 1) Stature at low percentiles; and 2) Precocious or delayed puberty. The statural problems in children with NF1 have been covered in the section on minor disease features. Here below we will describe the pubertal-related problems.

## Pubertal problems (precocious/delayed puberty)

Precocious puberty has been reported in 2% to 6% of patients with NF1 (Carmi et al. 1999, Cnossen et al. 1997, Habiby et al. 1994). Pascual-Castroviejo in his series of over than 600 NF1 patients (personal observation) recorded precocious puberty in females much more frequently than in males, and the same results have been often reported. However, there are NF1 series in which precocious puberty was recorded only in males or only in females. Precocious puberty associated with NF1 is most often associated with pathway glioma(s), followed by brainstem tumours, aqueduct stenosis with hydrocephalus, but it can be recorded as an isolated pathology in some cases as well. Tumours of the optic pathway and hypothalamus are the most frequent underlying lesions associated with precocious puberty (Listernick et al. 1995, North 1997).

*Puberty retardation* can be seen in patients with NF1 (Carmi et al. 1999, Friedman and Birch 1997), although it is most frequently observed after surgery or radiotherapy on the hypothalamus (Pascual-Castroviejo et al. 1988). The endocrinologists must control patients with NF1 and endocrinologic features.

## Neurological complications

The temptation to accept every neurological occurrence in a patient with NF1 as part of the NF1 phenotype should be avoided as the most recent population-based studies show that neurological involvement is less frequent than previously thought (Créange et al. 1999; Huson and Hughes 1994; Ruggieri 1999, 2007; Ruggieri et al. 2007).

## Cognitive impairment

The intellectual impairment in NF1 presents in childhood as learning difficulties and is relatively mild and non-progressive (North 1997, North et al. 1997). The majority of NF1 patients have a mean full-scale IQ in the low average range around 90 compared with age-matched or siblings controls. According to our experience only around 3% (8% in other literature series) of the children with NF1 may have true mental retardation (defined as an IQ <70). However, IQ of most patients with NF1 is between 68 and 100 and very few cases surpass 100 (Chapman et al. 1996). On psychological assessment patients with NF1 perform better on verbal than performance tests and have particular difficulties with visual/spatial orientation, attention span, short-term memory writing and calculation, most often leading to disruptive behaviour, poor reading and lack of organisation skills. The situation is further compounded by the high frequency (~40%) of impairment of gross and fine co-ordination in NF1. Cognitive impairment may improve with age but only early intervention can avoid functioning below one's own intellectual capabilities in adulthood. Few patients have severe mental retardation and autistic behaviour is very rare in patients with NF1 in contrast to what recorded in previous studies (Gilberg and Forsell 1984). Cognitive problems are present in as many as 30–60% of the NF1 children as compared to 6–9% of schoolchildren in the general population and are genetic in origin, albeit not fully penetrant, as shown in a mouse model of NF1 (Silva et al. 1997). However, no differences of intellectual level have been constated between patients with inherited NF1 and those caused by "the novo" mutations (Ferner et al. 1993). Academic difficulties are most common in patients with NF1 because of the many physical problems. However, the behaviour and psychosocial disorders have a higher contribution to the quality of life than the intellectual level (North et al. 2002). Several studies have examined the hypothesis that either the number of the high signal lesions typically seen on brain MRI in NF1 patients (discussed below), or the megalencephaly may account for cognitive deficits in NF1, but there has been no consensus of opinion among researchers (North et al. 1997, Ruggieri 2007).

All patients with NF1 should have full neuropsychological assessment before school entry. Those infants and toddlers presenting with delay in developmental milestones, hypotonia and incoordination require early referral for appropriate management (Ferner et al. 2007).

The role of the neurofibromin as the origin of learning difficulties of patients with NF1 is evident and it is constated in all tissues (Davies 2000, Gutman 2002). Experimental studies in animal models (mice) suggest that difficulties to learn associated with NF1 are caused by excessive activity of *Ras* that leads to an excessive increase of γ-aminobutitic acid (GABA) that increases the inhibition of the neuronal activity (Costa et al. 2002, Costa and Silva 2002). These findings suggest that strategies that decreased either *Ras* activity or GABA-mediated inhibition might be used to treat the learning deficits associated with NF1 (Costa et al. 2002). It has been also speculated on the possibility of subjects with macrocephaly (and underlying megalencephaly) and altered proportion of grey and white matter due to apoptosis disorder (Moore et al. 2000).

## Attention deficit hyperactivity disorder (ADHD) and psychiatric features

ADHS is a common feature (prevalence = 15–17%) in NF1 children. A prevalence of 50% (Eliason 1986) is more in accordance with our experience (Pascual-Castroviejo 2001a, b). Few papers on the psychiatric impact of NF1 on patients and their families do exist. Some type of mental disease has been found in a

33% of subjects (Samuelson and Samuelson 1989, Samuelson and Riccardi 1989). Low authoesteem, depression, ansiety and vegetative nervous system dysfunction are the main psychiatric manifestations.

## High signal lesions on T2-weighted MRI brain scan

High-signal-intensity lesions on $T_2$-weighted MRI images of the brain are a frequent finding in individuals with NF1 (Barkovich, 2005, Tortori-Donati et al. 2005). These lesions appear as well-circumscribed, poorly defined, round to ovular, non-enhancing hyperintense lesions that usually do not produce mass effect (Fig. 33). They are referred as "unidentified bright objects" (UBOs) and most commonly found in the basal ganglia (Fig. 33A), especially in the globus pallidus, internal capsule, thalamus, cerebellum, and brain-stem regions. They are generally asymmetrical (Fig. 33A) and can be diffuse (Fig. 33B) with cystic components (Fig. 33C) occurring by the age of 2–3 years in about 60–80% of children and young adults with NF1 who undergo MRI, but they tend to disappear in adulthood and are seldom observed in patients over 30 years of age. They do not cause overt neurological symptoms. Although they have been postulated to represent foci of abnormal neuronal dysplasia, hamartomas, abnormal myelination, low-grade gliomas or heterotopias their pathological correlation is yet unclarified. Pathologic analysis of limited tissue specimens have confirmed several of these histological findings in addition to intramyelinic areas of vacuolar or spongiotic changes with fluid-filled, coalesced or conflated vacuoles (from 5 to 100 um in diameter) (Di Paolo et al. 1995). Although these lesions are distinctive and associated with NF1, data on their specificity for NF1 are controversial; hence, there should be no reason to perform MR imaging to screen for the presence of UBOs, since they are (so for) neither a clinical diagnostic criterion nor have any prognostic or therapeutic significance. Nonetheless, when these high signal lesions are located in specific places (see above) are pathogenomonic of NF1 and their presence can assist the diagnosis of NF1, their radiological behaviour

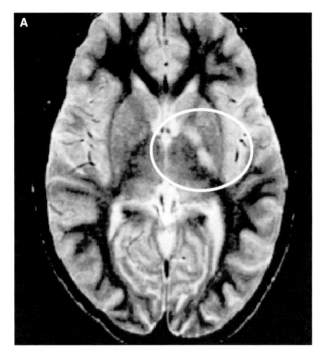

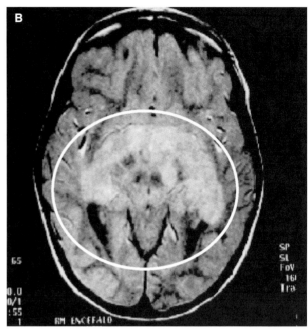

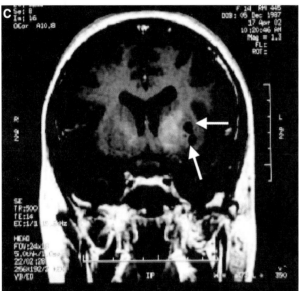

**Fig. 33.** Axial T$_2$-weighted (**A**, **B**) and coronal T$_1$-weighted (**C**) magnetic resonance images of the brain showing single ovular (**A**, circle) or large diffuse (**B**, circle) high signal lesions with a cystic component (**C**, white arrows) localised in the basal ganglia and thalami.

is heterogeneous and the lesions located in the brain stem, thalamus and cerebellar peduncles evolved into true masses in one study. These findings suggest the possibility that there may be different effects of neurofibromin on different CNS locations. Hypometabolism was demonstrated in UBOs in one study but not in others (reviewed in Barkovich 2005, and Tortori-Donati et al. 2005). UBOs must be distinguished from high signal lesions which displace neighbouring structures and are brighter on T$_2$-weighted images or more intensely enhance after intravenous injection of contrast medium as the latter may well be low grade gliomas and necessitate continuous monitoring as discussed below.

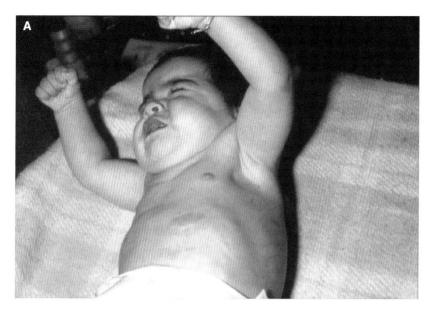

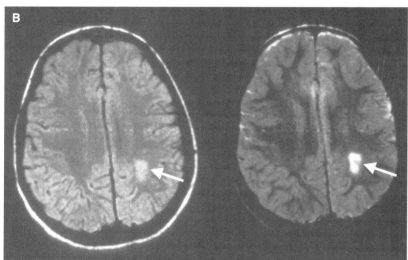

**Fig. 34.** (**A**) An infant with NF1 photographed during an episode of infantile spasms; (**B**) axial T$_2$-weighted magnetic resonance images of the brain in the same child show (atypical) high signal lesions in the subcortical white matter (arrows).

## Seizures and epilepsy

The occurrence of a seizure in a NF1 patient may well signal the existence of a recognised complication of NF1 such as tumours, hydrocephalus or cerebrovascular disease, but may, as for seizures in the general population, be idiopathic or a consequence of non-neurofibromatosis-related pathology (Kulkantrakon et al. 1999, Motte et al. 1993, Ruggieri et al. 2006a). There is an increasingly awareness that seizures may be relatively uncommon in NF1 and not fully explained by underlying CNS lesions (Ruggieri 1999, Ruggieri et al. 2007a). The prevalence of seizures according to our NF1 population based studies is around 3%, which is similar to the overall lifetime risk of epilepsy in the general population (2–5%). Other (hospital-based series) has recorded higher figures (Vivarelli et al. 2006). We could only record an increased prevalence of infantile spasms (Fig. 34A) in our NF1 populations as compared with the general population: interestingly these cases had atypical high signal lesions (Fig. 34B) (Ruggieri et al. 2007). Overall, the most common seizures patterns in NF1 are partial seizures followed by idiopathic generalised seizures and typical absences. Overall, the clinical course, causes, response to treatment and prognosis are similar to seizures in the general population (Ruggieri 1999).

## Headache

There is some suggestion in the literature and it is the experience of those who examine large num-

bers of NF1 patients that some individuals with NF1, especially children, may experience migraine headaches, characterised by either steady or throbbing cephalalgia, nausea or abdominal pain (Korf and Rubinstein 2005, Clementi et al. 1996). Abdominal pain can be accompanied by headache. These patients should have a careful physical and neurological examination to exclude any other underlying NF1 complication. By contrast, the use of neuroimaging or other diagnostic study will depend on the history, signs, and persistence of symptoms.

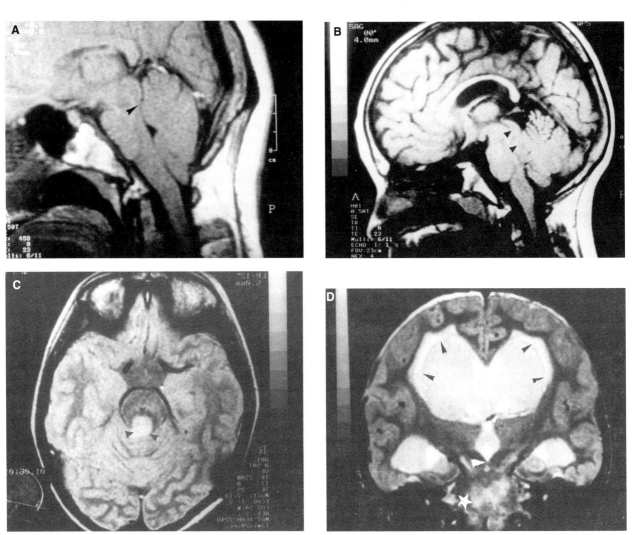

**Fig. 35.** (**A**) Sagittal T$_1$-weighted magnetic resonanced images show the obstruction of the aqueduct (arrowhead), a small fourth ventricle and a Chiari 1 malformation; (**B**) sagittal (**B**) and axial (**C**) T$_1$-weighted images show obstruction of the aqueduct (arrowheads) caused by an ependymal tumour; (**D**) Coronal T$_2$-weighted images show a diffuse benign brainstem tumour (asterisk), obstruction of the aqueduct (white arrowhead) and severe enlargement of the third and the lateral ventricles, with periventricular interstitial edema (black arrowhead).

## Aqueductal stenosis

Stenosis of the aqueduct is one of the most frequent complications of neurofibromatosis, following ADHD, tumours and skeletal disturbances which are observed more often. One of the problems in detecting the hydrocephalus by stenosis of the aqueduct in NF1 is the slow progression of the neurological disorder. MRI shows the obstruction of the aqueduct, better in the sagittal view (Fig. 35A, B). The incidence of aqueduct stenosis in patients with neurofibromatosis has been reported to be about 1 to 2.5% (Huson et al. 1988, North 1993). However, the prevalence of aqueduct stenosis associated with NF1 in our series of more than 600 patients was about 5% in patients aged below 16 years (Pascual-Castroviejo et al. 2001). The first described patient probably was made by Pennybacker (1940) in a young adult. Horwich et al. (1983) found 13 patients reported in the English literature adding 3 personal cases. Sajid and Copple (1968) described an adult with neurofibromatosis who began to have some difficulty in walking at 18 years of age; at 25 years he began to complain of poor vision and appeared depressed, his memory failing gradually; finally, he was diagnosed at 39 years of age when he was in a wheelchair unable to walk. Because of the progressive symptomatology, he was thought to have a white matter degenerative disease. His brother of 27 years of age began to present some symptoms of intracranial hypertension within the first years of age. The largest series reported to date is one of 11 patients in which 7 were under 14 years of age (Pou Serradell 1983). Although the neurological disease is commonly slowly progressive, cases with a short history of progression have been reported as well (Tashiro et al. 1975). Progressive aqueduct obstruction has been reported in monozygotic twins who also had optic glioma "in mirror image" (one with involvement of the left optic nerve and the other with the right optic nerve) (Pascual-Castroviejo et al. 1988). They presented hydrocephalus with a difference of 3 years (8 and 11 years of age respectively) (see Fig. 17). Aqueduct stenosis has been described in association with ependymal investment by glial conjuctival formations, with glial septum, and with growth of ependymal granulation tissue of polyplike type. Aqueduct stenosis

due to a pilocytic astrocitoma has been also found in patients with neurofibromatosis (Hosoda et al. 1986). Treatment of the hydrocephalus consists in the liberation of CSF by shunt or by ventriculostomy.

## Cortical malformation

Disorders of cortical development are relatively uncommon in NF1 and include hemimegalencephaly (Cusmai et al. 1990), cerebellar leptomeningeal heterotopias (Kato et al. 1995), occipital encephalocele (Bodhey and Gupta 2006), transmantle cortical dysplasia (Balestri et al. 2003), periventricular band of heterotopic gray matter (Balestri et al. 2003), pachygyria (Balestri et al. 2003), and unilateral (Balestri et al. 2003, Chang et al. 2006, Clark and Neville 2008) or bilateral polimicrogyria (Ruggieri et al. 2008).

## Spinal meningoceles

In NF1 these are predominantly lateral herniation of the theca in the thoracic or cervical regions (Barkovich 2005, Tortori-Donati 2005). Most are incidentally found during radiological investigations but neurological symptoms have been also reported.

## Neurofibromatous neuropathy

Rare cases of progressive sensorimotor peripheral neuropathy in association with NF1 have been reported: the neurological deficit was due to accumulation of multiple peripheral neurofibromas on the nerve roots (Ferner et al. 2000b, 2004). Electrophysiology can easily distinguish this occurrence from hereditary neuropathies (Huson and Hughes 1994). There are however few cases of NF1 patients with peroneal muscular atrophy due to an axonal form of hereditary motor and sensory neuropathy (neurofibromatous neuropathy) who present with foot drop and generalised weakness, mostly after intense exercise. Pathological findings reveals neurofibroma-like tissue in a subperineurial sleeve showing interlacing bundles of collagen fibrils with blood vessels surrounding a central core of more normal endoneurial tissue. The progression is slow (Ferner et al. 2004, 2007).

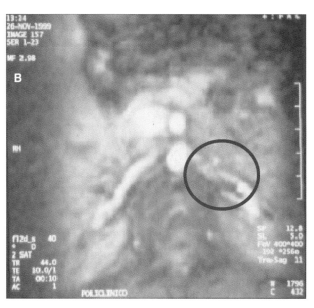

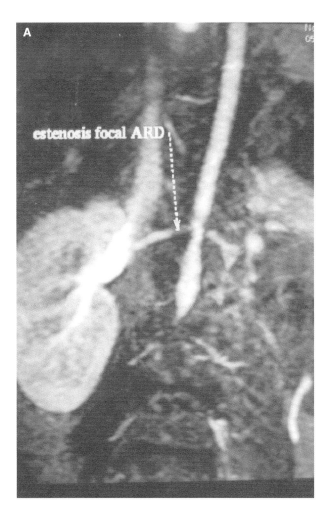

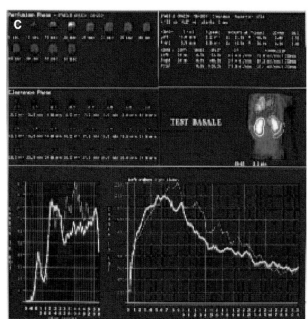

**Fig. 36.** Aortic magnetic resonance arteriography shows (**A**, arrowhead) right and (**B**, black circle) left renal artery stenosis; (**C**) the nuclear scintigraphy shows altered patterns in the dysplastic artery.

## Vascular, cardiac and peripheral arterial abnormalities

Vascular abnormalities are seen in about 9% of patients with NF1 (Brunner et al. 1974, Finman and Yakovac 1970). Clinical features caused by vascular abnormalities are often difficult to evaluate and hypertension secondary to progressive stenosis of renal arteries (Fig. 36) is the best-known disease (Kurien et al. 1997). Necropsic studies of patients with neurofibromatosis demonstrated some type of vascular lesions in an important number of patients (Salyer

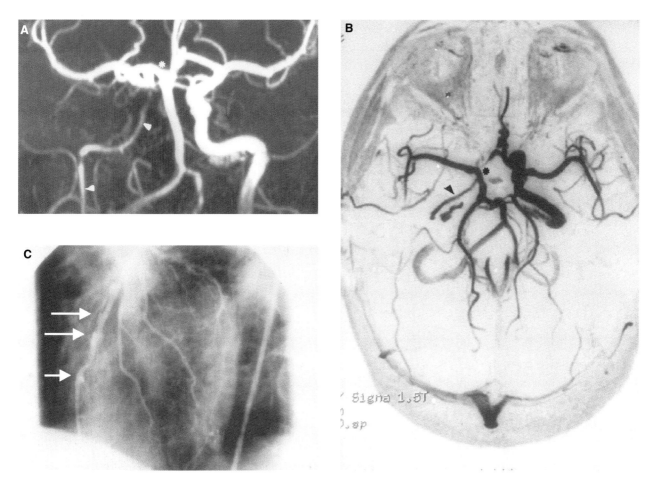

**Fig. 37.** Coronal (**A**) and axial (**B**) magnetic resonance arteriography images show severe right carotid artery hypoplasia (arrowheads), hyperplasia of the left carotid artery and of the posterior communicating artery (asterisk). Both anterior cerebral arteries originate from the left carotid artery; (**C**) heart arteriography shows multiple coronary artery aneurisms (arrows).

and Salyer 1974). Conventional arteriography and magnetic resonance arteriography (MRA) show various types of vascular abnormalities (Sabota et al. 1988): a) Occlusive lesions with moyamoya imaging. b) Isolated aneurysmatic dilatation. c) Aneurysmatic dilatation associated with arterial stenosis. Tomsick et al. (1976) described 14 patients with neurofibromatosis of all ages who had intracranial arterial occlusive disease, 9 of them showed moyamoya images. $T_2$-weighted MR enhanced with gadolinium can show the ischemic cerebral zones in patients of moyamoya-like syndrome (El-Koussy et al. 2002). Asymmetry with hypoplasia of one carotid or vertebral artery or their intracranial branches and vascular compensation with hypertrophy of the artery

of the other side can be seen (Fig. 37A). Intracranial aneurysms in NF1 has been detected in 5% of 39 patients (Fig. 37B) (Schievink et al. 2005) (prevalence in a control population is about 0%). Research papers that were published during the last years suggest that neurofibromin isoforms may play a role on the vessels formation (Norton et al. 1995, Stocker et al. 1995).

Cardiac malformations and lesions of middle or big size arteries are demonstrated in 1.6% (Friedman et al. 1997) to 5% (Riccardi 1987) of patients of any age with NF1. Cardiac disease is more frequent in adults, but it can be also seen in children and may appear as coronary obstruction (Halper and Factor 1984), multiple coronary artery aneurisms

(Fig. 37C) (Ruggieri et al. 2000), hypertrophic cardiomyopathy (Fitzpatrick and Emanuel 1988), sudden death (Halmiton et al. 2001), and spontaneous hemothorax with sudden death (Griffiths et al. 1998).

NF1 may present as a severe systemic vasculopathy (Lehrnebecher et al. 1994) involving any artery of the body. The veins rarely show changes. The association of renal stenosis and coarctation of the aorta in the thoracic and/or abdominal traject is very common (Greene et al. 1974, Tenschet et al. 1985). Angioplasty has been use to treatment of arterial stenosis, but recidive of the stenosis is common after a given time (Mallmann and Roth 1986).

## Ophthalmologic complications

Optic pathway gliomas aside, these include neurofibromas involving the eyelids or the orbit, sphenoid wing dysplasia often associated with disruption of the posterior and superior wall of the orbit leading in turn to herniation of the temporal lobe into the orbit and pulsating exophthalmos, idiopathic congenital ptosis [sometimes referred as part of the so-called Noonanoid phenotype (Noonan/NF1, see below NF1 related forms], congenital or acquired glaucoma (usually unilateral), choroidal hamartomas and diffuse or nodular enlargement of the corneal nerves (not pathogenomonic of the disease).

## Gastrointestinal problems

Carcinoid tumours, gastrointestinal neurofibromas, gangliocytic paraganglioma and ganglioneuromas have been, albeit rarely, reported in NF1. They may cause pain, dyspepsia, haematemesis and melaena, abdominal distension, discomfort or constipation, and they must be taken into high consideration when dealing with **gastrointestinal problems** in NF1 patient (Huson and Ruggieri 2006, Ruggieri 1999, Ruggieri and Huson 1999). Carcinoid tumours have a predilection for the duodenum where they give rise to facial flushing, diarrhoea, right sided cardiac lesions, facial telangiectasias, and bronchocostriction. The prognosis for this gut associated tumours is however good (Ferner et al. 2007).

## Pregnancy

Information of NF1 and pregnancy is limited. In a series of 105 pregnants, 60% showed increase of the subcutaneous neurofibromas and increase of the size of the previously existing neurofibromas in 52% (Dugoff and Sujansky 1996). Despite the many complications that patients with NF1 can show, such as scoliosis, pelvic neurofibromas, delivery by caesarean surgery is performed with similar frequency as in women without NF1 (Dugoff and Sujansky 1996). Pregnancy of women with NF1 has been associated with thrombosis of the renal artery, renovascular hypertension (Pilmore et al. 1997, Hagymasi et al. 1998) or other low frequent complications in few cases.

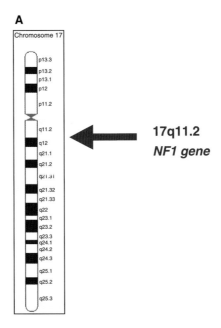

Fig. 38. (**A**) Chromosomal location of the NF1 gene; (**B**) exon sequence and organisation of the *NF1* gene. Exons are represented by boxes and the number above each is the exon size in base pairs. Alternatively spliced exons are distinguished by blue boxes. Introns are represented by broken lines and are to scale with the exception of intron 27b, which is over 60 kb in length. The green box represents the core promotor (–341bp to –261 bp). CPG denotes CPG island of the gone (–731 to 261bp); CSD, cysteine/serine-rich domain (Fahsold et al. 2000) as shown in yellow; GRD, GAP-related domain as shown in orange. Sec 14p; region of homology to a liqid-binding domain of the S. Cerevisiae phosphatidylinositol transfer protein *Sec 14p* (Aravind et al. 1999), *AK3;* adenylate kinase 3 pseudogene. The three embedded genes (*OMG, EV120 EVl2a*) are shown in bold, with the arrow indicating the direction of transcription.

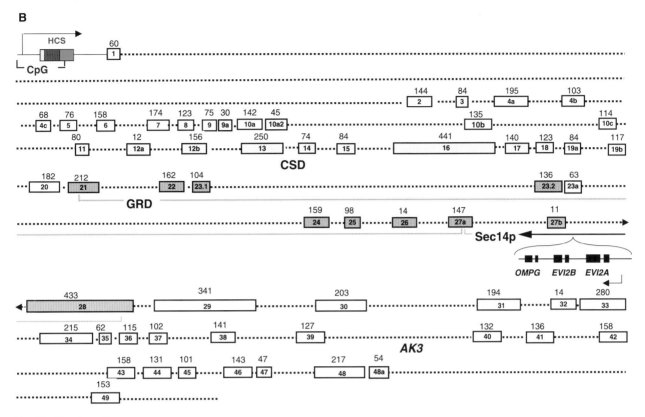

**Fig. 38.** (Continued)

## Pathogenesis & molecular genetics

### The *NF1* gene

The *NF1* gene is located at 17q11.2, spans 280 kb of genomic DNA, and contains 61 exons, that encodes a 12 kb mRNA transcript (Fig. 38A–C) (Viskochil 1998). The gene contains several large introns with introns 1 and 27b, both larger than 60 kb. Three genes (*EVI2A*, *EVI2B* and *OMG)* are located within intron 27b, each of which comprises two exons. *EVI2A* is a small gene, encoding a 232 amino acid polypeptide, which is expressed in the brain and bone marrow. The sequences of *EVI2A* are predicted to be a transmembrane protein. The *EVI2B* gene encodes a 448 amino acid protein; this is expressed exclusively in the bone marrow. The *OMG* gene encodes a 416 amino acid cell adhesion protein that is expressed primarily in oligodendrocytes. All three genes are transcribed in the opposite orientation to the *NF1* gene (Fig. 39). The role of these genes individually, or together in regulating *NF1* gene expression is however not known.

The *NF1* gene promoter is located within a CpG island and exhibits a high degree of sequence conservation with the *NF1* gene present in several organisms (Hajra et al. 1994). No pathogenic mutations of the *NF1* promoter have been reported (Horan et al. 2004, Osborn et al. 2001). Hypermethylation of the promoter may not be a common event in the inactivation of the normal *NF1* allele in NF1-related tumours (Luijten et al. 2000a, Horan et al. 2000). The 3′ untranslated region (UTR) of the human *NF1* gene is 3.5 kb in length and also demonstrates a high level of sequence conservation indicating that it may be functionally important either for mRNA stability or for controlling translational efficiency.

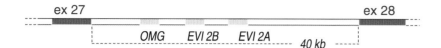

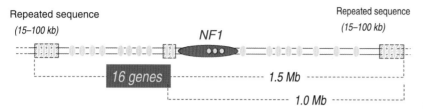

**Fig. 39.** Embedded introns and exons in the *NF1* gene.

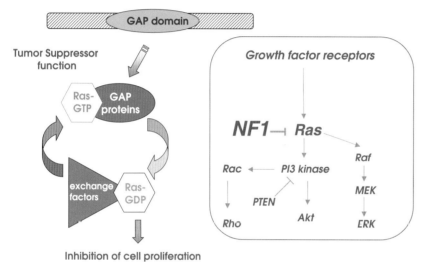

**Fig. 40.** The RAS-activating cycle and neurofibromin.

## Neurofibromin: the *NF1* gene product

Neurofibromin is a ubiquitously expressed large (2818 amino acid) protein, although usually only present at low level in most tissues (Wallace et al. 1990). The highest level of neurofibromin expression is found in the central nervous system, where it appears in association with tubulin (Gregory et al. 1993).

Neurofibromin exhibits structural and amino acid sequence similarity to a large family of evolutionarily conserved proteins, the mammalian GTPase activating protein (GAP)-related proteins (Fig. 40) (Xu et al. 1990a, b). The most highly conserved region of neurofibromin is the NF1 GAP-related domain (GRD), which is encoded by exons 21–27a. The

functional role of the NF1-GRD is stimulation of the intrinsic GTPase activity of GTP-bound Ras proteins (GAP activity). This GAP activity down-regulates activated Ras proteins, and loss of functional neurofibromin in different cell types leads to a loss of growth control in these cells. Activation of Ras is achieved via GTP-binding and the subsequent conformational change involved in the protein. The activating conversion from inactive GDP-bound Ras to active GTP-bound form is controlled by guanine nucleotide exchange factors. Conversely, the inactivating GTP to GDP conversion occurs through stimulation of the Ras GTPase activity by a variety of GTPase activating proteins (GAPs). The NF1-GRD stimulates this intrinsic GTPase activity of Ras by a factor greater than 1000-fold (Xu et al.

1990a, b). Ras proteins are involved in complex signal transduction pathways, and moderate cellular response to different factors, including mitogens and differentiation factors. The three main Ras effectors are PI3-K (phosphatidylinositol 3 kinase), RAL-GEFs and Raf kinase. Perhaps the best described signal transduction pathway, Raf activates a series of kinases in cascade in the MAPK kinase pathway leading to cell proliferation or differentiation. Thus, inactivation of neurofibromin might be predicted to lead to increased Ras signalling and cell proliferation. The *NF1* gene is therefore considered to function as tumour suppressor gene (Harber and Harlow 1997). In keeping with this postulate, studies in NF1-related malignant peripheral nerve sheath tumours (MPNSTs) have shown that lack of (or reduced) neurofibromin correlated with increased levels of activated Ras-GTP (Basu et al. 1992, deClue et al. 1992, Guha et al. 1996). In a murine NF1 model, introduction of *Nf1*-GRD in *Nf1*$^{-/-}$ cells

has also been shown to be sufficient to restore normal cell growth *in vitro* and *in vivo*, through direct interaction with Ras (Hiatt et al. 2001).

The role of activated Ras proteins in overall cell signalling process is complex (Figs. 40, 41). Activated Ras sends signals along the Raf-mitogen-activated protein (MAP) kinase pathway thereby promoting cellular proliferation. Activated Ras also sends signals through the PI3 kinase and PKB (protein kinase B, also known as Akt) complexes and nuclear factor-kappaB (NF-kappaB) thereby exerting an anti-apoptotic influence. Indeed the activation of the Ras pathway has been detected in many different human tumour types. In some NF1-deficient cells and tumours, the inappropriate activation of these downstream effectors has also been reported (Cichowski and Jacks 2001).

It was recently reported that the mTOR pathway is tightly regulated in neurofibromas (Fig. 41). In the absence of growth factors mTOR is activated

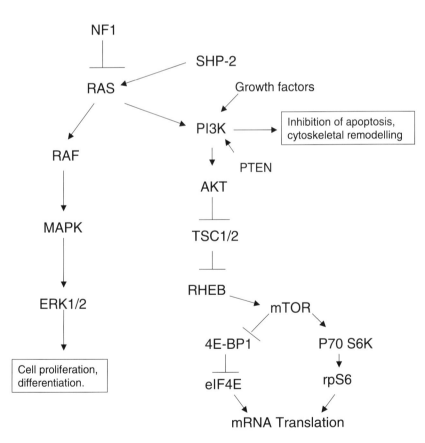

**Fig. 41.** Mammalian Target for Rapamycin (**mTOR**) mediates a signalling pathway that couples aminoacid availability to S6 kinase (S6K) activation, translational initiation and cell growth. mTOR is constitutively activated in NF1-deficient primary cells. Aberrant activation of Ras and PI3 kinase inactivate the TSC1/2 gene products via AKT. Cells derived from NF1 tumours exhibit a constitutive phosphorylation of TSC1/2 products.

in both NF1 tumours and in NF1-deficient primary cells (Johannessen et al. 2005, Dasgupta et al. 2005). In neurofibromin deficient cells, an aberrant activation of p21 as leads to the activation of PI3K, which phosphorylates protein kinase B (AKT or PKB). This phosphorylated protein kinase in turn phosphorylates and inactivates the TSC1-TSC2 complex. Inhibition of the TSC1-TSC2 complex leads to the activation of the small GAP protein Rheb (Ras homolog enriched in brain) and consequently to the activation of the kinase serine/threoninem TOR (mammalian target of rapamycin). The mTOR pathway is involved in regulating a number of key cellular activities such as cell growth, apoptosis and proliferation and it is also involved in the integration of a number of extracellular and intracellular signals into the control of these various processes (Wullschleger et al. 2006). This is also evolutionarily conserved. Cell lines derived from NF1-related tumours have been shown to be highly sensitive to the mTOR inhibitor rapamycin (Dasgupta et al. 2005, Johannessen et al. 2005).

Ras activity has also been suggested to be associated with NF1-related learning deficiencies, and suspected of leading to impairment in long-term potentiation caused due to increased GABA-mediated inhibition (Costa et al. 2002)

Ras-GAP is the only domain of neurofibromin for which a definite function has been ascribed. However, as the Ras-GAP domain comprises only 10% of the neurofibromin, we can assume that additional protein domains of neurofibromin may well be implicated in other disease related features. While the absence of neurofibromin and the concomitant elevation in activated Ras-GTP levels may explain tumour formation, it fails to account for many of the other NF1-associated clinical features, such as short stature and scoliosis.

Structural and biochemical data demonstrate that the main function of the GAP domain is the formation of an "arginine finger" that inserts into the active site of the Ras protein where it appears to stabilise the transition state of the GTPase reaction (Ahmadian et al. 1997, Scheffzek et al. 1999).

A second putative functional domain has been proposed upstream of the GRD, this was identified when a possible mutational hotspot was found involving exons 11–17 (Fahsold et al. 2000). The region of the protein encompasses a cysteine/serine-rich domain, with three potential cAMP-dependant protein kinase recognition sites, that are subject to phosphorylation by protein kinase, and also contains three cysteine pairs indicative of ATP binding (Izawa et al. 1996). Interestingly, mutations in the *Drosophila* neurofibromin orthologue were shown to inhibit both the cAMP (cyclic adenosine monophosphate) and protein kinase-signalling pathway, through regulation of adenylyl cyclase (AC), a process that may potentially be involved in learning deficits (Guo et al. 1997, 2000; The et al. 1997). In mammalian neurones, neurofibromin has been shown to positively regulate intracellular cAMP levels (Tong et al. 2002), which are probably involved in modulating cell growth and differentiation in the brain. Neurofibromin has also been implicated in the regulation of cAMP generation in astrocytes (Dasgupta and Gutmann 2003).

A third potential lipid-binding domain, Sec-14, located immediately adjacent to GRD domain, has recently been reported (D'Angelo et al. 2006). This represents a novel structural bipartite domain that is able to bind phospholipids. The tandem arrangement of GRD-Sec14 is also evolutionarily conserved.

Amino acid residues, which lie N-terminal to the GRD domain, are required for the neurofibromin ubiquitin-mediated proteolysis (Cichowski et al. 2003). These authors have shown that the ubiquitin-proteasome pathway dynamically regulatesneurofibromin.

While neurofibromin clearly down regulates Ras activity, co-localisation of neurofibromin and Ras has never been demonstrated. Neurofibromin has also been found to be involved with other cytoskeletal structures, including the kinesin-1 containing complex (Hakami et al. 2002), and the F-actin cytoskeleton (Li et al. 2001). Neurofibromin is found in association with microtubules (Gregory et al. 1993), with syndecan (Hsueh et al. 2001) and with caveolin (Boyanapalli et al. 2006). Analysis of neurofibromin primary structure identified four potential caveolin binding domains and in NF1 patients, missense mutations have been found to occur with high frequency in at least 3 of the 4 putative domains. It is suggested therefore that neurofibromin and caveolin co-ordinately regulate cell growth and differentiation (Boyanapalli et al. 2006).

## Alternative splicing

The *NF1* gene has four exons alternatively spliced: exons 9a, 10a-2, 23a and 48a and in each case the reading frame is not altered when these exonic sequences are included. The various *NF1* transcripts are often found to be differentially expressed in different tissues in normal individuals for example, the type II *NF1* transcript, which contains the alternatively spliced exon 23a, an inframe insertion of 63 nucleotides in the GAP-related domain (GRD) of neurofibromin is ubiquitously expressed (Suzuki et al. 1991). Andersen et al. reported that this type II *NF1* transcript, is conserved across several species (Andersen et al. 1993). Type II neurofibromin has reduced GAP activity but exhibits an increased affinity for Ras in comparison to a construct, which lacks the exon 23a. Most tissues seem to express an equal amount of both transcripts with and without exon 23a. Intriguingly, Costa et al. have produced mice that do not express exon 23a and these animals demonstrate a learning disability (Costa et al. 2001). Another alternatively spliced 3′ALT transcript exon (48a) which has an in-frame insertion of 54 nucleotides is abundantly expressed in muscle (Gutmann et al. 1993) while the 5′ALT2 transcript, with an in-frame insertion of 30 bp (forming exon 9a) between exons 9 and 10a, is highly expressed in the CNS (Danglot et al. 1995). An alternative splice product of the N-terminus of the *NF1* gene termed NF1-10a-2, comprises 45 bp inserted between exon 10a and 10b. The expression of this form was considerably lower than the wild type RNA in all human primary and tumour cells examined (Kaufmann et al. 2002).

A number of additional alternative transcripts have been reported, these include variants which show deletions of exons 4b, 29, 30, 33, 37, 43 and 45 (NF1-ΔE4b, NF1-ΔE29, NF1-ΔE30, NF1-ΔE29/30, NF1-ΔE33, NF1-ΔE37, NF1-Δ43, NF1-ΔE45) and an insertion of 31 bp between exons 4a and 4b (Park et al. 1998, Ars et al. 2000, Thomson et al.

2002, Vandenbroucke et al. 2002). Vandenbroucke et al. (2002) have postulated that quantitative differences between these variants might contribute to the phenotypic variability often observed in NF1 patients.

## Germline mutations of the *NF1* gene

The *NF1* gene exhibits one of the highest mutation rates reported in any human disorder, with approximately 1/10,000 mutation per gametes per generation and this is underlined by the finding that half of all patient represents *de novo* cases (Huson et al. 1989b, Li et al. 1995). The germline mutational spectrum of the *NF1* gene associated with disease expression in NF1 patients is well characterised. To-date more than 900 different germline mutations have been identified (http://www.hgmd.org) and the majority (~80%) of these are predicted to produce truncating lesions. No apparent clustering of mutations occurs within the *NF1* gene (Fahsold et al. 2000, Ars et al. 2000a, Messiaen et al. 2000, Castle et al. 2003, Upadhyaya et al. 2004). Missense mutations represent 5–10% of all micro-lesions (Fahsold et al. 2000), and it is often difficult to predict the pathogenecity of these mutations in the absence of functional *in vitro* tests. About 30% of all *NF1* mutations are predicted to cause alterations to mRNA splicing (Ars et al. 2000b) and a number of *NF1* nonsense mutations have also been demonstrated to result in exon skipping (Hoffmeyer et al. 1998). More recently, coding region mutations that disrupt exonic splicing enhancer elements have also been recognised and these may underlie the observed exon skipping sometimes associated with the presence of nonsense and missense mutations in the *NF1* gene (Zatkova et al. 2004). No mutations have been detected in the three embedded genes in NF1 patients.

About 5% of NF1 patients exhibit large 1.4 Mb genomic deletions that remove the entire *NF1* gene, in addition to as many as 17 flanking genes (Lopez-Correa et al. 2001). This common 1.4 Mb microdeletion is flanked by paralogous sequences (NF1-REPs), and these facilitate unequal homologous recombination between the two strands (Dorschner et al. 2000).

A 1.2 Mb deletion (Kehrer-Sawatzki et al. 2003) has also been reported and is mediated by recombination between *SVZ2* gene and its pseudogene *SVZ2*. The *SVZ2* gene is completely deleted in patients with 1.4 Mb deletion but is disrupted in patients with 1.2 Mb deletion.

Given the high mutation rate for the *NF1* gene, rare cases of multiple unrelated *NF1* mutations in the same NF1 family are to be expected and indeed we identified three separate *de novo* mutations of the *NF1* gene (a 1.5 Mb deletion, a nonsense mutation and a frameshift mutation) in a Portuguese NF1 family (Upadhyaya et al. 2003).

The identification and characterisation of mutations in the *NF1* gene has been a challenging task mainly due to the large size of the gene, the absence of any obvious mutational clustering and the wide diversity of mutation type found that disrupt the gene.

New *NF1* mutations, especially single base pair alterations tend to exhibit a bias towards paternal origin (Jadayel et al. 1990, Stephens et al. 1992, Upadhyaya et al. 1994, 1998), whereas large gene deletions are often of maternal origin (Lazaro et al. 1996, Ainsworth et al. 1997, Updhyaya et al. 1998).

The large size of the *NF1* gene does not itself however account for the observed high mutation rate (Upadhyaya et al. 1994, Rodenhiser et al. 1997) and several explanations have been proposed. The identification of numerous *NF1* pseudogene sequences located on several autosomes have been implicated as a mutational "reservoir" for the functional *NF1* gene (Marchuck et al. 1991), however, this postulate has yet to be validated. Another suggestion is the post-zygotic occurrence of disease-causing somatic mutations in patients who are clinically unaffected (Zlotogora 1993). These somatic mosaic individuals then produce mutational gametes and these result in fully affected offspring.

## NF1 Pseudogenes

Fluorescence *in situ* hybridisation (FISH) analysis using *NF1* cDNA sequences as probes identified a number of partial long processes pseudogenes on chromosomes 2q12-13, 12q11, 14p11-q11, 15q11.2, 18p11.2, 21p11-q11 and 22p11-q11 (Marchuk et al. 1991, Legius et al. 1992, Gasparini et al. 1993, Suzuki et al. 1994, Purandare et al. 1995, Hulsebos et al. 1996, Kehrer-Sawatzki et al. 1997, Barber et al. 1998, Luijten et al. 2000b, c, Fantes et al. 2002). The majority of pseudogene sequences display greater than 90% homology to the *NF1* sequence, although they also contain many nucleotide substitutions, insertions and deletions. Both chromosomes 15 and 22 exhibit more than one *NF1* homologous sequence (Legius et al. 1992, Gasparini et al. 1993). Luijten et al. (2001) postulated that some pseudogenes probably arose via sequential inter-chromosomal transposition events. In this manner, 640 kb sequence on 2q11 was first duplicated and then subsequently transposed to 14q11. The same mechanism, this time employing the 14q11 *NF1* pseudogene sequence as a template, gave rise to an *NF1* pseudogene at locus 22q11 (Luijten et al. 2001).

While none of the partial *NF1* pseudogene sequences would appear to encode a functional protein, it has been suggested that these sequences could act as a potential *NF1* mutational reservoir, thereby serving to increase the *NF1* mutation rate by inter-chromosomal gene conversion (Marchuk et al. 1992). However, as very few disease-causing *NF1* gene mutations appear to have their equivalents complete sequence in any identified pseudogene, this suggests that inter-chromosomal gene conversion makes only a very limited contribution to the *NF1* mutation rate (Luijten et al. 2001).

A cytogenetic study in 2002 reported a direct tandem duplication of the entire *NF1* gene at locus 17q11.2 as assessed by high-resolution FISH on stretched chromosomes and DNA fibres (Gervasini et al. 2002). If validated, this *NF1*-related sequence would be the first to be located on chromosome 17 and would represent the most complete copy of the *NF1* gene to date, as it lacked only exon 22. This putative new pseudogene, resulting from intrachromosomal duplication, claimed to shed new light on the contribution of gene conversion to the observed high mutation rate of the *NF1* gene. Unfortunately, other groups have so far failed to reproduce such findings despite extensive cytogenetic and molecular analysis (Kehrer-Sawatzki et al. 2002, 2003; De

Raedt et al. 2004). This *NF1* duplication, if it was confirmed would be of the utmost importance for future mutation detection, because PCR (polymerase Chain Reaction) primers should be designed to amplify only the true *NF1* gene. Similarly, it might warrant the re-examination of all mutations.

The use of *NF1* mRNA might circumvent the problem created by pseudogenes. Yu et al. (2005) investigated the possibility of expression from *NF1* pseudogenes. They demonstrated transcription of *NF1* pseudogenes located on chromosome 2, 15 and 21. This finding may complicate functional *NF1* mutational analysis at mRNA level and also the molecular diagnosis for NF1.

## Mosaicism

Evidence for germline mosaicism in an NF1 family has been demonstrated. Molecular studies in an *NF1* family with two affected siblings, but in whom neither parent was apparently affected, revealed that both affected children had the same 12 kb deletion involving the *NF1* gene on their paternally derived chromosome 17. Although this deletion was not identifiable in DNA from their father's blood, examination of his sperm DNA demonstrated that some 10% of his sperm carried the same large *NF1* deletion (Lazaro et al. 1994). Mosaicism for large deletions has been demonstrated in a number of typical NF1 patients using lymphocyte fluorescent *in situ* hybridisation (FISH) analysis (Wu et al. 1997). Patients with segmental NF1 manifest NF1 features that are confined to a particular part of the body. It is believed that the molecular basis of this condition may be the somatic mutation of the *NF1* gene in an early stage of fetal development (Ruggieri and Huson, 1999, 2001; Tinschert et al. 2000). Evidence of gonosomal mosaicism for the *NF1* gene in a segmental patient has recently been reported (Consoli et al. 2005). In this study they analysed DNA from a girl with generalised NF1, and her mother who has segmental NF1. A nonsense mutation (R1947X) was identified in the daughter's lymphocyte DNA. When skin tissue from the affected region of the mother was analysed, the same mutation was found in 20% of keratinocytes clones from the affected region and 9% of the fibroblasts from the affected region.

Twenty patients with sporadic NF1 in association with large microdeletions were found to exhibit an unexpected high frequency of somatic mosaicism (8/20 [40%]). This proportion of mosaic deletions is much higher than previously anticipated (Kehrer-Sawatzki et al. 2004). None of the eight patients with mosaic deletions exhibited the mental retardation and facial dysmorphism usually associated with NF1 microdeletions. In patients with mosaicism, the proportion of cells with the deletion was 91%–100% in peripheral leukocytes but was much lower (51%–80%) in buccal smears or peripheral skin fibroblasts. Therefore, the analysis of other tissues than blood is recommended, to exclude mosaicism with normal cells in patients with *NF1* microdeletions. In this study, a second major type of *NF1* microdeletion, which spans 1.2 Mb and affects 13 genes was identified. This type II deletion was found in 8 (38%) of 21 patients and is mediated by recombination between the *SVZ2* gene and its pseudogene. The *SVZ2* gene, which is completely deleted in patients with type I *NF1* microdeletions (1.5 Mb) and is disrupted in deletions of type II (1.2 Mb), is highly expressed in brain structures associated with learning and memory.

## *NF1* gene somatic mutations

Characterised somatic microlesions of the *NF1* gene have so far been reported in DNA from less than 100 NF1-associated tumours (Sawada et al. 1996; Serra et al. 1997, 2000, 2001a; Eisenbarth et al. 2000; John et al. 2000; Wiest et al. 2003; Upadhyaya et al. 2004). Similar somatic *NF1* gene lesions have also been identified in a number of tumour types that are not usually associated with NF1 patients (Li et al. 1992) It is however unclear, how such *NF1* gene mutations may contribute to the formation of tumours either in NF1 patients associated or in sporadic tumours not associated with NF1 (Li et al. 2002). Mitotic recombination is one of the mechanisms for NF1 tumour development (Serra et al.

2001b). Further information on the overall somatic mutational spectrum of the *NF1* gene that may be present in many different tumours could help to identify additional functional domains of neurofibromin. Such knowledge would also improve our currently inadequate understanding of genotype/phenotype relationships in NF1. A direct comparison of the spectrum of germline and somatic *NF1* mutations in tumours may help to elucidate whether the nature and location of the original *NF1* germline mutations has some determination on the type and location of the "second hit" of the *NF1* gene as has been reported in the *APC* gene involved in familial adenomatous polyposis (Lamlum et al. 1999).

Recently, DeRaedt et al. (2006) have demonstrated that in NF1 patients with large constitutional gene deletion, the somatic mutation in the neurofibroma derived from these patients is usually a small-scale mutation. Our findings on MPNST mutation analysis indicates that large genomic deletions represent the predominant 'second hits' in these tumours, the underlying germline mutations are mainly point mutations or small (<20 bp) deletions and insertions (Upadhyaya et al. 2007).

### *NF1* as a tumour suppressor gene

Extensive genetic and biochemical evidence indicates that the *NF1* gene functions as a tumour suppressor (Fig. 42) (Xu et al. 1992, Basu et al. 1992, Legius et al. 1993, Colman et al. 1995, Cappione et al. 1997). Molecular analysis of DNA from multiple benign neurofibromas isolated from an individual NF1 patient have demonstrated a variety of different somatic mutations, indicating that the process involved in the 'second hit' appears to be an independent molecular event in each neurofibroma (Serra et al. 1997, 2000; Upadhyaya et al. 2004). The somatic mutational spectrum of the *NF1* gene may thus have an important implication in the variable clinical expression often observed in NF1. It follows that the factors, which influence somatic mutation rates may be considered, at least in some sense as potential modifiers of NF1 (Wiest et al. 2003).

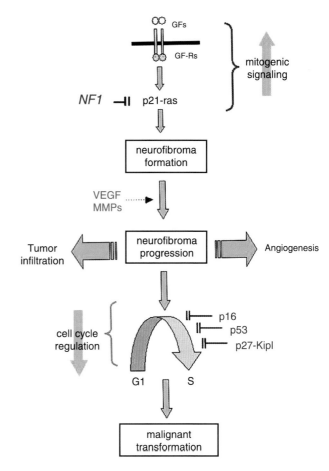

**Fig. 42.** Tumour suppressor sequence in the neurofibromin cascade (adapted from Packor and Rosser 2002).

Schwann cells are now accepted as being the key cellular components involved in dermal NF1 tumours, in which these cells constitute up to 80% of the neurofibroma tissue (Peltonen et al. 1988). Two genetically different Schwann cell populations, $NF1^{+/-}$ and $NF1^{-/-}$, have also been identified in tumours (Rosenbaum et al. 2000, Serra et al. 2000), it would appear that it is only Schwann cells which contain the somatic mutations in neurofibroma tissue (Serra et al. 2000).

A variety of different genetic mechanisms may result in the inactivation of the normal wild-type *NF1* allele in an NF1-associated tumour; these involve large or small DNA rearrangements, single base pair changes, insertions and deletions, genomic instability either at the nucleotide or chromosomal level or hyper-methylation of the gene promoter region. The acquisition of microsatellite instability may be a relatively late event in NF1-related malignancy, it is however comparatively infrequent in NF1 tumourigenesis (Upadhyaya et al. 2004).

It is still unclear whether cells that are only heterozygous for mutations at the *NF1* locus actually contribute to tumour formation, or whether tumour development is only initiated in those cells in which both *NF1* alleles are inactivated. Mutations of the wild-type allele are most likely to occur during cell division, however, adult nerve sheath cells, the obvious candidate cell for formation of neurofibromas, only show very low level of cell division. Whether the *NF1* somatic mutation is acquired at much earlier developmental stage, with another subsequent event required stimulating the growth of the cell and development of the tumour is unknown. Furthermore, the number of non-allelic gene lesions (subsequent to the initial *NF1* mutations), that are required for development of neurofibromas or for their progression to MPNSTs is also unclear. Although dermal neurofibromas never become malignant, second hit mutations at the *NF1* locus have been detected in these benign tumours. The nature of the other nongenetic factors that may also be involved in NF1 tumourigenesis is yet to be resolved. Local trauma and hormonal changes have both been suggested to be implicated in the development of neurofibromatosis in NF1 patients (Riccardi 1992). Interestingly related defects in mast cells and fibroblasts have been observed during the wound healing studies in *Nf1*$^{-/+}$ mice (Atit et al. 1999, Ingram et al. 2000). Thus, local wound when combined with *NF1* haploinsufficiency, may well potentiate neurofibroma formation.

Several reports have indicated that the *NF1* gene is one of the primary targets for somatic mutations in those rare individuals who are homozygous for mutations of mismatch repair genes (Wang et al. 1999, 2001; Whiteside et al. 2002, Menko et al. 2004; Bertholon et al. 2006).

The elucidation of molecular events that underly any tumourigenic pathway is a much more complex task than is the simple identification of a predisposing genetic lesion in a given gene. A complete understanding of this process will only come with the elucidation of the cellular consequences of those lesions in terms of the altered levels of expression of many other genes. Information on the gene expression patterns of cells in different developmental contexts, and in response to different environmental conditions or disease states, is currently being obtained using microarray-based expression analysis of tissue from NF1 patients.

## Malignant peripheral nerve sheath tumours (MPNSTs)

The majority of NF1-associated MPNSTs appear to develop within pre-existing plexiform neurofibromas however, some MFNSTs may be deep seated (Ferner and Gutmann 2002). The generation of mice with targeted mutations in the *Nf1* gene has confirmed that loss of *Nf1* expression does appear to be sufficient for the formation of tumours with pathological features of plexiform neurofibromas. MPNST development is however seemingly dependent on concominent functional inactivation of *Tp53* and a mouse model of MPNST development, involving both *NF1* and *Tp53* loss has been described (Cichowski et al. 1999, Vogel et al. 1999) in which mice carrying *Nf1* and *p53* mutations in *cis* eventually developed MPNSTs. Mouse models have further shown that NF1 malignancy is associated with homozygosity for mutations in the *Nf1* and *Tp53* genes. Epidermal growth factor receptor (EGFR), a protein that is not usually expressed in the Schwann cells is reported to be over expressed in MPNSTs (Li et al. 2002) Additional genetic mutations appear to represent later events in malignant transformation of Schwann cells as they are not observed in neurofibromas (Evans et al. 2002a, DeClue et al. 2000). Brain lipid binding protein (BLBP) gene is also overexpressed in some malignant Schwann cells and that may be induced by Ras-independent EGFR signalling (Miller et al. 2003). A cell adhesion molecule, CD44, is also overexpressed in MPNSTs. In addition mutations at the *INK4* locus, that inactivates both *p16* and *INK4a* and *p14ARF* tumour suppressor genes, have also been identified in MPNSTs (Berner et al. 1999, Upadhyaya et al. 2004, Sabah et al. 2006).

## Gastro-intestinal stromal tumours (GIST)

Molecular analysis of GIST from NF1 patients has indicated that these tumours do not have the *KIT* or *PDGFRA* mutations usually found in sporadic GISTS. It thus appears that unlike the molecular findings in most GIST tumours, somatic inactivation of wild type *NF1* allele underlies GIST formation and that JAK-STAT3 and PI3K-AKT pathways are less activated in NF1 related vs. sporadic GISTs (Maertens et al. 2006).

## Genotype/phenotype correlations

No clear relationship between the identified genotype and the observed clinical phenotype has been discerned for NF1 (Easton et al. 1993). This may be due either to the influence of unlinked modifier loci, or to the variable nature, location and developmental timing of the *NF1* somatic mutations, which may well determine the rate of progression and severity of disease in different tissues. Indeed genetic counselling for NF1 patients is often problematic owing to the marked inter- and intra-familial variation in NF1 expression observed in affected individuals. Identical *NF1* gene mutations have been identified in unrelated patients who exhibit very different phenotypes (Upadhyaya and Cooper 1998a). The first confirmed genotype/phenotype study demonstrated that NF1 patients with large genomic deletions tended to exhibit large number of neurofibromas for their age, dysmorphic features and develop learning disability (Kayes et al. 1994). NF1 patients with whole gene deletions are also at greater risk of developing MPNSTs (De Raedt et al. 2003, Kluwe et al. 2003), although another study has not confirmed this finding (Upadhyaya et al. 2006). We have found that NF1 individuals with missense germline

mutations had a relatively lower risk of developing Lisch nodules compared to NF1 patients with either nonsense or frameshift germline mutations (Castle et al. 2003). This preliminary finding awaits confirmation in much larger NF1 patient population. Recently we have identified 23 NF1 families, in which none of the affected individuals have developed the dermal neurofibromas which are once the hall mark features of NF1. Intriguingly each of the affected individuals was shown to have the same germline mutation, a 3 bp deletion in exon 17 of the *NF1* gene (Stevenson et al. 2006a, Upadhyaya et al. 2007).

Exploration of genotype-phenotype correlations in *NF1* is still however in its infancy mainly due to the extensive mutational heterogeneity observed in the gene, and because large-scale mutation screening is still quite laborious owing to the size and complexity of the gene. The exact nature of the *NF1* mutation does not appear to be a major determinant of any commonly observed NF1 disease features other than the study mentioned above. A corollary to this is that mutations in the *NF1* gene have also been identified in families who are classified as representing rare variants of NF1 these include Watson syndrome, neurofibromatosis-Noonan syndrome, familial café-au-lait spots, spinal neurofibromatosis, and Leopard syndrome (Viskochil 1994).

## Modifying genes

A role for modifier genes in NF1 disease phenotype expression (Easton et al. 1993, Bahuau et al. 2001, Szudek et al. 2000) was first proposed following the observation that monozygotic twins shared certain NF1 traits (e.g. café-au-lait spots, neurofibromas, head circumference) with high similarity. By contrast, distant relatives exhibited more variable clinical phenotypes (Easton et al. 1993). Genes influencing mitotic recombination, and thus the rate of LOH as a second hit, have also been proposed as modifier genes that might account for the observed variation in neurofibroma number (Serra et al. 2001b). Wiest et al. (2003) suggested that functional variants of genes involved in mismatch repair might also modulate the *NF1* mutation rate in a given patient. Various environmental and stochastic factors have also been proposed to explain the marked inter-individual clinical phenotypic variation observed in NF1 (Riccardi 1993).

Modifying genes may also influence tumour susceptibility and the modifying effect of the mouse genetic strain has been shown on the observed tumour phenotype (Reilly et al. 2004). These findings resulted in the identification of a genetic locus on chromosome 11 in the mouse that probably functions to modify the tumour spectrum and may explain the variability in the number and nature of tumour spectrum within a family.

## Animal models of NF1

Neurofibromin is highly conserved at the amino acid sequence level in human, mice, *Drosophila* and yeast. Indeed, the mouse and human *NF1* genes exhibit high levels of sequence homology in both the coding and non-coding region (Bernard et al. 1993). In order to help decipher the early development and the underlying mechanisms of development and tumour formation in NF1, a number of mouse models have been generated (Cichowski and Jacks 2001, Costa et al. 2002, Dasgupta and Gutmann 2003).

Heterozygous mice *(Nf1$^{+/-}$)* do not develop neurofibromas the hallmark features of NF1, but they do exhibit an enhanced predisposition to the development of phaeochromocytomas and myeloid leukaemia (Jacks et al. 1994). In these two tumour types, loss of the wild type *Nf1* allele is observed at a high frequency. Heterozygous *Nf1$^{+/-}$* mice also exhibit decreased learning ability, showing poor performance in tests involving spatial learning and memory.

Homozygous (*Nf1$^{-/-}$*) mice are severely affected and all die *in utero* between days 11.5 and 14 of gestation, with embryonic death attributed to severe malformation of the developing heart. Neurons harvested from the peripheral nervous systems of such homozygous animals demonstrate an increased

ability to survive in cell culture, even in the absence of any growth factor stimulation. The presence of myeloid leukaemia in *Nf1$^{+/-}$* mice indicates that the *Nf1* gene may play an important role in the haemopoietic cell development. In order to test the leukaemic potential of *Nf1$^{-/-}$* stem cells *in vivo*, fetal liver cells, (which contain haematopoietic stem cells), isolated from *Nf1$^{-/-}$* embryos were transplanted into lethally irradiated mice. These mice produced *Nf1$^{-/-}$* stem cells but also developed chronic myeloid leukaemia (Largaespada et al. 1996). These mice, when exposed to granulocyte/macrophage-colony stimulating factor (GM-CSF) exhibited a prolonged rise in Ras-GTP levels in their myeloid cells. A similar hypersensitivity to GM-CSF has also been described in human leukaemic cells derived from NF1 patients (Bollag et al. 1995). The reduction in NF1-GAP activity and the elevated levels of Ras-GTP are likely to be the cause of this GM-CSF hypersensitivity and subsequent development of myeloid leukaemia. The loss of neurofibromin in these mice would appear to be sufficient to produce the myeloproliferative symptoms associated with human JCML. The lack of any hallmark clinical features in *Nf1$^{+/-}$* mice, and the early lethality in homozygous *Nf1$^{-/-}$* mice, makes it difficult to study the late developmental stages of the disorder, and this has led to researchers to take several different approaches to try to resolve this problem.

One such study set out to determine whether a mutation of the wild type *NF1* allele is the critical rate-limiting event in neurofibroma formation in mice. Homozygous *Nf1$^{-/-}$* embryonic stem cell lines (ES), labelled with beta-galactosidase, were injected into normal mouse blastocysts (Cichowski et al. 1999). The resultant chimeric mice (*Nf1$^{-/-}$* *Nf1$^{+/+}$*) subsequently developed plexiform neurofibromas that were all derived from E cells that were *Nf1$^{-/-}$*, confirming that the complete loss of neurofibromin is indeed an obligate step in benign plexiform neurofibroma formation in mice. As all the different cell types in these mice were uniformly homozygous for *NF1* mutations, it was impossible to determine just which cell types was directly involved neurofibroma formation.

## Conditional *Nf1* knockout mice

The production of NF1 conditional knockout mice utilises Cre-LoxP technology to selectively abolish *NF1* expression in a specific tissue type. Using this system it was shown that mice with wild type *Nf1* alleles flanked by LoxP sequences (*Nf1*$^{flox/flox}$) continue to express normal levels of neurofibromin and appear phenotypically normal. When the bacteriophage Cre recombinase is inserted in such cells, an excision event occurs at both the flanking LoxP sites, which results in total excision and inactivation of the targeted *Nf1* gene. In these tissue specific animal studies, the normal *Nf1*$^{flox/flox}$ mice were crossed with a second transgenic mouse strains which only expresses Cre recombinase under the control of a number of different tissue-specific promoters. This directed genetic manipulation permits the generation of mice strains in which the *Nf1* gene may be specifically inactivated in a single cell type such as in the neurons, in Schwann cells, in astrocytes or in endothelial cells (Bajenaru et al. 2003, Gitler et al. 2003).

Schwann cell-specific *Nf1* knockout mice, which express one *Nf1*$^{mut}$ allele and one normal flox *Nf1* allele (*Nf1*$^{flox/mut}$; Krox 20-Cre mice) in all cells eventually develop plexiform neurofibromas (Zhu et al. 2002). However, Schwann cell-specific *Nf1* knockout mice, in which all cells in the surrounding tissues were genotypically wild-type (*Nf1*$^{flox/flox}$ Krox20-Cre), only ever developed small infrequent hyperplastic lesions in their cranial nerves. It would therefore appear that a haploinsufficient state of the cell tissue microenvironment is a critical factor for the formation of tumours. Those neurofibromas that developed in *Nf1*$^{flox/mut}$; Krox 20-Cre mice demonstrated an extensive infiltration of *Nf1*$^{+/-}$ mast cells (Zhu et al. 2002). Interestingly, *Nf1*$^{+/-}$ mast cells have been shown to hyperproliferate *in vitro* and *in vivo* in *Nf1*$^{+/-}$ mice (Ingram et al. 2000). It seems as though the loss of *Nf1* gene in Schwann cells provides a potent chemotactic stimulus for *Nf1*$^{+/-}$ mast cells through the secretion of the soluble kit ligand and activation of a specific Ras effector-signalling pathway (Yang et al. 2003). These findings emphasise the critical role of mast cells in the initiation of neurofibroma development.

Other tissue-specific *Nf1* knockout mice also demonstrate individual phenotype. Neuron-specific knock out mice develop neurotrophin-independent dorsal root ganglion neuron survival *in vitro* and an overall reduction in brain cortical thickness. Astrocyte-specific *Nf1* conditional knockout mice exhibit an increased astrocyte proliferation both *in vitro* and *in vivo* but they do not develop gliomas. In a more recent study however Bajenaru et al. demonstrated that *Nf1*$^{+/-}$ mice lacking *Nf1* (*Nf1*$^{-/-}$) in astrocytes did develop optic nerve gliomas (Bajenaru et al. 2003).

Endothelial-specific *Nf1* knockout mice develop multiple cardiovascular abnormalities that develop the endocardial cushions and myocardium (Gitler et al. 2003). This cardiopathogenic phenotype is associated with elevated levels of Ras signalling in *Nf1*$^{-/-}$ endothelial cells.

## Diagnosis

The diagnosis of NF1 can be made by a careful clinical examination and detailed history. Family history should be obtained and minimally include information on tumours and skin lesions in first- and second-degree relatives. One must remember however that approximately half of the NF1 sufferers are the first in their family to have the condition.

Physical examination is directed at determining whether NF1 diagnostic criteria (Table 1) are present and at different ages should be geared to particular complications (Table 2). These diagnostic criteria are robust and have stood the test of time well (Ferner et al. 2007). Clinicians should be aware that some individuals with mosaic/segmental NF1 (see below) might present with typical café-au-lait spots, skin-fold freckling or neurofibromas (fulfilling or not the diagnostic criteria) in restricted segments of the body (Ruggieri and Huson 2001).

Hyperintense lesions on T2-weighted brain MR images (formerly called UBOs) when located in specific places (see above neurological complications) are pathognomonic of NF1. The presence of thee lesions can assist the diagnosis of NF1 but MRI under aneasthetic is not warranted for this purpose in young children (Ferner et al. 2007). Laboratory or imaging tests should be dictated only by the findings on clinical examination. Thus, routine screening by any mean of investigation is not warranted in the diagnostic work-up of NF1 (Ruggieri 1999).

Children with six café-au-lait patches alone and no family history should be followed up as if they have the disease, as 95% of them will develop NF1 (Ferner et al. 2007). Children with 3–5 café-au-lait patches but no other signs of NF1 should be followed in a specialist neurofibromatosis clinic as they might have mosaic/segmental NF1 or NF2. The reader is referred to the section below on NF1 related forms for the NF1 subtypes in differential diagnosis with NF1.

Genetic counselling should be provided for all at risk family members.

*Molecular Diagnosis* – Owing to the extreme variability of clinical expression often observed in NF1 patients even with the same mutation, disease progression, and severity cannot be readily predicted. To-date there has been little demand for prenatal diagnosis in NF1 families possibly because majority of couples would wish to know the likely clinical severity of the disease in their baby, something which we cannot currently predict. There is still an urgent need however for the development of an inexpensive, rapid and accurate, DNA-based diagnostic test for NF1. The development of a preimplantation test for NF1 has also been initiated (Verlinski et al. 2002).

## Management

Clinicians familiar with neurofibromatosis should provide longitudinal care of NF1 patients. In our respective centres we run specialist neurofibromatosis clinics offering co-ordinated care and follow-up by a group of specialists, including a paediatrician, ophthalmologist, neurologist, dermatologist, neurosurgeon and neuroradiologist.

The recommended protocol for **children** with NF1 is to have an annual review to monitor disease progression, particularly with respect to the development of complications. Examination should be

**Table 3.** Assessment of children with NF1 (compare with Table 2)

| |
|---|
| Medical enquire (including development and progress at school) |
| Height |
| Weight |
| Head circumference |
| Pubertal development |
| General physical examination including evaluation of the skin and spine |
| Cardiovascular examination |
| Visual symptoms, visual acuity and fundoscopy until puberty* |
| Neurological examination |
| Blood pressure |

*One baseline assessment of colour vision and visual fields at the appropriate developmental age

geared appropriately, as the majority of NF1 complications present with symptoms either in childhood or not at all (Table 3).

Annual review at all ages must include blood pressure measurements. Young adults aged 16–25 years are at a vulnerable stage of life and require education about NF1 and its possible complications (Maria 2002, Listernick et al. 2004a Ferner et al. 2007).

Monitoring after the mid-twenties depends on patient preference and disease severity. Adults with mild disease have a much lower risk of complications. If they elect not to attend a specialist NF1 clinic, they should be fully conversant with the problem they might encounter (Ferner et al. 2007). The minimum requirements for follow-up of **adults** with uncomplicated NF1 should include annual review of symptoms (see Table 2) and blood pressure check. More frequent re-evaluation should only be dictated by unusual symptoms.

Laboratory or imaging tests should be dictated only by the findings on clinical examination. Baseline brain and spine MRI and routine imaging screening of the chest and abdomen by any mean of investigation to identify asymptomatic tumours is not recommended in NF1 as it does not influence management.

The mainstay of care is anticipatory guidance and surveillance for age specific treatable complications. As most of the patients with NF1 will never develop major complications it is not advocated that all patients need to attend a specialist clinic. Specialist assessment, however, can be helpful at the time of initial diagnosis, in the assessment of patients with unusual symptoms or complications or whose neurofibromatosis phenotype does not easily fall into the category of NF1 or NF2.

## Treatment

### Neurofibromas and plexiform neurofibromas

*Dermal neurofibromas* often catch on clothing and cause cosmetic problems, transient stinging and itching. Irritation sometimes responds to antihistamines whilst the benefit of mast cell stabilisers is uncertain; excessive heat should be avoided and the use of emollient is advised (Ferner et al. 2007). Cutaneous neurofibromas can be removed if they cause any of the problems mentioned above (Ferner et al. 2007). Referral to dermatologists and/or surgeons skilled in the removal of neurofibromas is advocated and plastic surgeons should be consulted for neurofibromas in the face or neck. Surgical removal is advocated for troublesome neurofibromas but laser may be helpful for some small lesions. There is a risk of post-surgical complications such as hypertrophic scarring and or recurrence of neurofibromas in the same area of removal (residual neurofibromas or new lesions, previously undetectable, within the same area).

If removal is contemplated for a *subcutaneous neurofibroma* (because of neurological symptoms or suspect/proven malignant transformation, expert advice should be sought from NF1 specialists or soft tissue/peripheral nerve surgeons as removal occasionally result in neurological deficits.

Surgical treatment of *plexiform neurofibromas* is difficult because of the massive involvement of soft (e.g., the tongue) or nervous tissues or both and because of the frequent "entrapment" of vital anatomic structures (e.g., blood vessels, muscles, trachea, oesophagus, bladder, gut, etc.) within the masses. There are few studies on large series of plexiform neurofibromas operated whose follow-up lasted many years. In the review of Needle et al. (1997) on 121 patients

who were operated of 168 tumours, it was observed that 94 (56%) did not present recurrences after 2 to 24.5 years (average 6.8 years). Ages of patients less than 10 years, location of the tumours in the head, face and neck, and the presence of tumoural rests after surgery, are unfavourable signs. At present, the therapeutical strategy for plexiform neurofibromas is first of all surgical, and, later, radiotherapy and chemotherapy (which are mostly employed in malignant tumours, with moderate effects to date).

Treatment of clitoromegaly in NF1 is clitoplasty with preservation of the neurovascular bundle and glandular tissue (Griebel et al. 1991, Kearse et al. 1993). The plexiform neurofibroma of the penis requires only excision, but those causing urinary obstruction, needs urinary diversion.

During the last years, many pharmacological substances have been used (as alternatives to surgery) to try to reduce the growth rate or to decrease the volume of plexiform neurofibromas (reviewed in Korf 2002, Rosser and Packer 2002, Packer et al. 2002) including:

(a) *Antihistamines, including ketotifen fumurate* (Riccardi 1987, 1993), employed (in children and adults) on the basis that mast cells, often found in plexiform neurofibromas were important in the pathogenesis of such lesions (Riccardi 1990). The first trial, a double-blind, crossover design was used on 20 patients selected on symptomatic compromise, including pruritus or dysesthetic pain (Riccardi 1987) and a follow-up study of 25 patients was performed using an open-label design (Riccardi 1993). In both (phase II) studies patients were evaluated for change in clinical symptomatology (using a disability score), and change in lesion size (either by direct or radiographic measurements) (Packer and Rosser 2002). Clear-cut radiographic and/or measurable "surface size" progression responses were not well documented and thus the studies' results were difficult to interpret (even thought the author claimed that the drug resulted in symptomatic relief of pruritus or dysesthetic pain in a subset of patients;

(b) *Conventional chemotherapy*, including a combination of *vincristine* and *methotrexate*, has provided little evidence of efficacy of any regimen (Packer and Rosser 2002).

(c) *Maturation agents*, including *retinoic acid*, have been used in a randomised, non-comparative phase II trial in 57(prevalently paediatric) patients (Phillips P, personal communication reported in Packer and Rosser 2002) with progressive lesions documented clinically or by means of imaging: after 18 months of follow-up 87% of cases were reported to be stable, 10% to 20% had reduction in surface measurement of the lesion with no patient however having a demonstrable radiographic response to treatment (only 3 patients also had symptomatic improvement);

(d) *Antiangiogenesis drugs*, including *interferon-α* (used also for its anti-inflammatory effects) (Kirsch et al. 1998, Kurtz and Martuza 2002, Takamiya et al. 1993) and *thalidomide*, have been used in NF1 children with radiographic progression of tumour or measurable tumour growth. In a paediatric trial of 57 patients treated with interferon-α, 96% were at least stable 18 months after study entry, five had symptomatic improvements and 10 to 20% reduction in surface measurement (Phillips PC, personal communication, 2001). A phase I study using thalidomide (Gupta et al. 2003) demonstrated good tolerability of the drug and decrease in size of the tumour in 4/20 patients who entered the study.

(e) *Oral Farnesyl Protein Transferase Inhibitors* (including *tipifarnib*) [used on the basis that the inhibition of Ras farnesylation may inhibit the growth of plexiform neurofibromas in NF1] (Gurujeyalakshmi et al. 1999) were recently demonstrated to be well tolerated in a phase I trial with no radiographic partial response(s) recorded so far: a phase II study using a randomised placebo-controlled crossover design is ongoing (Widemann et al. 2006).

(f) *Cytokine modulators*, including *pirfenidone* (5-methyl-1-phenyl-2-(1H)-pyridone) a broad spectrum antifibrotic drug that modulates the actions of cytokines, including several growth factors has been used in a phase 1 trial (Babovic-Vuksanovic et al. 2007) and in ongoing phase 2 trial in NF1 children and adults with plexiform neurofibromas.

In addition to pharmacological substances *radiofrequency* has been used with excellent tolerance, no major side effects and no pain in the postoperative course in a pilot study of 5 NF1 children with cranio-orbital plexiform neurofibromas (Baujat et al. 2006).

A diminution of the size of the lesion was noted clinically in four patients and on computed tomography in two patients. A biopsy performed in one case illustrated the effect of the treatment. The best effects were observed in the early stages of the disease.

## Optic pathway gliomas

Treatment of optic pathway gliomas is controversial because of their unpredictable evolution (e.g., tumour regression) even in symptomatic cases. Physicians must carefully balance the risks and benefits of any therapeutical intervention in these children attempting to preserve function and being harmless. When indicated, treatment options are surgery and chemotherapy (usually with vincristine and cisplatinum), alone or in combination (Kedar 1997, Packer et al. 1997). Surgical resection is usually indicated when the tumour: (1) progresses, either clinically or radiologically; (2) involves the optic nerve unilaterally or bilaterally, and causes proptosis, pain and/or visual loss (Rosser and Packer 2002). A blind or proptotic eye may be removed for cosmetic reasons. Another indication for surgery is to prevent the invasion (and mass compression) of local and/or more distant structures including the chiasm, although there is limited evidence to support this. Chiasmatic-hypothalamic gliomas in children with NF1 tend to be solid and infiltrative, making extensive surgical resection difficult. Evidence suggests that in total doses of 5000 cGy to 5400 cGy, given in daily dose fractions of 150 cGy to 180 cGy, radiation therapy will result in disease stabilisation or tumour shrinkage in 80% of patients (Garvey and Packer 1996). However, radiotherapy is not advocated in young children because of potential second malignancy, neuropsychological, vascular and endocrine consequences (Fig. 5) (Pierce et al. 1990, De Winter et al. 1999), and because does not consistently improve visual outcome or prolonged survival (Garvey and Packer 1996).

## Mosaic/segmental NF1

It is increasingly recognised that both NF1 and NF2 can arise from somatic mosaicism (Huson and Ruggieri 2006, Ruggieri and Huson 2001). For both forms of neurofibromatosis, patients with clinical generalised disease have been demonstrated to be mosaic at the molecular level and cases with localised/segmental manifestations of either form have been reported. Patients with the signs of the NF1 limited to one or more body segments are usually referred to as having segmental NF1 (Ruggieri 2001, Ruggieri and Huson 2001). Patients may also have typical NF2-related tumours localised to one part of the central (unilateral VSs with ipsilateral non-VS tumours) and/or peripheral nervous system and are referred as mosaic/segmental NF2. These conditions are being reported with increasing frequency. The calculated frequencies in our studies have been of 1 in 36,000–40,000 individuals in the general population, or 0.02% (segmental NF1) and 1 in 333,000 in the general population, or 0.0003% (segmental NF2) (Ruggieri and Huson 2001).

## Mosaic/segmental NF1

### Clinical manifestations

Any division of patients with mosaic/segmental manifestations of NF1 on clinical grounds is to some extent arbitrary. Ruggieri and Huson (2001) have categorised four groups according to the presence or absence of pigmentary changes or neurofibromas (including plexiform neurofibromas), or both. The clinical significance of this categorisation is that the groups tend to present at different ages and to different specialists (Huson and Ruggieri 2006, Ruggieri 2001, Ruggieri and Huson 2001). The disease features develop at the same time as in generalised NF1: pigmentary features and plexiform neurofibromas in childhood and neurofibromas in adulthood. What is different is that not all patients with pigmentary changes will develop neurofibromas in the affected area(s) as adults. This presumably reflects the cell lineage in which the mutation took place (see section on molecular genetics and pathogenesis)

Patients may have (Figs. 43–45) (reviewed in Huson and Ruggieri 2006, Listernick et al. 2003, Ruggieri and Huson 2001, Ruggieri et al. 2004):

1) *Pigmentary changes alone* (i.e., café-au-lait spots and/or freckling) (Fig. 43). In these patients

the natural history is similar to generalised NF1: the only remarkable difference is that the initial (but also definitive) number of larger macules could be limited (i.e., less than 6 café-au-lait spots) depending on the proportion of skin involved (see Fig. 43 A, B and D). The café-au-lait spots develop first (Fig. 43 D), then the freckling (Fig. 43 E). If freckling is present it is often very intense (Fig. 43 C) and develops in parts of the body not usually associated with dense freckles in the generalised disease (Fig. 43 A–C). Most affected persons with pigmentary changes only do not develop neurofibromas as adults. One of the most striking features seen in this group is that the area of skin involved has a darker background (see Figs. 43 A, circle; and 43 D–E, dotted area), which sometimes only becomes apparent with an ultraviolet light. The café-au-lait spots and/or freckles are all within the background-pigmented area (Fig. 43). This background pigmentation has been interpreted as the effect of the NF1 gene on skin colour (even in the heterozygous state) (Ruggieri and Huson 2001).

2) *Neurofibromas* alone (Fig. 44). This is the phenotype most frequently reported in the literature (>55%) (Reviewed in Huson and Ruggieri 2006). The appearance of the individual neurofibromas is exactly the same as when they occur in the generalised disease: i.e., with dermal (Fig. 44A) and/or nodular neurofibromas (Fig. 44 B–C). It is patients with localised nodular (subcutaneous) neurofibromas who most frequently present to neurologists or child neurologists. The clinical presentation varies depending on which nerve is involved.

3) *Neurofibromas and pigmentary changes* (Fig. 45 A). Patients may have both disease features in a circumscribed area, often in association with a darker background area in the affected part of the body. These patients are frequently diagnosed as having full-blown NF1, especially if the area(s) involved are multiple or widely distributed.

4) *Solitary plexiform neurofibromas* (Fig. 45 B). These patients present with a small to huge plexiform neurofibroma as the solely manifestation of their disease (see Fig. 6 C). The appearance and natural history of these lesions is the same as when they occur as a complication in NF1.

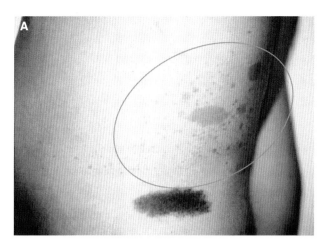
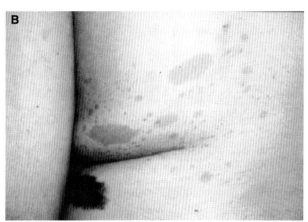
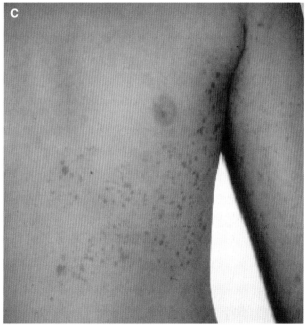
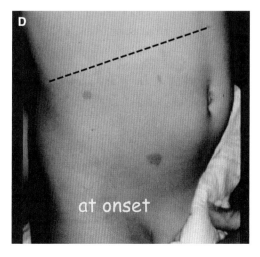
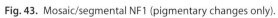
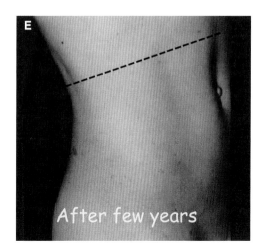

**Fig. 43.** Mosaic/segmental NF1 (pigmentary changes only).

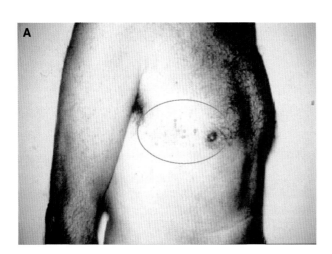

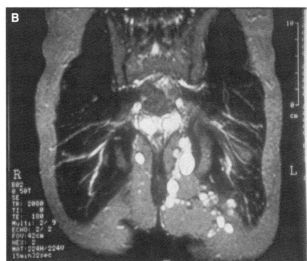

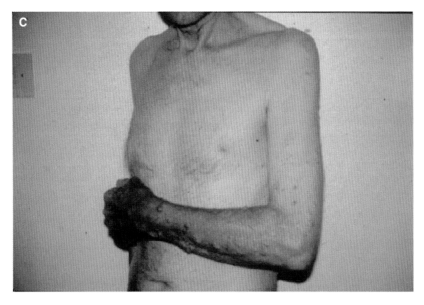

**Fig. 44.** Mosaic segmental/NF1 (neurofibromas only).

## Disease features

Age at onset. Age at onset of NF1 manifestations in localised NF1 phenotypes varies according to the presence of pigmentation anomalies (from birth until first 1–2 years of life) (see Fig. 43 D) or neurofibromas only (from around puberty to young adulthood) (see Fig. 44 A). In some patients the segment involved seem to be more severely affected than not usually seen in generalised disease (see Figs. 43 C; 44 B; 45 A).

Area of involvement. The area of involvement is variable (Figs. 43–45). In the majority of patients it is unilateral. The affected area varies from a narrow strip (Fig. 44 A, C) to one quadrant (Figs. 43 A–C) and occasionally one half (see Fig. 6C) or one section (Fig. 45 A) of the body. Some patients may have more than one segment involved on both sides of the midline, either in a symmetric or asymmetric arrangement, thus reflecting the patterns of skin mosaicism proposed by Happle (1993, 1997).

Other NF1 features and disease complications. Lisch nodules are rarely (if at all) seen (Listernick et al. 2003; Ruggieri et al. 2004). Minor disease features (e.g., macrocephaly, stature at lower percentiles,

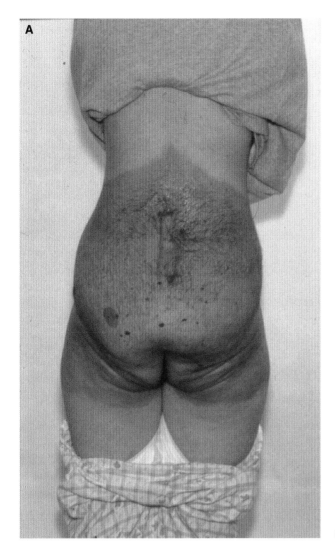

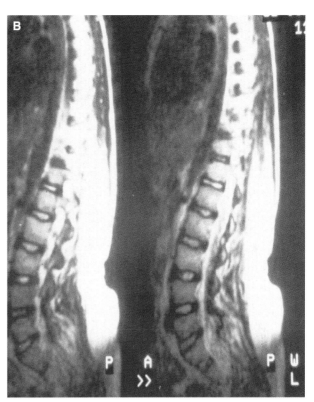

**Fig. 45.** Mosaic/segmental NF1 (plexiform neurofibromas only).

etc.) were not recorded in one large study (Ruggieri and Huson 2001). Specific *NF1 complications* are usually rare (rarer than in the generalised disease) (estimated at around 5–6% in one study) (Ruggieri and Huson 2001). These include learning difficulties, plexiform neurofibromas (see Fig. 45 A), optic pathway gliomas, and pseudarthrosis (reviewed in Ruggieri and Huson 2001).

Additional localised phenotypes. Patients with isolated optic pathways gliomas (Listernick et al. 2003, Ruggieri et al. 2004) and isolated dysplasia of the long bones (Listernick et al. 2003) have been reported. The peculiarity of these cases was that they

manifested these NF1 complications with the same features and natural history seen in the generalised disease as the solely manifestation of NF1.

## Genetic basis: Familial mosaic/segmental NF1

All authors reporting cases of localised NF1 phenotypes had agreed they reflected somatic mosaicism and this was later proven at the molecular level (Tinschert et al. 2000, Vandenbroucke et al. 2004, see also section on pathogenesis and molecular genetics).

The majority of reported patients with mosaic/segmental NF1 have no affected relatives with the disease. There are however a handful of reported instances in which parents with mosaic/segmental NF1 had children with full-blown disease (Boltshauser et al. 1989, Huson and Ruggieri 2006, Moss and Green 1994, Oguzcan et al. 2004, Rubenstein et al. 1983, Uhlin 1980): it was assumed that these patients were gonosomal mosaics, with involvement of both somatic and gonadal tissue and that was demonstrated by Consoli et al. (2004). It is important to note that in these patients the affected area can be anywhere, i.e., does not necessarily overlie the gonads.

More difficult to explain are the cases of vertical transmission of mosaic/segmental NF1 (Huson and Ruggieri 2006, Rubenstein et al. 1983, Segal 1993). Various possibilities exist: perhaps the NF1 gene in these families has variable expression within the same individual analogue to positional effect variegation. Alternatively, perhaps an inherited permutation become a full mutation only in certain body areas or there is a partial correction of a germ-line mutation in the offspring after somatic mutation in the patient as seen in revertant mosaicism (Consoli et al. 2004, Ruggieri and Huson 2001).

## Management and genetic counselling

There is no management specific for mosaic/segmental NF1 (Ingordo et al. 1995, Poyhonen 2000, Ruggieri and Huson 2001, Wolkenstein et al. 1995). Patients need to be advised they do not have generalised NF1 and are at low risk of developing any disease-associated complications. Those considering children need to be aware of the small risk of having a child with generalised NF1 (Consoli et al. 2004, Moss and Green 1994, Ruggieri and Huson 2001). The exact risk is not definable but, based on animal work is proportional to the percentage of body area involved.

## NF1 related forms (NF1 subtypes)

The outlying phenotypes and the molecular genetics of other, rare, types of neurofibromatosis have been recently delineated. The main clinical features and the genetic aspects are summarised show below.

## Familial spinal neurofibromatosis

Few families exhibiting a distinct clinical entity of hereditary neurofibromatosis, consisting of extensively and apparently symmetrically distributed, histologically proven, multiple spinal neurofibromas, in association with CAL spots and occasional axillary freckling have been reported to date. (Ars et al. 1998, Kaufmann et al. 2001, Méssiaen et al. 2003, Pascual-Castroviejo et al. 2007, Poyhonen et al. 1997, Pulst et al. 1991, Winner et al. 2002) Lisch nodules were detected only in two affected members of one family. No affected members in any family showed clinical features of Nf2. Ars et al. (1998) recorded in affected members of the family a frameshift mutation in the NF1 gene. In affected members of 2 families with spinal neurofibromas but no cafe-au-lait macules, Kaufmann et al. (2001) identified 2 different mutations in the NF1 gene: both NF1 mutations caused a reduction in neurofibromin of approximately 50%, with no truncated protein present in the cells. The findings demonstrated that typical NF1 null mutations could result in a phenotype that is distinct from classical NF1, showing only a small spectrum of the NF1 symptoms, such as multiple spinal tumours, but not completely fitting the current clinical criteria for spinal neurofibromatosis. Kaufmann et al. (2001) suggested that the spinal neurofibromatosis phenotype may be caused by a modifying gene that partially compensates for the effects of neurofibromin deficiency. In 4 affected members of the family with spinal neurofibromas and café-au-lait spots reported by Pulst et al. (1991), Messiaen et al. (2003) identified a mutation in the NF1 gene. In affected members of the family with spinal neurofibromas reported by Poyhonen et al. (1997), Messiaen et al. (2003) identified a mutation in the NF1 gene. Interestingly, the most recent familial cases of multiple, extensive spinal root neurofibromas were all associated to specific NF1 mutations (Pascual-Castroviejo et al. 2007, Wimmer et al. 2002) thus demonstrating that this might be a true NF1 subtype (Pascual-Castroviejo et al. 2007).

More recent clinical observations in individuals with multiple, extensive, bilateral spinal root neurofibromas at every level (Pascual-Castroviejo et al. 2007; Ruggieri, personal observation; Wimmer et al. 2002) recorded no cord symptoms but signs and symptoms of progressive nerve sheath neuropathy segmentally distributed. Typically patients manifest symptomatic peripheral nerve involvement at around or shortly after puberty or during adulthood. One of the most important features from a prognostic viewpoint is that the spinal roots are progressively involved initially segment-by-segment in a mosaic distribution (i.e., even starting in distant roots) and then leaving no intact segment (see Fig. 24). Recently, it has been suggested that spinal neurofibromatosis associated with Nf1 does occur more often than initially thought, its infrequent detection by other investigators being explained by the previous lack of routine spinal MRI studies.

## Familial intestinal neurofibromatosis

Neurofibromas of the intestine are a recognised though rare feature of Nf1 (Magro et al. 2000). Sporadic cases of multiple intestinal Nf without cutaneous features of Nf1 have been observed. Hashemian (1952) described "familial fibromatosis" of the small intestine, but two of the three cases had other stigmata of Nf1. *Lipton and Zuckerboard* (1966) described familial intestinal Nf (without other features of Nf1). Verhest et al. (1981) and subsequent *restudies* (Heimann et al. 1988, Verhest et al. 1988) described a family with localised intestinal neurofibromas with onset of symptoms in adulthood and some gene carriers asymptomatic into middle and late adulthood. This description might fit with a localised expression of phenotype that may be allelic and tissue specific.

## Autosomal dominant café-au-lait spots alone

There have been a handful of families reported world-wide with multiple CAL spots, indistinguishable from those commonly found in Nf1, as the only disease feature segregating as an autosomal domi-

nant. The segregation of DNA markers in the region of the Nf1 gene has been studied in three of these families. Two showed evidence of non linkage (Brunner et al. 1993, Charrow et al. 1993) and the other appeared to be linked to the Nf1 locus (Abeliovich et al. 1995). Hoo and Shrimpton (2005) excluded the NF1 locus in a family with café-au-lait spots and hypopigmented macules.

When assessing children with multiple CAL spots as the only feature and no family history, Nf1 is by far the most likely diagnosis, although the diagnosis cannot be confirmed until other disease features appear.

## Autosomal dominant neurofibromas alone

Korf et al. (personal communication, 1999) studied 12 affected individuals with multiple subcutaneous and deep peripheral nerve tumours from a kindred of 5 generations. Age of onset ranged over the first two decades. Detailed examination of affected individuals failed to identify clinical features of either Nf1 (CAL spots, freckling or Lisch nodules) or Nf2 (vestibular schwannomas, meningiomas, or cataracts). In addition, the affected individuals were intellectually normal, without evidence of developmental problems or learning disabilities.

Tumours from two members of the family were of nerve sheath origin with pathological features intermediate between neurofibroma and schwannoma.

Absence of linkage to the Nf1 as well as the Nf2 gene using polymorphic microsatellite markers was demonstrated.

## Watson syndrome

Watson (1967) described autosomal dominant inheritance of pulmonary stenosis, multiple CAL spots and intelligence at the lower end of the normal range. The features distinguishing the condition from Nf1 were the pulmonary stenosis and the fact that the intellectual problems were found in all family members in the original report. Allanson et al. (1999) followed up the original Watson patients and confirmed that their phenotype had remained distinct from Nf1. A few other Nf1 features namely Lisch nodules and dermal neurofibromas were present in some of the individuals studied by Watson, but at a very much lower frequency than is usually seen in Nf1 (Partington et al. 1985). Linkage with markers for the Nf1 gene and an Nf1 mutation were subsequently demonstrated in these families (Upadhyaya et al. 1989, 1990, 1992). The pathogenesis is so far unclear.

## Neurofibromatosis-Noonan syndrome

### Clinical manifestations

A few patients with NF1 have clinical features that overlap with mild *Noonan's syndrome* (NS) (OMIM # 163950) with mild ptosis and hypertelorism, down-slanting palpebral fissures, posteriorly rotated ears, midface hypoplasia, webbed neck, congenital heart disease (e.g., pulmonic stenosis) and muscle weakness. Pectus excavatum and learning disabilities can also occur in both conditions.

This association was first described by Allanson and colleagues (1985) in 4 unrelated patients with NF1. Despite the volume of work and number of cases and families (Abuelo and Meryash 1988, Colley et al. 1996, Kaplan and Rosenblatt 1985, Meinecke 1987, Mendez 1985, Saul 1985, Shuper et al. 1987, Stern 1992), including families transmitting the trait (Quattrin et al. 1987), controversy and conflict (Carey 1998; De Luca et al. 2005; Sarkozy et al. 2007) still surround the topic of what Opitz and Weaver (1985) called *Neurofibromatosis-Noonan syndrome* (NFNS) (OMIM # 601231).

According to the studies by Carey (1998) and De Luca et al. (2005) in affected individuals with NFNS: (1) *distinctive NF1 features* are the absence of Lisch nodules, the small number of dermal neurofibromas, the low incidence of plexiform neurofibromas, and the lack of the typical NF1 internal tumours; (2) *distinctive NS features* are typical dysmorphism including hypertelorism, ptosis, and low-set ears whereas short neck and stature and thoracic abnormalities are present in only half of patients (De Luca et al. 2005). Of note, both Stern

et al. (1992) and Colley et al. 1996) reported a few NFNS families in which only a fraction of affected members with NF1 exhibited some NS features.

## Pathogenesis and molecular genetics

*Hypotheses.* Various possibilities have been proposed to explain the coexistence of NF1 and NS in the same patient (reviewed in Carey 1998, De Luca et al. 2005 and OMIM 2007): (1) coincidence of two common autosomal dominant disorders with the traits and genes for NF1 and NS segregating independently (Abuelo and Meryash 1988; Bahuau et al. 1996, 1998; Colley et al. 1996); (2) the manifestations of NF1, specifically the café-au-lait spots, can occur as a component of the classical NS as reported in a family with NS and café-au-lait spots with no linkage to the NF1 locus; (3) the manifestations of NS in these patients are simply a variable manifestation of classic NF1, just like optic gliomas, scoliosis, etc. (Meinicke 1987, Quattrin et al. 1987, Huson and Ruggieri 2006); (4) NFNS may represent a discrete entity with the entire pattern running true in some kindred.

*Genetic basis.* Carey et al. (1997) first identified in a two-generation family, in which an affected mother had 4 of her 5 offspring affected with NFNS, a 3bp deletion in exon 17 of the NF1 gene. Stevenson et al. (2006), by performing a follow-up study of this family (Carey et al. 1997) recorded that all the affected family members had multiple features consistent with NS; the only features consistent with NF1 however were multiple café-au-lait spots and relative macrocephaly. None had neurofibromas or other diagnostic features or complications of NF1 (Stevenson et al. 2006). Subsequently, Baralle et al. 2003 examined the NF1 gene in six subjects with NFN and found mutations in two cases. Recently, Bertola et al. (2005) reported a patient with NF1 and NS features who carried a heterozygous mutation in both NF1 and PTPN11, the gene responsible for half of the cases of NS (Jamieson et al. 1994, Tartaglia et al. 2001).

A comprehensive study performed by De Luca et al. (2005) in a cohort of clinically well-characterised NFNS patients, screened or mutations in the entire coding sequence of the NF1 and PTPN11 genes, revealed heterozygous NF1 defects in 16 of the 17 unrelated subjects studied (vs. no defect in the PTPN11 gene), thus providing evidence that mutations in NF1 represent the major molecular event underlying this condition and supporting the view that NFNS is a variant of NF1 and is caused by mutations of the NF1 gene, some of which have been demonstrated to cause classic NF1 in other individuals. Huffmeier et al. (2006) provided further confirmation to such hypothesis recording heterozygous mutations and deletions of the NF1 gene (vs. no mutations in the PTPN11 gene) in seven NFNS patients from five unrelated families. From a molecular viewpoint, the clinical overlap between NF1 and NS is not surprising in that the NF1 and PTPN11 gene products, neurofibromin and SHP2 (a cytoplasmic protein tyrosinase phosphatase functioning as a transducer), elicit their modulatory (antagonistic) role in RAs signalling through a common transduction cascade pathway which control a number of developmental processes (Arun and Gutmann 2004, Tartaglia et al. 2004a) (see also fig. 41 in this chapter and fig. 8, chapter 66). Consistent with the crucial role of neurofibromin and SHP-2 in modulating cell proliferation, children with NF1 or NS are predisposed to distinct but overlapping spectra of haematologic malignancies (Shannon et al. 1994, Tartaglia et al. 2004b).

No mutation affecting PTPN11 gene has been identified in NFNS so far (Baralle et al. 2003, De Luca et al. 2005), strongly supporting the hypothesis that PTPN11 is not a major disease gene contributing to or causing NFNS and that NFNS and NS are distinct genetic disorders (De Luca et al. 2005). In addition, large clinical studies of NS make no references to patients with diagnostic NF1 features, which suggest that NF1 features do not occur frequently in classic NS. The co-occurrence of mutations in both NF1 and PTPN11 genes in a NFNS patient recorded by Bertola et al. (2005) reflects likely a rare event (an exception to the rule) accounting for a minority of NFNS cases.

## References

Abeliovich D, Gelman-Kohan Z, Silverstein S, Lerer I, Chemke J, Merlin S, Zlotogora J (1995) Familial cafe au lait spots: a variant of neurofibromatosis type 1. J Med Genet 32:985–986.

Abuelo DN, Meryash DL (1988) Neurofibromatosis with fully expressed Noonan syndrome. Am J Med Genet 29: 937–941.

Ahmadian MR, Hoffmann U, Goody RS, Wittinghofer A (1997) Individual rate constants for the interaction of Ras proteins with GTPase-activating proteins determined by fluorescence spectroscopy. Biochemistry 36: 4535–4541.

Ainsworth PJ, Chakraborty PK, Weksberg R (1997) Example of somatic mosaicism in a series of de novo neurofibromatosis type 1 cases due to a maternally derived deletion. Hum Mut 9: 452–457.

Akbarnia BA, Gabriel KR, Beckman E, Chalk D (1992) Prevalence of scoliosis in neurofibromatosis. Spine 17: S244–S248.

Akenside M (1768) Observations on cancers. Med Trans Coll Phys Lond 1: 64–92.

Albisi P, Balestri P, Bartalini G, Barardi A, Bergamaschi G, Bianchi E et al. (1993) Resultati dello studio collaborativo sulla neurofibromatosis tipe 1 (NF1) in Intalia. Riv Ital Pediatr 19: 138–151.

Aldrovandi U (1642) Monstruorum Historia: Cum Paralipomenis Historiae omnium Animalium. Bologna: Typis Nocolai Tibaldini.

Allan BT (1985) Plexiform neurofibroma in neurofibromatosis. Am J Radiol 144: 1300–1302.

Allanson JE, Hall JG, Van Allen MI (1985) Noonan phenotype associated with neurofibromatosis. Am J Med Genet 21: 457–462.

Allanson JE, Upadhyaya M, Watson GH, Partington M, MacKenzie A, Lahey D, MacLeod H, Sarfarazi M, Broadhead W, Harper PS, Huson SM (1991) Watson syndrome: is it a subtype of type 1 neurofibromatosis? J Med Genet 28: 752–756.

Alwan S, Tredwell SJ, Friedman JM (2005) Is osseous dysplasia a primary feature of neurofibromatosis 1 (NF1)? Clin Genet 67: 378–390.

Anagnostouli M, Piperingos G, Yapijakis G, Gourtzetidis P, Balafouta S, Zournas C Vassilopoulos D, Koutras D, Papageorgiou C (2002) Thyroid gland neurofibroma in a NF 1 patient. Acta Neurol Scand 106: 58–61.

Andersen LB, Ballester R, Marchuk DA, Chang E, Gutmann DH, Saulino AM, Camonis J, Wigler M, Collins FS (1993) A conserved alternative splice in the von Recklinghausen neurofibromatosis (NF1) gene produces two neurofibromin isoforms, both of which have GTPase-activating protein activity. Mol Cell Biol 13: 487–495.

Ars E, Kruyer H, Gaona A, Casquero P, Rosell J, Volpini V, Serra E, Lazaro C, Estivill X (1998) A clinical variant of neurofibromatosis type 1: familial spinal neurofibromatosis with a frameshift mutation in the NF1 gene. Am J Hum Genet 62: 834–841.

Ars E, Serra E, Garcia J, Kruyer H, Gaona A, Lazaro C, Estivill X (2000a) Mutations affecting mRNA splicing are the most common molecular defects in patients with neurofibromatosis type 1. Hum Mol Genet 9: 237–247.

Ars E, Serra E, De la Luna S et al. (2000b) Cold shock induces the insertion of a cryptic exon in the neurofibromatosis type 1 (NF1) mRNA. NAR 28: 1307–1312.

Artaza T, Garcìa JF, Gonzalez C, Amengual M, Mazarro A, Rodrìguez R (1999) Simultaneous involvement of the jejunum and the colon by type 1 neurofibromatosis. Scan J Gastroenterol 34: 331–334.

Arun D, Gutmann DH (2004) Recent advances in neurofibromatosis type 1. Curr Opin Neurol 17: 101–105.

Atit RP, Crowe MJ, Greenheigh DG, Wenetrup RJ, Ratner N (1999) The Nf1 tumor suppressor regulates mouse skin wound healing, fibroblast proliferation, and collagen deposited by fibroblasts. J Invest Dermatol 112: 835–842.

Babovic-Vuksanovic D, Widemann BC, Dombi E, Gillespie A, Wolters PL, Toledo Tamula MA, O'Neill BP, Fox E, MacDonald T, Beck H, Packer RJ (2007) Phase I trial of pirfenidone in children with neurofibromatosis 1 and plexiform neurofibromas. Pediatr Neurol 36. 293–300.

Bahuau M, Flintoff W, Assouline B, Lyonnet S, Le Merrer M, Prieur M, Guilloud-Bataille M, Feingold N, Munnich A, Vidaud M, Vidaud D (1996) Exclusion of allelism of Noonan syndrome and neurofibromatosis-type 1 in a large family with Noonan syndrome-neurofibromatosis association. Am J Med Genet 66: 347–355.

Bahuau M, Houdayer C, Assouline B, Blanchet-Bardon C, Le Merrer Ml, Lyonnet Sl, Giraud S, Recan D, Lakhdar H, Vidaud Ml, Vidaud D (1998) Novel recurrent nonsense mutation causing neurofibromatosis type 1 (NF1) in a family segregating both NF1 and Noonan syndrome. Am J Med Genet 75: 265–272.

Bahuau M, Pelet A, Vidaud D, Lamireau T, Bail B, Munnich A, Vidaud M, Lyonnet S, Lacombe D (2001) GDNF as a candidate modifier for neurofibromatosis enteric phenotype. J Med Gene 38: 638–643.

Bajenaru ML, Herandez MR, Perry A, Zhu Y, Parada LF, Garbow JR, Gutmann DH (2003) Optic nerve glioma in mice requires astrocyte Nf1 gene inactivation and brain heterozygosity. Cancer Res 63: 8573–8577.

Balestri P, Vivarelli R, Grosso S, Santori L, Farnetani MA, Galluzzi P, Vatti GP, Calabrese F, Morgese G (2003) Malformations of cortical development in neurofibromatosis type 1. Neurology 61: 1799–1801.

Baltrusaitis J (1960) Reveil et prodiges. Le gothique fantastique. Paris: Armand Colin, pp. 105–106, 349, nota 59.

Baralle D, Mattocks C, Kalidas K, Elmslie F, Whittaker J, Lees M, Ragge N, Patton MA, Winter RM, Affrench-Constant C (2003) Different mutations in the NF1 gene are associated with neurofibromatosis-Noonan syndrome (NFNS). Am J Med Genet 119A: 1–8.

Barber JC, Cross IE, Douglas F, Nicholson JC, Moore KJ, Browne CE (1998) Neurofibromatosis pseudogene amplification underlies euchromatic cytogenetic duplications and triplications of proximal 15q. Hum Gen 103: 600–607.

Barkovich AJ (2005) The Phakomatoses. In: Barkovich AJ (ed.) Pediatric neuroimaging. Philadelphia: Lippincott Williams & Wilkins, pp. 245–289.

Baser ME, Friedman JM, Wallace AJ, Ramsden RT, Joe H, Evans DG (2002) Evaluation of clinical diagnostic criteria for neurofibromatosis 2. Neurology 59: 1759–1765.

Bass JC, Korobkin M, Francis IR, Ellis JH, Cohan RH (1994) Retroperineal plexiform neurofibromas: CT findings. A J Radiol AJR 163: 617–620.

Basu TN, Gutmann DH, Fletcher JA, Glover TV, Collins FS, Downward J (1992) Aberrant regulation of ras proteins in malignant tumor cells from type 1 neurofibromatosis patients. Nature 356: 713–715.

Baujat B, Krastinova-Lolov D, Blumen M, Baglin AC, Coquille F, Chabolle F. (2006) Radiofrequency in the treatment of craniofacial plexiform neurofibromatosis: a pilot study. Plast Reconstr Surg 117: 1261-1268.

Bergin DJ, Johnson TE, Spencer WH, McCord D (1988) Ganglioglioma of the optic nerve. Am J Ophthalmol 105: 146–149.

Bernards A, Snijders AJ, Hannigan GE, Murthy AE, Gusella JF (1993) Mouse neurofibromatosis type 1 cDNA sequence reveals high degree of conservation of both coding and non-coding mRNA segments. Hum Mol Genet 2: 645–650.

Berner JM, Sorile T, Mertons F, Henriksen J, Saeter G, Mandahl N, Brogger A, Myklebost O, Lothe RA (1999) Chromosome band 9p21 is frequently altered in malignant peripheral nerve sheath tumors: studies of CDKN2A and other genes of the pRB pathway. Genes Chromosomes Cancer 26: 151–160.

Bertholon J, Wang Q, Galmarin C, Puisieux A (2006) Mutational targets in colorectal cancer cells with microsatellite instability. Fam Can 5: 29–34.

Bertola DR, Pereira AC, Passetti F, de Oliveira PS, Messiaen L, Gelb BD, Kim CA, Krieger JE (2005)

Neurofibromatosis-Noonan syndrome: molecular evidence of the concurrence of both disorders in a patient. Am J Med Genet A136: 242–245.

Birch R (1993) Peripheral nerve tumors. In: Dyck PJ, Thomas RK (eds.) Peripheral nerve tumors. Philadelphia: WB Saunders, pp. 1623–1640.

Blatt J, Jaffe R, Deutsch M, Adkins JC (1986) Neurofibromatosis in childhood tumours. Cancer 57: 1225–1229.

Bodhey NK, Gupta AK (2006) Neurofibromatosis type I with occipital encephalocele. Neurol India 54: 103-104.

Bognanno JR, Edwards MK, Lee TA, Dunn DW, Roos KL, Klatte EC (1988) Cranial MR imaging in neurofibromatosis. Am J Roentgenol 151: 381–388.

Bollag G, Clapp DW, Shih S, Adler F, Zhang YY, Thompson P, Lange BJ, Freedman MH, McCormick F, Jacks T, Shannon K (1995) Loss of NF1 results in activation of the Ras signalling pathway and leads to aberrant growth in growth heamatopoietic cells. Nature 12: 144–148.

Boltshauser E, Stocker H, Machler M (1989) Neurofibromatosis type 1 in a child of a parent with segmental neurofibromatosis (NF–5). Neurofibromatosis 2: 244–245

Boulanger JM, Larbrisseau A (2005) Neurofibromatosis type 1 in a pediatric population: Ste-Justine's experience. Can J Neurol Sci 32: 225–231.

Boyanapalli M, Lahoud OB, Messiaen L, Kim B, Anderle de Sylor MS, Duckett SJ, Somara S, Mikol DD (2006) Neurofibromin binds to caveolin-1 and regulates ras, FAK, and Akt. Biochem Biophys Res Commun 24(340): 1200–1208.

Broniscer A, Gajjar A, Bhargava R, Langston JW, Heideman R, Jones D (1997) Brain stem involvement in children with neurofibromatosis type 1: role of magnetic resonance imaging and spectroscopy in the detection from diffuse pontine glioma. Neurosurgery 40: 331–338.

Brunner H, Stacher G, Bankl H, Grabner G (1974) Chronic mesenteric arterial insufficiency caused by vascular neurofibromatosis. Am J Gastroenterol 62: 442–447.

Brunner HG, Hulsebos T, Steijlen PM, der Kinderen DJ, van den Steen A, Hamel BCJ (1993) Exclusion of the neurofibromatosis 1 locus in a family with inherited cafe-au-lait spots. Am J Med Genet 46:472–474.

Brzowski AE, Bazan C, Mumma JV, Ryan SG (1992) Spontaneous regression of optic glioma in a patient with neurofibromatosis. Neurology 42: 679–681.

Burgdorf WH, Zelger B (2004) JXG, NF1, and JMML: alphabet soup or a clinical issue? Pediatr Dermatol 21: 174–176.

Cakirer S, Karaarslan E (2004) Spontaneous involution of a non-optic astrocitoma in neurofibromatosis type 1: serial magnetic resonance imaging evaluation. Acta Radiol 45: 669–673.

Cambiaghi S, Restano L, Caputo R (2004) Juvenile xanthogranuloma associated with neurofibromatosis 1: 14 patients without evidence of hematologic malignancies. Pediatr Dermatol 21: 97–101.

Cappione AJ, French BL, Skuse GR (1997) A potential role for NF1 *m*RNA editing in the pathogenesis of NF1 tumors. Am J Hum Genet 60: 305–312.

Caprotti E (1980) Mostri. Draghi e Serpenti nelle Xilografie di Ulisse Aldrovandi e dei suoi Contemporanei. Milano: Mazzotta.

Carella A, Medicamento N (1997) Malignant evolution of presumed benign lesions in the brain in neurofibromatosis: case report. Neuroradiology 39: 639–641.

Carey JC (1998) Neurofibromatosis-Noonan syndrome. Am J Med Genet 75: 263–264.

Carey JC, Stevenson DA, Ota M, Neil S, Viskochil DH (1997) Is there an NF/Noonan syndrome: Part 2. Documentation of the clinical and molecular aspects of an important family. Proc Greenwood Genet Center 17: 152–153 (Abstract).

Carmi D, Shohat M, Meztker A, Dickerman Z (1999) Growth, puberty and endocrine functions in patients with sporadic or familial neurofibromatosis type 1: A longitudinal study. Pediatrics 103: 1257–1262.

Castillo M, Green C, Kwock L, Smith K, Wilson D, Schiro S, Greenwood R (1995) Proton M spectroscopy in patients with neurofibromatosis type 1: evaluation of hamartomas and clinical correlation. Am J Neuroradiol 16: 141–147.

Castle B, Baser ME, Huson SM, Cooper DN, Upadhyaya M (2003) Evaluation of genotype-phenotype correlations in neurofibromatosis type 1. J Med Genet 40: e109.

Ceard J (1971) Ambroise Parè. Des Monstres et prodiges. Edition critique e commentèe. Geneve: Librairie Droz: p. 101.

Chaglassian JH, Riseborough EJ, Hall JE (1976) Neurofibromatous scoliosis: natural history and results of treatment in thirty-seven cases. J Bone Joint Surg 58A: 695–702.

Chang BC, Mirabella G, Yagev R, Banh M, Mezer E, Parkin PC, Westall CA, Buncic JR (2007) Screening and diagnosis of optic pathway gliomas in children with neurofibromatosis type 1 by using sweep visual evoked potentials. Invest Ophthalmol Vis Sci 48: 2895–2902.

Chang BS, Apse KA, Caraballo R, Cross JH, Mclellan A, Jacobson D, Valente KD, Barkovich AJ, Walsh A (2006) A familial syndrome of unilateral polymicrogyria affecting the right hemisphere. Neurology 66: 133–135.

Chang-Lao M (1977) Laryngeal involvement in von Recklinghausen's disease: a case report and review of the literature. Laryngoscope 87: 435–442.

Chapman CA, Waber DP, Bassett N, Urion DK, Korf BR (1996) Neurobehavioral profiles of children with neurofibromatosis 1 referred for learning disabilities are sex-specific. Am J Med Genet Neuropsychiatric Genetics 67: 127–132.

Charrow J, Listernick R, Ward K (1993) Autosomal dominant multiple cafe-au-lait spots and neurofibromatosis-1: evidence of non-linkage. Am J Med Genet 45: 606–608.

Chen PC, Ball WS, Towbin RB (1989) Aggressive fibromatosis of the tongue: MR demonstration. J Comp Assist Tomogr 13: 343–345.

Choulant L (1963) Grapische Incunabeln fr Naturgeschichte und Medizin. Leipzig, 1858, reprinted Hildesheim: Georg Olms, p. 113.

Chow LT, Shum BS, Chow WH (1993) Intrathoracic vagus nerve neurofibroma and sudden death in a patient with neurofibromatosis. Thorax 48: 298–299.

Cichowski K, Shih TS, Schmitt E, Santiago S, Reilly K, McLaughlin ME, Bronson RT, Jacks T (1999) Mouse models of tumor development in neurofibromatosis type 1. Science 286: 2172–2176.

Cichowski K, Jacks T (2001) NF1 tumor suppressor gene function: narrowing the GAP. Cell 104: 593–604.

Cichowski K, Santiago S, Jardim M, Johnson BW, Jacks T (2003) Dynamic regulation of the Ras pathway via proteolysis of the NF1 tumor suppressor. Genes Dev 17: 449–454.

Clark M, Neville BG (2008) Familial and genetic associations in Worster-Drought syndrome and perisylvian disorders. Am J Med Genet A 146: 35-42.

Clausen N, Andersson P, Tommerup N (1989) Familial occurrence of neuroblastomas, von Recklinghausen's neurofibromatosis, Hirschprum's agangliosis and Jawwinking syndrome. Acta Pediatr Scan 78: 736–741.

Clementi M, Battistella PA, Rizzi L, Boni S, Tenconi R (1996) Headache in patients with neurofibromatosis type 1. Headache 36: 10.

Cnossen MH, Stam EN, Cociman LCMG, Simonz HJ, Stroink H, Oranje AP, Halley DJ, de Goede-Bolder A, Niermeijer MF, de Muinck Keizer-Schrama SM (1997) Endocrinologic disorders and optic pathway gliomas in children with neurofibromatosis type 1. Pediatrics 100: 667–670.

Cnossen MH, de Goede-Bolder A, van den Broek KM, Waasdorp CME, Oranje AP, Stroink H, Simonsz HJ, van den Ouweland AM, Halley DJ, Niermeijer MF (1998a) A prospective 10 years follow-up study of patients with neurofibromatosis type 1. Arch Dis Child 78: 408–412.

Cnossen MH, Moon KGM, Garssen MPJ, Pasmans NM, de Goede-Bolder A, Niermeijer MF, Grobbee DE (1998b) Minor disease features in neurofibromatosis

type 1 (Nf1) and their possible value in diagnosis of Nf1 children <6 years and clinically suspected of having Nf1. J Med Genet 35: 624–627.

Colledge L (1930) Two tumors of the peripheral nerves. I. Neurofibromas of the pharynx in the course of von Recklinghausen's disease. J Laryngol Otol 45: 409–410.

Colley A, Donnai D, Evans DGR (1996) Neurofibromatosis/Noonan phenotype: a variable feature of type 1 neurofibromatosis. Clin Genet 49: 59–64.

Colman SD, Williams CA, Wallace MR (1995) Benign neurofibromas in type 1 neurofibromatosis (NF1) show somatic deletions of the NF1 gene. Nat Genet 11: 90–92.

Consoli C, Moss C, Gren S, Balderson D, Cooper DN, Upadhyaya M (2004) Gonosomal mosaicism for a nonsense mutation (R1947X) in an individual with segmental neurofibromatosis type1 (SNF1). J Invest Dermatol 125: 463–466.

Corkill AGL, Ross CF (1969) A case of neurofibromatosis complicated by medulloblastoma, neurogenic sarcoma and radiation-induced carcinoma of thyroid. J Neurol Neurosurg Psychiatr 32: 43–47.

Costa RM, Yang T, Huynh DP, Pulst SM, Viskochil DH, Silva AJ, Brannan CI (2001) Learning deficits, but normal development and tumor predisposition, in mice lacking exon 23a of Nf1. Nat Genet 27: 399–405.

Costa RM, Silva AJ (2002) Molecular and cellular mechanisms underlying the cognitive deficits associated with neurofibromatosis 1. J Child Neurol 17: 622–626.

Costa RM, Federov NB, Kogan JH, Murphy GG, Stern J, Ohno M, Kucherlapati R, Jacks T, Silva AJ (2002) Mechanism for learning deficits in a mouse model of neurofibromatosis type 1. Nature 415: 526–530.

Crawford MJ, Buckler JMH (1983) Optic gliomata affecting twins with neurofibromatosis. Dev Med Child Neurol 25: 370–373.

Crawford AH, Bagamery N (1986) Osseous manifestations of neurofibromatosis in childhood. J Pediatr Orthop 6: 72–88.

Crawford AH, Schorry EK (1999) Neurofibromatosis in children: the role of the orthopaedist. J Am Acad Orthop Surg 7: 217–230.

Crawford AH, Schorry EK (2006) Neurofibromatosis update. J Pediatr Orthop 26: 413–423.

Crèange A, Zeller J, Rostaing-Rigattieri S, Brugieres P, Degos JD, Revuz J, Wolkenstein P (1999) Neurological complications of neurofibromatosis type 1 in adulthood. Brain 122: 473–481.

Crowe FW, Schull WJ, Neel JV (1956) Clinical, pathological, and genetic study of multiple neurofibromatosis. Springfield, III, Charles C Thomas, pp. 1–181.

Cusmai R, CurDe Luca atolo P, Mangano S, Cheminal R, Echenne B (1990) Hemimegalencephaly and neurofibromatosis. Neuropediatrics 21: 179-182.

Czyzyk E, Jozwiak S, Roszkowski M, Schwartz RA (2003) Optic pathway gliomas with and without neuofibromatosis 1. J Child Neurol 18: 471–478.

D'Ambrosio J, Langlais R, YRS (1988) Jaw and skull changes in neurofibromatosis. Oral Surg Oral Med Oral Pathol 66: 391–396.

D'Angelo I, Welti S, Bonneau F, Scheffzek K (2006) A novel bipartite phospholipids-binding module in neurofibromatosis type 1 protein. EMBO reports.

Danglot G, Regnier V, Fauvet D, Vassal G, Kujas M, Bernheim A (1995) Neurofibromatosis 1 (Nf1) mRNAs expressed in the central nervous system are differentially spliced in the 5' part of the gene. Hum Mol Genet 4: 915–920.

Dasgupta B, Gutmann DH (2003) Neurofibromatosis type 1: closing the GAP between mice and men. Curr Opin Genet Dev 13: 20–27.

Dasgupta B, Yi Y, Chen DY, Weber JD, Gutmann DH (2005) Proteomic analysis reveals hyperactivation of the mammalian target of rapamycin pathway in neurofibromatosis 1-associated human and mouse brain tumors. Can Res 5: 2775–2760.

Davies RL (2000) Neurofibromin progress on the fly. Nature 403: 846–847.

DeBella K, Szudek J, Friedman JM (2000) Use of the NIH criteria for diagnosis of NF1 in children. Pediatrics 105: 608–614.

DeClue JE, Papageorge AG, Fletcher JA, Diehl SR, Ratner N, Vass WC, Lowy DR (1992) Abnormal regulation of mammalian p21 Ras contributes to malignant tumour growth in neurofibromatosis type 1. Cell 89: 266–273.

DeClue JE, Heffelfinger S, Benvenuto G, Ling B, Li S, Rul W, Vess WC, Viskochil D, Ratner N (2000) Epidermal growth factor receptor expression in neurofibromatosis type 1-related tumors and NF1 animal models. J Clin Invest 105: 1233–1241.

De Luca A, Bottillo I, Sarkozy A, Carta C, Neri C, Bellacchio E, Schirinzi A, Conti E, Zampino G, Battaglia A, Majore S, Rinaldi MM, Carella M, Marino B, Pizzuti A, Digilio MC, Tartaglia M, Dallapiccola B (2005) NF1 gene mutations represent the major molecular event underlying neurofibromatosis-Noonan syndrome. Am J Hum Genet 77: 1092–1101.

Deniz E, Shimkus GJ, Weller CG (1966) Pelvic neurofibromatosis: localized von Recklinghausen's disease of the bladder. J Urol 96: 906–909.

De Raedt T, Brems H, Wolkenstein P, Vidaud D, Pilotti S, Perrone F, Mautner V, Frahm S, Sciot R, Legius E (2003) Elevated risk for MPNST in NF1 microdeletion patients. Am J Hum Genet 72: 1288–1292.

De Raedt T, Brems H, Lopez-Correa C, Vermeesch JR, Marynen P, Legius E (2004) Genomic organization and evolution of the NF1 microdeletion region. Genomics 84: 346–360.

De Raedt T, Maertens O, Brems H, Heyns I, Sciot R, Majounie E, Upadhyaya M, Speleman F, Messiaen L, Joris R, Vermeesch JR, Legius E (2006) Loss of heterozygosity in neurofibromas: comparison of NF1 microdeletion and non-microdeletion patients. Genes Chromosome Cancer 45: 893–904.

De Smet L, Sciot R, Legius E (2002) Multifocal glomus tumours of the fingers in two patients with neurofibromatosis type 1. J Med Genet 39: e45.

De Winter AE, Moore BD III, Slopis JM, Ater JL, Copeland DR (1999) Brain tumors in children with neurofibromatosis: additional neuropsychological morbidity? Neuro-Oncology: 1: 275–281.

Deux livres de chirurgie (1573) 1. De la generation de l'homme – 2. Des monstres tant terrestres, que marins, aveuc leurs portraits …. Par Ambroise Parè, premier chirurgien du Roy, et iurè a Paris. A Paris, chez Andrè Wechel, ……

DiPaolo DP, Zimmerman RA, Rorke LB, Zackai EH, Bilaniuk LT, Yachnis AT (1995) Neurofibromatosis type 1: pathologic substrate of high signal intensity foci in the brain. Radiology 195: 721–724.

Dorschner MO, Sybert VP, Weaver M, Pletcher BA, Stephens K (2000) NF1 microdeletion breakpoints are clustered at flanking repetitive sequences. Hum Mol Genet 9: 35–46.

Ducatman B, Scheithauer B, Piepgras D, Reiman H, Istrup D (1986) Malignant peripheral nerve sheath tumors: a clinicopathological study of 120 patients. Cancer 57: 2006–2021.

Dugoff L, Sujansky E (1996) Neurofibromatosis type 1 and pregnancy. Am J Med Genet 66: 7–10.

Dulai S, Briody J, Schindeler A, North KN, Cowell CT, Little DG (2007) Decreased bone mineral density in neurofibromatosis type 1: results from a pediatric cohort. J Pediatr Orthop 27: 472–475.

Duman O, Ozdem S, Turkkahraman D, Olgac ND, Gungor F, Haspolat S (2008) Bone metabolism markers and bone mineral density in children with neurofibromatosis type-1. Brain Dev Mar 24 [Epub ahead of print].

Dunn DW (1987) Neurofibromatosis in childhood. Curr Probl Pediatr 17: 451–497.

Duve S, Rakoski J (1994) Cutaneous melanoma in patient with neurofibromatosis: a case report and review of the literature. Br J Dermatol 131: 290–294.

Easton DF, Ponder MA, Huson SM, Ponder BA (1993) An analysis of variation in expression of neurofibromatosis (NF) type 1 (NF1): evidence for modifying genes. Am J Hum Genet 53: 305–313.

Egelhoff JC, Bates DJ, Ross JS, Rothner AD, Cohen BH (1992) Spinal MR findings in neurofibromatosis types 1 and 2. Am J Neuroradiol 13: 1071–1073.

Eisenbarth I, Beyer K, Krone W, Assum G (2000) Toward a survey of somatic mutation of the NF1 gene in benign neurofibromas of patients with neurofibromatosis type 1. Am J Hum Genet 66: 393–401.

Eliason MJ (1986) Neurofibromatosis: implications for learning and behaviour. Dev Behav Pediatr 7: 175–179.

El-Koussy M, Lövbland K-O, Steinlin M, Kiefer C, Schroth G (2002) Perfusion MRI abnormalities in the absence of diffusiön changes in a case of moyamoya-like syndrome in neurofibromatosis type 1. Neuroradiology 44: 938–941.

Enzinger FM, Weis SW (1988) Soft tissue tumors, 2nd ed. St Louis: Mosby, pp. 719–780.

Erbay SA, Oljeski SA, Bhadelia R (2004) Rapid development of optic glioma in a patient with hybrid phakomatosis: neurofibromatosis type 1 and tuberous sclerosis. Am J Neuroradiol 25: 1297–1298.

Evans DG, Baser ME, McGaughran J, Sharif S, Howard E, Moran A (2002a) Malignant peripheral nerve sheath tumours in neurofibromatosis 1. J Med Genet 39: 311–314.

Evans DRG, Baser ME, Mc Gaughran J, Sharif S, Howard E, Moran A (2002b) Malignant peripheral fluorodeoxyglucosa positron emission tomography (FDG PET) in the detection of malignant peripheral nerve sheath tumors arising from within plexiform tumors in neurofibromatosis 1. J Neurol Neurosurg Psychiatry 68: 353–357.

Fahsold R, Hoffmeyer S, Mischung C, Gille C, Ehlers C, Kucukceylan N, Abdel-Nour M, Gewies A, Peters H, Kaufmann D, Buske A, Tinschert S, Nurnberg P (2000) Minor lesion mutational spectrum of the entire NF1 gene does not explain its high mutability but points to a functional domain upstream of the GAP-related domain. Am J Hum Genet 66: 790–818.

Fantes JA, Mewborn SK, Lese CM, Hedrick J, Brown RL, Dyomin V, Chaganti RS, Christian SL, Ledbetter DH (2002) Organisation of the pericentric region o chromosome 15: at least four partial gene copies are amplified in patients with a proximal duplication of 15q. J Med Genet 39: 170–177.

Ferner RE, Chaudhuri R, Bingham J, Cox T, Hughes RAC (1993) MRI in neurofibromatosis 1-the nature and evolution of increased intensity $T_2$ weighted lesions and their relationship to intellectual impairment. J Neurol Neurosurg Psychiatry 56: 492–495.

Ferner RE, Lucas JD, O'Doherty MJ, Hughes RA, Smith MA, Cronin BF, Bingham J (2000a) Evaluation of (18) fluorodeoxyglucose positron emission tomography ((18)FDG PET) in the detection of malignant peripheral nerve sheath tumours arising from within plexiform neurofibromas in neurofibromatosis 1. J Neurol Neurosurg Psychiatry 68: 353–357.

Ferner RE, Lucas JD, O'Doherty MJ, Hughes RAC, Smith MA, Cromin BF (2000b) Evaluation of (18) nerve sheath tumors in neurofibromatosis. J Med Genet 39: 311–314.

Ferner RE, Gutmann DH (2002) International consensus statement on malignant peripheral nerve sheath tumors in neurofibromatosis. Cancer Res 62: 1573–1577.

Ferner RE, Hughes RA, Hall SM, Upadhyaya M, Johnson MR (2004) Neurofibromatous neuropathy in neurofibromatosis 1 (NF1). J Med Genet 41: 837–841.

Ferner RE (2007a) Neurofibromatosis 1. Eur J Hum Genet 15: 131–138.

Ferner RE (2007b) Neurofibromatosis 1 and neurofibromatosis 2: a twenty first century perspective. Lancet Neurol 6: 340–351.

Ferner RE, Huson SM, Thomas N, Moss C, Willshaw H, Evans DG, Upadhyaya M, Towers R, Gleeson M, Steiger C, Kirby A (2007) Guidelines for the diagnosis and management of individuals with neurofibromatosis 1. J Med Genet 44: 81–88.

Finley JL, Dabbs BJ (1988) Renal vascular smooth muscle proliferation in neurofibromatosis. Hum Pathol 19: 107–110.

Finman NL, Yakovac WC (1970) Neurofibromatosis in childhood. J Pediatr 76: 339–346.

Fitzpatrick AP, Emanuel RW (1988) Familial neurofibromatosis hypertrophic cardiomyopathy. Br Heart 60: 247–261.

Friedman JM, Birch PH (1997) Type 1 neurofibromatosis: a descriptive analysis of the disorder in 1728 patients. Am J Med Genet 70: 138–143.

Friedman JM, Birch PH, and the NNFF International Database Participants (1997) Cardiovascular malformations in NF1 (abstract) Am J Hum Genet 61: A98.

Friedman JM, Gutmann DH, MacCollin M, Riccardi V (1999) Neurofibromatosis: phenotype, natural history, and pathogenesis. Baltimore: Johns Hopkins University Press.

Friedrich RE, Giese M, Schmelzle R, Mautner VF, Scheuer HA (2003) Jaw malformations plus displacement and numerical aberrations of teeth in neurofibromatosis type 1: a descriptive analysis of 48 patients based on panoramic radiographs and oral findings. J Craniomaxillofac Surg 31: 1–9.

Fuller CE, Williams GT (1991) Gastrointestinal manifestations of type 1 neurofibromatosis (von Recklinghausen's disease. Histopathology 19: 1–11.

Fuller LC, Cox B, Gardner RJ (1989) Prevalence of von Recklinghausen neurofibromatosis in Dunedin, New Zealand. Neurofibromatosis 2: 278–288.

Gabriele AL, Grifa D, Thomas NS, Ruggieri M, Carella M, Larizza L, Clementi M, Bonioli E, De Luca A, Pavone P, Polizzi A, Origone P, Riva P, Peluso G, Sprovieri T, Patitucci T, Magariello A, Muglia M, Mazzei R, Conforti FL, Augello B, Stanziale P, Muscarella L, Iannetti P, Pascali MP, Bavastrelli M, Dallapiccola B, Upadhyaya M, Quattrone A, Zelante L (2007) Molecular testing in neurofibromatosis type 1 (NF1) : The mutational spectrum, patterns of recurrence and correlations with clinical features in a large cohort of Italian NF1 patients. Hum Mutat (in press).

Gadner H, Haas OA (1992) Experience in pediatric myelodysplastic syndromes. Hematol Oncol Clin North Am 6: 655–672.

Garty BZ, Laor A, Danon YL (1994) Neurofibromatosis type 1 in Israel: survey of young adults. J Med Genet 31: 853–857.

Garvey M, Packer RJ (1996) An integrated approach to the treatment of chiasmatic-hypothalamic gliomas. 28: 167–183.

Gasparini P, Grifa A, Origone P, Coviello D, Antonacci R, Rocchi M (1993) Detection of a neurofibromatosis type 1 homologous sequence by PCR: implications for the diagnosis and screening of genetic disease. Mol Cell Probes 7: 415–418.

Gervanasini C, Bentivegna A, Venturin M, Corrado L, Larizza L, Riva P (2002) Tandem duplication of the NF1 gene detected by high-resolution FISH in the 17q11.2 region. Hum Genet 110(4): 314–321.

Gilberg C, Forsell C (1984) Childhood psychosis and neurofibromatosis more than a coincidence. J Autism Dev Disord 14: 1–8.

Gitler AD, Zhu Y, Ismat FA, Lu M, Yamauchi Y, Parada L, Epstein JA (2003) NF1 has an essential role in endothelial cells. Nat Genet 33: 75–79.

Gorlin R, Cohen MM Jr, Levine M (2005) The neurofibromatoses [NFI Recklinghausen type, NFII acoustic type, other types]. In: Gorlin R, Cohen MM Jr, Levine M: Syndromes of the head and neck. Oxford: Oxford University Press, pp. 392–399.

Greager JA, Reichard KW, Campana JP, Das Gupta TK (1992) Malignant schwannoma of the head and neck. Am J Surg 163: 440–442.

Greene JF, Fitzwater JE, Burgess J (1974) Arterial lesions associated with neurofibromatosis. Am J Clin Pathol 62: 481–487.

Gregory PE, Gutmann DH, Mitchell A, Park S, Boguski M, Jacks T, Wood DL, Jove R, Collins FS (1993) Neurofibromatosis type 1 gene product (Neurofibromin) associates with microtubules. Somat Cell Molec Genet 19: 265–274.

Griebel ML, Redman JF, Kemp SF, Elders MJ (1991) Hypertrophy of clitoral hood: presenting sign of neurofibromatosis in female child. Urology 37: 337–339.

Griffiths AP, White J, Dawson A (1998) Spontaneous hemithorax: a cause of sudden death in von Recklinghausen's disease. Postgra Med J 74: 679–681.

Grill F, Bollini C, Dungl P (2000) Treatment approaches for congenital pseudoarthrosis of tibia: results of the EPOS multicenter study. Eur Paediatr Othopaed Soc J Pediatr Orthop B 9: 75–89.

Guha A, Lau N, Huvar I, Gutmann D, Provian J, Pawson T, Boss G (1996) Ras-GTP levels are elevated in human NF1 peripheral nerve tumours. Oncogene 12: 507–513.

Guillamo JS, Créange A, Kalifa C, Grill J, Rodriguez D, Doz F, Barbarot S, Zerah M, Sanson M, Bastuji-Garin S, Wolkenstein P; RÈseau NF France (2003) Prognostic factors of CNS tumours in neurofibromatosis 1 (NF1). A retrospective study of 104 patients. Brain 126: 152–160.

Guo HF, The I, Hannan F, Bernards A, Zhong Y (1997) Requirement of Drosophila NF1 for activation of adenylyl cyclase by PACAP38-like neuropeptides. Science 276: 795–798.

Guo HF, Tong J, Hannan F, Luo L, Zhong Y (2000) A neurofibromatosis-1-regulated pathway is required for learning in Drosophila. Nature 403: 895–898.

Gupta A, Cohen BH, Ruggieri P, Packer RJ, Phillips PC (2003) Phase I study of thalidomide for the treatment of plexiform neurofibroma in neurofibromatosis 1. Neurology 60: 130–132.

Gurney JG, Shannon KM, Gutmann DH (1996) Juvenile xanthogranuloma neurofibromatosis 1 and juvenile chronic myeloid leukaemia. Arch Dermatol 132: 1390.

Gurujeyalakshmi G, Hollinger MA, Giri SN (1999) Perfenidone inhibits PDGF isoforms in bleomycin hamster model of lung fibrosis at the translational level. Am J Psysiol 276: L311–L318.

Gutmann D, Andersen L, Cole J (1993) An alternatively spliced mRNA in the carboxy terminus of the neurofibromatosis type 1 (NF1) gene is expressed in muscle. Hum Mol Genet 2: 989–992.

Gutman DH, Aynsworth A, Carey JC, Korf B, Marks J, Pyeritz RE, Rubenstein A, Viskochil D (1997) The diagnostic evaluation and multidisciplinary management of neurofibromatosis 1 and neurofibromatosis 2. JAMA 278: 51–57.

Gutman DH (2002) Neurofibromin in the brain. J Child Neurol 17: 592–601.

Gutzmer R, Herbst RA, Mommert S, Kiehl P, Matiaske F, Rütten A, Kapp A, Weiss J (2000) Allelic loss at the neurofibromatosis type 1 (NF1) gene locus is frequent in dermoplastic neurotropic melanoma. Hum Genet 107: 357–361.

Habiby R, Silverman B, Listernick R, Charrow J (1994) Precocious puberty in children with neurofibromatosis type 1. J Pediatr 125: 63–66.

Hagymasi L, Toth M, Szucs N, Rigo J Jr (1998) Neurofibromatosis type 1 with pregnancy associated renovascular hypertension and the syndrome of hemolysis, elevated liver enzymes, and low platelets. Am J Obst Gynecol 179: 272–274.

Hajra A, Martin-Gallardo A, Tarle SA, Freedman M, Wilson-Gunn S, Bernards A, Collins FS (1994) DNA sequences in the promoter region of the NF1 gene are highly conserved between human and mouse. Genomics 21: 649–652.

Hakami MA, Speicher DW, Shiekhattar R (2002) The motor protein kinesin-1 links neurofibromin and merlin in a common cellular pathway of neurofibromatosis. J Boil Chem 277: 36909–36912.

Halliday AL, Sobel RA, Martuza RL (1991) Benign spinal nerve sheath tumours: their occurrence sporadically and in neurofibromatosis types 1 and 2. J Neurosurg 74: 248–253.

Halper J, Factor SM (1984) Coronary lesions in neurofibromatosis associated with vasospasms and myocardial infarction. Am Heart J 108: 420–422.

Hamilton SJ, Allard MF, Friedman JM (2001) Cardiac findings in an individual with neurofibromatosis 1 and sudden death. Am J Med Genet 100: 95–99.

Happle R (1993) Mosaicism in human skin. Understanding the patterns and mechanisms. Arch Dermatol 129: 1460–1470.

Happle R (1997) A rule concerning the segmental manifestation of autosomal dominant skin disorders. Review of clinical examples providing evidence for dichotomous types of severity. Arch Dermatol 133: 1505–1509.

Harber D, Harlow E (1997) Tumour-supressor genes: evolving definitions in the genomic age. Nature Gen 16: 320–332.

Hashemian H (1952) Familial fibromatosis of small intestine. Brit J Surg 40: 346–350.

Hecht F (1989) Recognition of neurofibromatosis before von Recklinghausen. Neurofibromatosis 2: 180–184.

Heimann R, Verhest A, Verschraegen J, Grosjean W, Draps JP, Hecht F (1988) Hereditary intestinal neurofibromatosis. I. A distinctive genetic disease. Neurofibromatosis 1: 26–32.

Hess E (1938) Sarcoma of the prostate and adjacent retrovesical structures. J Urol 40: 629–640.

Hiatt KK, Ingram DA, Zhang Y, Bollag G, Clapp DW (2001) Neurofibromin GTPase-activating protein-related domains restore normal growth in Nf1 −/− cells. J Biol Chem 276(10): 7240–7245.

Hochberg FA, Dasilva AB, Galdabini J, Richardson EP (1974) Gastrointestinal involvement in von Recklinghausen's neurofibromatosis. Neurology 24: 1144–1151.

Hochstrasser H, Boltshauser E, Valavanis A (1988) Brain tumors in children with von Recklinghausen neurofibromatosis. Neurofibromatosis 1: 233–238.

Hoffman HJ, Humphreys RP, Drake JM, Rutka JT, Becker lE, Jenkin D, Greenbery M (1993) Optic pathway/hypothalamic gliomas: a dilemma in management. Pediatr Neurosurg 19: 186–195.

Hoffmeyer S, Nunberg P, Ritter H, Fahsold R, Leistner W, Kaufmann D, Krone W (1998) Nearby stop codons in exons of the neurofibromatosis type 1 gene are disparate splice effectors. Am J Hum Genet 62: 269–277.

Holt JF (1977) Neurofibromatosis in children. Edward BD Neuhaser lecture. Am J Radiol 130: 615–639.

Hoo JJ, Shrimpton AE (2005) Familial hyper- and hypopigmentation with age-related pattern change. Am J Med Genet 132A: 215–218.

Hope DG, Mulvihill JJ (1981) Malignancy in neurofibromatosis. Adv Neurol 29: 33–36.

Horan M, Cooper DN, Upadhyaya M (2001) Site-specific methylation of the neurofibromatosis type 1 gene promoter bis rarely involved in *NF1* gene inactivation in NF1-specific tumours. Hum Genet 107: 33–39.

Horan M, Osborm M, Cooper DN, Upadhyaya M (2004) Functional analysis of polymorphic variation within the promoter and 5' untranslated region of the neurofibromatosis type 1 (NF1) gene. Am J Med Genet 131A: 227–231.

Horwich A, Riccardi VM, Francke U (1983) Aqueductal stenosis leading to hydrocephalus – an unusual manifestation of neurofibromatosis. Am J Med Genet 14: 577–581.

Hosoda K, Kanazawa Y, Tanaka J, Tamaki N, Matsumoto S (1986) Neurofibromatosis presenting with aqueductal stenosis due to a tumor of the aqueduct: case report. Neurosurgery 19: 1035–1037.

Hoyt WF, Baghdassarian SA (1969) Optic glioma of childhood: natural history and rationale for conservative management. Br J Ophthalmol 53: 793–798.

Hrban RH, Shiu MH, Senie RT, Woodrun JM (1990) Malignant peripheral nerve sheath tumours of the buttockand lower extremity. A study of 43 cases. Cancer 66: 1253–1265.

Hsueh YP, Roberts AM, Volta M, Sheng M, Roberts RG (2001) Bipartite interaction between neurofibromatosis type I protein (neurofibromin) and syndecan transmembrane heparan sulfate proteoglycans. J Neurosci 21: 3764–3770.

Hulsebos TJ, Bijleveld EH, Riegman PH, Smink LJ, Dumham I (1996) Identification and characterisation of NF1-related loci on human chromosomes 22, 14 and 2. Hum Gemet 98: 7–11.

Huson SM, Harper PS, Compston DAS (1988) Von Recklinghausen neurofibromatosis: a clinical and population study in southeast Wales. Brain 111: 1355–1381.

Huson SM (1989) Recent developments in the diagnosis and management of neurofibromatosis type 1. Arch Dis Child 64: 745–749.

Huson SM, Compston DAS, Harper PS (1989a) A genetic study of von Recklinghausen neurofibromatosis in southeast Wales. 1: Guidelines for genetic counselling. J Med Genet 26: 712–721.

Huson SM, Compston DAS, Clark P, Harper PS (1989b) A genetic study of von Recklinghausen neurofibromatosis in south east Wales. I. Prevalence, fitness, mutation rate, and effect of parental transmission on severity. J Med Genet 26: 704–711.

Huson SM (1994) Neurofibromatosis 1: a clinical and genetic overview. In: Huson SM, Hughes RAC (eds.) The neurofibromatosis: a pathogenic and clinical overview. London. Chapman and Hall Medical: 160–204.

Huson SM, Hughes RAC (1994) The neurofibromatoses: pathogcnetic and clinical overview. London: Chapman & Hall.

Huson SM, Ruggieri M (2006) The neurofibromatoses. In: Harper J, Oranje JM, Rose M (eds.) Textbook of paediatric dermatology. Oxford: Blackwell Science Publishers, pp. 1345–1385.

Il Teatro della Natura di Ulisse Aldrovandi (2001) Bologna: Editrice Compositori.

Illes T, Halmai V, de Jonge T, Dubousset J (2001) Decreased bone mineral density in eurofibromatosis-1 patients with spinal deformities. Osteoporos Int 12: 823–827.

Ingordo V, D'Andria G, Mendicini S, Grecucci M, Baglivo A (1995) Segmental neurofibromatosis: is it uncommon or underdiagnosed? Arch Dermatol 131: 959–960.

Ingram DA, Yang FC, Travers JB, Wenning MJ, Hiott K, New S, Hood A, Shannon K, Williams DA, Clapp DW (2001) Genetic and biochemical evidence that haploinsufficiency of the NF1 tumor suppressor gene modulates melanocyte and mast cell fates in vivo. J Exp Med 191: 181–188.

Ishkanian AS, Malloff CA, Watson SK, DeLeeuw RJ, Chi B, Snijders A, Albertson DG, Pinkel D, Marra MA, Ling V, MacAuley C, Lew WL (2004) A tiling resolution DNA microarray with complete coverage of the human genome. Nat Gen 36: 299–303.

Izawa I, Tamaki N, Saya H (1996) Phosphorylation of neurofibromatosis type 1 gene product (neurofibromin) CAMP-dependent protein kinase. FEBS Lett 382: 53–59.

Jacks T, Shih TS, Schmitt EM, Bronson RT, Bernards A, Weinberg RA (1994) Tumor predisposition in mice heterozygous for a targeted mutation in Nf1. Nat Genet 7: 353–361.

Jacquemin C, Bosley TM, Liu D, Svedberg H, Buhalique A (2002) Reassessment of sphenoid dysplasia associated with neurofibromatosis type 1. Am J Neuroradiol 23: 644–648.

Jadayel D, Fain O, Upadhyaya M, Ponder MA, Huson SM, Carrey J, Fryer A, Mathew CGP, Barker DF, Ponder BAJ (1990) Paternal origin of new mutations in von Recklinghausen neurofibromatosis. Nature 343: 558–559.

Jamieson CR, van der Burgt I, Brady AF, van Reen M, Elsawi MM, Hol F, Jeffery S, Patton MA, Mariman E (1994) Mapping a gene for Noonan syndrome to the long arm of chromosome 12. Nature Genet 8: 357–360.

Johannessen CM, Reczek EE, James MF, Brems H, Legius E, Cichowski K (2005) The NF1 tumor suppressor critically regulates TSC2 and mTOR. PNAS 102: 8573–8580.

John A, Ruggieri M, Ferner R, Upadhyaya M (2000) A search for evidence of somatic mutation of the NF1 gene. J Med Genet 37: 44–49.

Johnson MR, Ferner RE, Bobrow M, Hughes RA (2000) Detailed analysis of the oligodendrocyte myelin glycoprotein gene in four patients with neurofibromatosis 1 and primary progressive multiple sclerosis. J Neurol Neurosurg Psychiatry 68: 643–646.

Kaefer M, Adams MC, Rink RC, Kaeting MA (1997) Principles in management in complex pediatric genitourinary plexiform neurofibroma. Urology 49: 936–940.

Kato M, Takashima S, Houdou S, Miyahara S (1995) Cerebellar leptomeningeal astroglial heterotopia in neurofibromatosis type 1. Clin Neuropathol 14: 175-178.

Kaufmann D, Muller R, Bartelt B, Wolf M, Kunzi-Rapp K, Hanemann CO, Fahsold R, Hein C, Vogel W, Assum G (2001) Spinal neurofibromatosis without cafe-au-lait macules in two families with null mutations of the NF1 gene. Am J Hum Genet 69: 1395–1400.

Kaufmann D, Muller R, Kenner O, Leistner W, Heim C, Vogel W, Bartlett B (2002) The N-terminal splice product NF1-10a-2 of the NF1 codes for a transmembrane segment. Biochim Biophys Res Commun 294: 496–503.

Kayes LM, Burke W, Riccardi VM, Bennet R, Ehrlich P, Rubenstein A, Stephens K (1994) Deletions spanning the neurofibromatosis 1 gene: identification and phenotype of five patients. Am J Hum Genet 54: 424–436.

Kearse WS Jr, Ritchey ML (1993) Clitoral enlargement secondary to neurofibromatosis. Clin Pediatr 32: 303–304.

Kedar A (1997) Chemotherapy for pediatric brain tumors. Semin Pediatr Neurol 4: 320–332.

Kehrer-Sawatzki H, Schwickardt T, Assum G, Rocchi M, Krone W (1997) A third neurofibromatosis type 1 pseudogene at chromosome 15q11.2. Hum Genet 100: 595–600.

Kehrer-Sawatzki H, Assum G, Hameister H (2002) Molecular characterisation of t(17; 22)(q11.2; q11.2) is not consistent with NF1 gene duplication. Hum Genet 111: 465–467.

Kehrer-Sawatzki H, Tinschert S, Jenne DE (2003) Heterogeneity of breakpoints in constitutional deletions of the 17q11.2 NF1 tumour suppressor region. J Med Gen 40: 116.

Kehrer-Sawatzki H, Kluwe L, Sandig C, Kohn M, Wimmer M, Krammer U, Peyrl A, Jenne DE, Hansmann I, Mautner VF (2004) High Frequency of Mosaicism among Patients with Neurofibromatosis Type 1 (NF1) with Microdeletions Caused by Somatic Recombination of the *JJAZ1* Gene. Am J Hum Genet 75: 410–423.

Keller RT, Logan GM Jr (1977) Adenocarcinoma of the pancreas associated with neurofibromatosis. Cancer 39: 1264–1266.

King AA, De Baun MR, Riccardi VM, Gutmann DH (2000) Malignant peripheral nerve sheath tumors in neurofibromatosis 1. Am J Hum Genet 93: 388–392.

Kirsch M, Strasser J, Allende R, Bello L, Zhang JMP (1998) Angiostatin suppresses malignant glioma growth in vivo. Cancer Res 58: 4654–4659.

Kluwe L, Friedrich RE, Peiper M, Friedman J, Mautner VF (2003) Constitutional NF1 mutations in neurofibromatosis 1 patients with malignant peripheral nerve sheath tumors. Hum Mutat 22: 420.

Korf BR (2002a) Clinical features and pathobiology of neurofibromatosis 1. J Child Neurol 17: 573–577.

Korf BR (2002b) Determination of end points for treatment of neurofibromatosis 1. J Child Neurol 17: 642–645.

Korf BR, Rubinstein A (2005) Neurofibromatosis type 1. A handbook for patients, families and health care professionals. Berlin: Thieme Publishing Group.

Kornreich L, Blaser S, Schwarz M, Shuper A, Vishne TH, Cohen IJ, Faingold R, Michovitz S, Koplewitz B, Horev G (2001) Optic pathway glioma: correlation of imaging findings with the presence of neurofibromatosis. Am J Neuroradiol 22: 1963–1969.

Kousseeff BG, Hoover DL (1999) Penile neurofibromas. Am J Med Genet 87: 1–5.

Kuenzle C, Weissert M, Roulet E, Bode H, Schefer S, Huisman T, Landau K, Boltshauser E (1994) Follow-up of optic pathway gliomas in children with neurofibromatosis type 1. Neuropediatrics 25: 295–300.

Kulkantrakorn K, Geller TJ (1999) Seizures in neurofibromatosis type 1(NF1). Ped Neurol 19: 347–350.

Kuorilehto T, Poyhonen M, Bloigu R, Heikkinen J, Vaananen K, Peltonen J (2005) Decreased bone mineral density and content in neurofibromatosis type 1: lowest local values are located in the load-carrying parts of the body. Osteoporos Int 16: 928–936.

Kurien A, John PR, Mildford DV (1997) Hypertension secondary to progressive vascular neurofibromatosis. Arch Dis Child 76: 454–455.

Kurtz A, Martuza RL (2002) Antiangiogenesis in Neurofibromatosis 1. J Child Neurol 17: 578–584.

Labardini MM, Kallet HA, Cerny JC (1968) Urogenital neurofibromatosis simulating an intersex problem. J Urol 98: 627–632.

Lamlum H, Ilyas M, Rowan A, Clark S, Johnson V, Bell J, Frayling I, Efstathiou J, Pack K, Payne S, Roylance R, Gorman P, Sheer D, Neale K, Phillips R, Talbot I, Bodmer W, Tomlinson I (1999) The type of somatic mutation at APC in familial adenomatous polyposis is determined by the site of the germline mutation: a new facet to Knudson's 'two-hit' hypothesis. Nat Med 5: 1071–1075.

Lammert M, Kappler M, Mautner VF, Lammert K, Storkel S, Friedman JM, Atkins D (2005) Decreased bone mineral density in patients with neurofibromatosis 1. Osteoporos Int 16: 1161–1166.

Largaespada DA, Brannan CI, Jenkins A, Copeland NG (1996) NF1 deficiency causes Ras-mediated granulocyte/macrophage colony stimulating factor hypersensitivity and chronic myeloid leukaemia. Nat Genet 12: 137–143.

Laue L, Comite F, Hench K, Loriaux L, Cutler GB, Pescovitz GH (1985) Precocious puberty associated with neurofibromatosis and optic gliomas. Am J Dis Child 139: 1097–1100.

Lázaro C, Ravella A, Gaona A, Volpini V, Estiville X (1994) Neurofibromatosis type 1 due to germline mosaicism in a clinically normal father. New Engl J Med 331: 1403–1407.

Lázaro C, Gaona A, Ainsworth P, Tenconi R, Kruyer H, Ars E, Volpini V, Estivill X (1996) Sex differences in mutational rate and mutational mechanism in the NF1 gene in neurofibromatosis type 1 patients. Hum Genet 98: 696–699.

Lederman SM, Martin EC, Laffey KT, Lefkowith JH (1987) Hepatic neurofibromatosis malignant schwannoma and angiosarcoma in von Recklinghausen's disease. Gastroenterology 92: 234–239.

Lee M, Rezai AR, Freed D, Epstein FJ (1996) Intramedullary spinal cord tumours in neurofibromatosis. Neurosurgery 38: 32–37.

Legius E, Marchuk DA, Hall BK, Anderson LB, Wallace MR, Collins FS, Glover TW (1992) NF1-related locus on chromosome 15. Genomics 13: 1316–1318.

Legius E, Merchuk DA, Collins FS, Glover TW (1993) Somatic deletion of the neurofibromatosis type 1 gene in a neurofibrosarcoma supports a tumor suppressor gene hypothesis. Nat Genet 3: 122–126.

Lehman WB, Atar D, Feldman DS (2000) Congenital pseudoarthrosis of the tibia. J Pediatr Orthop B 9: 103–107.

Lehrnebecher T, Gassel AM, Rauh V, Kirchner T, Huppertz HI (1994) Neurofibromatosis presenting a severe systemic vasculopathy. Eur J Pediatr 153: 107–109.

Les Oeuvres d'Ambroise Parè (1585) *Conseiller et premier Chirurgien du Roy. Divisèes en vingt huit Livres. Avec les figures et portraicts, tant de l'Anatomie, que des instruments de Chirurgie, et de plusiers Monstres.....* A Paris, chez Gabriel Buon.

Li Y, Bollag G, Clark R, Stevens J, Conroy L, Fults D, Ward K, Friedman E, Samowitz W, Robertson M, Bradley P, McCormick F, White R, Cawthon R (1992) Somatic mutations in the neurofibromatosis 1 gene in human tumors. Cell 69: 275–281.

Li Y, O'Connell P, Breidenbach HH, Cawthon R, Stevens J, Xu G, Neil S, Robertson M, White R, Viskochil D (1995) Genomic organization of the neurofibromatosis 1 gene (NF1). Genomics 25: 9–18.

Li C, Cheng Y, Gutmann DA, Mangoura D (2001) Differential localization of the neurofibromatosis 1 (NF1) gene product, neurofibromin, with the F-actin or microtubule cytoskeleton during differentiation of telencephalic neurons. Brain Res Dev 130: 231–248.

Li H, Velasco-Miguel S, Vass WC, Parada LF, DeClue JE (2002) Epidermal growth factor receptor signaling pathways are associated with tumorigenesis in the Nf1:p53 mouse tumor model. Cancer Res 62: 4507–4513.

Lipton S, Zuckerbrod M (1966) Familial enteric neurofibromatosis. Med Times 94: 544–548.

Listernick R, Charrow J, Greenwald MJ, Sterly NB (1989) Optic gliomas in children with neurofibromatosis type 1. J Pediatr 114: 788–799.

Listernick R, Darling C, Greenwald M, Strauss L, Charrow J (1995) Optic pathway in children. The effect of neurofibromatosis type 1 on clinical manifestations and natural history. J Pediatr 127: 718–722.

Listernick R, Louis DN, Packer RJ, Gutman DH (1997) Optic pathways gliomas in children with neurofibromatosis type 1: consensus statement from the NF1 optic pathway glioma task force. Ann Neurol 41: 143–149.

Listernick R, Charrow J, Gutmann DH (1999) Intracranial gliomas in neurofibromatosis type 1. Am J Med Genet 89: 38–44.

Listernick R, Gutman DH (1999) Tumors of optic pathway: In: Friedman JM, Gutman DH, Mc Collin M, Riccardi VM (eds.) Neurofibromatosis. Phenotype, natural history and pathogenesis. Baltimore and London: The John Hopkins University Press, pp. 203–230.

Listernick R, Mancini AJ, Charrow J (2003) Segmental neurofibromatosis in childhood. Am J Med Genet A 121: 132–135.

Listernick R, Ferner R, Piersall L, Sharig S, Gutmann DH, Charrow J (2004) Late onset optic pathway tumours in children with neurofibromatosis 1. Neurology 63: 1944–1946.

Listernick R, Charrow J (2004a) Knowledge without truth: screening for complications of neurofibromatosis type 1 in childhood. Am J Med Genet 127A: 221–223.

Listernick R, Charrow J (2004b) Neurofibromatosis type 1 in childhood. Adv Dermatol 20: 75–115.

Liu GT, Lessell S (1992) Spontaneous visual improvement in chiasmal gliomas. Am J Ophthalmol 114: 193–201.

Lopez-Correa C, Dorscher M, Brems H, Lazaro C, Clementi M, Upadhyaya M, Dooijes D, Moog U, Kehrer-Sawatzki H, Rutkowski JL, Fryns JP, Marynen P, Stephens K, Legius E (2001) Recombination hotspot in NF1 microdeletion patients. Hum Mol Genet 10: 1387–1392.

Luijten M, Redeker S, van Noesel MM, Troost D, Westveld A, Hulsebos TJ (2000a) Microsatellite instability and promoter methylation as possible causes of NF1 gene inactivation in neurofibromas. Eu J Hum Genet 8: 939–949.

Luijten M, Wang Y, Smith BT, Westerveld A, Smink LJ, Dunham I, Roe BA, Hulsebos TJ (2000b) Mechanism of spreading of highly related neurofibromatosis type 1 (Nf1) pseudogenes on chromosome 2, 14 and 22. Eur J Hum Genet 8: 209–214.

Luijten M, Redeker S, Minoshima S, Shimizu N, Westerveld A, Hulsebos T (2000c) Duplication and transposition of the NF1 pseudogene regions on chromosomes 2, 14, and 22. Hum Gen 109: 109–116.

Luijten M, Fahsold R, Mischung C, Westerveld A, Nürnberg P, Hulsebos TJM (2001) Limited contribution of interchromosomal gene conversion to *NF1* gene mutation. J Med Genet 38: 481–485.

Luria D, Avigad S, Cohen IJ, Stark B, Weitz R, Zaizov R (1997) p[53] mutation as the second event in juvenile chronic myelogenous leukaemia in a patient with neurofibromatosis type 1. Cancer: 2013–2018.

Maertens O, Prenen H, Debiec-Rychter M, Wozniak A, Sciot R, Pauwels P, Wever I, Vermeesch JR, de Raedt T, Paepe A, Speleman F, Oosterom A, Messiaen L, Legius E (2006) Molecular pathogenesis of multiple gastrointestinal stromal tumors in NF1 patients. Human Mol Genet 15: 1015–1023.

Macaluso M, Russo G, Cinti C, Bazan V, Gebbia N (2002) A Ras family genes: an interesting link between cell cycle and cancer. J Cellular Phys 192: 125–130.

MacCollin M, Chiocca EA, Evans DG, Friedman JM, Horvitz R, Jaramillo D, Lev M, Mautner VF, Niimura M, Plotkin SR, Sang CN, Stemmer-Rachamimov A, Roach ES. Diagnostic criteria for schwannomatosis. Neurology 64: 1838–1845.

Madigan P, Masello MJ (1989) Report of a neurofibromatosis-like case: Monstrorum Historia, 1642. Neurofibromatosis 2: 53–56.

Magro G, Piana M, Venti C, Lacagnina A, Ruggieri M (2000) Solitary neurofibroma of the mesentery: report of a case and review of the literature. Pathol Res Pract 196: 713-718.

Mallmann R, Roth FJ (1986) Treatment of neurofibromatosis associated renal artery stenosis with hypertensión by percutaneous transluminal angioplasty. Clin Exp Hypertens 8: 893–899.

Manoli A, Potter RT, Perfetto J, Coleman A (1969) Thoracic manifestations of Recklinghausen's disease. NY State J Med 69: 3014–3018.

Marchuk DA, Saulino AM, Tavakkol R, Swaroop M, Wallace MR, Andersen LB, Mitchell AL, Gutmann DH, Boguski M, Collins FS (1991) cDNA cloning of the type 1 neurofibromatosis gene: complete sequence of NF1 gene product. Genomics 11: 931–940.

Marchuk DA, Tavakkol R, Wallace MR, Brownstein BH, Taillon-Miller P, Fong CT, Legius E, Anderson LB, Glover TW, Collins FS (2001) A yeast artificial chromosome contig encompassing the type 1 neurofibromatosis gene. Genomics 13: 672–680.

Maria B (2002) Neurofibromatosis. J Child Neurol 17: 547–653.

Maris JM, Wiersma SR, Mahgoub N, Thomson P, Geyer J, Hurwitz CG, Lange BJ, Shannon KM (1997) Monosomy 7 myelodysplastic syndrome and other second malignant neoplasms in children with neurofibromatosis type 1. Cancer 79: 1438–1446.

Martin-Gallardo A, Tarle SA, Freedman M, Wilson-Gunn S, Bernards A, Collins FS (1994) DNA sequences in the promoter region of the NF1 gene are highly conserved between human and mouse. Genomics 3: 649–652.

Masip MJ, Esteban E, Alberto C, Menor F, Cortina H (1996) Laryngeal involvement in pediatric neurofibromatosis: a case report and review of the literature. Pediatr Radiol 26: 488–492.

Mautner VF, Friedich RE, von Deimling A, Hagel C, Korf B, Knöfel MT, Wenzel R, Funsterer C (2003) Malignant peripheral nerve sheath tumours in neurofibromatosis type 1: MR1 supports the diagnosis of malignant plexiform neurofibroma. Neuroradiology 45: 618–625.

Mc Donnell CH (1936) Neurofibromatosis of the bladder and prostate. Amer J Surg 34: 90.

Mc Gaughran JM, Harris DI, Donnai D, Teare D, Mc Leod R, Westerbeek R et al. (1999) A clinical study of type 1 neurofibromatosis in north west England. J Med Genet 36: 197–203.

Mc Grath PC, Sloan DA, Schwartz RW, Kenady DE (1998) Advances in the diagnosis and treatment of adrenal tumors. Curr Opin Oncol 10: 52–57.

Mc Keen EA, Bodurtha J, Meadows AT, Douglas EC, Mulvihill JJ (1978) Rhabdomyosarcoma complicating multiple neurofibromatosis. J Pediatr 93: 992–993.

Mcfarlane R, Levin AV, Weksswerg R, Blaser S, Rutka JT (1995) Absence of the greater sphenoid wing in neurofibromatosis type 1: congenital or acquired: case report. Neurosurgery 37: 129–133.

Meadows AT, D'Angio GF, Mike V, Banfi A, Harris C, Jenkin RDT, Schwartz A (1977) Pattern of second malignant neoplasms in children. Cancer 40. 1903–1911.

Meinecke P (1987) Evidence that the neurofibromatosis-Noonan syndrome is a variant of von Recklinghausen neurofibromatosis. Am J Med Genet 26: 741–745.

Menko FH, Kaspers GL, Meijer GA, Claes K, van Hagen JM, Gille JJ (2004) A homozygous MSH6 mutation in a child with cafe-au-lait spots, oligodendroglioma and rectal cancer. Fam Cancer 3: 123–127.

Messiaen L, Callens T, Mortier G, Beysen D, Vandenbroucke I, Van Roy N, Speleman F, Paepe AD (2000) Exhaustive mutation analysis of the NF1 gene allows identification of 955 of mutations and reveals a high frequency of unusual splicing defects. Hum Mut 15: 541–555.

Messiaen L, Riccardi V, Peltonen J, Maertens O, Callens T, Karvonen SL, Leisti EL, Koivunen J, Vandenbroucke I, Stephens K, Poyhonen M (2003) Independent NF1 mutations in two large families with spinal neurofibromatosis. J Med Genet 40: 122–126.

Miller SJ, Li H, Rizvi TA, Huang Y, Johansson G, Bowersock J, Sidani A, Vitullo J, Vogel K, Parysek LM, DeClue JE, Ratner N (2003) Brain lipid binding protein in axon-Schwann cell interactions and peripheral nerve tumorigenesis. Mol Cell Biol 23: 2213–2224.

Molloy PT, Bilaniuk LT, Vaughan SN, Needle MN, Lin GT, Zackai EH, Phillips PC (1995) Brainstem tumors in patients with neurofibromatosis type 1: a distinct clinical entity. Neurology 45: 1897–1902.

Moore BD III, Slopis JM, Jackson FF, De Winter AE, Leeds NE (2000) Brain volume in children with neurofibromatosis type 1. Relation to neuropsychological status. Neurology 54: 914–920.

Morse RP (1999) Neurofibromatosis type 1. Arch Neurol 6: 364–365.

Moss C, Green SH (1994) What is segmental neurofibromatosis? Br J Dermatol 130: 106–110.

Motte J, Billard C, Fejerman N, Sfaello Z, Arroyo H, Dulac O (1993) Neurofibromatosis type 1 and west syndrome: a relatively benign association. Epilepsia 34: 723–726.

Mulvihill JJ (1988) Neurofibromatosis: history, nomenclature, and natural history. Neurofibromatosis 1(2): 124–131.

National Institutes of Health Consensus Development Conference Statement (1988) Neurofibromatosis. Arch Neurol 45: 575–578.

Needle MN, Cnaan A, Dattilo J, Chatten J, Phillips PC, Shochat S, Sutton LN, Vaughan SN, Zackai EH, Zhao H, Molloy PT (1997) Prognostic signs in the surgical management of plexiform neurofibroma – The Children's Hospital of Philadelphia experience, 1974–1994. J Pediatr 131: 678–682.

Negoro M, Nakaya T, Terashima K, Sugita K (1990) Extracranial vertebral artery aneurysm with neurofibromatosis. Neuroradiology 31: 533–536.

North K (1993) Neurofibromatosis type 1: review of the first 200 patients in an Australian clinic. J Child Neurol 8: 395–402.

North K, Cochineas C, Tang E, Fagan E (1994) Optic gliomas in neurofibromatosis type 1: role of evoked potentials. Pediatr Neurol 10: 117–123.

North K (1997) Neurofibromatosis type 1 in childhood. International Review of Child Neurology Series. London: McKeith, pp. 36.

North KN, Riccardi VM, Samango-Sprouse C et al. (1997) Cognitive function and academic performance in neurofibromatosis type 1. Neurology 48: 1121–1127.

North K (2000) Neurofibromatosis type 1. Am J Med Genet (Sem Med Genet) 97: 119–127.

North K, Hyman S, Barton B (2002) Cognitive deficits in neurofibromatosis 1. J Child Neurol 17: 605–612.

Norton KK, Xu J, Gutmann DH (1995) Expression of the neurofibromatosis 1 gene product, neurofibromin, in blood vessels, endothelial cells and smooth muscle. Neurobiol Dis 2: 13–21.

Ogawa A, Watanabe K (1986) Genitourinary neurofibromatosis in a child presenting with enlarged penis and scrotum. J Urol 135: 755–757.

Ogawa T, Mitsukawa T, Ishikawa T, Tamura K (1994) Familial pheochromocytoma associated with von Recklinghausen's disease. Int Med 33: 110–114.

Oguzkan S, Cinbis M, Ayter S, Anlar B, Aysun S (2004) Familial segmental neurofibromatosis. J Child Neurol 19: 392–394.

Opitz JM, Weaver DD (1985) The neurofibromatosis-Noonan syndrome. Am J Med Genet 21: 477–490.

Osborn M, Cooper DN, Upadhyaya M (2001) Molecular analysis of the 5'- flanking region of the neurofibromatosis type 1(NF1) gene: identification of five sequence variants in NF1 patients. Clin Genet 57: 221–224.

Packer RJ, Ater J, Allen J, Phillips P, Geyer R, Nicholson HS, Jakacki R, Kurczynski E, Needle M, Finlay J, Reaman G, Boyett JM (1997) Carboplatin and vincristine chemotherapy for children with newly diagnosed progressive low-grade gliomas. J Neurosurg 86: 747–754.

Packer RJ, Rosser T (2002) Therapy for plexiform neurofibromas in children with neurofibromatosis 1: an overview. J Child Neurol 17: 638–641.

Packer RJ, Gutmann DH, Rubenstein A, Viskochil D, Zimmerman RA, Vezina G, Small J, Korf B (2002) Plexiform neurofibromas in NF1: toward biologic-based therapy. Neurology 58: 1461–1470.

Parazzini C, Triulzi F, Bianchini E, Agnetti V, Conti M, Zanolini C, Maninetti MM, Rossi LN, Scotti G (1995) Spontaneous involution of optic pathway lesions in neurofibromatosis type 1: serial contrast MR evolution. Am J Neurorradiol 16: 1711–1719.

Parizel PM, Martin JJ, Van Vyve M, van den Hauwe L, De Schepper AM (1991) Cerebral ganglioglioma and neurofibromatosis type 1. Case report and review of the literature. Neuroradiology 33: 357–359.

Park VM, Kenwright KA, Sturtevant DB, Pivmick EK (1998) Alternative splicing of exons 29 and 30 in the neurofibromatosis type 1 gene. Hum Genet 103: 382–385.

Parsa CF, Hoyt CS, Lesser RL, Weinstein JM, Strother CM, Muci-Mendoza R, Ramella M, Manor RS, Fletcher WA, Repka MX, Garrity JA, Ebner RN, Monteiro ML, McFadzean RM, Rubtsova IV, Hoyt WF (2001) Spontaneous regression of optic gliomas: thirteen cases documented by serial neuroimaging. Arch Ophthalmol 119: 516–529.

Partington MW, Burggraf GW, Fay JE, Frontini E (1985) Pulmonary stenosis, cafe au lait spots and dull intelligence: the Watson syndrome revisited. (Abstract) Proc Greenwood Genet Center 4: 105.

Pascual-Castroviejo I, Velez A, De la Cruz Medina M, Verdú A, Villarejo F, Pèrez-Higueras A (1986) Neurofibromatosis y tumores del sistema nervioso central. Neurologìa 1: 6–10.

Pascual-Castroviejo I, Verdú A, Román M, De la Cruz-Medina M, Villarejo F (1988) Optic glioma with progressive occlusion of the aqueduct of Sylvius in monozygotic twins with neurofibromatosis. Brain Dev 10: 24–29.

Pascual-Castroviejo I (1992) Complications of neurofibromatosis type 1 in a series of 197 children. In: Fukuyama Y, Suzuki Y, Kamoshita S, Casaer P (eds.) Fetal and perinatal neurology. Basel: Karger, pp. 162–173.

Pascual-Castroviejo I, Martìnez Bermejo A, Lopez Martìn V, Roche C, Pascual-Pascual SI (1994) Optic gliomas in neurofibromatosis type 1 (NF1). Presentation of 31 cases. Neurologia 9: 173–177.

Pascual-Castroviejo I, Pascual-Pascual SI, Viaño J, Martìnez V (2000) Generalized nerve sheath tumors in neurofibromatosis type 1 (NF1). A case report. Neuropediatrics 31: 211–213.

Pascual-Castroviejo I, Pascual-Pascual SI, Rafia S (2001) Tumores. In: Pascual-Castroviejo I (ed.) Neurofibromatosis. Madrid: Escuela Libre Editorial, pp. 133–182.

Pascual-Castroviejo I (2001a) Estenosis del acueducto de Silvio. In: Pascual-Castroviejo I (ed.) Neurofibromatosis. Madrid: Escuela Libre Editorial, pp. 66–70.

Pascual-Castroviejo I (2001b) Sìndrome de dèficit de atención con hiperactividad (SDAHA). In: Pascual-Castroviejo I (ed.) Neurofibromatosis. Madrid: Escuela Libre Editorial, pp. 198–199.

Pascual-Castroviejo I, Cortés P, Fernández-Cuadrado J, De la Flor-Crespo M, Pascual-Pascual SI (2002) Hemangioma cutáneo asociado a hemangioma hepático y neurofibromatosis tipo 1 (NF1). Rev Neurol 34: 652–654.

Pascual-Castroviejo I, Pascual-Pascual SI, Velazquez-Fragua R, Botella P, Viano J. (2007) Familial spinal neurofibromatosis. Neuropediatrics 38: 105–108.

Payne MS, Nadell JM, Lacassie Y, Tilton AH (2003) Congenital glaucoma and neurofibromatosis in a monozygotic twin: case report and review of the literature. J Child Neurol 18: 504–508.

Peltonen J, Jaakola S, Lebwohl M, Renvall S, Risteli L, Virtanen I, Uitto J (1998) Cellular differentiation and expression of matrix genes in type 1 neurofibromatosis. Lab Invest 59: 760–771.

Pennybacker J (1940) Stenosis of the aqueduct of Sylvius. Proc R Soc Med 33: 507–512.

Perez-Grueso FJ (2001) La columna vertebral en la neurofibromatosis. In: Pascual-Castroviejo I (ed.) Neurofibromatosis. Madrid: Escuela Libre Editorial, pp. 113–120.

Perrin RG, Guha A (2004) Malignant peripheral nerve sheath tumors. Neurosurg Clin N Am15: 203–216.

Pierce SM, Barnes PD, Loeffler JS, McGinn C, Tarbell NJ (1990) Definitive radiation therapy in the management of symptomatic patients with optic glioma. Cancer 65: 45–52.

Pilmore HL, Nagara MP, Walker RJ (1997) Neurofibromatosis and renovascular hypertension presenting in early pregnancy. Nephrol Dial Transplant 12: 187–189.

Pohymen M, Leisti EL, Kytola S, Leisti J (1997) Hereditary spinal neurofibromatosis: a rare form of NF1? J Med Genet 34: 184–187.

Pollack IF, Shultz B, Mulvihill JJ (1996) The management of brainstem gliomas in patients with neurofibromatosis 1. Neurology 46: 1652–1660.

Poole MD (1989) Experiences in the surgical treatment of cranio-orbital neurofibromatosis. Br J Plast Surg 42: 155–162.

Pou Serradell A (1983) Hidrocefalia no-tumoral y neurofibromatosis. Rev Neurol 11: 231–255.

Poyhonen M, Leisti EL, Kytola S, Leisti J (1997) Hereditary spinal neurofibromatosis: a rare form of NF1? J Med Genet 34: 184–187.

Poyhonen M (2000) A clinical assessment of neurofibromatosis type 1 (NF1) and segmental NF in Northern Finland. J Med Genet 37: E43.

Pulst SM, Riccardi VM, Fain P, Korenberg JR (1991) Familial spinal neurofibromatosis: clinical and DNA linkage analysis. Neurology 41: 1923–1927.

Purandare S, Cawthon R, Nelson LM, Sawada S, Watkins WS, Ward K, Jorde LB, Viskochil DII (1996) Genotyping of PCR based polymorphisms and linkage-disequilibrium analysis at the NF1 locus. Am J Hum Genet 59: 159–166.

Quattrin T, McPherson E, Putnam T (1987) Vertical transmission of the neurofibromatosis/Noonan syndrome. Am J Med Genet 26: 645–649.

Raffel C, McComb JG, Bodner S, Gilles FE (1989) Benign brainstem lesions in pediatric patients with neurofibromatosis: case report. Neurosurgery 25: 959–964.

Rasmusen SA, Friedman JM (2000) NF1 gene and neurofibromatosis 1. Am J Epidemiol 151: 33–40.

Rasmusen SA, Yang Q, Friedman JM (2001) Mortality in neurofibromatosis 1: an analysis using U.S. death certificates. Am J Hum Genet 68: 1110–1118.

Reilly KM, Tuskan RG, Christy E, Loisel DA, Ledger J, Bronson RT, Smith CD, Tsang S, Munroe DJ, Jacks T (2004) Susceptibility to astrocytoma in mice mutant for *Nf1* and *Trp53* is linked to chromosome 11 and subject to epigenetic effects. PNAS 101(35): 13008–13013.

Riccardi VM (1982) Neurofibromatosis: clinical heterogeneity. Curr Probl Cancer 7: 1–34.

Riccardi VM (1987) Neurofibromatosis. In: Gomez MR (ed.) Neurocutaneous diseases. A practical approach. Stoneham: Butterworths, pp. 11–29.

Riccardi VM (1992) Neurofibromatosis. Phenotype, natural history, and pathogenesis, 2nd ed. Baltimore-London: The Johns Hopkins University Press.

Ricciardone MD, Ozcelik T, Cevher B, Ozdag H, Tuncer M, Gürgey A, Uzunalimoglu O, Cetinkaya H, Tanyeli A, Erken E, Oztürk M (1999) Human MLH1 deficiency predisposes to hematological malignancy and neurofibromatosis type 1. Cancer Res 59: 290–293.

Richetta A, Giustini S, Recupero SM, Pezza M, Carlomagno V, Amoruso G, Calvieri S (2004) Lisch nodules of the iris in neurofibromatosis type 1. J Eur Acad Dermatol Venereol 18: 342–344.

Rink RC, Mitchell MR (1983) Genitourinary neurofibromatosis in childhood. J Urol 130: 1176–1179.

Rodenhiser DI, Andrews JD, Mancini DN, Jung JH, Singh SM (1997) Homonucleotide tracts, short repeats and CpG/CpNpG motifs are frequent sites for heterogeneous mutations in the neurofibromatosis type 1 (NF1) tumour-suppressor gene. Mutat Res 373: 185–195.

Rodriguez FJ, Perry A, Gutmann DH, O'Neill BP, Leonard J, Bryant S, Giannini C (2008) Gliomas in neurofibromatosis type 1: a clinicopathologic study of 100 patients. J Neuropathol Exp Neurol 67: 240–249.

Rosenbaum T, Rosenbaum C, Winner U, Müller HW, Lenard H-G, Hanemann CO (2000) Long-term culture and characterization of human neurofibroma-derived Schwann cells. J Neuro Res 61: 524–531.

Rosser T, Packer RJ (2002) Intracranial neoplasms in children with neurofibromatosis 1. J Child Neurol 17: 630–637.

Rubenstein A, Bader JL, Aron AA, Wallace S (1983) Familial transmission of segmental neurofibromatosis. Neurology 33(Suppl 2): 76 (Abstract).

Ruggieri M (1999) The different forms of neurofibromatosis. Child's Nerv Syst 15: 295–308.

Ruggieri M, Huson SM (1999) The neurofibromatoses. An overview. Ital J Neurol Sci 20: 89–108.

Ruggieri M, Pavone V, De Luca D, Franzò A, Tinè A, Pavone L (1999) Congenital bone malformations in patients with neurofibromatosis type 1. J Pediatr Orthop 19: 301–305.

Ruggieri M, Dárrigo G, Abate M, Distéfano A, Upadhyaya M (2000) Multiple coronary artery aneurysms in a child with neurofibromatosis type 1. Eur J Pediatr 159: 477–480.

Ruggieri M (2001) Mosaic (segmental) neurofibromatosis type 1 (NF1) and type 2 (NF2): no longer neurofibromatosis type 5 (NF5). Am J Med Genet 101: 178–180.

Ruggieri M, Huson SM (2001) The clinical and diagnostic implications of mosaicism in the neurofibromatoses. Neurology 56: 1433–1443.

Ruggieri M, Packer J (2001) Why do benign astrocytomas become malignant in NF1? Neurology 56: 827–829.

Ruggieri M, Polizzi A (2003) From Aldrovandi's Homuncio (1592) to Buffon's girl (1749) and the Wart Man of Tilesius (1793): antique illustrations of mosaicism in neurofibromatosis? J Med Genet 40: 227–232.

Ruggieri M, Pavone P, Polizzi A, Di Pietro M, Scuderi A, Gabriele A, Spalice A, Iannetti P (2004) Ophthalmological manifestations in segmental neurofibromatosis type 1. Br J Ophthalmol 88: 1429–1433.

Ruggieri M, Iannetti P, Polizzi A, La Mantia I, Spalice A, Giliberto O, Platania N, Gabriele AL, Albanese V, Pavone L (2005) Earliest clinical manifestations and natural history of neurofibromatosis type 2 (NF2) in childhood: a study of 24 patients. Neuropediatrics 36: 21–34.

Ruggieri M, Iannetti P, Clementi M, Polizzi A, Incorpora G, Spalice A, Elia M, Gabriele A, Tenconi R, Pavone L (2008) Neurofibromatosis type 1 and infantile spasms (in press).

Ruggieri M, Mastrangelo M, Spalice A, Mariani R, Bottillo I, Torrente I, Iannetti P (2008) A further case of Neurofibromatosis type 1 and polymicrogyria (in press).

Ruggieri M, Upadhyaya M, Pascaul-Castroviejo I (2008) The different forms of neurofibromatosis: update 2008 (in press).

Sabah MM, Cummins RBS, Leader MF, Kay EF (2006) Loss of p16INK4A expression is associated with allelic imbalance/loss of heterozygosity of chromosome 9p21 in microdissected malignant peripheral nerve sheath tumors. Appl Immunohistochem M M 14: 97–102.

Sadun F, Hinton DR, Sadun AA (1996) Rapid growth of optic nerve ganglioglioma in a patient with neurofibromatosis 1. Ophthalmology 103: 794–799.

Sajid MH, Copple PJ (1968) Familial aqueductal stenosis and basilar impression. Neurology 18: 260–262.

Salyer WR, Salyer DC (1974) The vascular lesion of neurofibromatosis. Angiology 25: 510–519.

Samuelson B, Samuelson S (1989) Neurofibromatosis in Gothenburg. Sweden. I. Background, study design and epidemiology. Neurofibromatosis 2: 6–22.

Samuelson B, Riccardi VM (1989) Neurofibromatosis in Gothenburg. Sweden. III. Psychiatric and social aspects. Neurofibromatosis 2: 84–106.

Sarkozy A, Schirinzi A, Lepri F, Bottillo I, De Luca A, Pizzuti A, Tartaglia M, Digilio MC, Dallapiccola B (2007) Clinical lumping and molecular splitting of LEOPARD and NF1/NF1-Noonan syndromes. Am J Med Genet A 143: 1009–1011.

Savasan S, Smith L, Scheer C, Dansey R, Abella E (2005) Successful bone marrow transplantation for life threatening xanthogranuloma disseminatum in neurofibromatosis type-1. Pediatr Transplant 9: 534–536.

Sawada S, Florell S, Purandare SM, Ota M, Stephens K, Viskochil D (1996) Identification of NF1 mutations in both alleles of a dermal neurofibroma. Nat Genet 14: 110–112.

Scheffzek K, Lautwein A, Kabsch W, Ahmadian MR, Wittinghofer A (1999) Crystal structure of the GTPase-activating domain of human p120GAP and implications for the interaction with Ras. Nat 384: 591–596.

Schievink WI, Riedinger M, Maya MM (2005) Frequency of incidental intracranial aneurysms in neurofibromatosis type 1. Am J Med Genet 134A: 45–48.

Schindeler A, Little DG (2008) Recent insights into bone development, homeostasis, and repair in type 1 neurofibromatosis (NF1). Bone 42: 616–622.

Schorry EK, Crawford AH, Egelhoff JC, Lovell AM, Saal HM (1997) Thoracic tumors in children with neurofibromatosis 1. Am J Med Genet (Neuropsychiatr Genet) 74: 533–537.

Segal R (1993) Segmental neurofibromatosis of the sciatic nerve: case report. Neurosurgery. 33: 948.

Serra E, Plug S, Otero D, Gaons A, Kruyer H, Ars E, Estivill X, Lazaro C (1997) Confirmation of a double-hit model for the NF1 gene in benign neurofibromas. Am J Hum Genet 51: 512–519.

Serra E, Rosenbaum T, Winner U, Aldeo R, Ars E, Estivill X, Lenard HG, Lazaro C (2000) Schwann cells harbor the somatic NF1 mutation in neurofibromas: evidence of two Schwann cells subpopulations. Hum Mol Genet 9: 3055–3084.

Serra E, Ars E, Ravella A, Sanchez A, Puig S, Rosenbaum T, Estivill X, Lazaro C (2001a) Somatic NF1 mutational spectrum in benign neurofibromas: mRNA splice defects are common among point mutations. Hum Genet 108: 416–429.

Serra E, Rosenbaum T, Nadal M, Winner U, Ars E, Estivill X, Lazaro C (2001b) Mitotic recombination effects homozygosity for NF1 germline mutations in neurofibromas. Nat Genet 28: 294–296.

Shannon KM, Watterson J, Johnson P, O'Connell P, Lange B, Shah N et al. (1992) Monosomy 7 myeloproliferative disease in children with neurofibromatosis type 1: epidemiology and molecular analysis. Blood 79: 1311–1318.

Shannon KM, O'Connel P, Martin GA, Paderanga D, Olson K, Dinndorf P, McCormick F (1994) Loss of the normal NF1 allele from the bone marrow of children with type 1 neurofibromatosis and malignant myeloid disorders. N Engl J Med 330: 597–601.

Silva AJ, Franckland PW, Marowitz Z, Friedman E, Laszlo GS, Cioffi D, Jacks T, Bourtchuladze R (1997) A

mouse model for the neurological deficits associated with neurofibromatosis type 1. Nature Genet 15: 281–284.

Singh K, Samartzis D, An HS (2005) Neurofibromatosis type I with severe dystrophic kyphoscoliosis and its operative management via a simultaneous anterior-posterior approach: a case report and review of the literature. Spine J 5: 461–466.

Sobata E, Ohkuma H, Suzuki S (1988) Cerebrovascular disorders associated with von Recklinghausen's neurofibromatosis: a case report. Neurosurgery 22: 544–549.

Sorensen SA, Mulvihihill JJ, Nielsen A (1986) Long-term follow-up of von Recklinghausen neurofibromatosis. Survival and malignant neoplasms. N Engl J Med 314: 1010–1015.

Specht CS, Smith TW (1988) Uveal malignant melanoma and von Recklinghausen's neurofibromatosis. Cancer 62: 812–817.

Stay EJ, Vawter G (1977) The relationship between neuroblastoma and neurofibromatosis (von Recklinghausen's disease) Cancer 39: 2250–2255.

Stephens K, Kayes L, Riccardi VM, Rising M, Sybert VP, Pagon RA (1992) Preferential mutation of the neurofibromatosis type 1 gene in paternally derived chromosomes. Hum Genet 88: 279–282.

Stevenson DA, Viskochil DH, Rope AF, Carey JC (2006a) Clinical and molecular aspects of an informative family with neurofibromatosis type 1 and Noonan phenotype. Clin Genet 69: 246–253.

Stevenson DA, Zhou H, Ashrafi S, Messiaen LM, Carey JC, D'Astous JL, Santora SD, Viskochil DH (2006b) Double inactivation of NF1 in tibial pseudoarthritis. Am J Hum Genet 79: 143–148.

Stevenson DA, Moyer-Mileur LJ, Murray M, Slater H, Sheng X, Carey JC, Dube B, Viskochil DH (2007) Bone mineral density in children and adolescents with neurofibromatosis type 1. J Pediatr 150: 83–88.

Suh JS, Abenoza P, Galloway HR, Everson LI, Griffiths HJ (1992) Peripheral (extracranial) nerve tumors: correlation of MR imaging and histology findings. Radiology 183: 341–346.

Sutphen R, Galán-Gómez E, Kousseff BG (1995) Clitoromegaly in neurofibromatosis. Am J Med Genet 55: 325–330.

Suzuki V, Suzuki H, Kayama T et al. (1991) Brain tumours predominantly express NF1 gene transmembrane containing the 63 base in the region coding for GTPase activating protein related domain. Biochem Biophys Res Commun 181: 955–961.

Suzuki H, Takahashi K, Kubota Y, Shibahara S (1992) Molecular cloning of a cDNA coding for neurofibromatosis type 1 protein isoform lacking the domain related to ras GTPase-activating protein. Biochem Biophys Res Commun 187: 984–990.

Suzuki H, Ozawa N, Taga C, Kano T, Hattori M, Sakati Y (1994) Genomic analysis of a NF1-related pseudogene on human chromosome 21. Gene 147: 247–250.

Szudek J, Birch SJ, Friedman JM (2000) The national neurofibromatosis foundation international database participants. Growth in North American white children with neurofibromatosis 1 (NF1). J Med Genet 37: 933–938.

Szudek J, Joe H, Friedman JM (2002) Analysis of intrafamilial phenotypic variation in neurofibromatosis type 1 (NF1). Genet Epidemiol 23: 150–164.

Taboada D, Alonso A, Moreno J, Muro D, Mulas F (1979) Occlusion of the cerebral arteries in Recklinghausen's disease. Neuroradiology 18: 281–284.

Takamiya Y, Friendlander RM, Brem H, Malick A, Martuza RL (1993) Inhibition of angiogenesis and growth of human nerve-sheath tumors by AGM-1470. J Neurosurg 78: 470–476.

Tartaglia M, Mehler EL, Goldberg R, Zampino G, Brunner HG, Kremer H, van der Burgt I, Crosby AH, Ion A, Jeffery S, Kalidas K, Patton MA, Kucherlapati RS, Gelb BD (2001) Mutations in PTPN11, encoding the protein tyrosine phosphatase SHP-2, cause Noonan syndrome. Nat Genet 29: 465–468.

Tartaglia M, Niemeyer CM, Shannon KM, Loh ML (2004a) SHP-2 and myeloid malignancies. Curr Opin Hematol 11: 44–50.

Tartaglia M, Martinelli S, Cazzaniga G, Cordeddu V, Iavarone I, Spinelli M, Palmi C, Carta C, Pession A, Arico M, Masera G, Basso G, Sorcini M, Gelb BD, Biondi A. (2004b) Genetic evidence for lineage-related and differentiation stage-related contribution of somatic PTPN11 mutations to leukemogenesis in childhood acute leukemia. Blood 104: 307–301.

Tashiro K, Nakagawa T, Ito T (1975) An autopsy case of Von Recklinghausen's disease with aqueductal occlusion due to septum formation and gliosis associated with subtentorial cyst formation (in Japanese). No To Shinkei 27: 333–342.

Tega W (2002) Guide to Palazzo Poggi Museum. Science and Art. Bologna: Editrice Compositori, pp. 18–25.

Tenny RT, Laws ER Jr, Younge BR, Rush JA (1982) The neurosurgical management of optic glioma. Results in 104 patients. J Neurosurg 57: 452–458.

The I, Hannigan GE, Cowley GS, Reginald S, Zhong Y, Guesella JF, Harriharan IK, Bernards A (1997) Rescue of a Drosophila NF1 mutant by protein kinase A. Science 276: 791–794.

Thomas PK, King RHM, Chiang TR, Scaravalli F, Sharma AK, Downie AW (1990) Neurofibromatosis neuropathy. Muscle Nerve 13: 93–101.

Thomson PD, Harty YI, Koper D (1992) Neurofibroma of the penis. Urology 40: 555–556.

Thomson SA, Wallace MR (2002) RT-PCR splicing analysis of the NF1 open reading frame. Hum Genet 110: 495–502.

Tilesius von Tilenau WG (1793) Historia pathologica singularis Cutis Turpitudinis: Jo Gondofredi Rheinardi viri Lannorum. Leipzig: Germanny, SL Crusius.

Tinschert W, Holdener EE, Haertel MM, Senn H, Vetter W (1985) Secondary hypertension and neurofibromatosis: bilateral renal artery stenosis and coarctation of the abdominal aorta. Klin Wochens 63: 593–596.

Tinschert S, Naumann I, Stegmann E, Buske A, Kaufmann D, Thiel G, Jenne DE (2000) Segmental neurofibromatosis is caused by somatic mutation of the neurofibromatosis type 1 (NF1) gene. Eur J Hum Genet 8: 455–459.

Tomsick TA, Lukin RR, Chambers AA, Benton C (1976) Neurofibromatosis and intracranial arterial occlusive disease. Neuroradiology 11: 229–234.

Tong J, Hannan F, Zhu Y, Bernards A, Zhong Y (2002) Neurofibromin regulates G protein stimulating adenylyl cyclase activity. Nat Neurosci 5: 95–96.

Tortori-Donati P, Rossi A, Biancheri R, Andreula CF (2005) Phakomatoses. In: Tortori-Donati P (ed.) Pediatric neuroradiology. Brain. Berlin New York: Springer, pp. 763–818.

Tow SL, Chandela S, Miller NR, Avellino AM (2003) Long-term outcome in children with gliomas of the anterior visual pathway. Pediatr Neurol 28: 262–270.

Traub JA, O'Connor W, Masso PD (1999) Congenital pseudoarthrosis of the tibia: a retrospective review. J Pediatr Orthop 19: 735–738.

Tudisco C, Bollini C, Dungel P (2000) Functional results at the end of skeletal growth in 30 patients affected by congenital pseudoarthrosis of the Tibia. J Pediatr Orthop 9: 94–102.

Uhlin SR (1980) Segmental neurofibromatosis. South Med J 73: 526–567.

Upadhyaya M, Sarfarazi M, Broadhead W, Huson SM, Allanson J, Fryer AE, Harper PS (1989) Linkage of Watson's syndrome to chromosome 17 markers. (Abstract) Cytogenet Cell Genet 51: 1094.

Upadhyaya M, Sarfarazi M, Huson S, Broadhead W, Allanson J, Fryer A, Harper PS (1990) Linkage of Watson's syndrome to chromosome 17 markers. (Abstract) J Med Genet 27: 209.

Upadhyaya M, Shen M, Cherryson A, Farnham J, Maynard J, Huson SM, Harper PS (1992) Analysis of mutations at the neurofibromatosis 1 (NF1) locus. Hum Molec Genet 1: 735–740.

Upadhyaya M, Cooper DN (1998a) Neurofibromatosis type 1. From genotype to phenotype. Oxford: Bios Scientific Publishers.

Upadhyaya M, Cooper DN (1998b) The mutational spectrum in neurofibromatosis type 1 and its underlying mechanisms. In: Upadhyaya M, Cooper DN (eds.) NF1: from genotype to phenotype. Oxford: BIOS Publishers.

Upadhyaya M, Shaw DJ, Harper PS (1994) Molecular basis of neurofibromatosis type1 (*NF1*): mutation analysis and polymorphisms in the *NF1* gene. Hum Mutation 4: 83–101.

Upadhyaya M, Ruggieri M, Maynard J, Osborn M, Hartog C, Mudd S, Penttinen M, Cordeiro A, Ponder M, Ponder B, Krawczak M, Cooper DN (1998) Gross deletions of the neurofibromatosis type 1 (NF1) gene are predominantly of maternal origin and commonly associated with a learning disability, dysmorphic features and developmental delay. Hum Genet 102: 591–597.

Upadhyaya M, Majounie E, Thompson P, Han S, Consoli C, Krawczak M, Cordeiro I, Cooper DN (2003) Three different pathological lesions in the NF1 gene originating de novo in a family with neurofibromatosis type 1. Hum Genet 112: 12–17.

Upadhyaya M, Han S, Consoli C, Majounie E, Horan M, Thomas N, Potts C, Griffiths S, Ruggieri M, von Deimling A, Cooper DN (2004) Characterisation of somatic mutational spectrum of neurofibromatosis type 1 (NF1) gene in neurofibromatosis patients with benign and malignant tumours. Hum Mut 23: 134–146.

Upadhyaya M, Spurlock G, Majounie E, Griffiths S, Forrester N, Baser M, Huson SM, Evans G, Ferner R (2006) The heterogeneous nature of germlinemutations in NF1 patients with malignant peripheral nerve sheath tumours (MPNSTs). Hum Mut 27: 716.

Upadhyaya M, Huson SM, Davies M, Thomas N, Chuzhanova N, Giovannini S, Evans DG, Howard E, Kerr B, Griffiths S, Consoli C, Side L, Adams D, Pierpont M, Hachen R, Barnicoat A, Li H, Wallace P, Van Biervliet JP, Stevenson D, Viskochil D, Baralle D, Haan E, Riccardi V, Turnpenny P, Lazaro C, Messiaen L. (2007) An absence of cutaneous neurofibroma associated with a 3-bp in-frame deletion in exon 17 of the *NF1* gene (c.2970_2972 delAAT): Evidence of a clinically significant NF1 genotype-phenotype correlation. Am J Hum Genet 80(1): 140–151.

Vandenbroucke I, Doorn R, Callens, T, Cobben J, Starink T, Messiaen L (2004) Genetic and clinical mosaicism in a patient with neurofibromatosis type 1. Hum Genet 114: 284–290.

Verhest A, Verschraegen J, Grosjean W, Heimann R (1981) Transmissible chromosome abnormality in familial intestinal neurofibromatosis. (Abstract) Sixth Int. Cong. Hum. Genet., Jerusalem, p. 176.

Verhest A, Verschraegen J, Grosjean W, Draps JP, Vamos E, Heimann R, Hecht F (1988) Hereditary intestinal neurofibromatosis. II. Translocation between chromosomes 12 and 14. Neurofibromatosis 1: 33–36.

Viskochil D, Carey JC (1992) Nosological considerations of the neurofibromatosis. J Dermatol 19: 873–880.

Viskochil D, Carey J (1994) Alternate and related forms of neurofibromatosis. In The Neurofibromatoses: A Pathogenic and Clinical Overview. Eds S Huson And R Hughes, Chapman and Hall Medical, p. 445.

Viskochil, DH (1998) Gene structure and function. In Neurofibromatosis Type 1: From Genotype to Phenotype (Upadhyaya, M.A.C., ed.), 39–56, BIOS Scientific Publications Limited.

Vivarelli R, Grosso S, Calabrese F, Farnetani M, Di Bartolo R, Morgese G, Balestri P (2003) Epilepsy in neurofibromatosis 1. J Child Neurol 18: 338–342.

Vogel KS, Klesse LJ, Velasco-Miguel S, Meyers K, Rushing EJ, Parade LF (1999) Mouse tumor model for neurofibromatosis type 1. Science 286: 2176–2179.

Von Deimling A, Krone W, Menon AG (1995) Neurofibromatosis type 1: pathology, clinical features and molecular genetics. Brain Pathol 5: 153–162.

Waldassen FV (1998) Foundation Library. Passau: Peda-Kunstfuhrer.

Wallace MR, Marchuk DA, Andersen LB, Letcher R, Odeh HM, Seulino AM, Fountain JW, Brereton A, Nicholson J, Mitchell AL, et al (1990) Type 1 neurofibromatosis gene: identification of a large transcript disrupted in three NF1 patients. Science 249: 181–186.

Wang Q, Lasset C, Desseigne F, Frappaz D, Bergeron C, Navarro C, Ruano E, Puisieux A (1999) Neurofibromatosis and early onset of cancers in hMLH1-deficient children. Cancer Res 59: 294–297.

Wang Q, Montmain G, Ruano E, Upadhyaya M, Dudley S, Liskay MR, Thibodeau SN, Puisieux A (2003) The neurofibromatosis type 1 gene as a mutational target in mismatch repair-deficient cells. Hum Genet 112: 117–123.

Watson GH (1967) Pulmonary stenosis, cafe-au-lait spots, and dull intelligence. Arch Dis Child 42: 303–307.

Weinberg RA (1991) Tumor suppressor genes. Science 254: 1138–1146.

Whiteside D, McLeod R, Graham G, Steckley JL, Booth K, Somerville MJ, Andrew SE (2002) A homozygous germ-line mutation in the human *MSH2* gene predisposes to hematological malignancy and multiple café-au-lait spots. Cancer Res 62: 359–362.

Widemann BC, Salzer WL, Arceci RJ, Blaney SM, Fox E, End D, Gillespie A, Whitcomb P, Palumbo JS, Pitney A, Jayaprakash N, Zannikos P, Balis FM (2006) Phase I trial and pharmacokinetic study of the farnesyltransferase inhibitor tipifarnib in children with refractory solid tumors or neurofibromatosis type I and plexiform neurofibromas. J Clin Oncol 24: 507–516.

Wiest V, Eisenbarth I, Schmegner C, Krone W, Assum G (2003) Somatic NF1 mutation spectra in a family with neurofibromatosis type 1 toward a theory of genetic modifiers. Hum Mutat 22: 423–427.

Wimmer K, Eckart M, Stadler PF, Rehder H, Fonatsch C (2000) Three different premature stop codons lead to skipping of exon 7 in neurofibromatosis type 1 patients. Hum Mutat 16: 90–91.

Wimmer K, Muhlbauer M, Eckart M, Callens T, Rehder H, Birkner T, Leroy JG, Fonatsch C, Messiaen L (2002) A patient severely affected by spinal neurofibromas carries a recurrent splice site mutation in the NF1 gene. Eur J Hum Genet 10: 334–338.

Wittkower R (1942) Marvels of the East. A study in the history of monsters. Warburg Courtauld Inst 5: 159.

Witzleben CL, Landy RA (1974) Disseminated neuroblastoma in a child with von Recklinghausen disease. Cancer 34: 786–790.

Woodruff JM, Perino G (1994) Non-germ cell or teratomateus malignant tumors showing additional rhabdomyoblastic differentiation, with emphasis on the malignant Triton tumor. Sem Diagn Surg Pathol 11: 69–81.

Woodruff JM (1999) Pathology of tumors of the peripheral nerve sheath in type 1 neurofibromatosis. Am J Med Genet (Sem Med Genet) 89: 23–30.

Wolkenstein P, Mahmoudi A, Zeller J, Revuz J (1995) More on the frequency of segmental neurofibromatosis. Arch Dermatol 131: 1465.

Wolkenstein P, Freche B, Zeller J, Revuz J (1996) Usefulness of screening investigations in neurofibromatosis type 1. A study of 152 patients. Arch Dermatol 132: 1333–1336.

Wu BL, Boles RG, Yaari H, Weremowicz S, Schneider GH, Korf BR (1997) Somatic mosaicism for deletion of the entire NF1 gene identified by FISH. Hum Genet 99: 209–213.

Wullschleger S, Loewith R, Hall MN (2006) TOR signaling in growth and metabolism. Cell 124: 471–484.

Xu GF, O'Connell P, Viskochil DH, Cawthon R, Robertson M, Culver M, Dunn D, Stevens J, Gesteland R, White R, et al (1990a) The neurofibromatosis type 1 gene encodes a protein related to GAP. Cell 62: 599–608.

Xu GF, Lin B, Tanaka K, Dunn D, Wood D, Gesteland R, White R, Weiss R, Tamanoi F (1990b) The catalytic domain of the neurofibromatosis type 1 gene product stimulates ras GTPase and complements ira mutants of S. cerevisiae. Cell 63: 853–841.

Xu GF, Mulligan LM, Ponder MA, Llu L, Smith BA, Mathew CG, Ponder BA (1992) Loss of NF1 alleles in phaeochromocytomas form patients with type 1 neurofibromatosis. Genes Chromosome Cancer 4: 337–342.

Yang KH, Rim H, Cho OK, Ko BH (2002) Segmental colonic involvement of plexiform neurofibroma in neurofibromatosis type 1. J Comp Assist Tomogr 26: 129–131.

Yang FC, Ingram DA, Chen S, Hingtgen CM, Ratner N, Monk KR, Clegg T, White H, Mead L, Wenning MJ, Williams DA, Kapur R, Atkinson SJ, Clapp DW (2003) Neurofibromin-deficiant Schwann cells secrete a potent migratory stimuli for Nf1 +/− mast cells. J Clin Invest 122: 1851–1861.

Yilmaz K, Ozmen M, Bora Goksan S, Eskiyurt N (2007) Bone mineral density in children with neurofibromatosis 1. Acta Paediatr 96:1220–1222.

Yu X, Milas J, Watanabe N, Rao N, Murthy S, Potter OL, Wenning MJ, Clapp WD, Hock JM (2006) Neurofibromatosis type 1 gene haploinsufficiency reduces AP-1 gene expression without abrogating the anabolic effect of parathyroid hormone. Calcif Tissue Int 78: 162–170.

Yüksel H, Odabasi AR, Kalkas S, Omur E, Turgut M (2003) Clitoromegaly in type 2 neurofibromatosis: a case report and review of the literature. Eur J Gynaecol Oncol 24: 447–451.

Yumoto E, Nakamura K, Mori T, Yanagihara N (1996) Parapharyngeal vagal neurilemmoma extending to the jugular foramen. J Laryngol Otol 10: 485–489.

Zanca A, Zanca A (1980) Antique illustrations of neurofibromatosis. Int J Dermatol 19: 55–58.

Zatkova A, Messiaen L, Vandenbroucke I, Wieser R, Fonatsch C, Krainer AR, Wimmer K (2004) Disruption of exonic splicing enhancer elements is the principal cause of exon skipping associated with seven nonsense or missense alleles of NF1. Hum Mut 24: 491–501.

Zhu Y, Ghosh P, Charnay P, Burns DK, Parada LF (2002) Neurofibromas in NF1: Schwann cell origin and role of tumor environment. Science 296: 920–922.

Zlotogora J (1993) Mutations in von Recklinghausen neurofibromatosis: an hypothesis. Am J Med Genet. 46: 182–184.

Zvulunov A, Barak Y, Metzker A (1995) Juvenile xanthogranuloma, neurofibromatosis and juvenile chronic myelogenous leukaemia. World statistical analysis. Arch Dermatol 131: 904–908.

# Chapter 4

# NEUROFIBROMATOSIS TYPE 2 AND RELATED DISORDERS

Scott Randall Plotkin

Department of Neurology, Massachusetts General Hospital and Harvard Medical School, Boston, USA

## Introduction

Neurofibromatosis 1 (NF1), neurofibromatosis 2 (NF2), and schwannomatosis comprise the neurofibromatoses. NF2 (MIM 101000) is an autosomal dominant neurogenetic disorder characterized by the presence of schwannomas, meningiomas, ependymomas, and ocular abnormalities. For many years, NF2 was confounded with the more common syndrome NF1 from which it derives its name. In the 1980's, these two disorders were finally differentiated when tumor studies and linkage analysis localized the genes to different chromosomes. The introduction of gadolinium contrast for MRI scanning in June, 1988, significantly improved detection of small tumors, particularly near the skull base. The cloning of the NF2 gene in 1993 ushered in a period of intense research activity in which mutational analysis was used to establish genotype-phenotype correlations and to study the role of *NF2* inactivation in NF2-associated tumors. More recently, a consortium of hospitals completed the Natural History of Neurofibromatosis Type 2 Study, which prospectively tracked the growth of tumors in patients with NF2. Looking forward, the primary goal of the research community is to identify an effective treatments for patients with NF2.

## Historical perspective and terminology

### Initial clinical description

The first clinical description of NF2 dates to 1822 when the Scottish surgeon J. H. Wishart presented an unusual case to the Royal College of Surgeons of Edinburgh. He described a 21-year-old man with amblyopia and macrocephaly who became deaf at age 19 (Wishart 1822). The patient subsequently developed seizures and was found to have a tumor that protruded from the occipital eminence. An attempt to resect the lesion was unsuccessful and the patient died from a wound infection. At autopsy, multiple tumors arising from the skull base were identified. His description of a severely affected patient led to the denomination of Wishart subtype for NF2 with an early and severe clinical course.

### Delineation of NF2 from NF1

In 1882, von Recklinghausen published his landmark monograph on the disease that would later become known as NF1 (Crump 1981). In the following years, patients with skin and spinal cord tumors were diagnosed with neurofibromatosis. As early as 1903, clinicians began to distinguish NF2 from NF1. In that year, Henneberg and Koch described a distinct form of neurofibromatosis that involved the eighth cranial nerves bilaterally but spared the skin. They introduced the term "central" neurofibromatosis to distinguish these patients from those with the more common "peripheral" neurofibromatosis described by von Recklinhausen. The distinction between central and peripheral neurofibromatosis was further confounded after publication of *Tumors of the nervus acusticus and the syndrome of the cerebellopontile angle* by Harvey Cushing in 1917. In it, he writes "when the acoustic tumors are bilateral they are very apt to be merely a local expression of a more widespread process (central or general neurofibromatosis) of the von Recklinghausen type". (Cushing 1917). Subsequently, NF2 was seen as manifestation of von Recklinghausen's disease rather than as an independent entity. Given Cushing's lofty reputation, it took almost seven decades for the two diseases to be fully separated again. The unique identity of these conditions was confirmed in the 1980's when linkage analysis localized NF1 to chromosome 17 and NF2 to chromosome 22.

## Genetic inheritance

The heritability of neurofibromatosis was established around 1900 but detailed information about the transmission of NF2 was not available for many years. In 1930, Gardner and Frazier described a family with 38 affected family members over five generations. They noted that affected members had early onset deafness and balance problems and often died prematurely (Gardner and Frazier 1930). Autopsy was performed on two affected family members and revealed bilateral cerebellopontine angle (CPA) tumors. They observed that the condition was transmitted with an autosomal dominant pattern with 50% of individuals at risk developing the condition. No evidence of incomplete penetrance or sex specificity was noted (Gardner and Frazier 1930). Ultimately, Gardner published on 97 members of the index family and noted that the majority of patients had a relatively mild clinical course (Young et al. 1970). His description of a mildly affected family led to the denomination of Gardner subtype for NF2 with a mild clinical course.

## Incidence and prevalence

The present knowledge about the prevalence and incidence of NF2 comes from large population-based studies in the United Kingdom (UK) and Finland. In a recent study from the UK, the annual incidence of NF2 was estimated at 1 in 1,312,000, the birth incidence at 1 in 24,844, and the prevalence at 1.14 per 100,000 persons (Evans et al. 2005). In the Finnish study, the annual age-adjusted incidence of NF2 was estimated at 1 per 2,004,000 and the birth incidence at 1 in 87,410 (Antinheimo et al. 2000). The differences in estimates between the two studies may be explained by differences in ascertainment of subjects. For example, in the UK study, subjects were ascertained through practitioners and through a tumor registry, and asymptomatic relatives were screened by cranial CT or MRI scans. In the Finnish study, subjects were identified only by pathology reports in medical records and in a cancer registry.

## Clinical manifestations

### Presentation of NF2

Several large studies have documented the clinical and radiographic findings of patients with NF2. The results are summarized in Table 1 and will be discussed further below. In patients with NF2, the average age of onset of symptoms is between 17 and 21 and typically precedes a formal diagnosis by 5–8 years. Deafness, tinnitus, or imbalance are the most common presenting symptoms, occurring in up to 50% of patients, and reflect dysfunction of the eighth cranial nerve. Less commonly, patients present with symptoms related to other CNS tumors (20%), painful or growing skin lesions (up to 25%), or visual changes (13%) (Evans et al. 1992, Parry et al. 1994, LoRusso et al. 1995). About 10% of patients are asymptomatic at diagnosis and are detected through screening of first-degree relatives of known cases.

### Pediatric presentation of NF2

Pediatric patients comprise about 16–18% of cases in large databases in Europe and the U.S. (Evans et al. 1999a, Nunes and MacCollin 2003, Ruggieri et al. 2005). In these patients, dysfunction of the eighth cranial nerve (hearing loss, tinnitus, or imbalance) is less frequent than in adults and occurs in 8–40% of children diagnosed with NF2 (Mautner et al. 1993, Evans et al. 1999a, Nunes and MacCollin 2003, Ruggieri et al. 2005) (Figs. 1–6). Other presenting symptoms include cranial (Fig. 2A) or peripheral nerve dysfunction (Figs. 2B–C), myelopathy (Figs. 3A–C), seizures, skin tumors (Fig. 4A), café-au-lait macules, and juvenile cataracts (Fig. 4B) (Mautner et al. 1993, Evans et al. 1999a, Nunes and MacCollin 2003, Ruggieri et al. 2005, Bosch et al. 2006b). Stroke has also been reported (Ng et al.

**Table 1.** Clinical findings in individuals with NF2

| Reference | All subjects | | | Pediatric subjects | | |
|---|---|---|---|---|---|---|
| | Evans et al. (1992) | Parry et al. (1994) | Mautner et al. (1996) | Mautner et al. (1993) | Nunes et al. (2003) | Ruggieri et al. (2005) |
| Number cases | 120 | 63 | 48 | 9 | 12 | 24 |
| Number families | 75 | 32 | | | | 5 |
| Sporadic cases | 45 | 17 | | | | 19 |
| Mean age at onset (years) | 21.2 | 20.3 | 17 | 5.9 | 6.5 | 5.5 |
| Mean age deafness (years) | 24.3 | | | | | |
| Cranial nerve schwannoma (%) | | 24 | 48 | 33 | 83 | 90 |
| Intracranial meningiomas (%) | 45 | 49 | 58 | 22 | 83 | 60 |
| Spinal tumors (%) | 26 | 67 | 90 | 78 | 75 | 88 |
| Skin tumors (%) | 68 | 68 | 64 | 56 | 67 | 92 |
| >10 skin tumors (%) | 10 | 14.5 | | | | 0 |
| Optic sheath meningioma (%) | 4.1 | 4.8 | 8 | 0 | | 0 |
| Lens opacities (%) | 38 | 81 | 63 | 44 | 75 | 36 |
| Retinal hamartoma | | 9 | | 0 | 42 | 24 |
| Astrocytoma (%) | 4.1 | 1.6 | 14.6 | 0 | 0 | 24 |
| Ependymoma (%) | 2.5 | 3.2 | 6.3 | 11 | 25 | 12 |
| Peripheral neuropathy (%) | 6 | 2 | | 0 | 0 | 42 |
| Any CAL macules (%) | 43 | 47.5 | 42 | 0 | | 100 |
| Lisch nodules (%) | 4 | 3 | | 22 | 0 | |

2008). Due to this variable presentation of NF2 in children, a high index of suspicion is required for diagnosis of a patient without a known family history.

## Skin abnormalities

Skin abnormalitites are a common feature of NF2. Skin tumors occur in 60–70% of patients with NF2 and is the presenting sign in 12% of pediatric patients and 27% of adult patients (Mautner et al. 1993, 1997; Evans et al. 1999a; Nunes and MacCollin 2003; Ruggieri et al. 2005). Two presentations are most common: a well-circumscribed, raised area that is slightly hyperpigmented and may contain hair follicles, or a subcutaneous, spherical mass that occur along peripheral nerves (Fig. 4A) (Mautner et al. 1997). Histologically, the vast majority of these tumors are schwannomas although a minority are neurofibromas (Mautner et al. 1997). Up to 20% of patients have greater than 10 skin tumors on presen-

tation; these patients are more likely to have a severe clinical course of their disease (Mautner et al. 1997). Skin tumors are more likely to be a cause for evaluation in children than in adults (Evans et al. 1999a, Nunes and MacCollin 2003).

Café-au-lait (CAL) macules are hyperpigmented skin lesions with well-demarcated borders. CAL macules are found in genetically normal individuals as well as in patients with genetic conditions such as NF1. Increased numbers (>6) of CAL macules are a diagnostic criterion for NF1 and are found in >90% of patients with NF1. CAL macules are present in up to 40% of adult patients with NF2, although fewer than 5% of patients have more than 4 CAL macules on close inspection (Mautner et al. 1997). Interestingly, in one series, CAL macules were reported in 100% of pediatric patients, with 8% having greater than four macules (Ruggieri et al. 2005). The reason for this discrepancy is not known but may reflect decreased visibility of CAL macules in adults or particular attention to skin examination in these subjects.

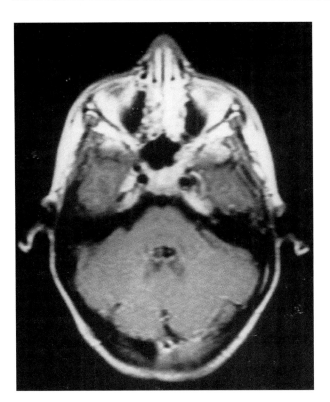

**Fig. 1.** Axial T1-weighted brain MR image in a child with NF2 showing no intracranial lesion [reprinted with permission from Ruggieri et al. 2005].

## Ophthalmic abnormalities

The association between posterior lens opacities (ie, cataracts) and NF2 was first reported in 1969 and later confirmed in the 1980's (Lee and Abbott 1969, Kaiser-Kupfer et al. 1989). Lens opacities occur in 70–90% of patients with NF2 (Bouzas et al. 1993a, b; Ragge et al. 1995). Less than 40% of opacities are cortical in location; the remainder involves the posterior capsular (involving the posterior capsule) region, the posterior subcapsular (anterior to and not involving the posterior capsule) region, or a combination of these regions (Fig. 4B). Only a minority of patients experience diminished visual acuity (20/40 or less) or increased sensitivity to glare. Surgical intervention for lens opacities is rarely necessary. Genotype-phenotype correlations suggest that patients with mosaic disease and those with large deletions have a significantly reduced risk of developing cataracts compared to patients with classic NF2 (Baser et al. 2003).

Epiretinal membranes have been detected in 80% of patients undergoing comprehensive ophthalmologic testing and in 100% of eyes examined dur-

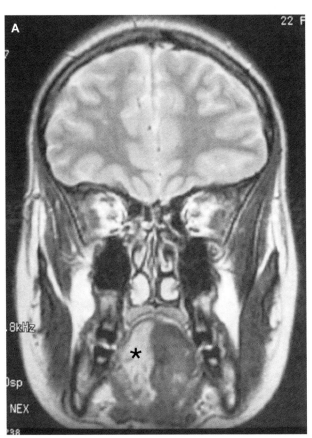

**Fig. 2.** (**A**) Coronal T1-weighted head MR image demonstrating right tongue atrophy (asterisk) secondary to XII cranial nerve schwannoma – this girl's first NF2 manifestations were two lumps in the right hand misdiagnosed as plexiform neurofibromas the diagnosis being postponed until tongue atrophy and brain MR scanning showed multiple cranial schwannomas and meningiomas; (**B**) coronal T1-weighted spinal MR image of the same child in (Fig. 3B) showing a large paravertebral plexiform schwannoma extending from C1 to T1 which distorts the spine and protrudes in the left thoracic wall (white arrows); (**C**) coronal CT scan images showing two large pelvic masses (white arrows) occupying the entire pelvic region. These masses, which were palpable at physical examination and dislocated the urinary bladder, led the general pediatrician to refer the child to a pediatric oncologist and in turn to the suspicion of "a form of NF" because of café-au-lait spots – the diagnosis of NF2 was then clinically raised because of the presence of typical NF2-plaques and confirmed at MRI because of a bilateral vestibular schwannomas and spinal meningiomas and schwannomas [reprinted with permission from Ruggieri et al. 2005].

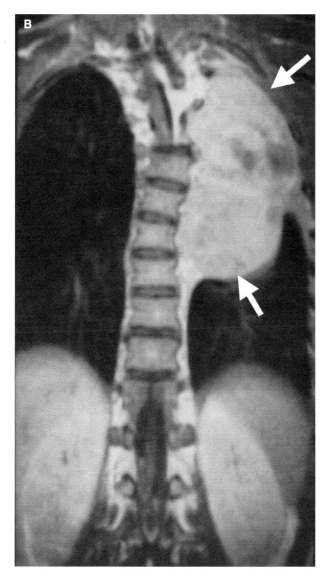

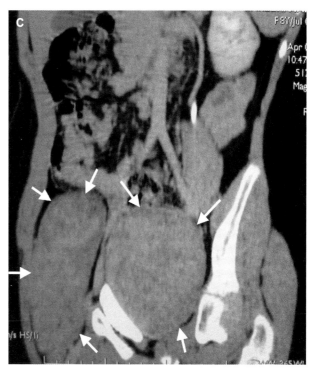

**Fig. 2.** (Continued)

ing autopsy (Meyers et al. 1995, Chan et al. 2002). Pigment epithelial or retinal hamartomas are benign growths that are located in the peripapillary, macular, or peripheral retinal areas. These hamartomas are derivatives of glial, vascular, and/or melanocytic tissue within the retina and occur in up to 25% of patients with NF2. In a minority of patients, retinal or pigment epithelial hamartomas can cause decreased visual acuity, amblyopia, or strabismus in the affected eye (Bouzas et al. 1993b, Ragge et al. 1995). Epiretinal membranes and pigment epithelial/retinal hamar-

tomas are associated with inactivation of chromosome 22 and loss of expression of merlin (Chan et al. 2002).

Optic sheath meningiomas occur in 4–8% of patients with NF2 and are a disproportionate cause of decreased visual acuity (Evans et al. 1992; Parry et al. 1994; LoRusso et al. 1995; Ragge et al. 1995; Bosch et al. 2006a, b). Compression of the optic nerve can produce optic atrophy. Lisch nodules occur in less than 5% of patients with NF2 and, if present, typically occur as a single nodule (Evans et al. 1992, Parry et al. 1994).

Exposure keratopathy is an important cause of visual impairment in patients with NF2. This condition usually arises after surgery for vestibular schwannomas and is caused by dysfunction of trigeminal (sensory) and facial (motor) nerves. Diligent care can reduce the incidence of exposure keratopathy and close follow-up by an experienced ophthalmologist is recommended.

## Nervous system abnormalities

### Cranial schwannomas

Vestibular schwannomas (VS) are the hallmark of NF2. A diagnosis of NF2 should be reconsidered in patients who do not have evidence of bilateral VS on a high resolution MRI scan. Unilateral hearing loss, tinnitus, and/or imbalance are common initial presentation for adult patients with NF2. These symptoms typically occur during the third decade of life but can begin as early as the first decade (Fig. 6A, B) or as late as the seventh decade (Evans et al. 1992,

Nunes and MacCollin 2003). Vestibular schwannomas typically develop within the internal auditory canal and grow centrally along the nerve. If tumors are not removed surgically, they can indent the pons and lead to compression of the brainstem (Fig. 8). As tumors expand into the cerebellopontine angle, patients may experience other cranial nerve deficits such as facial weakness, dysphagia, pyramidal tract signs (eg, weakness and spasticity), or headache due to obstructive hydrocephalus. The growth rate of vestibular schwannomas is highly variable. In patients with NF2, the growth rate of VS, expressed as a time to tumor doubling, ranges from 11 days to 70 years with a median value of 13.6 years (Mautner et al. 2002, Baser et al. 2002b). In general, the growth rate of VS is greater in younger patients than in older patients (Mautner et al. 2002, Baser et al. 2002b). Growth rates for left- and right-sided tumors are highly correlated even when tumors are different sizes. This finding supports the hypothesis that tumor initiation is a stochastic (ie, random) event (Mautner et al. 2002, Baser et al. 2002b). Intrafamilial variability in growth rates is high even

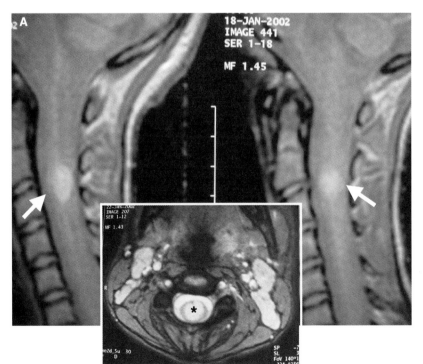

Fig. 3. (A) Sagittal T1-weighted spinal MR image, obtained at age 7 years in the same child with NF2 in Fig. 1, showing a cervical high signal lesion (histologically an astrocytoma) (white arrows); the window in **A** shows an axial T2-weighted image of the same lesion shown in the sagittal planes (asterisk); (**B**) Sagittal T1-weighted spinal MR images showing a cervical meningioma indenting the spinal cord (white arrow) in a child with NF2; (**C**) Sagittal FLAIR (fluid attenuated inverse recovery) image from an MRI scan of cervical spine demonstrating multiple intramedullary lesions consistent with ependymomas [Figs. 3A, 3B reprinted with permission from Ruggieri et al. 2005].

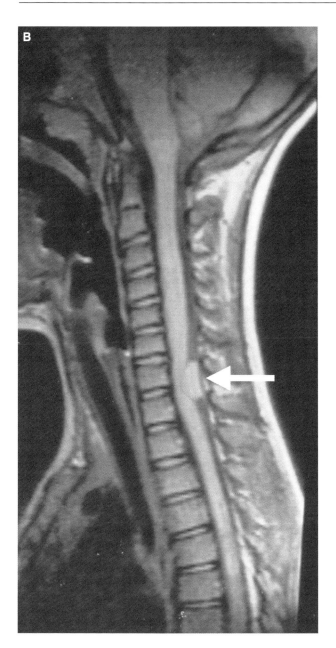

**Fig. 3.** (Continued)

lence among pediatric patients is roughly the same as among adults (Mautner et al. 1993, Nunes and MacCollin 2003). The trigeminal nerve is the most commonly involved (about 30% of cases) but almost any nerve can be affected (Fig. 2A) (LoRusso et al. 1995). Neurologic symptoms related to non-vestibular schwannomas are uncommon and the tumors are usually detected incidentally during cranial imaging for vestibular schwannomas or meningiomas.

Schwannomas in patients with NF2 are almost always histologically benign. Compared with unilateral sporadic tumors, NF2-related VS more frequently demonstrate a lobular growth pattern, Verocay bodies, high cellularity, and meningeal cell proliferation or meningioma cells (Sobel 1993). In addition, NF2-related schwannomas are more likely to have embedded nerves than are sporadic schwannomas. Schwannomas typically grow eccentric to the nerve and cause symptoms by compression rather than by direct invasion. For this reason, surgical resection is possible in some cases. Gross and microscopic analysis of autopsy specimens suggests that Schwann cell tumorlets are present in patients with NF2. Histologically, tumorlets are expansions of nerve fibers and for many years, it was unclear whether they represented a benign form of Schwann cell hyperplasia or an initial step in schwannoma formation (Fig. 5A–C). Loss of heterozygosity analysis of tumorlets and schwannomas in a patient with germline frameshift mutation confirms that tumorlets represent an early phase of schwannomagenesis (Stemmer-Rachamimov et al. 1998).

**Intracranial meningiomas**

among individuals with similar disease severity. For this reason, caution should be used in extrapolating the clinical behavior of VS even among members of the same family that share a common mutation (Baser et al. 2002b).

Twenty-five to 50% of patients with NF2 have schwannomas of non-vestibular cranial nerves (Parry et al. 1994, LoRusso et al. 1995). The preva-

About half of all patients with NF2 develop intracranial meningiomas (Evans et al. 1992, Parry et al. 1994, LoRusso et al. 1995). These tumors can arise from any surface lined by dura including the skull base, falx, and convexity (Fig. 8A). Occasionally, they can arise from arachnoid cells located in the choroids plexus of the lateral ventricle (Figs. 8A–B). Meningiomas associated with NF2 are almost universally benign histologically. These tumors are a common cause of death among patients with NF2

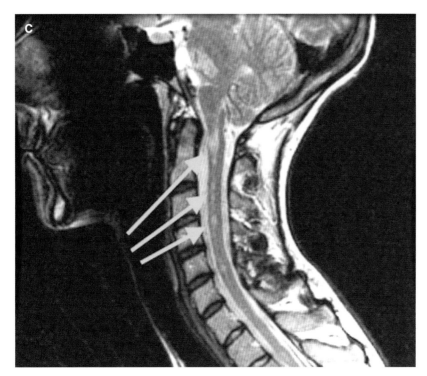

**Fig. 3.** (Continued)

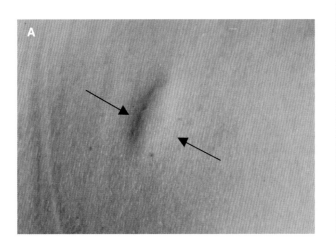

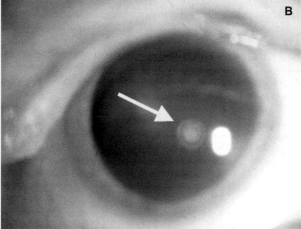

**Fig. 4.** (**A**) Typical cutaneous NF2 plaque (black arrows); (**B**) Photograph of a subcapsular lenticular opacity (arrow) in a patient with NF2. The reflection from the flash is lateral to the opacity (Courtesy of Dr. Simmons Lessell, Massachusetts Eye and Ear Infirmary, Boston, MA).

as reflected by a 2.5-fold increase in the relative risk of death in these patients compared with those lacking intracranial meningiomas (Baser et al. 2002a). Symptoms from intracranial meningiomas are generally related to local mass effect and include headache, seizures, weakness, sensory abnormalities, and obstructive hydrocephalus.

## Spinal cord schwannomas and meningiomas

Spinal cord tumors are common in patients with NF2. If the entire spinal cord is imaged, between 67 and 90% of patients will have evidence of at least one spinal tumor (Figs. 3B–C). Schwannomas and meningiomas typically present as intradural extramedullary lesions. In general, patients have more than one spinal tumor. For example, in a series of 27 patients, a total of 177 schwannomas (88%) and 24 meningiomas (12%) were identified. The mean number of schwannomas and meningiomas per patient was 6.8 and 2.6, respectively (Patronas et al. 2001). Despite the heavy burden of spine tumors in these patients, slightly less than 50% of patients showed radiographic evidence of cord compression (Patronas et al. 2001). Progression is more likely in tumors >5 mm in size than in those smaller in size.

## Spinal cord gliomas: ependymomas and astrocytomas

Spinal ependymomas and astrocytomas in patients with NF2 present as intramedullary spinal cord lesions and occur in up to 53% of patients (Mautner et al. 1995, Patronas et al. 2001). Two-thirds of patients with ependymomas have multiple tumors. The cervicomedullary junction or cervical spine is most commonly involved (Fig. 3C) (63–82%) followed by the thoracic spine (36–44%) (Mautner et al.

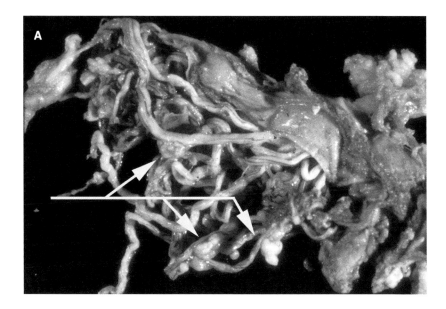

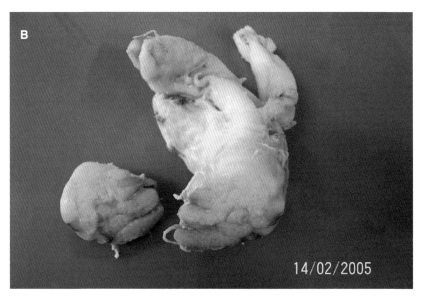

Fig. 5. (**A**) Gross pathologic specimen of a cauda equima from a patient with NF2. Arrows denote schwannoma tumorlets (Courtesy of Dr. Anat Stemmer-Rachamimov, Massachusetts General Hospital, Boston, MA); (**B**) Gross pathologic specimen of a plexiform schwannoma removed in the NF2 girl shown in Fig. 3C; (**C**) histological appearance of the plexiform schwannoma in Fig. 5B (see text for explanation) (courtesy of G. Magro, Institute of Anatomic pathology, University of Caternia).

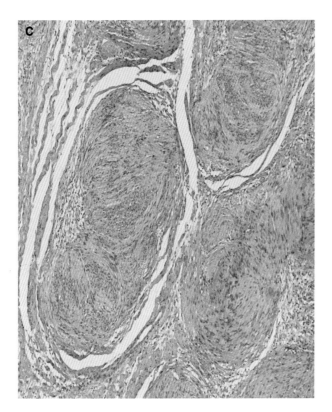

**Fig. 5.** (Continued)

1995, Patronas et al. 2001). The brain and lumbar spine are rarely involved. Radiographic evidence of tumor progression occurs in less than 10% of patients and progressive neurologic dysfunction requiring surgical intervention occurs in 12–20% of patients (Patronas et al. 2001) (F. Nunes, personal communication).

Since surgery is rarely necessary for intramedullary spinal cord tumors, little pathologic data is available. In three small series comprising 13 patients, ependymomas were most common (69%), followed by astrocytomas (15%) and intramedullary schwannomas (15%) (Mautner et al. 1995, Lee et al. 1996, Patronas et al. 2001).

## Neuromuscular abnormalities

Peripheral neuropathy and monomelic atrophy have been reported in patients with NF2. In a clinical study of 100 patients with NF2 in the UK, 3% of patients demonstrated clinical findings consistent with a symmetric sensorimotor neuropathy which was confirmed by electrodiagnostic testing, and an additional 3% had clinical evidence of asymmetric sensorimotor neuropathy (Evans et al. 1992). In a similar study performed in the US, 1 in 63 patients (1.6%) with NF2 had clinical and EMG findings consistent with a peripheral neuropathy (Parry et al. 1994). A dedicated study of peripheral neuropathy in patients with NF2 suggests that this condition may be underrecognized. Fifteen patients with NF2 (mean age at evaluation 37.9 years) were investigated by clinical exam, electrophysiology, and sural biopsy (Sperfeld et al. 2002). Seven of 15 patients (47%) showed evidence for a motor and/or sensory distal periphal neuropathy. Neuropathy was mild in four, moderate in two, and severe in one. Ten of 15 patients had evidence of symmetric polyneuropathy by nerve conduction and EMG of which seven were axonal, one demyelinating, and two mixed axonal-demyelinating (Sperfeld et al. 2002). MRI scans revealed no evidence of tumors that could explain the clinical or electrophyiological findings.

More recently, focal amyotrophy has been documented in patients with NF2. Although the prevalence of this finding has not been firmly established, wasting of a single limb was noted in 4% of patients in a registry of NF2 patients in the UK (Evans et al. 1992). Detailed examination of four different patients by MRI and electrodiagnostic studies excluded compression of proximal nerves or roots by tumors as a cause (Trivedi et al. 2000). The etiology of focal amyotrophy in NF2 is not known but is thought to arise from neurofibromatous changes in peripheral nerves (Trivedi et al. 2000).

## Other intracranial lesions

**Intracranial calcifications** on CT scans not due to tumors and somewhat similar to those seen in tuberous sclerosis have been reported in a number of NF2 patients (Fig. 9A) (reviewed in Friedman et al. 1999, Short et al. 1994). In addition, either periventricular (Fig. 9B) or cortical (Fig. 9C) high signal lesions resembling **cortical dysplasia** can be recorded. The latter finding has been reported in association to NF2

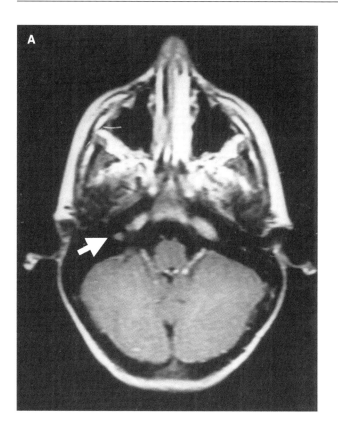
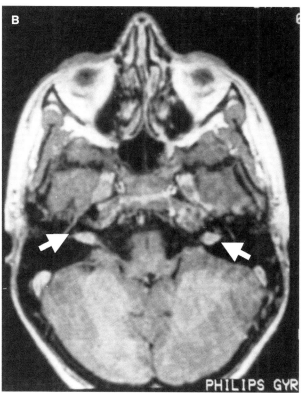

**Fig. 6. (A–B)** axial T2-weighted brain MR images showing the progression of a vestibular schwannoma from a single (right) lesion (**A**, white arrow) to a bilateral middle sized lesions (**B**, white arrows).

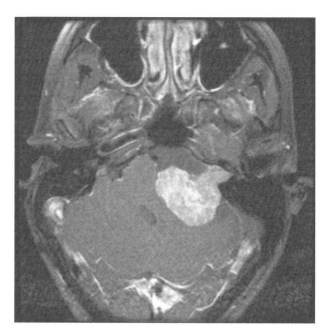

**Fig. 7.** Gadolinium-enhanced cranial MRI scan of a vestibular schwannoma in a patient with NF2. Note significant compression of the brainstem with effacement of the fourth ventricle.

and attributed either to meningoangiomatosis or to hamartomatous lesions. Of interest, the high signal lesions recorded in one series (Ruggieri et al. 2005) were asymptomatic as reported in four of 11 NF2 cases who had meningoangiomatosis (Huson and Hughes 1994).

## Molecular genetics and Pathogenesis

### Molecular biology

In 1987, the *NF2* gene was mapped to chromosome 22 by tumor studies of vestibular schwannomas (Seizinger et al. 1986) and by linkage analysis in patients with NF2 (Rouleau et al. 1987, Wertelecki et al. 1988). In 1993, two groups independently published the identity of the *NF2* gene. One group named the protein "merlin" (<u>m</u>oezin, <u>e</u>zrin, <u>r</u>adixin-<u>li</u>ke protein) to emphasize its relationship to various cytoskeletal proteins (Trofatter et al. 1993). The other

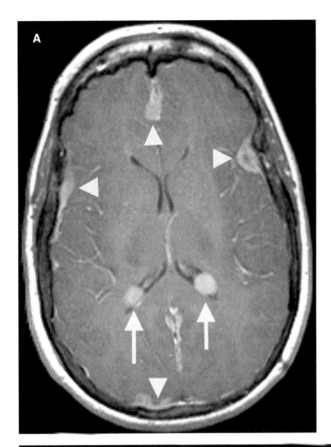

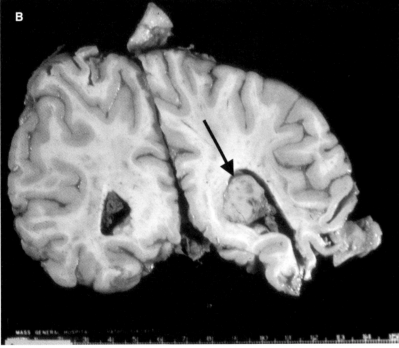

Fig. 8. (A) Axial T1-weighted image from a gadolinium-enhanced cranial MRI scan demonstrating bilateral intraventricular meningiomas (arrows) and multiple dural-based meningiomas (arrowheads). (B) Gross pathologic specimen of brain from a patient with NF2 demonstrating an intraventricular meningioma.

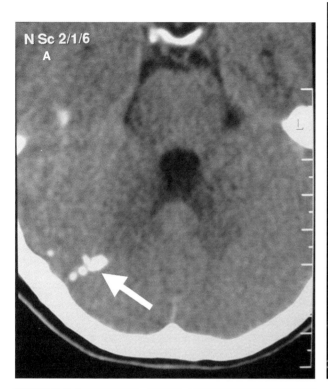

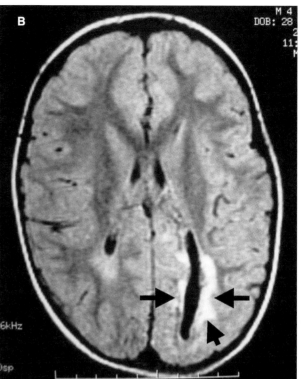

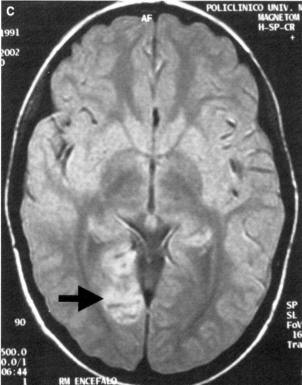

**Fig. 9.** (**A**) Axial CT scan of the brain showing occipital lobe calcifications (white arrow); (**B**) axial T2-weighted brain MR images showing diffuse left periventricular high signal lesions suggestive of cortical dysplasia; (**C**) other aspects of abnormal brain signal lesions in NF2 suggestive of cortical dysplasia (posterior periventricular high signal lesion along the sulci and convolutions: black arrow) [reprinted with permission from Ruggieri et al. 2005].

group named the protein "schwannomin" to emphasize its role in suppression of schwannoma formation (Rouleau et al. 1993). The *NF2* gene is composed of 17 exons spanning 110 kb. There are three alternative messenger RNA species (7 kb, 4.4 kb, and 2.6 kb) due to variable length of the 3'untranslated region. The predominant *NF2* gene product is a 595 amino-acid protein and is a member of the 4.1 family of cytoskeletal proteins. The protein links membrane-associated proteins and the actin cytoskeleton, thereby acting as an interface with the extracellular environment (McClatchey and Giovannini 2005).

The *NF2* protein acts as a true tumor suppressor: loss of both copies of the gene results in tumor growth. Inactivation of the *NF2* gene can be detected in the vast majority of sporadic schwannoma (Jacoby et al. 1996) and in about 50–60% of sporadic meningiomas. *NF2* mutations have been found in unrelated tumors such as melanoma and malignant mesothelioma (Bianchi et al. 1994). In NF2, loss of the first copy occurs in the egg or sperm and usually involves a coding sequence mutation or deletion. Loss of the second copy occurs as a somatic event, often as loss of part or all of the trans chromosome. Molecularly, this event can be visualized as loss of heterozygosity of nearby polymorphic markers. Despite significant progress in understanding the role of the *NF2* gene product, the molecular mechanism by which loss of the NF2 protein leads to tumorgenesis has not been fully elucidated. Recent data suggests that the protein has an important role in the regulation of receptor tyrosine kinases and in maintenance of contact-dependent inhibition of proliferation (McClatchey and Giovannini 2005).

All families with affected members in more than one generation show linkage to the *NF2* gene and there is no evidence for locus heterogeneity (Evans et al. 1998a). Using exon scanning and single strand conformation polymorphism (SSCP), detection rates for germline mutation in patients with vestibular schwannomas varies between 40 and 66% (Parry et al. 1996, Evans et al. 1998a). The presence of large deletions, mutations in promoter or intronic regions, and somatic mosaicism may explain the

difficulty in identifying a causative mutation in all patients. More recently, use of multiplex ligation-dependent probe amplification (MLPA) assays has improved the ability to detect deletions of one to a few exons (Diebold et al. 2005, Kluwe et al. 2005). The most common type of gene alteration identified in NF2 patients are frameshift and nonsense mutations, although point mutations, deletions, and insertions have also been found (MacCollin et al. 1994). The majority of these mutations lead to truncation of the gene product which are predicted not to function either due to loss of the C-terminus of the protein or to instability of the protein product.

## Genotype/phenotype correlations

Genotype/phenotype correlations have been published by multiple groups. All studies are limited by the small number of patients with mutations identified. In a German study using number of tumors identified by MRI scan as a measure of disease severity, frameshift and nonsense mutations were associated with severe disease while missense mutations were associated with mild disease (Kluwe et al. 1996a). Splice site mutations were associated with both mild and severe phenotype, suggesting the possible importance of additional determinants such as stochastic, epigenetic, or environmental factors (Kluwe et al. 1996a). In a US study, frameshift or nonsense mutations were associated with a younger age at onset and diagnosis and with a larger mean number of tumors than were splice-site mutations (MacCollin et al. 1994). Interestingly, an association between nonsense mutations and retinal hamartomas and/or epiretinal membranes has been found (Parry et al. 1996). Finally, in UK series, truncating mutations, as compared with other mutations, were associated with an early age at onset and diagnosis, with symptomatic CNS tumors besides vestibular schwannomas, and with spinal tumors (Evans et al. 1998a). Point mutations are rare in patients with NF2 and have been associated with mild, moderate, and severe disease (Kluwe and Mautner 1996b).

Detailed clinical studies of patients with NF2 suggest that phenotypic variability is smaller within families than between families. This is in contrast to patients with NF1 where there is significant variability within families. Mathematical modeling of intrafamilial correlation supports these clinical impressions. In a study of 390 patients from 153 families in the UK NF2 registry, age at onset of diagnosis, age at onset of hearing loss, and number of intracranial meningiomas was correlated within families (Zhao et al. 2002). A significant intrafamiliar correlation was noted for age at onset (correlation coefficient, 0.35), age at onset of hearing loss (correlation coefficient, 0.51), and number of meningiomas (correlation coefficient, 0.29) (Zhao et al. 2002). This study supports the notion of familial homogeneity but also demonstrates the importance of other uncharacterized factors.

## Mosaic/segmental NF2

Mutations in the *NF2* gene have been detected in up to 70% of affected subjects (MacCollin et al. 1994; Ruttledge et al. 1996; Parry et al. 1996; Kluwe and Mautner 1998, Kluwe et al. 2005). The detection rate for mutations is 20–30% lower for founders (i.e., patients without a family history of NF2) (Kluwe and Mautner 1998, Evans et al. 1998b). In part, the low rate of detection for mutations in sporadic cases is due to somatic mosaicism. Somatic mosaicism develops when a mutation occurs during postzygotic embryonic development. In these patients, only a subpopulation of cells carry the constitutional mutation and analysis of blood leukocytes is often unremarkable.

Indirect evidence suggests that mosaicism exerts a mitigating effect on the NF2 phenotype such that patients may experience a later time of onset and milder course of disease (Evans et al. 1998b, Kluwe et al. 2003) on a unilateral involvement of central nervous system (Fig. 10) (Ruggieri and Huson 2001). Historically, a precise estimate of the rate of mosaicism in these patients has been difficult to establish. The most definitive numbers come from a study of 233 NF2 founders with bilateral vestibular schwannomas. In this study, the authors estimated the rate of mosaicism to be 16.7% to 24.8% (MacCollin et al. 1994, Evans et al. 1998a, Kluwe et al. 2003). Recurrence risk to offspring of mosaic patients is significantly lower than the 50% expected rate for an autosomal dominant disorder (Evans et al. 1998b) and is probably on the order of 5–10%.

## Diagnosis, follow-up, and management

### Diagnosis

Clinical criteria for the diagnosis of NF2 were first formulated at the National Institutes of Health Consensus Conference on NF1 and NF2 in 1987 (1988) and revised in 1991 (Mulvihill et al. 1990). These criteria emphasize the presence of bilateral vestibular schwannomas in a high percentage of patients with NF2 (Table 2). Alternatively, patients can qualify for a diagnosis of NF2 with a family history of NF2 and either a unilateral vestibular schwannoma or any two other tumors typically associated with NF2 (Table 1). Under NIH criteria, patients without bilateral vestibular schwannomas or a family history of NF2 cannot qualify for a diagnosis of NF2.

Revised criteria were proposed by the Manchester group in 1992 (Evans et al. 1992), and by the National Neurofibromatosis Foundation (NNFF) in 1997 (Gutmann et al. 1997). The goal of these revisions was to improve the sensitivity for patients with features associated with NF2 but who did not reach formal NIH criteria. None of the criteria can distinguish perfectly normal individuals from those with NF2 and each has its strengths and weaknesses. Unfortunately, mutational analysis cannot replace clinical criteria for diagnosis of NF2 since a causative mutation cannot be identified in about 30% of affected patients.

### Initial evaluation

Initial evaluation of patients who have or are at risk for NF2 should include testing to confirm a diagnosis and to identify potential problems. A medical

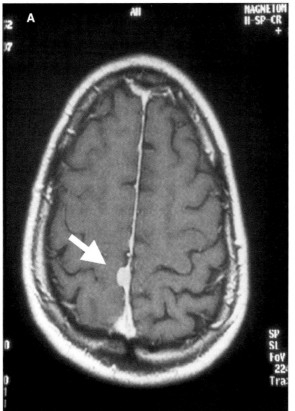

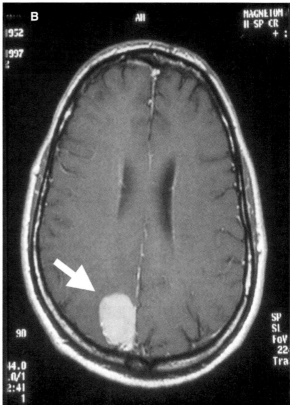

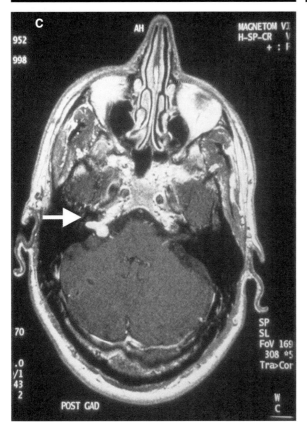

Fig. 10. (A–C) Axial T1-weighted images of the brain showing a right meningioma of the falx (A), a right meningioma of the occipital lobe (B) and a right vestibular schwannoma (C) (white arrows) in a patient with mosaic NF2 [reprinted with permission from Ruggieri and Huson 2001].

**Table 2.** Clinical criteria for diagnosis of NF2

| NIH criteria | Manchester criteria | NNFF criteria |
| --- | --- | --- |
| **Definite or confirmed NF2** | | |
| • Bilateral vestibular schwannoma<br>• 1st degree family relative with NF2 and either unilateral VS or any one of: meningioma, schwannoma, glioma, neurofibroma, juvenile posterior subcapsular lens opacity | • Bilateral vestibular schwannoma<br>• 1st degree family relative with NF2 and either unilateral VS or any two individual manifestations including: meningioma, schwannoma, glioma, neurofibroma, posterior subcapsular lens opacity<br>• Unilateral VS and any two individual manifestations including: meningioma, schwannoma, glioma, neurofibroma, posterior subcapsular lens opacity<br>• Multiple meningiomas ($\geq$2) and either unilateral VS or any two individual manifestations including: schwannoma, glioma, neurofibroma, cataract | • Bilateral vestibular schwannoma<br>• 1st degree family relative with NF2 and either unilateral VS at <30 years of age or any two of: meningioma, schwannoma, glioma, juvenile lens opacity |
| **Presumptive or probable NF2** | | |
| | | • Unilateral VS < 30 years of age and at least one of: meningioma, schwannoma, glioma, juvenile lens opacity<br>• Multiple meningiomas and either unilateral VS < 30 years of age or at least one of: schwannoma, glioma, juvenile lens opacity |

history should include questions about auditory and vestibular function, focal neurologic symptoms, skin tumors, seizures, headache, and visual symptoms. A family history should explore unexplained neurological and audiological symptoms in all first-degree relatives.

MRI scan of the brain should include gadolinium and include axial and coronal thin cuts through the brainstem to identify vestibular schwannomas. MRI scan of the cervical spine should be performed given the predilection of ependymoma for this site. Some clinicians recommend imaging of the thoracic and lumbar spine whereas others reserve these exams for patients with neurologic symptoms referable to these locations. Ophthalmologic examination serves to identify characteristic lesions such as lens opacities, retinal hamartomas, or epiretinal membranes.

A complete neurological examination serves as a baseline for future comparison and may assist in the selection of sites within the nervous system that require further imaging studies. Audiology (including pure tone threshold and word recognition) and brainstem evoked responses document eighth cranial nerve dysfunction related to vestibular schwannomas and set a baseline for future comparisons. Abnormalities of pure tone thresholds are present in 90% of patients between 10 and 72 years with NF2. Word recognition serves as a measure of functional hearing. Brainstem auditory evoked responses are a more sensitive measure of auditory function and is abnormal in 100% of patients with symptomatic vestibular schwannomas. In cases where the diagnosis is uncertain, review of any pathologic material may be helpful.

## Follow-up

After initial diagnosis, patients should be seen relatively frequently (every 3–6 months) until the growth rate and biologic behavior of tumors are determined. Consultation with an experienced surgeon after initial diagnosis is often helpful for presymptomatic patients (ie, those with adequate hearing) to discuss the feasibility of hearing-sparing surgery. Most patients without acute problems can be followed on an annual basis. Evaluation at these visits should include complete neurological examination, MRI scans of the brain with thin cuts through the brainstem, MRI scans of symptomatic lesions outside the brain if present, audiology, and brainstem evoked responses. Ophthalmologic evaluation should be performed in selected patients with visual impairment or facial weakness. Yearly audiology serves to document changes in pure tone threshold and word recognition. This information can be helpful in planning early surgical intervention for vestibular schwannomas and in counseling patients about possible deafness. Changes in brainstem auditory evoked responses may precede hearing loss. The frequency with which routine spinal imaging is obtained varies among clinics, but is clearly indicated in patients with new or progressive symptoms referable to the spinal cord.

## Management

The approach to management of NF2-associated tumors differs from that of sporadic tumors. Because patients with NF2 develop multiple cranial and spinal tumors, surgical removal of every lesion is not possible or advisable. Instead, the primary goal is to preserve function and to maximize quality of life.

## Surgery

Surgery is the mainstay for treatment of NF2-related tumors. Patients with NF2 typically have multiple tumors in the brain and spinal cord and surgical extirpation of all lesions is not a practical goal. Surgery is clearly indicated for patients with significant brainstem or spinal cord compression or with obstructive hydrocephalus. In patients with little or no neurologic

dysfunction related to their tumors, watchful waiting may allow patients to retain neurologic function for many years (Liu and Fagan 2001). For this reason, timing of intervention is often a difficult decision for patients and physicians. Superior short-term outcomes and shorter length of stay for VS surgery has been associated with higher volume hospitals and surgeons (Barker et al. 2003). For this reason, surgery, if indicated, should be performed at hospitals by surgeons with expertise in management of these patients.

The approach to vestibular schwannomas has been the best studied. Surgical extirpation of vestibular schwannomas can be accomplished using middle cranial fossa, posterior suboccipital, and translabyrinthine approaches. The goal of presymptomatic surgery is retention of hearing with a minimum of post-operative complications such as facial weakness or dysphagia. In patients with a documented change in hearing, bony decompression of the internal auditory canal through a middle cranial fossa can stabilize hearing for a period of time. A middle cranial fossa approach for tumor resection can preserve measurable hearing is in 65–70% of adult patients (Doyle and Shelton 1993, Slattery III et al. 1998, Brackmann et al. 2001). Pre-operative tumor size has been shown to be an important indicator of outcome in some series (Doyle and Shelton 1993), but not in others (Slattery III et al. 1998). In general, patients with vestibular schwannomas related to NF2 have comparable surgical outcomes to patients with sporadic lesions (Slattery III et al. 1997). A suboccipital approach for small tumors can result in hearing preservation although precise numbers using this technique have not been published. Alternatively, a translabyrinthine approach with placement of an auditory brainstem implant (ABI) can provide auditory sensations in some patients (Otto et al. 2002). Patients opting for this approach should be counseled that about 10% of patients do not receive auditory sensations, that ABI's do not provide normal sound quality, that processor optimization requires regular follow-up, and that maximal benefit is often not achieved for many years (Otto et al. 2002). For most patients with ABI's, the primary benefit occurs when the implant is used in conjunction with lip reading. In a recent study on a small NF2 cohort (Vincenti et al. 2008) coclear implant patients performed better than ABI's patients even if variability in auditory performance was observed with both devices. At the present time, little information is available about the efficacy of hearing sparing surgery in pediatric patients but outcomes appear to be inferior to that for adults (Nunes and MacCollin 2003).

The decision to proceed with hearing-sparing surgery must be individualized for each patient. Options include observation without surgical intervention and hearing-sparing surgery; stereotactic radiation has not yielded comparable results for preservation of hearing (see below). For those with tumors that are multilobulated or greater than 1.5 cm in greatest dimension, the risk of peri-operative complications (including hearing loss and cranial nerve dysfunction) likely outweight the potential benefits. In these patients, tumor resection should be deferred until another indication for surgery such as increased intracranial pressure, impending hydrocephalus, or new neurologic symptoms develops.

Indications for surgical resection of other tumors are less well defined. In general, schwannomas of other cranial nerves are slow growing and produce few symptoms. Surgical resection in these patients should be reserved for those with unacceptable neurologic symptoms or rapid tumor growth. Patients with meningiomas typically have more than one tumor and resection of all lesions is often not advisable. The benefit of surgery must be carefully weighed against potential complications. As a general rule, indications for resection include rapid tumor growth and worsening neurologic symptoms. Spinal cord tumors are present in about 90% of patients with NF2 and have no site of predilection. Intervention is necessary in a minority of patients (Mautner et al. 1995). Surgery is more often required in patients with extramedullary tumors (59%) than for intramedullary tumors (12%) (Patronas et al. 2001). In general, spinal meningiomas behave more aggressively than schwannomas and require surgery more frequently.

## Radiation

Radiation is often used as adjuvant therapy for treatment of sporadic brain tumors. Treatment outcomes for patients with NF2-related vestibular schwannomas are worse than for patients with sporadic tumors (Fuss et al. 2000). In early studies of stereotactic radiosurgery, 18–20 Gy were delivered to tumors. Local control was achieved in 90% of patients but no serviceable hearing was preserved in patients with serviceable hearing pre-operatively (Linskey et al. 1992). For this reason, the dose of radiation to the tumor margin was reduced to 12–16 Gy. Using modern regimens, treatment with stereotactic radiosurgery results in tumor control in 98% of patients with NF2 with preservation of useful hearing in 40–67% (Subach et al. 1999, Rowe et al. 2003). Decreased facial and trigeminal function occurs in 5–16% and 10% of patients, respectively (Subach et al. 1999, Rowe et al. 2003). The risk of deafness in patients with serviceable hearing pre-operatively is about 20% (Rowe et al. 2003). More recently, fractionated stereotactic radiotherapy has been advocated to minimize the risk of hearing loss. The actuarial 5-year local control rate using this technique is 93% and the hearing-preservation rate is 64% (Combs et al. 2005).

The role of adjuvant radiation in other tumors such as meningiomas and ependymomas is not established but the majority of these tumors demonstrates benign histology and can be controlled surgically. No case series have been published on treatment of NF2-related meningiomas. In general, treatment of sporadic tumors with stereotactic radiosurgery results in local control in 90–95% of cases (Flickinger et al. 2003, DiBiase et al. 2004). Peritumoral cerebral edema develops in up to 25% of patients, but symptoms referable to cerebral edema develop in less than 10% of patients (Flickinger et al. 2003, Chang et al. 2003).

Most clinicians prefer surgical extirpation of tumors when possible and reserve radiation treatment for tumors that are not surgically accessible. This practice is based on the experience that radiation therapy makes subsequent resection of VS and function of ABI's more difficult (Slattery III and Brackmann 1995). In addition, there are anectodal reports of malignant transformation of NF2-associated schwannomas after radiation treatment and indirect evidence of increased numbers of malignancy in NF2 patients who have received radiation (Baser et al. 2000, Thomsen et al. 2000).

## Chemotherapy

At the present time, there is no effective chemotherapy for treatment of NF2-related tumors. Sporadic meningiomas represent the best-studied tumor at the present time. Typically, patients with refractory or non-surgical tumors have been included in chemotherapy trials. Although some initial reports suggested efficacy of hydroxyurea in treating meningiomas (Schrell et al. 1997), more recent reports do not support this view (Loven et al. 2004). Furthermore, there seems to be little role for use of tamoxifen or temozolomide for recurrent tumors (Chamberlain et al. 2004). No trials of chemotherapy for treatment of vestibular schwannomas or ependymomas have been reported. Gene therapy remains a potential option for the future as injection of oncolytic recombinant herpes virus into schwannomas in mice results in significant tumor shrinkage (Messerli et al. 2005).

### Mortality in NF2

Patients with NF2 have diminished lifespan compared to non-affected family members. In a study of 74 Japanese patients with bilateral vestibular schwannomas, the overall 5-, 10-, and 20-years survival rates after diagnosis were 85, 67, and 38%, respectively (Otsuka et al. 2003). Younger age at diagnosis was correlated with poor survival (Otsuka et al. 2003). In a UK study, the mean actuarial survival for patients with NF2 was 62 years (Evans et al. 1992). Of 368 people from 261 families registered in the UK NF registry as of February 15, 2002, 74 (20%) died during follow-up (Baser et al. 2002a). The cause of death in these patients was tumor burden (69%), peri-operative complications (19%), malignancy from NF2-related tumor (4%), traffic accident (3%), suicide (3%), falls (1%), and myocardial infarction (1%) (Baser et al. 2002a). Cox proportional hazards models revealed increased relative risk of mortality associated with decreasing age of diagnosis (relative risk, 1.13-fold per year decrease below 27 years of age) and presence of intracranial meningiomas (relative risk, 2.51). A decreased risk of mor-

tality was associated with treatment at a specialty medical center (relative risk, 0.34) and with presence of a missense mutation compared with nonsense or frameshift (relative risk, 0.08) (Baser et al. 2002a).

## Differential diagnosis

The diagnosis of NF2 is generally straightforward when a patient has a family history. In sporadic cases, other diagnostic possibilities must be considered.

### Bilateral cerebellopontine angle masses

Vestibular schwannomas are the hallmark of NF2. Any disease that presents with bilateral cerebellopontine angles masses can resemble NF2 at initial presentation. Case reports of such mimic syndromes include patients with glioblastoma multiforme, metastases, and petrous apex cholesterol granulomas. A detailed history and examination coupled with a high-quality MRI scan is usually sufficient to differentiate these entities from NF2. Only rarely is a brain biopsy required to confirm a diagnosis in the presence of bilateral vestibular schwannomas.

### Unilateral vestibular schwannoma

Vestibular schwannomas are relatively common and represent about 7% of all primary central nervous system tumors. The vast majority of these tumors are unilateral and sporadic in nature. However, between 10 and 20% of patients with NF2 initially present with unilateral VS (Evans et al. 2005). Thus, when evaluating a young patients with unilateral VS, one should consider the possibility of NF2. Using epidemiologic data, the average risk (per decade) of having NF2 has been calculated for patients presenting with a unilateral vestibular schwannoma (Evans et al. 1999b). For a patient who presents in the second decade, the average risk of having NF2 is 6%. This average risk declines to 2.7% in the third decade, to 0.9% in the fourth decade, and to 0.36% in the fifth decade (Evans et al. 1999b). In younger patients with unilateral vestibular schwannomas, particular attention should be given to identification of other manifestations of NF2 such as meningiomas, ependymomas, skin tumors, and lens opacities.

Patients with unilateral vestibular schwannomas and other NF2-related tumors (e.g., meningioma) represent a unique phenotype (Aghi et al. 2006). These patients tend to present with symptoms later in life than those with classic NF2 and are less likely to have ophthalmologic findings (Fig. 10) (Ruggieri and Huson 2001). Cranial and spinal tumors are common with a mean of 2.9 intracranial nonunilateral schwannomas and 2.3 spinal tumors. Contralateral vestibular schwannoma can develop with an actuarial chance of 2.9% at 17 years, 11% at 24 years and 29% at 40 years. Molecular analysis has confirmed somatic mosaicism in 18% of these patients. Transmission to offspring is rare with only 2 of 63 children of subjects exhibiting NF2-related findings such as unilateral VS or cataracts.

## Multiple meningiomas

Multiple meningiomas are found in up to 10% of patients with meningiomas (Davis et al. 1998, Antinheimo et al. 2000). In such patients, diagnostic considerations include NF2, non-contiguous spread of a single meningioma, or familial multiple meningiomas. Analysis of tumor and blood samples from patients with multiple meningiomas without a family history of NF2 usually supports a somatic and clonal origin for these tumors (Stangl et al. 1997). In rare circumstances, multiple meningiomas are familial but the identity of this tumor suppressor gene has not been identified (Heinrich et al. 2003). The initial work-up should include a contrast-enhanced cranial MRI scan with axial and coronal thin cuts through the brainstem to identify any possible VS. The presence of bilateral vestibular schwannomas confirms a diagnosis of NF2 whereas a unilateral vestibular schwannoma ipsilateral to multiple meningiomas suggests a diagnosis of mosaic NF2.

## Genetic counseling

Genetic counseling is an essential component of the care of the patient with NF2. All patients and families with NF2 should have access to genetic testing to facilitate presymptomatic diagnosis of individuals at risk. If a causative mutation in the *NF2* gene can be identified, molecular testing with 100% specificity will be available for that family. Mosaicism is a common cause of non-informative testing in sporadic NF2 patients. For these individuals, tumor specimens should be frozen for analysis, if possible. If two genetic alterations (e.g., one mutation and one allele loss of the *NF2* gene) can be identified in a tumor, one is inferred to be the constitutional mutation. Haplotype analysis can then be used to screen at risk individuals for the mutation in constitutional DNA. (Kluwe et al. 2002). In families with two or more affected individuals, linkage analysis using intragenic markers or markers flanking the *NF2* gene can be used for presymptomatic diagnosis with >99% certainty of affected status. As with other genetic diseases, genetic counseling by an experienced provider is essential prior to embarking on prenatal or presymptomatic diagnosis.

## Schwannomatosis

Schwannomatosis (OMIM 162091) is a recently recognized form of neurofibromatosis. In early clinical reports, these patients were described as having multiple schwannomas, multiple neurilemomas, multiple neurilemmomas, or neurilemmomatosis. Historically, these patients have been difficult to distinguish from those with NF2 due to the overlap in their phenotypes.

No estimate of the prevalence of schwannomatosis has been reported. The annual incidence is estimated to be 0.58 cases per 1,000,000 persons, which is similar to that of NF2 (0.50 cases per 1,000,000) from the same study (Antinheimo et al. 2000). Two percent of patients with schwannomas qualify for a diagnosis of schwannomatosis (Antinheimo et al. 2000). Data from German and US clinics suggest that 15% of cases of schwannomatosis are familial whereas data from the UK suggest that up to 50% of cases may be familial (MacCollin et al. 2005).

Schwannomatosis is characterized by the predisposition to develop multiple schwannomas (Figs. 11, 12). In contrast to patients with NF2, patients with

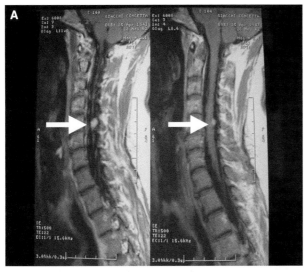

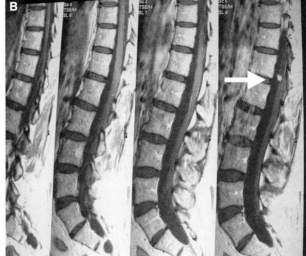

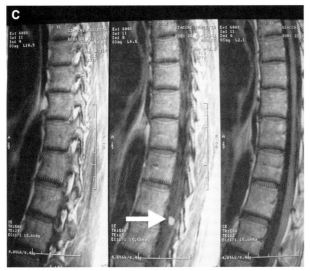

**Fig. 11.** Sagittal T-weighted images of the cervical (**A**), thoracic (**B**) and lumbar (**C**) spine showing multiple schwannomas (white arrows) in a patient with schwannomatosis.

schwannomatosis do not have vestibular or intradermal schwannomas on other NF2 features (Baser et al. 2006). Patients with schwannomatosis most commonly develop symptoms in the second or third decade of life. Pain is the hallmark of schwannomatosis and is the most common initial complaint. Neurologic dysfunction related to schwannomas is uncommon and, when present, is often a complication of surgery. One-third of patients with schwannomatosis have evidence of anatomically limited disease. The MRI appearance of schwannomatosis is characterized by multiple, discrete lesions along peripheral or spinal nerves. The lesions have low to in-

termediate signal intensity on T1 sequence and high signal intensity on T2- and short T1 inversion recovery (STIR) sequences (Fig. 12). Pathologically, schwannomas in patients with schwannomatosis resemble those from patients with NF2 and sporadic lesions. Although no single feature can reliably distinguish schwannomatosis-associated schwannomas, they tend to have more peritumoral edema in the adjacent nerve, intratumoral myxoid changes, and intraneural growth patterns than other schwannomas (MacCollin et al. 2005).

The pathogenesis of schwannomatosis is an area of active research. A minority of patients with

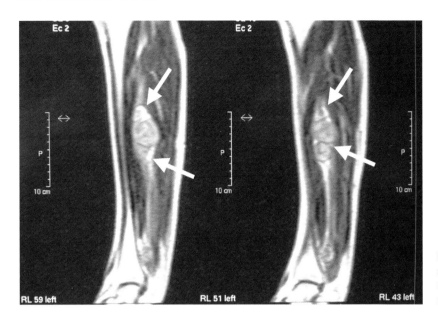

**Fig. 12.** Coronal T2-weighted image of the leg showing an isolated multilobular schwannoma (white arrow) in a patient with schwannomatosis.

**Table 3.** Clinical criteria for diagnosis of schwannomatosis

| Definite schwannomatosis* | Possible schwannomatosis* |
|---|---|
| *Presence of all the following criteria* | *Presence of all the following criteria* |
| Age <30 years, 2 or more non intradermal schwannomas of which at least on histologically proven, lack of vestibular tumor after high quality MR study, lack of constitutional mutations of the NF2 gene | Age <30 years, 2 or more non intradermal 2 or more non intradermal histologically proven, lack of vestibular schwannoma after high quality MR study, lack of constitutional mutations of the NF2 gene |
| *or* | *or* |
| 1 non-vestibular schwannoma histologically proven, one 1st degree parent satisfying the above criteria | Age >45 years, 2 or more non intradermal 2 or more non intradermal histologically proven, lack of symptoms of eight nerve dysfunction, lack of constitutional mutations of the NF2 gene |
| | *or* |
| | Radiological evidence of non-vestibular Schwannoma, 1st degree parent satisfying the above criteria |

Adapted and modified from MacCollin et al. (2005)
*According to the **revised criteria** for schwannomatosis (Baser et al. 2006) all patients with **definite** or **possible** schwammomatosis must not fulfill any of the existing sets of diagnostic criteria for NF2 (see Table 2) and have no evidence of vestibular schwannoma on high quality MRI scan, no first-degree relative with NF2, and no known constitutional NF2 mutation.

sporadic schwannomatosis have been shown to have mosaic NF2 (Jacoby et al. 1997). Truncating mutations in the *NF2* gene are present in the vast majority of schwannomatosis-associated schwannomas. However, multiple tumors from the same patient do not share a common mutation. The underlying cause for somatic instability in the *NF2* gene in schwannomatosis is not known. Mutational analysis of tumors from affected families has excluded germline inactivation of *NF2* gene as the cause of schwannomatosis (MacCollin et al. 2003). Hulsebos et al. (2007) identified on inactivating germline mutation in exon 1 of the tumor suppressor gene INI1/SMARCB1 (OMIM 601607) on chromosome 22q12.2 in a father and daughter who both had schwannomatosis. In 2 of 4 investigated schwannomas from these patients, inactivation of the wildtype INI1 allele by a second mutation in exon 5 of the gene on by loss of the gene was found, consistent with the Kondson 2-hit hypothesis and suggesting that INI1 might be the predisposing gene in familial schwonnomatosis (Hulsebos et al. 2007). More recently, two studies (Hadfield et al. 2008, Sestini et al. 2008) identified germline SMARCB1 mutations in patients with schwonnomatosis along with somatic NF2 mutations in the same patients' tumours suggesting a four-hit mechanism involving the SMARCB1 and NF2 genes in schwonnomatosis-related tumorigenesis.

Consensus criteria for diagnosis of schwannomatosis have been published (Table 3) (MacCollin et al. 2005) and, more recently modified (Baser et al. 2006). Initial evaluation of patients who have or are at risk for schwannomatosis should include testing to confirm a diagnosis (usually exclusion of NF1 and NF2) and to identify potential problems. A medical history should include questions about auditory and vestibular function, focal neurologic symptoms, skin tumors or hyperpigmented lesions, seizures, headache, and visual symptoms. A family history should explore unexplained neurological, dermatological, and audiological symptoms in all first-degree relatives. MRI scan of the brain with attention to the internal auditory canals should be performed to exclude vestibular schwannomas on other NF2 features (Baser et al. 2006). MRI scans of other body parts should be obtained based on the history and clinical exam. A combination of MRI scan and pathologic analysis is used to establish a diagnosis of definite or possible schwannomatosis. Management of patients with schwannomatosis is primarily symptom oriented. As noted above, pain is the hallmark of this disorder. Surgery should be reserved for patients with symptomatic tumors or rapidly expanding lesions in the spinal cord. Most patients require pain medication; these patients may benefit from referral to a Pain Clinic with experience in managing neuropathic pain.

The differential diagnosis for schwannomatosis includes other disorders characterized by multiple nerve sheath tumors including NF1, NF2, Carney complex (characterized by skin pigmentation, myxomas, and endocrine tumors), and an unnamed syndrome characterized by the presence of multiple schwannomas, multiple nevi, and multiple vaginal leiomyomas. A combination of history, pathologic diagnosis of tumor tissue, and imaging is usually sufficient to distinguish between these competing diagnoses.

## References

Aghi M, Kluwe L, Webster MT, Jacoby LB, Barker FG, Ojemann RG, Mautner VF, MacCollin M (2006) Unilateral vestibular schwannoma with other neurofibromatosis Type 2-related tumors: clinical and molecular study of a unique phenotype. J Neurosurg 104: 201–207.

Antinheimo J, Sankila R, Carpen O, Pukkala E, Sainio M, Jaaskelainen J (2000) Population-based analysis of sporadic and type 2 neurofibromatosis-associated meningiomas and schwannomas. Neurology 54: 71.

Barker FG, Carter BS, Ojemann RG, Jyung RW, Poe DS, McKenna MJ (2003) Surgical excision of acoustic neuroma: patient outcome and provider caseload. Laryngoscope 113: 1332–1343.

Baser ME, Evans DG, Jackler RK, Sujansky E, Rubenstein A (2000) Neurofibromatosis 2, radiosurgery and malignant nervous system tumours. Br J Cancer 82: 998.

Baser ME, Friedman JM, Aeschliman D, Joe H, Wallace AJ, Ramsden RT, Evans DG (2002a) Predictors of the risk of mortality in neurofibromatosis 2. Am J Hum Genet 71: 715–723.

Baser ME, Makariou EV, Parry DM (2002b) Predictors of vestibular schwannoma growth in patients with neurofibromatosis Type 2. J Neurosurg 96: 217–222.

Baser ME, Kuramoto L, Joe H, Friedman JM, Wallace AJ, Ramsden RT (2003) Genotype-phenotype correlations for cataracts in neurofibromatosis 2. J Med Genet 40: 758–760.

Baser ME, Friedman JM, Evans DG (2006) Increasing the specificity of diagnostic criteria for schwonnomatosis. Neurology 66: 730–732.

Berg JC, Scheithauer BW, Spinner RJ, Allen CM, Koutlas IG (2008) Plexiform schwannoma: a clinicopathologic overview with emphasis on the head and neck region. Hum Pathos 39: 633–640.

Bianchi AB, Hara T, Ramesh V, Gao J, Klein-Szanto AJ, Morin F, Menon AG, Trofatter JA, Gusella JF, Seizinger BR, et al. (1994) Mutations in transcript isoforms of the neurofibromatosis 2 gene in multiple human tumour types. Nat Genet 6: 185–192.

Bosch MM, Wichmann WW, Boltshanser E, Landan K (2006a) Optic nerve sheath meningiomas in patients with neurofibromatosis type 2. Arch Ophthal Mol 124: 379–385.

Bosch MM, Boltshanser E, Harper P, Landan K (2006b) Ophtholmologic findings and long-term course in patients with neurofibromatosis type 2. Am J Ophthalmol 141: 1068–1077.

Bouzas EA, Freidlin V, Parry DM, Eldridge R, Kaiser-Kupfer MI (1993a) Lens opacities in neurofibromatosis 2: further significant correlations. Br J Ophthalmol 77: 354–357.

Bouzas EA, Parry DM, Eldridge R, Kaiser-Kupfer MI (1993b) Visual impairment in patients with neurofibromatosis 2. Neurology 43: 622–623.

Brackmann DE, Fayad JN, Slattery WH III, Friedman RA, Day JD, Hitselberger WE, Owens RM (2001) Early proactive management of vestibular schwannomas in neurofibromatosis type 2. Neurosurgery 49: 274–280.

Chamberlain MC, Tsao-Wei DD, Groshen S (2004) Temozolomide for treatment-resistant recurrent meningioma. Neurology 62: 1210–1212.

Chan CC, Koch CA, Kaiser-Kupfer MI, Parry DM, Gutmann DH, Zhuang Z et al. (2002) Loss of heterozygosity for the NF2 gene in retinal and optic nerve lesions of patients with neurofibromatosis 2. J Pathol 198: 14–20.

Chang JH, Chang JW, Choi JY, Park YG, Chung SS (2003) Complications after gamma knife radiosurgery for benign meningiomas. J Neurol Neurosurg Psychiatry 74: 226–230.

Combs SE, Volk S, Schulz-Ertner D, Huber PE, Thilmann C, Debus J (2005) Management of acoustic neuromas with fractionated stereotactic radiotherapy (FSRT): long-term results in 106 patients treated in a single institution. Int J Radiat Oncol Biol Phys 63: 75–81.

Crump T (1981) Translation of case reports in *Ueber die multplen fibrome der haut und ihre beziehung zu den multiplen neuromen* by F.v. Recklinghausen. In: Riccardi VM, Mulvihill JJ (eds.) Neurofibromatosis (von Recklinghausen Disease). New York: Raven Press, pp. 259–275.

Cushing H (1917) Bilateral tumors and generalized neurofibromatosis. Tumors of the nervus acusticus and the syndrome of the cerebellopontile angle. New York: Hafner Publishing Company, pp. 210–216.

Davis FG, Freels S, Grutsch J, Barlas S, Brem S (1998) Survival rates in patients with primary malignant brain tumors stratified by patient age and tumor histological type: an analysis based on Surveillance, Epidemiology, and End Results (SEER) data, 1973–1991. J Neurosurg 88: 1–10.

DiBiase SJ, Kwok Y, Yovino S, Arena C, Naqvi S, Temple R, Regine WF, Amin P, Guo C, Chin LS (2004) Factors predicting local tumor control after gamma knife stereotactic radiosurgery for benign intracranial meningiomas. Int J Radiat Oncol Biol Phys 60: 1515–1519.

Diebold R, Bartelt-Kirbach B, Evans DG, Kaufmann D, Hanemann CO (2005) Sensitive Detection of Deletions of One or More Exons in the Neurofibromatosis Type 2 (NF2) Gene by Multiplexed Gene Dosage Polymerase Chain Reaction. J Mol Diagn 7: 97–104.

Doyle KJ, Shelton C (1993) Hearing preservation in bilateral acoustic neuroma surgery. Am J Otol 14: 562–565.

Evans DG, Huson SM, Donnai D, Neary W, Blair V, Newton V, Harris R (1992) A clinical study of type 2 neurofibromatosis. Q J Med 84: 603–618.

Evans DG, Trueman L, Wallace A, Collins S, Strachan T (1998a) Genotype/phenotype correlations in type 2 neurofibromatosis (NF2): evidence for more severe disease associated with truncating mutations. J Med Genet 35: 450–455.

Evans DG, Wallace AJ, Wu CL, Trueman L, Ramsden RT, Strachan T (1998b) Somatic mosaicism: a common cause of classic disease in tumor-prone syndromes? Lessons from type 2 neurofibromatosis. Am J Hum Genet 63: 727–736.

Evans DG, Birch JM, Ramsden RT (1999a) Paediatric presentation of type 2 neurofibromatosis. Arch Dis Child 81: 496–499.

Evans DG, Lye R, Neary W, Black G, Strachan T, Wallace A, Ramsden RT (1999b) Probability of bilateral disease in people presenting with a unilateral vestibular schwannoma. J Neurol Neurosurg Psychiatry 66: 764–767.

Evans DG, Moran A, King A, Saeed S, Gurusinghe N, Ramsden R (2005) Incidence of vestibular schwannoma and neurofibromatosis 2 in the North West of England over a 10-year period: higher incidence than previously thought. Otol Neurotol 26: 93–97.

Flickinger JC, Kondziolka D, Maitz AH, Lunsford LD (2003) Gamma knife radiosurgery of imaging-diagnosed intracranial meningioma. Int J Radiat Oncol Biol Phys 56: 801–806.

Friedman JM, Gutmann DH, MacCollin M, Riccardi VM (1999) Neurofibromatosis. Phenotype, Natural History, and Pathogensis, 3rd ed. Baltimore: Johns Hopkins University Press.

Fuss M, Debus J, Lohr F, Huber P, Rhein B, Engenhart-Cabillic R, Wannenmacher M (2000) Conventionally fractionated stereotactic radiotherapy (FSRT) for acoustic neuromas. Int J Radiat Oncol Biol Phys 48: 1381–1387.

Gardner WJ, Frazier CH (1930) Bilateral acoustic neurofibromas. Arch Neurol Psychiat 23: 266–302.

Gutmann DH, Aylsworth A, Carey JC, Korf B, Marks J, Pyeritz RE, Rubenstein A, Viskochil D (1997) The diagnostic evaluation and multidisciplinary management of neurofibromatosis 1 and neurofibromatosis 2. JAMA 278: 51–57.

Hadfield KD, Newman WG, Bowers NL, Wallace A, Bolger CM, Colley A, McCann E, Trump D, Prescott T, Evans G (2008) Molecular characterisation of SMARCB1 and NF2 in familial and sporadic schwannomatosis. J Med Genet Feb 29 [Epub ahead of print].

Heinrich B, Hartmann C, Stemmer-Rachamimov AO, Louis DN, MacCollin M (2003) Multiple meningiomas: investigating the molecular basis of sporadic and familial forms. Int J Cancer 103: 483–488.

Hulsebos TJ, Plomp AS, Wolterman RA, Robanus-Maandag EO, Baas F, Wesseling P (2007) Germline mutations of INI1/SMARCB1 in familial schwannomatosis. Am J Hum Genet 80: 805–810.

Jacoby LB, MacCollin M, Barone R, Ramesh V, Gusella JF (1996) Frequency and distribution of NF2 mutations in schwannomas. Genes Chromosomes Cancer 17: 45–55.

Jacoby LB, Jones D, Davis K, Kronn D, Short MP, Gusella J et al. (1997) Molecular analysis of the NF2 tumor-suppressor gene in schwannomatosis. Am J Hum Genet 61: 1293–1302.

Kaiser-Kupfer MI, Freidlin V, Datiles MB, Edwards PA, Sherman JL, Parry D, McCain LM, Eldridge R (1989) The association of posterior capsular lens opacities with bilateral acoustic neuromas in patients with neurofibromatosis type 2. Arch Ophthalmol 107: 541–544.

Kluwe L, Bayer S, Baser ME, Hazim W, Haase W, Funsterer C, Mautner VF (1996a) Identification of NF2 germline mutations and comparison with neurofibromatosis 2 phenotypes. Hum Genet 98: 534–538.

Kluwe L, Mautner VF (1996b) A missense mutation in the NF2 gene results in moderate and mild clinical phenotypes of neurofibromatosis type 2. Hum Genet 97: 224–227.

Kluwe L, Mautner VF (1998) Mosaicism in sporadic neurofibromatosis 2 patients. Human Molecular Genetics 7: 2051–2055.

Kluwe L, Friedrich RE, Tatagiba M, Mautner VF (2002) Presymptomatic diagnosis for children of sporadic neurofibromatosis 2 patients: a method based on tumor analysis. Genet Med 4: 27–30.

Kluwe L, Mautner V, Heinrich B, Dezube R, Jacoby LB, Friedrich RE, MacCollin M (2003) Molecular study of frequency of mosaicism in neurofibromatosis 2 patients with bilateral vestibular schwannomas. J Med Genet 40: 109–114.

Kluwe L, Nygren AO, Errami A, Heinrich B, Matthies C, Tatagiba M et al. (2005) Screening for large mutations of the NF2 gene. Genes Chromosomes Cancer 42: 384–391.

Lee DK, Abbott ML (1969) Familial central nervous system neoplasia. Case report of a family with von Recklinghausen's neurofibromatosis. Arch Neurol 20: 154–160.

Lee M, Rezai AR, Freed D, Epstein FJ (1996) Intramedullary spinal cord tumors in neurofibromatosis. Neurosurgery 38: 32–37.

Linskey ME, Lunsford LD, Flickinger JC (1992) Tumor control after stereotactic radiosurgery in neurofibromatosis patients with bilateral acoustic tumors. Neurosurgery 31: 829–838.

Liu R, Fagan P (2001) Facial nerve schwannoma: surgical excision versus conservative management. Ann Otol Rhinol Laryngol 110: 1025–1029.

LoRusso P, Foster BJ, Poplin E, McCormick J, Kraut M, Flaherty L, Heilbrun LK, Valdivieso M, Baker L (1995) Phase I clinical trial of pyrazoloacridine NSC366140 (PD115934). Clin Cancer Res 1: 1487–1493.

Loven D, Hardoff R, Sever ZB, Steinmetz AP, Gornish M, Rappaport ZH, Fenig E, Ram Z, Sulkes A (2004) Non-resectable slow-growing meningiomas treated by hydroxyurea. J Neurooncol 67: 221–226.

MacCollin M, Ramesh V, Jacoby LB, Louis DN, Rubio MP, Pulaski K, Trofatter JA, Short MP, Bove C, Eldridge R, et al. (1994) Mutational analysis of patients with neurofibromatosis 2. Am J Hum Genet 55: 314–320.

MacCollin M, Willett C, Heinrich B, Jacoby LB, Acierno JS Jr, Perry A, Louis DN (2003) Familial schwannomatosis: exclusion of the NF2 locus as the germline event. Neurology 60: 1968–1974.

MacCollin M, Chiocca EA, Evans DG, Friedman JM, Horvitz R, Jaramillo D, Lev M, Mautner VF, Niimura M, Plotkin SR, Sang CN, Stemmer-Rachamimov A, Roach ES (2005) Diagnostic criteria for schwannomatosis. Neurology 64: 1838–1845.

Mautner VF, Tatagiba M, Guthoff R, Samii M, Pulst SM (1993) Neurofibromatosis 2 in the pediatric age group. Neurosurgery 33: 92–96.

Mautner VF, Tatagiba M, Lindenau M, Funsterer C, Pulst SM, Baser ME, Kluwe L, Zanella FE (1995) Spinal tumors in patients with neurofibromatosis type 2: MR imaging study of frequency, multiplicity, and variety. Am J Roentgenol 165: 951–955.

Mautner VF, Lindenau M, Baser ME, Hazim W, Tatagiba M, Haase W, Samii M, Wais R, Pulst SM (1996) The neuroimaging and clinical spectrum of neurofibromatosis 2. Neurosurgery 38: 880–885.

Mautner VF, Lindenau M, Baser ME, Kluwe L, Gottschalk J (1997) Skin abnormalities in neurofibromatosis 2. Arch Dermatol 133: 1539–1543.

Mautner VF, Baser ME, Thakkar SD, Feigen UM, Friedman JM, Kluwe L (2002) Vestibular schwannoma growth in patients with neurofibromatosis Type 2: a longitudinal study. J Neurosurg 96: 223–228.

McClatchey AI, Giovannini M (2005) Membrane organization and tumorigenesis–the NF2 tumor suppressor, Merlin. Genes Dev 19: 2265–2277.

Messerli SM, Prabhakar S, Tang Y, Mahmood U, Giovannini M, Weissleder R, Bronson R, Martuza R, Rabkin S, Breakefield XO (2005) Treatment of Schwannomas with an Oncolytic Recombinant Herpes Simplex Virus in Murine Models of Neurofibromatosis Type 2. Hum Gene Ther.

Meyers SM, Gutman FA, Kaye LD, Rothner AD (1995) Retinal changes associated with neurofibromatosis 2. Trans Am Ophthalmol Soc 93: 245–252.

Mulvihill JJ, Parry DM, Sherman JL, Pikus A, Kaiser-Kupfer MI, Eldridge R (1990) NIH conference. Neurofibromatosis 1 (Recklinghausen disease) and neurofibromatosis 2 (bilateral acoustic neurofibromatosis). An update. Ann Intern Med 113: 39–52.

National Institutes of Health Consensus Development Conference (1988) Neurofibromatosis. Conference statement. Arch Neurol 45: 575–578.

Ng J, Mordekar SR, Connolly DJ, Baxter P (2008) Stroke in a child with neurofibromatosis type 2. Eur J Paediatr Neurol Apr 10 [Epub ahead of print].

Nunes F, MacCollin M (2003) Neurofibromatosis 2 in the pediatric population. J Child Neurol 18: 718–724.

Otsuka G, Saito K, Nagatani T, Yoshida J (2003) Age at symptom onset and long-term survival in patients with neurofibromatosis type 2. J Neurosurg 99: 480–483.

Otto SR, Brackmann DE, Hitselberger WE, Shannon RV, Kuchta J (2002) Multichannel auditory brainstem implant: update on performance in 61 patients. J Neurosurg 96: 1063–1071.

Parry DM, Eldridge R, Kaiser-Kupfer MI, Bouzas EA, Pikus A, Patronas N (1994) Neurofibromatosis 2 (NF2): clinical characteristics of 63 affected individuals and clinical evidence for heterogeneity. Am J Med Genet 52: 450–461.

Parry DM, MacCollin MM, Kaiser-Kupfer MI, Pulaski K, Nicholson HS, Bolesta M, Eldridge R, Gusella JF (1996) Germ-line mutations in the neurofibromatosis 2 gene: correlations with disease severity and retinal abnormalities. Am J Hum Genet 59: 529–539.

Patronas NJ, Courcoutsakis N, Bromley CM, Katzman GL, MacCollin M, Parry DM (2001) Intramedullary and spinal canal tumors in patients with neurofibromatosis 2: MR imaging findings and correlation with genotype. Radiology 218: 434–442.

Ragge NK, Baser ME, Klein J, Nechiporuk A, Sainz J, Pulst SM, Riccardi VM (1995) Ocular abnormalities in neurofibromatosis 2. Am J Ophthalmol 120: 634–641.

Rouleau GA, Wertelecki W, Haines JL, Hobbs WJ, Trofatter JA, Seizinger BR, Martuza RL, Superneau DW, Conneally PM, Gusella JF (1987) Genetic linkage of bilateral acoustic neurofibromatosis to a DNA marker on chromosome 22. Nature 329: 246–248.

Rouleau GA, Merel P, Lutchman M, Sanson M, Zucman J, Marineau C, Hoang-Xuan K, Demczuk S, Desmaze C, Plougastel B, et al. (1993) Alteration in a new gene encoding a putative membrane-organizing protein causes neuro-fibromatosis type 2. Nature 363: 515–521.

Rowe JG, Radatz MW, Walton L, Soanes T, Rodgers J, Kemeny AA (2003) Clinical experience with gamma knife stereotactic radiosurgery in the management of vestibular schwannomas secondary to type 2 neurofibromatosis. J Neurol Neurosurg Psychiatry 74: 1288–1293.

Ruggieri M, Huson SM (2001) The clinical and diagnostic implications of mosaicism in the neurofibromatosis. Neurology 56: 1433–1443.

Ruggieri M, Iannetti P, Polizzi A, La MI, Spalice A, Giliberto O, Platania N, Gabriele AL, Albanese V, Pavone L (2005) Earliest clinical manifestations and natural history of neurofibromatosis type 2 (NF2) in childhood: a study of 24 patients. Neuropediatrics 36: 21–34.

Ruttledge MH, Andermann AA, Phelan CM, Claudio JO, Han FY, Chretien N, Rangaratnam S, MacCollin M, Short P, Parry D, Michels V, Riccardi VM, Weksberg R, Kitamura K, Bradburn JM, Hall BD, Propping P, Rouleau GA (1996) Type of mutation in the neurofibromatosis type 2 gene (NF2) frequently determines severity of disease. Am J Hum Genet 59: 331–342.

Schrell UM, Rittig MG, Anders M, Koch UH, Marschalek R, Kiesewetter F, Fahlbusch R (1997) Hydroxyurea for treatment of unresectable and recurrent meningiomas. II. Decrease in the size of meningiomas in patients treated with hydroxyurea. J Neurosurg 86: 840–844.

Seizinger BR, Martuza RL, Gusella JF (1986) Loss of genes on chromosome 22 in tumorigenesis of human acoustic neuroma. Nature 322: 644–647.

Sestini R, Bacci C, Provenzano A, Genuardi M, Papi L (2008) Evidence of a four-hit mechanism involving SMARCB1 and NF2 in schwannomatosis-associated schwannomas. Hum Mutat 29: 227–231.

Short PM, Martuza RL, Huson SM (1994) Neurofibromatosis 2: clinical features, genetic counselling and management issues. In: Huson SM, Hughes RAC (eds.) The neurofibromatosis a pathogenetic and clinical overview. London: Chapman and Hall medical, pp. 414–444.

Slattery WH III, Brackmann DE (1995) Results of surgery following stereotactic irradiation for acoustic neuromas. Am J Otol 16: 315–319.

Slattery WH III, Brackmann DE, Hitselberger W (1997) Middle fossa approach for hearing preservation with acoustic neuromas. Am J Otol 18: 596–601.

Slattery WH III, Brackmann DE, Hitselberger W (1998) Hearing preservation in neurofibromatosis type 2. Am J Otol 19: 638–643.

Sobel RA (1993) Vestibular (acoustic) schwannomas: histologic features in neurofibromatosis 2 and in unilateral cases. J Neuropathol Exp Neurol 52: 106–113.

Sperfeld AD, Hein C, Schroder JM, Ludolph AC, Hanemann CO (2002) Occurrence and characterization of peripheral nerve involvement in neurofibromatosis type 2. Brain 125: 996–1004.

Stangl AP, Wellenreuther R, Lenartz D, Kraus JA, Menon AG, Schramm J, Wiestler OD, von Deimling A (1997) Clonality of multiple meningiomas. J Neurosurg 86: 853–858.

Stemmer-Rachamimov AO, Ino Y, Lim ZY, Jacoby LB, MacCollin M, Gusella JF, Ramesh V, Louis DN (1998) Loss of the NF2 gene and merlin occur by the tumorlet stage of schwannoma development in neurofibromatosis 2. J Neuropathol Exp Neurol 57: 1164–1167.

Subach BR, Kondziolka D, Lunsford LD, Bissonette DJ, Flickinger JC, Maitz AH (1999) Stereotactic radiosurgery in the management of acoustic neuromas associated with neurofibromatosis Type 2. J Neurosurg 90: 815–822.

Thomsen J, Mirz F, Wetke R, Astrup J, Bojsen-Moller M, Nielsen E (2000) Intracranial sarcoma in a patient with neurofibromatosis type 2 treated with gamma knife radiosurgery for vestibular schwannoma. Am J Otol 21: 364–370.

Trivedi R, Byrne J, Huson SM, Donaghy M (2000) Focal amyotrophy in neurofibromatosis 2. J Neurol Neurosurg Psychiatry 69: 257–261.

Trofatter JA, MacCollin MM, Rutter JL, Murrell JR, Duyao MP, Parry DM, Eldridge R, Kley N, Menon AG, Pulaski K, et al. (1993) A novel moesin-, ezrin-, radixin-like gene is a candidate for the neurofibromatosis 2 tumor suppressor. Cell 75: 826.

Vincenti V, Pasanisi E, Guida M, Di Trapani G, Sanna M (2008) Hearing rehabilitation in neurofibromatosis type 2 patients: Cochlear versus auditory brainstem implantation. Audiol Neurootol 13: 273–280.

Wertelecki W, Rouleau GA, Superneau DW, Forehand LW, Williams JP, Haines JL, Gusella JF (1988) Neurofibromatosis 2: clinical and DNA linkage studies of a large kindred. N Engl J Med 319: 278–283.

Wishart JH (1822) Case of tumours in the skull, duraq mater, and brain. Edinburgh Med Surg J 18: 393–397.

Young DF, Eldridge R, Gardner WJ (1970) Bilateral acoustic neuroma in a large kindred. JAMA 214: 347–353.

Zhao Y, Kumar RA, Baser ME, Evans DG, Wallace A, Kluwe L, Mautner VF, Parry DM, Rouleau GA, Joe H, Friedman JM (2002) Intrafamilial correlation of clinical manifestations in neurofibromatosis 2 (NF2). Genet Epidemiol 23: 245–259.

# Chapter 5

# THE TUBEROUS SCLEROSIS COMPLEX

**Sergiusz Jóźwiak, Nicola Migone, and Martino Ruggieri**

Department of Neurology and Epileptology, Children's Memorial Health Institute, Warsaw, Poland (SJ);
Department of Genetics Biology and Biochemistry, Section of Genetics, University of Torino, Torino, Italy (NM); Institute of Neurological
Science, National Research Council, Catania, and Department of Paediatrics, University of Catania, Catania, Italy (MR)

## Introduction

Tuberous sclerosis complex (TSC) is the now preferred name for the autosomal dominant condition also known as tuberous sclerosis (OMIM # 191100). The addition of the term *complex* (first introduced in 1942 by the pathologist Moolten) emphasizes the multisystem involvement and variable expression of the disease, which "may affect any human organ with well-circumscribed, benign, non-invasive lesions known as hamartias and hamartomas" (Gomez 1999). The skin, brain, retina, heart, kidney, lung and liver are the organs most often involved, usually with the lesions called *hamartomas* (i.e., well-circumscribed groups of disorganized/dysplastic cells that, in addition, have a propensity to multiply excessively, thus growing as benign tumours that may or may not cause symptoms e.g., cardiac rhabdomyomas and renal angiomyolipomas) (Wilson et al. 2005) or with the other characteristic TSC lesion, the *hamartias* (i.e., well-circumscribed, misaligned or misarranged groups of dysplastic cells that nevertheless are appropriate for the organ or tissue involved and do not multiply or grow more rapidly than the normal cells of the affected organ e.g., hypomelanotic maculae in the skin, depigmented spots in the retina and cortical tubers in the brain). Other tissues that may be affected include bone, dental enamel, gums, oral, nasal and rectal mucosa, pituitary gland, thyroid, adrenals, thymus, gonads, uterus, vagina, pancreas, spleen, lymph nodes, lymphatics, synovia, aorta, and other large-caliber arteries. The spinal cord is rarely involved (e.g., spinal cordoma). Neither the skeletal muscles nor the peripheral nerves have been reported to be affected in TSC individuals so far. Except for the limited dysplastic lesions, the remaining parenchyma of the affected organs is normal in TSC (for reviews see Curatolo 2004, Gomez et al. 1999, Huson and Korf 2002, Osborne 2006). Central nervous system tumours are the leading cause of morbidity and mortality below 20 yrs, while renal disease is the main cause of death after the second decade (Northrup and Au 2006).

TSC is best known for its association with seizures, cognitive and behavioural impairment and skin manifestations. Until recently it was regarded as a rare disease and always associated with neuropsychiatric impairment. It is now apparent that TSC is not so rare and that only half of symptomatic mutation carriers have cognitive and behavioural difficulties, a further quarter have seizures but not intellectual impairment while the remainder have neither, being asymptomatic neurologically but having skin and/or visceral lesions (Osborne 2006, Schwartz et al. 2007).

Recent advances in molecular genetics have shed light into the pathogenesis and complex nature of this intriguing disease, and have been instrumental in the development of new treatment modalities. TSC results from mutations in one of two genes, *TSC1* (encoding *hamartin*) (OMIM # 605284) or *TSC2* (encoding *tuberin*) (OMIM # 191092). The activity of *TSC1* and *TSC2* is regulated by both inhibitory and activating phosphorylation events at specific amino acid residues. The TSC1-TSC2 protein complex interacts with several proteins: the clinical relevance of these interactions however is not yet well understood.

## Historical background and eponyms

For thorough reviews see also Curatolo (2004), Gomez (1987, 1995) and Wikipedia (2007).

### 19<sup>th</sup> century: the earliest pathological descriptions

The earliest writing on TSC is a brief necropsy description made by the German pathologist **Friedrich Daniel von Recklinghausen** on March 25<sup>th</sup> *1862* at the Obstetrical Society of Berlin: a newborn infant who (had) "died after taking a few breaths", had "several myomata" protruding "on the cardiac surface…into the cardiac chambers…and embedded in the ventricular walls" and "a great number of scleroses" of the brain.

An earlier (possible) illustration of TSC is given by the French dermatologist *Pierre François Rayer* in his *1835* atlas of skin disorders: a young man's face is dotted with clusters of small, erythematous papules with a characteristic distribution and similar appearance to the typical TSC facial angiofibromas.

It was not until *1880* however that the French physician, writer and politician **Désiré-Magloire Bourneville** (1840–1909), gave the first detailed report of the typical skin and neurological TSC abnormalities and gross cerebral and renal pathology in a 15–year-old epileptic and mentally handicapped inmate girl at *La Pitié Salpetrièr* who died in her bed at 3 o' clock in the morning on May 7<sup>th</sup> 1879: clinically she presented with skin tags (of the "molluscum pendulum" type) of the neck and "confluent vesiculopapular eruption of the nose, cheeks and forehead"; she had suffered of (partial and generalised) seizures most of her life and frequent episodes of status epilepticus and developed right spastic hemiplegia. On post-mortem examination of the brain Bourneville found "hard, raised, whitish ("opaque") areas of greater density ("sclerotic") than the surrounding cortex in some of the cerebral circumvolutions" and "white nodular tumours embedded in the corpus striatum and protruding into the lateral ventricles". Bourneville coined the term *tuberous sclerosis* (because of the "potato-like consistency" of the sclerotic areas

in many convolutions) *of the cerebral convolutions*. Notably, he also found small yellowish white tumours in the kidney which he thought were unrelated to the cerebral pathology.

A year later (1881) **Bourneville** and **Brissaud** reported on a second child who died at *La Biçêtre* of status epilepticus at age 4 years with similar cerebral (and kidneys) pathological findings. Between the years 1880 and 1900 the same authors (Bourneville and Brissaud 1881, 1900) reported on a total of ten patients and emphasised the association of cerebral TSC with renal tumours.

Désiré-Magloire Bourneville was the son of a small Normandy landowner born on 20 October 1840 in the little village of Garanciéres (Eure) (Jansen et al 2004; Poirier and Signoret 1991). He studied in Paris and became interne des hôpitaux at the Bicêtre, the Salpêtrière, the Hôpital St. Louis and the Pitié. During the Franco-Prussian War he was surgeon to the 160<sup>th</sup> Battalion of the Garde Nationale. Later he became assistant medical officer at the field hospital of the Jardin des Plantes. Finally, even though he was a well-established physician, he resumed his internship at the Pitié, which was then covered by fire from German artillery. During the Paris Commune in 1871, when the violent revolutionaries wanted to execute their wounded political enemies, Bourneville personally intervened and saved several of his patients. He received his doctorate in 1870 in Paris. He was physician at the paediatric service at Bicêtre with the title of Médecin des services d'aliénés from 1879 to 1905, and upon his retirement still held the directorship of the Foundation Vallée at the Bicêtre. In 1873 Bourneville founded the journal "Progrés Médical"; in 1880 the "Archives de neurologie"; he also established the "Revue photographique des hôpitaux de Paris". Besides his own works he arranged for the publication of an edition of the works of Jean Martin Charcot (1825-1893). He was the founder of the first school for mentally retarded children (Reyre 1989). In addition to his description of tuberous sclerosis, he made observations on myxoedema, cretinism, and mongolism. He retired as physician at the Bicêtre in 1905, and then was entrusted the directorship of the Fondation Vallée, concentrating his efforts on the treatment of mentally retarded children. He founded the first day school for special instruction of defective children in Paris, a movement that later took hold in many countries (Who named it? 2007). On Saturdays he held open-house at the Bicêtre in which his charges performed exercises and dances to the accompaniment of a band composed of idiots, epileptics, and spastics; the thrombonist had wooden legs. From 1876 he was a member of the Paris city council and in 1873 became a member of parliament, both positions an enthusiastic advocate of reforms of the health system (Brais 1993; Gateaux-Mennecier 2002). Paris owes him for the expansion of its hospitals. He championed the worldliness of the care of the sick and created public school for the education of nurses, he founded isolatory departments for contagious diseases, special wards for sick children (Gateaux-Mennecier 2003; Who named it? 2007). He died on 29th May 1909 at his home, 14 rue des Carmes in Paris (Poirier and Signoret 1991).

In the same period of these first descriptions *Hardegen* (1881) described the brain cutting findings of a 2-day old infant who died in status epilepticus: his "areas of sclerosis throughout the cerebral cortex" and the "small tumours protruding into the lateral ventricles" contained giant ganglionic cells and giant hyperplasia that Hartdegen supposed to be a "congenital gangliocellular glioma" offering a tumour aetiology hypothesis later supported by Vogt (1908) and Bielschkowsky (1914).

During the remainder of the 19th century, dermatologists led by *Balzer* and *Ménétrier* (1885) and *Hallopeau* and *Lerede* (Gomez 1999) in France and by **Pringle** (1890) in Great Britain recognised and named "*adenoma sebaceum*" a characteristic facial lesion found in some individuals (and also running in some families) with seizures and mental handicap.

## Clinical, pathological and early genetics developments of the 20th century

Histopathological studies of the cerebral lesions began with *Pellizzi* (1901) in the 20th century who emphasised the dysplastic nature of the cerebral lesions (disordered cortical architecture, heterotopias

and defective myelination) and went on with *Perusini* (1905) who drew similar conclusions and also observed the association of cerebral, renal and cardiac lesions with facial angiofibromas ("adenoma sebaceum") in TSC patients.

In 1905 *Campbell* described the TSC-associated ocular findings and in 1908 *Heinrich Vogt* diagnosed TSC apparently for the first time on a living patient who had seizures, mental handicap and "adenoma sebaceum" and thus this "triad" was named after him. He also noted that heart and kidney tumours were part of the disease.

*Kirpicznik* (1910) and *Berg* (1913) first noted and emphasised the hereditary nature of TSC by studying multiple generation TSC families (Berg 1913, Kirpicznik 1910) and describing the condition in identical (and fraternal) twins (Kirpicznik 1910). *Schuster* (1914) reported on a unique case of a TSC individual with only the "adenoma sebaceum" component of the classic Vogt triad (i.e., without intellectual impairment and seizures) and coined the term *forme fruste* (from the French *fruste* = defaced). *Nieuwenhuise* in 1912 first drew attention to the long life span of TSC patients. At the same time the British physician *Sherlock* (1911) coined the unfortunate term (used mainly in the UK for the severe TSC phenotypes) of "*epiloia*" (reflecting the combination of *epilepsy* and *anoia* or mindlessness (Critchley 1988)).

**Van der Hoeve**, in 1920, called attention to the retinal astrocytic hamartomas and other well-circumscribed organ lesions in TSC patients listing the varieties of these lesions in TSC. Noting the similarities between TSC, neurofibromatosis and von Hippel-Lindau disease in the spotty distribution of these lesions and their tendency to grow as benign tumours, he introduced the term *phakoma* and the concept of *phakomatosis*. In the first decades of the 20th century it was soon realised that TSC was not as rare disease as previously thought the majority of reported patients however were inmates of hospitals, asylums or (similar) homes for mentally handicapped or epileptic individuals. By counting these inmates the first TSC population-based studies recorded prevalence figures of 1 in 30,000 or 1 in 100,000 inhabitants (Nevin and Pearce 1968).

In 1932 *Critchley* and *Earl* published a thoroughly description of 29 TSC cases emphasising for the first time the clinical value of white spots (hypomelanotic macules) in diagnosing the disease, a feature that was subsequently emphasised by *Gold* and *Freeman* (1965), *Harris* and *Moynahan* (1966) and *Fitzpatrick et al.* (1968). Critchley also noted (years before the first description of "infantile autism" by Kanner) the association of autistic behaviour with TSC.

It was however earlier, in 1924, and then in 1935 that *Marcus* (1924) and *Dalsgaard-Nielsen* (1935) described intracranial calcifications by means of X-rays. In the meantime *Berkowitz et al.* (1934) demonstrated intraventricular subependimal nodules by pneumoencephalography in a living patient (the so-called "candle-guttering" sign taken from the resemblance of nodules to the drippings of a burning candle). As a consequence of both these discoveries, the number of patients diagnosed increased dramatically.

The landmark for the understanding of natural history of TSC was however achieved by the study of **Lagos** and **Gomez** in 1967: these authors demonstrated, in a series of 71 TSC patients from the Mayo clinic, that only 62% had intellectual handicap while 38% had normal or near normal intelligence. More interestingly was the finding that all the mentally retarded TSC patients had had seizures but among those with average cognitive capacities, some had had seizures and some had not.

## Impact of the new technologies

The introduction and progressive improvement of imaging methods which began in the mid-1970s with computed tomography followed by echocardiography and abdominal ultrasound and in the 80s by magnetic resonance imaging provided reliable non-invasive methods of diagnosis that aided in establishing new and more extensive criteria for diagnosis of TSC. The number of TSC new diagnoses increased and new prevalence estimates in the general population varied between 1 in 6,000 to 1 in 10,000 (Sampson et al. 1989, Osborne et al. 1991). Milder phenotypes and patients lacking neurologic symptoms, mostly relatives of index cases, were increasingly recognised. Then

came the first linkage studies localising one *TSC* gene at chromosome 9q34 (called *TSC1* gene) (Fryer et al. 1987) and a second *TSC* gene on chromosome 16p13.3 (called *TSC2* gene) (Kandt et al. 1992).

In 1993 the **TSC2 gene** (42 exons) was cloned and its product (a 1807 aminoacid protein called tuberin) identified by the European Chromosome 16 consortium (1993) and a few years later, the **TSC1 gene** (23 exons) and its protein product (hamartin, 1164 aminoacids) (van Slegtenhorst 1997). In the very last few years, the first comprehensive genotype-phenotype studies have been published (Dabora et al. 2001).

To underline the complexity of the clinical presentation the term *tuberous sclerosis complex* obtained a general favour, so that its acronim became the official name of the two genes. Presently, both terms *tuberous sclerosis* and *tuberous sclerosis complex* are equally used to define the disease.

## Incidence and prevalence

The incidence of TSC at birth cannot be assessed since a still undefined fraction of mutation carriers are either free of neurologic symptoms (seizures and intellectual/behavioural deficit), or show mild phenotypes that do not prompt them to ask for medical assistance. The generally reported prevalence of 1 in 6000 has been estimated from the screening of children attending the primary schools. Three-quarters of patients are sporadic (Dabora et al. 2001, Jóźwiak et al. 2000), the remaining have one or more affected relatives.

Among familial cases, about half are due to a defect of the *TSC1* and half to the *TSC2* gene. On the other hand, sporadic cases, thought to represent new mutations, are five times more commonly caused by *TSC2* than to *TSC1* gene mutations (Dabora et al. 2001).

## Clinical manifestations

The clinical features of TSC involve several body systems (Table 1) and most importantly develop at different ages. In addition, not all clinical signs and symptoms appear in every patient. This means that, as in NF1 (see Chapter 3), the assessments should vary according to the age of affected individuals. For many years it was believed that the classic triad of features identified by Vogt (1908) of mental re-

**Table 1.** Revised diagnostic criteria for tuberous sclerosis complex

*Major features*
Facial angiofibromas or forehead plaque
Nontraumatic ungual or periungual fibroma
Hypomelanotic macule (three or more)
Shagreen patch (connective tissue nevus)
Multiple retinal nodular hamartomas
Cortical tuber[#]
Subependymal nodule
Subependymal giant cell astrocytoma
Cardiac rhabdomyoma, single or multiple
Lymphangiomyomatosis[*]
Renal angiomyolipoma[*]

*Minor features*
Multiple, randomly distributed pits in dental enamel
Hamartomatous rectal polyps[§]
Bone cysts [&]
Cerebral white matter radial migration lines [#,&]
Gingival fibromas
Nonrenal hamartomas [§]
Retinal achromic patch
"Confetti" skin lesions
Multiple renal cysts [§]

**Definite tuberous sclerosis complex:**
Either two major features or one major feature plus two minor features.
**Probable tuberous sclerosis complex:**
One major plus one minor feature.
**Possible tuberous sclerosis complex:**
Either one major feature or two or more minor features.

[#]When cerebral cortical dysplasia and cerebral white matter migration tracts occur together, they should be counted as one rather than two features of tuberous sclerosis.
[*]When both lymphangiomyomatosis and renal angiomyolipomas are present, other features of tuberous sclerosis should be present before a definite diagnosis is assigned.
[§]Histologic confirmation is suggested.
[&]Radiographic confirmation is suggested.

tardation, epilepsy, and "adenoma sebaceum" (now called "facial angiofibroma") had to be present for the diagnosis of TSC. However as this triad is only present in less than 30% of cases many patients were undiagnosed. We now know that milder phenotypes exist and cases with single (or few) lesions harbour TSC mutations; in addition, clinical expression and severity are variable between families and even within the same family. This led to a dramatic revision of diagnostic criteria (see Roach et al. 1992, 1998; Gomez et al. 1999) and to reconsideration of previously established diagnostic workups. Even with current imaging techniques however the diagnosis of TSC can be difficult in individuals with subtle findings.

## Skin manifestations

Due to their long list and clinical accessibility dermatological manifestations belong to the most important diagnostic markers of TSC. A careful skin examination of patients at risk for TSC continues to be the easiest method of establishing the diagnosis. Some of them are pathognomonic, but some are not and may be seen in healthy persons. The careful examiner may reveal some skin manifestations of TSC even in the neonatal period. As the child grows additional cutaneous lesions may appear and the diagnosis becomes frequently evident. Because about 30% of cases are familial, and some skin manifestations are better seen in adults, it should be stressed that in all suspected paediatric cases careful skin examination should be done not only in the child, but also in the parents (Jóźwiak et al. 1998a, Jóźwiak and Schwartz 2003). The knowledge about the incidence of the lesions, specificity for TSC and typical age of presentation may be crucial for the proper diagnosis.

## Hypomelanotic macules

The most characteristic type of hypomelanotic macule is leaf-shaped or lance ovate, resembling the leaf of the European mountain ash tree (Fig. 1). However, other shapes such as round macules are also observed in TSC patients (Fig. 1A, B). Their margins are usually

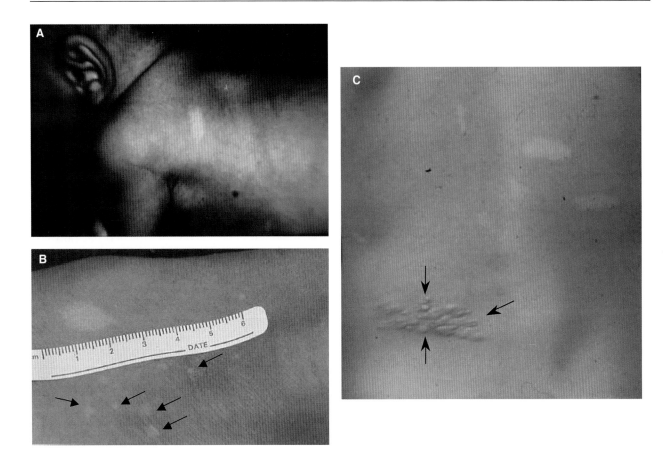

**Fig. 1.** Different aspects of hypomelanotic macules in the skin in TSC patients: (**A**) large, leaf-shaped macules in the trunk of an infant; (**B**) a large (2 cm across) rounded to ovalar macule associated to multiple "confetti-like" lesions (black arrows) in a toddler; (**C**) multiple, large, leaf-shaped macules in the posterior trunk associated to a shagreen patch (black arrows) in a 10-year-old boy.

well demarcated; their size can range from a few millimeters to several centimeters and their number can range from 2 or 3 to over 40. They are asymmetrically distributed over the body, especially over the trunk and buttocks and are rarely evident on the face. The involvement of the scalp may produce areas of poliosis.

Hypomelanotic spots are frequently seen in newborns and infants with TSC and thus are regarded as the earliest visible sign of the disease. Hypomelanotic macules may be the only skin finding in infants and, if coupled with the presence of infantile spasms, they strongly allude to the diagnosis of TSC. Overall, hypomelanotic macules are observed in approximately 90% of children below 2 years of age and in about 95–97% of older patients (Jóźwiak et al. 1998a).

The hypomelanotic macules may be found in 4.7% of the general population, so the presence of less then 3 macules does not indicate the necessity of an extensive evaluation to confirm TSC. The use of ultraviolet light (Wood's lamp, 365 nm) can reveal lesions that are invisible on skin examination under the normal light.

Skin biopsy specimens taken from hypomelanotic macules of patients with TSC usually demonstrate a normal number of melanocytes with reduction in intensity of histochemical reaction as compared to the surrounding normal skin. Electron microscopic studies, showing reduced number, diameter and melanization of melanosomes in melanocytes in TSC patients, may be necessary to differentiate a hypomelanotic macule from vitiligo, nevus anemicus, nevus depigmentosus, piebaldism or Vogt-Koyanagi-Harada syndrome (Schwartz and Janniger 1997).

## Confetti-like lesions

These small lesions are the second type of hypomelanocytic macules associated with TSC (Fig. 1B). They are regarded as a separate diagnostic feature from the other types hypomelanocytic macules in the clinical criteria of tuberous sclerosis (Roach et al. 1998). Webb et al. (1996) reported them in 28% of patients with TSC. In our experience they are more common in the second decade of life and adulthood and in cases with a more severe neurocutaneous phenotype. Confetti-like macules present as multiple, 1-2 mm white spots symmetrically distributed over the extremities. Their histopathology is similar to that of the hypomelanotic macules.

## Forehead fibrous plaques

Forehead fibrous plaques are yellowish-brown or flesh-colored patches of raised skin of variable size and shape from a few millimeters to several centimeters in diameter (Fig. 2). The lesion is usually located on the forehead or scalp, is soft, medium or hard in consistency, and may have a smooth or rough surface. Single large or sometimes multiple lesions can be seen. Because of a lesser vascular component as compared to facial angiofibromas, forehead fibrous plaque is not altered by warm weather or when the child cries. Contrary to facial angiofibromas, forehead plaque may become evident at any age (Jóźwiak et al. 1998a). In some patients they can be seen at birth. In newborns and infants they are hyperpigmented, flat and soft in consistency and gradually grow becoming raised and solid after many years (Fig. 2B).

As forehead fibrous plaques and facial angiofibromas share a similar histological appearance, Roach et al. (1998) suggested that these two lesions should be regarded as a single entity for the diagnostic criteria of TSC.

Forehead fibrous plaques may be noted in about 20% of children and more than 40% of adult patients (Jóźwiak et al. 1998a, Webb et al. 1996).

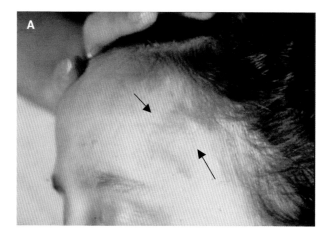

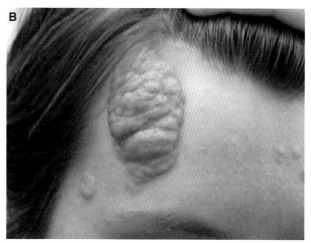

Fig. 2. (**A, B**) Forehead plaques in two children with TSC (black arrows).

There is a higher incidence of forehead plaques in patients harbouring TSC2 versus TSC1 mutations (Dabora et al. 2001).

Laser treatment of these lesions may be recommended. Removal of large disfiguring forehead fibrous plaques may be necessary especially in adolescents and adults with fair mental development.

## Shagreen patches

They represent the third most common skin feature of TSC, after hypomelanotic macules and angiofibromas (see below). They are firm yellowish-red or pink nodules slightly elevated above the surrounding skin, with their surface resembling in texture the skin of the orange (Figs. 1C and 3). These lesions are usually found on the dorsal body surfaces, especially the lumbosacral area. In the majority of patients the lesions are multiple and small, from few millimeters to 1 centimeter in size and might be easily overlooked in younger children. Usually appearing in clusters in a few patients they become large lesions (more then 10 centimeters in diameter). Their first appearance usually takes place soon before or around puberty, but we observed several patients with shagreen patches being present from

early infancy. Their incidence increases with age reaching about 50% in adult patients (Jóźwiak et al. 2000). Multiple, small lesions may be observed and may easily be overlooked in early childhood.

The shagreen patch is a connective tissue hamartoma composed of excess collagen and elastic tissue. Rogers (1988) delineates two main types of shagreen patches. In the first, more common type, a band of superficial dermis is normal but its deeper layers are composed of a haphazard arrangement of collagen fibers. In the second type a uniform hamartomatous proliferation of collagen throughout the whole section of dermis is seen. The general appearance of both types is that of excess collagen and elastic tissue in disproportion to the amount of muscle, adipose tissue, appendages, and vascular structures (Rogers 1988).

The shagreen patch is difficult to differentiate both clinically and histopathologically from other connective tissue nevi. The differential diagnosis should include connective tissue nevi with osteopoikilosis (Buschke-Ollendorf syndrome). Large shagreen patches may require cosmetic treatment.

## Facial angiofibromas

The earliest illustration of the lesion was displayed in the color atlas of skin diseases of Rayer in 1835 (Rayer 1835). The author described and illustrated a man with facial erythematous papules: "vascular vegetations … a rare and little known condition … characterized by little red vascular persistent papules, single or in groups … occurring most often on the face". In 1880 Bourneville (1880) described similar lesions in his patients with TSC but considered them as coincidental and not related with cerebral and renal pathology. The name of the lesions is usually linked with the name of Pringle, as "Pringle's sign", who reported: "indolent, firm, whitish, or yellowish, sago-grain like, solid papules or little tumours imbedded in the skin at different depths, or projecting from it … intermingled with these lesions and transgressing their limits in every direction, especially over the cheeks, toward the ears, innumerable capillary dilatations and stellate telangiectases" (Pringle 1890). Pringle and other authors of that

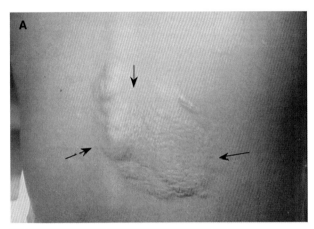

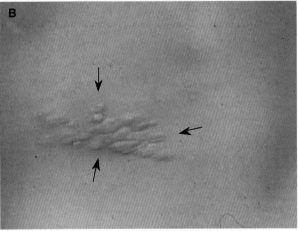

**Fig. 3.** (**A, B**) Different aspects of the shagreen patches (black arrows) in the posterior trunk: note the size and more homogeneous tissue texture of one plaque (**A**) as compared to the more irregular aspect of the other plaque (**B**).

times inaccurately labelled the lesions "adenoma sebaceum". This term is sometimes erroneously used even in nowadays publications.

The typical facial angiofibromas are red to pink papules or nodules with a smooth, glistening surface imbedded in the skin at different depths (Fig. 4). They are symmetrically and bilaterally distributed over the centrofacial areas, especially over the nasolabial folds, cheeks and chin. Interestingly, these lesions tend to spare the upper lip. Angiofibromas with a prominent vascular component are more obvious when the child is irritated or in warm weather. Early angiofibromas are red due to an excessive vascular proliferation.

It is a peculiar skin lesion in TSC with a clearly defined age of presentation. Angiofibromas usually become apparent between the second and fifth year of life and become more prominent with age. We found them in 74.5% (79 out of 106) of paediatric patients (Jóźwiak et al. 1998a). Webb et al. (1996) recorded facial angiofibromas in 88% of patients aged more than 30 years. In pubertal children the lesions should be differentiated with *acne vulgaris.*

Some reports have shown an association between facial angiofibromas and MEN 1, suggesting that facial angiofibromas are not characteristic for TSC (Darling et al. 1997). However, these studies did not mention sufficiently results of examinations to exclude the diagnosis of TSC. As it is known that some patients with TSC present MEN1 manifestations we believe that the aforementioned studies described rather patients with TSC and MEN1 features, rather then patients with MEN1 and isolated angiofibromas.

Histopathological studies revealed that the term *angiofibroma* seems to be more proper and acceptable, than *adenoma sebaceum*, as there is hyperplasia of both connective tissue and vascular elements of the dermis (Fig. 4D). The multitude of vessels results in some patients in a red colouring of the lesions. Large angiofibromas may be polypoid and are characterised by the presence of dense fibrous tissue with collagen bundles often arranged in layers around adnexal structures. In perivascular areas can be found multinucleated giant cells. With increasing age the collagen becomes sclerotic and layered.

The diagnostic significance of facial angiofibromas has never been questioned. Since 1908 the facial angiofibromas (as "adenoma sebaceum") were included by Vogt (1908) in the diagnostic triad of TSC (with mental retardation and epilepsy). In the recent classifications of diagnostic criteria from 1992 (Roach et al. 1992) and 1998 (Roach et al. 1998) multiple, bilateral lesions in characteristic distribution are regarded as primary or characteristic of TSC and do not require histopathological confirmation. In adults, facial angiofibromas are often misdiagnosed as acne rosacea.

Various modalities have been used in the treatment of facial angiofibromas including shave excision, cryosurgery, dessication, dermabrasion, carbon and argon laser (Papadavid et al. 2002, Bittencourt et al. 2001).

There is no consensus about the most suitable time of the treatment. Some authors suggest removal of early angiofibromas, being convinced that such approach should prevent the development of full-fledged, fibrous angiofibromas. Still, as the lesions may continue to grow until adulthood and faster growth during puberty may be noted, the postponement of the treatment until then may be justified. The decision must be balanced by the serious psychosocial problems seen in adolescents with fair mental development and extensive angiofibromas. Especially in these group of children cosmetic treatment of the lesions is strongly recommended.

## Ungual or periungual fibromas

Ungual or periungual fibromas are regarded as very characteristic or pathognomonic for TSC. According to the last diagnostic criteria of TSC by Roach et al. (1998) periungual fibromas are regarded as a major sign of TSC. The lesions are known also as Koenen's tumours since their description by Koenen (1932) in members of a Dutch TSC family. These fibromas are skin colored or reddish nodules usually arising from the finger or toe nail bed, appearing clinically over the lateral nail groove, nail plate or along the proximal nail folds (Fig. 5). Their size

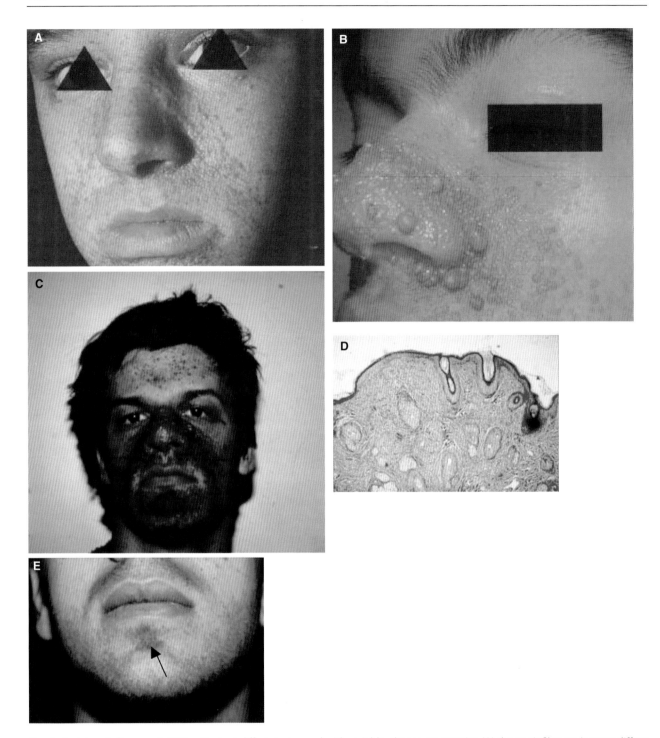

**Fig. 4.** Facial angiofibromas in TSC patients at different ages and with variable phenotype severity: (**A**) the angiofibroma is more diffuse and (relatively) milder at age 8 years (**A**); the lesions are more pronounced (**B**) and much more diffuse (**C**) in patients with more severe neurocutaneous phenotypes; (**D**) histopathological aspect of an angiofibroma (see text for explanation); (**E**) a solitary facial angiofibroma of the chin (black arrow) in a 30-year-old TSC patient who had (otherwise) normal skin appearance, normal intellect and no other TSC lesions besides few cortical tubers in the brain: this proband was referred because he asked to remove the chin lesions which in turn (at histology, see **D**) turned out to be an angiofibroma and prompted investigation in the proband and in his family (16 asymptomatic members of this family harbouring a TSC1 mutation were diagnosed with TSC).

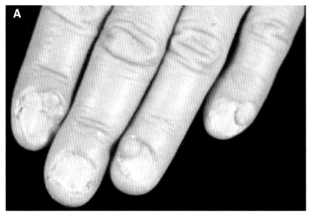
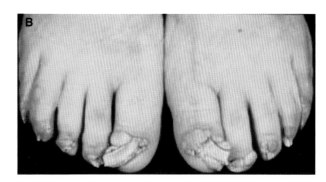
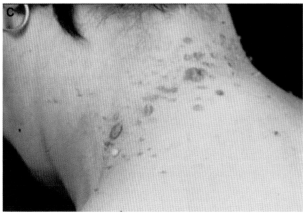

**Fig. 5.** Ungual fibromas of the hands (**A**) and feet (**B**) and diffuse firbromas of the neck (molluscum fibrosum pendulum) (**C**).

ranges from several millimeters to about 1 centimeter. They are more commonly found on the toes than on the fingers.

These lesions usually present at puberty or soon after and become more common with increasing age. They are usually absent in younger patients with TSC. Webb et al. (1996) found them in none of their TSC children before the age of 5 years, but in 68% between the ages of 15 and 29 years. In our paediatric population of TSC patients we have seen them in 16 out of 106 children (15.1%) – in one child aged 2 to 5 years, in 3 patients aged 5 to 9, in 8 children aged 9 to 14 years and in 4 children over 14 years (Jóźwiak et al. 1998a).

It has been suggested that tight shoes may stimulate fibroma growth, especially on the lateral aspect of the fifth toe. Usually, these fibromas tend to regrow after their removal. Special attention should be paid to single lesions which may arise spontaneously or after trauma, and may not be related to TSC. Practically, in our opinion, multiple lesions without any history of trauma can be regarded as pathognomonic to TSC. We found them also helpful in making the diagnosis in young children, when ungual fibromas are demonstrated in their apparently non-affected parents.

Histologically, these lesions are fibromas or angiofibromas, similar to the fibrous forehead plaques and the facial angiofibromas.

Excision of large or symptomatic ungual fibromas is the choice method of treatment, although recurrences are common (Berlin and Billick 2002).

## Other skin lesions

In TSC many other non specific skin lesions have been reported, among them – cafè au lait spots and molluscum fibrosum pendulum (see Fig. 5C). Because of their high prevalence in the general population and uncertain frequency in the TSC population, it is difficult to judge whether these lesions represent a coincidental finding or are the result of the hyperproliferative nature of TSC. So far these cutaneous findings are not included in the clinical diagnostic criteria for TSC.

## Oral manifestations

Gingival fibromas and dental pitting (Fig. 6) are included in the diagnostic criteria for TSC (Sparling et al. 2007). Oral fibromas are common in adults with TSC: these are usually gingival (>50%) or at other oral mucosal sites (40%) including the buccal mucosa (inside the angular commissure), the labial mucosa, the superior labial frenulum, and palate and tongue. Oral fibromas also can occur sporadically in the general population but at a much lower frequency (e.g., 12/1000).

Another common (drug induced) oral complication of TSC is gingival overgrowth (hyperplasia or hypertrophy) usually secondary to the use of phenytoin.

Dental enamel pitting (Fig. 6) is observed in up to 100% of patients with TSC. Dental pits can also be observed in the general population but at lower frequency and with fewer lesions than in TSC.

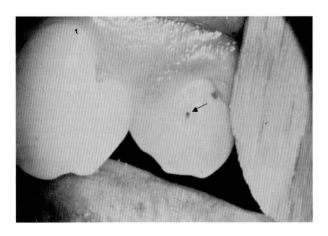

**Fig. 6.** Dental pitting (black arrow) in a TSC child. Courtesy of Dr. Rudolf Happle, Marburg, Germany. From: Vakilzadeh F, Happle R (1980) Schmelzdefekte bei tuberöser sklerose. Hautarzt 31: 336–337.

## Neurological manifestations

There is considerable heterogeneity in the neurological manifestations. The spectrum includes patients with normal intellect and no seizures and extends to those with severe mental retardation and incapacitating seizures (Leung et al. 2007). However, when present, neurological complications are the most common causes of mortality and morbidity and the most likely to affect the quality of life.

## Epilepsy

The most frequent neurological feature, epilepsy, is diagnosed in 60–90% of TSC patients during their lifetime (Curatolo et al. 2005, Holmes et al. 2007). Seizures occurred in 96% of patients aged 9–14 years referred to a child neurology clinic (Jóźwiak et al. 2000). In a recent retrospective epidemiological study on the prevalence of TSC in Northern Ireland, it was noted that 93.2% had epilepsy (Devlin et al. 2006). However, in an unbiased genetic linkage study only 62% of the patients developed seizures (Webb and Osborne 1991): it must be noted that these patients were not followed throughout their lifespan and therefore the incidence figures may be low (Holmes et al. 2007).

Seizures are the presenting sign in 67% of patients and in most patients the onset of epilepsy is between the 4th and 6th month of life. The most common type of seizures in the first months of life are infantile spasms: the other commonest seizures types are complex partial, generalized tonic-clonic and myoclonic (Holmes et al. 2007). There is a relationship between epilepsy and mental retardation (Jóźwiak et al. 1998b). Patients with early onset of epilepsy (<6th month of life) and unremitting seizures are more prone to develop severe mental retardation. Patients with a sustained remission are more likely to have normal intelligence. Overall poor prognostic factors include multiple seizure types, seizures onset before one year of age, and multifocal EEG abnormalities. The clinical challenge is to predict seizure intractability and intervene before it occurs (Holmes et al. 2007). There is an increasing body of evidence that some in same infants with confirmed diagnosis of TSC and epileptic discharges in EEG, the introduction of antiepileptic treatment even before the appearance of clinical seizures may prevent from epilepsy and subsequent mental retardation (Jozwiak et al. 2007, Stafstrom et al. 2007).

Infantile spasms are particularly prevalent among children with TSC (Curatolo and Cusmai 1987, O'Callaghan et al. 2004, Thiele 2004), and TSC accounts for up to 25% of infantile spasms cases (Young 2002). Data is accumulating that infantile spasms and associated EEG findings in TSC are somewhat different than those seen in classic West syndrome. In TSC, focal seizures can precede, coexist with, or evolve into infantile spasms (Curatolo et al. 2005). EEG features of focal or multifocal spikes are most common when seizures are first identified, with hypsarrhytmia (often with focal features) evolving later (Holmes et al. 2007).

Epilepsy in children with TSC tends to be progressive, with increasing seizure frequency and pharmacological intractability over time. Despite the multifocal occurrence of tubers and hence multifocal nature of epileptic foci in TSC, many children are considered for epilepsy surgery, especially if a single tuber acts as a predominant focus. The success of tuber resection is encouraging enough to warrant an aggressive approach (Bebin et al. 1993; Guerreiro et al. 1998; Koh et al. 2000; Weiner et al. 2004, 2006). In addition to EEG, epileptogenic areas can be identified using magnetic resonance imaging (MRI) and positron emission tomography (PET) scans (Asano et al. 2000, Kagawa et al. 2005, Jansen et al. 2006). A multimodality approach is most helpful in identifying the epileptic focus (Lachhwani et al. 2005).

The surgical outcome varies: recent studies indicated 60% surgically treated children seizure-free at a median follow-up of 15 months (Kagawa et al. 2005). However, seizures can recur after removal of an offending tuber. Similarly, the effect of surgical resection on cognitive and behavioural outcome is unclear (Holmes et al. 2007).

## Learning disabilities and mental retardation

These are very common in TSC, affecting from 40% to 80% of patients (Jambaque et al. 1991, Osborne and Webb 1993, O'Callaghan et al. 2004). Cognitive disabilities tend to be moderate or severe in degree. Children with a TSC2 mutation generally have a greater cognitive disability. A higher number of tubers correlated with a poorer cognitive outcome in some studies (Jambaque et al. 1991, O'Callaghan et al. 2004), but not in others (Doherty et al. 2005). There is no direct association between cognitive impairment, brain tuber localization, infantile spasms or focal EEG abnormalities and autism in TSC. However, the presence of cortical tubers in frontal and temporal lobes as opposed to a history of infantile spasms was associated with TSC in a recent study (Raznahan et al. 2007).

Attention deficit, hyperactivity, and sleep problems are the most frequent behavioural disorders. Cognitive disabilities of various degrees of severity are recorded in adulthood (Pulsifer et al. 2007, Winterkorn 2007). De Vries et al. (2007) in a postal survey of physical and behavioural abnormalities in children and adolescents with TSC in UK reported that patients with mental retardation were significantly more likely to have an autism spectrum disorder, attention deficit-related symptoms and speech and language difficulties. They were more likely to have a history of epilepsy, facial angiofibromas and shagreen patches and tended to have a greater number of physical features of the disorder. However, about one third of the children without mental retardation had features suggestive of a developmental disorder. Anxiety symptoms, depressed mood and aggressive outbursts occurred at equally high rates in those with and without mental retardation and were often not recognised (de Vries et al 2007). A consensus panel for the evaluation of cognitive and behavioural profiles has been recently proposed (de Vries et al 2005) for being incorporated in the overall formulation of the needs of the persons with TSC to plan educational, social and clinical management strategies. Assessments should be documented so that individual regular longitudinal progress can be monitored.

## Autism

The exact proportion of autistic patients suffering from TSC is not well established, however, the risk of autism in TSC is much higher than in general population. Several studies tried to establish the prevalence of TSC in the autism spectrum disorder population and estimates varied from 0.9 to 1.1% (Frombonne et al. 1997; Wong 2006) to 9% (Gillberg et al 1994) whereas features of autism were present in 5% (Webb et al. 1996) to 61% (Gillberg et al. 1994) of patients with TSC (see also the studies by Baker et al. 1998, Bolton and Griffiths 1997, Calderon Gonzalez et al. 1994, Curatolo et al. 1991, Gutierrez et al. 1998, Hunt and Dennis 1987, Hunt and Shepherd 1993, Riikonen and Simell 1990, Smalley et al. 1992, Wiznitzer et al. 2004).

Despite considerable progresses in the last few years, the neurobiological basis of autism in TSC is still largely unknown and its clinical management represents a major challenge for the physicians involved in taking care of TSC patients. Recent evidence suggests that early-onset refractory epilepsy (Deonna et al. 2007, Humphrey et al. 2006) and/or functional deficits associated with the anatomical lesions in the temporal lobes (Chou et al. 2007) or in the cerebellum (Eluvathingal et al 2006) or the overall load of the cerebral lesions (Chou et al. 2007, Wong and Khong 2006) may be associated with autism. The emerging evidence is consistent with the notion that early onset electrophysiological disturbances within the temporal lobes (and perhaps other locations) (Deonna et al. 2006, Waltz et al. 2002) has a deleterious effect on the development and establishment of key social cognitive representations concerned with processing social information, perhaps especially from faces (Bolton 2004). No one factor alone (cognitive impairment, tuber localization, occurrence of infantile spasms, focal EEG abnormalities), can be causally linked with the abnormal behaviour. Autism may also reflect a direct effect of the abnormal genetic program (Au et al. 2007, Holmes et al. 2007). In this respect, the likelihood of a child with TSC developing autism is greater if the child harbours a mutation in the TSC2 gene, although autism also develops in children with TSC1 mutations (Bolton and Griffiths 1997, Holmes et al. 2007).

## Neuroimaging

There are several types of intracranial lesions found on imaging studies in TSC patients: cortical tubers, periventricular (subependymal) nodules and subependymal giant cell astrocytomas, white matter abnormalities, parenchymal cysts and vascular lesions (Barkovich 2005, Luat et al. 2007, Tortori-Donati et al. 2005).

## Cortical tubers (cerebral hamartomas)

These are the most pathologically characteristic lesions in TSC. Macroscopically they are smooth, whitish, slightly raised nodules that appears as enlarged, atypically shaped gyri; they may be either round or polygonal. Histologically, they consist of bizarre giant cells, dense fibrillary gliosis, and diminished, disordered myelin sheaths; ballon cells may be seen, making these lesions indistinguishable from focal cortical dysplasia with balloon cells. Any single patient may have as few as one to two or as many as 20 to 30 or more tubers. They are most commonly supratentorial, although 8% to 15% of affected patients have cerebellar tubers. The proportion that calcifies has not been reliably determined. The number of calcified cortical tubers seen on CT increases with age (by age 10 years, calcified cortical tubers are present in up to 50% of TSC patients). The cortical calcifications may be gyriform, simulating the appearance of Sturge-Weber syndrome on CT.

In infants, cortical hamartomas can be seen on transfontanelle ultrasound where they appear as focal hyperechogenicity. Neonatal and infantile tubers appear on CT as lucencies within broadened cortical gyri. The lucency diminishes with age, making the noncalcified cortical hamartomas difficult to identify in older children and adults. The MRI appearance of cortical tubers also changes with age: in neonates, they appear as gyri that are hyperintense as compared to the surrounding unmyelinated white matter on T1-weighted images and

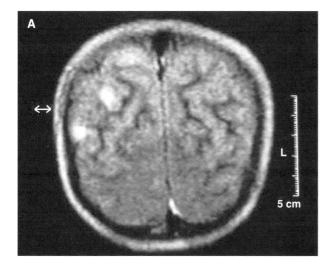

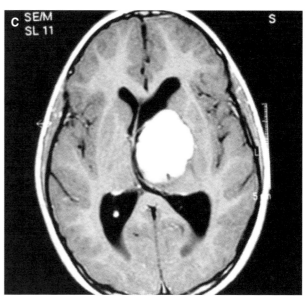

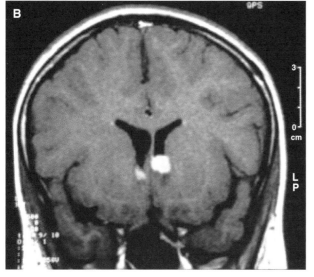

**Fig. 7.** Coronal T2-weighted (**A**) and T1-weighted (**B**) and axial T1-weighted magnetic resonance images of the brain in TSC showing right hemisphere cortical tubers (**A**); two intraventricular subependymal nodules (**B**); and (**C**) a large intraventricular giant cell tumour infiltrating the surrounding brain parenchyma and displacing the basla ganglia and septum pellucidum (**C**).

hypointense on T2-weighted images (Fig. 7A); about 20% of affected gyri are enlarged and T1 or T2 shortening may extent through the cerebral mantle to the ventricle from the tuber. The appearance changes as the white matter myelinates: the signal of the lesion slowly becomes isointense. In older infants tubers have a low-intensity center on T1-weighted images and high signal intensity on T2-weighted and FLAIR images (see Barkovich 2005 and Tortori-Donati et al. 2005 for review of imaging features).

Cortical tubers are regarded as highly epileptogenic, and thus their large number is considered a poor prognostic factor for drug-resistant epilepsy (Curatolo et al. 2006, Wu et al. 2006). Cyst-like cortical tubers can be found in the majority of patients below 7 years of age on FLAIR MRI images (Jurkiewicz et al. 2006). Sometimes, the tubers can be found in fetuses on MRI examination. Recent molecular studies revealed that some patients with focal cortical dysplasia type IIb and absence of other manifestations of TSC may represent a focal form of TSC restricted only to the brain (Jóźwiak et al. 2006a).

Chandra et al. (2007) in a study of children with and without infantile spasms, determined brain volumes and cell densities in epilepsy surgery patients with TSC and cortical dysplasia with balloon cells. Patients with tuberous sclerosis without spasms showed microencephaly associated with decreased cortical neuronal densities. In contrast, cortical dysplasia patients without spasms were normocephalic with increased cell densities. The authors inferred that their findings supported the concept that TSC and cortical dysplasia have different pathogenetic mechanisms despite similarities in refractory epilepsy and postnatal histopathology. Furthermore, a history of infantile spasms was associated with reduced cerebral volumes in both cortical dysplasia and TSC patients, suggesting that spasms or their treatment may contribute to microencephaly independent of aetiology.

## Subependymal hamartomas (nodules)

These tend to be located along the ventricular surface of the caudate nucleus, most often on the lamina of the sulcus thalamostriatus immediately posterior to the foramen of Monro. Less commonly, the nodules may be detected along the frontal and temporal horns, the lateral ventricular bodies, the third venricle, or the fourth ventricle.

In neonates, subependymal nodules can be detected by transfontanelle sonography, on which they appear as echogenic subependymal masses. They cannot be differentiated from germinal matrix haemorrhages or gray matter heterotopia by cranial sonography alone. The imaging appearance on CT and MRI changes with age: they are rarely calcified in the first year of life; the number of calcification typically increases with age. On MRI they typically appear as irregular subependymal nodules that protrude into the adjacent ventricle (Fig. 7B). In infants (who have unmyelinated white matter), the hamartomas are relatively hyperintense on T1-weighted images and hypointense on T2-weighted images; in premature babies they can be mistaken for subependymal haemorrhages (Barkovich 2005). They are detectable in 95–98% of patients. There is no direct correlation between the number of the nodules and severity of disease.

## Giant cell tumours

In 5–12% of patients, prevalently in the first and second decade of life, intraventricular tumours may develop: the term giant cell tumour is given to the enlarging subependymal nodules that are usually situated near the foramen of Monro (Fig. 7C). Anatomically, they differ from the subependymal nodule by their size and their rendency to enlarge. Histopathologically are subependymal giant cell astrocytoma (SEGA). On imaging studies they are identified by the demonstration of tumour growth on serial studies (Fig. 8). Most giant cell tumours are located near the foramen of Monro; however, they can occur anywhere along the ependymal surface. Progressive enlargement of a nodule is the more reliable criterion for diagnosis. They tend to grow into the ventricle and only rarely invade the parenchyma. Occasionally, degeneration into higher grade, or infiltrating neoplasms can occur. The tumours frequently obstruct flow of the CSF and produce symptoms of intracranial hypertension.

Neonatal subependymal giant cell astrocytomas may also occur (Hussain et al. 2006, Medkhour et al. 2002, Mirkin et al. 1999, Raju et al. 2007, Ramenghi et al. 1996) – their natural history and prognosis are poorly understood (Raju et al. 2007).

The mainstay treatment strategy for subependymal giant cell tumours in TSC is still surgery. In the series of Torres et al. (1998) surgical criteria included: (1) presence of hydrocephalus; (2) interval increase in tumour size; (3) new focal neurological deficit attributable to the tumour; and/or (4) symptoms of increased intracranial pressure. According to de Ribaupierre et al. (2007) any lesion fulfilling the criteria for a subependymal giant-cell astrocytoma as previously described in the literature (i.e., lesion around the foramen of Monro, greater than 5 mm, with incomplete calcifications) (Nabbout et al. 1999, O'Callaghan et al. 1999) should be removed as soon as clear evidence of growth has been confirmed. Oral rapamycin therapy has recently proven to induce regression of subependymal giant cell astrocytomas associated with TSC offering an alternative to operative therapy of these lesions

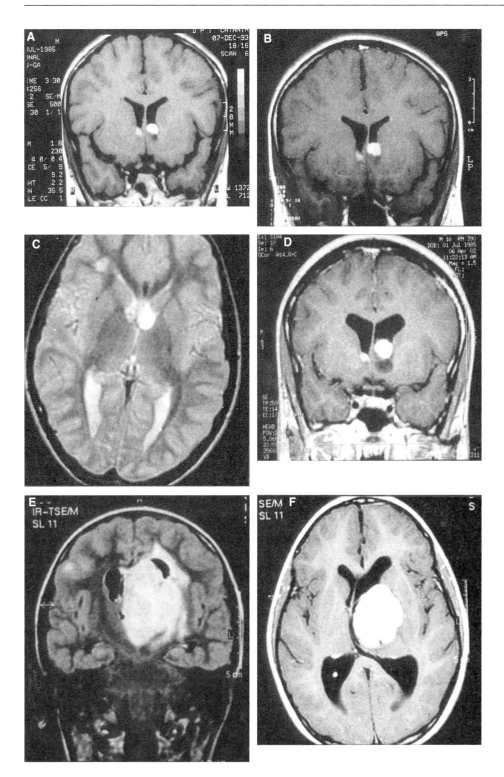

**Fig. 8.** (**A–G**) Natural history of a growing subependymal nodule transforming into a giant cell tumour. Coronal T1-weighted (**A, B, D, E**), axial T2-weighted (**C**) and T1-weighted (**F**) and sagittal T1-weighted (**G**) magnetic resonance images of the brain show the progression of one subependymal nodule (located near the left foramen of Monro: right aspect of the figures) which starts as a "larger" subependymal nodule with a minor cystic component in the lower aspect of the lesion (**A, B**) and grows up (**C, D**) to displace the surrounding tissues with cystic lesions within the mass (**E–G**).

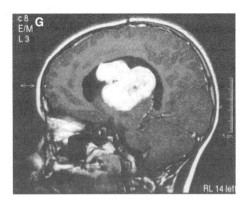

**Fig. 8.** (Continued)

(Franz et al. 2006). In the series of five TSC patients by Franz et al. (2006) all lesions exhibited regression and, in one case, necrosis. Interruption of therapy resulted in regrowth of subependymal giant cell astrocytomas in one patient. Resumption of therapy resulted in further regression. Treatment was well tolerated.

## White matter lesions

Islets consisting of grouping of neurons and glial cells are invariably present in the white matter of TSC patients. Microscopically, they contain bizarre cells including neurons and ballon cells (i.e., giant dysplastic cells with intermediate features between neurons and glia). These white matter foci also contain areas of hypomyelination similar to those seen in cortical tubers. Many of these clusters are microscopic and therefore they do not appear on imaging studies. Those large enough have variable imaging characteristics most similar however to cortical tubers (Fig. 9A).

## Parenchymal cysts

An unknown percentage of TSC patients have cystic-like structures in the cerebral hemispheric white matter. The cysts are more commonly periventricu-

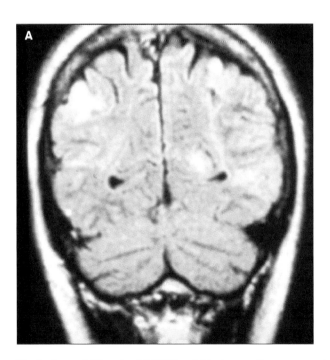

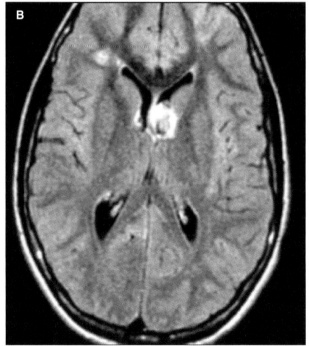

**Fig. 9.** Coronal (**A**) and axial (**B**) T1-weighted magnetic resonance images of the brain showing (**A**) rounded high signal lesions in the cortical (tubers) and radial (TSC white matter abnormalities) high signal lesions in the subcortical white matter and a cystic lesion (**B**) within a subependymal nodule which is transforming in a giant cell tumour.

lar, but may occur nearly anywhere aven within known brain hamartomas (Fig. 9B). Their clinical significance is uncertain.

## Vascular lesions

These are rare in TSC although angiographic studies have demonstrated aneurysms in the kidney, liver, aorta, and distal extremities in affected patients. Involvement of the cerebral vasculare is very rare, but aneurysms have been reported in the internal carotid arteries or in the anterior cerebral arteries.

## Spinal cord involvement

Recently, some cases showing spinal cord involvement in tuberous sclerosis have been reported. Hydrosyringomyelia in TSC was found in cervical and dorsal-lumbar part of spinal cord. It can either produce typical symptoms, like pes cavus and scoliosis, or remain clinically silent (Coppola et al. 2006).

## Renal involvement

It is estimated that more than 80% of affected individuals with TSC may develop some form of renal manifestation during their lifetime. Renal involvement is second to neural involvement as a cause of morbidity and mortality in TSC patients (Shepherd et al. 1991). Two renal abnormalities are regarded as very characteristic for TSC: angiomyolipomas (AMLs) and renal cysts (Fig. 10).

Bilateral, multiple renal AMLs are found n 80–90% of adult patients and, when present, increase with age. Renal symptoms or signs of angiomyolipomas rarely appear before the third decade of life. Symptoms include flank pain, nausea and vomiting, hypertension, uremia and fever. There are also reports of sudden bleeding into the kidney from ruptured aneurysmatic vessels within the angiomyolipoma followed by bleeding into the retroperitoneal space. However, bleeding or rupture seldom occur in children, and are usually related to larger tumours appearing in adolescents and adults. Large

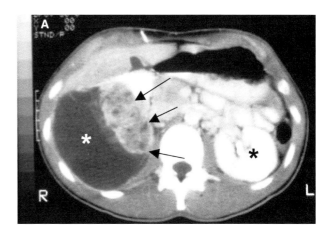

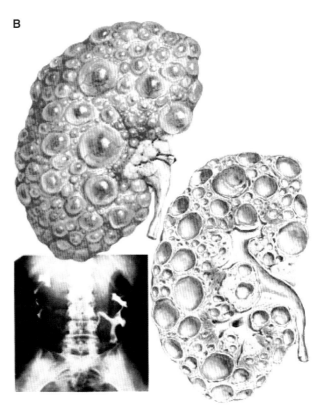

**Fig. 10.** Kidney lesions in TSC: (**A**) CT scan study of the abdomen showing a large angiomyolipoma located aside the right kidney (shown in the left side of the figure) (white asterix) and multiple cystic lesions of the left kidney (black arrows) (compare with the contralateral normal kidney, black asterix). (**B**) A drawing showing the most severe aspects of multicystic kidney in TSC (in the box is shown the X-ray aspect of the lesions with urinary pathway dilatation).

renal AMLs are much more frequent in patients with TSC2 gene mutations (Dabora et al. 2001). End-stage renal insufficiency caused by replacement of renal parenchyma by tumour masses may be observed in adult patients with multiple and large AMLs and may necessitate renal transplantation. Some of the tumours undergoes malignant transformation into renal clear cell carcinoma (RCC). Therefore the differential diagnosis of renal AMLs includes mostly renal malignancies. In patients with the classic triad of flank pain, painless hematuria and palpable abdominal mass the differentiation of a renal neoplasm from unilateral AML may be particularly difficult. The presence of fever and weight loss, observed in 30% of cases of renal malignancies, are unusual in renal AMLs, unless there is an associated retroperitoneal haemorrhage.

Microscopically, renal AMLs contain varying proportions of blood vessels, adipose tissue and smooth muscle cells, justifying the name "angiomyolipoma". Depending on which tissue predominates, the tumour may also be identified as myolipoma or angiomyoma. There are few descriptions of renal AMLs with retroperitoneal lymph node involvement, suggesting the continuum between AML and renal cell carcinoma. Recent immunohistochemical reports hypothesized that some AMLs may undergo malignant transformation to malignant AMLs. Malignant AMLs histologically may resemble sarcomatoid renal cell carcinomas.

Immunostaining for HMB-45 and cytokeratin may represent a useful staining in distinguishing AML from other tumours of the kidney and liver, especially from renal cell carcinoma and hepatocellular carcinoma (Al-Saleem et al. 1998). Contrary to sporadic RCC, benign AMLs in TSC patients are HMB-45 positive and cytokeratin negative (Koide et al. 1998).

However, TSC-associated RCCs differ distinctly from sporadic RCC. Four of the seven tumours reported by Bjornsson et al. (1999) immunostained positively for a melanocyte-associated marker, HMB-45. None of 10 sporadic RCCs from a control group stained with this marker and all stained with cytokeratin markers, which tended to be negative in TSC-associated tumours.

Patients with TSC require regular periodic sonographies to assess renal AMLs growth. Lesions exceeding 4 cm in diameter may require more frequent examinations, every 6–12 months, because of a high risk of rapid enlargement and bleeding. Such an approach should allow identification of individuals that can be treated with arterial embolisation or nephron-sparing surgery preventing the patients from development of symptoms and life-threatening bleeding (Harabayashi et al. 2004, Hsu et al. 2002, Shiroyanagi et al. 2002, Simmons et al. 2003). Arterial embolisation is regarded by some authors as a treatment of choice in all renal AMLs that are symptomatic and measure more than 4 cm. There is an increasing number of reports about interventional selective embolisation of haemorrhagic AMLs (Williams et al. 2006). Pain and fever lasting for several days after embolisation may be observed in about 90% of patients. To reduce the symptoms associated with the postembolisation syndrome a tapering dose of prednisone over a 2-week period has been administered by some authors (Bissler et al. 2002, Kothary et al. 2005).

Multiple and large renal cysts associated with polycystic kidney disease are found in 2–3% of patient of any age (see Fig. 10B). These patients harbour TSC2 mutation with large deletions involving the PKD gene. Such lesions should be differentiated from very small and solitary cysts found incidentally on control sonography of abdomen. They are much more frequent (up to 30%) in children aged 14 to 18 years and are thought to appear in TSC patients as a result of AMLs formation. They usually do not produce any symptoms.

## Hepatic involvement

Until recently hepatic hamartomas had been rarely reported in patients with TSC, probably in part due to their usually asymptomatic course. Their benign nature, coexistence with renal AMLs and angiomyolipomatous appearance in relatively few pathological studies suggest that the vast majority (if not all) of hepatic hamartomas are AMLs. Liver angiomyolipomas are found in 45% of patients over the age of 10 (Jóźwiak et al. 1992). They are more common in girls than in boys.

The hepatic hamartomas in TSC do not usually cause hepatic dysfunction or other symptoms or signs. The serum levels of liver enzymes are normal. These tumours are found incidentally or during the periodic follow up of TSC patients. Sonographically the liver lesions are highly echogenic, round to ovoid in shape and sharply demarcated from the surrounding normal parenchyma. Contrast enhanced CT is able to provide greater detail by demonstrating low density areas that represent fatty tissue (Fig. 11). In addition, magnetic resonance imaging may demonstrate a hyperintense signal on T2-weighted images indicating better than ultrasonography areas of fat within the tumour. Frequently these tumours are multiple and localised in both liver lobes. The average size of the lesion is 0.5 to 1.0 cm.

There are only two symptomatic hepatic hamartomas reported in the literature presenting with flank pain, spontaneous haemorrhage or rapid growth (Huber et al. 1996, Kristal and Sperber 1989). Both of them proved to be hepatic AMLs. In contrast to renal lesions, hepatic AMLs grow slower and were not mentioned as a possible cause of death in a large study of 355 patients with TSC (Shepherd et al. 1991).

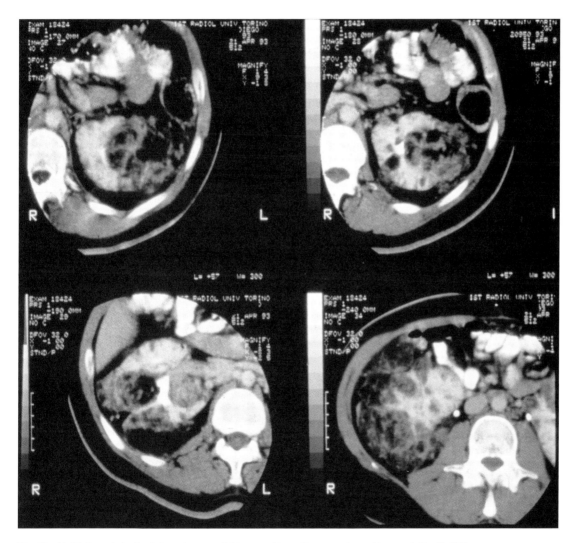

Fig. 11. Multiple cysts in the internal organs (kidney and hepatic parenchyma) in an adult with TSC.

Usually renal AMLs precede the development of hepatic AMLs in TSC patients and are frequent coexisting lesions. They were noted in 9 of 12 children with hepatic AMLs in our series (Jóźwiak et al. 1992) and in all 16 individuals with hepatic lesions reported by Sheffield et al. (1998).

On gross examination the hepatic AMLs are yellow to light tan, depending upon the amount of fat tissue. Histologically, these neoplasms are characterised by a mixture of mature fat cells, blood vessels and smooth muscle cells, with occasional foci of extramedullary hematopoiesis. There are also aneurysmatic dilatations of thick-walled blood vessels, which may facilitate spontaneous bleeding.

Recent immunohistochemical studies demonstrated that hepatic lesions in TSC patients may represent monotypic epithelioid AMLs with pronounced presence of epithelioid PEC (Bonetti et al. 1997). Positive HMB-45 staining has been proposed as a defining criterion of hepatic AML (Tsui et al. 1999).

## Cardiac involvement

Cardiac rhabdomyomas represent the earliest detectable hamartoma in TSC and, interestingly, are the only lesion in TSC which may regress with age (Fig. 12). Cardiac rhabdomyomas are found in 47–67% of all patients with TSC (Jóźwiak et al. 2006). There is a higher incidence of cardiac tumours in infants and newborns with TSC (80%) even disclosed prenatally (Bader et al. 2003, Fesslova et al. 2004, Pipitone et al. 2002). The incidence decreases with age to 20% in *2- to 9-year-old* children with TSC and slightly increases again in the pubertal age (Jóźwiak et al. 2000, 2006).

Conversely, the prevalence of TSC in patients with cardiac rhabdomyomas may be close to 100% as very often the tumours are the first manifestation of the disease, being diagnosed in newborns and very young infants, when the majority of symptoms of TSC cannot be noted. We reported a child with multiple cardiac rhabdomyomas diagnosed prenatally, who had not manifested other symptoms of TSC during six years of follow up. Molecular stud-

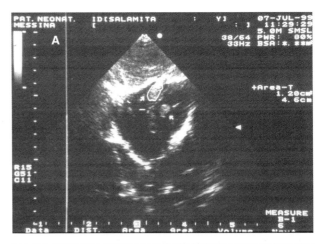

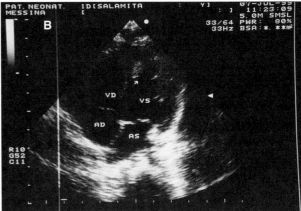

**Fig. 12.** (**A, B**) Ultrasonographic aspect of multiple cardiac rhabdomyomas (white circles).

ies confirmed a mutation in the TSC2 gene (Jóźwiak et al. 2005).

Most tumours are asymptomatic. If cardiac symptoms occur, these are largely a consequence of the tumour size or location within the heart. These symptoms and signs may be explained by one or more of the following three mechanisms: obstruction of inflow or outflow tract, secondary to an obstructing intracavitary tumour; myocardial involvement with secondary deterioration of ventricular function; and cardiac rhythm abnormalities.

The tendency of cardiac rhabdomyomas toward spontaneous resolution, particularly in infancy and early childhood, dictates a conservative approach in the majority of patients. According to the latest recommendations periodic echocardiography of all asymptomatic patients is unnecessary (Roach et al. 1999). Occasionally asymptomatic children may require follow-up echocardiography when the initial study raised specific concerns about the size or location of a rhabdomyoma or in patients considered to be at relative risk of tumour enlargement e.g., patients on ACTH treatment.

In patients with congestive heart failure the treatment with digitalis, diuretics and salt restriction may be utilised. Cardiac rhythm disturbances are usually treated with antidysrhythmic drugs. In children with dysrhythmia refractory to medication a cardiac pacemaker or the division of the abnormal conduction pathway may be considered.

Due to spontaneous regression of the tumours the surgical excision of tumour in infancy is justified only in the presence of a life-threatening hemodynamic condition. These patients, frequently newborns, usually have multiple obstructing masses (Ruggieri et al. 1997). The operative risk depends on the number, size and location of the tumours, but in this group of patients is very high. Still, the prognosis for survival without surgical intervention in these critically ill children is very poor.

An association of arterial aneurysms and TSC has been reported in a number of patients (Jurkiewicz and Jóźwiak 2006). Such a coincidence led some authors to the conclusion that a congenital defect of the arterial wall was part of the condition.

## Ocular manifestations

Retinal hamartomas, retinal pigmentary and vascular changes, optic nerve atrophy, glaucoma and coloboma of the iris, lens, choroid and retina have been described in TSC (Fig. 13). However, the most common ophthalmologic sign is the retinal hamartoma (RA) which is often multiple. Three basic morphological forms of retinal hamartomas are recognized: noncalcified, calcified mulberry-like and transitional type, the latter sharing morphologic features of both previously mentioned types. Since all these lesions are mostly located in the periphery and loose early their growth capacity, they are generally asymptomatic. Nevertheless, aggressive hamartomas have been observed (Shields et al. 2005).

The wide range of prevalence (4% to 76%) of retinal hamartomas reported so far in TSC can account in part for the differences in the patient's age distribution (retinal hamartomas can be overlooked in infancy and generally in non-compliant patients) or for different ratios of TSC1 vs TSC2 patients.

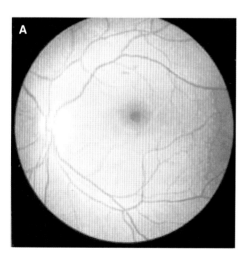
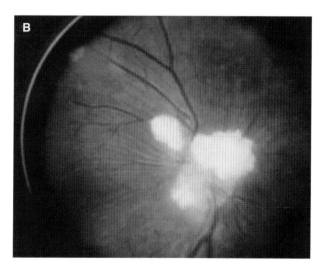

**Fig. 13.** Retinal hamartomas as demonstrated by fundoscopy (**A, B**). Note the red lesion (initial stages of the hamartoma which is not calcified) (**A**) and the yellowish lesions (calcified hamartomas) (**B**) seen at fundoscopy.

Recent data from large series of patients indicate that one third to one half of adult TSC probands have one or more retinal hamartoma (Robertson 1999).

## Pulmonary manifestations

Symptomatic lung involvement in TSC patients is rare, the onset is after the second decade of life and is virtually restricted to females, with an estimated incidence between 1% and 6% (Polosa 1996). Two pulmonary lesions with different histopathologic features have been described in TSC: the well known lymphangioleiomyomatosis (LAM) (Fig. 14), and the less common multifocal micronodular hyperplasia of type II pneumocytes (MMPH) (Popper HH et al. 1991, Guinee D et al. 1995, Nagar et al. 2008). The two manifestations, LAM and MMPH, can coexist or appear as a pure, monomorphic lung disease. The major difference is that LAM affects only females, with only rare exceptions, and may progress to cause serious respiratory complications, whereas MMPH occurs in both sexes, is often recognized in subjects without any pulmonary disfunctions and appears to have a more favourable evolution. Both LAM and MMPH have been described as isolated lung diseases in subjects who did

not fulfill the TSC diagnostic criteria. A retrospective analysis of CT scans of the chest, abdomen and pelvis in a large series of LAMs with and without TSC has suggested that lymphatic involvement, such as thoracic duct dilatation, chylous pleural effusion, and ascites are less common in LAM with TSC (Avila et al. 2007). The pathogenesis of pulmonary involvement is still not clear. Exacerbation during pregnancy and estrogen supplementation has been reported.

# Pathogenesis/molecular genetics

## Molecular genetics

TSC is an autosomal dominant disorder in which sporadic cases account for about two-thirds of all patients, and reflect the occurrence of new mutations (Kwiatkowski et al. 2004). Within families there is a wide variation in the extent and degree of clinical manifestations, indicating that there is no rigid correlation between specific TSC gene mutation and clinical outcome.

### *TSC1* and *TSC2* genes

Linkage analysis in multigenerational families and positional cloning has been used to map both the *TSC1* and *TSC2* genes (Fig. 15). Linkage of the first TSC locus (*TSC1*) to 9q34, near the AB0 blood groups, was reported in 1987 (Fryer et al. 1987, Northrup et al. 1987). Subsequent studies provided strong evidence for locus heterogeneity (Janssen et al. 1990, 1994; Northrup et al. 1992; Sampson et al. 1989, 1992; Povey et al. 1994) and led to the identification of the second locus, *TSC2*, at 16p13.3, near the autosomal dominant polycystic kidney disease major gene (Kandt et al. 1992). Although the OMIM catalog lists other two putative *TSC* loci, at 12q and 11q, on the basis of the breakpoints of de novo translocations found in two patients with TSC, presently there is no convincing experimental evidence for a third locus. Indeed, all multigeneration TSC families reported so far showed linkage to

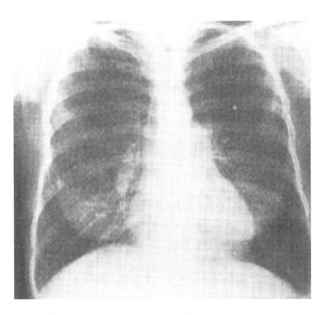

**Fig. 14.** X-ray appearance of pulmonary limphangioleyomyomatosis.

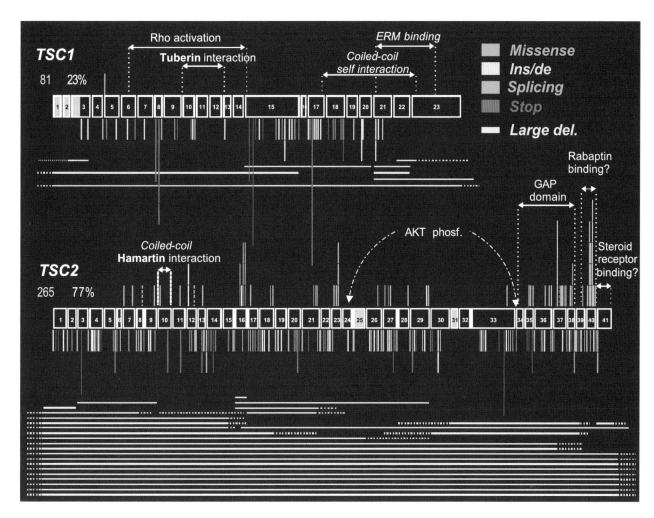

**Fig. 15.** The *TSC1* and *TSC2* genes.

either *TSC1* or *TSC2*, the few exceptions being eventually solved by the finding of two different *TSC1* and *TSC2* mutations, independently originated in two relatives. Nevertheless, genetic and epigenetic variations in other genes, either related or unrelated to the biochemical pathways of the two known *TSC* genes, are expected to modify or even mimic at least in part the pleiomorphic TSC phenotype.

The *TSC1* transcript is 8.6-kb long and contains 23 exons (Fig. 15), (the first two are non-coding and alternatively spliced), encompassing 55 kb of genomic DNA (van Slegtenhorst et al. 1997). The gene has no known structural homologies to other known gene families.

The *TSC2* transcript is 5.6-kb long, contains 41 coding exons (plus an upstream non-coding exon) (Fig. 15), encompassing 40 kb of genomic DNA (European Chromosome 16 Tuberous Sclerosis Consortium 1993). Exons 25 and 31, the only two *TSC2* exons not showing so far any mutation, are alternatively spliced (Xu et al. 1995); the functional significance of the transcripts showing both, one or neither exons 25 and 31 is not known.

More than 900 different micro-mutations, nearly 100 rare variants of uncertain pathogenicity and 350 polymorphisms have been identified in the two *TSC* genes (http://consortium.liacs.nl/lovd/index.php?-select_db=TSC1 or db=TSC2 and personal data).

Except for the CpG mutational hot spots and short nucleotide repeats, there are no particular regions within the two genes in which mutations occur at a higher rate. Overall, the most recurrent mutation (18-bp deletion in exon 40 of *TSC2*) is found in less than 3% of the patients. If the wide variety of *TSC* mutations can be accounted for the length and structural complexity of the two genes, more intriguing is the dramatic difference between *TSC1* and *TSC2* in the occurrence of in frame mutations (3% vs. 30%). In particular, missense mutations are extremely rare in *TSC1*, whereas 1/4 of *TSC2* mutations are missenses ($P < 10^{-4}$). Large genomic rearrangements, such as partial or full deletions of either *TSC* gene and, rarely, duplications and inversions, have been reported. The prevalence of large deletions is not statistically different between TSC1 and TSC2 patients (9% and 11%, respectively). A subgroup of large genomic deletions or rearrangements affect both *TSC2* and the adjacent *PKD1* gene, frequently mutated in the adult variety of polycystic kidney disease, causing early-onset, multiple renal cysts associated with the TSC phenotype (OMIM # 600273). The *PKD1* and *TSC2 contiguous gene deletion syndrome* may be recognized at birth or shortly thereafter for the enlarged and polycystic kidneys (characterized by a multitude of variably sized cysts closely resembling those more commonly seen in later life in the advanced stages of autosomal dominant polycystic kidney disease, or PKD1; OMIM # 173900) (Brook-Carter et al. 1994, O'Callaghan et al. 1975, Sampson et al. 1997, Stapleton et al. 1980, Wenzel et al. 1970).

In agreement with Knudson's two-hit tumour suppressor gene model (Knudson 1971), inactivation of both alleles of either *TSC1* or *TSC2* gene appears to be required for the development of hamartomas in TSC. Somatic defect of the second allele has been clearly documented in a variety of proliferative TSC lesions, such as renal AML, pulmonary LAM, cardiac rabdomiomas, and brain subependimal giant cell astrocytomas (SEGA). The difficulty of finding a biallelic defect in cortical tubers initially suggested that *TSC1* or *TSC2* haploinsufficiency per se might cause aberrant cortical lamination (Henske et al. 1996, Niida et al. 2001). Later it has been unequivocally shown that a biallelic defect is present, but re-

stricted to a small fraction of the heterogeneous and dysmorphic cells contained in the tubers, i.e., to poligonal or ovoid giant cells with eosinophilic cytoplasm and thickened processes (Crino 2004), identical to the major cell component of the SEGA.

It is reasonable to conclude that the TSC hamartomas prevalent pathogenic mechanism is that already described or that the inactivation of the second allele might be preferentially obtained, at least in the tubers, by epigenetic mechanisms. Indeed, Han et al. (2004) found that in tubers, but not in angiomyolipomas, tuberin is expressed and phosphorylated in an specific residue known to cause its inactivation (see below pathogenesis).

At present, the prevailing opinion is that the mTOR/p70S6K/S6 signal pathway is activated in giant cells, suggesting that the surrounding neurons acquire dismorphic features similar to those of the adjacent dismorphic neurons. Nevertheless, it is reasonable to assume that also epigenetic mechanisms, such as the abnormal tuberin phosphorylation reported in tubers (Han et al. 2004) might interfere with tumour suppressor activity or other critical, yet unknown, TSC functions. Overall, the most reasonable mechanism in classic hamartomas in TSC would be that of second-hit mutations occurring in limited numbers of cells. These mutations are referred to as loss of heterozygosity, since they affect neighbouring heterozygous polymorphic markers. Loss of heterozygosity in *TSC1* or *TSC2* has been consistently observed in the majority of TSC-associated angiomyolipomas, cardiac rhabdomyomas, subependymal giant-cell tumours, and lymphangiomyomatosis cells but has only rarely been found in cerebral cortical tubers (Chan et al. 2004, Henske et al. 1996, Niida et al. 2001, Crino et al. 2006).

## Molecular genetic testing

The clinical use of genetic testing in TSC is aimed: (a) to confirm a clinical diagnosis; (b) to offer genetic counselling to probands and family members relatives, including prenatal diagnosis.

The genetic testing for TSC is complicated by the large size of the two genes, the necessity to screen for both point mutations and large deletions, and the presence of somatic mosaicism (Emmerson et al. 2003, Sampson et al. 1997, Verhoef et al. 1999). As TSC1 mutations are primarily small deletions and insertions and nonsense mutations these are better detected by sequence analysis; TSC2 mutations also include significant numbers of large deletions and rearrangements that cannot be detected by sequence analysis (Nellist et al. 2005, Northrup and Au 2006). In the major studies so far published the mutation detection rate varied from 62.4% (Au et al. 2004; using SSCA and direct sequencing and including approximately 10% of cases not meeting diagnostic criteria for TSC) to 70% (Sancak et al. 2005; using SSCP, DHPLC, DGGE, direct sequencing, Southern blotting, and FISH analysis), 74% (Dabora et al. 2001), 76% (Hung et al. 2006), 80% (Jones et al. 1999), 83% (Kwiatkowski et al. 2004) and 95.8% (Devlin et al. 2006). Overall, the mutation detection rate by means of sequence analysis varies from 15% (TSC1 gene) to 60–70% (TSC2 gene) in sporadic cases and from 30% (TSC1 gene) to 50% (TSC2 gene) in familial cases (Jones et al. 2000, Northrup and Au 2006).

## Genotype-phenotype correlations

Linkage studies initially suggested that there would be equivalent numbers of families with mutations in each TSC gene (Povey et al. 1994). However, the frequency of mutations reported in TSC2 is consistently higher than in TSC1: TSC1 mutations account for only 10 to 30% of the families identified with probands with TSC (Jones et al. 1997, 1999; Kwiatkowska et al. 1998; Niida et al. 1999; Sancak et al. 2005; van Slegtenhorst et al. 1999). In sporadic cases of TSC, there is an even greater excess of mutations in TSC2 (Crino et al. 2006) whilst identification of TSC1 mutations appears to be twice as likely in familial cases as in sporadic cases. The disparity in mutational frequency may reflect an increased rate of germ-line and somatic mutations in TSC2 as compared with TSC1, as well as ascertainment bias, since mutations in TSC2 are associated with more severe disease (Crino et al. 2006; Jones et al. 1997, 1999; Kwiatkowski et al. 2004; Sancak et al. 2005).

Except for the contiguous gene deletion syndrome (PKDTS), the phenotypes caused by mutations in TSC1 and TSC2 were initially considered to be identical; however with more genotype/phenotype data available, it appears that TSC1 mutations produce a less severe phenotype than TSC2 mutations (Jones et al. 1997, 1998, 1999; Au et al. 1998; Dabora et al. 2001; Lewis et al. 2004; Sancak et al. 2005). The exception is that some missense TSC2 mutations are associated with milder disease phenotypes (Khare et al. 2001). In individuals harboring TSC2 mutations: (1) Al-Saleem et al. (1998) reported a greater risk of renal malignancy; (2) Jones et al. (1997, 1998, 1999) found a higher frequency of intellectual disability [however, other series have not replicated this finding (Kwiatkowska et al. 1998, Niida et al. 1999, van Slegtenhorst et al. 1999, Young et al. 1998)]; (3) Dabora et al. (2001) found that 8 out of 16 clinical features investigated occurred at a significantly higher frequency and/or with greater severity including seizures, moderate to severe learning disability, mean number of subependymal nodules, tuber count, kidney angiomyolipomas, mean grade of facial angiofibromas, forehead plaque and retinal hamartomas; (4) Lewis et al. (2004) recorded more commonly autistic disorders, low IQ and infantile spasms; and (5) Devlin et al. (2006) observed a more severe phenotype including epilepsy and learning disabilities; (6) Hung et al. (2006) found a higher incidence of intellectual disability and mental retardation but no significant differences in all the remaining clinical features of TSC. (7) Strizheva et al. (2001) suggested that females with mutations on the carboxy terminus of the TSC2 gene product (tuberin) may have increased incidence and/or severity of lymphangiomyomatosis. (8) Au et al. (2007) showed that patients with TSC2 mutations have significantly more hypomelanotic macules and learning disability and overall more severe symptoms. In addition they found that male patients have more frequent neurological and eye symptoms, renal and ungual fibromas.

## Mosaicism

Among patients meeting the clinical criteria for a diagnosis of TSC, 15 to 20% have no identifiable mutations (Dabora et al. 2001, Sancak et al. 2005). These persons generally have milder clinical disease (i.e., a lower incidence of mental retardation, seizures, and dermatological manifestations) than patients with identified *TSC1* or *TSC2* mutations (Crino et al. 2006). Mosaicism for a mutation in the first allele of either *TSC1* or *TSC2* has been reported in probands or in the first affected relative of the family, i.e. in a proband's parent or grandparent. It is not known how many de novo TSC mutations of the first allele are generated during the gametogenesis of a healthy parent (germinal mutation) or during the embryonic development of a normal zygote (somatic mutation). In principle, individuals with a post-zygotic mutation should be somatic mosaics, having two cell populations, one with and one without that mutation. It is reasonable to assume that the quantity of "mutated" cells in critical organs such as the brain and kidneys will determine at least in part the severity of the phenotype. Since the sensitivity threshold of the techniques for mutation detection-currently used is low ($\geq 5\%$), and a single tissue – the peripheral leukocytes  – is normally tested, only a fraction is available for screening reasons. In principle, mosaic post-zygotic mutations of the first allele are thought to account for a milder clinical phenotype (Jones et al. 2001; Roberts et al. 2004; Verhoef et al. 1995; 1999; Rose et al. 1999; Emmerson et al. 2003). Germ-line mosaicism has been also confirmed in families with affected siblings and unaffected (Yates et al. 1997) or mildly affected parents. Mosaicism is also a credible explanation for the failure to detect a mutation (Kwiatkowski 2005; Kwiatkowski et al. 1999, 2004). The highest level of mosaicism (7/27 unrelated families, or 26%) was reported in a series of patients with the contiguous gene syndrome due to deletion of both *TSC2* and *PKD1* genes (Sampson et al. 1997).

Cases with solitary, typical TSC lesions which developed from two somatic hit mutations in the TSC genes (in this case *TSC2* gene), rather than being part of a phenotype manifesting with very small fraction of somatic mosaicism have been recorded (e.g., solitary SEGA; Ichikawa et al. 2005).

## Penetrance

After careful, detailed evaluation of each individual known to have a *TSC1* or *TSC2* mutation, the penetrance of TSC is now thought to be 100%. Rare cases of seemingly non-penetrance have been reported; however, molecular studies have resolved these cases, revealing two different TSC mutations in the family and the existence of germ-line mosaicism in others (Connor et al. 1986, Webb and Osborne 1991).

There are no other genetically related (allelic) disorders associated with mutations in *TSC1* and *TSC2*. In some cases, DNA extracted from lung tissue in individuals with sporadic pulmonary lymphangioleiomyomatosis (LAM) harbors mutations of *TSC2* or *TSC1* not present in the germ-line (Carsillo et al. 2000, Smolarek et al. 1998): the role of *TSC1* and *TSC2* genes in this process is not yet fully determined. Several lines of evidence support the conclusion that the actions of *TSC1* and *TSC2* are probably limited in the complex process of LAM development (see also below, pathogenesis).

## Anticipation

Anticipation has not been observed in TSC.

## Pathogenesis (Functions of *TSC1* and *TSC2*)

### Animal models

Homologs to the *TSC* genes in model organisms (e.g., rat, mouse, *Drosophila*, *Fugu*, and, more distantly, fission yeast) were identified and found to be highly conserved, suggesting similar, if not identical, evolutionary functions (Au et al. 2004, Piedimonte et al. 2006, Scheidenhelm and Gutmann 2004). Similarly to many evolutionary conserved genes, engineered homozygous *TSC* gene mutants are embryonic lethal in these models (e.g., TSC1 null embryos die at mid-gestation from a failure of liver development; *TSC2* null embryos die at mid-gestation as well displaying dysraphia and papillary overgrowth of the neuroepithelium) (Kobayashi et al.

2001, Kwiatkowski et al. 2002, Rennebeck et al. 1998, Uhlmann et al. 2002).

The *Eker* rat (Eker 1954), a spontaneous mutant predisposed to autosomal dominant renal carcinoma, was the first animal model found to contain an insertion mutation in the *TSC2* gene (Hino et al. 1994, Kobayashi et al. 1995, Kubo et al. 1995, Yeung et al. 1994, 2004). Several engineered *TSC1* and *TSC2* gene disruptions created in the mouse have been shown to have renal pathology similar to that of humans affected with TSC but, interestingly do not have significant brain pathology (Hino et al. 1994; Jin et al. 1996; Kenerson et al. 2005; Kobayashi et al. 1995, 1999; Onda et al. 1999; Takahashi et al. 2004; Wolf et al. 1998). Also, $TSC1^{\pm}$ and $TSC2^{\pm}$ mice have some phenotypic differences [e.g., development of renal cystadenomas, early onset bilateral polycystic kidney disease and extra-renal tumours such as hepatic hemangiomas (Kleymenova et al. 2001, Kobayashi et al. 2001), or anaplastic ganglioglioma (Kwiatkowski et al. 2002, Mizuguchi et al. 2000). A conditional deletion of the *TSC1* gene in heterozygosity (and/or homozygousity) limited/restricted to astrocytes in mice exhibited abnormal neuronal organization in the hippocampus, age-dependent increase of astrocyte proliferation, seizures and death: these findings suggested that the increase in astrocyte proliferation precedes the neuronal abnormalities, causing mass effect changes or disturbance of complex astrocyte-neuron interactions (Uhlmann et al. 2002, Wenzel et al. 2004). $TSC2^{\pm}$ rats exhibits a marked reduction of different forms of hyppocampal synaptic plasticity (e.g., loose of their potential for activity-dependent synaptic modification) (von der Brelie et al. 2006) and enhanced episodic-like memory and kindling epilepsy (Waltereit et al. 2006) and $TSC1^{\pm}$ or $TSC2^{\pm}$ mice and rats exhibit perturbed dendritic spine structures (Tavazoie et al. 2005) and spatial memory impairment (Dash et al. 2006).

Studies on mutations in the *Drosophila TSC1* and *TSC2* (*gigas*) genes revealed an identical *Drosophila* phenotype characterized by enhanced growth and increased cell size with no changes in ploidy (Potter et al. 2001, Tapon et al. 2001). Thus, although the mammalian models have been and will continue to be useful in studying TSC (El-Hashemite et al. 2004, Ess et al. 2005, Hino et al. 2001, Lee et al. 2005, Meikle et al. 2005, Mizuguchi et al. 2004, Momose et al. 2002, Wilson et al. 2005), the studies in *Drosophila* homologs established the role of *TSC1* and *TSC2* genes in regulating cell size, morphology and proliferation (Gao et al. 2001, Potter et al. 2001). This discovery led to localize the function of the *TSC1* and *TSC2* genes in the PI3K-AKT-mTOR (mammalian target of rapamycin) pathway or AKT pathway paving the way to several investigations on potential therapies (Gino et al. 2006) (see below).

## TSC products and their functions (hamartin-tuberin structure)

*TSC1* encodes TSC1 (*hamartin*) a 140-kDa protein with no homology to TSC2. *TSC2* encodes TSC2 (*tuberin*), a 200-kDa protein with a GAP domain near the carboxy terminal. Tuberin, through its C-terminal GAP domain, is the major regulator of the small G-protein RHEB and downstream protein translation pathway, essential to the cell growth (Inoki et al. 2003). This C-terminal GAP domain is a frequent target of missense mutations in TSC (Sancak et al. 2005).

Hamartin and tuberin interact physically with high affinity to form heterodimers (Fig. 16), suggesting that they may act in concert to regulate cell proliferation (Ess 2006, Plank et al. 1998, van Slegtenhorst et al. 1998) an observation that is consistent with the similar clinical features of patients harboring either *TSC1* or *TSC2* mutations. A shared motif of these proteins is the coiled-coil domain. These domains mediate protein–protein binding and likely permit hamartin and tuberin to interact, although the exact borders of these domains are not known (Hodges et al. 2001). It appears that the hamartin binding stabilizes tuberin, preventing its degradation (Benvenuto et al. 2000). Additional functions assigned to hamartin are the regulation of cytoskeleton-mediated processes through its interaction with the ezrin-radixin-moesin (ERM) family of actin-binding proteins (Lamb et al. 2000) and with

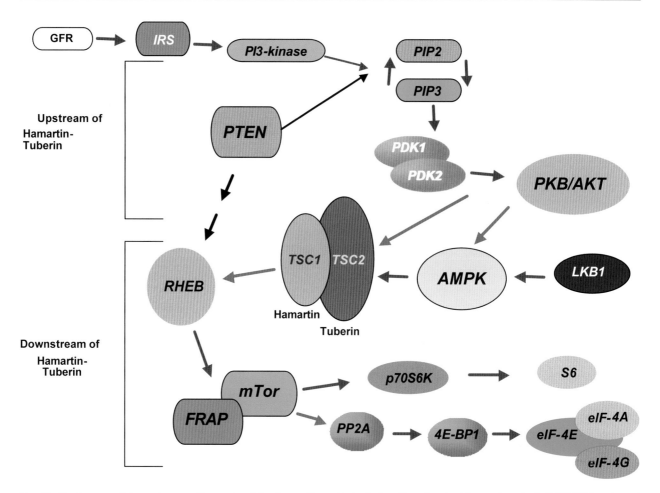

**Fig. 16.** Upstream and downstream pathways involving hamartin and tuberin functions (see text for explanation). *AMPK* AMP-activated protein kinase; *FRAP* FKBP12-rapamycin associated protein; *GFR* growth factor receptor; *IRS* insulin receptor substrate; *LKB1* serin-threonin protein kinase; *mTOR* mammalian target of rapamycin; *p70S6K* p70 ribosomal S6 subunit-kinase; *PI3-kinase* phosphoinositide 3-kinase; *PIP2* phosphatidytl-inositol (4,5) biphosphate; *PIP3* phosphatidyl-inositol (3,4,5) triphosphate; *PP2A* protein phosphatase 2 A, alpha isoform; *PTEN* phosphatase and tensin homolog; *PDK1* phosphoinositide-dependent kinase 1; *PDK2* phosphoinosititde-dependent kinase 2; *PKB/AKT* protein kinase B/Akt; *RHEB* RAS homolog enriched in brain; *TSC1* tuberous sclerosis complex 1; *TSC2* tuberous sclerosis complex 2; *4E-BP1* eukaryotic initiation factor 4E binding protein 1.

neurofilament-L (Haddad et al. 2002). Moreover, it has been suggested that hamartin regulates the cell cycle through the interaction with CDK (Astrinidis et al. 2003).

Hamartin and tuberin are expressed in all tissues. The intracellular localization of the two proteins is more complex than initially thought (Nellist et al. 1999, Murthy et al. 2000, Yamamoto et al. 2002), i.e., they are not confined to cytosol and nucleus, being detected also in nucleoli and mitochondria (Clements et al. 2006). Moreover, the latter

authors, using synchronized cultures of human airways smooth muscle cells, clarified the inconsistent findings on nuclear localization: tuberin and hamartin enter the nucleus at the G1-S phase of the cell cycle (Clements et al. 2006). Tuberin and hamartin have been shown to be key regulators of several cell-signalling pathways including (see Fig. 16): (1) a growth and translation regulatory pathway (PI3K/PKB pathway) involving the "mammalian target of rapamycin" (mTOR) cascade; (2) a cell adhesion/migration/protein transport pathway (glycogen synthase kinase 3 [GSK3]/β-catenin/focal adhesion kinase [FAK]/Ras-related homolog [Rho] pathway); and (3) a cell growth and proliferation pathway (mitogen-activated protein kinase [MAPK] pathway) (Astrinidis et al. 2003, Au et al. 2004, Birchenall-Roberts et al. 2004, Crino et al. 2006, El-Hashemite et al. 2003, Ess 2006, Harris and Lawrence 2003, Kozma and Thomas 2002, Li et al. 2004, Mak and Yeung 2004, Yeung 2003). In most cases the clinical relevance of these TSC1-TSC2 complex interactions is not yet well understood.

## Tuberin and Hamartin as growth and translation regulators

The function of tuberin and hamartin in the protein translation cascade involving PI3K/PKB/mTOR is not yet established (Jozwiak et al. 2008).

## mTOR

A serine-threonine kinase, mTOR has a central role in the regulation of cell growth and proliferation in response to growth factors, amino acids, and nutrients. First, mTOR phosphorylates and activates the p70S6 kinase 1 to enhance ribosomal protein translation and ribosome biogenesis. Secondly, it phosphorylates and inactivates the eukaryotic initiation translation factor 4E (eIF4E)-binding protein 1 (4E-BP1), the suppressor of protein eIF4E (Fig. 16). Release of eIF4E from phosphorylated 4E-BP1 enables the formation of the eIF4F complex, which is required for cap-dependent translation of mRNAs, such as Cyclin D1 and c-*MYC*, which have extensive secondary structures in their 5´-untranslated region.

## AKT, AMPK and PTEN

In normal cells, in presence of insulin or other growth factors, tuberin activity can be suppressed upon via direct phosphorylation (*upstream of hamartin-tuberin*) (see Fig. 16) by AKT protein kinase (also known as PKB). Phosphorylation of tu-

berin at amino acids serine 939, 981 or threonine 1462 inactivates the tuberin-hamartin complex, likely by disassembling the dimer. Without a functional tuberin-hamartin complex, suppression of S6 kinase 1, mTOR, and translation initiation factor 4E will be released (*downstream of hamartin-tuberin*) (Fig. 16) to facilitate assembly of 40S and 60S ribosomal subunits and other translational initiation factors (A, G and B) on capped messenger RNA to start the protein translation process. Thus, loss of hamartin or tuberin results in increased mTOR-dependent phosphorylation of p70S6 kinase, ribosomal protein S6, and 4E-BP1.

Additional studies revealed that the genetic loss - of the phosphorylated PTEN(a tyrosine phosphatase) in animal models (with biallelic *PTEN* mutations in somatic cells) produced alterations of cell size and proliferation that closely mimicked those seen with loss of the *TSC* genes (Corradetti et al. 2004). These findings support a model in which growth factor binding and receptor activation leads to enhanced PI3-kinase activity that converts phosphatidylinositol 4,5-biphosphate to phosphatidylinositol 3,4,5-triphosphate (*upstream of AKT/hamartin-tuberin*) (Fig. 16). This reaction is reversible and catalysed by PTEN. Loss of PTEN activity then allows the second messenger phosphatidylinositol 3,4,5-triphosphate to increase and activate AKT.

In addition to phosphorylation by AKT, tuberin is also a substrate for the AMPK kinase (see also below) (Inoki et al. 2003). Unlike AKT, tuberin phosphorylation by AMPK potentiates its inhibitory effect on downstream targets. AMPK is inactivated by AKT phosphorylation but is stimulated by the LKB1 kinase (Corradetti et al. 2004). It is worth to note that germline defects of PTEN and LKB1 leads to human diseases that share with TSC features of hamartomatous growth. PTEN defects are associated with Cowden syndrome, and Bannayan-Riley-Ruvalcaba syndrome (Liaw et al. 1997, Nelen et al. 1997, Marsh et al. 1977). A further neurological phenotype caused by a PTEN germline defect is the adult variety of dysplastic gangliocytoma of the cerebellum or Lhermitte-Duclos disease (Liaw et al. 1997). In addition, PTEN is also frequently lost in glioblastoma and other central nervous system tumours (Bonneau and Longy 2000). Loss of LKB1 causes the autosomal dominant genetic disorder Peutz-Jeghers syndrome (Hemminki et al. 1998). The striking confluence between Cowden/Lhermitte-Duclos syndrome, Bannayan-Riley-Ruvalcaba syndrome, Peutz-Jeghers syndrome and tuberous sclerosis to a common signal transduction pathway suggests that the hamartomatous cell proliferation seen in all these disorders may be due at least in part to the hyper activation of the mTOR pathway. However the severe neurological involvement in TSC suggests that additional roles for the hamartin-tuberin complex remain to be elucidated.

## RHEB

So far, most if not all experimentally documented functions of hamartin/tuberin complex of the mTOR pathway appear mediated by RHEB (RAS-homologue expressed in brain) (*downstream of hamartin-tuberin*) (Fig. 16), a member of the RAS-like super-family of GTPases. GTPases cycle between an active GTP-bound state and an inactive GDP-bound state. Tuberin through its GAP domain accelerates the conversion of the active RHEB-GTP to the inactive RHEB-GDP. Loss of tuberin increases Rheb-GTP/GDP and mTOR activation. Since patients with germ-line *TSC1* mutations and those with *TSC2* mutations have similar phenotypes but with significantly different severity, it seems likely that hamartin should have specific roles beyond the before mentioned tuberin stabilization via ethero-dimerization. Tuberin participates in the regulation of tuberin-related GAP activity with respect to Rheb, but its precise role is not yet clear. In addition, other recent findings suggest that the phenotypic findings in TSC might occur secondary to mechanisms other than hyperactivation of S6 kinase 1 through mTOR (Au et al. 2004)

Analysis of surgically resected tubers have revealed cell-specific activation of the mTOR cascade in giant cells, as evidenced by the expression of activated (phosphorylated) components of the mTOR cascade (*downstream of hamartin-tuberin*), including phosphorylated p70S6 kinase and phosphorylated ribosomal protein S6. Since mTOR is a critical regulator of cell size, it is logical to infer that the activation of mTOR is responsible for cytomegaly in tubers and subependymal giant cell tumours. One hypothesis to explain giant cell formation is the second hit mechanism: a neural progenitor cell has one normal *TSC* allele and one existing *TSC* mutation (Fig. 17). A second-hit mutation occurs and there is inactivation of the normal allele so that the cells contain two mutated *TSC* genes. The progenitor cell with two mutations can give rise to a giant cell only or to a mixed population of GC and dysplastic neurons. These cells exhibit abnormal morphology, make aberrant synaptic connections, and migrate to inappropriate cortical layers. In addition, giant cells (or dysplastic neurons) may interfere with migratory pathways of adjacent "normal" neurons containing only one mutated *TSC* gene, and further disrupt the formation of appropriate synaptic connections during brain development (Gino 2004, Gino et al. 2006).

## Role of tuberin and hamartin in cell adhesion, migration, and protein trafficking

Loss of heterozygosity at the *TSC1* or *TSC2* locus and hyperphosphorylation of ribosomal protein S6 have been documented in each of the three components of angiomyolipomas (vessels, smooth muscle, and fat), suggesting that all three components arise from a common progenitor and that the tuberin-hamartin complex regulates the differentiation of cells that are derived from mesenchyme (Gino et al. 2006).

Notably, the smooth muscle component of angiomyolipomas is histologically and immunophenotypically identical to the smooth muscle cells of lymphangiomyomatosis. Approximately 60% of women with the sporadic form of lymphangiomyomatosis have renal angiomyolipomas: some of these individuals, in addition, harbor somatic *TSC2* mutations in the abnormal lung and kidney cells but not in the normal cells suggesting that lymphangiomyomatosis and angiomyolipomas are genetically related and most likely arise from a common progenitor cell. These data

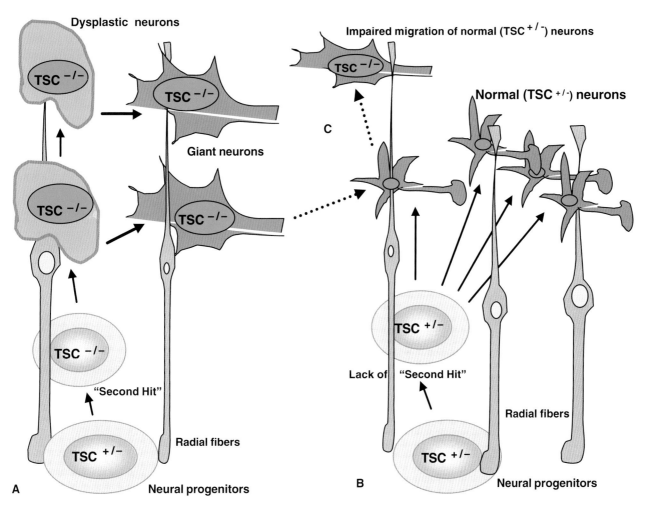

**Fig. 17.** Diagram showing what occurs to the brain neurons in TSC after the second hit mutations (**A**) and without second hit mutations (**B**) (see text for explanation).

have led to the "*benign metastasis*" hypothesis for the pathogenesis of lymphangiomyomatosis which proposes that histologically benign cells with mutations in *TSC1* or *TSC2* may have the ability to travel to the lungs from angiomyolipomas in the kidney (Gino 2004, Gino et al. 2006). This ability might be linked to an altered (increased in this case) capacity for motility and migration expressed by cells lacking tuberin or hamartin, which is associated with the activation of Rho, a small GTPase that regulates the actin cytoskeleton and focal adhesions. Thus, tuberin and hamartin seems to function to promote cell adhesion and correct migration of precursors cells via the activation of focal adhesion kinase and Rho-guanosine

triphosphate. The fact that pulmonary lymphangiomyomatosis occurs only in women has suggested a role for estrogens in regulating TSC signalling and perhaps also cell migration.

## Role of tuberin and hamartin in growth and cell proliferation

There is also evidence to indicate that tuberin and hamartin regulate the MAPK signal pathway in controlling cell proliferation. Tuberin phosphorylated at amino acid serine 1210 is mediated by p38 mitogen-activated protein (MAP) kinase, and the phosphorylated tuberin-hamartin complex is subsequently sequestered from their functional sites by 14-3-3 protein. Notably, the expression of 14-3-3 protein is regulated by tuberin and hamartin, suggesting a tightly interregulated mechanism. On the other hand the tuberin-hamartin complex can function to regulate p42/44 Map kinase activity. Suppressing the phosphorylation of p42/44 MAP kinase results in a decrease in vascular endothelial growth factor production and inhibited growth of TSC2Ang1 tumour cells. Additional roles of tuberin are the upstream regulation of the Erk (Mapk1 and Mapk3) pathway to activate a battery of transcription factors and proto-oncogenes to stimulate cell growth and proliferation (Fig. 17).

Other factors (i.e., platelet-derived growth factor receptor, estrogen receptor, and calmodulin binding) have been suggested to play a role in the function of the tuberin-hamartin complex, suggesting that this complex can be involved in even more cellular functions that have yet to be uncovered.

## Natural history

The natural course of the disorder is slow but progressive. All inner organ tumours, except for cardiac rhabdomyomas, enlarge with increasing age. Only cardiac rhabdomyomas usually regress in the first years of life.

## Diagnosis

The early recognition of the disease is essential for TSC patients due to: 1) possible devastating effect of visceral lesions requiring frequent control studies, and 2) necessary genetic counselling.

The first diagnostic criteria of TSC were established by the German physician, Vogt, in 1908 (Vogt 1908). This author published the classic diagnostic triad of TSC: seizures, mental retardation and adenoma sebaceum (former term for angiofibromas). However, more recent studies made by M. R. Gomez revealed that all three features of Vogt's triad were found in only 29% of patients, and in 6% of them none of these three findings were observed.

In subsequent years new necessary modifications to the original diagnostic criteria were done. After several editions of proposed sets a consensus conference held at Annapolis in 1998 announced the latest version of diagnostic criteria (Roach et al. 1998). The revised clinical criteria were simplified into two main categories, major and minor, based on the diagnostic importance and degree of specificity for TSC of each clinical and radiographic feature (see Table 1). The definite diagnosis of TSC is established when two major features or one major feature and two minor features are demonstrated.

Despite the long number of clinical features listed in the criteria, the diagnosis of TSC may be extremely difficult early in life. It needs to be understood that the diagnostic criteria in TSC are age dependent. Many features of TSC are absent in infants and become apparent in late childhood or adulthood. Such natural course of TSC limits the value of clinical diagnostic criteria for early diagnosis and prompt management of TSC (Jóźwiak et al. 2000).

In young children or asymptomatic cases genetic testing may now aid in making the diagnosis. Direct sequencing is able to determine the causative mutation in either *TSC1* or *TSC2* gene in approximately 80% of cases (Cheadle et al. 2000). However, universal use of molecular genetics testing for diagnosis of TSC has thus far not been feasible because of genetic variation, limited availability, undetermined sensitivity, and high costs. Therefore, the role of thorough skin, full eye and neurological evaluation coupled with nervous system and systemic imaging will remain essential to the diagnosis of TSC.

## Differential diagnosis

Different disorders should be considered in differential diagnosis of TSC. Facial angiofibromas in teenager should be differentiated with acne vulgaris. Depigmented spots should be differentiated with vitiligo or isolated (not-TSC associated) depigmentations. Renal cysts should be differentiated with PKD1.

## Treatment, follow-up and management

Presently there is no available causative treatment for TSC. There are two main symptomatic treatment strategies required in the majority of patients with TSC: epilepsy treatment and management of visceral tumours and their complications.

There is no specific treatment of epilepsy in TSC, except for the good effect of vigabatrin in infantile spasms (Curatolo et al. 2005). Due to the increasing number of patients with diagnosed prenatally, one could consider the chance to start antiepileptic treatment very early. Jozwiak et al. (2007) proposed that in order to prevent mental decline in the first years of life, all young infants with active epileptic discharges on EEG should be proposed for an antiepileptic treatment, even before the onset of clinical seizures. Recently, evidence is growing for the high effectiveness of surgical treatment of epilepsy in tuberous sclerosis (Curatolo et al. 2006).

Early identification of visceral lesions in patients with TSC may help their effective management. Due to their possibly life threatening complications renal, cardiac and cerebral lesions are paid particular attention. The Tuberous Sclerosis Consensus Conference held in Annapolis in 1998 developed the latest recommendations for diagnostic follow up of internal lesions (Roach et al. 1999) (Table 2).

Large renal angiomyolipomas (>4.5 cm) may require surgery. Embolization and/or renal sparing surgery are treatment options currently available.

As cardiac tumours regress with age, they usually do not require surgery.

Special attention should be paid to subependymal giant cell astrocytomas (Madhavan et al. 2007, O'Callaghan et al. 2008). They should be early removed as prolonged intracranial hypertension frequently causes optic atrophy and blindness. This is a special problem in mentally handicapped children as in this group of patients the symptoms of growing tumour may be easily overlooked.

Disfiguring dermatological lesions deserve special attention, especially in young patients without mental retardation. The treatment methods currently available for patients with facial angiofibromas include cryosurgery, dermabrasion, chemical peeling, excision and laser. If lesions affect large areas of the face, dermabrasion is a very effective treatment. Surgical excision is a reasonable option only in case where few lesions are present. During the last decade, lasers have become a popular treatment option.

The discovery of the rapamycin effects on growth inhibition of TSC lesions in animal models of the disease raised the possibility of using this drug for treatment of TSC patients (Zeng et al. 2008). Preliminary results of few clinical trials are promising (Bissler et al. 2008, Davies et al. 2008, Paul et al. 2008) showing regression of angiomyolipomas during therapy with tendency of increase of volume after the therapy was stopped and improvement of spirometric measurements and gas trapping that persisted after treatment.

**Table 2.** Testing recommendations (according to Roach et al. 1999)

| Assessment | Initial testing | Repeat testing |
| --- | --- | --- |
| Neurodevelopmental testing | at diagnosis and at school entry | as indicated |
| Ophthalmic examination | at diagnosis | as indicated |
| EEG | if seizures occur | as indicated for seizures management |
| ECG | at diagnosis | as indicated |
| Echocardiography | if cardiac symptoms occur | if cardiac dysfunction occurs |
| Renal ultrasonography | at diagnosis | every 1–3 years |
| Chest computed tomography | at adulthood (women only) | if pulmonary dysfunction occurs |
| Cranial computed tomography* | at diagnosis | children/adolescents: every 1–3 years |
| Cranial MRI* | at diagnosis | children/adolescents: every 1–3 years |

* Either cranial CT or MRI, but usually not both.

## Genetic counselling

TSC is inherited in an autosomal dominant manner. About one-third of probands with TSC have an affected parent. Overall, two-thirds of TSC probands carry a de novo mutation in either TSC gene (Northrup and Au 2006). More precisely, a denovo mutation occur in approximately 80% of TSC2 and 50% of TSC1 probands.

### Risk to family members: parents of a proband

Recommendations for the evaluation of parents of a child with no apparent family history of TSC include thorough skin examination, retinal examination, brain imaging, renal ultrasound examination, and molecular genetic testing if the disease-causing mutation has been identified in the proband. Molecular genetic testing plays an important role whenever asymptomatic parents of a TSC child, or other family members, desire to plan a pregnancy. In these cases, gene testing is particularly helpful if the parents are healthy and wants to determine their own TSC genotype without undergoing extensive diagnostic work-up. Unaffected parents have a 12% chance of having gonadal mosaicism (Verhoef et al. 1999). A careful clinical investigation of the parents, or genetic testing, may disclose TSC lesions missed by previous controls by health care professionals because of a milder phenotypic presentation. Therefore, an apparently negative family history, or a negative physical examination by physicians with no direct experience on TSC should be confirmed by appropriate evaluations.

### Risk to family members: sibs of a proband

The risk to the sibs of the proband depends on the genetic status of the parents: if a parent is affected or has the disease-causing mutation identified in the family, the risk to the sibs is 50%; if neither parent has any findings indicative of TSC or if neither parent has the disease-causing mutation detectable in DNA extracted from leukocytes, sibs of a proband have a 1 to 2% recurrence risk because of the possibility of gonadal mosaicism.

### Risk to family members: offspring of a proband

Each child of an individual with TSC has a 50% chance of inheriting the mutation.

### Risk to family members: other family members of a proband

The risk to other family members depends upon the genetic status of the proband's parents. If a parent is found to be affected or to have the disease-causing mutation, family members of the parent are at risk.

### High-risk pregnancies

Prenatal diagnosis by chorionic villi sampling (CVS) at the 10–12th week of gestation should be offered to high risk couples with an ongoing pregnancy if the disease-causing mutation has been previously identified in one affected relative. The process of *TSC1* and *TSC2* mutation screening usually requires a few months, thus the testing should initiate far in advance of the desired pregnancy. On the other hand, the search for a known mutation can be completed in a week. For families who present too late for a prenatal TSC test high-resolution ultrasound examination for cardiac rhabdomyomas can be performed in a reference center at the 20th week of gestation, followed by a second examination at the 28th week. Even in the best centers using the highest resolution available, cardiac rhabdomyomas are rarely detectable earlier than the 20th week. Moderately large brain displastic areas, particularly if associated to ventricular asymmetries can be revealed by fetal MRI, thus this investigation may be offered to high risk pregnancies. However, the parents must be informed that normal results of the heart and brain fetal examinations do not significantly reduce the a priori probability to be a carrier of a TSC gene defect. Pre-implantation genetic diagnosis is available and has been utilized by families in which the disease-causing mutation had been previously identified.

### References

Al-Saleem T, Wessner LL, Scheithauer BW, Patterson K, Roach ES, Dreyer SJ, Fujikawa K, Bjornsson J, Bernstein J, Henske EP (1998) Malignant tumors of the kidney, brain, and soft tissues in children and young adults with the tuberous sclerosis complex. Cancer 83: 2208–2216.

Antonarakis ES, Sampson JR, Cheadle JP (2002) Temperature modulation of DHPLC analysis for detection of coexisting constitutional and mosaic sequence variants in TSC2. J Biochem Biophys Methods 51: 161–164.

Asano E, Chugani DC, Muzik O, Shen C, Juhasz C, Janisse J, Ager J, Canady A, Shah JR, Shah AK, Watson C, Chugani HT (2000) Multimodality imaging for improved detection of epileptogenic foci in tuberous sclerosis complex. Neurology 54: 1976–1984.

Astrinidis A, Senapedis W, Coleman TR, Henske EP (2003) Cell cycle-regulated phosphorylation of hamartin, the product of the tuberous sclerosis complex 1 gene, by cyclin-dependent kinase 1/cyclin B. J Biol Chem 278: 51372–51379.

Au KS, Pollom GJ, Roach ES, Delgado MR, Northrup H (1998a) TSC1 and TSC2 gene mutations: detection and genotype/phenotype correlation. Am J Hum Genet 63S: 350.

Au KS, Rodriguez JA, Finch JL, Volcik KA, Roach ES, Delgado MR, Rodriguez E Jr, Northrup H (1998b) Germ-line mutational analysis of the TSC2 gene in 90 tuberous-sclerosis patients. Am J Hum Genet 62: 286–294.

Au KS, Williams AT, Gambello MJ, Northrup H (2004) Molecular genetic basis of tuberous sclerosis complex: from bench to bedside. J Child Neurol 19: 699–709.

Au KS, Williams AT, Roach ES, Batchelor L, Sparagana SP, Delgado MR, Wheless JW, Baumgartner JE, Roa BB, Wilson CM, Smith-Knuppel TK, Cheung MY, Whittemore VH, King TM, Northrup H (2007) Genotype/phenotype correlation in 325 individuals referred for a diagnosis of tuberous sclerosis complex in the United States. Genet Med 9: 88–100.

Avila NA, Dwyer AJ, Rabel A, Moss J (2007) Sporadic lymphangioleiomyomatosis and tuberous sclerosis complex with lymphangioleiomyomatosis: comparison of CT features. Radiology 242: 277–285.

Bader RS, Chitayat D, Kelly E, Ryan G, Smallhorn JF, Toi A, Hornberger LK (2003) Fetal rhabdomyoma: prenatal diagnosis, clinical outcome, and incidence of associated tuberous sclerosis complex. J Pediatr 143: 620–624.

Baker P, Piven J, Sato Y (1998) Autism and tuberous sclerosis complex: prevalence and clinical features. J Autism Dev Disord 28: 279–285.

Balzer F, Menetrier P (1885) Etude sur un cas d'adénomes sébacés de la face et du cuir chevelu. Arch Physiol Norm Pathol (série III) 6: 564–576.

Barkovich AJ (2005) The Phakomatoses. I: Barkovich AJ (ed.) Pediatric Neuroimaging. 4th ed. Boston: Lippincott Williams & Wilkins, pp. 245–289.

Bebin EM, Kelly PJ, Gomez MR (1993) Surgical treatment for epilepsy in cerebral tuberous sclerosis. Epilepsia 34: 651–657.

Benvenuto G, Li S, Brown SJ, Braverman R, Vass WC, Cheadle JP, Halley DJ, Sampson JR, Wienecke R, DeClue JE (2000) The tuberous sclerosis-1 (TSC1) gene product hamartin suppresses cell growth and augments the expression of the TSC2 product tuberin by inhibiting its ubiquitination. Oncogene 19: 6306–6316.

Berg H (1913) Vererbung der tuberösen Sklerose durch zwei bzw. drei Generationen. Z ges Neurol Psychiatr 19: 528–539.

Berkowitz NJ, Rigler LG (1934) Tuberous sclerosis diagnosed with cerebral pneumography. Arch Neurol Psychiatr 35: 833–838.

Berlin AL, Billick RC (2002) Use of $CO_2$ laser in the treatment of periunqual fibromas associated with tuberous sclerosis. Dermatol Surg 28: 434–436.

Bielschowsky M (1914) Uber tuberose Sklerose und ihre Beziehungen zur Recklinghausenschen Krankheit. Z Ges Neurol Psychiatr 26: 133–135.

Birchenall-Roberts MC, Fu T, Bang OS, Dambach M, Resau JH, Sadowski CL, Bertolette DC, Lee HJ, Kim SJ, Ruscetti FW (2004) Tuberous sclerosis complex 2 gene product interacts with human SMAD proteins. A molecular link of two tumor suppressor pathways. J Biol Chem 279: 25605–25613.

Bissler JJ, McCormack FX, Young LR, Elwing JM, Chuck G, Leonard JM, Schmithorst VJ, Laor T, Brody AS, Bean J, Salisbury S, Franz DN (2008) Sirolimus for angiomyolipoma in tuberous sclerosis complex or lymphangioleiomyomatosis. N Engl J Med 10;358: 140–151.

Bissler JJ, Racadio J, Donnelly LF, Johnson ND (2002) Reduction of postembolization syndrome after ablation of renal angiomyolipoma. Am J Kidney Dis 39: 966–971.

Bittencourt RC, Huilgol SC, Seed PT, Calonje E, Markey AC, Barlow RJ (2001) Treatment of angiofibromas with a scanning carbon dioxide laser: a clinicopathological study with long-term follow-up. J Am Acad Dermatol 45: 731–735.

Bjornsson J, Henske EP, Bernstein J (1999) Renal manifestations. In: Gomez MR, Sampson JR, Whittemore VH (eds.) Tuberous Sclerosis Complex. New York: Oxford University Press, pp 181–193.

Bolton PF, Griffiths PD (1997) Association of tuberous sclerosis of temporal lobes with autism and atypical autism. Lancet 349: 392–395.

Bolton PF (2004) Neuroepileptic correlates of autistic symptomatology in tuberous sclerosis. Ment Retard Dev Disabil Res Rev 10: 126–131.

Bonetti F, Pea M, Martignoni G (1997) The perivascular epithelioid cell and related lesions. Adv in Anat Pathol 4: 343–358.

Bourneville DM (1880) Sclérose tubéreuse des circonvolutions cérébrales: Idiotie et épilepsie hémiplégique. Arch Neurol (Paris) 1: 81–91.

Bourneville DM, Brissaud E (1881) Encéphalite ou sclérose tuberouse des circonvolutions cérébrales. Arch Neurol 1: 390–412.

Bourneville DM, Brissaud E (1900) Idiotie et epilepsie symptomatique de sclérose tuberouse ou hypertrophique. Arch Neurol 10: 29–39.

Brais B (1993) Désiré Magloire Bourneville and French anticlericalism during the Third Republic. Clio Med 23:107–139.

Brook-Carter PT, Peral B, Ward CJ, Thompson P, Hughes J, Maheshwar MM, Nellist M, Gamble V, Harris PC, Sampson JR (1994) Deletion of the TSC2 and PKD1 genes associated with severe infantile polycystic kidney disease a contiguous gene syndrome. Nat Genet 8: 328–332.

Calderón González R, Treviño Welsh J, Calderón Sepúlveda A (1994) Autism in tuberous sclerosis. Gac Med Mex 130: 374–379.

Campbell AW (1906) Cerebral sclerosis. Brain 28: 382–396.

Carbonara C, Longa L, Grosso E, Mazzucco G, Borrone C, Garre ML, Brisigotti M, Filippi G, Scabar A, Giannotti A, Falzoni P, Monga G, Garini G, Gabrielli M, Riegler P, Danesino C, Ruggieri M, Magro G, Migone N (1996) Apparent preferential loss of heterozygosity at TSC2 over TSC1 chromosomal region in tuberous sclerosis hamartomas. Genes Chromosomes Cancer 15: 18–25.

Carsillo T, Astrinidis A, Henske EP (2000) Mutations in the tuberous sclerosis complex gene TSC2 are a cause of sporadic pulmonary lymphangioleiomyomatosis. Proc Natl Acad Sci USA 97: 6085–6090.

Chan JA, Zhang H, Roberts PS, Jozwiak S, Wieslawa G, Lewin-Kowalik J, Kotulska K, Kwiatkowski DJ (2004) Pathogenesis of tuberous sclerosis subependymal giant cell astrocytomas: biallelic inactivation of TSC1 or TSC2 leads to mTOR activation. J Neuropathol Exp Neurol 63: 1236–1242.

Chandra PS, Salamon N, Nguyen ST, Chang JW, Huynh MN, Cepeda C, Leite JP, Neder L, Koh S, Vinters HV, Mathern GW (2007) Infantile spasm-associated microencephaly in tuberous sclerosis complex and cortical dysplasia. Neurologo 68: 438–445.

Cheadle JP, Reeve MP, Sampson JR, Kwiatkowski DJ (2000) Molecular genetic advances in tuberous sclerosis. Hum Genet 107: 97–114.

Choi JE, Chae JH, Hwang YS, Kim KJ (2006) Mutational analysis of TSC1 and TSC2 in Korean patients with tuberous sclerosis complex. Brain Dev 28: 440–446.

Chou IJ, Lin KL, Wong AM, Wang HS, Chou ML, Hung PC, Hsieh MY, Chang MY (2007) Neuroimaging correlation with neurological severity in tuberous sclerosis complex. Eur J Paediatr Neurol Sep 13 [Epub ahead of print].

Clements D, Mayer RJ, Johnson SR (2007) Subcellular distribution of the TSC2 gene product tuberin in human airways smooth muscle cells is driven by multiple localization sequences and is cell cycle dependent. Am J Physiol Lang Cell Moll Physiol 292: 258–266.

Connor JM, Stephenson JB, Hadley MD (1986) Non-penetrance in tuberous sclerosis. Lancet 2: 1275

Coppola G, Cerminara C, Spigapiena R et al (2006) Tuberous sclerosis complex and syringomyelia: report of two cases. Eur J Paediatr Neurol 10(1): 37–40.

Corradetti MN, Inoki K, Bardeesy N, DePinho RA, Guan KL (2004) Regulation of the TSC pathway by LKB1: evidence of a molecular link between tuberous sclerosis complex and Peutz-Jeghers syndrome. Genes Dev 18: 1533–1538.

Crino PB (2004) Molecular pathogenesis of tuber formation in tuberous sclerosis complex. J Child Neurol 19: 716–725.

Crino PB, Nathanson KL, Henske EP (2006) The tuberous sclerosis complex. N Engl J Med 355: 1345–1356.

Critchley M, Earl CJC (1932) Tuberous sclerosis and allied conditions. Brain 55: 311–346.

Curatolo P, Cusmai R (1987) Autism and infantile spasms in children with tuberous sclerosis. Dev Med Child Neurol 29: 551.

Curatolo P, Cusmai R, Cortesi F, Chiron C, Jambaque I, Dulac O (1991) Neuropsychiatric aspects of tuberous sclerosis. Ann N Y Acad Sci 615: 8–16.

Curatolo P (2004) Historical background. In: Curatolo P (ed.) Tuberous Sclerosis Complex: From Basic Science to Clinical Phenotypes. London: McKeith Press, pp. 1–10.

Curatolo P, Porfirio MC, Manzi B, Seri S (2004) Autism in tuberous sclerosis. Eur J Paediatr Neurol 8: 327–332.

Curatolo P, Bombardieri R, Cerminara C (2006) Current management for epilepsy in tuberous sclerosis complex. Curr Opin Neurol 19: 119–123.

Curatolo P, Bombardieri R, Verdecchia M, Seri S (2005) Intractable seizures in tuberous sclerosis complex: from molecular pathogenesis to the rationale for treatment. J Child Neurol 20(4): 318–325.

Curatolo P, Porfirio MC, Manzi B, Seri S (2004) Autism in tuberous sclerosis. Eur J Paediatr Neurol 8: 327–332.

Dabora SL, Jozwiak S, Franz DN, Roberts PS, Nieto A, Chung J, Choy YS, Reeve MP, Thiele E, Egelhoff JC, Kasprzyk-Obara J, Domanska-Pakiela D, Kwiatkowski DJ (2001) Mutational analysis in a cohort of 224 tuberous sclerosis patients indicates increased severity of TSC2, compared with TSC1, disease in multiple organs. Am J Hum Genet 68: 64–80.

Darling TN, Skarulis MC, Steinberg SM, Marx SJ, Spiegel AM, Turner M (1997) Multiple facial angiofibromas and collagenomas in patients with multiple endocrine neoplasia type 1. Arch Dermatol 133: 853–857.

Dash PK, Orsi SA, Moore AN (2006) Spatial memory formation and memory-enhancing effect of glucose involves activation of the tuberous sclerosis complex-Mammalian target of rapamycin pathway. J Neurosi 26: 8048–8056.

Davies DM, Johnson SR, Tattersfield AE, Kingswood JC, Cox JA, McCartney DL, Doyle T, Elmslie F, Saggar A, de Vries PJ, Sampson JR (2008) Sirolimus therapy in tuberous sclerosis or sporadic lymphangioleiomyomatosis. N Engl J Med 10;358: 200–203.

Deonna T, Roulet E (2006) Autistic spectrum disorder: evaluating a possible contributing or causal role of epilepsy. Epilepsia 47 (Suppl 2): 79–82.

Deonna T, Roulet-Perez E, Chappuis H, Ziegler AL (2007) Autistic regression associated with seizure onset in an infant with tuberous sclerosis. Dev Med Child Neurol 49: 320.

Devlin LA, Shepherd CH, Crawford H, Morrison PJ (2006) Tuberous sclerosis complex: clinical features, diagnosis, and prevalence within Northern Ireland. Dev Med Child Neurol 48: 495–499.

Doherty C, Goh S, Young Poussaint T, Erdag N, Thiele EA (2005) Prognostic significance of tuber count and location in tuberous sclerosis complex. J Child Neurol 20: 837–841.

de Ribaupierre S, Dorfmuller G, Bulteau C, Fohlen M, Pinard JM, Chiron C, Delalande O (2007) Subependymal giant-cell astrocytomas in pediatric tuberous sclerosis disease: when should we operate? Neurosurgery 60: 83–89.

de Vries P, Humphrey A, McCartney D, Prather P, Bolton P, Hunt A; TSC Behaviour Consensus Panel (2005) Consensus clinical guidelines for the assessment of cognitive and behavioural problems in Tuberous Sclerosis. Eur Child Adolesc Psychiatry 14: 183–190.

de Vries PJ, Hunt A, Bolton PF (2007) The psychopathologies of children and adolescents with tuberous sclerosis complex (TSC): a postal survey of UK families. Eur Child Adolesc Psychiatry 16: 16–24.

El-Hashemite N, Zhang H, Henske EP, Kwiatkowski DJ (2003) Mutation in TSC2 and activation of mammalian target of rapamycin signalling pathway in renal angiomyolipoma. Lancet 361: 1348–1349.

El-Hashemite N, Zhang H, Walker V, Hoffmeister KM, Kwiatkowski DJ (2004) Perturbed IFN-gamma-Jak-signal transducers and activators of transcription signaling in tuberous sclerosis mouse models: synergistic effects of rapamycin-IFN-gamma treatment. Cancer Res 64: 3436–3443.

Eker R (1954) Familial renal adenomas in Wistar rats; a preliminary report. Acta Pathol Microbiol Scand 34: 554–5562.

Eluvathingal TJ, Behen ME, Chugani HT, Janisse J, Bernardi B, Chakraborty P, Juhasz C, Muzik O, Chugani DC (2006) Cerebellar lesions in tuberous sclerosis complex: neurobehavioral and neuroimaging correlates. J Child Neurol 21: 846–851.

Emmerson P, Maynard J, Jones S, Butler R, Sampson JR, Cheadle JP (2003) Characterizing mutations in samples with low-level mosaicism by collection and analysis of DHPLC fractionated heteroduplexes. Hum Mutat 21: 112–115.

Ess KC, Kamp CA, Tu BP, Gutmann DH (2005) Developmental origin of subependymal giant cell astrocytoma in tuberous sclerosis complex. Neurology 64: 1446–1449.

European Chromosome 16 Tuberous Sclerosis Consortium (1993) Identification and characterization of the tuberous sclerosis gene on chromosome 16. Cell 75: 1305–1315.

Fesslova V, Villa L, Rizzuti T, Mastrangelo M, Mosca F (2004) Natural history and long-term outcome of cardiac rhabdomyomas detected prenatally. Prenat Diagn 24: 241–248.

Fombonne E, Du Mazaubrun C, Cans C, Grandjean H (1997) Autism and associated medical disorders in a French epidemiological survey. J Am Acad Child Adolesc Psychiatry 36: 1561–1569.

Franz DN, Leonard J, Tudor C, Chuck G, Care M, Sethuraman G, Dinopoulos A, Thomas G, Crone KR (2006) Rapamycin causes regression of astrocytomas in tuberous sclerosis complex. Ann Neurol 59: 490–498.

Fryer AE, Chalmers A, Connor JM, Fraser I, Povey S, Yates AD, Yates JR, Osborne JP (1987) Evidence that the gene for tuberous sclerosis is on chromosome 9. Lancet 21: 659–661.

Gao X, Pan D (2001) TSC1 and TSC2 tumor suppressors antagonize insulin signaling in cell growth. Genes Dev 15: 1383–1392.

Gillberg C (1992) Subgroups in autism: are there behavioural phenotypes typical of underlying medical conditions? J Intellect Disabil Res 36: 201–214.

Gillberg IC, Gillberg C, Ahlsen G (1994) Autistic behaviour and attention deficits in tuberous sclerosis: a population-based study. Dev Med Child Neurol 36: 50–56.

Gateaux-Mennecier J (2002) Bourneville, humanist and reformer. Rev Prat 52: 1517–1521.

Gateaux-Mennecier J (2003) Bourneville's medico-social work. Hist Sci Med 37: 13–30.

Gold AP, Freeman JM (1965) Depigmented nevi: the earliest sign of tuberous sclerosis. Pediatrics 35: 1003–1005.

Gomez MR (1987) Tuberous Sclerosis. In: Neurocutaneous Diseases. A Practical Approach. Boston: Butterworths, pp. 30–52.

Gomez MR (1988) Tuberous Sclerosis, 2nd edn. New York: Raven Press.

Gomez MR (1991) Phenotypes of the tuberous sclerosis complex with a revision of diagnostic criteria. Ann NY Acad Sci 615: 17.

Gomez MR (1995) History of the Tuberous Sclerosis Complex. Brain Dev 17: 55–57.

Gomez MR (1999) History of Tuberous Sclerosis Complex. In: Gomez MR, Sampson JR, Whittemore VH (eds.) Tuberous Sclerosis Complex. Developmental Perspectives in Psychiatry, 3rd ed. New York: Oxford University Press, pp. 1–9.

Guerreiro MM, Andermann F, Andermann E, Palmini A, Hwang P, Hoffman HJ, Otsubo H, Bastos A, Dubeau F, Snipes GJ, Olivier A, Rasmussen T (1998) Surgical treatment of epilepsy in tuberous sclerosis: strategies and results in 18 patients. Neurology 51: 1263–1269.

Guinee D, Singh R, Azumi N, Singh G, Przygodzki RM, Travis W, Koss M (1995) Multifocal micronodular pneumocyte hyperplasia: a distinctive pulmonary manifestation of tuberous sclerosis. Mod Pathos 8: 902–926.

Gutierrez GC, Smalley SL, Tanguay PE (1998) Autism in tuberous sclerosis complex. J Autism Dev Disord 28: 97–103.

Haddad LA, Smith N, Bowser M, Niida Y, Murthy V, Gonzalez-Agosti C, Ramesh V. (2002) The TSC1 tumor suppressor hamartin interacts with neurofilament-L and possibly functions as a novel integrator of the neuronal cytoskeleton. J Biol Chem 277: 44180–44186.

Haines JL, Short MP, Kwiatkowski DJ, Jewell A, Andermann E, Bejjani B, Yang CH, Gusella JF, Amos JA (1991) Localization of one gene for tuberous sclerosis within 9q32-9q34, and further evidence for heterogeneity. Am J Hum Genet 49: 764–772.

Han SH, Santos TM, Puga A, Roy J, Thiele EA, McCollin M, Stemmer-Rachamimov A, Ramesh V (2004) Phosphorylation of tuberin as a novel mechanism of somatic inactivation of the tuberous sclerosis complex in brain lesions. Cancer Res 64: 81–816.

Harabayashi T, Shinohara N, Katano H, Nonomura K, Shimizu T, Koyanagi T (2004) Management of renal angiomyolipomas associated with tuberous sclerosis complex. J Urol 171: 102–105.

Harris TE, Lawrence JC Jr (2003) TOR signaling. Sci STKE 2003: re15.

Hartdegen A (1881) Ein Fall von multipler Verhartung des Grosshirns nebst histologisch eigenartigen harten Geschwulsten der Seitenventrikel (Glioma gangliocellulare) bei einem Neugeborenen. Arch Psychiatr Nervenkr 11: 117–131.

Henske EP, Neumann HP, Scheithauer BW, Herbst EW, Short MP, Kwiatkowski DJ (1995) Loss of heterozygosity in the tuberous sclerosis (TSC2) region of chromosome band 16p13 occurs in sporadic as well as TSC-associated renal angiomyolipomas. Genes Chromosomes. Cancer 13: 295–298.

Henske EP, Scheithauer BW, Short MP, Wollmann R, Nahmias J, Hornigold N, van Slegtenhorst M, Welsh CT, Kwiatkowski DJ (1996) Allelic loss is frequent in tuberous sclerosis kidney lesions but rare in brain lesions. Am J Hum Genet 59: 400–406.

Hino O, Kobayashi T, Tsuchiya H, Kikuchi Y, Kobayashi E, Mitani H, Hirayama Y (1994) The predisposing gene of the Eker rat inherited cancer syndrome is tightly linked to the tuberous sclerosis (TSC2) gene. Biochem Biophys Res Commun 203: 1302–1308.

Hino O, Majima S, Kobayashi T, Honda S, Momose S, Kikuchi Y, Mitani H (2001) Multistep renal carcinogenesis as gene expression disease in tumor suppressor TSC2 gene mutant model genotype, phenotype and environment. Mutat Res 477: 155–164.

Hodges AK, Li S, Maynard J, Parry L, Braverman R, Cheadle JP, DeClue JE, Sampson JR (2001) Pathological mutations in TSC1 and TSC2 disrupt the interaction between hamartin and tuberin. Hum Mol Genet 10: 2899–2905.

Holmes GL, Stafstrom CE; Tuberous Sclerosis Study Group (2007) Tuberous sclerosis complex and epilepsy: recent developments and future challenges. Epilepsia 48: 617–630.

Hsu TH, O'Hara J, Mehta A, Levitin A, Klein EA (2002) Nephron-sparing nephrectomy for giant renal angiomyolipoma associated with lynphangioleiomyomatosis. Urology 59: 138.

Huber C, Treutner KH, Steinau G, Schumpelick V (1996) Ruptured hepatic angiolipoma in tuberous sclerosis complex. Langenbecks Arch Chir 381: 7–9.

Humphrey A, Neville BG, Clarke A, Bolton PF (2006) Autistic regression associated with seizure onset in an infant with tuberous sclerosis. Dev Med Child Neurol 48: 609–611.

Hunt A, Dennis J (1987) Psychiatric disorder among children with tuberous sclerosis. Dev Med Child Neurol 29:190–198

Hunt A, Shepherd C (1993) A prevalence study of autism in tuberous sclerosis. J Autism Dev Disord 23: 323–339.

Huson SM, Korf BR (2002) The Phakomatoses. In: Rimoin D, Connor JM, Pyeritz RE, Korf BR (eds.) Emery and Rimoin's Principles and Practice of Medical Genetics. 4th ed. London: Churchill Livingstone: pp. 3162–3202.

Hussain N, Curran A, Pilling D, Malluci CL, Ladusans EJ, Alfirevic Z, Pizer B (2006) Congenital subependymal giant cell astrocytoma diagnosed on fetal MRI. Arch Dis Child 91: 520.

Hung CC, Su YN, Chien SC, Liou HH, Chen CC, Chen PC, Hsieh CJ, Chen CP, Lee WT, Lin WL, Lee CN (2006) Molecular and clinical analyses of 84 patients with tuberous sclerosis complex. BMC Med Genet 7: 72.

Ichikawa T, Wakisaka A, Daido S, Takao S, Tamiya T, Date I, Koizumi S, Niida Y (2005) A case of solitary subependymal giant cell astrocytoma: two somatic hits of TSC2 in the tumor, without evidence of somatic mosaicism. J Mol Diagn 7: 544–549.

Inoki K, Li Y, Xu T, Guan KL (2003) Rheb GTPase is a direct target of TSC2 GAP activity and regulates mTOR signaling. Genes Dev 17: 1829–1834.

Jambaque I, Cusmai R, Curatolo P, Cortesi F, Perrot C, Dulac O (1991) Neuropsychological aspects of tuberous sclerosis in relation to epilepsy and MRI findings. Dev Med Child Neurol 33: 698–705.

Janssen B, Sampson J, van der Est M, Deelen W, Verhoef S, Daniels I, Hesseling A, Brook-Carter P, Nellist M, Lindhout D, Sandkuijl L, Halley D (1994) Refined localization of TSC1 by combined analysis of 9q34 and 16p13 data in 14 tuberous sclerosis families. Hum Genet 94: 437–440.

Jansen FE, van Nieuwenhuizen O, van Huffelen AC (2004) Tuberous Sclerosis Complex and its founders. J Neurol Neurosurg Psychiatr 75: 770.

Jansen FE, Huiskamp G, van Huffelen AC, Bourez-Swart M, Boere E, Gebbink T, Vincken KL, van Nieuwenhuizen O (2006) Identification of the epileptogenic tuber in patients with tuberous sclerosis: a comparison of high-resolution EEG and MEG. Epilepsia 47: 108–114.

Janssen LA, Sandkuyl LA, Merkens EC, Maat-Kievit JA, Sampson JR, Fleury P, Hennekam RC, Grosveld GC, Lindhout D, Halley DJ (1990) Genetic heterogeneity in tuberous sclerosis. Genomics 8: 237–242.

Jin F, Wienecke R, Xiao GH, Maize JC Jr, DeClue JE, Yeung RS (1996) Suppression of tumorigenicity by the wild-type tuberous sclerosis 2 (Tsc2) gene and its C-terminal region. Proc Natl Acad Sci USA 93: 9154–9159.

Johnson SR, Clelland CA, Ronan J, Tattersfield AE, Knox AJ (2002) The TSC-2 product tuberin is expressed in lymphangioleiomyomatosis and angiomyolipoma. Histopathology 40: 458–463.

Jones AC, Daniells CE, Snell RG, Tachataki M, Idziaszczyk SA, Krawczak M, Sampson JR, Cheadle JP (1997) Molecular genetic and phenotypic analysis reveals differences between TSC1 and TSC2 associated familial and sporadic tuberous sclerosis. Hum Mol Genet 6: 2155–2161.

Jones AC, Shyamsundar MM, Thomas MW, Maynard J, Idziaszczyk S, Tomkins S, Sampson JR, Cheadle JP (1999) Comprehensive mutation analysis of TSC1 and TSC2-and phenotypic correlations in 150 families with tuberous sclerosis. Am J Hum Genet 64: 1305–1315.

Jones AC, Sampson JR, Hoogendoorn B, Cohen D, Cheadle JP (2000) Application and evaluation of denaturing HPLC for molecular genetic analysis in tuberous sclerosis. Hum Genet 106: 663–668.

Jones AC, Sampson JR, Cheadle JP (2001) Low level mosaicism detectable by DHPLC but not by direct sequencing. Hum Mutat 17: 233–234.

Jóźwiak S, Pedich M, Rajszys P, Michałowicz R (1992) Incidence of hepatic hamartomas in tuberous sclerosis. Arch Dis Childh 67: 1363–1365.

Jóźwiak S, Schwartz RA, Janniger CK, Michalowicz R, Chmielik J (1998a) Skin lesions in children with tuberous sclerosis complex: their prevalence, natural course, and diagnostic significance. Int J Dermatol 37: 911–917.

Jóźwiak S, Goodman M, Lamm SH (1998b) Poor mental development in patients with tuberous sclerosis complex: clinical risk factors. Arch Neurol 55: 379–384.

Jóźwiak S, Schwartz RA, Janniger CK, Bielicka-Cymerman J (2000) Usefulness of diagnostic criteria of tuberous sclerosis complex in pediatric patients. J Child Neurol 15: 652–659.

Jóźwiak S, Schwartz R (2003) Dermatological and stomatological manifestations. In: Paolo Curatolo (ed.) Tuberous sclerosis complex: from basic science to clinical phenotypes. London: Mac Keith Press, pp. 136–169.

Jóźwiak S, Domańska-Pakieła D, Kwiatkowski DJ, Kotulska K (2005) Multiple cardiac rhabdomyomas as a sole symptom of tuberous sclerosis complex: case report with molecular confirmation. J Child Neurol 20: 988–989.

Jóźwiak J, Jóźwiak S (2005) Giant cells: contradiction to two-hit model of tuber formation? Cell Mol Neurobiol 25: 795–805.

Jóźwiak J, Kotulska K, Jozwiak S (2006) Similarity of balloon cells in focal cortical dysplasia to giant cells in tuberous sclerosis. Epilepsia 47: 805.

Jóźwiak S, Kotulska K, Kasprzyk-Obara J, Domanska-Pakiela D, Tomyn-Drabik M, Roberts P, Kwiatkowski D (2006) Clinical and genotype studies of cardiac tumors in 154 patients with tuberous sclerosis complex. Pediatrics 118: e1146–1151.

Jóźwiak J, Jóźwiak S, Oldak M (2006) Molecular activity of sirolimus and its possible application in tuberous sclerosis treatment. Med Res Rev 26: 160–180.

Jóźwiak J, Kotulska K, Jóźwiak S (2006a) Similarity of balloon cells in focal cortical dysplasia to giant cells in tuberous sclerosis. Epilepsia 47: 805.

Jóźwiak S, Domanska-Pakiela D, Kotulska K, Kaczorowska M (2007) Treatment before seizures: new indications for antiepileptic therapy in children with tuberous sclerosis complex. Epilepsia 48: 1632.

Józwiak J, Józwiak S, Wlodarski P (2008) Possible mechanisms of disease development in tuberous sclerosis. Lancet Oncol 9: 73–79.

Jurkiewicz E, Józwiak S (2006) Giant intracranial aneurysm in a 9-year-old boy with tuberous sclerosis. Pediatr Radiol 36: 463.

Jurkiewicz E, Józwiak S, Bekiesinska-Figatowska M, Pakula-Kosciesza I, Walecki J (2006) Cyst-like cortical tubers in patients with tuberous sclerosis complex: MR imaging with the FLAIR sequence. Pediatr Radiol 36: 498–501.

Kagawa K, Chugani DC, Asano E, Juhasz C, Muzik O, Shah A, Shah J, Sood S, Kupsky WJ, Mangner TJ, Chakraborty PK, Chugani HT (2005) Epilepsy surgery outcome in children with tuberous sclerosis complex evaluated with alpha-[11C]methyl-L-tryptophan positron emission tomography (PET). J Child Neurol 20: 429–438.

Kandt RS, Haines JL, Smith M, Northrup H, Gardner RJ, Short MP, Dumars K, Roach ES, Steingold S, Wall S, Blanton SH, Flodman P, Kwiatkowski DJ, Jewell A, Weber Jl, Roses AD, Pericak-Vance MA (1992) Linkage of an important gene locus for tuberous sclerosis to a chromosome 16 marker for polycystic kidney disease. Nat Genet 2: 37–41.

Kenerson H, Dundon TA, Yeung RS (2005) Effects of rapamycin in the Eker rat model of tuberous sclerosis complex. Pediatr Res 57: 67–75.

Khare L, Strizheva GD, Bailey JN, Au KS, Northrup H, Smith M, Smalley SL, Henske EP (2001) A novel missense mutation in the GTPase activating protein homology region of TSC2 in two large families with tuberous sclerosis complex. J Med Genet 38: 347–349.

Kirpicznik J (1910) Ein Fall von Tuberoser Sklerose und gleichzeitigen multiplen Nierengeschwülsten. Virchow's Archiv für pathologische Anatomie und Physiologie und für klinische Medicin 202: 258.

Kleymenova E, Ibraghimov-Beskrovnaya O, Kugoh H, Everitt J, Xu H, Kiguchi K, Landes G, Harris P, Walker C (2001) Tuberin-dependent membrane localization of polycystin-1: a functional link between polycystic kidney disease and the TSC2 tumor suppressor gene. Mol Cell 7: 823–832.

Knudson AG Jr (1971) Mutation and cancer: statistical study of retinoblastoma. Proc Natl Acad Sci USA 68: 820–823.

Kobayashi T, Hirayama Y, Kobayashi E, Kubo Y, Hino O (1995) A germline insertion in the tuberous sclerosis (Tsc2) gene gives rise to the Eker rat model of dominantly inherited cancer. Nat Genet 9: 70–74.

Kobayashi T, Minowa O, Kuno J, Mitani H, Hino O, Noda T (1999) Renal carcinogenesis, hepatic hemangiomatosis, and embryonic lethality caused by a germ-line Tsc2 mutation in mice. Cancer Res 59: 1206–1211.

Kobayashi T, Minowa O, Sugitani Y, Takai S, Mitani H, Kobayashi E, Noda T, Hino O (2001) A germ-line Tsc1 mutation causes tumor development and embryonic lethality that are similar, but not identical to, those caused by Tsc2 mutation in mice. Proc Natl Acad Sci USA 98: 8762–8767.

Kobayashi T, Satoh K, Ohkawa M (2005) Multifocal micronodular pneumocyte hyperplasia associated with tuberous sclerosis. Acta Radiol 46: 37–40.

Koh S, Jayakar P, Dunoyer C, Whiting SE, Resnick TJ, Alvarez LA, Morrison G, Ragheb J, Prats A, Dean P, Gilman J, Duchowny MS (2000) Epilepsy surgery in children with tuberous sclerosis complex: presurgical evaluation and outcome. Epilepsia 41: 1206–1213.

Koide O, Matsuzaka K, Tanaka Y (1998) Multiple giant angiomyolipomas with a polygonal epithelioid cell component in tuberous sclerosis: an autopsy case report. Pathol Internat 48: 998–1002.

Kothary N, Soulen MC, Clark TW et al (2005) Renal angiomyolipoma: long-term results after arterial embolization. J Vasc Interv Radiol 16: 45–50.

Kozma SC, Thomas G (2002) Regulation of cell size in growth, development and human disease: PI3K, PKB and S6K. Bioessays 24: 65–71.

Kristal H, Sperber F (1989) Hepatic angiomyolipoma in a tuberous sclerosis patient. Isr J Med Sci 25: 412–414.

Kubo Y, Kikuchi Y, Mitani H, Kobayashi E, Kobayashi T, Hino O (1995) Allelic loss at the tuberous sclerosis (Tsc2) gene locus in spontaneous uterine leiomyosarcomas and pituitary adenomas in the Eker rat model. Jpn J Cancer Res 86: 828–832.

Kwiatkowski D (2005) TSC1, TSC2, TSC3? Or mosaicism? Eur J Hum Genet 13: 695–696.

Kwiatkowski DJ (2003) Tuberous sclerosis: from tubers to mTOR. Ann Hum Genet 67: 87–89.

Kwiatkowski DJ (2003a) Rhebbing up mTOR: new insights on TSC1 and TSC2, and the pathogenesis of tuberous sclerosis. Cancer Biol Ther 2: 471–476.

Kwiatkowski DJ, Reeve MP, Chaeadle JP, Sampson JR (2004) Molecular genetics. In: Curatolo P (ed.) Tuberous Sclerosis Complex: from Basic Science to Clinical phenotypes. London: Mac Keith Press, pp. 228–263.

Kwiatkowski DJ, Zhang H, Bandura JL, Heiberger KM, Glogauer M, el-Hashemite N, Onda H (2002) A mouse model of TSC1 reveals sex-dependent lethality from liver hemangiomas, and up-regulation of p70S6 kinase activity in Tsc1 null cells. Hum Mol Genet 11: 525–534.

Kwiatkowska J, Jozwiak S, Hall F, Henske EP, Haines JL, McNamara P, Braiser J, Wigowska-Sowinska J, Kasprzyk-Obara J, Short MP, Kwiatkowski DJ (1998)

Comprehensive mutational analysis of the TSC1 gene: observations on frequency of mutation, associated features, and nonpenetrance. Ann Hum Genet 62: 277–285.

Kwiatkowska J, Wigowska-Sowinska J, Napierala D, Slomski R, Kwiatkowski DJ (1999) Mosaicism in tuberous sclerosis as a potential cause of the failure of molecular diagnosis. N Engl J Med 340: 703–707.

Lachhwani DK, Pestana E, Gupta A, Kotagal P, Bingaman W, Wyllie E (2005) Identification of candidates for epilepsy surgery in patients with tuberous sclerosis. Neurologo 64: 1651–1654.

Lagos JC, Gómez MR (1967) Tuberous sclerosis: reappraisal of a clinical entity. Mayo Clinic Proc 42: 26–49.

Lamb RF, Roy C, Diefenbach TJ, Vinters HV, Johnson MW, Jay DG, Hall A (2000) The TSC1 tumour suppressor hamartin regulates cell adhesion through ERM proteins and the GTPase Rho. Nat Cell Biol 2: 281–287.

Lee L, Sudentas P, Donohue B, Asrican K, Worku A, Walker V, Sun Y, Schmidt K, Albert MS, El-Hashemite N, Lader AS, Onda H, Zhang H, Kwiatkowski DJ, Dabora SL (2005) Efficacy of a rapamycin analog (CCI-779) and IFN-gamma in tuberous sclerosis mouse models. Gene Chromosome Canc 42: 213–227.

Leung AK, Robson WL (2007) Tuberous sclerosis complex: a review. J Pediatr Health Care 21: 108–114.

Lewis JC, Thomas HV, Murphy KC, Sampson JR (2004) Genotype and psychological phenotype in tuberous sclerosis. J Med Genet 41: 203–207.

Li Y, Corradetti MN, Inoki K, Guan KL (2004) TSC2: filling the GAP in the mTOR signaling pathway. Trends Biochem Sci 29: 32–38.

Luat AF, Makki M, Chugani HT (2007) Neuroimaging in tuberous sclerosis complex. Curr Opin Neurol 20: 142–150.

Madhavan D, Schaffer S, Yankovsky A, Arzimanoglou A, Renaldo F, Zaroff CM, LaJoie J, Weiner HL, Andermann E, Franz DN, Leonard J, Connolly M, Cascino GD, Devinsky O (2007) Surgical outcome in tuberous sclerosis complex: a multicenter survey. Epilepsia 48: 1625–1628.

Maheshwar MM, Cheadle JP, Jones AC, Myring J, Fryer AE, Harris PC, Sampson JR (1997) The GAP-related domain of tuberin, the product of the TSC2 gene, is a target for missense mutations in tuberous sclerosis. Hum Mol Genet 6: 1991–1996.

Mak BC, Yeung RS (2004) The tuberous sclerosis complex genes in tumor development. Cancer Invest 22: 588–603.

Marcus H (1924) *Svenska Làk Sallsk Forth*. (As cited by Dickerson WW (1945). "Characteristic roentgenog-raphic changes associated with tuberous sclerosis". Arch Neurol Psychiat 199–220.

Martignoni G, Bonetti F, Pea M, Tardanico R, Brunelli M, Eble JN (2002) Renal disease in adults with TSC2/PKD1 contiguous gene syndrome. Am J Surg Pathol 26: 198–205.

Medhkour A, Traul D, Husain M (2002) Neonatal subependymal giant cell astrocytoma. Pediatr Neurosurg 36: 271–274.

Meikle L, McMullen JR, Sherwood MC, Lader AS, Walker V, Chan JA, Kwiatkowski DJ (2005) A mouse model of cardiac rhabdomyoma generated by loss of Tsc1 in ventricular myocytes. Hum Mol Genet 14: 429–435.

Mirkin LD, Ey EH, Chaparro M (1999) Congenital subependymal giant-cell astrocytoma: case report with prenatal ultrasonogram. Pediatr Radiol 29: 776–780.

Mizuguchi M, Mori M, Nozaki Y, Momoi MY, Itoh M, Takashima S, Hino O (2004) Absence of allelic loss in cytomegalic neurons of cortical tuber in the Eker rat model of tuberous sclerosis. Acta Neuropathol (Berl) 107(1): 47–50.

Mizuguchi M, Takashima S, Yamanouchi H, Nakazato Y, Mitani H, Hino O (2000) Novel cerebral lesions in the Eker rat model of tuberous sclerosis: cortical tuber and anaplastic ganglioglioma. J Neuropathol Exp Neurol 59: 188–196.

Momose S, Kobayashi T, Mitani H, Hirabayashi M, Ito K, Ueda M, Nabeshima Y, Hino O (2002) Identification of the coding sequences responsible for Tsc2-mediated tumor suppression using a transgenic rat system. Hum Mol Genet 11: 2997–3006.

Murthy V, Haddad LA, Smith N, Pinney D, Tyszkowski R, Brown D, Ramesh V (2000) Similarities and differences in the subcellular localization of hamartin and tuberin in the kidney. Am J Physiol Renal Fluid Electrolyte Physiol 278: F737–F746.

Nabbout R, Santos M, Rolland Y, Delalande O, Dulac O, Chiron C (1999) Early diagnosis of subependymal giant cell astrocytoma in children with tuberous sclerosis. J Neurol Neurosurg Psychiatry 66: 370–375.

Nagar AM, Teh HS, Khoo RN, Morani AC, Vrishni K, Raghuram J (2008) Multifocal pneumocyte hyperplasia in tuberous sclerosis. Thorax 63: 186.

Nellist M, Sancak O, Goedbloed MA, van Veghel-Plandsoen M, Maat-Kievit A, Lindhout D, Eussen BH, de Klein A, Halley DJ, van den Ouweland AM (2005) Large deletion at the TSC1 locus in a family with tuberous sclerosis complex. Genet Test 9: 226–230.

Nellist M, van Slegtenhorst Ma, Goedbloed M, van den Ouwenland AMW, Halley DJJ, van der Sluijs P (1999) Characterization of the Cytosolic Tuberin Hamartin Complex. J Biol Chem 274: 35647–35652.

Nevin NC, Pearce WG (1968) Diagnostic and genetical aspects of tuberous sclerosis. J Med Genet 5: 273–280.

Niida Y, Lawrence-Smith N, Banwell A, Hammer E, Lewis J, Beauchamp RL, Sims K, Ramesh V, Ozelius L (1999) Analysis of both TSC1 and TSC2 for germline mutations in 126 unrelated patients with tuberous sclerosis. Hum Mutat 14: 412–422.

Niida Y, Stemmer-Rachamimov AO, Logrip M, Tapon D, Perez R, Kwiatkowski DJ, Sims K, MacCollin M, Louis DN, Ramesh V (2001) Survey of somatic mutations in tuberous sclerosis complex (TSC) hamartomas suggests different genetic mechanisms for pathogenesis of TSC lesions. Am J Hum Genet 69: 493–503.

Northrup H, Au KS (2006) Tuberous sclerosis complex. Genet Rev. http://www.genetests.org.

Northrup H, Beaudet AL, O'Brien WE, Herman GE, Lewis RA, Pollack MS (1987) Linkage of tuberous sclerosis to ABO blood group. Lancet 3 (credo sia 2): 804–805.

Northrup H, Kwiatkowski DJ, Roach ES, Dobyns WB, Lewis RA, Herman GE, Rodriguez E Jr, Daiger SP, Blanton SH (1992) Evidence for genetic heterogeneity in tuberous sclerosis: one locus on chromosome 9 and at least one locus elsewhere. Am J Hum Genet 51: 709–720.

Northrup H, Wheless JW, Bertin TK, Lewis RA (1993) Variability of expression in tuberous sclerosis. J Med Genet 30: 41–43.

O'Callaghan TJ, Edwards JA, Tobin M, Mookerjee BK (1975) Tuberous sclerosis with striking renal involvement in a family. Arch Intern Med 135: 1082–1087.

O'Callaghan FF, Martyn CN, Renowden S, Noakes M, Presdee D, Osborne JP (2008) Sub-ependymal nodules, giant cell astrocytomas and the tuberous sclerosis complex: a population based study. Arch Dis Child May 2 [Epub ahead of print].

O'Callaghan FJ, Shiell AW, Osborne JP, Martyn CN (1998) Prevalence of tuberous sclerosis estimated by capture-recapture analysis. Lancet 351: 1490.

O'Callaghan FJ, Lux A, Osborne J (2000) Early diagnosis of subependymal giant cell astrocytoma in children with tuberous sclerosis. J Neurol Neurosurg Psychiatry 68: 118.

O'Callaghan FJ, Harris T, Joinson C, Bolton P, Noakes M, Presdee D, Renowden S, Shiell A, Martyn CN, Osborne JP (2004) The relation of infantile spasms, tubers, and intelligence in tuberous sclerosis complex. Arch Dis Child 89: 530–533.

Okamoto T, Hara A, Hino O (2003) Down-regulation of cyclooxygenase-2 expression but up-regulation of cyclooxygenase-1 in renal carcinomas of the Eker (TSC2 gene mutant) rat model. Cancer Sci 94: 22–25.

Onda H, Lueck A, Marks PW, Warren HB, Kwiatkowski DJ (1999) Tsc2(±) mice develop tumors in multiple sites that express gelsolin and are influenced by genetic background. J Clin Invest 104: 687–689.

Osborne JP, Fryer A, Webb D (1991) Epidemiology of tuberous sclerosis. Ann N Y Acad Sci 615: 125–127.

Osborne J, Webb D (1993) Seizures and intellectual disability associated with tuberous sclerosis. Dev Med Child Neurol 35: 276.

Osborne JP, Jones AC, Burley MW, Jeganathan D, Young J, O'Callaghan FJ, Sampson JR, Povey S (2000) Non-penetrance in tuberous sclerosis. Lancet 355: 1698.

Osborne J (2006) Tuberous Sclerosis. In: Harper J, Oranje A, Prose N (eds.) Textbook of Pediatric Dermatology, 2nd ed. Oxford: Blackwell Science, pp. 1491–1502.

Papadavid E, Markey A, Bellaney G, Walker NP (2002) Carbon dioxide and pulsed dye laser treatment of angiofibromas in 29 patients with tuberous sclerosis. Br J Dermatol 147: 337–342.

Paul E, Thiele E (2008) Efficacy of sirolimus in treating tuberous sclerosis and lymphangioleiomyomatosis. N Engl J Med 358: 190–192.

Pellizzi GB (1901) Contributo allo studio dell'idiozia: rivisita sperimentale di freniatria e medicina legale delle alienazioni mentali. Riv Sper Freniat **27**: 265–269.

Perusini G (1903) Uber einen Fall von Sclerosis Tuberosa hypertrophica. Monatsschr Psychiatr Neurol 17: 69–255.

Piedimonte LR, Wailes IK, Weiner HL (2006) Tuberous sclerosis complex: molecular pathogenesis and animal models. Neurosurg Focus 20: E4.

Pipitone S, Mongiovi M, Grillo R, Gagliano S, Sperandeo V (2002) Cardiac rhabdomyoma in intrauterine life: clinical features and natural history. A case series and review of published reports. Ital Heart J 3: 48–52.

Plank TL, Yeung RS, Henske EP (1998) Hamartin, the product of the tuberous sclerosis 1 (TSC1) gene, interacts with tuberin and appears to be localized to cytoplasmic vesicles. Cancer Res 58: 4766–4770.

Poirier J, Signoret JL (1991) De Bourneville a la Sclérose Tubéreuse. Un homme – Une époque – Une maladie. Paris: Médecine-Sciences Flammarion.

Polosa R (1996) Pulmonary lymphangioleiomyomatosis and tuberous sclerosis. Respir Med 90: 121–122.

Popper HH, Juettner-Smolle FM, Pongratz MG (1991) Micronodular hyperplasia of type II pneumocytes – a new lung lesion associated with tuberous sclerosis. Histopathology 18: 347–354.

Potter CJ, Huang H, Xu T (2001) Drosophila Tsc1 functions with Tsc2 to antagonize insulin signaling in regulating cell growth, cell proliferation, and organ size. Cell 105: 357–368.

Povey S, Burley MW, Attwood J, Benham F, Hunt D, Jeremiah SJ, Franklin D, Gillett G, Malas S, Robson EB, Tippett P, Edwards Jh, Kwiatkowski DJ, Super M,

Mueller R, Fryer A, Clarke A, Webb D, Osborne J (1994) Two loci for tuberous sclerosis: one on 9q34 and one on 16p13. Ann Hum Genet 58: 107–127.

Pringle JJ (1890) A case of congenital adenoma sebaceum. Br J Dermatol 2: 1–14.

Pulsifer MB, Winterkorn EB, Thiele EA (2007) Psychological profile of adults with tuberous sclerosis complex. Epilepsy Behav 10: 402–406.

Raju GP, Urion DK, Sahin M (2007) Neonatal subependymal giant cell astrocytoma: new case and review of literature. Pediatr Neurol 36: 128–131.

Ramenghi LA, Verrotti A, Domizio S, Di Rocco C, Morgese G, Sabatino G (1996) Neonatal diagnosis of tuberous sclerosis. Childs Nerv Syst 12: 121–123.

Rayer PFO (1835) Traité théorique et pratique des maladies de la peau. 2nd ed. Paris: JB Bailiére.

Raznahan A, Higgins NP, Griffiths PD, Humphrey A, Yates JR, Bolton PF (2007) Biological markers of intellectual disability in tuberous sclerosis. Psychol Med 37: 1293–1304.

Rennebeck G, Kleymenova EV, Anderson R, Yeung RS, Artzt K, Walker CL (1998) Loss of function of the tuberous sclerosis 2 tumor suppressor gene results in embryonic lethality characterized by disrupted neuroepithelial growth and development. Proc Natl Acad Sci USA 95: 15629–15634.

Reyre G (1989) Bourneville: "an attempt at control of madness in the schools". Soins Psychiatr (104–105): 55–59.

Riikonen R, Simell O (1990) Tuberous sclerosis and infantile spasms. Dev Med Child Neurol 32: 203–209.

Roach ES, DiMario FJ, Kandt RS, Northrup H (1999) Tuberous Sclerosis Consensus Conference: recommendations for diagnostic evaluation. J Child Neurol 14: 401–407.

Roach ES, Gomez MR, Northrup H (1998) Tuberous sclerosis complex consensus conference: revised clinical diagnostic criteria. J Child Neurol 13: 624–628.

Roach ES, Smith M, Huttenlocher P, Bhat M, Alcorn D, Hawley L (1992) Diagnostic criteria: tuberous sclerosis complex. J Child Neurol 7: 221–224.

Roberts PS, Dabora S, Thiele EA, Franz DN, Jozwiak S, Kwiatkowski DJ (2004) Somatic mosaicism is rare in unaffected parents of patients with sporadic tuberous sclerosis. J Med Genet 41: e69.

Robertson DM (1999) Ophthalmic findings. In: Gomez MR, Sampson JR, Whittemore VH (eds.) Tuberous Sclerosis Complex. New York: Oxford University Press, pp. 145–159.

Rogers RS (1988) Dermatologic manifestations. In: Gomez MR (ed.) Tuberous Sclerosis. New York: Raven Press, pp. 111–131.

Rose VM, Au KS, Pollom G, Roach ES, Prashner HR, Northrup H (1999) Germ-line mosaicism in tuber-

ous sclerosis: how common? Am J Hum Genet 64: 986–992.

Ruggieri M, Carbonara C, Magro G, Migone N, Grasso S, Tine A, Pavone L, Gomez MR (1997) Tuberous sclerosis complex: neonatal deaths in three of four children of consan guineous, non-expressing parents. J Med Genet 34: 256–260.

Sampson JR, Scahill SJ, Stephenson JB, Mann L, Connor JM (1989) Genetic aspects of tuberous sclerosis in the west of Scotland. J Med Genet 26: 2831.

Sampson JR, Janssen LA, Sandkuijl LA (1992) Linkage investigation of three putative tuberous sclerosis determining loci on chromosomes 9q, 11q, and 12q. The tuberous sclerosis collaborative group. J Med Genet 29: 861–866.

Sampson JR, Maheshwar MM, Aspinwall R, Thompson P, Cheadle JP, Ravine D, Roy S, Haan E, Bernstein J, Harris PC (1997) Renal cystic disease in tuberous sclerosis: role of the polycystic kidney disease 1 gene. Am J Hum Genet 61: 843–851.

Sancak O, Nellist M, Goedbloed M, Elfferich P, Wouters C, Maat-Kievit A, Zonnenberg B, Verhoef S, Halley D, van den Ouweland A (2005) Mutational analysis of the TSC1 and TSC2 genes in a diagnostic setting: genotype phenotype correlations and comparison of diagnostic DNA techniques in tuberous sclerosis complex. Eur J Hum Genet 13: 731–741.

Scheidenhelm DK, Gutmann DH (2004) Mouse models of tuberous sclerosis complex. J Child Neurol 19: 726–733.

Schwartz RA, Janniger CK (1997) Vitiligo. Cutis 60: 239–244.

Schwartz RA, Fernandez G, Kotulska K, Jozwiak S (2007) Tuberous sclerosis complex: advances in diagnosis, genetics, and management. J Am Acad Dermatol 57: 189–202.

Schuster P (1914) Beiträge zur Klinik der tuberösen Sklerose des Gehirns. Dtsch Z Nervenheilk 50: 96–133.

Sepp T, Yates JR, Green AJ (1996) Loss of heterozygosity in tuberous sclerosis hamartomas. J Med Genet 33: 962–964.

Sheffield EG, Sparagana SP, Batchelor LL et al (1998) The incidence and natural history of hepatic angiomyolipomas in tuberous sclerosis complex in the pediatric population. Abstracts of World Congress on Tuberous Sclerosis, Goeteborg, S12 p.

Shepherd CW, Gomez MR, Lie JT, Crowson CS (1991) Causes of death in patients with tuberous sclerosis. Mayo Clin Proc 66: 792–796.

Sherlock EB (1911) The Feeble-minded, A Guide to Study and Practice. Macmillan & Co.

Shields JA, Eagle RC, Shields C, Marr BP (2005) Aggressive retinal astrocytomas in 4 patients with tuberous sclerosis complex. Arch Ophthalmol 123(6): 856–863.

Shiroyanagi Y, Kondo T, Tomita E, Onitsuka S, Ryoji O, Ito F, Nakazawa H, Toma H (2002) Nephron-sparing tumorectomy for a large benign renal mass: a case of massive bilateral renal angiomyolipomas associated with tuberous sclerosis. Int J Urol 9: 117–119.

Simmons JL, Hussain SA, Riley P, Wallace DM (2003) Management of renal angiomyolipoma in patients with tuberous sclerosis complex. Oncol Rep 10: 237–241.

Smalley SL, Tanguay PE, Smith M, Gutierrez G (1992) Autism and tuberous sclerosis. J Autism Dev Disord 22: 339–355.

Smolarek TA, Wessner LL, McCormack FX, Mylet JC, Menon AG, Henske EP (1998) Evidence that lymphangiomyomatosis is caused by TSC2 mutations: chromosome 16p13 loss of heterozygosity in angiomyolipomas and lymph nodes from women with lymphangiomyomatosis. Am J Hum Genet 62: 810–815.

Smulders YM, Eussen BH, Verhoef S, Wouters CH (2003) Large deletion causing the TSC2-PKD1 contiguous gene syndrome without infantile polycystic disease. J Med Genet 40: E17.

Sparling JD, Hong CH, Brahim JS, Moss J, Darling TN (2007) Oral findings in 58 adults with tuberous sclerosis complex. J Am Acad Dermatol 56: 786–790.

Stafstrom CE, Holmes GL (2007) Can preventative antiepileptic therapy alter outcome in infants with tuberous sclerosis complex? Epilepsia 48: 1632–1634.

Stapleton FB, Johnson D, Kaplan GW, Griswold W (1980) The cystic renal lesion in tuberous sclerosis. J Pediatr 97: 574–579.

Strizheva GD, Carsillo T, Kruger WD, Sullivan EJ, Ryu JH, Henske EP (2001) The spectrum of mutations in TSC1 and TSC2 in women with tuberous sclerosis and lymphangiomyomatosis. Am J Respir Crit Care Med 163: 253–258.

Takahashi DK, Dinday MT, Barbaro NM, Baraban SC (2004) Abnormal cortical cells and astrocytomas in the Eker rat model of tuberous sclerosis complex. Epilepsia 45: 1525–1530.

Tapon N, Ito N, Dickson BJ, Treisman JE, Hariharan IK (2001) The Drosophila tuberous sclerosis complex gene homologs restrict cell growth and cell proliferation. Cell 105: 345–355.

Tavazoie SF, Alvarez VA, Ridenour DA, Kwiatkowski DJ, Sabatini BL (2005) Regulation of neuronal morphology and function by the tumor suppressors Tsc1 and Tsc2. Nat Neurosci 8: 1727–1734.

Thiele EA (2004) Managing epilepsy in tuberous sclerosis complex. J Child Neurol 19:680–686.

Tortori-Donati P, Rossi A, Biancheri R, Andreula CF (2005) Phakomatoses. In Tortori-Donati P (ed). Pediatric Neuroradiology. Brain. Berlin-New York: Springer-Verlag, pp. 763–818.

Torres OA, Roach ES, Delgado MR, Sparagana SP, Sheffield E, Swift D, Bruce D (1998) Early diagnosis of subependymal giant cell astrocytoma in patients with tuberous sclerosis. J Child Neurol 13: 173–177.

Tsui WM, Colombari R, Portmann BC, Bonetti F, Thung SN, Ferrell LD, Nakanuma Y, Snover DC, Bioulac-Sage P, Dhillon AP (1999) Hepatic angiomyolipoma: a clinico-pathologic study of 30 cases and delineation of unusual morphologic variants. Am J Surg Pathol 23: 34–48.

Uhlmann EJ, Apicelli AJ, Baldwin RL, Burke SP, Bajenaru ML, Onda H, Kwiatkowski D, Gutmann DH (2002) Heterozygosity for the tuberous sclerosis complex (TSC) gene products results in increased astrocyte numbers and decreased p27-Kip1 expression in TSC2± cells. Oncogene 21: 4050.

Vakilzadeh F, Happle R (1980) Schmelzdefekte bei tuberöser sklerose. Hautarzt 31: 336–337.

Van der Hoeve J (1920) Eye symptoms in tuberous sclerosis of the brain. Trans Ophthalmol Soc UK 40: 329–334.

Von Recklinghausen F (1862) Ein Herz von einem Neugeborenen welches mehrere. Theils nach aussen, Theils nach den hohlen prommirende Tumoren (Myomen) trug. Verh Ges Geburtsh 25 Marz. Monasschr Geburtskd 20: 1–2.

van Slegtenhorst M, de Hoogt R, Hermans C, Nellist M, Janssen B, Verhoef S, Lindhout D, van den Ouweland A, Halley D, Young J, Burley M, Jeremiah S, Woodward K, Nahmias J, Fox M, Ekong R, Osborne J, Wolfe J, Povey S, Snell RG, Cheadle JP, Jones AC, Tachataki M, Ravine D, Kwiatkowski DJ et al (1997) Identification of the tuberous sclerosis gene TSC1 on chromosome 9q34. Science 277: 805–808.

van Slegtenhorst M, Nellist M, Nagelkerken B, Cheadle J, Snell R, van den Ouweland A, Reuser A, Sampson J, Halley D, van der Sluijs P (1998) Interaction between hamartin and tuberin, the TSC1 and TSC2 gene products. Hum Mol Genet 7: 1053–1057.

van Slegtenhorst M, Verhoef S, Tempelaars A, Bakker L, Wang Q, Wessels M, Bakker R, Nellist M, Lindhout D, Halley D, van den Ouweland A (1999) Mutational spectrum of the TSC1 gene in a cohort of 225 tuberous sclerosis complex patients: no evidence for genotype-phenotype correlation. J Med Genet 36: 285–289.

Verhoef S, Bakker L, Tempelaars AM, Hesseling-Janssen AL, Mazurczak T, Jozwiak S, Fois A, Bartalini G, Zonnenberg BA, van Essen AJ, Lindhout D, Halley DJ, van den Ouweland AM (1999) High rate of mosaicism in tuberous sclerosis complex. Am J Hum Genet 64: 1632–1637.

Verhoef S, Vrtel R, van Essen T, Bakker L, Sikkens E, Halley D, Lindhout D, van den Ouweland A (1995) Somatic mosaicism and clinical variation in tuberous sclerosis complex. Lancet 345: 20.

Vogt H (1908) Zur Diagnostik der tuberosen sklerose. Z Erforsch Behandl Jugeudl Schwachsinns 2: 116.

von der Brelie C, Waltereit R, Zhang L, Beck H, Kirschstein T (2006) Impaired synaptic plasticity in a rat model of tuberous sclerosis. Eur J Neurosci 23: 686–692.

Von Recklinghausen F (1862) Ein Herz von einem Neugeborenen welches mehrere theils nach aussen, Theils nach den Höhlen prominirende Tumoren (Myomen) trug. Verh Ges Geburtsh Monatschr Geburtsk 20: 12.

Waltereit R, Welzl H, Dichgans J, Lipp HP, Schmidt WJ, Weller M (2006) Enhanced episodic-like memory and kindling epilepsy in a rat model of tuberous sclerosis. J Neurochem 96: 407–413.

Walz NC, Byars AW, Egelhoff JC, Franz DN (2002) Supratentorial tuber location and autism in tuberous sclerosis complex. J Child Neurol 17: 830–832.

Ward PE, McCarthy DJ (1990) Periungual fibroma. Cutis 46: 118–124.

Webb DW, Clarke A, Fryer A, Osborne JP (1996) The cutaneous features of tuberous sclerosis: a population study. Br J Dermatology 135: 15.

Webb DW, Osborne JP (1991) Non-penetrance in tuberous sclerosis. J Med Genet 28: 417–419.

Wenzel HJ, Patel LS, Robbins CA, Emmi A, Yeung RS, Schwartzkroin PA (2004) Morphology of cerebral lesions in the Eker rat model of tuberous sclerosis. Acta Neuropathol (Berl) 108: 97–108.

Who named it? (2007) A comprehensive dictionary of medical eponyms. http://www.whonamedit.com

Wienecke R, Konig A, DeClue JE (1995) Identification of tuberin, the tuberous sclerosis-2 product. Tuberin possesses specific Rap1GAP activity. J Biol Chem 270: 16409–16414.

Weiner HL, Ferraris N, LaJoie J, Miles D, Devinsky O (2004) Epilepsy surgery for children with tuberous sclerosis complex. J Child Neurol 19: 687–689.

Weiner HL, Carlson C, Ridgway EB, Zaroff CM, Miles D, LaJoie J, Devinsky O (2006) Epilepsy surgery in young children with tuberous sclerosis: results of a novel approach. Pediatrics 117: 1494–1502.

Wikipedia (2007) Timeline for Tuberous Sclerosis. http://en.wikipedia.org/wiki/Timeline_of_tuberous_sclerosis

Williams JM, Racadio JM, Johnson ND, Donnelly LF, Bissler JJ (2006) Embolization of renal angiomyolipomata in patients with tuberous sclerosis complex. Am J Kidney Dis 47: 95–102.

Wilson C, Idziaszczyk S, Parry L, Guy C, Griffiths DF, Lazda E, Bayne RA, Smith AJ, Sampson JR, Cheadle JP (2005) A mouse model of tuberous sclerosis 1 showing background specific early post-natal mortality and

metastatic renal cell carcinoma. Hum Mol Genet 14: 1839–1850.

Winterkorn EB, Pulsifer MB, Thiele EA (2007) Cognitive prognosis of patients with tuberous sclerosis complex. Neurology 68: 62–64.

Wiznitzer M (2004) Autism and tuberous sclerosis. J Child Neurol 19: 675–679.

Wolf DC, Goldsworthy TL, Donner EM, Harden R, Fitzpatrick B, Everitt JI (1998) Estrogen treatment enhances hereditary renal tumor development in Eker rats. Carcinogenesis 19: 2043–2047.

Wong V (2006) Study of the relationship between tuberous sclerosis complex and autistic disorder. J Child Neurol 21: 199–204.

Wong V, Khong PL (2006) Tuberous sclerosis complex: correlation of magnetic resonance imaging (MRI) findings with comorbidities. J Child Neurol 21: 99–105.

Wu JY, Sutherling WW, Koh S, Salamon N, Jonas R, Yudovin S, Sankar R, Shields WD, Mathern GW (2006) Magnetic source imaging localizes epileptogenic zone in children with tuberous sclerosis complex. Neurology 66: 1270–1272.

Xiao GH, Shoarinejad F, Jin F, Golemis EA, Yeung RS (1997) The tuberous sclerosis 2 gene product, tuberin, functions as a Rab5 GTPase activating protein (GAP) in modulating endocytosis. J Biol Chem 272: 6097–6100.

Xu L, Sterner C, Maheshwar MM, Wilson PJ, Nellist M, Short PM, Haines JL, Sampson JR, Ramesh V (1995) Alternative splicing of the tuberous sclerosis 2 (TSC2) gene in human and mouse tissues. Genomics 27: 475–480.

Yamamoto Y, Jones KA, Mak BC, Muehlenbachs A, Yeung RS (2002) Multicompartimental distribution of the tuberous sclerosis gene products, hamartin and tuberin. Arch Biochem Biophys 404: 210–207.

Yates JR, van Bakel I, Sepp T, Payne SJ, Webb DW, Nevin NC, Green AJ (1997) Female germline mosaicism in tuberous sclerosis confirmed by molecular genetic analysis. Hum Mol Genet 6: 2265–2269.

Yeung RS, Xiao GH, Jin F, Lee WC, Testa JR, Knudson AG (1994) Predisposition to renal carcinoma in the Eker rat is determined by germ-line mutation of the tuberous sclerosis 2 (TSC2) gene. Proc Natl Acad Sci U S A 91: 11413–11416.

Yeung RS (2003) Multiple roles of the tuberous sclerosis complex genes. Gene Chromosome Canc 38: 368–375.

Yeung RS (2004) Lessons from the Eker rat model: from cage to bedside. Curr Mol Med 4: 799–806.

Zeng LH, Xu L, Gutmann DH, Wong M (2008) Rapamycin prevents epilepsy in a mouse model of tuberous sclerosis complex. Ann Neurol 63: 444–453.

# Chapter 6

# VON HIPPEL-LINDAU DISEASE

S. Taylor Jarrell, Edward H. Oldfield, and Russell R. Lonser

Surgical Neurology Branch, National Institute of Neurological Disorders and Stroke, National Institutes of Health, Bethesda, USA

## Introduction

von Hippel-Lindau disease (VHL) is an autosomal dominant familial neoplasia syndrome that results from a germline mutation of the *VHL* gene on the short arm of chromosome 3. It is characterized by the development of central nervous system (CNS) and visceral lesions. CNS lesions include retinal, cerebellar, brainstem and spinal hemangioblastomas, and endolymphatic sac tumors (ELSTs). Visceral lesions include renal cell carcinomas (RCC), renal cysts, pheochromocytomas, pancreatic cysts and neuroendocrine tumors, as well as cystadenomas of the epididymis and broad ligament (Fig. 1).

Certainly, from a clinical point of view VHL is a somewhat different condition from classical neurocutaneous diseases (e.g., there are no known associated cutaneous abnormalities; see below). However, from a pathogenic point of view it overlaps with many other well-known neurocutaneous disorders. In addition, it features (and is often first diagnosed because of) typical ocular "phakomas" and systemic "hamartomas" and tumours. Thus, for these and other reasons (e.g., historical) we have maintained its handling in this book.

## Historical perspective and terminology

Although the contribution of von Hippel and Lindau were decisive, many others played an important part in the description of clinical manifestations of VHL (Richard et al. 2004). In 1872, Jackson first described a cerebellar haemangioblastoma whilst retinal haemangioblastoma was described by Panas and Rémy in 1879 (Richard et al. 2004). The first recorded case of a probable patient with VHL was a 35-year-old woman who died in 1864 with eye and brain tumors (Galezowski 1987). In 1885, Pye-Smith showed that a cerebellar cystic tumor was associated with several renal and pancreatic cysts (Richard et al. 2004). The first histological description of VHL is credited to Edward Treacher Collins (1862–1932), an eminent British ophthalmologist at the Royal London Eye Hospital, Moordfields, who described bilateral retinal haemangioblastomas of enucleated eyes from two affected siblings in 1894 (Collins 1894). He judged the retinal lesions to be true vascular neoformations, which he named capillary nevus (Beighton and Beighton 1986, Richard et al. 2004).

**Eugen Von Hippel** (1867–1939) was born in Konigsberg (non Kaliningrad), Germany, son of Arthur von Hippel (1841–1916) professor of ophthalmology in that town and a pioneer in the field of corneal grafting (Beighton and Beighton 1986). Eugen received his MD in Gottingen in 1890 and two years later endeavored his specialization in ophthalmology with Theodore von Leber becoming professor of ophthalmology at Halle, Germany, at the turn of the century. He gained international recognition for his work on the pathological anatomy and congenital malformations of the eye. In 1895, he first described the fundoscopy findings in the eye of a 23-year-old man, Otto Mayer, who had presented two years earlier with visual loss (Von Hippel 1896). In 1904, presented further details on the same patient, who had developed three additional retinal lesions, as well as another similar case of a 28-year-old patient (Von Hippel 1904), and after careful analysis of the histological characteristics of the right eye of patient Mayer concluded, in 1911, that the retinal lesion was a congenital cystic capillary angiomatosis which he termed *angiomatosis retinae* (Richard et al. 2004, Von Hippel 1911).

In 1921, Brandt published autopsy results of the 47-year-old Mayer died after having had various neurological disturbances: he was found to also have tumors of the cerebellum and conus medullaris, and

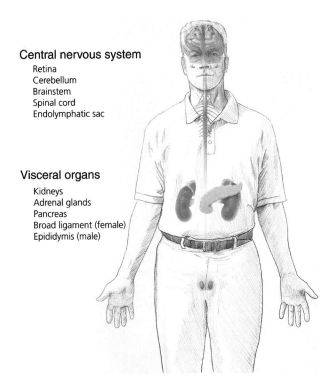

**Central nervous system**
Retina
Cerebellum
Brainstem
Spinal cord
Endolymphatic sac

**Visceral organs**
Kidneys
Adrenal glands
Pancreas
Broad ligament (female)
Epididymis (male)

Fig. 1. Affected organs. Central nervous system lesions include hemangioblastomas, retinal angiomas, and endolymphatic sac tumors. Visceral lesions include renal cell carcinoma, pheochromocytoma, pancreatic cysts and neuroendocrine tumors, and cystadenomas of the epididymis and broad ligament (from Lonser et al. 2003a).

cystic lesions of the kidneys, pancreas, and epididymis (Brandt 1921).

However, it was **Arvid Lindau** (1892–1958), in 1926, that made the critical link between retinal haemangioblastomas, cerebellar haemangioblastomas, and visceral tumors in the syndrome he called *"Angiomatosis des Zentralnervenssystems"* (Richard et al. 2004). Lindau was the son of a military surgeon who completed his medical training in Lund prior to specialize in pathology and bacteriology at the Karolinska Institute in Stockholm and at the University of Lund (Richard et al. 2004). He continued his education in various centers in Europe and United States being as fellow under von Hippel (in 1925), Ludwig Ashoff, Cushing and Percival holding a concurrent appointment as a military doctor in years 1924–1933 and then as a professor of pathology in Lund (Beighton and Beighton 1986, Richard et al. 2004). It was his power of observation and intuition that helped draw

the different features of VHL into a single recognizable entity. In a 1928 monograph, Cushing and Bailey provided detailed descriptions of 11 patients with what they described as "Lindau's disease". These descriptions included detailed clinical, surgical and histopathological findings (Cushing 1928). Later, in 1936, Davison honored both von Hippel and Lindau by giving VHL the name it bears today (Davison 1936). In 1964, Melmon and Rosen published the first major review with diagnostic criteria for VHL (Melmon and Rosen 1964). The *VHL* gene was fully identified and cloned in 1993 (Latif et al. 1993).

## Incidence and prevalence

VHL has an incidence of 1 in 36,000 people (Maher et al. 1991). Penetrance is nearly complete by the age of 60 years (Maher et al. 1990). Maher et al. estimated that 84%, 70%, and 69% of VHL patients will develop cerebellar hemangioblastoma, retinal hemangioblastoma, or renal cell carcinoma, respectively, by age 60 (Maher et al. 1990). Because it is an autosomal dominant transmitted syndrome, males and females are affected equally.

## Childhood presentations of VHL

There are no distinct pediatric presentations of VHL. Many pediatric cases are discovered during genetic testing of family members of VHL patients, and are treated similarly to adult cases.

## Clinical manifestations

### Skin abnormalities

There are no known associated cutaneous lesions.

### Nervous system abnormalities

### CNS Hemangioblastomas

**General Features.** CNS hemangioblastomas in VHL are often multiple, and most often arise in the cerebellum (75%), followed by the spinal cord (15%), brainstem (10%), and lumbosacral nerve roots (Neumann et al. 1989, Richard et al. 1998). Supratentorial brain lesions are infrequent (less than 1%). Spinal cord hemangioblastomas may be intramedullary, extramedullary, or both. They tend to be more frequent in rostral portions of the spinal cord, with 43%, 47% and 11% occurring at cervical, thoracic, and lumbar levels, respectively (Lonser et al. 2003b, Wanebo et al. 2003). Ninety-three percent of spinal cord hemangioblastomas are located posterior to the dentate ligament (most frequently in the dorsal root entry zone) (Lonser et al. 2003b, Wanebo et al. 2003). Brainstem hemangioblastomas are most frequently found at the obex. Though histologically benign, hemangioblastomas are a significant source of morbidity and mortality in VHL due to their size, occurrence in eloquent locations, associated edema/cysts, and multiplicity.

**Clinical Findings**. Presenting symptoms of hemangioblastoma depend on the site of the tumor. Cerebellar lesions may present with headache, nausea, ataxia, or dizziness. Brainstem hemangioblastomas may present with dysarthria, dysphagia, hiccups, chronic cough, ophthalmoplegia or long tract signs. Spinal cord hemangioblastomas can present with pain, motor or sensory deficit, spasticity, gait instability, and/or bowel or bladder incontinence.

**Diagnosis**. The optimal imaging modality for hemangioblastomas is post-contrast T1-weighted magnetic resonance (MR)-imaging (Fig. 2). Tumors are iso- to hypointense on uncontrasted T1-weighted MR-imaging, but enhance brightly with contrast. Hemangioblastomas are frequently associated with edema and/or cysts (Fig. 2). Edema is easily visualized as a hyperintense region on T2-weighted or FLAIR MR-imaging, and cysts are isointense to cerebrospinal fluid on MR-imaging.

Hemangioblastomas typically go through phases of rapid growth followed by prolonged quiescent phases (Wanebo et al. 2003). Most instances of symptom development or progression result from development or enlargement of tumor-associated edema and cysts rather than from enlargement of the tumor itself (Slater et al. 2003, Wanebo et al. 2003).

**Pathology**. Grossly, hemangioblastomas are highly vascular, bright-red and thinly encapsulated tumors. Microscopically, they are composed of endothelium-lined vascular channels forming a rich vascular plexus with intervening polyhedral stromal cells and pericytes (Fig. 2) (Grossniklaus et al. 1992). The neoplastic cell is the stromal cell (Berkman et al. 1993, Vortmeyer et al. 1997). Stromal cells closely resemble those of clear cell renal carcinoma, and have a characteristic vacuolated or foamy-appearing cytoplasm (Sano and Horiguchi 2003).

**Treatment**. The definitive treatment for symptomatic hemangioblastomas is surgical excision (Bostrom et al. 2008). Asymptomatic tumors may be followed clinically and radiographically. Brainstem, cerebellar, spinal cord, and nerve root tumors may be safely removed microsurgically (Jagannathan et al. 2008, Lonser et al. 2003b, Murota and Symon 1989, Van Velthoven et al. 2003, Wang et al. 2001, Weil et al. 2003). Preoperative arteriography and embolization is generally not considered necessary (Lonser et al. 2003a). A tumor-associated edema and cysts require no specific treatment, and resolve after the associated tumor is removed (Lonser et al. 2003b, Weil et al. 2003).

Stereotactic radiosurgery has been used to treat cerebellar hemangioblastomas (Chandler and Friedman 1994, Chang et al. 1998, Niemela et al. 1996, Patrice et al. 1996). Radiosurgery may be useful to treat these vascular tumors, and can potentially reduce the morbidity associated with multiple surgeries. However, the long-term effectiveness of this therapy needs to be determined and it is unclear at this time if the absence of growth seen in some treated tumors is not merely reflective of the quiescent phase that naturally occurs.

## Retinal hemangioblastomas

**General Features**. Retinal hemangioblastomas are a common cause of morbidity in VHL, and one of the earliest manifestations (Wong and Chew 2008). Mean age at diagnosis in one study was 21 years, with 68% of patients presenting with multiple lesions (Kreusel et al. 2000). The cumulative probability of developing a retinal hemangioblastoma during the life of a VHL patient may be as high as 80% (Maher et al. 1990). Lesions are nonrandomly distributed in the retina. Most occur peripherally, with

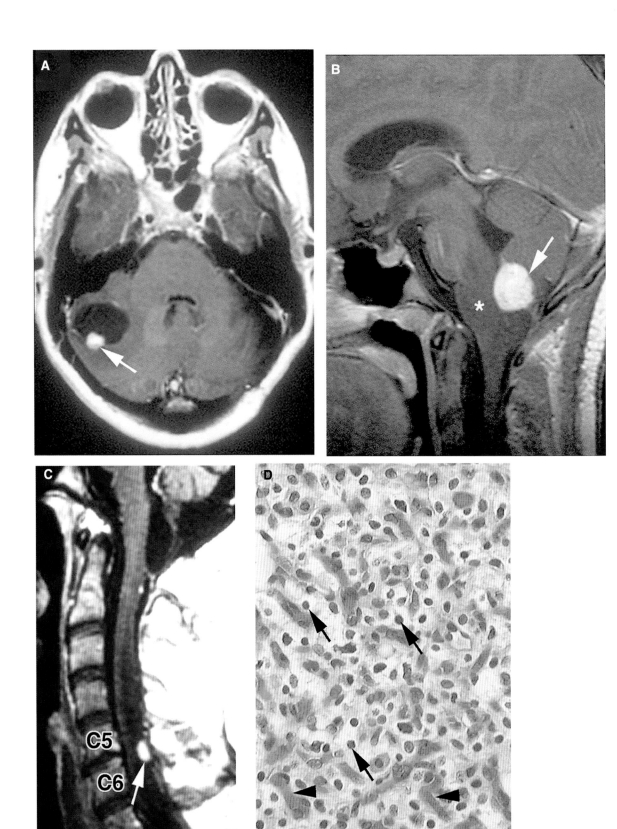

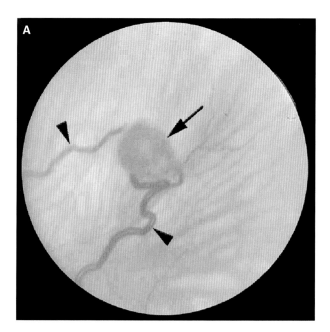

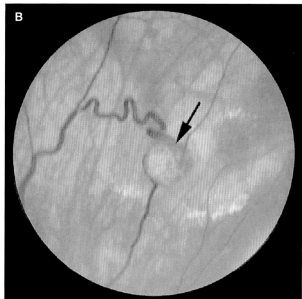

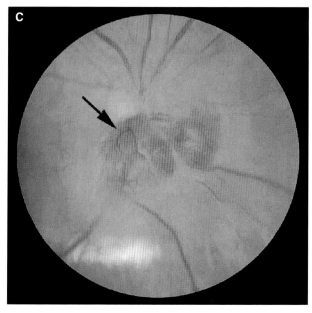

**Fig. 3.** Ophthalmoscopic view of retinal hemangioblastomas. (**A**) Peripheral retinal hemangioblastoma (arrow) with an enlarged vessel (arrowheads) in a 22-year-old woman. (**B**) Peripheral retinal hemangioblastoma (arrow) with fibrous changes, hard exudates, and retinal edema in the surrounding region in a 24-year-old man. (**C**) Retinal hemangioblastoma (arrow) on the optic nerve head with yellow retinal hard exudates below it in a 32-year-old man (from Lonser et al. 2003a).

←————————————————————————————————————————

**Fig. 2.** Magnetic resonance imaging and histological features of central nervous system hemangioblastomas. (**A**) Axial T1-weighted contrast-enhanced magnetic resonance imaging of a cerebellar hemangioblastoma (arrow) with an associated cyst (homogeneous associated dark region) in a 40-year-old woman. (**B**) Mid-sagittal T1-weighted postcontrast magnetic resonance imaging of a medullary hemangioblastoma (arrow) with associated brainstem edema (star) in a 12-year-old girl. (**C**) Mid-sagittal postcontrast T1-weighted magnetic resonance imaging of the spinal cord of a 50-year-old man. The hemangioblastoma is located in the posterior portion of the spinal cord at C5 and C6 (arrow), and is associated with a large syrinx (dark intraspinal region extending rostral and caudal to the lesion). (**D**) Hematoxylin and eosin staining of a hemangioblastoma showing the lipid-laden stromal cells (arrows) distributed within a capillary network (arrowheads) (from Lonser et al. 2003a).

only 1% occurring at the posterior pole, while the optic disc is involved in 8% of affected eyes (30 times the predicted incidence based on surface area) (Webster et al. 1999).

**Clinical Findings**. Retinal hemangioblastomas that are not discovered incidentally during serial screening may present with decreased visual acuity or a visual field defect due to macular edema, retinal or vitreous exudates and hemorrhage, and/or retinal detachment.

**Diagnosis**. Diagnosis is made by dilated fundoscopy, slit-lamp examination, or with Goldman three-mirror lens (in cases of extreme peripheral lesions) (Fig. 3). Flourescein angiography may be a useful adjunct in the diagnosis of early lesions, and to evaluate the vascular pattern before treatment (Wittebol-Post et al. 1998). Lesions vary in size from microscopic up to three disc diameters in width (Webster et al. 1999).

Early retinal hemangioblastomas may appear as a small discoloration on the retina, and may take decades to progress to a raised, red nodule. Feeding vessels become prominent, and exudates and vitreous hemorrhage may occur with tumor progression. Eventually, tumor-associated retinal hemorrhages and exudate may lead to retinal detachment and visual loss.

**Pathology**. Retinal angiomas are grossly and histologically identical to hemangioblastomas of the cerebellum, brainstem and spinal cord (Grossniklaus et al. 1992). The neoplastic cell is the stromal cell.

**Treatment**. Retinal angiomas are treated to prevent visual loss. Laser photo-coagulation is typically the first-line therapy. Cryoablation is reserved for eyes in which media opacities, extreme peripheral lesions, and retinal detachment prohibit laser photocoagulation (Palmer and Gragoudas 1997). Multiple treatments are often necessary to arrest tumor growth. Side effects of therapy may include hemorrhage, retinal detachment, increased fluid exudate into the retina, retinal holes, visual field loss, and distortion of the retinal surface. Retinal detachment, either as a consequence of the angioma or treatment, can progress to development of painful glaucoma that may necessitate enucleation. Optic disc, macular, and para-macular angiomas are usually not treated, as therapy to those regions may be more

damaging than the natural history of the disease (Webster et al. 1999, Wittebol-Post et al. 1998).

## Endolymphatic sac tumours (ELSTs)

**General Features**. Although rare in the general population, unilateral or bilateral ELSTs occur frequently in VHL. ELSTs are locally invasive, slow-growing tumors of the *pars rugosa* of the endolymphatic duct or sac (Heffner 1989). MR- or CT-imaging evidence of ELST may be found in 11–16% of VHL patients, with up to 30% of patients with ELST having bilateral tumors (Choo et al. 2004, Manski et al. 1997). The average age at diagnosis is 22 years (Manski et al. 1997).

**Clinical Findings**. The mean duration of symptoms is approximately 15 years (Manski et al. 1997). Clinical findings of ELST commonly include audiovestibular symptoms, such as high-frequency sensorineural hearing loss (95%), tinnitus (81%), vertigo (67%), disequilibrium (24%) or aural fullness 24% (Choo et al. 2004). Most patients (62%) with ELSTs suffer hearing loss as the first manifestation (Manski et al. 1997). The majority of ELST patients will have complete or measurable hearing loss on the affected side, and many will report complete or incremental loss of auditory function, suggesting that the natural history of ELST is progression to total deafness (Manski et al. 1997). Hearing loss is sudden in 43%, progressive and stepwise in 43%, or insidious in 14% (Choo et al. 2004). Audiovestibular symptoms in the absence of imaging evidence of tumor may occur in up to 65% of all VHL patients, suggesting the presence of microscopic (infraradiologic) ELST's in these patients. (Manski et al. 1997).

Hearing loss is believed to be a result of tumor invasion of middle ear structures, intralabyrinthine hemorrhage and/or inflammation, hydrops (due to tumor fluid production or obstruction of the flow/resorption of endolymph), or a combination of these factors (Lonser et al. 2004). The severity of hearing deficit has been associated with duration of symptoms, but not with tumor size, indicating that even smaller tumors can cause severe aural deficit (Kim et al. 2005, Lonser et al. 2004, Manski et al. 1997). Late findings of larger tumors are often related to contiguous structure invasion or mass effect and may

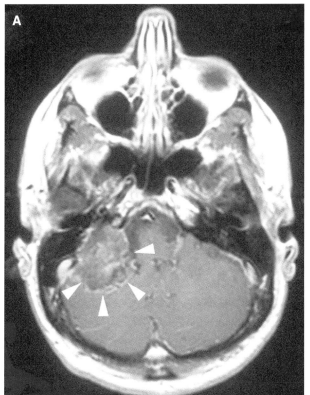

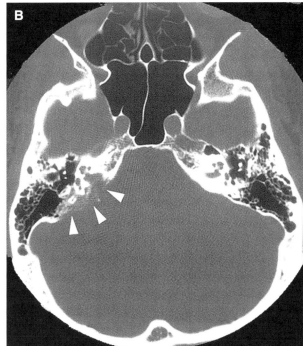

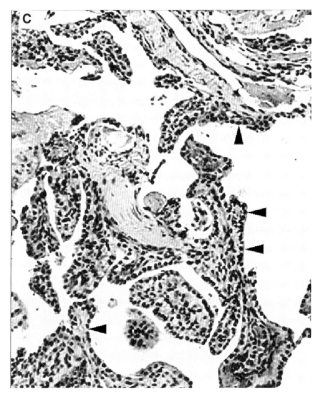

Fig. 4. Imaging and histological characteristics of endolymphatic sac tumor in a 33-year-old man with right-sided hearing loss. (A) Axial T1-weighted postcontrast magnetic resonance imaging shows a large heterogeneously enhancing tumor in the right mastoid region (indicated by arrows). (B) Axial computed tomographic scan through the same region showing the bony erosion of the posterior petrous region that often occurs in these tumors (indicated by arrowheads). (C) Hematoxylin and eosin-stained section showing the typical histological features of this neoplasm, including cuboidal epithelium (arrowheads) in a papillary pattern (from Lonser et al. 2003a).

include facial nerve paresis, facial hypoesthesia or brainstem compression with hemiparesis or lower cranial nerve findings.

**Diagnosis**. Radiographic studies for ELST evaluation include high-resolution CT- and MR-imaging through the temporal bones. CT-imaging may demonstrate a destructive or expanding posterior petrous bone lesion in the region of the endolymphatic duct and sac (Fig. 4). MR-imaging usually shows a ragged tumor with variable enhancement (Fig. 4). A focus of intralabyrinthine hyperintensity due to hemorrhage on T1-weighted MR-imaging may be the only imaging manifestation of an ELST.

Audiograms are essential to supplement the radiological data, and to document the presence or progression of hearing loss. Typical audiogram findings in ELSTs include high-frequeny sensorineural hearing loss in VHL patients. Angiography demonstrates the highly vascular nature of these tumors, and endovascular embolization of external carotid feeders is infrequently necessary (Ferreira et al. 2002, Richards and Clifton 2003).

**Pathology**. Pathologic examination of ELSTs reveals a firm, reddish mass composed of cuboidal tumor cells in a papillotubular pattern without mitotic figures, local bone erosion, an extensive inflammatory response, and frequently hemosiderin (Fig. 4) (Ferreira et al. 2002, Lonser et al. 2004, Richards and Clifton 2003).

**Treatment**. ELSTs are treated by complete surgical removal. The surgical approach is guided by the hearing status of the patient. Surgery is curative, and can be performed with preservation of hearing and relief of vestibular symptoms (Kim et al. 2005, Lonser et al. 2004). Because of the frequent association with permanent hearing loss and the increased morbidity associated with removal of larger lesions, surgery is performed as soon as ELST is diagnosed. In deaf patients, surgery may be delayed until other neurolog-ical impairments attributed to the tumor are present, or tumor compression of surrounding structures necessitates resection. It is still undetermined whether patients with demonstrable audiovestibular symptoms, but negative imaging studies, should undergo exploratory surgery for ELST to prevent hearing loss or vestibular symptoms. Recurrence or incomplete resection has been treated with stereotactic radiosurgery and conventional radiotherapy, but the efficacy is unproven (Ferreira et al. 2002, Hansen and Luxford 2004, Heffner 1989, Megerian et al. 1995).

## Visceral abnormalities

### Renal cell carcinoma (RCC)

**General Features**. RCCs and renal cysts occur in 24–45% of VHL patients (Roupret et al. 2003). Up to 95% of VHL patients over the age of 60 have a renal lesion (Roupret et al. 2003). It is estimated that there are 600 neoplastic lesions and 1100 cysts in the average 37-year-old VHL patient's kidney (Walther et al. 1995). Cysts may be simple and benign or have an associated solid region that is more likely to harbor neoplastic cells. RCC occurs at a younger age (mean 37.2 years) in VHL than in the sporadic population, and tends to be bilateral and multicentric (Roupret et al. 2003). VHL patients are also more likely to have recurrences of their RCC (51%) after surgical extirpation than sporadic cases (4–9%) (Morgan and Zincke 1990, Novick et al. 1989, Steinbach et al. 1992, Steinbach et al. 1995). However, the presence of metastases at recurrence is much lower in VHL-associated cases than in sporadic cases, perhaps reflecting a lower malignant potential of RCC in VHL (Novick et al. 1989, Steinbach et al. 1995).

Renal cysts are generally considered benign lesions in VHL patients, though neoplastic cells may

---

**Fig. 5.** Axial postcontrast computed tomography and histological characteristics of various visceral tumors. (**A**) Bilateral multifocal renal cell carcinoma with both solid (arrows) and cystic (arrowheads) disease in a 22-year-old man. (**B**) Bilateral pheochromocytomas (arrows) with rim enhancement in the adrenal glands of a 29-year-old woman. (**C**) Pancreatic neuroendocrine tumor (arrows) in the head of the pancreas of a 26-year-old woman. (**D**) Renal cell carcinoma of the clear-cell subtype (arrows) with acinar and tubular architecture embedded in fibrovascular stroma (arrowheads). (**E**) Pheochromocytomas are composed of chromaffin cells. The tumor cells are arranged in rounded clusters, separated by endothelial-lined spaces, and have vesicles containing norepinephrine and epinephrine. (**F**) Pancreatic neuroendocrine tumors show trabecular architecture, small nuclei, and abundant eosinophilic cytoplasm. Nests of tumor cells show focal nuclear atypia with surrounding stromal collagen bands (arrows) (from Lonser et al. 2003a).

be found in their lining. Cysts can be lined by a single layer of epithelium, or less commonly can be complex, with a solid component to the wall. A seri-al imaging study of VHL patients with renal involvement found 74% of all renal lesions to be cysts rather then solid lesions. The majority of cysts

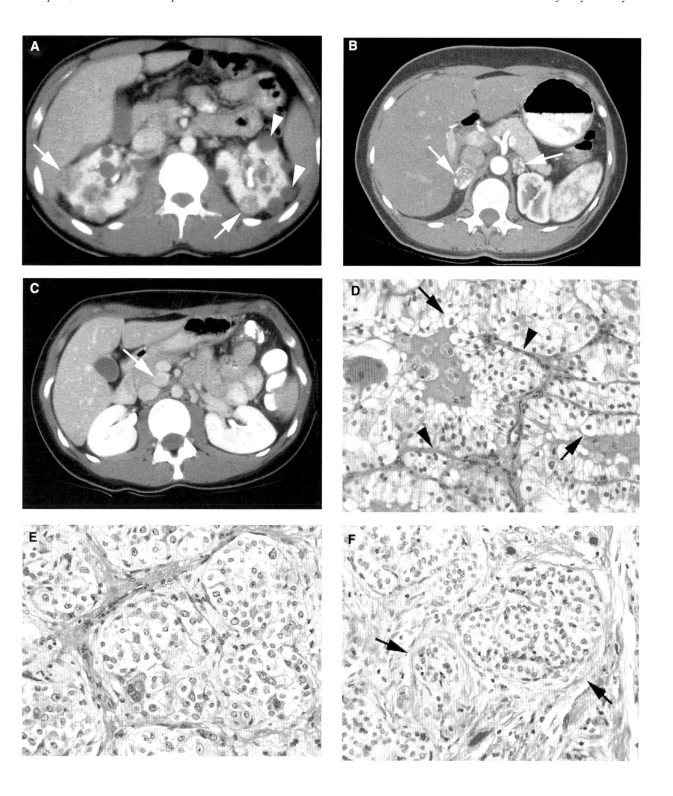

remained stable in size (Choyke et al. 1992). Because the appearance of cysts tends to precede that of solid lesions by 3–7 years (Choyke et al. 1992) and neoplastic cells can often be found in their walls, it has been suggested that renal cysts are a precursor lesion to RCC's (Solomon and Schwartz 1988, Tory et al. 1989); however, conversion from cystic to solid lesion occurred in only 1.1% of simple cysts (Choyke et al. 1992). The vast majority of renal tumors appear to arise as solid tumors, rather than as a transformed cyst (Choyke et al. 1992). More complex solid/cystic structures behave more unpredictably, with 17% of these lesions showing an increase in the solid component on serial imaging (Choyke et al. 1992).

**Clinical Findings**. Rarely, very large RCCs present with hematuria, flank pain or mass, or metastasis. Classically (two-thirds of VHL-related cases), RCCs are discovered incidentally on imaging studies (Homma et al. 1995).

**Diagnosis**. Contrast-enhanced abdominal CT-imaging is the standard for detection and surveillance of renal lesions in VHL (Fig. 5). Solid tumors appear hyperdense, and enhance uniformly after contrast infusion. Cysts can be easily differentiated from solid tumors by CT-imaging. MR-imaging may be used in patients with allergy to CT contrast media or advanced renal insufficiency. Renal ultrasound may be valuable as a screening tool, but does not provide the anatomic detail of CT-imaging.

**Pathology**. RCCs are usually yellow to orange, and clearly demarcated from normal renal parenchyma both grossly and microscopically. They are usually confined by a pseudocapsule (Poston et al. 1995). Pathologic examination reveals clear cell carcinoma in all cases (Fig. 5).

**Treatment**. Surgical treatment of RCC is indicated to prevent the occurrence of metastatic disease. There is a strong positive correlation between tumor size and propensity to metastasis. Duffey et al. followed patients with tumors smaller than 3 cm for an average of 58 months with no metastases (Duffey et al. 2004). Alternatively, 27.4% of patients with RCCs larger than 3 cm developed metastatic disease (Duffey et al. 2004). Because of the low likelihood of RCCs smaller than 3 cm to metastasize, many centers have advocated watchful waiting for RCCs less than 3 cm in diameter (Duffey et al. 2004, Walther et al. 1999a).

If surgical treatment is warranted, options for RCC include radical nephrectomy, partial nephrectomy, enucleation (nephron sparing surgery), or ablative procedures. Bilateral radical nephrectomy is rarely used and is generally reserved for large, very advanced tumors. In cases of smaller tumors, enucleation can preserve renal function and still provide adequate cancer control. Indeed, the well-circumscribed nature of RCC's often lends itself to parenchyma-sparing procedures. In cases of metastatic RCC, cytoreductive nephrectomy may be performed to increase the effectiveness of systemic medical therapy (Finelli et al. 2004). Surgical treatment of RCC may be performed in a single stage with treatment of adrenal, pancreatic or other visceral tumors of VHL (Hwang et al. 2003).

Ablative procedures for RCC include cryoablation and radiofrequency ablation. These continue to be experimental procedures, but evidence is mounting that they may be safe and effective treatments for smaller renal cancers (Johnson et al. 2004). Ablation can be performed percutaneously or laparoscopically (Delworth et al. 1996; Gill et al. 1998; Shingleton and Sewell 2001, 2002). Most ablative series report a decrease in size or cessation of enhancement in the majority of cases (Hwang et al. 2004b; Moon et al. 2004; Pavlovich et al. 2002; Shingleton and Sewell 2001, 2002). There are as yet no randomized trials comparing cryoablation or RF ablation to surgical extirpation.

## Pheochromocytoma

**General Features**. Pheochromocytoma, a tumor of chromaffin cells of the adrenal medulla or sympathetic ganglia, is a major cause of correctable hypertension and is a common manifestation in VHL (Opocher et al. 2003). Overall, it is estimated that 80% of pheochromocytomas are sporadic, while the remainder are associated with familial conditions including VHL, multiple endocrine neoplasia 2 (MEN-2), and neurofibromatosis 1 (Opocher et al.

2003). Compared with sporadic cases, fewer VHL-associated pheochromocytomas are malignant (Baghai et al. 2002, Lonser et al. 2003a, Yip et al. 2004), but are more frequently bilateral or multiple (29–47%) (Baghai et al. 2002, Walther et al. 1999c). VHL-associated pheochromocytomas are found earlier than sporadic cases (29 versus 39.7 years) (Richard et al. 1994, Walther et al. 1999c).

**Clinical Findings**. Signs and symptoms of pheochromocytoma result from an abundance of circulating catecholamines and include headache, sweating, palpitations, arrhythmias, chest pain, and anxiety (Baghai et al. 2002, Opocher et al. 2003). Hypertension may be paroxysmal or sustained, and may predictably lead to morbidity and mortality from cardiovascular or cerebrovascular complications. Up to 41% of patients with VHL-associated pheochromocytoma are asymptomatic (Baghai et al. 2002). Tumor size has been correlated with catecholamine levels and presence of symptoms (Eisenhofer et al. 2001).

**Diagnosis**. The diagnosis of pheochromocytoma relies on imaging and laboratory testing. Traditional laboratory testing for pheochromocytoma, including urinary measurements of catecholamines, vanillylmandelic acid and metanephrines, suffer from a lack of sensitivity and specificity. More recently, these tests have been replaced by high-performance liquid chromatography for plasma normetanephrine and metanephrine, which have a sensitivity and specificity of 97% and 96%, respectively (Eisenhofer et al. 1999, Lenders et al. 2002). VHL-associated pheochromocytomas usually express norepinephrine, leading to high levels of its metabolite, normetanephrine (Eisenhofer et al. 1999, 2001).

The imaging technique of choice to localize pheochromocytoma is pre- and post-contrast CT-imaging (Fig. 5). MR-imaging of the abdomen is an alternative technique in patients that cannot tolerate CT contrast, and $^{123}$I-metaiodobenzylguanidine scintigraphy may be helpful in detection of small or extra-adrenal tumors.

**Pathology**. Grossly, pheochromocytomas are spongy, reddish tumors with a well-defined capsule. Microscopically, pheochromocytomas are composed of pink cells arranged in nests, with an intervening vascular network (Fig. 5).

**Treatment**. Due to the rarity of malignant or metastatic disease in VHL-associated pheochromocytoma, complete surgical resection of these tumors is curative. Previously, many pheochromocytomas were treated with total adrenalectomy, or bilateral adrenalectomy (in bilateral cases), and subsequently required adrenocortical replacement with fludrocortisone and corticosteroids. Cortical-sparing partial adrenalectomy, usually by laparoscopic approach, has become the most commonly used technique, with the benefits of preserved adrenocortical function outweighing the low risk of incomplete tumor removal or recurrence (Baghai et al. 2002, Walther et al. 2000, Yip et al. 2004). Accessible extra-adrenal tumors may also be approached using minimally invasive techniques (Hwang et al. 2004a).

Surgical treatment of pheochromocytoma requires careful preparation by the operative and anesthetic teams. To prevent morbid hypertensive crisis during intubation or intraoperative tumor manipulation, catecholamine storm can be blunted with 2 to 3 weeks of metyrosine, which inhibits an early step of catecholamine biosynthesis, and alpha blockade with phenoxybenzamine or prazosin, followed by beta-blockers if the patient is persistently tachycardic. Perioperatively, sodium nitroprusside drips may be necessary to control rapid elevations in blood pressure (Hoshino et al. 1987, Opocher et al. 2003).

Pheochromocytomas should be removed as soon as convenient after diagnosis, as larger size may be associated with increased perioperative morbidity and risk of loss of adrenocortical function (Walther et al. 1999b). Postoperatively, patients are followed for biochemical evidence of recurrence, as well as for adequacy of adrenocorticotropic hormone responsiveness of remaining adrenocortical tissue.

## Pancreatic neuroendocrine tumors, cystadenomas, and cysts

**General Features**. Pancreatic involvement in VHL is quite common, occurring in 56–77% of patients (Hammel et al. 2000, Hough et al. 1994, Mukhopadhyay et al. 2002). Manifestations of pancreatic disease may take the form of cysts (91.1%), serous cystadenomas (12.3%), neuroendocrine (islet cell) tumors (12.3%), or a combination of lesions (11.5%) (Hammel et al. 2000).

**Clinical Features**. Pancreatic lesions in VHL are frequently clinically silent, but may become symptomatic due to mass effect and compression of surrounding structures including the common bile duct, duodenum or the mesenterico-portal venous system. Other patients may present with pancreatic duct obstruction and pancreatitis (Hammel et al. 2000). Development of diabetes due to pancreatic involvement is rare (2.4%), even in patients with extensive parenchymal replacement (Hammel et al. 2000). Neuroendocrine tumors rarely cause clinical symptoms of hormonal hypersecretion (Hammel et al. 2000, Lubensky et al. 1998, Marcos et al. 2002, Mukhopadhyay et al. 2002).

**Diagnosis**. Radiological investigation of pancreatic lesions in VHL is best performed with pre- and post-contrast CT- or MR-imaging (Fig. 5). True cysts appear as nonenhancing hypodense lesions, while serous cystadenomas are multicystic with a partially enhancing rim. Neuroendocrine tumors are solid and show strong early-phase contrast enhancement. Larger neuroendocrine tumors (>3 cm), however, may appear ragged and enhance heterogeneously (Marcos et al. 2002). Scant calcification may be present in any of the 3 types of lesions (i.e. cysts, cystadenomas, or neuroendocrine tumors). Somatostatin receptor scintigraphy and endoscopic ultrasound are useful adjuncts in the diagnosis of pancreatic neuroendocrine tumors.

**Pathology**. Pancreatic neuroendocrine tumors are composed of cuboidal to columnar cells with eosinophilic or clear cytoplasm and salt-and-pepper chromatin. Though mitoses are rare, nuclear atypia is not uncommon. Cells are arranged in nests or cords with prominent collagen bands outlining the nests (Lubensky et al. 1998).

**Treatment**. Definitive treatment of symptomatic cysts, cystadenomas and neuroendocrine tumors is surgical. Surgical treatment of pancreatic cysts, cystadenomas and neuroendocrine tumors is generally reserved for patients with symptoms of compression. Neuroendocrine tumors do carry a risk of malignant transformation and have been noted to metastasize

to the liver (Libutti et al. 1998, Marcos et al. 2002). Specifically, tumors over 3 cm in diameter (Hammel et al. 2000, Libutti et al. 2000) and those carrying germline mutations in exon 3 of the *VHL* gene (Libutti et al. 2000) have a propensity to metastasize.

Lubutti and colleagues outlined their criteria for surgical excision of pancreatic neuroendocrine tumors: (1) no evidence of metastatic disease, (2) lesion diameter >3 cm, or >2 cm in the pancreatic head, or (3) patient undergoing laparotomy for management of another pathological manifestation of VHL (Libutti et al. 1998). Surgical options for neuroendocrine tumors include open or laparoscopic enucleation, distal pancreatectomy in tumors of the tail, and total pancreatectomy or pancreaticoduodenectomy (Whipple's procedure) with more extensive involvement of the pancreas (Akerstrom et al. 2004; Libutti et al. 1998, 2000). Metastatic disease may be treated with a combination of systemic chemotherapy (Akerstrom et al. 2004), isolated hepatic chemotherapeutic perfusion (Grover et al. 2004) and ablative therapies (Hellman et al. 2002).

## Epididymal cystadenomas

**General Features**. Epididymal papillary cystadenomas are benign lesions of the head of the epididymis noted in 54% of male VHL patients, with two-thirds having bilateral tumors (Choyke et al. 1997). They are believed to originate from efferent ductules of the testis, which are a derivative of the embryonic mesonephric duct. About one-third of epididymal cystadenomas are associated with VHL.

**Clinical Features**. These lesions typically present as firm scrotal masses and are rarely symptomatic (Choyke et al. 1997). Seventeen percent of lesions were nonpalpable and diagnosed by ultrasound alone (Choyke et al. 1997). One case presenting with infertility has been documented in the literature (de Souza Andrade et al. 1985).

**Diagnosis**. Scrotal ultrasound is used to evaluate epididymal cystadenomas. Ultrasound typically shows heterogeneous hyperechoic masses with cystic foci and, in some cases, dilation of efferent ductules secondary to obstruction (Choyke et al. 1997).

Proposed diagnostic criteria are: (1) predominantly solid tumor greater than 10 by 14 mm, (2) occurrence in VHL, and (3) slow growth (Choyke et al. 1997). Differentiation from epididymal cyst or spermatocele is not difficult, and history and serial examination can help distinguish epididymal cystadenoma from epididymal carcinomas, adenomatoid tumors, leiomyomas, lymphomas, and metastases.

**Pathology**. Microscopic examination reveals cystic regions intermixed with papillary structures composed of uniform clear cells around a fibrovascular core (Choyke et al. 1997, Gruber et al. 1980).

**Treatment**. Epididymal cystadenomas are benign tumors and removal is generally not warranted. Serial ultrasound can be used to monitor these lesions.

## Broad ligament cystadenomas

**General Features**. Papillary cystadenomas of the broad ligament are a rare and probably underestimated manifestation of VHL (Gaffey et al. 1994). They are homologous to papillary cystadenomas of the epididymis in males, though they appear to be much less common. The frequency and age at presentation of broad ligament cystadenomas is not clear.

**Clinical Findings**. Broad ligament cystadenomas are typically asymptomatic.

**Diagnosis**. These tumors may be detected by CT- or MR-imaging, or ultrasound of the pelvis.

**Pathology**. Broad ligament cystadenomas are histologically identical to epididymal cystadenomas. Microscopic examination reveals a cystic tumor with a complex papillary pattern, and bland-appearing, cuboidal cells around a fibrovascular core (Funk and Heiken 1989, Gersell and King 1988).

**Treatment**. These benign lesions are followed with serial ultrasound in VHL patients and removed when symptomatic.

## Natural history

The mean age at diagnosis of VHL is 26.3 years, with 97% of patients presenting by the age of 60 (Maher et al. 1990). The most frequent presenting manifestation is retinal hemangioblastoma (43%), followed by cerebellar hemangioblastoma (39%) and renal cell carcinoma (10%) (Maher et al. 1990, Richard et al. 1998). However, systematic screening of the families of affected patients has led

**Table 1.** Frequency of lesions and age at onset of von Hippel-Lindau lesions

| Location | Mean age of onset (years) | Age range (years) | Frequency of patients (%) |
| --- | --- | --- | --- |
| Central nervous system | | | |
| Retinal hemangioblastomas | 25 | 1–67 | 25–60% |
| Endolymphatic sac tumors | 22 | 12–50 | 10% |
| Craniospinal hemangioblastomas | | | |
| Cerebellum | 33 | 9–78 | 44–72% |
| Brainstem | 32 | 12–46 | 10–25% |
| Spinal cord | 33 | 12–66 | 13–50% |
| Lumbosacral nerve roots | unknown | unknown | rare |
| Supratentorial | unknown | unknown | rare |
| Visceral | | | |
| Renal cell carcinoma/cysts | 39 | 16–67 | 25–60% |
| Pheochromocytomas | 30 | 5–58 | 10–20% |
| Pancreatic tumor/cyst | 36 | 5–70 | 35–70% |
| Epididymal cystadenoma | unknown | unknown | 25–60% |
| Broad ligament cystadenoma | unknown | 16–46 | unknown |

*Adapted from Lonser et al. 2003a.

to the identification of a number of patients presymptomatically.

Median survival in a 1990 study was approximately 49 years of age, with a mean survival of 41 years (Maher et al. 1990). The most frequent cause of death historically has been CNS hemangioblastomas; however, with improved screening and treatment of these lesions, metastatic renal cell carcinoma now appears to be the most common underlying cause of death (Horton et al. 1976, Maher et al. 1990). The incidence and age of presentation of the complications of VHL are presented in Table 1 (Lonser et al. 2003a).

Based upon the presence or absence of pheochromocytoma, VHL patients may be categorized as type 1 (no pheochromocytoma), or type 2 (pheochromocytoma present). Type 2 patients may have either a low risk (type 2A) or high risk (type 2B) of renal cell carcinoma. Type 2C patients have pheochromocytoma only (Brauch et al. 1995, Hoffman et al. 2001, Neumann and Wiestler 1991). Despite these categorizations, the extent and number of lesions within families can be quite variable.

## Molecular genetics and pathogenesis

### VHL gene and gene product

The *VHL* gene was localized by linkage analysis in 1988 to chromosome 3p25–26 by Seizinger et al. (1988), and fully identified and cloned by Latif et al. (1993). Spanning 14.5 kbp, it is composed of three exons which encode a 30 kDa protein and, by translation at an alternate initiation site, an 18 kDa protein (Blankenship et al. 1999). The *VHL* gene product (pVHL) is widely expressed in the body (Corless et al. 1997) and in all three germ layers of the developing embryo (Richards et al. 1996).

The *VHL* gene behaves as a tumor suppressor and according to Knudson's "two-hit hypothesis" requires that both copies of the gene be inactivated to induce tumorigenesis (Knudson 1986). Generally, all cells in a VHL patient have a germline mutation in one copy of the gene. Subsequent inactivation of the second copy must occur by somatic mutation to produce a tumor. Moreover, VHL is a tissue-specific disease and only those cells in certain tissues (e.g. CNS, retina, adrenals, kidneys, pancreas, broad ligament and epididymis) with two inactivated genes are prone to develop tumor. The *VHL* gene locus may be regarded as an important tumor suppressor in VHL as well as for cancers in general, as *VHL* gene inactivation has been identified not only in patients with VHL (Stolle et al. 1998), but also patients with sporadic hemangioblastomas, renal cell carcinomas, and pheochromocytomas (Kaelin 2002).

## Neoplastic mechanisms

Though incompletely understood, loss of pVHL may lead to neoplasia by several different mechanisms. By binding to Elongin C, Elongin B and Cullin 2 (Cul2) in the so-called VCB-Cul2 complex, pVHL acts to target certain molecules for destruction via ubiqitination. Key among these molecules is the alpha subunit of the hypoxia inducible factor (HIF) heterodimer (Maxwell et al. 1999). HIF proteins are activated by low oxygen tension

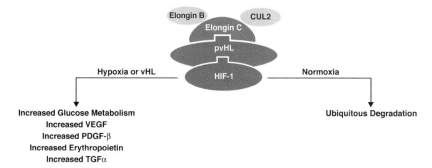

**Fig. 6.** Interaction of pVHL with other proteins including elongin B, elongin C, and CUL2, to form the VCB-CUL2 complex. Glut-1=glucose transporter 1 (from Lonser et al. 2003a).

and cause the upregulation of a number of growth factors, including VEGF, platelet derived growth factor-fl (PDGF-fl), erythropoietin, and transforming growth factor-a (TGF-a). In the setting of normoxia, HIF is quickly targeted for degradation in proteosomes by pVHL. Loss of the negative influence of pVHL on HIF, however, mimics the hypoxic condition, and leads to an upregulation of VEGF, PDGF-fl and other growth factors, leading to angiogenesis and tumor formation (Kaelin 2002).

There are other, HIF-independent, ways that pVHL loss might cause cell transformation. pVHL has been shown to be directly involved in the suppression of the VEGF promoter, which is upregulated in its absence (Cohen et al. 1999). pVHL has also been demonstrated to participate in formation of a normal fibronectin extracellular matrix, loss of which may be important in carcinogenesis (Hoffman et al. 2001, Ohh et al. 1998). Moreover, pVHL loss may also play a part in preventing mutant cells from exiting the cell cycle (Pause et al. 1998). High levels of TGF-a (in the pVHL-deficient condition) can cause it to upregulate its own receptor, resulting in an autocrine loop and stimulation of tumor growth (Kaelin 2002, Reifenberger et al. 1995).

## Diagnosis, follow-up and management

### Clinical diagnostic criteria

In the presence of a positive family history, one typical VHL-associated tumor (retinal, cerebellar or spinal hemangioblastoma; renal cell carcinoma; pheochromocytoma) establishes the diagnosis. In cases with no known family history of VHL, either two central nervous system hemangioblastomas, or one hemangioblastoma in association with either renal cell carcinoma or pheochromocytoma is diagnostic (Maher and Kaelin 1997, Melmon and Rosen 1964). While ELST and multicystic pancreatic disease are reliable indicators of VHL due to the rarity of sporadic cases, they are not considered diagnostic VHL tumors according to current criteria. Renal and epididymal cysts are frequent in the general population and are not included in the diagnostic criteria for VHL.

### Genetic testing

Clinical diagnosis may prompt genetic testing, both in the patient and willing first-degree family members. Direct gene sequencing, quantitative Southern Blot analysis, and fluorescence in-situ hybridization are used to efficiently detect abnormalities of the *VHL* gene (Stolle et al. 1998). To date there are over 700 mutations recorded in the Universal VHL-Mutation Database (http://www.umd.necker.fr:2005). Large or partial germline deletions are detected in 20–37%, missense mutations in 30–38%, and nonsense or frameshift mutations are discovered in 23–27% (Maher and Kaelin 1997, Stolle et al. 1998). Germline mutations of *VHL* are extremely heterogeneous and may occur throughout the sequence, excepting that mutations rarely occur in the first 50 codons of the gene (Zbar et al. 1996).

### Clinical screening

Initial screening of at-risk individuals should be designed for early detection of all VHL-associated le-

**Table 2.** Recommended intervals for screening tests in at-risk individuals with von Hippel-Lindau disease*

| Test | Start age (frequency) |
|---|---|
| Ophthalmoscopy | Infancy (yearly) |
| Plasma or 24-hour urinary catecholamines and metanephrines | 2 years of age (yearly and when blood pressure is elevated) |
| Magnetic resonance imaging of craniospinal axis** | 11 years of age (yearly) |
| Computed tomography and magnetic resonance imaging of internal auditory canals** | Onset of symptoms (hearing loss, tinnitus, vertigo, or unexplained balance difficulties) |
| Ultrasound of abdomen | 8 years of age (yearly; magnetic resonance imaging as clinically indicated) |
| Computed tomography of abdomen** | 18 years of age or earlier if clinically indicated (yearly) |
| Audiologic function tests | When clinically indicated |

*Adapted from Choyke et al. (1995).
**Imaging studies that are often recommended before and after contrast infusion.

sions. Recommended screening studies and screening intervals are summarized in Table 2.

## Genetic counseling

First-degree family members may be tested to identify patients early to improve surveillance, permit earlier treatment, and prevent unnecessary testing in unaffected individuals. Since VHL is transmitted in an autosomal dominant fashion, parents must be well informed of the 50% risk of transmission to their children.

## References

Akerstrom G, Hellman P, Hessman O, Osmak L (2004) Surgical treatment of endocrine pancreatic tumours. Neuroendocrinology 80 (Suppl 1): 62–66.

Baghai M, Thompson GB, Young WF Jr, Grant CS, Michels VV, van Heerden JA (2002) Pheochromocytomas and paragangliomas in von Hippel-Lindau disease: a role for laparoscopic and cortical-sparing surgery. Arch Surg 137: 682–688; discussion 688–689.

Beighton P, Beighton G (1986) The man behind the syndrome. Berlin: Springer.

Berkman RA, Merrill MJ, Reinhold WC, Monacci WT, Saxena A, Clark WC, Robertson JT, Ali IU, Oldfield EH (1993) Expression of the vascular permeability factor/vascular endothelial growth factor gene in central nervous system neoplasms. J Clin Invest 91: 153–159.

Blankenship C, Naglich JG, Whaley JM, Seizinger B, Kley N (1999) Alternate choice of initiation codon produces a biologically active product of the von Hippel Lindau gene with tumor suppressor activity. Oncogene 18: 1529–1535.

Boström A, Hans FJ, Reinacher PC, Krings T, Bürgel U, Gilsbach JM, Reinges MH (2008) Intramedullary hemangioblastomas: timing of surgery, microsurgical technique and follow-up in 23 patients. Eur Spine J Apr 4 [Epub ahead of print].

Brandt R (1921) Zur Frage der Angiomatosis retinae. A von Graefe's Arch Ophthalmol 106: 127–165.

Brauch H, Kishida T, Glavac D, Chen F, Pausch F, Hofler H, Latif F, Lerman MI, Zbar B, Neumann HP (1995) Von Hippel-Lindau (VHL) disease with pheochromocytoma in the Black Forest region of Germany: evidence for a founder effect. Hum Genet 95: 551–556.

Chandler HC Jr, Friedman WA (1994) Radiosurgical treatment of a hemangioblastoma: case report. Neurosurgery 34: 353–355; discussion 355.

Chang SD, Meisel JA, Hancock SL, Martin DP, McManus M, Adler JR Jr (1998) Treatment of hemangioblastomas in von Hippel-Lindau disease with linear accelerator-based radiosurgery. Neurosurgery 43: 28–34; discussion 34–35.

Choo D, Shotland L, Mastroianni M, Glenn G, van Waes C, Linehan WM, Oldfield EH (2004) Endolymphatic sac tumors in von Hippel-Lindau disease. J Neurosurg 100: 480–487.

Choyke PL, Glenn GM, Walther MM, Zbar B, Weiss GH, Alexander RB, Hayes WS, Long JP, Thakore KN, Linehan WM (1992) The natural history of renal lesions in von Hippel-Lindau disease: a serial CT study in 28 patients. AJR Am J Roentgenol 159: 1229–1234.

Choyke PL, Glenn GM, Walther MM, Patronas NJ, Linehan WM, Zbar B (1995) von Hippel-Lindau disease: genetic, clinical, and imaging features. Radiology 194: 629–642.

Choyke PL, Glenn GM, Wagner JP, Lubensky IA, Thakore K, Zbar B, Linehan WM, Walther MM (1997) Epididymal cystadenomas in von Hippel-Lindau disease. Urology 49: 926–931.

Cohen HT, Zhou M, Welsh AM, Zarghamee S, Scholz H, Mukhopadhyay D, Kishida T, Zbar B, Knebelmann B, Sukhatme VP (1999) An important von Hippel-Lindau tumor suppressor domain mediates Sp1-binding and self-association. Biochem Biophys Res Commun 266: 43–50.

Collins ET (1894) Intra-ocular growths (two cases, brother and sister, with peculiar vascular new growth, probably retinal, affecting both eyes). Trans Ophthalmol Soc UK 14: 141–149.

Corless CL, Kibel AS, Iliopoulos O, Kaelin WG Jr (1997) Immunostaining of the von Hippel-Lindau gene product in normal and neoplastic human tissues. Hum Pathol 28: 459–464.

Cushing HBP (1928) Tumors arising from blood vessels of the brain: angiomatous malformations and hemangioblastomas. Charles C. Thomas Publisher, Springfield, Ill.

Davison C (1936) Retinal and central nervous system hemangioblastomas with visceral changes (von Hippel-Lindau's disease). Bull Neurol Instit NY 5: 72–93.

de Souza Andrade J, Bambirra EA, Bicalho OJ, de Souza AF (1985) Bilateral papillary cystadenoma of the epididymis as a component of von Hippel-Lindau's syndrome: report of a case presenting as infertility. J Urol 133: 288–289.

Delworth MG, Pisters LL, Fornage BD, von Eschenbach AC (1996) Cryotherapy for renal cell carcinoma and angiomyolipoma. J Urol 155: 252–254; discussion 254–255.

Duffey BG, Choyke PL, Glenn G, Grubb RL, Venzon D, Linehan WM, Walther MM (2004) The relationship between renal tumor size and metastases in patients with von Hippel-Lindau disease. J Urol 172: 63–65.

Eisenhofer G, Lenders JW, Linehan WM, Walther MM, Goldstein DS, Keiser HR (1999) Plasma normetanephrine and metanephrine for detecting pheochromocytoma in von Hippel-Lindau disease and multiple endocrine neoplasia type 2. N Engl J Med 340: 1872–1879.

Eisenhofer G, Walther MM, Huynh TT, Li ST, Bornstein SR, Vortmeyer A, Mannelli M, Goldstein DS, Linehan WM, Lenders JW, Pacak K (2001) Pheochromocytomas in von Hippel-Lindau syndrome and multiple endocrine neoplasia type 2 display distinct biochemical and clinical phenotypes. J Clin Endocrinol Metab 86: 1999–2008.

Ferreira MA, Feiz-Erfan I, Zabramski JM, Spetzler RF, Coons SW, Preul MC (2002) Endolymphatic sac tumor: unique features of two cases and review of the literature. Acta Neurochir (Wien) 144: 1047–1053.

Finelli A, Kaouk JH, Fergany AF, Abreu SC, Novick AC, Gill IS (2004) Laparoscopic cytoreductive nephrectomy for metastatic renal cell carcinoma. BJU Int 94: 291–294.

Funk KC, Heiken JP (1989) Papillary cystadenoma of the broad ligament in a patient with von Hippel-Lindau disease. AJR Am J Roentgenol 153: 527–528.

Gaffey MJ, Mills SE, Boyd JC (1994) Aggressive papillary tumor of middle ear/temporal bone and adnexal papillary cystadenoma. Manifestations of von Hippel-Lindau disease. Am J Surg Pathol 18: 1254–1260.

Galezowski X (1987) Traité iconographique d'ophthalmoscopie. In: Balliere (ed.) Diagnostique et traitment des affections oculaires par les docteurs. Paris, Baillieres.

Gersell DJ, King TC (1988) Papillary cystadenoma of the mesosalpinx in von Hippel-Lindau disease. Am J Surg Pathol 12: 145–149.

Gill IS, Novick AC, Soble JJ, Sung GT, Remer EM, Hale J, O'Malley CM (1998) Laparoscopic renal cryoablation: initial clinical series. Urology 52: 543–551.

Grossniklaus HE, Thomas JW, Vigneswaran N, Jarrett WH 3rd (1992) Retinal hemangioblastoma. A histologic, immunohistochemical, and ultrastructural evaluation. Ophthalmology 99: 140–145.

Grover AC, Libutti SK, Pingpank JF, Helsabeck C, Beresnev T, Alexander HR Jr (2004) Isolated hepatic perfusion for the treatment of patients with advanced liver metastases from pancreatic and gastrointestinal neuroendocrine neoplasms. Surgery 136: 1176–1182.

Gruber MB, Healey GB, Toguri AG, Warren MM (1980) Papillary cystadenoma of epididymis: component of von Hippel-Lindau syndrome. Urology 16: 305–306.

Hammel PR, Vilgrain V, Terris B, Penfornis A, Sauvanet A, Correas JM, Chauveau D, Balian A, Beigelman C, O'Toole D, Bernades P, Ruszniewski P, Richard S (2000) Pancreatic involvement in von Hippel-Lindau disease. The Groupe Francophone d'Etude de la Maladie de von Hippel-Lindau. Gastroenterology 119: 1087–1095.

Hansen MR, Luxford WM (2004) Surgical outcomes in patients with endolymphatic sac tumors. Laryngoscope 114: 1470–1474.

Heffner DK (1989) Low-grade adenocarcinoma of probable endolymphatic sac origin: a clinicopathologic study of 20 cases. Cancer 64: 2292–2302.

Hellman P, Ladjevardi S, Skogseid B, Akerstrom G, Elvin A (2002) Radiofrequency tissue ablation using cooled tip for liver metastases of endocrine tumors. World J Surg 26: 1052–1056.

Hoffman MA, Ohh M, Yang H, Klco JM, Ivan M, Kaelin WG Jr (2001) von Hippel-Lindau protein mutants linked to type 2C VHL disease preserve the ability to downregulate HIF. Hum Mol Genet 10: 1019–1027.

Homma Y, Kawabe K, Kitamura T, Nishimura Y, Shinohara M, Kondo Y, Saito I, Minowada S, Asakage Y (1995) Increased incidental detection and reduced mortality in renal cancer – recent retrospective analysis at eight institutions. Int J Urol 2: 77–80.

Horton WA, Wong V, Eldridge R (1976) Von Hippel-Lindau disease: clinical and pathological manifestations in nine families with 50 affected members. Arch Intern Med 136: 769–777.

Hoshino Y, Obara H, Mikawa K, Iwai S (1987) Anesthesia and von Hippel-Lindau disease associated with pheochromocytoma. J Anesth 1: 195–198.

Hough DM, Stephens DH, Johnson CD, Binkovitz LA (1994) Pancreatic lesions in von Hippel-Lindau disease: prevalence, clinical significance, and CT findings. AJR Am J Roentgenol 162: 1091–1094.

Hwang J, Shoaf G, Uchio EM, Watson J, Pacak K, Linehan WM, Walther MM (2004a) Laparoscopic management of extra-adrenal pheochromocytoma. J Urol 171: 72–76.

Hwang JJ, Uchio EM, Pavlovich CP, Pautler SE, Libutti SK, Linehan WM, Walther MM (2003) Surgical management of multi-organ visceral tumors in patients with von Hippel-Lindau disease: a single stage approach. J Urol 169: 895–898.

Hwang JJ, Walther MM, Pautler SE, Coleman JA, Hvizda J, Peterson J, Linehan WM, Wood BJ (2004b) Radio frequency ablation of small renal tumors: intermediate results. J Urol 171: 1814–1818.

Jagannathan J, Lonser RR, Smith R, DeVroom HL, Oldfield EH (2008) Surgical management of cerebellar hemangioblastomas in patients with von Hippel-Lindau disease. J Neurosurg 108: 210–222.

Johnson DB, Solomon SB, Su LM, Matsumoto ED, Kavoussi LR, Nakada SY, Moon TD, Shingleton WB, Cadeddu JA (2004) Defining the complications of cryoablation and radio frequency ablation of small renal tumors: a multi-institutional review. J Urol 172: 874–877.

Kaelin WG Jr (2002) Molecular basis of the VHL hereditary cancer syndrome. Nat Rev Cancer 2: 673–682.

Kim HJ, Butman JA, Brewer C, Zalewski C, Vortmeyer AO, Glenn G, Oldfield EH, Lonser RR (2005) Tumors of the endolymphatic sac in patients with von Hippel-Lindau disease: implications for their natural history, diagnosis, and treatment. J Neurosurg 102: 503–512.

Knudson AG Jr (1986) Genetics of human cancer. Annu Rev Genet 20: 231–251.

Kreusel KM, Bechrakis NE, Heinichen T, Neumann L, Neumann HP, Foerster MH (2000) Retinal angiomatosis and von Hippel-Lindau disease. Graefes Arch Clin Exp Ophthalmol 238: 916–921.

Latif F, Tory K, Gnarra J, Yao M, Duh FM, Orcutt ML, Stackhouse T, Kuzmin I, Modi W, Geil L et al. (1993) Identification of the von Hippel-Lindau disease tumor suppressor gene. Science 260: 1317–1320.

Lenders JW, Pacak K, Walther MM, Linehan WM, Mannelli M, Friberg P, Keiser HR, Goldstein DS, Eisenhofer G (2002) Biochemical diagnosis of pheochromocytoma: which test is best? Jama 287: 1427–1434.

Libutti SK, Choyke PL, Bartlett DL, Vargas H, Walther M, Lubensky I, Glenn G, Linehan WM, Alexander HR (1998) Pancreatic neuroendocrine tumors associated with von Hippel Lindau disease: diagnostic and management recommendations. Surgery 124: 1153–1159.

Libutti SK, Choyke PL, Alexander HR, Glenn G, Bartlett DL, Zbar B, Lubensky I, McKee SA, Maher ER, Linehan WM, Walther MM (2000) Clinical and genetic analysis of patients with pancreatic neuroendocrine tumors associated with von Hippel-Lindau disease. Surgery 128: 1022–1027; discussion 1027–1028.

Lonser RR, Glenn GM, Walther M, Chew EY, Libutti SK, Linehan WM, Oldfield EH (2003a) von Hippel-Lindau disease. Lancet 361: 2059–2067.

Lonser RR, Weil RJ, Wanebo JE, DeVroom HL, Oldfield EH (2003b) Surgical management of spinal cord hemangioblastomas in patients with von Hippel-Lindau disease. J Neurosurg 98: 106–116.

Lonser RR, Kim HJ, Butman JA, Vortmeyer AO, Choo DI, Oldfield EH (2004) Tumors of the endolymphatic sac in von Hippel-Lindau disease. N Engl J Med 350: 2481–2486.

Lubensky IA, Pack S, Ault D, Vortmeyer AO, Libutti SK, Choyke PL, Walther MM, Linehan WM, Zhuang Z (1998) Multiple neuroendocrine tumors of the pancreas in von Hippel-Lindau disease patients: histopathological and molecular genetic analysis. Am J Pathol 153: 223–231.

Maher ER, Yates JR, Harries R, Benjamin C, Harris R, Moore AT, Ferguson-Smith MA (1990) Clinical features and natural history of von Hippel-Lindau disease. Q J Med 77: 1151–1163.

Maher ER, Iselius L, Yates JR, Littler M, Benjamin C, Harris R, Sampson J, Williams A, Ferguson-Smith MA, Morton N (1991) Von Hippel-Lindau disease: a genetic study. J Med Genet 28: 443–447.

Maher ER, Kaelin WG Jr (1997) von Hippel-Lindau disease. Medicine (Baltimore) 76: 381–391.

Manski TJ, Heffner DK, Glenn GM, Patronas NJ, Pikus AT, Katz D, Lebovics R, Sledjeski K, Choyke PL, Zbar B, Linehan WM, Oldfield EH (1997) Endolymphatic sac tumors. A source of morbid hearing loss in von Hippel-Lindau disease. Jama 277: 1461–1466.

Marcos HB, Libutti SK, Alexander HR, Lubensky IA, Bartlett DL, Walther MM, Linehan WM, Glenn GM, Choyke PL (2002) Neuroendocrine tumors of the pancreas in von Hippel-Lindau disease: spectrum of appearances at CT and MR imaging with histopathologic comparison. Radiology 225: 751–758.

Maxwell PH, Wiesener MS, Chang GW, Clifford SC, Vaux EC, Cockman ME, Wykoff CC, Pugh CW, Maher ER, Ratcliffe PJ (1999) The tumour suppressor protein VHL targets hypoxia-inducible factors for oxygen-dependent proteolysis. Nature 399: 271–275.

Megerian CA, McKenna MJ, Nuss RC, Maniglia AJ, Ojemann RG, Pilch BZ, Nadol JB Jr (1995) Endolymphatic sac tumors: histopathologic confirmation, clinical characterization, and implication in von Hippel-Lindau disease. Laryngoscope 105: 801–808.

Melmon KL, Rosen SW (1964) Lindau's Disease. Review of the literature and study of a large kindred. Am J Med 36: 595–617.

Moon TD, Lee FT Jr, Hedican SP, Lowry P, Nakada SY (2004) Laparoscopic cryoablation under sonographic guidance for the treatment of small renal tumors. J Endourol 18: 436–440.

Morgan WR, Zincke H (1990) Progression and survival after renal-conserving surgery for renal cell carcinoma: experience in 104 patients and extended followup. J Urol 144: 852–857; discussion 857–858.

Mukhopadhyay B, Sahdev A, Monson JP, Besser GM, Reznek RH, Chew SL (2002) Pancreatic lesions in von Hippel-Lindau disease. Clin Endocrinol (Oxf) 57: 603–608.

Murota T, Symon L (1989) Surgical management of hemangioblastoma of the spinal cord: a report of 18 cases. Neurosurgery 25: 699–707; discussion 708.

Neumann HP, Eggert HR, Weigel K, Friedburg H, Wiestler OD, Schollmeyer P (1989) Hemangioblastomas of the central nervous system. A 10-year study with special reference to von Hippel-Lindau syndrome. J Neurosurg 70: 24–30.

Neumann HP, Wiestler OD (1991) Clustering of features of von Hippel-Lindau syndrome: evidence for a complex genetic locus. Lancet 337: 1052–1054.

Niemela M, Lim YJ, Soderman M, Jaaskelainen J, Lindquist C (1996) Gamma knife radiosurgery in 11 hemangioblastomas. J Neurosurg 85: 591–596.

Novick AC, Streem S, Montie JE, Pontes JE, Siegel S, Montague DK, Goormastic M (1989) Conservative surgery for renal cell carcinoma: a single-center experience with 100 patients. J Urol 141: 835–839.

Ohh M, Yauch RL, Lonergan KM, Whaley JM, Stemmer-Rachamimov AO, Louis DN, Gavin BJ, Kley N, Kaelin WG Jr, Iliopoulos O (1998) The von Hippel-Lindau tumor suppressor protein is required for proper assembly of an extracellular fibronectin matrix. Mol Cell 1: 959–968.

Opocher G, Schiavi F, Conton P, Scaroni C, Mantero F (2003) Clinical and genetic aspects of phaeochromocytoma. Horm Res 59 (Suppl 1): 56–61.

Palmer JD, Gragoudas ES (1997) Advances in treatment of retinal angiomas. Int Ophthalmol Clin 37: 159–170.

Patrice SJ, Sneed PK, Flickinger JC, Shrieve DC, Pollock BE, Alexander E 3rd, Larson DA, Kondziolka DS, Gutin PH, Wara WM, McDermott MW, Lunsford LD, Loeffler JS (1996) Radiosurgery for hemangioblastoma: results of a multiinstitutional experience. Int J Radiat Oncol Biol Phys 35: 493–499.

Pause A, Lee S, Lonergan KM, Klausner RD (1998) The von Hippel-Lindau tumor suppressor gene is required for cell cycle exit upon serum withdrawal. Proc Natl Acad Sci USA 95: 993–998.

Pavlovich CP, Walther MM, Choyke PL, Pautler SE, Chang R, Linehan WM, Wood BJ (2002) Percutaneous radio frequency ablation of small renal tumors: initial results. J Urol 167: 10–15.

Poston CD, Jaffe GS, Lubensky IA, Solomon D, Zbar B, Linehan WM, Walther MM (1995) Characterization of the renal pathology of a familial form of renal cell carcinoma associated with von Hippel-Lindau disease: clinical and molecular genetic implications. J Urol 153: 22–26.

Reifenberger G, Reifenberger J, Bilzer T, Wechsler W, Collins VP (1995) Coexpression of transforming growth factor-alpha and epidermal growth factor receptor in capillary hemangioblastomas of the central nervous system. Am J Pathol 147: 245–250.

Richards FM, Schofield PN, Fleming S, Maher ER (1996) Expression of the von Hippel-Lindau disease tumour suppressor gene during human embryogenesis. Hum Mol Genet 5: 639–644.

Richards PS, Clifton AG (2003) Endolymphatic sac tumours. J Laryngol Otol 117: 666–669.

Richard S, Chauveau D, Chretien Y, Beigelman C, Denys A, Fendler JP, Fromont G, Paraf F, Helenon O, Nizard S et al. (1994) Renal lesions and pheochromocytoma in von Hippel-Lindau disease. Adv Nephrol Necker Hosp 23: 1–27.

Richard S, Campello C, Taillandier L, Parker F, Resche F (1998) Haemangioblastoma of the central nervous system in von Hippel-Lindau disease. French VHL Study Group. J Intern Med 243: 547–553.

Richard S, Graff J, Lindau J, Resche F (2004) Von Hippel-Lindau disease. Lancet 363: 1231–1234.

Roupret M, Hopirtean V, Mejean A, Thiounn N, Dufour B, Chretien Y, Chauveau D, Richard S (2003) Nephron sparing surgery for renal cell carcinoma and von Hippel-Lindau's disease: a single center experience. J Urol 170: 1752–1755.

Sano T, Horiguchi H (2003) Von Hippel-Lindau disease. Microsc Res Tech 60: 159–164.

Seizinger BR, Rouleau GA, Ozelius LJ, Lane AH, Farmer GE, Lamiell JM, Haines J, Yuen JW, Collins D, Majoor-Krakauer D et al. (1988) Von Hippel-Lindau disease maps to the region of chromosome 3 associated with renal cell carcinoma. Nature 332: 268–269.

Shingleton WB, Sewell PE Jr (2001) Percutaneous renal tumor cryoablation with magnetic resonance imaging guidance. J Urol 165: 773–776.

Shingleton WB, Sewell PE Jr (2002) Percutaneous renal cryoablation of renal tumors in patients with von Hippel-Lindau disease. J Urol 167: 1268–1270.

Slater A, Moore NR, Huson SM (2003) The natural history of cerebellar hemangioblastomas in von Hippel-Lindau disease. AJNR Am J Neuroradiol 24: 1570–1574.

Solomon D, Schwartz A (1988) Renal pathology in von Hippel-Lindau disease. Hum Pathol 19: 1072–1079.

Steinbach F, Stockle M, Muller SC, Thuroff JW, Melchior SW, Stein R, Hohenfellner R (1992) Conservative surgery of renal cell tumors in 140 patients: 21 years of experience. J Urol 148: 24–29; discussion 29–30.

Steinbach F, Novick AC, Zincke H, Miller DP, Williams RD, Lund G, Skinner DG, Esrig D, Richie JP, deKernion JB et al. (1995) Treatment of renal cell carcinoma in von Hippel-Lindau disease: a multicenter study. J Urol 153: 1812–1816.

Stolle C, Glenn G, Zbar B, Humphrey JS, Choyke P, Walther M, Pack S, Hurley K, Andrey C, Klausner R, Linehan WM (1998) Improved detection of germline mutations in the von Hippel-Lindau disease tumor suppressor gene. Hum Mutat 12: 417–423.

Tory K, Brauch H, Linehan M, Barba D, Oldfield E, Filling-Katz M, Seizinger B, Nakamura Y, White R, Marshall FF et al. (1989) Specific genetic change in tumors associated with von Hippel-Lindau disease. J Natl Cancer Inst 81: 1097–1101.

Van Velthoven V, Reinacher PC, Klisch J, Neumann HP, Glasker S (2003) Treatment of intramedullary hemangioblastomas, with special attention to von Hippel-Lindau disease. Neurosurgery 53: 1306–1313; discussion 1313–1314.

Von Hippel E (1896) Vorstellung eines Patienten mit einer sehr ungewohnlichen Netzhaut. XXIV Verstellung der ophthalmologischen Gesellschaft (Heidelberg, 1895). JF Bergman Verlag, Wiesbaden, 269.

Von Hippel E (1904) Ueber eine sehr seltene Erkrankung der Netzhaut. Klinische Beobachtungen. A von Graefe Arch Ophthalmol 59: 83–106.

Von Hippel E (1911) Die anatomische Grundlage der von mir beschriebenen "sehr seltene Erkrankung der Netzhaut". A von Graefe's Arch Ophthalmol 79: 350–377.

Vortmeyer AO, Gnarra JR, Emmert-Buck MR, Katz D, Linehan WM, Oldfield EH, Zhuang Z (1997) von Hippel-Lindau gene deletion detected in the stromal cell component of a cerebellar hemangioblastoma associated with von Hippel-Lindau disease. Hum Pathol 28: 540–543.

Walther MM, Lubensky IA, Venzon D, Zbar B, Linehan WM (1995) Prevalence of microscopic lesions in grossly normal renal parenchyma from patients with von Hippel-Lindau disease, sporadic renal cell carcinoma and no renal disease: clinical implications. J Urol 154: 2010–2014; discussion 2014–2015.

Walther MM, Choyke PL, Glenn G, Lyne JC, Rayford W, Venzon D, Linehan WM (1999a) Renal cancer in families with hereditary renal cancer: prospective analysis of a tumor size threshold for renal parenchymal sparing surgery. J Urol 161: 1475–1479.

Walther MM, Keiser HR, Choyke PL, Rayford W, Lyne JC, Linehan WM (1999b) Management of hereditary pheochromocytoma in von Hippel-Lindau kindreds with partial adrenalectomy. J Urol 161: 395–398.

Walther MM, Reiter R, Keiser HR, Choyke PL, Venzon D, Hurley K, Gnarra JR, Reynolds JC, Glenn GM, Zbar B, Linehan WM (1999c) Clinical and genetic characterization of pheochromocytoma in von Hippel-Lindau families: comparison with sporadic pheochromocytoma gives insight into natural history of pheochromocytoma. J Urol 162: 659–664.

Walther MM, Herring J, Choyke PL, Linehan WM (2000) Laparoscopic partial adrenalectomy in patients with hereditary forms of pheochromocytoma. J Urol 164: 14–17.

Wanebo JE, Lonser RR, Glenn GM, Oldfield EH (2003) The natural history of hemangioblastomas of the central nervous system in patients with von Hippel-Lindau disease. J Neurosurg 98: 82–94.

Wang C, Zhang J, Liu A, Sun B (2001) Surgical management of medullary hemangioblastoma. Report of 47 cases. Surg Neurol 56: 218–226; discussion 226–227.

Webster AR, Maher ER, Moore AT (1999) Clinical characteristics of ocular angiomatosis in von Hippel-Lindau disease and correlation with germline mutation. Arch Ophthalmol 117: 371–378.

Weil RJ, Lonser RR, DeVroom HL, Wanebo JE, Oldfield EH (2003) Surgical management of brainstem hemangioblastomas in patients with von Hippel-Lindau disease. J Neurosurg 98: 95–105.

Wittebol-Post D, Hes FJ, Lips CJ (1998) The eye in von Hippel-Lindau disease. Long-term follow-up of screening and treatment: recommendations. J Intern Med 243: 555–561.

Wong WT, Chew EY (2008) Ocular von Hippel-Lindau disease: clinical update and emerging treatments. Curr Opin Ophthalmol 19: 213–217.

Yip L, Lee JE, Shapiro SE, Waguespack SG, Sherman SI, Hoff AO, Gagel RF, Arens JF, Evans DB (2004) Surgical management of hereditary pheochromocytoma. J Am Coll Surg 198: 525–534; discussion 534–535.

Zbar B, Kishida T, Chen F, Schmidt L, Maher ER, Richards FM, Crossey PA, Webster AR, Affara NA, Ferguson-Smith MA, Brauch H, Glavac D, Neumann HP, Tisherman S, Mulvihill JJ, Gross DJ, Shuin T, Whaley J, Seizinger B, Kley N, Olschwang S, Boisson C, Richard S, Lips CH, Lerman M et al. (1996) Germline mutations in the Von Hippel-Lindau disease (VHL) gene in families from North America, Europe, and Japan. Hum Mutat 8: 348–357.

# Chapter 7

# KLIPPEL–TRANAUNAY, PARKES WEBER AND STURGE–WEBER SYNDROMES (INCLUDING KASABACH–MERRIT PHENOMENA)

Martino Ruggieri, Orhan Konez, and Ignacio Pascual-Castroviejo

Institute of Neurological Science, National Research Council, Catania, and Department of Paediatrics, University of Catania, Catania, Italy (MR); Department of Radiology, Vascular and Interventional Radiology, St. John West Shore Hospital; University Hospitals Case Medical Center, Westlake, Ohio, USA (OK); Paediatric Neurology Service, University Hospital La Paz, University of Madrid, Madrid, Spain (IPC)

## Introduction

The following chapters consider Klippel–Tranaunay syndrome (OMIM # 149000), Parkes Weber syndrome and Sturge–Weber syndrome (OMIM # 185300) together because all three have various types of vascular malformations and overgrowth involving the limbs in Klippel–Tranaunay and Parkes Weber syndromes and the head (but also other body regions) in Sturge–Weber syndrome (Cohen 2006, Cohen et al. 2002). Besides Sturge–Weber syndrome the other two conditions (or three if one includes Kasabach–Merrit syndrome) are not truly neurocutaneous disorders because their nervous system involvement is of limited extent if any and extremely infrequent. In these chapters however we have treated them all in consideration of their relevance for differential diagnosis.

These disorders have been also said to overlap with each other (Happle 1993, 2003; Vissers et al. 2003, reviewed in Gorlin et al. 2001), but they should be considered separate clinical entities that for the most part occur sporadically and have different clinical manifestations and types of complications (Cohen 2000, 2002, 2006; Cohen et al. 2002). In this connection, some authors (Cohen 2002, 2006; Cohen et al. 2002; Gorlin et al. 2001; Hand and Frieden 2002) find it essential to discuss along with the three main syndromes vascular tumours vs. vascular malformations and also the Kasabach–Merrit phenomenon.

## Current terminology

*Klippel–Tranaunay syndrome* consists of a complex constellation of anomalies that includes (a) combined vascular malformations of the capillary, venous, and lymphatic types, (b) varicosities of unusual distribution, in particular a lateral venous anomaly observed during infancy or childhood, and (c) limb enlargement (Berry et al. 1998; Cohen 2000, 2002, 2006; Cohen et al. 2002; Gorlin et al. 2001).

The main clinical features of *Parkes Weber syndrome* are enlarged arteries and veins, capillary or venous malformations, and enlargement of a limb (Cohen 2002, 2006; Cohen et al. 2002; Gorlin et al. 2001).

*Sturge–Weber syndrome* also known as encephalofacial or encephalotrigeminal angiomatosis or meningofacial angiomatosis is characterised by a capillary malformation involving the brain and meninges with or without choroid (and/or episclera or conjunctive) and skin (facial V1–V3 territory including the mouth, pharynx and nasal mucosa or often the rest of the body) involvement (Baselga 2004, Cohen 2006, Gorlin et al. 2001, Thomas-Sohl et al. 2004).

*Kasabach–Merrit syndrome* is better designated "*Kasabach–Merrit phenomenon*" because it is likely to be pathogenetically variable (as one of its features, thrombocytopenia occurs in various types of vascular neoplasms) and has variable therapeutic response. The term is frequently applied (incorrectly) to patients with extensive venous or lymphatic venous malformations who develop a localised intravascular coagulopathy (chronic consumptive coagulopathy) in which the platelet count is minimally depressed (varying from 50,000 to 150,000/mm$^3$). In contrast, thrombocytopenia is profound varying from 3,000 to 60,000/mm$^3$ with an average of <25,000/mm$^3$ (Cohen 2006, Sarker et al. 1997). This distinction has important treatment implications as for example, heparinisation might be indicated in consumptive coagulopathy in vascular malformations, particularly with thrombotic complications, but is contraindicated in Kasabach–Merrit thrombocytopenia found with vascular tumours (Sarkar et al. 1997; Cohen 2002, 2006). Similar diagnostic implications are applied to Kasabach–Merrit phenomenon vs. Klippel–Tranaunay syndrome (see below) (Cohen 2002, 2006; Cohen et al. 2002; Gorlin et al. 2001).

## Nosologic considerations on vascular confusion

The terminology describing congenital vascular birthmarks has been a source of confusion in the medical literature. Discrepant terms still exist (Hand and Frieden 2002, Vissers et al. 2003) and physicians have used multiple names to characterise the same anomaly. This persistent ambiguity has generated a increasing taxonomy (Cohen 2002, 2006; Happle 1993, 2003). Resolving vascular confusion has been a primary mission of John Mulliken and his co-workers (Burns et al. 1991; Cheung et al. 1997; Enjorlas and Mulliken 2000; Enjolras et al. 2001; Grevelink and Mulliken 1999; Martinez-Perez et al. 1995; Mulliken 1993, 1997, 1998; Mulliken and Burrows 2001; Mulliken and Glowacki 1982; Mulliken and Young 1988; Mulliken et al. 2006; Sarkar et al. 1997; Takahashi et al. 1994; Vikkula et al. 1998, 2001; reviewed in Hand and Frieden 2002; Cohen 2002, 2006; and Mulliken et al. 2006).

Mulliken and Glowacki (1982), Mulliken and Young (1988)and Mulliken et al. (2006) published a biological classification system which has become the most widely accepted (Cohen 2002, 2006; Hand and Frieden 2002) framework for classifying vascular birthmarks and is accepted as the official classification schema by the International Society for the Study of Vascular Anomalies (ISSVA) (Enjolras and Mulliken 2000, Mulliken et al. 2006). In the Mulliken classification (Mulliken 1993, Mulliken and Glowacki 1982, Mulliken et al. 2006) a distinction is made between vascular tumours and vascular malformations based on cellular kinetics and clinical behaviour. *Vascular tumours* have endothelial hyperplasia with rapid postnatal growth followed by slow involution. In contrast, *vascular malformations* are characterised by flat endothelium, and growth of the lesion is commensurate with growth of the child. An additional category, introduced by Burns et al. (1991) are *macular stains* (commonly knows as nevus flammeus) which are flat, pink, and irregularly outlined vascular lesions that are transient and disappear (Cohen 2006). The ISSVA classes for *tumours* include: (a) haemangioma of infancy (PHACE syndrome, diffuse neonatal haemangiomas and lumbosacral haemangiomas); (b) Kaposiformi haemangioendothelioma (with or without Kasabach–Merrit phenomenon); (c) Tufted angioma (with or without Kasabach–Merrit phenomenon); and (d) other vascular tumours. Vascular *malformations* of the skin can be assigned to one of five groups based on histological and clinical appearance: (a) *simple malformations (pure types)* [*fast flow*: arterial (AM) or arteriovenous (AVM) including also arteriovenous fistulas (AVF); *slow flow*: capillary (CM) including Cobb syndrome, Sturge–Weber syndrome, Cutis marmorata telangiectatica congenital, Phakomatosis pigmentovascularis, Robert-SC Phocomelia, Wiedemann-Beckwith syndrome and Hereditary neurocutaneous angioma; lymphatic (LM); and venous (VM) including Blue-rubber Bleb Nevus syndrome and glomangiomas]; or (b) *combined lesions (complex types)* which can be localised or syndromic [CLM including Klippel–Tranaunay syndrome and Proteus syndrome; CVM including Hyperkeratotic cutaneous capillary-venous malformations; CLVM including Parkes Weber syndrome and LVM] (Cohen 2002, 2006; Mulliken and Glowacki 1982; Mulliken 1993; Mulliken et al. 2006). All the above conditions are extensively treated in the present and other chapters and therefore we refer the reader to these sections. It must be noted however that these malformations can be isolated or be accompanied by soft tissue or bone hyper- or hypotrophy and other soft tissue abnormalities or tumours and extra-vascular malformations (Cohen 2001, Mulliken 1988). It is sometimes the combination of these associated features which better characterises a syndromic spectrum.

By using this classification system physicians are able to classify 90% of vascular anomalies seen in infants, which can be distinguished from one another by history taking and physical examination, without the need for ancillary studies such as ultrasonographic studies, computerised tomography (CT), magnetic resonance imaging (MRI) or histological examination (Hand and Friedman 2002, Vissers et al. 2003). In this respect however Hand and Frieden (2002) and Happle (1993, 2000, 2003) have been also careful to point out that in rare instances, vascular lesions may not behave in accordance with the modern classification of vascular anomalies (Cohen 2002, 2006). There are examples of clinical and histological overlaps between vascular tumours and malformations (Garzon et al. 2000) or rare congenital haemangiomas that do not involute (Enjolras et al. 2001) or histologically diagnosed haemangiomas of adulthood that do not regress (Mulliken and Burrows 2001). In addition, diagnostic difficulties exist when vascular anomalies present after infancy or the features which should distinguish tumours from malformations may not be evident on a single exam. In these cases laboratory tests (North et al. 2000) or imaging (Cohen 2002, 2006) may help. MRI is the most informative modality for studying odd vascular malformations and can demonstrate flow characteristics and the extent of involvement within tissue planes. In addition, an MRI with gadolinium administration can distinguish lymphatic from venous malformations, MR venograms or phlebography/venography can document accessory (deep) venous anomalies in the limbs. CT and/or MRI can also demonstrate arteriovenous malformations, intraosseous vascular malformations or leptomeningeal abnormalities (Cohen 2002, Konez et al. 2003).

Several case reports published in the last 20 years, claimed that often there is no clear distinction between some disorders with clinical and biological overlaps (Happle 2003, Vissers et al. 2003) and umbrella terms (such as for example Sturge–Weber–Klippel–Tranaunay syndrome) have been proposed to encompass mixing and coexisting phenotypes. Patients with Sturge–Weber syndrome have been described with other vascular abnormalities including the spectrum of Klippel–Tranaunay syndrome or associated pigmentary anomalies such as the blue nevus of phakomatosis pigmentovascularis (Al Robaee et al. 2004, Cho et al. 2001, Diociaiuti et al. 2005, Hagiwara et al. 1998, Lee et al. 2005, Saricaoglu et al. 2002, Uysal et al. 2000). The coexistence of clinical and/or imaging features of Sturge–Weber syndrome, Klippel–Trenaunay syndrome and phacomatosis pigmentovascularis in the same patient is not an exceptional event. In this respect and in agreement with other authors (Cohen 2000, 2002, 2006; Cohen et al. 2002; Gorlin et al. 2001) we believe that this conventional thinking can be seriously challenged. As it occurred with the different forms of neurofibromatosis (Ruggieri 1999, 2000, 2001; Ruggieri and Huson 1999, 2001) after careful literature review none of these mixed phenotypes stood up as a separate disorder (with the exception of true newly recognised disorders which however present with their own unique features). However, it could be that the loci of the responsible genes for all (or some of) these conditions (e.g., Sturge–Weber, Klippel–Trenaunay and Parkes Weber syndromes) might be probably close neighbours (see below and Tian et al. 2004) on that the protein products of the defective gene(s) share common pathways or cooperate with each other.

Here below we analyse this important topic with regard to Klippel–Trenaunay, Parkes Weber and Sturge–Weber syndromes tabulating the criteria for distinction between the three disorders.

## Klippel–Tranaunay vs. Parkes Weber vs. Sturge–Weber: overlaps or variations on a theme?

The multiple, combined vascular malformations and skeletal asymmetry characteristics of Klippel–

Tranaunay syndrome and Parkes Weber syndrome and the capillary malformation (nevus flammeus) typical of Sturge–Weber syndrome often occur in the same patients, establishing them as overlapping disorders (Happle 1993, 2000, 2003; Vissers et al. 2003; Wilson 2004).

Conventional wisdom about *Klippel–Tranaunay syndrome* and *Sturge–Weber syndrome* include reviewed in (Cohen 2002, 2006): 1) overlap between Klippel–Tranaunay and Sturge–Weber syndromes; 2) addition of arteriovenous fistulas and renaming of the disorder as Klippel–Tranaunay-Weber syndrome; 3) the presence of a bleeding diathesis of the Kasabach–Merrit type in Klippel–Tranaunay syndrome; and 4) familial aggregation in either syndrome with various genetic interpretations (Cohen et al. 2002, Gorlin et al. 2001). *Sturge–Weber syndrome* is defined as a capillary malformation of the leptomeninges with or without choroid and facial V1 or V1–V3 involvement (Cohen 1998). Capillary malformations of the skin may extend to appear anywhere on the body, including the upper and lower limbs. Presumed cases of "*merged*" *Klippel–Tranaunay syndrome* and *Sturge–Weber syndrome* most always represent Sturge–Weber syndrome with capillary malformations only below the head and neck. Few of these cases however could represent "combined cases" because of the presence of essential manifestations of Klippel–Tranaunay syndrome such as lymphatic malformations, lateral venous anomaly, lymphatic vesicles, and venous flares within the capillary malformation, limb enlargement, and macrodactyly (Cohen 2006). On the other hand, most large surgical series of Klippel–Tranaunay syndrome patients do not include patients with capillary malformations involving the face (Lindenauer 1965, Mulliken 1999, Serville 1985, Young 1998). Hemiparesis, present in some cases of Sturge–Weber syndrome, may result in a hypotrophic limb. Overgrowth may occur in Sturge–Weber syndrome but tends to be minor and is always secondary to the vascular anomaly. Hypertrophy of the area with the capillary malformation in the face may occur with time and overgrowth of the bony maxillae is common in Sturge–Weber syndrome. When the capillary malformation involves the ear, its length may be greater than that of the contralateral ear. Rarely, a digit may be enlarged. In contrast, overgrowth in Klippel–Tranaunay syndrome is striking and macrodactyly may occur in the "uninvolved" limb (reviewed in Cohen 2002, 2006).

*Parkes Weber* and *Klippel–Tranaunay syndromes* are similar but some important distinctive features exist: 1) slow-flow venous malformations are predominant in Klippel–Tranaunay syndrome (vs. fast-flow vascular malformations in Parkes Weber syndrome), but arteriovenous (AV) fistulas are always found in Parkes-Weber syndrome; 2) the colour of the cutaneous malformation in Parkes-Weber syndrome is

**Table 1.** Criteria for distinction between Klippel–Tranaunay, Parkes Weber and Sturge–Weber syndromes

| | |
|---|---|
| **Klippel–Tranaunay** | Slow-flow, combined vascular (capillary, lymphatic and venous) involving limb(s) and/pr trunk. Bluish to purplish colour of vascular malformation. Insignificant arteriovenous fistula. Very common lateral venous anomaly. Lymphatic vesicles and venous flares found. Disproportionate limb enlargement involving soft tissue and bone; macrodactyly (particularly of toes). Good prognosis (occasional pulmonary embolia). |
| **Parkes Weber** | Fast follow, combined vascular (capillary, arterial, and venous) involving upper/lower limbs; usually pink and more diffuse colour of vascular malformation. Significant arteriovenous fistula. Lateral venous anomaly, lymphatic vesicles and venous flares not found. Arm or leg length discrepancy. More problematic prognosis (bradycardia, cardiac enlargement with limb amputation). |
| **Sturge–Weber** | Capillary malformation of leptomeninges with or without choroid (episclera/conjunctive) and facial (V1–V3) involvement. Capillary malformations can occur elsewhere in the body. Glaucoma. Common associated neurological manifestations including seizures, neurological deficits, stroke-like episodes, headache, developmental delay, lower limb(s) hemihyperplasia. |

Adapted from Cohen 2002, 2006 and Cohen et al. 2002.

usually more diffuse and pinker than that observed in Klippel–Tranaunay syndrome; 3) lymphatic malformations do not occur and no lymphatic vessels are found in the discoloured skin of Parkes Weber syndrome; and 4) the prognosis in Parkes Weber syndrome is more problematic particularly in those developing bradycardia leading to cardiac failure, cardiac enlargement and cutaneous ischemia requiring limb amputation. We summarise the main differences in Table 1.

By applying these simple diagnostic criteria (e.g., capillary malformation of leptomeninges and/or choroid and/or facial trigeminal regions vs. combined vascular lesions) overlaps and mixed phenotypes become almost always untenable. For instance in a recent case reported by Vissers et al. (2003) Sturge–Weber syndrome was claimed to coexist with Klippel–Tranaunay syndrome. However, careful and critical review of clinical summary and accompanying illustrations shows this was a Sturge–Weber syndrome because of "widespread capillary malformation on the face", neuroimaging demonstration of "leptomeningeal dysplasia at the level of the right occipital lobe with ipsilateral enlarged choroid plexus and subsequent "cortical atrophy in the same anatomical region" associated to "glaucoma of the right eye occurred at the age of 11 years", "complex partial seizures" and "psychomotor retardation". Additional areas of vascular (capillary) malformation in a mosaic pattern over the buttock and left leg and soft tissue overgrowth (and bone hyperplasia) in the areas within the vascular anomaly in the leg. Assignment of this patient to two different clinical entities (Vissers et al. 2003) or designation of new terms (such as Sturge–Weber–Klippel–Tranaunay syndrome) (Happle 2003) may be unjustified on clinical and imaging grounds.

One important issue in favour of possible overlaps between Klippel–Tranaunay, Parkes Weber and/or Sturge–Weber syndromes or a continuum spectrum of disorders is the recently proposed *angiogenic/vasculogenic model* which has been applied to Klippel–Tranaunay syndrome (Klessinger and Christ 1996) (see also chapter on Klippel–Tranaunay syndrome). This model suggests that the distinctive midline demarcation in Klippel–Tranaunay syndrome may be due to defined boundaries for endothelial

migration (bounded by the notocord) which cause defects in axial blood vessel formation (Sumoy et al. 1997). The genetic alteration that results in Klippel–Tranaunay syndrome may be located in endothelial cells altered in the process of vessels formation and the cellular lesion leading to the manifestations of Klippel–Tranaunay syndrome may be related to persistence of foetal structures (i.e., the foetal dermal capillary web an foetal vasculature) (Baskerville et al. 1985). The morphogenetic defect causing Klippel–Tranaunay syndrome thus may affect the normal process of remodelling of developing vascular structures as *vasculogenesis* (the process of generation of primitive vasculature networks which involves the differentiation of endothelial cells from mesenchimal progenitors to form a primary vascular plexus or network) and *angiogenesis* (the process that occurs once the primary plexus is established and new capillaries are formed by sprouting/budding and non sprouting/intussusception, or splitting) occur, perhaps by an interference with apoptosis required for vessel remodelling during embryogenesis. A series of ligands appear to be critical regulators of angiogenesis and vasculogenesis including members of the vascular endothelial growth factor (VEGF) (Cohen 2006, Klagsbrun and D'Amore 1996). Recently, an elegant combination of human genetics and functional analysis allowed the discovery of the first *susceptibility gene* for Klippel–Tranaunay syndrome (Tian et al. 2004, Whelan et al. 1995): the VG5Q (angiogenic factor VG5Q) gene (on chromosome 5q13.3) expressed strongly in blood vessels and secreted upon initiation of angiogenesis. Over expression of VG5Q stimulates angiogenesis and suppression of VG5Q by RNA or anti sense inhibits vessel formation. On the basis of the model of Tian et al. (2004) and according to the hypothesis of paradominance of Happle (1993, 2000, 2003) patients with the VG5Q E113K mutation may carry a second mutational hit in VG5Q or another gene within the affected tissue (Tian et al. 2004).

Thus, it could be that susceptibility genes may cause localised phenotypes characterised by either simple [Sturge–Weber syndrome with lesions confined to one or more tissues (i.e., skin, eye and leptomeninges) in the head only] or mixed

(Klippel–Tranaunay or Parkes Weber syndromes) vascular malformations or more generalised phenotypes (Sturge–Weber syndrome with head and trunk involvement) or ultimately to "merged" (overlapping) types of vascular malformations such as phakomatosis vasculovascularis or mixed epidermal/vascular malformations such as phakomatosis pigmentovascularis.

## References

Al Robaee A, Banka N, Alfadley A (2004) Phakomatosis pigmentovascularis type IIb associated with Sturge–Weber syndrome. Pediatr Dermatol 21: 642–645.

Baselga E (2004) Sturge–Weber syndrome. Semin Cut Med Surg 23: 87–98.

Baskerville PA, Ackroyd JS, Browse NL (1985) The etiology of the Klippel–Tranaunay syndrome. Ann Surg 202: 624–627.

Berry SA, Peterson C, Mize W, Bloom K, Zachary C, Blasco P, Hunter D (1998) Klippel–Tranaunay syndrome. Am J Med Genet 79: 319–326.

Burns AJ, Kaplan LC, Mulliken JB (1991) Is there an association between hemangioma and syndromes with dysmorphic features? Pediatrics 88: 1257–1267.

Cheung DSM, Warman MI, Mulliken JB (1997) Hemangioma in twins. Ann Plast Surg 38: 269–274.

Cho S, Choi JH, Sung KJ, Moon KC, Koh JK (2001) Phakomatosis pigmentovascularis type IIb with neurologic abnormalities. Pediatr Dermatol 18: 263.

Cohen MM Jr (2000) Klippel–Tranaunay syndrome. Am J Med Genet 93: 171–175.

Cohen MM Jr (2002) Vasculogenesis, angiogenesis, hemangiomas, and vascular malformations. Am J Med Genet 108: 265–274.

Cohen MM Jr (2006) Vascular update: morphogenesis, tumors, malformations, and molecular dimensions. Am J Med Genet A 140A: 2013–2038.

Cohen MM Jr, Neri G, Weksberg R (2002) Klippel–Tranaunay syndrome, Parkes Weber syndrome, and Sturge–Weber syndrome. In: Cohen MM Jr, Neri G, Weksberg R (eds.) Overgrowth Syndromes. New York: Oxford University Press, pp. 111–124.

Diociaiuti A, Guidi B, Aguilar Sanchez JA, Feliciani C, Capizzi R, Amerio P (2005) Phakomatosis pigmentovascularis type IIb: a case associated with Sturge–Weber and Klippel–Tranaunay syndrome. J Am Acad Dermatol 53: 536–539.

Enjorlas O, Wassef M, Mazoyer E, Frieden IJ, Rieu PN, Drouet L, Taieb A, Stalder JF, Escande JP (1997) Infants with Kasabach–Merrit syndrome do not have "true" heangiomas. J Pediatr 130: 631–640.

Enjorlas O, Mulliken JB (1998) Vascular tumors and vascular malformations. Adv Dermatol 13: 375–422.

Enjorlas O, Mulliken JB, Boon LM, Wassef M, Kozakevich HPW, Burrows PE (2001) Noninvoluting congenital hemangiomas: a rare cutaneous vascular anomaly. Plast Reconstr Surg 107: 1647–1654.

Enjorlas O, Mulliken JB (2006) Vascular birthmarks. In: Harper J, Oranje AP, Prose NS (eds.) Textbook of Pediatric Dermatology. pp. 1345–1377.

Garzon MC, Enjorlas O, Frieden IJ (2000) Vascular tumors and vascular malformations: evidence for an association. J Am Acad Dermatol 42: 275–279.

Gorlin RJ, Cohen MM Jr, Hennekam RCM (2001) Klippel–Tranaunay syndrome, Parkes Weber syndrome, and Sturge–Weber syndrome. In: Gorlin RJ, Cohen MM Jr, Hennekam M (eds.) Syndromes of the Head and Neck, 4th ed. New York: Oxford University Press, pp. 453–460.

Grevelink SV, Mulliken JB (1999) Vascular anomalies. In: Fitzpatrick TB (ed.) Dermatology in General Medicine, 5th ed. New York: Mc Graw Hill, pp. 1175–1194.

Hagiwara K, Uezato H, Nonaka S (1998) Phacomatosis pigmentovascularis type IIb associated with Sturge–Weber syndrome and pyogenic granulom. J Dermatol 25: 721–729.

Hand JL, Frieden IJ (2002) Vascular birthmarks of infancy: resolving nosologic confusion. Am J Med Genet 108: 257–264.

Happle R (1993) Mosaicism in human skin. Understanding the patterns and mechanisms. Arch Dermatol 129: 1460–1470.

Happle R (2003) Sturge–Weber-Klippel–Tranaunay syndrome: what's in a name? Eur J Dermatol 13: 237.

Happle R (2006) Mosaicism in human skin. In: Harper J, Oranje AP, Prose NS (eds.) Textbook of Pediatric Dermatology, pp. 1321–1335.

Hennekam RCM (ed.) Syndromes of the Head and Neck, 4th ed. New York: Oxford University Press, pp. 453–460.

Klessinger S, Christ B (1996) Axial structures control laterality in the distribution pattern of endothelial cells. Anat Embryol (Berl) 193: 39–330.

Konez O, Burrows PE, Mulliken JB, Fishman SJ, Kozakewich HP (2003) Angiographic features of rapidly involuting congenital hemangioma (RICH). Ped Radiol 33: 15–19.

Lee CW, Choi DY, Oh YG, Yoon HS, Kim JD (2005) An infantile case of Sturge–Weber syndrome in association with Klippel–Tranaunay–Weber syndrome and phakomatosis pigmentovascularis. J Korean Med Sci 20: 1082–1084.

Lindenauer SM (1965) The Klippel–Tranaunay-Weber syndrome: varicosity, hypertrophy, and hemangioma with no arteriovenous fistula. Ann Surg 162: 303–314.

Martinez-Perez D, Fein NA, Boon LM Mulliken JB (1995) Not all hemangiomas look like strawberries: uncommon presentations of the most common tumor in infancy. Pediatr Dermatol 12: 1–6.

Mulliken JB (1993a) Cutaneous vascular anomalies. Semin Vasc Surg 6: 204–218.

Mulliken JB (1993b) A biologic classification of vascular birthmarks. In: Boccalon H (ed.) Amsterdam: Elsevier Science Publisher, pp. 613–614.

Mulliken JB (1997) Vascular anomalies. In: Aston SJ, Beasley RW, Thorne CHM (eds.) Grabb and Smith's Plastic Surgery, 5th ed. Philadelphia: Lippincott-Raven, pp. 191–203.

Mulliken JB (1999) Personal communication.

Mulliken JB, Glowacki J (1982) Hemangiomas and vascular malformations in infants and children: a classification based on endothelial characteristics. Plast Reconstr Surg 69: 412–420.

Mulliken JB, Young AE (1988) Vascular Birthmarks: Haemangiomas and Malformations. Philadelphia: WB Saunders Company, pp. 246–264.

Mulliken JB, Burrows PE (2001) Vascular malformations. In: Golwyn RM, Cohen MN (eds.) The Unfavourable Results in Plastic Surgery, 3rd ed. Philadelphia: Lippincott-Raven, pp. 271–287.

Mulliken JB, Fishman SJ, Bunows PE (2006) Vascular anomalies, hemangiomas, and malformations. New York: Oxford University Press.

North PE, Warner M, Mizeracki A, Mihm MC (2000) GLUT1: a newly discovered immunohistochemical marker for juvenile hemangiomas. Hum Pathol 31: 11–22.

OMIM™ (2006) Online Mendelian Inheritance in Man. Baltimore: Johns Hopkins University Press. http://www.ncbi.nlm.nih.gov/omim

Ruggieri M (1999) The different forms of neurofibromatosis. Child's Nerv Syst 15: 295–308.

Ruggieri M (2001) Mosaic (segmental) neurofibromatosis type 1 (NF1) and type 2 (NF2) – no longer neurofibromatosis type 5. Am J Med Genet 101: 178–180.

Ruggieri M, Huson SM (2001) The clinical and diagnostic implications of mosaicism in the neurofibromatoses. Neurology 56: 1433–1443.

Saricaoglu MS, Guven D, Karakurt A, Sengun A, Ziraman I (2002) An unusual case of Sturge–Webers syndrome in association with phakomatosis pigmentovascularis and Klippel–Tranaunay-Weber syndrome Retina 22: 368–371.

Sarkar M, Mulliken JB, Kozakewich HP, Robertson RL, Burrows PE (1997) Thrombocytopenic coagulopathy (Kasabach–Merritt phenomenon) is associated with Kaposiform hemangioendothelioma and not with common infantile hemangioma. Plast Reconstr Surg 100: 1377–1386.

Servelle M (1985) Klippel and Trenaunay's syndrome. 768 operated acses. Ann Surg 201: 365–373.

Sumoy L, Keasey JB, Dittman TD, Kimelman D (1997) A role for notochord in axial vascular development revealed by analysis of phenotype and the expression of VEGR-2 in zebrafush flh and ntl mutant embryos. Mech Dev 63: 15–27.

Takahashi K, Mulliken JB, Kozakevich HPW, Rogers RA, Folkman J, Ezekowitz RAB (1994) Cellular markers that distinguish the phases of hemangioma during infancy and childhood. J Clin Invest 93: 2357–2364.

Thomas-Sohl KA, Vaslow DF, Maria BL (2004) Sturge–Weber syndrome: a review. Pediatr Neurol 30: 303–310.

Uysal G, Guven A, Ozhan B, Ozturk MH, Mutluay AH, Tulunay O (2000) Phakomatosis pigmentovascularis with Sturge–Weber syndrome. J Dermatol 27: 467–470.

Vikkula M, Boon LM, Mulliken JB, Olsen BR (1998) Molecular basis of vascular anomalies. Trends Cardiovasc Med 8: 281–292.

Vikkula M, Boon LM, Mulliken JB (2001) Molecular genetics of vascular malformations. Matrix Biol 20: 327–335.

Vissers W, Van Steensel M, Steijlen P, Van der Kerkhof P, Van der Vleuten C (2003) Klippel–Tranaunay syndrome and Sturge–Weber syndrome: variations on a theme? Eur J Dermatol 13: 238–241.

Whelan AJ, Watson MS, Porter FD, Steiner RD (1995) Klippel–Tranaunay-Weber syndrome associated with a 5:11 balanced translocation. Am J Med Genet 59: 492–494.

Young AE (1988) Hemangiomas and malformations. In: Mulliken JB, Young AE (eds.) Vascular birthmarks. Philadelphia: WB. Saunders.

# Chapter 8

# KLIPPEL–TRENAUNAY SYNDROME

**Martino Ruggieri, Concezio Di Rocco, and Orhan Konez**

Institute of Neurological Science, National Research Council, Catania, and Department of Paediatrics, University of Catania, Catania, Italy (MR); Section of Paediatric Neurosurgery, Department of Paediatrics, Catholic University of Sacred Heart, Rome, Italy (CDR); Department of Radiology, Vascular and Interventional Radiology, St. John West Shore Hospital, University Hospitals Case Medical Center, Westlake, OHIO, USA (OK)

## Introduction

*Klippel–Trenaunay syndrome* is characterised by (a) combined vascular malformations of the capillary, venous, and lymphatic types, (b) varicosities of unusual distribution, in particular a lateral venous anomaly observed during infancy or childhood, and (c) limb enlargement with limb asymmetry (Berry et al. 1998; Cohen 2000, 2002, 2006; Cohen et al. 2002; Gorlin et al. 2001; Huang and Creath 1994).

## Historical perspective and terminology

**Maurice Klippel** was born on 30 May 1858, in Mulhouse, France to a well-established family. He undertook medical studies in Paris where he was resident at the Hospitaux de Paris in 1884 and obtained his doctorate in 1889. Klippel was elevated to the attending staff at the same hospital in 1896 and appointed to a senior post, as chief of the service, at the Hospice Debrousse in 1901. The following year he became chief of the general medical service at the Hopital Tenon, Paris. He remained in this post until his retirement in January 1924. He published prodigiously, his last articles being submitted in 1942, the year of his death in Vevey, France. He wrote 340 papers and several monographs concerning histology, pathology, and congenital disorders, but he was best known for his publications on neurology and psychiatry. When Klippel died at the age of 84 years in his obituary (Obituary 1942) he was described as "a philosopher, poet, historian and one of the most prominent masters of French medicine" (Beighton and Beighton 1986). Among his areas of interest there were histology, general pathology, gross pathol-

ogy, neurology, psychiatry, neuropathology, psychopathology, and congenital hereditary and familial illnesses and malformations. To his scientific interests he added philosophy and poetry publishing books on these topics as well. His name is attached to several medical conditions (besides Klippel–Trenaunay) including Klippel–Feil syndrome, and Klippel–Feldstein syndrome (simple familial cranial hypertrophy) (Patel and Lauerman 1995).

**Paul Trenaunay**, born in 1875, was a Parisian physician and a junior colleague of Klippel's at the time of their case description (Beighton and Beighton 1986) published in 1900 (Klippel and Trenaunay 1900). At that time the two French physicians (Klippel and Trenaunay 1900) first noted the combination of capillary nevus, early onset of varicosities, and hypertrophy of tissues and bones of the affected limb. That paper (Klippel and Trenaunay 1900) shows that "Trenaunay" not "Trénaunay" is correct; there is no accent é, although many articles have added the accent (Cohen et al. 2002, 2006). The original three findings constituted the primary diagnostic criteria of the *Klippel–Trenaunay syndrome*.

In their original paper (Klippel and Trenaunay 1900) however these authors mention that in 1869, Trelat and Monod (1869) described the same disorder in six patients. Geoffry Saint-Hilaire (1942) on discussing hemi hypertrophy advised not to overlook extensive hemiangiomas. Friedberg in 1867 described a 10-year-old girl with hypertrophy of the right leg, phlebectasias, and varicosities (Stickler 1987).

*Weber* in 1907 (Weber 1907) reported patients with hypertrophic limbs and in a later publication (Weber 1918) pointed out their association with arteriovenous fistulas (anastomoses), and the additional name Weber is sometimes added to describe those individuals who also have clinical significant arteriovenous malformations as a component of their Klippel–Trenaunay syndrome (Berry et al. 1998, Cohen et al. 2002, Gorlin et al. 2001). Kramer (1972) discussed the historical aspects in greater detail (see also Beighton and Beighton 1986 and the historical background in the chapter on Parkes Weber syndrome).

Conventional thinking about Klippel–Trenaunay syndrome includes the following: 1) addition of arteriovenous fistulas and renaming of the disorder as Klippel–Trenaunay–Weber syndrome; 2) overlap between Sturge–Weber syndrome; 3) the presence of a bleeding diathesis of the Kasabach-Merrit type; and 4) familial aggregation with various genetic interpretations (Cohen et al. 2002, 2006; Gorlin et al. 2001). As mentioned in the previous chapter this conventional thinking can be seriously challenged.

Among the *eponyms* used (in the past) for this disorder are naevus variquex ostéohypertrophique, angiomatosis osteohypertrophica, angio-osteohypertrophy, nevus vasculosus osteohypertrophicus, haemangiectasia hypertrophicans, telangiectasia and angioelephantiasis and angioplastic macrosomia (Stickler 1987, Taybi and Lachman 1996).

## Incidence and prevalence

The prevalence of Klippel–Trenaunay syndrome is unknown. Stickler (1987) writing on Klippel–Trenaunay syndrome in Gomez's book on neurocutaneous diseases acknowledged at least 400–500 patients and well over 1500 cases have been recorded more recently (Cohen et al. 2002, 2006; Huang et al. 1994; Mulliken and Glowacki 1982; Samuel and Spitz 1995; Young 1978). Servelle (1985) alone documented 768 operated patients. Aelvoet et al. (1992) calculated the frequency of familial Klippel–Trenaunay syndrome as high as 1 in 880 first- and second-degree family members.

## Clinical manifestations

Usually monomelic (lower limb in about three fourth of the cases), this condition is characterised by the classical defining triad of capillary-venous malformation (CVM) or capillary-venous-lymphatic malformation (CVLM), superficial varicosities and soft-tissue/bone hypertrophy (Berry et al. 1998, Huang et al. 1994, Mulliken et al. 2006, Taybi and Lachman 1996). Capillary-lymphatic-arteriovenous malformation (CLAVM) have been recorded even though rather uncommonly (Berry et al. 1998).

### Skin abnormalities

#### Capillary malformations

The primary cutaneous manifestation of Klippel–Trenaunay syndrome is a diffuse superficial capillary malformation, bluish to purplish in colour, typically present on an affected limb although skin changes can be seen on any body part (Figs. 1–4). These

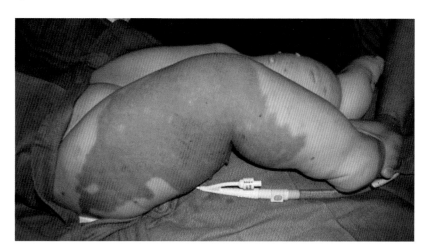

Fig. 1. An infant with a large stain on the leg.

often have an irregular, but relatively linear, border (Fig. 1). Common distribution patterns include lower limb(s) (Fig. 1) or mosaic lesions diffused over the trunk and limbs. When found on the trunk, the malformation rarely crosses the midline, sometimes exhibiting a sharp demarcation (Berry et al. 1998). According to Maari and Frieden (2004) cutaneous vascular stains can be classified into: 1) *geographic* which are extremely sharply demarcated, with irregular shape (resembling a country or a continent), dark red/purplish in colour (Fig. 1); or 2) *blotchy/segmental* having indistinct demarcation from normal skin in at least some areas (often with sharp demarcation from normal skin at midline), often large, typically with a segmental distribution and light pink or red-pink in colour. These vascular malformations are typically combined with cutaneous capillary malformation and persistence of abnormal superficial veins (Figs. 2–4) associated with deep venous hypoplasia, duplications, and abnormal venous valve formation (Berry et al. 1998, Cohen et al. 2002). Histopathological examination shows no specific morphological changes: subcutaneous tissue, muscle, synovium and other tissues contain blood-filled "cavernous" channels lined by single layers of endothelial cells (the latter thinned out or even absent in some places or lacking a basal membrane) with no cellular extravasation but with perivascular oedema (Stickler 1987). Vessel walls contain collagens and sparse smooth muscle. The rare arteries are of small caliber and seem to float in the midst of the cavernous spaces.

Most large surgical series of Klippel–Trenaunay syndrome patients do not include patients with capillary malformations involving the face on craniofacial region (Cohen 2006). Capillary malformations may be studded with lymphatic vesicles and venous flares.

## Secondary skin malformations

These may include eczema, hyperhidrosis, atrophy, ulceration, and cellulites. Among the cutaneous changes related to chronic venous insufficiency are oedema, hyperpigmentation, poor healing and ulceration.

## Vascular abnormalities

### Varicosities

Varicosities in Klippel–Trenaunay syndrome differ from commonly occurring varicose veins in that the distribution is different (being more extensive), and the age of onset is different (first being manifest during infancy or childhood). The classic lesion (found in about 80% of cases) is the lateral

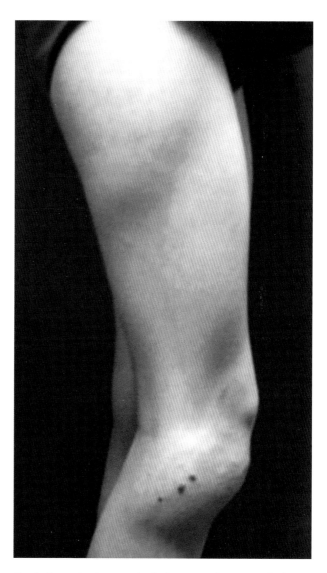

**Fig. 2.** Large focal areas of soft tissue prominence on the lateral side of the upper thigh and knee representing large venous anomalies.

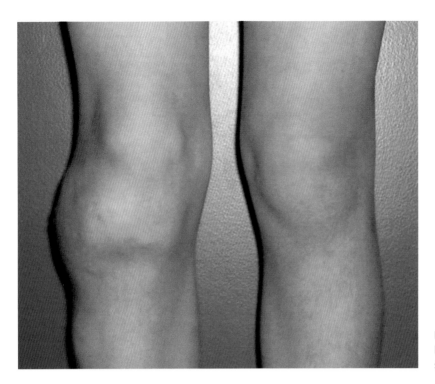

**Fig. 3.** Large soft tissue prominence on the lateral and frontal aspect of the knee representing a large varicoid venous anomaly.

venous anomaly and is known among surgeons as the vein of Servelle (Figs. 2 and 3). The malformations begin as a plexus of veins on the dorsum and lateral side of the foot and extends superiorly for various distances. Termination may occur in the popliteal vein (11%), superficial femoral vein (17%), deep femoral vein (19%), and external iliac vein (6%); full length extension is found in 33% of patients (Berry et al. 1998; Cohen et al. 2002, 2006). Veins may have a valve or may be valve-less. Ectatic veins may appear as studded venous flares in capillary malformation of the skin resulting from reflux of venous blood secondary to hypertension in the main venous anomaly. Intermittent episodes of thrombophlebitis in the affected limb have been reported in about 50% of cases often associated with pain.

Abnormalities of the deep veins may be common and defects include agenesis, atresia, hypoplasia, valvular incompetence, or aneurismal dilatations.

Significant arteriovenous communications of the type found in Parkes Weber syndrome are never found in Klippel–Trenaunay syndrome.

## Lymphatic malformations

These abnormalities are found in more than 70% of Klippel–Trenaunay patients. Cutaneous capillary malformations may be studded with lymphatic vesicles that leak lymph. Lymphoedema of the lower limb is particularly common. Micro- and macro cystic lymphatic malformations often involve the groin, genitalia, and retroperitoneum.

## Limb enlargement

Lower limb(s) enlargement is found in almost all cases. The affected limb may be thicker and longer (Figs. 1, 3 and 4). Thickness results from soft tissue enlargement (Figs. 5 and 6) and is especially pronounced with lymphatic involvement. Increased adiposity is found in some patients. When the long bones are involved, the affected limb is increased in length and bone thickness is also increased. With leg length discrepancy, compensatory scoliosis may ensue. In some cases there is atrophic instead of hypertrophic limb.

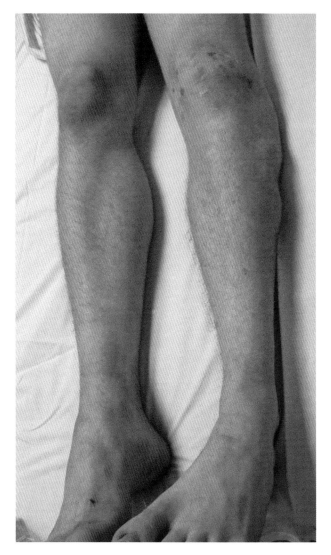

**Fig. 4.** There are large varicosities in the lateral upper calf.

Macrodactyly may involve toes on the affected foot but may be present on both feet. Other miscellaneous defects may include cutaneous syndactyly (which rarely involves more than two toes), polydactyly, clinodactyly, talipes equinovarus, talipes calcaneovarus, lobster claw hands, hammer toes, clubbed feet, and metatarsus varus (Cohen 2006, Cohen et al. 2002, Taybi and Lachman 1996).

## Eye abnormalities

These include conjunctive telangiectasias, retinal varicosities, choroidal angioma and glaucoma (probably due to misdiagnosis with Sturge–Weber syndrome), orbital varix, heterochromia iridis, iritic coloboma, abnormal discs, oculosympathetic paralysis, buphthalmos, Marcus Gunn pupil and strabismus (reviewed by O'Connor and Smith 1978 and Stickler 1987).

## Nervous system involvement

In one case Klippel–Trenaunay syndrome was associated with congenital nystagmus, anisomyopia and hemigalencephaly (Burke et al. 1991, Huang et al. 1994). Berry et al. (1998) recorded one child with extensive skin involvement including all four limbs, the scalp and face who had intracranial blood noted at delivery and developmental delay (probably a misdiagnosis) and another with macrocephaly and accelerated head circumference growth.

Vascular malformations of the brain have been recorded (Stickler 1987). Alberti (1976) described a

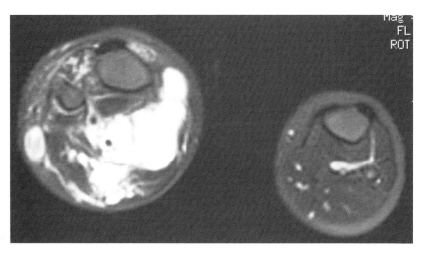

**Fig. 5.** T2 weighted axial MRI shows a large low-flow vascular anomaly (bright signal area) involving multiple muscle groups (see left part of the figure). Small rounded dark signal areas in the posterior calf represent normal tibial arteries. Please note that the diseased extremity is significantly larger than the other leg.

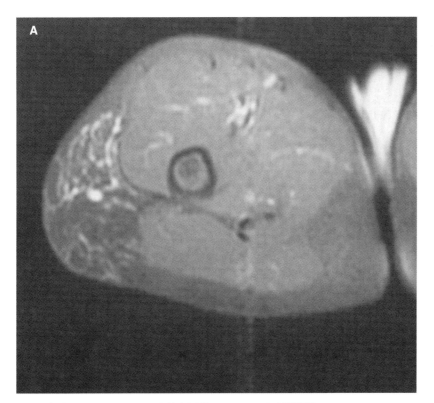

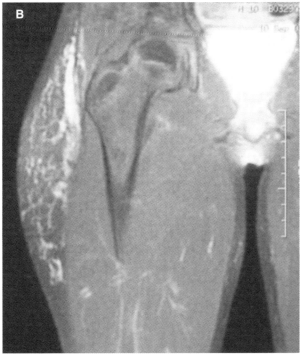

**Fig. 6.** Axial (**A**) and coronal (**B**) post-contrast MR images demonstrate a large soft tissue abnormality in the thigh laterally demonstrating streaky areas of abnormal contrast enhancement. This form of contrast enhancement is generally seen in lymphatic or lymphatic venous type low-flow anomalies. Note the large marginal vein opacify with contrast in the lateral upper thigh.

25-year-old man with right-sided extremity lesions of the Klippel–Trenaunay type who died of ischaemic infarct of the brain (he had multiple intracranial aneurismal dilatation of the basilar artery and of the junction of the right vertebral artery with the basilar artery). In some reported cases there was documentation of angiomatosis of the cerebellum and the medulla oblongata (Stickler 1987), of spinal arteriovenous malformations including fistulas (Rohany et al. 2007), of spinal intramedullary convernous angioma (Pichierri et al. 2006) and of peripheral neuropathy due to epineural microscopic arteriovenous anastomoses (Di Iorio et al. 2005).

Other recorded abnormalities have been micro- and acrocephaly, cerebral and cerebellar hemihypertrophy (with increased thickness of the white matter; reviewed by Torregrosa et al. 2000), cerebral atrophy, cerebral calcifications, angiomatous leptomeningeal enlargement and markedly enhancing choroid plexus (probably due to misdiagnosis with Sturge–Weber syndrome), aplasia of the cervical internal carotid artery and malformation of the circle of Willis, cerebral arteriovenous fistula cerebral haemangiopericytoma, Arnold-Chiari type 1 malformation, spinal cord arteriovenous fistula and spinal cord arteriovenous malformations (Anlar et al. 1998, Chen and Shu 1996, Cristaldi et al. 1995, Mathews et al. 2008, Matsubara et al. 1993, Valde's et al. 2007, Wolpert et al. 1994, You et al. 1983, reviewed in Taybi and Lachman 1996).

In our 19 children with the classical findings of Klippel–Trenaunay syndrome only one had nervous system involvement (unilateral hypoplasia of the circle of Wills) irrespective of extension of skin involvement (unreported data).

## Disease complications

Most complications of the condition are related to abnormal vasculature (Berry et al. 1998, Taybi and Lachman 1996). These include thrombosis, coagulopathy, pulmonary embolism (found in 10% of children or higher in adults) with secondary pulmonary hypertension, heart failure (in the presence of significant AVM), and bleeding from abnormal vessels in the gut, kidney, or genitalia. Gastrointestinal bleeding can be severe and its occurrence in these patients

should prompt an aggressive evaluation using non-invasive imaging and endoscopy. When the region of the trunk is involved with vascular lesions lymphatic anomalies of the intestine may be associated with a protein-losing enteropathy.

Internal organ involvement include recurrent nodular haemangiomas located on the trunk associated with visceral vascular malformations; chronic renal failure; hematuria; rectal bleeding.

Hemifacial hypertrophy has been also recorded as well as malocclusion and early eruption of permanent teeth.

Infection is a particular risk for those patients with abnormal lymphatic drainage. Some older children or adults also have pain due to venous insufficiency or lymphoedema.

Women with Klippel–Trenaunay syndrome may have complicated pregnancies (e.g., pulmonary embolism) (Rebarber et al. 2004) depending on the location of their vascular anomalies. According to the most recent studies however careful management of affected mothers during pregnancy achieves successful pregnancies (Rebarber et al. 2004).

Miscellaneous abnormalities include systemic hypertension, hypospadia, basal cell and squamous cell carcinoma of the affected limb and pseudo-sarcoma of Kaposi (reviewed in Taybi and Lachman 1996).

In their retrospective analysis of 40 cases of Klippel–Trenaunay syndrome (28 females, 12 males; aged 1 month to 58 years) seen over 12 years at the University of California San Francisco Maari and Frieden (2004) demonstrated that the presence of a geographic vascular stain is a predictor of the risk of associated lymphatic malformation and complications (including among the most frequent – 5/35% – leg length discrepancy, cellulites, severe pain, recurrent bleeding in the stain, and vaginal bleeding). Presence of at least one of the disease complications occurred in 86% of Klippel–Trenaunay patients with a geographic stain vs. 41% with a blotchy/segmental stain (p < 0.003).

## Natural history

The age of presentation to clinicians in the largest series (Berry et al. 1998, Huang et al. 1994, Maari and Frieden 2004) ranged from birth to 65 years. Although the findings of Klippel–Trenaunay syndrome are usually evident in infancy, approximately 30% of patients in one series (Berry et al. 1998) were not referred before age 10.

Ultimately, the vascular and bone lesions of Klippel–Trenaunay syndrome are not remarkably progressive or proliferative on postnatal life (Berry et al. 1998). There is also considerable variation among patients on the amount of hypertrophy and this discrepancy increases with age. Prognosis is largely dictated by ensuing disease complications (see above) which are more common with vascular lesions involving the trunk or chest (Stickler 1987). Death has occurred in some cases (Stickler 1987) either because of unrelated complications or because of pulmonary complications.

## Molecular genetics and pathogenesis

*Familial occurrence.* Klippel–Trenaunay syndrome is almost always sporadic in appearance. In the series of Berry et al. (1998) none had relatives with Klippel–Trenaunay syndrome except for one child with limb enlargement and deep venous hypoplasia (not the classical triad) and a mother with hemihypertrophy (and normal ultrasound exam). Some authors have described pedigrees where family members had capillary malformations (Craven and Wright 1995) or severe varicosities (Ceballos-Quintal et al. 1996). Koch (1956) cited a number of familial cases: relatives of probands however had isolated varicosities or birthmarks of the posterior neck and some examples of neurofibromatosis were also included (Cohen et al. 2002).

Familial cases have been critically reviewed by Aelvoet et al. (1992), Cohen (2006) and Cohen et al. (2002). Lian and Alhomme (1945) reported congenital varicose veins in three generations of a family in which the propositus had Klippel–Trenaunay syndrome. Norwood and Everett (1964) noted an affected propositus whose brother and mother had macular stains scattered over the face and trunk. Bessone (1950) and Wellens (1961) found two affected mothers and sons. Besson (1950) recorded

also two sisters with Klippel–Trenaunay syndrome. Lindenauer (1965) observed a brother and sister with well-documented identical lesions of the Klippel–Trenaunay type. In the family of Craven and Wrigth (1995) the patient with Klippel–Trenaunay syndrome was said to have an affected grandmother and in that of Ceballos-Quintalos (1996) the 3-year-old girl affected by Klippel–Trenaunay syndrome had a mother with capillary malformations on her back who developed varicose veins in both leg (the maternal grandmother also had varicosities but no vascular malformations). Further cases had affected second-degree relatives: Babboneix (1931) (an uncle and his nephew), Bessone (1950) (a maternal aunt and his nephew) and van der Molen (1954) and Wellens (1961) (two paternal aunts and their nieces).

Aelvoet et al. (1992) sent a questionnaire to 114 Dutch and Belgian patients with Klippel–Trenaunay syndrome of whom 91 responded. After exclusion of cases with incomplete disease features the results of 86 patients (47 males, 39 females; aged 2–37 years) were analysed indicating that the occurrence of Klippel–Trenaunay syndrome was recorded in both a propositus and second-degree relative in two different families: in the first family both the aunt and a nephew suffered from typical disease lesions of the left leg with accompanying spider naevi all over the body; in the second family a paternal grandfather had Klippel–Trenaunay syndrome lesions involving the left leg with an associate naevus flammeus in the back and his grandson extensive naevus flammeus on the face, left arm and left lumbosacral region, and hypertrophy of the left leg. In addition, 19 "naevi flammei" and 5 "angiomatous nevi" were noted in 24 family members of 15 Klippel–Trenaunay patients. Varicosities were also found in many families (unspecified number). Aelvoet et al. (1992) also indicated that the calculated frequency of familial cases of Klippel–Trenaunay syndrome in their series was 1/880 first- and second-degree family members.

As suggested by Cohen (2006) and Cohen et al. (2002) careful scrutiny of published "familial cases" indicates (as in other conditions; see Ruggieri 2000, Ruggieri and Huson 2001, Ruggieri and Pavone 2000) one or more of the following problems: (1) inadequate documentation of cases; (2) over interpretation of minor manifestations in relatives, including "nevus flammeus", haemangiomas, and varicosities, all of which occur commonly in the general population (for example in Klippel–Trenaunay syndrome varicose veins have early onset in infancy or childhood with more extensive distribution than classical varicose veins in the general population); (3) erroneous definition of Klippel–Trenaunay syndrome in cases with capillary malformation not associated with "hypertrophy" or lymphatic malformations or venous flares within the capillary malformation or macrodactyly. The only well documented case of Klippel–Trenaunay syndrome in a brother and sister apparently remains that of Lindenauer (1965).

*Paradominant inheritance.* Happle (1993a) in reviewing the data of Aelvoet et al. (1992) concluded that *paradominant inheritance* could be an explanation of (a) why Klippel–Trenaunay syndrome occurs virtually always sporadically; (b) why the lesions of Klippel–Trenaunay syndrome are arranged in a mosaic distribution; (c) why relatives with Klippel–Trenaunay syndrome are so rare, and when recorded, do not exhibit the Mendelian inheritance; and (d) why "naevi flammei" show an increased incidence in relatives of Klippel–Trenaunay syndrome patients (see also Happle 2000, 2003b, c). According to Happle concept (1993a, b, c, 2000) Klippel–Trenaunay would be caused by a single gene defect. Hetrozygous individuals would be, as a rule phenotypically normal, and therefore the allele would be transmitted imperceptibly through many generations. The trait would only be expressed when a somatic mutation occurs at an early stage of embryogenesis, giving rise to a clonal population of cells that display loss of heterozygosity for the Klippel–Trenaunay syndrome mutation (Happle 1993a). This model has been recently supported by the observation of a set of identical monozygotic male twins discordant for Klippel–Trenaunay syndrome (Hofer et al. 2005).

*Angiogenic/vasculogenic models.* Klessinger and Christ (1996) suggested that the distinctive midline demarcation in Klippel–Trenaunay syndrome may be due to defined boundaries for endothelial migration bounded by the notocord. Moreover, in zebra fish mutant for notochordal formation,

there were defects in axial blood vessels formation (Sumoy et al. 1997). This suggests that the genetic alteration that results in Klippel–Trenaunay syndrome may be located in endothelial cells altered in the process of vessels formation. It has been also speculated that the cellular lesion leading to the manifestations of Klippel–Trenaunay syndrome may be related to persistence of foetal structures (i.e., the foetal dermal capillary web an foetal vasculature) (Baskerville et al. 1985). The morphogenetic defect causing Klippel–Trenaunay syndrome thus may affect the normal process of remodelling of developing vascular structures as vasculogenesis and angiogenesis occur, perhaps by an interference with apoptosis required for vessel remodelling during embryo genesis.

Embryonic vascular morphogenesis involves two processes: vasculogenesis and angiogenesis (see also Cohen 2006). *Vasculogenesis* is the process of generation of primitive vasculature networks and involves the differentiation of endothelial cells from mesenchimal progenitors to form a primary vascular plexus or network. Once the primary plexus is established, new capillaries are formed by sprouting (budding) and non-sprouting (intussusception, or splitting) *angiogenesis.* During maturation peri endothelial support cells (pericytes, smooth muscle cells and myocardial cells) are recruited to encase the endothelial tubes. All these processes are determined by endothelial cell activity (Berry et al. 1998, Cohen 2002, Hanahan 1997). A series of ligands is necessary for angiogenesis and vasculogenesis. Of these, members of the vascular endothelial growth factor (VEGF) family appear to be critical regulators of both angiogenesis and vasculogenesis (Klagsbrun and D'Amore 1996). VEGF action is mediated by binding to a series of receptor-tyrosine kinases (VEGF-R1, -R2 and -R3) that mediate endothelial proliferation and vessel tube formation (vasculogenesis). They also stimulate angiogenesis in balance with the action of other factors angiopoietin-1 (Ang-1) to angiopoietin-4 (Ang-4) and their receptors, Tie-1 and Tie-2. Essential to the remodelling process is an antagonist, angiopoietin-2 (Ang-2), which appear to disrupt angiogenesis perhaps in part as an apoptotic factor. These processes are delicately balanced in the developing embryo. One could speculate that the origin of the vascular disturbances in Klippel–Trenaunay syndrome may be due to an alteration in this tightly regulated remodelling (Berry et al. 1998; Cohen 2002, 2006).

*Transcriptional de-repression: a unifying hypothesis.* Recently an elegant combination of human genetics and functional analysis allowed the discovery of the first susceptibility gene for Klippel–Trenaunay syndrome. In one child affected by Klippel–Trenaunay syndrome, the disease was reported to be associated with a balanced translocation between chromosomes 5 and 11 (Whelan et al. 1995). Somatic cell hybrids containing only the rearranged chromosomes were used to map the precise translocation breakpoints (Tian et al. 2004). Interestingly, a novel gene, VG5Q (the angiogenic factor VG5Q gene), was mapped at the 5q13.3 breakpoint and its transcription was found to be up regulated as a result of the translocation. Mutational analysis of VG5Q in five independent Klippel–Trenaunay patients found a single non-conservative E133K mutation (substitution of a glutamic acid residue by a lysine residue), which results in an enhanced angiogenic effect of the VG5Q protein (Tian et al. 2004). VG5Q is expressed strongly in blood vessels and is secreted upon initiation of angiogenesis. The VG5Q protein binds to endothelial cells and promotes their proliferation. Over expression of VG5Q stimulates angiogenesis and suppression of VG5Q by RNA or anti sense inhibits vessel formation. Even though it remains unclear whether other genes are involved in the disease (Wexler et al. in 1992 identified chromosomal mosaicism for a 1:20 translocation in a patient with Klippel–Trenaunay syndrome) the results of Tian et al. (2004) establish VG5Q as a (or one of the) causative gene(s) for Klippel–Trenaunay syndrome and show that increased angiogenesis is a molecular mechanism for this condition (Gabellini et al. 2004). In addition, on the basis of the model of Tian et al. (2004) and according to the hypothesis of Happle (1993, 2000, 2003a) patients with the VG5Q E113K mutation may carry a second mutational hit in VG5Q or another gene within the affected tissue (Tian et al. 2004). Alternatively, the sporadic nature of Klippel–Trenaunay syndrome may be explained by a model of autosomal dominant inheritance with incomplete penetrance or phenotypic variability.

Recently, Barker et al. (2006) provided evidence suggesting that the activating mutation E133K in the VG59 factor is a relatively common polymorphism in the general population, thus bringing into question the role of VG59 in causing Klippel–Trenaunay syndrome. Hershkovitz et al. (2008) found RASA1 gene mutations causing capillary malformation and limits enlargement and Revenuc et al. (2008) reported RASA1 gene mutations in a wide spectrum of fast-flow vascular malformations including the Parker Weber syndrome.

The postulated pathogenic mechanism or mechanisms leading to overgrowth of the affected limb have been either venous hypertension following congenital deep vein abnormalities or increased blood flow through the abnormal capillary network and cutaneous vessels promoting overgrowth in foetal life.

## Inverse Klippel–Trenaunay syndrome

There are a number of cases (reviewed by Danarti et al. 2007) of Klippel–Trenaunay syndrome associated with deficient growth (e.g., shortening or hypoplastic muscle mass of the affected extremity. These paradoxical cases have been named "inverse Klippel–Trenaunay syndrome" (Danarti et al. 2007). The postulated cause for such unusual deficient growth has been a state of compound heterozygons carriers with a "plus" and a "minus" allele at the responsible gene locus with postzygotic recombination giving rise to two different all clones heterozygons for either allele (Danarti et al. 2007).

## Diagnosis, management and follow-up

*Prenatal diagnosis* has been documented by ultrasonographic demonstration of limb asymmetry (Yankowitz et al. 1993, Yang et al. 2005, Chen et al. 2007), hemihypertrophy, visceral and peripheral vascular anomalies (Meizner et al. 1994), macrocephaly, non-immune hydrops and cardiomegaly (Drose et al. 1991, Meholic et al. 1991, Yancey et al. 1993) and thoracic (Yang et al. 2005) on subcutaneous (Chen et al. 2007) multi as ca-

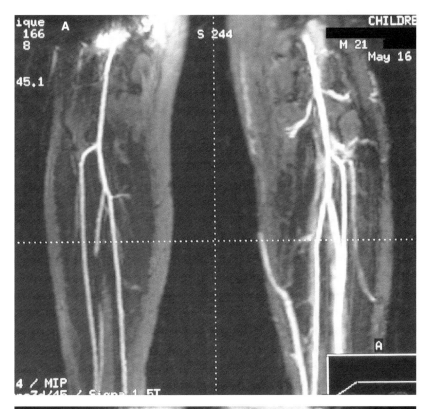

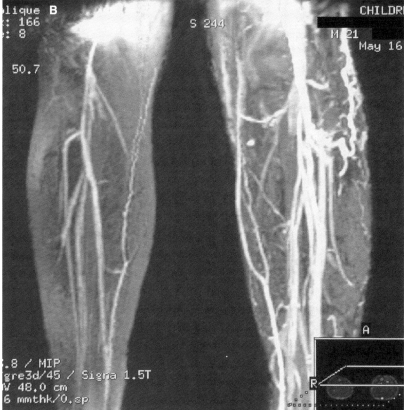

**Fig. 7.** Early (**A**) and slightly delayed (**B**) phases of contrast-enhanced MR angiography show relatively rapid opacification of the normal and varicoid veins of the diseased leg, which is not unusual despite the fact that this is a low-flow anomaly.

lated cysts. However such observations are serendipitous because Klippel–Trenaunay syndrome is almost sporadic in appearance (Berry et al. 1998).

When the clinical impression is suggestive of Klippel–Trenaunay syndrome the *postnatal diagnostic* and *ongoing evaluation work up* should include a combination of various imaging modalities (Berry et al. 1998, Enjolras and Mulliken 2000, Oduber et al. 2008, Taybi and Lachman 1996) including colour duplex ultrasonography, magnetic resonance imaging, lymphoscintigraphy using radio nuclide tracers and plain radiographs of bones (Figs. 5–10). These non-invasive methods have some limitations in the very young child. In particular cases (especially when arteriovenous shunting of arteriovenous malformation or Parkes Weber syndrome needs to be ruled out) contrast angiography may be necessary.

In many patients, it is important to distinguish Klippel–Trenaunay syndrome from arteriovenous malformation and Parkes Weber syndrome since this changes the therapeutic approach significantly. Ultrasonography combined with gray-scale and colour Doppler can be used to rule out arteriovenous shunting of arteriovenous malformation or Parkes Weber syndrome. Additionally, ultrasonographic examination gives valuable information about the venous anatomy of the diseased extremity and also the venous drainage pattern of Klippel–Trenaunay syndrome. Numerous venous varicosities and dilated marginal veins with or without patent deep veins are recognized in Klippel–Trenaunay syndrome. An arteriovenous (AVM) or Parkes Weber syndrome can easily be distinguished from Klippel–Trenaunay syndrome by heterogeneously echogenic and ex-

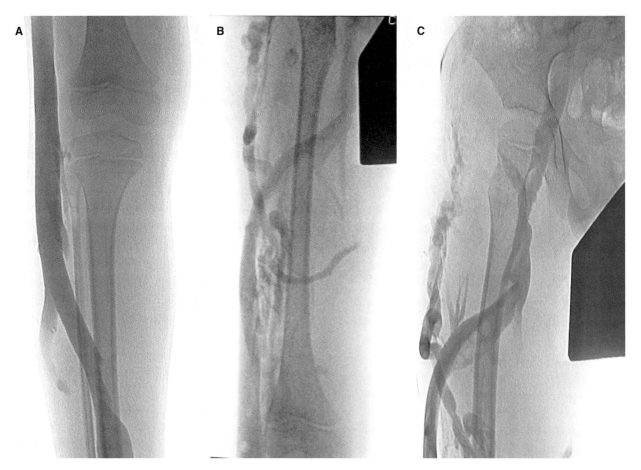

**Fig. 8.** (Continued)

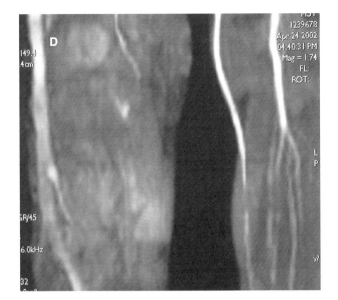

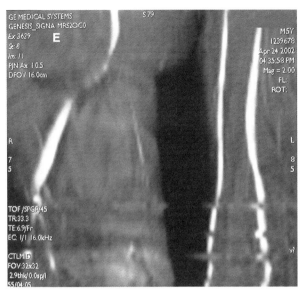

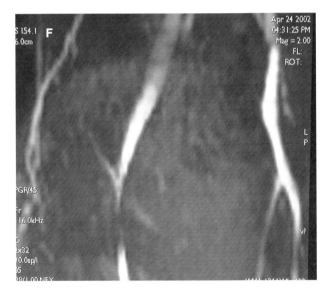

**Fig. 8.** Conventional venogram (**A**, **B** and **C**) of the leg demonstrates a large abnormal draining vein in the lateral aspect of the calf extending superiorly. This abnormal draining vein then drains into the deep veins in the upper calf and also partially fills the venous varicosities in the lateral aspect of the upper thigh. MR venography ("time-of-flight" technique) (**D**, **E** and **F**) findings correlate well with the conventional venography findings. However, MR venography demonstrated venous stenoses incorrectly, which is due to flow turbulence at the venous junctions. It is not uncommon to see false or exaggerated vascular stenoses on MR angiographies, particularly when non-contrast MR angiography techniques are used.

hibits numerous dilated arteries and veins with fast-flow and low resistance. Pulsed Doppler quantitates arterial output (e.g., from the carotid, axillary or femoral arteries) as compared with the uninvolved side, which gives valuable information about the flow dynamics of the diseased extremity. This method should be applied in every infant with a suspect Klippel–Trenaunay phenotype by recommending repeated studies between 12 and 18 months of age for more precise evaluation of venous structures (more subtle changes in venous caliber may not be noted at very young ages) (Berry et al. 1998). Evaluation by

magnetic resonance venography (MRV) could resolve this issue but it can be delayed (because typically no intervention is needed during infancy) until no sedation is needed (as the child has grown up).

Leg lengths could be monitored radiographically if there is clinical evidence of discrepancy. Lymphoscintigraphy is typically done in children with girth discrepancy more than 4 cm (Berry et al. 1998) (primarily to provide information about increased risks of infection due to abnormal lymphatic drainage). However as Enjolras and Mulliken (1993, 2000) suggest "accurate diagnosis and follow-up can

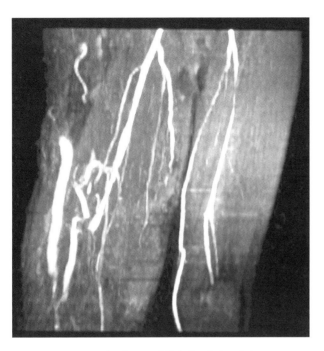

**Fig. 9.** MR venography ("time-of-flight" technique) demonstrates patent deep veins and venous varicosities, as well as a large marginal vein.

be done by clinical and non-invasive assessment of the vascular anomalies, with no need for arteriography or phlebography".

Computerized tomography (CT) has limited use in Klippel–Trenaunay syndrome. CT with contrast certainly demonstrates the gross extent of a vascular anomaly but (unlike MRI) cannot make a differentiation between high flow (AVM, Parkes Weber syndrome or arteriovenous fistula/AVF) and low flow anomalies (e.g., venous malformation/VM, lymphatic malformation/LM). However, recently implemented multi-detector CT scanners (e.g., 16 channel scanners) in common medical practice allow one to obtain excellent angiographic images in a very short period of time (less than 20–30 seconds), particularly arteriograms. The technique is somewhat limited to image venous or lymphatic anomalies of Klippel–Trenaunay syndrome, but it can be used effectively to rule out high flow anomalies. Since the scan is very rapid, sedation is less of a concern than that of MRI or MRA or MRV and can be utilized at an earlier age.

MRI clearly shows large areas of soft tissue signal abnormality in the diseased extremity, in some cases extending into the pelvis or trunk. Non-visualization of flow voids (corresponding to fast-flow vessels) in all sequences is typical. Depending on the nature of the underlying low-flow anomaly, there may or may not be parenchymal staining. MRI is also used in the work-up of Klippel–Trenaunay pa-

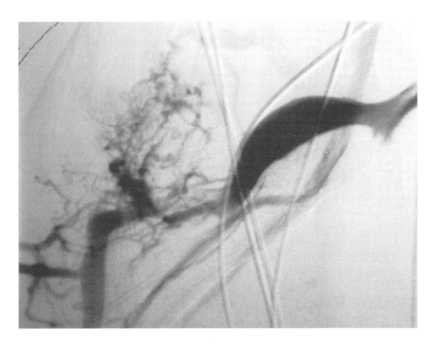

**Fig. 10.** Conventional venogram shows significant stenosis in the marginal vein. Depending on symptomatology, a venous intervention (angioplasty and/or stenting) may be needed in selected cases.

tients for evaluating pelvis or cranial structures not easily examined with ultrasonography. Head MRI is strongly advised even in absence of neurological signs or symptoms to evaluate the eventual associated nervous system (vascular) anomalies. MR angiography (MRA), performed with administration of intravenous contrast medium (called "contrast-enhanced MR angiography") or without injection of contrast medium by utilizing techniques such as "time-of-flight" (angiographic image is being solely created based on the flow dynamics of the vasculature), portrays the anomalous vasculature network. It is particularly important to tailor the MR scan in Klippel–Trenaunay syndrome patients so that the scan is optimized to rule out fast-flow anomalies and to image the deep veins and venous anomalies, in some cases requiring intravenous contrast injection via the diseased extremity ("contrast-enhanced MR venography").

Conventional venography to map out the extremity veins and conventional arteriography remain indispensable tools in the work-up of challenging cases and are used to depict the angioarchitecture in more detail, especially prior to surgical or percutaneous intervention.

Although the general rule for patients with Klippel–Trenaunay syndrome is that there is increased risk for Wilms tumor, it has been reported that patients with Klippel–Trenaunay syndrome are not at an increased risk for developing Wilms tumor (Greene et al. 2004). Therefore, routine ultrasonographic screening to rule out Wilms tumor is unnecessary in these patients.

Maari and Frieden (2004), retrospectively evaluating patients with Klippel–Trenaunay syndrome with geographic vascular stain versus "blotchy/segmental" vascular stain, concluded that the presence of a geographic vascular stain is a predictor of the risk of both associated lymphatic malformation and complications in patients with Klippel–Trenaunay syndrome and suggested that closer observation is needed in those patients.

## Differential diagnosis

Essentially the differential is with the conditions which are characterized or associated with vascu-

lar malformations such as Parkes Weber syndrome, limb hypertrophy due to plexiform neurofibromas in neurofibromatosis type 1, dystrophia lipomatosa, Beckwith–Wiedemann syndrome, Bannayan–Riley-Ruvalcaba syndrome, Proteus syndrome, Maffucci syndrome, Macrodactyly-cutis marmorata syndrome and lymphoedema. As regards to Parkes Weber syndrome (see following chapter) the two conditions should be separated clinically (see Table 1 in previous chapter). Although geneticists, dermatologists and many other clinicians have merged the two conditions under the term "Klippel–Trenaunay–Weber syndrome", surgeons who deal with large numbers of Klippel–Trenaunay patients all separate the two disorders (Samuel et al. 1995, Servelle 1985). Increased limb girth and macrodactyly may be found in hemihyperplasia.

In the series of Berry et al. (1998) diagnoses of patients not found to have Klippel–Trenaunay syndrome included isolated lymphatic malformations, isolated AVMs, hemihypertrophy without demonstrable vascular malformations, cutaneous capillary malformation only, and other isolated or complex vascular malformations.

## Treatment

Patients with minor involvement require no treatment but if there is leg length discrepancy and complicated vascular changes a combined strategy is advised. According to Jacob et al. (1998) the clearest indication for operation in their series of 116 male patients with Klippel–Trenaunay syndrome was leg length discrepancy projected to exceed 2.0 cm at skeletal maturity, which could be treated with epiphysiodesis in the growing child. If a functioning deep venous system is present, removal of symptomatic varicosities or localized superficial venous malformations (mostly by stripping of varicose veins or venous malformations, excision of vascular malformations) in selected patients yielded good results (Jacob et al. 2001). Surgical intervention includes excision of associated vascular anomalies, vein ligation, vein stripping, vein resection, and in rare cases, amputation.

The most common intervention used is compression, typically using a custom garment (Berry et al. 1998) with additional gradient pump when necessary (though acceptance of these garments by parents of very young children is often limited). Alternatively, manual lymphatic drainage could be combined along with garments.

Pulse-day laser treatment can reduce the redness of the capillary malformation to some extent and usually in limited areas.

Sclerotherapy is an excellent alternative to surgery in the treatment of associated venous and/or lymphatic malformations of Klippel–Trenaunay syndrome, as well as in the treatment of associated venous varicosities. However, it is very important to assess the venous architecture of the extremity fully before percutaneous (sclerotherapy) or surgical intervention to treat venous varicosities or anomalies so that the treatment would not compromise the venous drainage of the extremity. Percutaneous therapeutic approach should be tailored depending on the flow dynamics of the extremity. Sclerotherapy and/or coiling venous anomalies may be needed in some patients, whereas angioplasty or stenting of a marginal vein or one of the deep veins may be needed in some patients if there is a hemodynamically significant stenosis. Percutaneous intervention should only be performed by an experienced interventional radiologist in this field.

Leg length discrepancy and macrodactyly may require orthopaedic procedures for debulking of hands or feet by removals of digits (or ray reduction) and epiphysiodesis in late puberty (Berry et al. 1998). Special concern is warranted in monitoring healing after surgery as this can be significantly delayed in cases of abnormal lymphatic drainage.

Systemic antibiotic therapy should be used in the face of cellulites, surgery, or injury in an affected limb to prevent infections. Compression garments can be useful in many of the cases with lymphoedema.

# References

Aelvoet GE, Jorens PG, Roelen LM (1992) Genetic aspects of the Klippel–Trenaunay syndrome. Br J Dermatol 126: 603–607.

Anlar B, Yalaz K, Erzen C (1988) Klippel–Trenaunay–Weber syndrome: a case with cerebral and cerebellar hemihypertrophy. Neuroradiology 30: 360.

Babonneix L (1931) Nevus variqueux otéohypertrophique d'un member inferieur. Arch Med Enfants 34: 457.

Barker KT, Foulker WD, Schwartz CE, Labadie C, Mansell F, Houlton RS, Harper J (2006) Is the E133K allele on VG59 associated with Klippel–Trenaunay and other overgrowth syndromes. J Med Genet 43: 613–614.

Baskerville PA, Ackroyd JS, Browse NL (1985) The etiology of the Klippel–Trenaunay syndrome. Ann Surg 202: 624–627.

Beballos-Quintal JM, Pinto-Escalante D, Castillo-Zapata I (1996) A new case of Klippel–Trenaunay–Weber (KTW) syndrome: evidence of autosomal dominant inheritance. Am J Med Genet 63: 426–427.

Beighton P, Beighton G (1986) The man behind the syndrome. Berlin: Springer, pp. 191–215.

Berry SA, Peterson C, Mize W, Bloom K, Zachary C, Blasco P, Hunter D (1998) Klippel–Trenaunay syndrome. Am J Med Genet 79: 319–326.

Bessone L (1950) Angiectasia hypertrophicans dei Klippel–Trenaunay-Parkes–Weber. Arch Ital Derm Siph Vener 23: 133–139.

Boris M, Weindorf S, Lasinski B, Boris G (1994) Lymphedema reduction by non-invasive complex lymphedema therapy. Oncology 8: 95–106.

Burke JP, West NF, Strachan IM (1991) Congenital nystagmus, anisomyopia, and hemimegalencephaly in the Klippel–Trenaunay syndrome. J Pediatr Ophthalmol Strabismus 28: 41–44.

Chen PC, Shu WC (1996) Klippel–Trenaunay–Weber syndrome: report of one case. Acta Paediatr Sin 37: 138–141.

Chen CP, Lin SP, Chang TY, Lee HC, Hung HY, Lin HY, Huang JP, Wang W (2007) Prenatal sonographic findings of Klippel–Trenaunay syndrome. J Clin Ultrasound Mar 20 [Epub ahead of print].

Cohen MM Jr (2000) Klippel–Trenaunay syndrome: a critical analysis. Am J Med Genet 93: 171–175.

Cohen MM Jr, Neri G, Weksberg R (2002) Klippel–Trenaunay syndrome, Parkes Weber syndrome, and Sturge–Weber syndrome. In: Cohen MM Jr, Neri G, Weksberg R (eds.) Overgrowth Syndromes. New York: Oxford University Press, pp. 111–124.

Cohen MM Jr (2006) Vascular update: morphogenesis, tumors, malformations, and molecular dimensions. Am J Med Genet 140A: 2013–2038.

Craven N, Wright AL (1995) Familial Klippel–Trenaunay syndrome: a case report. Clin Exp Dermatol 20: 76–79.

Cristaldi A, Vigevano F, Antoniazzi G, di Capua M, Andreuazzi A, Morselli G, Iorio F, Fariello G, Trasimeni G, Gualdi GF (1995) Hemimegalencephaly, hemihypertrophy and vascular lesions. Eur J Pediatr 154: 134–137.

Danarti R, Konig A, Bittar M, Happle R (2007) Inverse Klippel–Trenaunay syndrome: review of cases showing deficient growth. Dermatology 214: 130–132.

Di Iorio G, Sanges G, Sannino V, De Cristofaro M, D'Ambrosio MR, Budillon A, Sampaolo S (2005) Peripheral nervous system involvement in Klippel-Trenaunay syndrome. Clin Neuropathol 24: 42–47.

Drose JA, Thickman D, Wiggins J, Haverkamp AB (1991) Foetal echographic findings in Klippel–Trenaunay–Weber syndrome. J Ultrasound Med 10: 525–527.

Enjolras O, Mulliken JB (1993) The current management of vascular birthmarks. Pediatr Dermatol 10: 311–333.

Enjolras O, Mulliken JB (2000) Vascular malformations. In: Harper J, Oranje A, Prose N (eds.) Textbook pf Pediatric Dermatology. Vol. 2. Oxford: Blackwell Science, pp. 975–996.

Friedberg H (1867) Riesenwuchs des rechten Beines. Virchows Arch 40: 353–379.

Gabellini D, Green MR, Tupler R (2004) When enough is enough: genetic diseases associate with transcriptional derepression. Curr Opin Genet Develop 14: 310–307.

Geoffroy Saint-Hilaire E (1942) Hisotire génerale et particulaire des anomalies de l'organisation chex l'homme et les animaux. Paris.

Gorlin RJ, Cohen MM Jr, Hennekam RCM (2001) Klippel–Trenaunay syndrome, Parkes Weber syndrome, and Sturge–Weber syndrome. In: Gorlin RJ, Cohen MM Jr, Hennekam RCM (eds.) Syndromes of the Head and Neck, 4th ed. New York: Oxford University Press, pp. 453–460.

Gloviczki P, Hollier LH, Telander RL, Kaufman B, Bianco J, Stickler GB (1983) Surgical implications of Klippel–Trenaunay syndrome. Ann Surg 197: 353–362.

Greene AK, Kieran M, Burrows PE, Mulliken JB, Kasser J, Fishman SJ (2004) Wilms tumor screening is unnecessary in Klippel–Trenaunay syndrome. Pediatrics 113: 326–329.

Hanahan D (1997) Signaling vascular morphogenesis and maintenance. Science 277: 48–59.

Happle R (1987) Lethal genes surviving by mosaicism: a possible explanation for sporadic birth defects involving the skin. J Am Acad Dermatol 16: 899–906.

Happle R (1993a) Klippel–Trenaunay syndrome: is it a paradominant trait? Br J Dermatol 128: 465.

Happle R (1993b) Pigmentary patterns associated with human mosaicism: a proposed classification. Eur J Dermatol 3: 170–174.

Happle R (1993c) Mosaicism in human skin: understanding the patterns and mechanisms. Arch Dermatol 129: 1460–1470.

Happle R (1996) Segmental forms of autosomal dominant skin disorders: different types of severity reflects different states of zygosity. Am J Med Genet 66: 241–242.

Happle R (1997) A rule concerning the segmental manifestations of autosomal dominant skin disorders: review of clinical examples providing evidence for dichotomous types of severity. Am J Med Genet 133: 1905–1909.

Happle R (2000) Principles of Genetics, Mosaicism and Molecular Biology. In: Harper J, Oranje A, Prose N (eds.) Textbook pf Pediatric Dermatology. Vol. 2. Oxford: Blackwell Science, pp. 1037–1056.

Happle R (2003) Sturge–Weber-Klippel–Trenaunay syndrome: what's in a name? Eur J Dermatol 13: 223.

Hershkovitz D, Bergman R, Sprecher E (2008) A novel mutation in RASA1 causes capillary malformation and limb enlargement. Arch Dermatol Res Mar 8 [Epub ahead of print].

Hofer T, Frank J, Itin PH (2005) Klippel–Trenaunay syndrome in a monozygotic male twin: supportive evidence for the concept of paradominant inheritance. Eur J Dermatol 15: 341–343.

Huang WJ, Creath CJ (1994) Klippel–Trenaunay syndrome: literature review and case report. Pediatr Dent 16: 231–235.

Jakob AG, Driscoll DJ, Shaughnessy WJ, Stanson AW, Clay RP, Gloviczki P (1998) Klippel–Trenaunay syndrome: spectrum and management. Mayo Clin Proc 73: 28–36.

Klagsbrun M, D'Amore PA (1996) Vascular endothelial growth factor and its receptors. Cytokine Growth factor Rev 7: 259–270.

Klessinger S, Christ B (1996) Axial structures control laterality in the distribution pattern of endothelial cells. Anat Embryol (Berl) 193: 39–330.

Klippel M, Trenaunay P (1900) Du nevus variqueux ostèo-hypertrophique. Arch Gen Med (Paris) 185: 641–672.

Kramer W (1972) Klippel–Trenaunay syndrome. In: Vinken PJ, Bruyn GW (eds.) Handbook of Clinical Neurology. New York: Elsevier, pp. 390–404.

Koch G (1956) Zur Klinik, Symptomatologie, Pathogenese und Erbpathologie des Klippel–Trenaunay–Weberschen Syndrome. Acta Genet Med Gemellol 5: 326–370.

Lian C, Alhomme P (1945) Les varices congenitale par dysembryoplasie (syndrome de Klippel–Trenaunay). Arch Mal Coeur 38: 176.

Lindenauer SM (1965) The Klippel–Trenaunay syndrome: varicosity, hypertrophy and haemangioma with no arterio-venous fistula. Ann Surg 162: 303–314.

Maari C, Frieden IJ (2004) Klippel–Trenaunay syndrome: the importance of "geographic stains" in identifying lymphatic disease and risk of complications. J Am Acad Dermatol 51: 391–398.

Mathews MS, Kim RC, Chang GY, Linskey ME (2008) Klippel-Trenaunay syndrome and cerebral haemangiopericytoma: a potential association. Acta Neurochir (Wien) 150: 399–402.

Matsubara O, Tanaka M, Ida T, Okada R (1993) Hemimegalencephaly with hemihypertrophy (Klippel–Trenaunay–Weber syndrome). Virchows Arch 400: 155–162.

Meizner J, Rosenak D, Nadjari M, Maor E (1994) Sonographic diagnosis of Klippel–Trenaunay–Weber syndrome presenting a a sacrococcygeal mass at 14–15 week's gestation. J Ultrasound Med 13: 901–904.

Meholic AJ, Freimanis AK, Stucka J, Lo Piccolo ML (1991) Sonographic in utero diagnosis of Klippel–Trenaunay–Weber syndrome. J Ultrasound Med 10: 111–114.

Mueller-Lessmann V, Behrendt A, Wetzel WE, Peteresen K, Anders D (2001) Orofacial findings in the Klippel–Trenaunay syndrome. Int J Pediatr Den 11: 225–229.

Mulliken JB (1993) Cutaneous vascular anomalies. Semin Vasc Surg 6: 204–218.

Mulliken JB, Glowacki J (1982) Haemangiomas and vascular malformations in infants and children. A classification based on endothelial characteristics. Plast Reconstr Surg 69: 412–420.

Mulliken JB, Young AE (1988) Vascular birthmarks: haemangiomas and malformations. Philadelphia: WB Saunders Company, pp. 246–264.

Mullikcn JB, Fishman SJ, Burrows PF (2006) Vascular anomalies, hemangiomas, and malformations. New York: Oxford University Press.

Norwood OT, Everett MD (1964) cardiac failure due to endocrine dependent haemangiomas. Arch Dermatol 89: 759–760.

Obituary (1942) Presse Méd 46: 654.

O'Connor P, Smith JL (1978) Optic nerve variant in Klippel–Trenaunay–Weber syndrome. Ann Ophthalmol 10: 131–134.

Oduber CE, van der Horst CM, Hennekam RC (2008) Klippel-Trenaunay syndrome: diagnostic criteria and hypothesis on etiology. Ann Plast Surg 60: 217–223.

Patel PR, Lauerman WC (1995) Historical perspective: Maurice Klippel. Spine 20: 2157–2160.

Pichierri A, Piccirilli M, Passacantilli E, Frati A, Santoro A, (2006) Klippel–Trenaunay–Weber syndrome and intramedullary cervical cavemoma: a very rare association. Case report. Surg Neural 66: 203–206.

Rebarber A, Roman AS, Roshan D, Blei F (2004) Obstetric management of Klippel–Trenaunay syndrome. Obstet Gynecol 104: 1205–1208.

Revencu N, Boon LM, Mulliken JB, Enjolras O, Cordisco MR, Burrows PE, Clapuyt P, Hammer F, Dubois J, Baselga E, Brancati F, Carder R, Quintal JM, Dallapiccola B, Fischer G, Frieden IJ, Garzon M, Harper J, Johnson-Patel J, Labrèze C, Martorell L, Paltiel HJ, Pohl A, Prendiville J, Quere I, Siegel DH, Valente EM, Van Hagen A, Van Hest L, Vaux KK, Vicente A, Weibel L, Chitayat D, Vikkula M (2008) Parkes Weber syndrome, vein of Galen aneurysmal malformation, and other fast-flow vascular anomalies are caused by RASA1 mutations. Hum Mutat Apr 29 [Epub ahead of print].

Rohany M, Shaibani A, Arafat O, Walker MT, Russell EJ, Batjer HH, Getch CC (2007) Spinal arteriovenous malformations associated with Klippel–Trenaunay–Weber syndrome: a literature search and report of two cases. AM J Neuroradial 28: 584–589.

Ruggieri M (2001) Mosaic (segmental) neurofibromatosis type 1 (NF1) and type 2 (NF2) – no longer neurofibromatosis type 5. Am J Med Genet 101: 178–180.

Ruggieri M, Pavone L (2000) Hypomelanosis of Ito: clinical syndrome or just phenotype? J Child Neurol 15: 635–644.

Ruggieri M, Huson SM (2001) The clinical and diagnostic implications of mosaicism in the neurofibromatoses. Neurology 56: 1433–1443.

Servelle M (1985) Klippel and Trenaunay's syndrome. 768 operated acses. Ann Surg 201: 365–373.

Stickler GB (1987) Klippel–Trenaunay syndrome. In Gomez MR (ed.) Neurocutaneous Diseases. Boston: Butterworths, pp. 368–375.

Sumoy L, Keasey JB, Dittman TD, Kimelman D (1997) A role for notochord in axial vascular development revealed by analysis of phenotype and the expression of VEGR-2 in zebrafush flh and ntl mutant embryos. Mech Dev 63: 15–27.

Taybi H, Lachman RS (1996) Klippel–Trenaunay syndrome. In: Taybi H, Lachman RS (eds.) Radiology of Syndromes, Metabolic Disorders, and Skeletal Dysplasia. 4th ed. St. Louis: Mosby, pp. 276–279.

Tian XL, Kadaba R, You SA, Liu M, Timur AA, Yang L, Chen Q, Szafranski P, Rao S, Wu L, Housman DE, DiCorleto PE, Drsicoll DJ, Borrow J, Wang Q (2004) Identification of an angiogenic factor that when mutated causes susceptibility to Klippel–Trenaunay syndrome. Nature 127: 640–648.

Timur AA, Sadgenphour A, Graf M, Schwartz S, Libby ED, Driscoll I, Wang Q (2004) Identification and molecular characterisation of a de novo supernumerary ring chromosome 18 in a patient with Klippel–Trenaunay syndrome. Ann Hum Genet 68: 353–361.

Torregrosa A, Marti-Bonmati L, Higueras V, Poyatos C, Sanchìs A (2000) Klippel–Trenaunay syndrome: frequency of cerebral and cerebellar hemihypertrophy on MRI. Neuroradiology 42: 420–423.

Trelat U, Monod A (1869) De l'hypertrophie unilatérale partielle or totale du corps. Arch Gen Med 13: 536–558.

Valdés F, Vadillo FJ, Martínez A (2007) Klippel-Trénaunay syndrome and Arnold-Chiari type I malformation. Actas Dermosifiliogr 98: 441–442.

Van Der Molen HR (1954) Angiopathie a retentissement osseux ou dysembrioplasie a la fois vasculaire et osseux? A propos de quelque cas de maladie de Klippel et Trenaunay. Rev Franc Rhumatol 4: 161–173.

Vissers W, Van Steensel M, Steijlen P, Renier W, Van Der Kerkhof P, Van Der Vleuten C (2003) Klippel–Trenaunay syndrome and Sturge–Weber syndrome: variations on a theme. Eur J Dermatol 13: 238–241.

Weber PF (1907) Angioma formation in connection with hypertrophy of limbs and hemihypertrophy. Br J Dermatol 19: 231–235.

Weber PF (1918) Hemangiectatic hypertrophy og lombs – congenital phlebarteriectasis and so-called varicose veins. Br J Child Dis 15: 13.

Wellens W (1961) Triade de Klippel–Trenaunay: à propos de 23 case. Phlebologie 14: 21–35.

Wexler P, McGavran L, Sujanski E (1992) Unilateral chromosomal mosaicism in Klippel–Trenaunay–Weber syndrome with short stature. 13th Annual David W. Smith Workshop on Malformations and Morphogenesis. August 59. Wake Forest University, Winstom-Salem, North carolina.

Whelan AJ, Watson MS, Porter FD Steiner RD (1995) Klippel–Trenaunay–Weber syndrome associated with a 5:11 balanced translocation. Am J Med Genet 59: 492–494.

Wolpert SM, Cohen A, Libenson MH (1994) Hemimegalencephaly: a longitudinal MR study. AJNR 15: 1479–1482.

Yancey MK, Lasley D, Richard DS (1993) An unusual neck mass in a foetus with Klippel–Trenaunay–Weber syndrome. J Ultrasound Med 12: 779–782.

Yang JI, Kim HS, Ryu HS (2005) Prenatal sonographic diagnosis of Klippel–Trenaunay–Weber syndrome: a case report. J Repord Med 50: 291–294.

Yankowitz J, Slagel DD, Williamson R (1994) Prenatal diagnosis of Klippel–Trenaunay–Weber syndrome by ultrasound. Prenat Diagn 14: 745–749.

You CK, Rees J, Gillis DA, Stevens J (1983) Klippel–Trenaunay syndrome: a review. Can J Surg 26: 399–403.

# Chapter 9

# PARKES WEBER SYNDROME

Orhan Konez, Martino Ruggieri, and Concezio Di Rocco

Department of Radiology, Vascular and Interventional Radiology, St. John West Shore Hospital, University Hospitals Case Medical Center, Westlake, OHIO, USA (OK); Institute of Neurological Science, National Research Council, Catania, and Department of Paediatrics, University of Catania, Catania, Italy (MR); Section of Paediatric Neurosurgery, Department of Paediatrics, Catholic University of Sacred Heart, Rome, Italy (CDR)

## Introduction

*Parkes Weber syndrome* (OMIM # 608355) is characterised by a cutaneous flush with underlying multiple micro arteriovenous fistulas (AVF) with enlarged arteries and veins and capillary/venous malformations in association with soft tissue and skeletal hypertrophy of a limb (Cohen 2000, 2006; Cohen et al. 2002; Gorlin et al. 2001; Mulliken and Young 1988).

## Historical perspective and terminology

This syndrome was described by the same F. Parkes Weber (Parkes Weber 1907, 1908, 1918) whose name is also attached to Klippel–Trenaunay–Weber syndrome, Sturge–Weber syndrome, Hutchinson–Weber–Peutz–Jeghers syndrome, Weber–Christian disease and Osler–Rendu–Weber syndrome (Bodensteiner and Roach 1999). Parkes Weber syndrome is commonly hyphenated as Parkes–Weber syndrome: however, in Parkes Weber's own papers (Parkes Weber 1907, 1908, 1918), no hyphen is used (Cohen 2006).

**Frederick Parkes Weber**, who was born in 1863, matriculated at Cambridge University and St. Bartholomew's Hospital, London. His father, Sir Hermann Weber, had come to England from Germany and served as physician to Queen Victoria. Weber and his family retained their German connections, emphasised by his persistent pronunciation of his surname with the continental "V" sound, now long forgotten since his death. Weber was legendary in the Royal Society of Medicine by virtue of his remarkable knowledge of rare disorders, for his clear and meticulous diction, and for his prolific contributions of more than 1200 medical articles over a span of 50 years of active medical practice. He was a prodigious describer of new or unique entities, many of them dermatologic, and his name has been attached to several disorders (see above).

Parkes Weber described patients with enlarged arteries and veins, capillary or venous malformations, and enlargement of a limb.

## Incidence and prevalence

All reported cases have been sporadic and the larger series are those of Robertson (1956) and Young (1988).

## Clinical manifestations

Upon physical examination the involved limb is warm. The colour of the cutaneous vascular malformation is usually more diffuse and pinker than that observed in Klippel–Trenaunay syndrome. Lymphatic malformations do not occur and no lymphatic vesicles are found in the discoloured skin. The main differences between Klippel–Trenaunay and Parkes Weber syndrome are contrasted in Table 1 (see also Cohen 2006, Taybi and Lachman 1996).

Because Klippel–Trenaunay syndrome has combined (mixed) type capillary, lymphatic, and venous malformations, lymphatic vesicles may appear on the surface of the cutaneous capillary malformation and may ooze lymph. The lateral venous anomaly in Klippel–Trenaunay syndrome may sometimes have

**Table 1.** Comparison of Klippel–Trenaunay syndrome and Parkes Weber syndrome

|  | Klippel–Trenaunay | Parkes Weber |
| --- | --- | --- |
| Types of vascular malformation | Slow flow<br>capillary, lymphatic, venous | Fast flow<br>capillary, arterial, venous |
| Colour of cutaneous malformation | Bluish to purplish, localised | Pinkish to red, diffuse |
| Arteriovenous fistulas | Insignificant | Significant |
| Lateral venous anomaly | Very common | Not found |
| Lymphatic vesicles | Present | Not found |
| Venous flares | Present | Not found |
| Limb involved |  |  |
| Upper | 5% | 23% |
| Lower | 95% | 77% |
| Limb enlargement | Usually disproportionate<br>Soft tissues, bone<br>Macrodactyly (toes), common | arm/leg length discrepancy |
| Prognosis | Usually good<br>Pulmonary embolism (10% children)<br>Postoperative risk of embolism | More problematic (fistulas)<br>Heart failure<br>Cardiac enlargement<br>Cutaneous ischemia<br>Limb amputation |

Adapted from Cohen (2002, 2006).

protrusions known as venous flares on the surface of the cutaneous capillary malformation (Cohen et al. 2002, Robertson 1956, Samuel and Spitz 1995, Young 1978).

## Molecular genetics and pathogenesis

In the studies of Eerola et al. (2002, 2003) on familial capillary malformation/arteriovenous malformation (CM-AVM) (OMIM # 608354) six of the 17 reported families had either arteriovenous malformation, arteriovenous fistula or Parkes Weber syndrome and were found to have RASA1 gene mutations on chromosome 5q13.1. Further studies (Revencu et al. 2008) demonstrated that a number of fast-flow vascular malformations including Parker Weber syndrome are caused by RASA1 gene mutations. The RASA1 gene encodes for a p120-RasGAP protein which promote signalling for various growth factor receptors that control proliferation, migration, and survival of several cell types, including vascular endothelial cells (Cohen 2006, Eerola et al. 2003).

Recently, a familial case of Parkes Weber has been reported in a boy who had an extensive vascu-

lar malformation of the right lower limb and right lower part of the back and abdomen with hypertrophy and aneurysmal varies and in his 10-year-old first cousin who had Parkes Weber syndrome in the right upper limb (Courivand et al. 2006).

## Diagnostic imaging

Although a detailed clinical assessment suffices for accurate diagnosis in the majority of patients, plain radiography to evaluate leg length discrepancy and magnetic resonance imaging (MRI) are the mainstay of imaging similar to other overgrowth syndromes that involve the limbs. MRI is important to assess the deep lymphatic, venous and adipose components in the affected limb, since the presence of each is highly variable. In atypical cases, MRI allows one to distinguish the condition from other similar anomalies, typically Klippel–Trenaunay syndrome and rarely large extremity infantile hemangiomas. The gold standard imaging modality is the conventional catheter based arteriogram, but it is an invasive procedure requiring deep sedation in children. This has

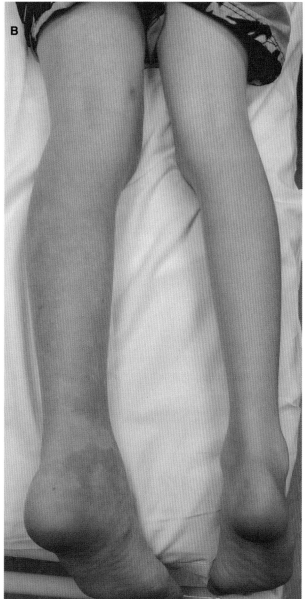

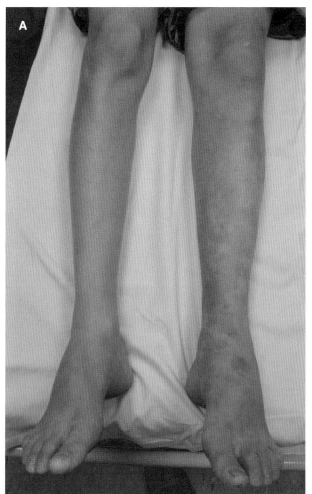

**Fig. 1.** Parkes Weber syndrome. (**A**) and (**B**) show enlarged left lower extremity with areas of brownish skin discoloration. (**C**) and (**D**) are axial CT images with intravenous contrast demonstrating enlarged left leg with prominent vasculature (femoral arteries and veins proximally and tibial arteries and veins more distally). There are also prominent superficial veins seen in the diseased extremity (**D**). (**E**) and (**F**) are CTA of the lower extremities, demonstrating an obvious increased vascularity in the left leg. The technique allows rapid imaging of the entire leg in less than a minute with relatively high resolution. (**G**) (early phase) and (**H**) (delayed phase) are post contrast MRA images demonstrating enlarged extremity arteries and rapid contrast opacification of the prominent extremity veins due to arteriovenous shunts. Timing of the scan following contrast administration is very important to obtain satisfactory imaging in both CTA and MRA.

been replaced by non-invasive imaging modalities in most tertiary centers, either computerised tomography (CT) angiography (CTA) or MR angiography (MRA). With the advantages of high image resolution and rapid imaging (typically less than a minute versus 30 minutes to 1 hour with MRA), CTA has a

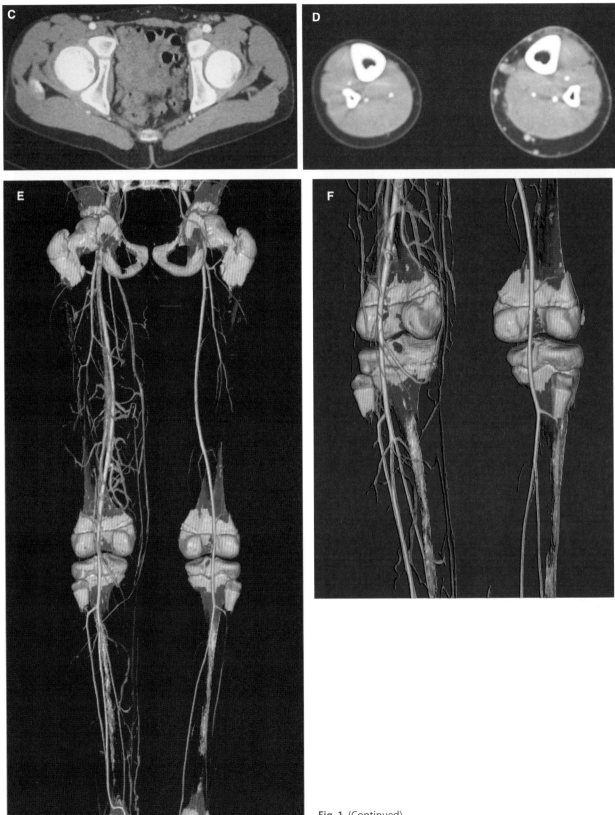

**Fig. 1.** (Continued)

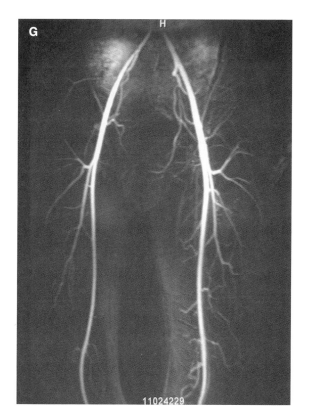

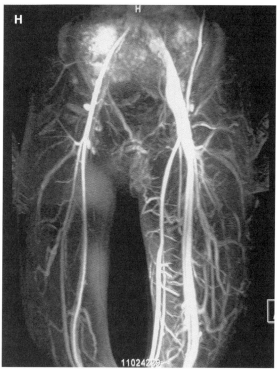

Fig. 1. (Continued)

clear advantage over MRA. With additional conventional MRI sequences, MRA, on the other hand, has the advantage of no radiation exposure to the patients and allows assessment of the soft tissues in more detail (soft tissue contrast resolution of MR is significantly better than that of CT). While conventional leg venography is the gold standard in Klippel–Trenaunay syndrome, it has a limited value in Parkes Weber syndrome.

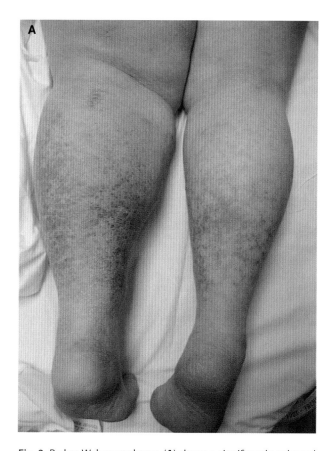

Fig. 2. Parkes Weber syndrome. (**A**) shows a significantly enlarged left leg with nonspecific skin changes. Some small varicosities are seen, most likely due to increased venous pressure secondary to arteriovenous shunts. (**B**) is a CT scan demonstrating increased fatty tissue in the area with involvement of the muscle groups. (**C**) and (**D**) are T1 and T2 weighted coronal MR images demonstrate multiple small abnormal vessels in the area, resulting in an inhomogeneous appearance. (**E**) is a contrast-enhanced MRA demonstrating a large femoral artery and arteriovenous shunts in the involved leg, as well as early opacification of the extremity veins. (**F**) is a conventional selective arteriogram with contrast injection in one of the arterial feeders demonstrating arteriovenous shunts.

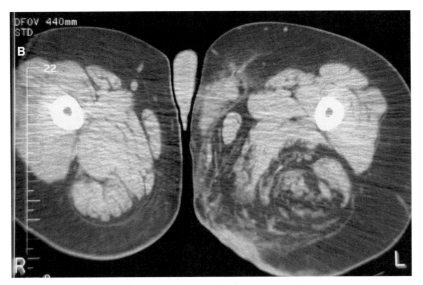

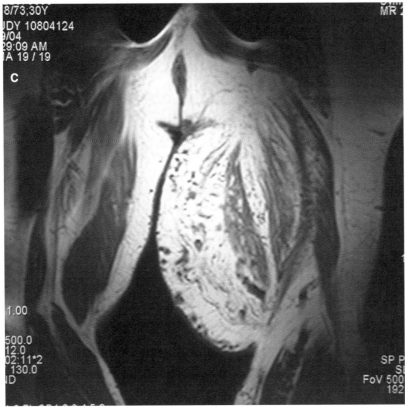

Fig. 2. (Continued)

Most patients with Parkes Weber syndrome have generalized enlargement of the arteries and veins, as well as true hypertrophy of the muscles of the affected limb. Rapid contrast opacification of the draining veins is typically seen on all angiographic imaging studies. Therefore, using an imaging modality that has a high temporal resolution (best would be a conventional catheter based arteriogram) is advantageous to assess the arteriovenous fistulae. For example, it may be problematic to assess the fis-

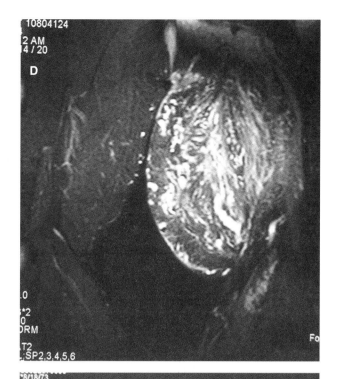

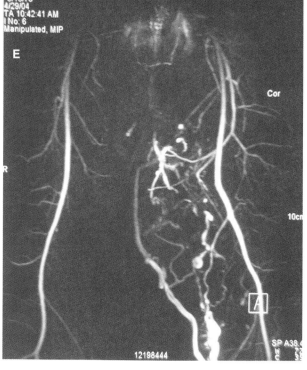

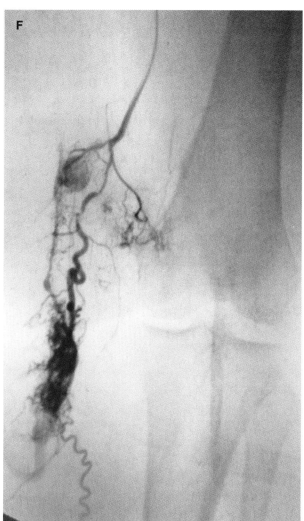

**Fig. 2.** (Continued)

tulae with MRA due to its slow image acquisition. This is somewhat less problematic with CTA due to its rapid image acquisition. However, when the timing of the image acquisition is selected well, these non-invasive imaging techniques would be adequate to assess the arteriovenous fistulae.

On MRI (typically T1 and T2 weighted images), signal voids (dark small rounded areas) are seen in the vessels that have a high flow, such as arteries, arteriovenous shunts, as well as in some veins depending on the degree of the blood flow in the veins and also based on the setting of the sequence being used. T2-weighted and post gadolinium sequences often show patchy increased signal in some of the muscles. They may, in addition, have focal arteriovenous (AV) shunts, increased subcutaneous fat, and lymphedema. These changes commonly result in inhomogeneous appearing soft tissues on MRI. This may be associated with an enlarged extremity, but this is significantly less striking compared to Klippel–Trenaunay syndrome. On MRA and CTA, enlargement of the main extremity arteries and veins (e.g., iliac and femoral in a typical leg involvement) are typically seen due to increased arteriovenous circulation in the diseased extremity. With intravenous contrast administration, abnormal enhancement can be seen in the soft tissues.

## Differential diagnosis

Main differential diagnostic considerations include Klippel–Trenaunay syndrome, extensive infantile hemangioma with arteriovenous shunting, rapidly involuting congenital hemangioma (RICH) and non-involuting congenital hemangioma (NICH) (Konez et al. 2003). In hemangiomas, there is extensive cutaneous involvement, usually present at birth or rapidly after birth. This may be associated with structural abnormalities. High-output cardiac failure may be a presenting condition in both Parkes Weber syndrome and in some extensive hemangiomas. In Klippel–Trenaunay syndrome, there is a dilated marginal vein typically identified, in addition to easily noticeable enlargement of the limb and relatively large soft tissue involvement of the extremity with a vascular anomaly of a low-flow pattern (capillary lymphatico-venous malformation).

## Outcome

The prognosis in Parkes Weber syndrome is more problematic due to the fast flow vascular malfor-mation/fistulas that could alter the vascular dynamics leading to cardiac failure and in turn to cardiac enlargement and cutaneous ischemia, requiring limb amputation. However, with appropriate embolizations, the limb can be saved and high-output cardiac failure can be improved. Since there are numerous shunting in the majority of patients, multiple embolization sessions may be needed. It is very important to approach these patients in a multidisciplinary fashion. If arteriovenous shunts are tiny and numerous, then embolization becomes more difficult.

## References

Bodensteiner JB, Roach ES (1999) Sturge–Weber syndrome. Mt. Freedom: The Sturge Weber Foundation.

Cohen MM Jr (2000) Klippel-Tranaunay syndrome: a critical analysis. Am J Med Genet 93: 171–175.

Cohen MM Jr, Neri G, Weksberg R (2002) Klippel–Trenaunay syndrome, Parkes Weber syndrome, and Sturge–Weber syndrome. In: Cohen MM Jr, Neri G, Weksberg R (eds.) Overgrowth Syndromes. New York: Oxford University Press, pp. 111–124.

Cohen MM Jr (2006) Vascular update: morphogenesis, tumors, malformations, and molecular dimensions. Am J Med Genet 140A: 2013–2038.

Courivand D, Delerue A, Delerue C, Boom L, Piette F, Modieno P (2006) Familial case of Parkes Weber syndrome. Ann Dermatol Venereol 133: 445–457.

Eerola I, Boon L, Watanabe S, Grynberg H, Mulliken JB, Vikkula M (2002) Locus for susceptibility for familial capillary malformation ("port-wine stain") maps to 5q. Eur J Hum Genet 10: 375–380.

Eerola I, Boon L, Mulliken JB, Burrows PE, Dompmartin A, Watanabe S, Vanwijck R, Vikkula M (2003) Capillary malformation-arteriovenous malformation, a new clinical and genetic disorder caused by RASA1 mutations. Am J Hum Genet 73: 1240–1249.

Gorlin RJ, Cohen MM Jr, Hennekam RCM (2001) Klippel–Trenaunay syndrome, Parkes Weber syndrome, and Sturge–Weber syndrome. In: Gorlin RJ, Cohen MM Jr, Hennekam RCM (eds.) Syndromes of the Head and Neck, 4th ed. New York: Oxford University Press, pp. 453–460.

Konez O, Burrows PE, Mulliken JB, Fishman SJ, Kozakewich HP (2003) Angiographic features of rapidly involuting congenital hemangioma (RICH). Ped Radiol 33: 15–19.

Mulliken JB, Young AE (1988) Vascular birthmarks: haemangiomas and Malformations. Philadelphia: WB Saunders Company, pp. 246–264.

Parkes Weber F (1907) Angioma formation in connection with hypertrophy of limbs and hemihypertrophy. Br J Dermatol 19: 231.

Parkes Weber F (1908) Haemangiectatic hypertrophy of the foot and lower extremity. Med Press (London) 136: 261.

Parkes Weber F (1918) Haemangiectatic hypertrophy of the limbs – congenital phlebarteriectasis and so-called congenital varicose veins. Br J Chil Dis 15: 13.

Revencu N, Boon LM, Mulliken JB, Enjolras O, Cordisco MR, Burrows PE, Clapuyt P, Hammer F, Dubois J, Baselga E, Brancati F, Carder R, Quintal JM, Dallapiccola B, Fischer G, Frieden IJ, Garzon M, Harper J, Johnson-Patel J, Labrèze C, Martorell L, Paltiel HJ, Pohl A, Prendiville J, Quere I, Siegel DH, Valente EM, Van Hagen A, Van Hest L, Vaux KK, Vicente A, Weibel L, Chitayat D, Vikkula M (2008) Parkes Weber syndrome, vein of Galen aneurysmal malformation, and other fast-flow vascular anomalies are caused by RASA1 mutations. Hum Mutat Apr 29 [Epub ahead of print].

Robertson DJ (1956) Congenital arteriovenous fistulae of the extremities. Ann R Coll Surg Engl 18: 73.

Samuel M, Spitz L (1995) Klippel–Tranaunay syndrome. Clinical features, complications and management in children. Br J Surg 82: 757–761.

Taybi H, Lachman RS (1996) Klippel–Trenaunay syndrome. In: Taybi H, Lachman RS (eds.) Radiology of Syndromes, Metabolic Disorders, and Skeletal Dysplasia, 4th ed. St. Louis: Mosby, pp. 276–279.

Young AE (1978) Mixed vascular deformities. M Chir Thesis, University of Cambridge, Cambridge, England.

# Chapter 10

# STURGE-WEBER SYNDROME

Ignacio Pascual-Castroviejo, Orhan Konez, Concezio Di Rocco, and Martino Ruggieri

Paediatric Neurology Service, University Hospital La Paz, University of Madrid, Madrid, Spain (IPC); Department of Radiology,

Vascular and Interventional Radiology, St. John West Shore Hospital, University Hospitals Case Medical Center, Westlake, OHIO, USA (OK);

Section of Paediatric Neurosurgery, Department of Paediatrics, Catholic University of Sacred Heart, Rome, Italy (CDR);

Institute of Neurological Science, National Research Council, Catania, and Department of Paediatrics, University of Catania, Catania, Italy (MR)

## Introduction

*Sturge–Weber syndrome* (SWS) (OMIM # 185300), also known as encephalofacial or encephalotrigeminal angiomatosis or meningofacial angiomatosis, is a (usually) sporadic congenital neurocutaneous disorder affecting the cephalic venous microvasculature. The hallmark anomaly is a capillary malformation affecting: (a) the brain and meninges with or without involvement of (b) the choroid and/or episclera or conjunctive and (c) the skin (the latter typically in the cranial nerve V1–V3 territory including the mouth, pharynx and nasal mucosa or elsewhere in the body) (Baselga 2004, Gorlin et al. 2001, Thomas-Sohl et al. 2004, Di Rocco and Tamburrini 2006). Many incomplete forms, lacking one or more features of this triad exist (Baselga 2004). Other clinical features associated with SWS are seizures, glaucoma, headache, transient stroke-like neurological deficits, and behavioural problems. Hemiparesis, hemiatrophy, and hemianopia may occur contralaterally to the cortical abnormality (Thomas-Sohl et al. 2004).

## Historical background and terminology

The initial documentable description of an association of an infantile bilateral facial port-wine nevus "angiomatosis" with other features including glaucoma and unilateral buphthalmos is attributed to the German physician *Schirmer* from Berlin in 1860 (Schirmer 1860). The credit, however, belongs to the British physician and neurologist Sturge who gave also in 1879 a clear description of this condition and predicted its cerebral pathology (Gomez and Bebin 1987).

**William A. Sturge** (1850–1919) was born in 1850 into a Quaker family in Bristol, England, where his father was a surveyor. After obtaining his medical degree at University College, London, in 1873, Sturge undertook higher training at the Salpetrière in Paris with Jean Martin Charcot, the founder of the discipline of neurology. Sturge then returned to private practice in Wimpole Street, London, in partnership with his wife who was also medically qualified, and obtained concurrent appointments at several hospitals in London. Sturge was a proponent of women's education and lectured at the Royal Free Hospital. He was also active in neurological research and published several articles in this discipline including a vivid account of progressive muscular atrophy, for which he was awarded the Silver Medal of the Medical Society of London. In 1879, he presented at that Society a $6^{1}/_{2}$ -year-old girl, who had a deep purple "mother's mark" on the right side of the head and face including the lips, gums, tongue, floor of mouth, palate, uvula, pharynx, and back of neck extending "as low as the third and fourth dorsal vertebrae behind and the second costal cartilage in front". The right eye was larger than the left. The child had "attacks of twitching in her left side affecting the face, arm and leg", lasting 10 or 12 minutes since the age of 6 months. As she grew older the seizures became stronger and were followed by temporary weakness. By age 5 years she had loss of consciousness with the attacks. Sturge cleverly deduced that the underlying flat vascular nevus over the cerebral cortex gave rise to the partial seizures. Sturge's wife suffered ill-health and in 1880 they moved to enjoy the more salubrious climate of Nice, on the French Riviera. He practised successfully in Nice for the next 27 years before retiring in Suffolk in 1907. He then had the time to pursue his hobby of archaeology and was founder and president of the local society. Sturge died in 1919 at the age of 68 years.

*Kalischer* (1897) confirmed at autopsy the intracranial vascular lesions predicted by Sturge. *Cushing* (1906) described after craniotomy "meningeal angiomas" in three patients with cutaneous nevus within the region of distribution of the trigeminal nerve. Weber (1922) described some of the radiological abnormalities (calcifications) in the affected cerebral hemisphere.

**Frederick Parkes Weber**, who was born in 1863, matriculated at Cambridge University and St. Bartholomew's Hospital, London. His father, Sir Hermann Weber, had come to England from Germany and served as physician to Queen Victoria. Weber and his family retained their German connections, emphasised by his persistent pronunciation of his surname with the continental "V" sound, now long forgotten since his death. Weber was legendary in the Royal Society of Medicine by virtue of his remarkable knowledge of rare disorders, for his clear and meticulous diction, and for his prolific contributions of more than 1200 medical articles over a span of 50 years of active medical practice. He was a prodigious describer of new or unique entities, many of them dermatological, and his name has been attached to several disorders, including Klippel-Trenaunay-Weber syndrome, Hutchinson-Weber-Peutz-Jeghers syndrome, and Osler-Rendu-Weber syndrome. In 1922, he reported the first radiological features of brain "atrophy" in the SWS, but did not mention the now classic intracranial calcifications (Bodensteiner and Roach 1999). In a later account of the same patient, however, he amended the description with a much better film of the skull (Weber 1929).

*Dimitri* (1923) described the characteristic double-contoured lines, and *Krabbe* (1934) correctly interpreted, by clinicopathological studies, these lines as calcifications of the cerebral cortex, not of the walls of cerebral vessels. *Van der Hoeve* (1937) classified SWS as another phakomatosis thus muddling a concept that he had introduced earlier to encompass tuberous sclerosis, neurofibromatosis, and von Hippel-Lindau disease.

Choroidal "angioma", first reported by *Jennings Milles* in 1884, was extensively described by Rosen (1950). Cerebral hemisphere hypoplasia was reported in 1901 by Kalisher in his second paper on the subject (Kalisher 1901), and focal microgiria by Hebold in 1913.

Several eponyms have been used to describe SWS (in addition to "Sturge-Weber syndrome" that is practically the only used now) including encephalofacial angiomatosis, angio-encephalo-cutaneous syndrome, vascular neuro-oculo-cutaneous syndrome, encephalotrigeminal angiomatosis, Sturge-Weber-Krabbe syndrome, Sturge-Weber-Dimitri syndrome or Sturge-Kalisher-Weber syndrome (Gomez and Bebin 1987).

## Incidence and prevalence

SWS is the fifth most frequent neurocutaneous disorder, surpassed only by "cutaneous hemangiomas: vascular anomaly complex" (Pascual-Castroviejo type II syndrome), neurofibromatosis type 1, tuberous sclerosis, and hypomelanosis of Ito. An estimated frequency of 1 per 50,000 live births have SWS, although experts believe many more people have the disorder but have not yet been identified (Thomas-Sohl et al. 2004). The syndrome affects both sexes and all the races with a slight male preponderance (Gomez and Bebin 1987).

## Clinical manifestations

### Skin manifestations

The cutaneous lesion is a capillary malformation (*nevus flammeus*) that affects the facial area innervated by the first sensory branch of the trigeminal nerve and possibly other facial areas on the same or opposite side or anywhere else on the skin of the body (Fig. 1) or the mucosa of the palate, pharynx, larynx, tongue, gums, or cheeks ipsilateral to the cutaneous nevus. Patients with a nevus solely on another part of the body have little chances of having

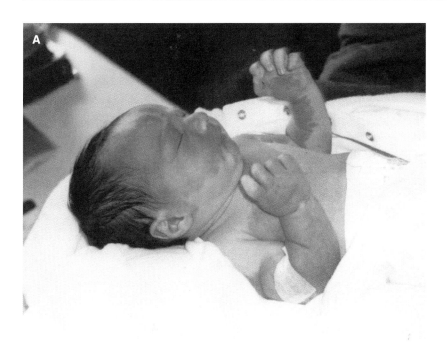

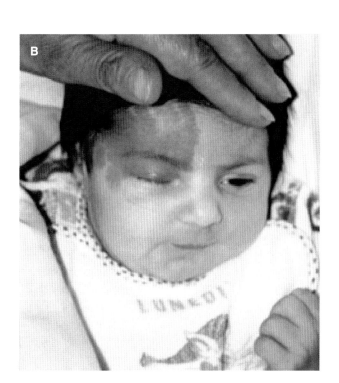

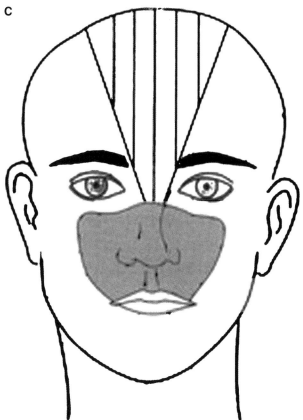

**Fig. 1.** Nevus flammeus extending over the right hemifacies (**A**) and other cutaneous areas elsewhere in the face (**B**); (**C**) the typically trigenominal (VI–V3) territory affected: the solid area represents the opital facial region; the striped area represents the opital forhead region; all other areas are considered peripheral [(C) adapted from Mguyen et al. 1998].

the ophthalmologic or brain complications of SWS (Riela and Roach 2004).

The nevus pigmentation appears initially as pale red and evolves into a dark port-wine colour. Some authors believe that the nevus flammeus may represent a telangiectatic condition of the capillaries which corresponds more to a congenital weakness of the walls than to the nature of a true capillary malformation (Barsky et al. 1980). The nevus flammeus is a congenital vascular anomaly that manifests from birth and usually increases progressively. More important than the size, degree of pigmentation, and unilaterality or bilaterality of the facial nevus is the neuroimaging abnormality in both cerebral hemispheres, changes in other regions of the brain be-

sides the classic one in the occipital area, as well as the very early appearance of these changes. Some cases with SWS show hypertrophy of the soft tissues underlying the areas covered by the nevus flammeus. This most frequently occurs after adolescence and, particularly in cases of dark coloured nevi (Fig. 2).

Some cases are accepted and classified as SWS with typical neurological features and leptomeningeal vascular malformation, but without facial nevus. A high proportion of cases truly without facial port-wine nevus has been reported in some series. Lund (1949) found seven patients without facial nevus with two proven at surgery in a review of 144 cases of SWS; Peterman et al. (1958) five out of 35; Tonnis and Friedman (1964) four out of 23;

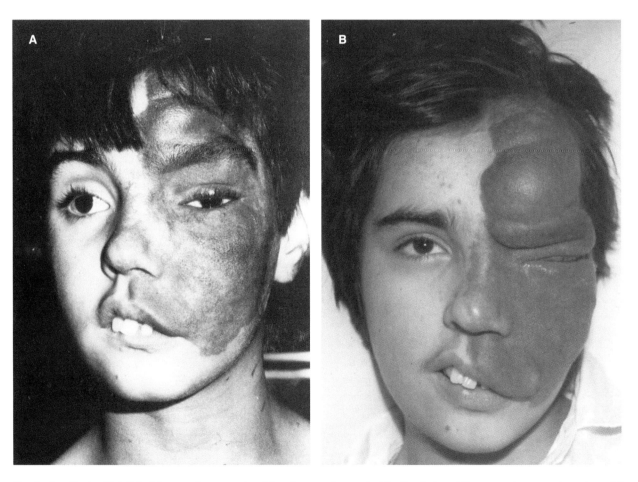

**Fig. 2.** A patient with left facial nevus flammeus involving the area innervated by the first and the second sensory branches of the trigeminal nerve. (**A**) At the age of 8 years there is a discrete hypertrophy of the soft tissues. (**B**) At 11 years of age the patient shows great hypertrophy of the area involved by the nevus flammeus.

Gomez and Bebin (1987) 13 of the total 101 patients seen at the Mayo Clinic 30 years after the study of Peterman et al. (1958); and Pascual-Castroviejo et al. (1995) one in 40 cases (the latter demonstrated by skull ray-X, MR enhanced with Gd-DPTA, MR angiography, and Tc99m SPECT). These cases with absent port-wine stain had been classified in the past (Roach 1988, 1992) as *SWS type 3* and considered as true variants of SWS opposed to *SWS type 1 or "classic" SWS* with both facial and intracranial disease manifestations and *SWS type 2* with only facial lesions (the latter considered probably a pure dermatological condition rather than a variant of SWS) (Roach 1992).

Patients with SWS may have other vascular abnormalities including those in the spectrum of Klippel-Trenaunay syndrome or associated pigmentary anomalies such as the blue nevus of phakomatosis pigmentovascularis.

The skin within the nevus flammeus area is firm during the first years and youth, but then becomes dry, hypertrophic, nodular and pruriginous.

## Ocular manifestations

Heterochromia of the iris, with ipsilateral hyperpigmentation is often seen in some cases. Buphthalmos (hydrophthalmia) or glaucoma associated with a choroidal capillary malformation occurs in at least 30% of cases (Iwach et al. 1990), although some studies have shown a prevalence as high as 60% in adults (Sujansky and Conradi 1995) or 71% (Sullivan et al. 1992). The age at onset of glaucoma is usually (a) during the first year of life; (b) between age 5 and 9 years; and (c) after age 20. Because of the chance of later onset of glaucoma (20% in the series of Sujansky and Conradi 1995), the true prevalence of glaucoma in SWS may be closer to 60% than to the 48% as was recorded in a previous study of SWS patients of all ages by the same authors (Sujansky and Conradi 1995). Glaucoma is associated with the nevus involving both the upper and lower lids (Enjolras et al. 1985, Pascual-Castroviejo et al. 1993, Stevenson et al. 1974, Tallman et al. 1991). The association of glaucoma and seizures that has been frequently

recorded (Sujansky and Conradi 1995, Tallman et al. 1991) is understandable because of the high prevalence of either complication in SWS. The choroidal vascular malformation is most frequently seen at fundoscopy, and is better documented by MR with Gd-DTPA as also occurs with the leptomeningeal malformation (Griffiths et al. 1996, Pascual-Castroviejo et al. 1993). Besides fundoscopy, enhanced MR with Gd-DTPA allows a better visualization of the unilateral (Fig. 3B–C) or bilateral localisation of the choroidal malformation which is always associated with the nevus flammeus affecting the lids and possibly with haemorrhages of the retina that can occur in some patients with SWS (Fig. 3C).

The pathogenesis of glaucoma has been tentatively explained by several mechanisms: 1) increased production of aqueous humour by the choroidal vascular malformation; 2) increased production of aqueous humour by increased permeability of the capillaries; and 3) a breakdown of the blood-aqueous barrier in the capillary malformation which produces a plasmoid aqueous humour that blocks the angle.

The ocular involvement usually causes loss of vision on the same side of the facial nevus and the contralateral eye also may be affected because of the brain lesion that most frequently involves the occipital lobe.

Abnormal conjunctival and/or episcleral vascularity can be seen hidden beneath the upper or lower lip (Fig. 4) (Bodensteiner and Roach 1999).

## Bones and teeth

Skeletal alterations may also occur aside the skin, ocular and brain manifestations. Generalized or localized decrease in size of the hemiplegic or hemiparetic side is most frequently observed. This usually causes a moderate scoliosis that may need orthopaedic treatment. Skull radiographs demonstrate all the signs of cerebral hemiatrophy after the first year of life: the most significant findings include cranial asymmetry with a smaller hemicranium on the involved side; overall decrease of one hemicra-

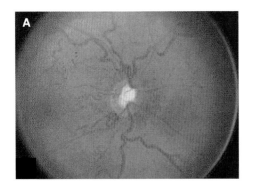

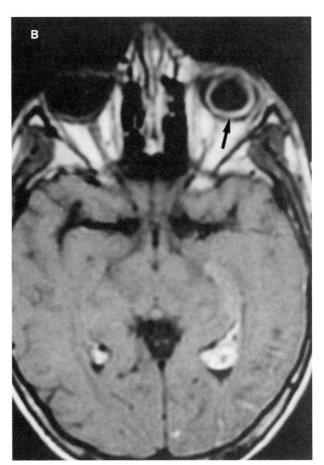

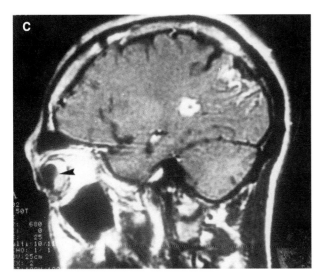

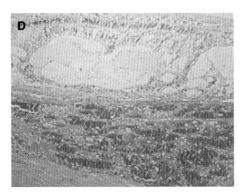

**Fig. 3.** (**A**) Retinal vascular malformation as seen at fundoscopy; (**B**) MRI enhanced with Gd-DTPA in a patient with SWS. Axial image discloses hypersignal of the left eye retina (arrow) and leptomeningeal capillary malformation in the ipsilateral hemisphere; (**C**) Enhanced MRI with Gd-DTPA. Sagittal image reveals hemorrhage of the retina (arrowhead) and the presence of occipital leptomeningeal capillary malformation and hypersignal of the left choroidal plexus; (**D**) Histology of a choroidal vascular malformation. In the upper part is visible the retina with its multiple layers detached (in this preparation) from the choroid which is tickened and contains the abnormal vascular channels; beneath the choroid lies the sclera (**D**) reprinted with permission from Bodenteiner and Roach 1999.

nium size or, occasionally, ipsilateral enlargement of a hemicranium; thickening of the cranial diploes; increased size of the frontal, ethmoidal and sphenoidal sinuses on the side of the nevus; enlarged vascular channels of the skull; double-contour "gyriform" patterns of intracranial calcifications in the subcortical region, primarily in the parietal and occipital regions (Taybi 1996).

It is common to see the eruption of the primitive (Fig. 5) and the definitive teeth some time earlier (months to years) on the side of the facial nevus (Pascual-Castroviejo et al. 1978). The presence of

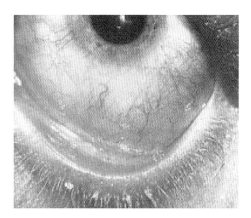

**Fig. 4.** Abnormal conjunctival and episclerel vessels [reprinted with permission from Bodensteiner and Roach 1999].

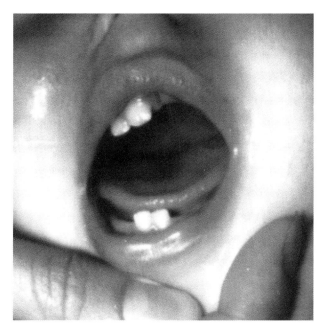

**Fig. 5.** Nevus flammeus on the right hemifacial side and presence of primitive teeth only on the right side in a patient a few months of age.

one or two teeth in the upper gum on the side of the nevus flammeus at birth is frequently seen.

## Connective tissue

The skin thickness and that of the underlying soft tissues tend to increase in those patients having the darkest pigmentation. This finding is particularly evident after 10–12 years of age, while the hard tissues (i.e., bones and teeth) exhibit hypertrophy at earlier ages.

## Central nevus system (CNS) manifestations

Intracranial abnormalities usually influence the neurologic deficit, mental level, seizures, behaviour, intracranial pressure, brain and leptomeninges anatomy, and vascularization. All the mentioned features and organs play an important role in the neurodevelopment of the patients and their outcome in adult life.

### Seizures

Seizures are one of the main features of SWS. Convulsions have been reported in 62% (Bebin and Gomez 1988), 75% (Breuner and Sharbrough 1976), 80% (Pascual-Castroviejo et al. 1993), 83% (Sujansky and Conradi 1995) and 89% (Peterman et al. 1958) of patients with SWS and are mostly of focal motor onset. Generalized onset (or better quick generalisation), however, can be observed as well. Occasionally, the initial type of seizure is infantile spasms or tonic, atonic, or myoclonic. These are usually related to severe cerebral lesions and have a very early presentation. Focal and generalized seizures may occur with febrile episodes in about a third of patients with SWS (Pascual-Castroviejo 1993). Fever can also trigger subsequent seizures at any time during life. This finding is observed equally in patients having either a favourable or poor clinical course. Seizures start before the age of 1 year in 75% of patients with epilepsy (Sujansky and Conradi 1995). The mean age at seizures onset, however, was 15 months (range: newborn to 6 years) in an important series (Pascual-Castroviejo et al. 1993). In the series of Sujansky and Conradi (1995), 12% of patients did not develop seizures until the third decade. Patients having more severe epileptic disorders (i.e., unilateral or bilateral lesions, resistance to antiepileptic drugs and worse course and outcome) manifest an earlier onset of seizures (most frequently before 6 months of age). The severity of the cerebral lesion, seizures of difficult control and severe psychomotor delay most frequently are related.

Patients with bilateral SWS have higher prevalence of seizures (89%) than those with unilateral SWS (74%) (Sujansky and Conradi 1995). Children most at risk for psychological problems are those with seizure disorders and those with more frequent seizures (Chapieski et al. 2000).

## EEG findings

The prevalent EEG finding is asymmetry of the background amplitude during the waking record, usually involving the entire affected hemisphere (Breuner and Sharbrough 1976, Pascual-Castroviejo et al. 1978). This asymmetry can be observed from the first months of life, but is more noticeable as cerebral hemiatrophy becomes more severe and can be seen both in patients who continue to have partial or generalized seizures and in those who have achieved seizure control by medication. Focal paroxysms occur mainly in the cerebral hemisphere with the lesion. However, these can also appear on the contralateral hemisphere in a significant number of patients (Fukuyama and Tsuchiya 1979). The severity of the electrical abnormalities is closely related to the extent and severity of cerebral atrophy and calcifications, and to a poor response to antiepileptic medications (Hatfield et al. 2007).

## Neurological vs. neuroimaging findings

More important than the size, degree of pigmentation, and unilaterality or bilaterality of the facial nevus is the imaging abnormality of both cerebral hemispheres, changes in other areas of the brain besides the classic occipital area, as well as the very early appearance of these changes. Patients who have cortical and/or subcortical changes in the first months of life usually develop an important progressive cerebral hemiatrophy. Cases with prenatal onset of the disease may show cortical/subcortical calcification

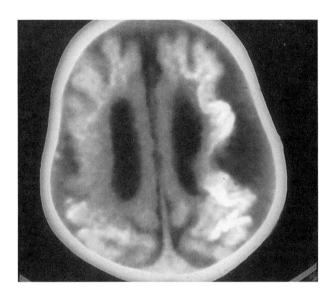

**Fig. 6.** Prenatal onset of SWS. MRI of a neonate. The axial view shows severe cortico-subcortical atrophy and increased signal and cortical dysplasia in both cerebral hemispheres.

and developmental dysplasia of the cerebral mantle (Yeakley et al. 1992). An association of cortical anomalies (Fig. 6) with the typical leptomeningeal vascular anomaly as also been demonstrated (Portilla et al. 2002).

Typical cortical/subcortical calcifications, most frequently found in the occipital area, appear after age 1 year on skull radiographs (Fig. 7A), while CT and MR studies may show these lesions as hyperdensity of the affected hemisphere in the newborn (Alonso et al. 1978, Kitahara and Maki 1978, Pascual-Castroviejo et al. 1993). CT and MR may also document important progressive changes in the cortex and subcortical parenchyma which parallels the increased development of the vascular malformation affecting the meninges. Extensive serial examination of these patients usually reveals an increase in density and extension of the calcified zones as well as in the appearance of the cerebral cortical/subcortical atrophy which has a progressive character, especially during the first years of life (Fig. 7). These radiological changes appear to have a vascular origin (Alonso et al. 1979, Di Trapani et al. 1982, Guseo 1975, Kitahara and Maki 1978) and are probably caused by alterations in the vessel wall

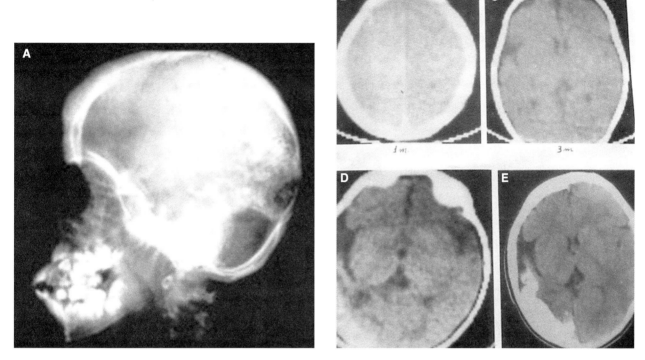

**Fig. 7.** (**A**) lateral skull X-ray study showing the typical double contour lesions; (**B–E**) unenhanced axial CT of the same patient at different ages: **B** At age one month, moderate hyperdensity of the left cerebral hemisphere is noted. **C** At age 3 months, corticosubcortical hematrophy in the same hemisphere is observed. **D** At 18 months of age, hemiatrophy is severe and the occipito-parietal brain parenchyma has hyperdensity on the left side. **E** At 6 years of age, the left cerebral hemisphere is still more atrophic and the hyperdensity of the occipito-parietal region has increased.

permeability and stasis in the vascular lumen which provokes an anoxic lesion of the endothelium (Schnyder 1957), an observation that coincides with the angiographic findings (Chamberlain et al. 1989). In adults, chronic cerebral ischaemia of SWS has been related to migraine attacks (Cambon et al. 1987), hemiplegia without cerebral infarction in term pregnancy (Chabriat et al. 1996), and other neurological abnormalities.

Gd-DTPA – enhanced MR improves the diagnostic value of standard MR (Benedikt et al. 1993, Pascual-Castroviejo et al. 1993, Sugama et al. 1997, Vogl et al. 1993) and can be used to recognize thrombotic changes in the leptomeningeal malformation as well as the subsequent cerebral injury (Sperner et al. 1990). MR with Gd-DTPA also allows observation of the extension of the leptomeningeal lesion which, in

some SWS patients, may extend over the entire hemisphere. The choroid plexus is enlarged early in the course of SWS in both unilateral (Fig. 8A, B) and bilateral cases (Fig. 8C) and there is positive correlation between choroid plexus size and the extent of leptomeningeal involvement (Griffiths 1996, Whischel and Font 1976).

In some cases, particularly those with the nevus flammeus extended on the neck as well, the leptomeningeal angioma may be also seen in the homolateral cerebellar hemisphere (Fig. 9).

A pattern of accelerated myelination in the affected cerebral hemisphere has been observed in small children (Fig. 8D) (Adamsbaum et al. 1996, Jacoby et al. 1987, Sperner et al. 1990). This finding has been interpreted as secondary to ischaemia subjacent to the leptomeningeal malformation (Jacoby

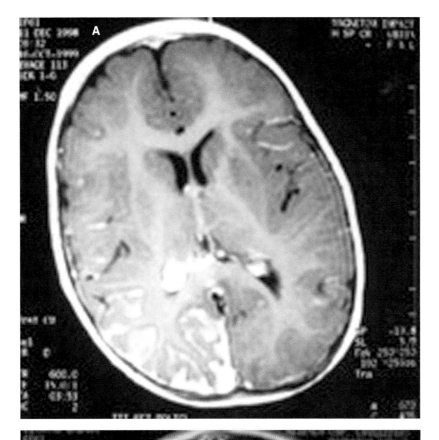

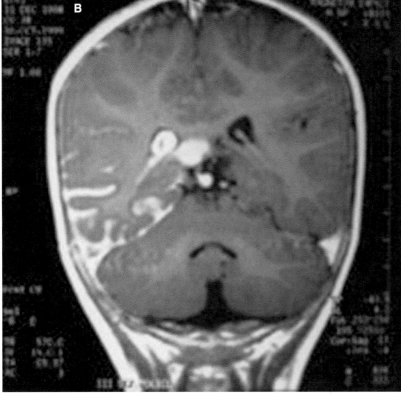

**Fig. 8.** Enhanced MRI with Gd-DTPA. Axial (**A**, **E**) and coronal (**B**, **C**, **D**) images show unilateral (right) (**A**, **B**) and bilateral (**C**) leptomeningeal capillary malformation; (**A–C**) enlarged choroidal plexus; (**C**) (right) white matter anomalies; (**E**) (left) cortical atrophy.

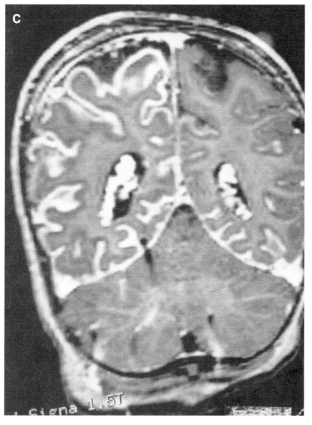

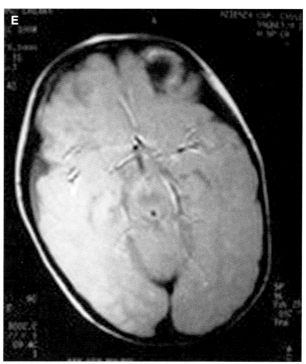

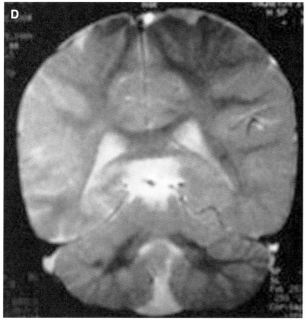

**Fig. 8.** (Continued)

et al. 1987), although it is most probable that, in infancy, it is due to a paradoxical increase in the metabolism of the affected hemisphere (Sperner et al. 1990) as has been demonstrated by positron emission tomography (PET) (Chugani et al. 1989). Accelerated myelination in infants with SWS, however,

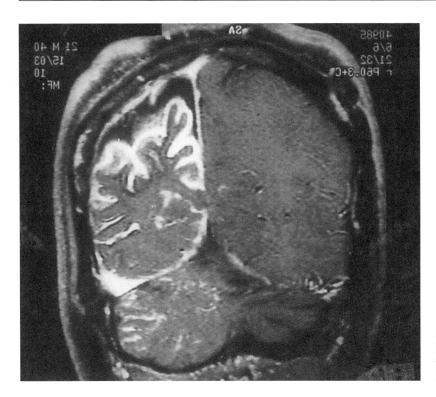

**Fig. 9.** Enhanced MRI with Gd-DTPA. Coronal image shows leptomeningeal vascular malformation in the right cerebral and cerebellar hemispheres.

appears to be transient because longitudinal MR studies have shown usually resolution of myelination asymmetry after 9 months of age (Adamsbaum et al. 1996). The mechanisms underlying this transient and seemingly paradoxical phenomenon have yet to be elucidated. High resolution MR and PET studies demonstrated that the grey-matter volumes ipsilateral to the angioma are smaller in the regions underneath the angioma. In infants, the white matter volumes were increased in the region of the angioma, whereas in the regions remote from the angioma, large decreases in white matter volume were found in the older children (Pfund et al. 2003). The PET studies showed severe hypometabolism in the region underneath the vascular anomaly. Both structural and functional abnormalities extend well beyond the capillary anomaly, indicating widespread abnormalities of growth and development of the affected hemisphere (Pfund et al. 2003). SPECT study revealed similar alterations in a case of SWS without facial capillary malformation but with occipital leptomeningeal malformation (Fig. 10) (Pascual-Castroviejo et al. 1995).

Hypoperfusion in the area of the leptomeningeal malformation is a common finding (Chiron et al. 1989, Evans et al. 2006, Juhasz et al. 2007, Yu et al. 2007). Some cases of SWS with decreased blood flow in the affected hemisphere may show a significantly increased blood flow in the unaffected hemisphere (Riela et al. 1985, Kelley et al. 2005).

Angiographic changes are very well documented by arteriography and MR angiography. These consist of smaller sized intracranial arteries secondary to cerebral atrophy in the affected hemisphere, even with interruption of the arterial lumen in some segments in patients having the most severe atrophy and venous abnormalities (Bentson et al. 1971, Garcìa et al. 1981, Pascual-Castroviejo et al. 1993). These abnormalities consist of a lack of superficial veins, associated non filling of the superior sagittal sinus (Fig. 11), thickening and tortuosity of the deep subependymal and medullary veins, and, occasionally, bizarre course of cerebral veins. The basis of this abnormal cerebral venous drainage pattern appears to be the non-functioning or absence of cortical veins beneath the SWS leptomeningeal

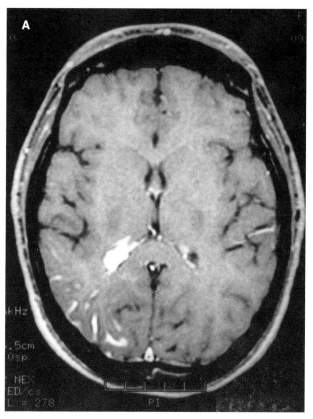

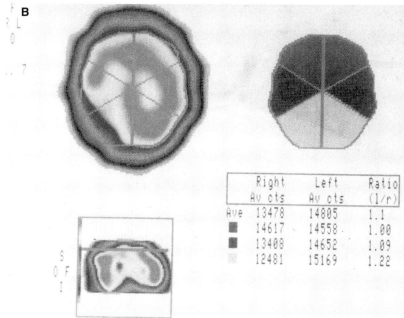

| | Right<br>Av cts | Left<br>Av cts | Ratio<br>(l/r) |
|---|---|---|---|
| Ave | 13478 | 14805 | 1.1 |
| ■ | 14617 | 14558 | 1.00 |
| ■ | 13408 | 14652 | 1.09 |
| ▒ | 12481 | 15169 | 1.22 |

**Fig. 10.** SWS without facial nevus flammeus. **A** Enhanced MRI wit Gd-DTPA, discloses hypersignal of the right occipital cortex-leptomeninges and an enlarged choroidal plexus. **B** Axial view of quantitative technetium Tc99m SPECT study shows a wide area of hypoperfusion in the right occipital area. The table presents an important difference of perfusion between both parieto-occipital areas, severely decreased in the right side.

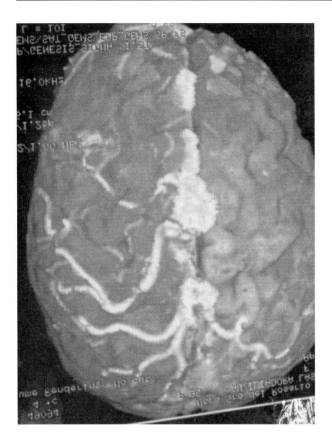

**Fig. 11.** MR angiography shows lack of superficial veins in the left cerebral hemisphere, that is smaller than the contralateral one, and presents cortical atrophy. The superior sagittal sinus shows non continuous filling.

malformation with collateral flow centrally to the subependymal veins (Bentson et al. 1971).

MR enhanced with Gd-DTPA permits to differentiate cases of SWS without facial nevus that show the typical leptomeningeal lesions (Pascual-Castroviejo et al. 1995) from the rare cases of gluten sensitive patients with celiac disease, which present with epilepsy and occipital cerebral calcifications (Gobbi et al. 1992), but without leptomeningeal vascular malformations. It must be noted however that few of these cases at pathology were found to have minimal (but true) vascular anomalies in the leptomeninges aside cortical architectural malformations (Gobbi 2005).

Although only rarely, persistent trigeminal artery has been associated with SWS (Loevner and Quint 1992). This association is seen in about 30% of cases

of Pascual-Castroviejo type II syndrome (the so-called "cutaneous hemangiomas: vascular anomaly complex") (Pascual-Castroviejo et al. 1996, Pascual-Castroviejo 2004) and suggests the possibility of some relationship between both disorders.

## Pathology

In gross section, the leptomeninges appear thickened and discoloured by the pial capillary malformation. Enlargement of the choroid plexus is common. Calcifications are observed in meningeal arteries and in cortical and subcortical veins underlying the pial malformation. Laminar cortical necrosis can accompany calcifications, suggesting ischaemic damage secondary to venous stasis in leptomeninges and in the cerebral vascular bed. With continued progression, neuronal loss and gliosis can occur.

Malformation(s) of cortical development with altered architectural layering have been reported throughout the entire cortex in isolated cases of severe SWS (reviewed in Simonati et al. 1994) or, most frequently, in the area underlying the vascular leptomeningeal malformation (Bodensteiner and Roach 1999). The lack of evidence of heterotopic neurons in the subjacent white matter in a SWS case with microgyria (Simonati et al. 1994) was suggestive of an early post-migratory vascular pathological event likely explained by ischaemic effects affecting the process of corticogenesis.

## Pathogenesis and molecular genetics

*Pathogenesis.* It has been suggested that SWS results from failure of the primitive cephalic venous plexus to regress during the 1st trimester of pregnancy (Comi 2003, Parsa 2008). During the 6th week of development, a vascular plexus forms around the cephalic portion of the neural tube and beneath the ectoderm destined to become the facial skin. Normally, this vascular plexus regresses during the 9th week of gestation, but in SWS, it persists, resulting in capillary malformation of the leptomeninges overlying the cerebral cortex together with a facial capillary malformation ("port-wine" stain) of the ipsilateral side (Cohen et al. 2002). At this stage, in embryogenesis, the close proximity of the ectoderm destined to form the facial skin to the portion of the neural tube destined to form the parietooccipital area of the brain may explain the association of facial and leptomeningeal capillary malformation (Baselga 2004, Comi 2003). Variations of the persistence or regression of the vascular plexus accounts for cases with unilateral or bilateral involvement and also for cases with capillary malformation of the leptomeninges with absence of facial involvement (Cohen 1998, Cohen et al. 2002, Simonati et al. 1994, Sujanski and Conradi 1995).

Other authors have suggested that there is either a failure of superficial cortical veins to develop or early thrombosis of these veins. As a result, there is redirection of blood to the developing leptomeninges and into the deep venous system. Despite this reduction there is insufficient venous drainage, leading to progressive venous stasis and vessel dilatation producing chronic hypoxia (Griffiths 1996).

More recent molecular studies suggest that abnormal brain blood vessel vasoactive and extracellular matrix molecule expression as well as absent brain vascular innovation, contribute to the vascular malformation and its consequences (reviewed in Comi 2006).

The pathogenesis of the capillary malformation of the skin (the port-wine stain or nevus flammeus) remains controversial (Baselga 2004). It seems clear that there is only dilatation of blood vessels without proliferation. The cause of blood vessels ectasie does not seem to be secondary to defective vessel wall but may be related to a deficiency in sympathetic innervations to the vessel and failure to regulate vasoconstriction (Smoller and Rosen 1987).

Recently, Comati et al. (2007) demonstrated increased hypoxia-inducible factor (HIF)-1alpha and -2alpha in SWS vessels with concomitant enhancement of endothelial cells tumours and apoptosis indicating dynamic (not static) modelling in SWS vessels.

*Familial occurrence.* SWS occurs sporadically with equal frequency in boys and girls. There are only a couple of familial cases reported in the literature: a father and a son both affected by SWS and a mother with port-wine stain in the distribution of the 3rd branch of the trigeminal nerve, whose son had SWS (Debicka et al. 1979, Pascual-Castroviejo et al. 1978). For several years it has been proposed that SWS (and also other neurocutaneous disorders) were the result of a somatic mutation in the affected area (Happle 1987). Discordance in monozygotic twins in SWS is consistent with this hypothesis (Baselga 2004). Evidence of somatic mosaicism (chromosomal rearrangements and trisomy in chromosomes 4 and 10) has been demonstrated in tissues from affected areas (facial and leptomeningeal capillary malformation) in selected patients with SWS who lacked these findings in normal skin and blood (Huq et al. 2002). This may suggest a gene dosage effect for genes on chromosome 10 or inactivation of a gene on chromosome 4q. Alternatively, it may suggest chromosomal instability in the affected tissue (Huq et al. 2002) or coincidental mosaicism (a rather common finding in areas with pathological lesions in any medical condition). The origin of SWS, however, remains unknown at present and deserves further study.

Familial occurrence of port-wine stain/capillary malformation (CMAL) (OMIM # 163000) and capillary malformation/arteriovenous malformation (CM-AVM) (OMIM # 608354) have been described in the literature (Breugen et al. 2002; Eerola et al. 2002, 2003; Shuper et al. 1984; van der Horst et al. 1999). Of the 60 subjects with (autosomal dominant) inherited CM-AVM from 13 families studied by Eerola et al. (2003) all the affected members manifested atypical capillary malformations that were multiple, small, round to oval in shape, pinkish red in colour and localised on the face, neck region or in other parts of the body. APP the capillary malformations were associated with either arteriovenous malformation, arteriovenous fistula, or Parkes Weber syndrome (Eerola et al. 2003). A susceptibility locus for this hereditary form was identified on chromosome 5q14q21 (Eerola et al. 2002) and termed CMC1. This locus was later narrowed to 5q13.3 (Eerola et al. 2003). Heterozygous inactivating RASA1 gene mutations were detected in several families with CM-AVM and Eerola et al. (2003) suggested that the phenotypic variability in this syndrome could be explained by the involvement of the p120-RasGAP protein (encoded by the RASA1 gene) which promote signalling for various growth factor receptors that control proliferation, migration, and survival of several cell types, including vascular endothelial cells. Notably, in one of the families studied by Eerola et al. (2002, 2003) with no RASA1 gene mutations there were two individuals with Klippel-Trenaunay syndrome and in another family one individual had SWS.

## Management

Cosmetic facial alterations caused by the nevus flammeus can best be treated by sophisticated laser therapeutic techniques. The results are satisfactory in cases with capillary malformations of low pigmentation, with lightening of the pigmented zones (Tan et al. 1989). The degree of decrease in pigmentation, however, depends on its intensity at the onset of treatment (Pascual-Castroviejo et al. 1993): in cases with highly pigmented vascular malformation of the skin although the treated skin becomes clearer after laser administration (Fig. 12) the previous colour usually returns after few months.

Seizures in SWS patients have been treated similarly to those in patients without SWS. Carbamazepine or oxicarbamazepine, valproic acid, topiramate, levetiracetam, hydantoins and clonazepam are the most used antiepileptic drugs. Patients with intractable seizures, especially those with permanent paralysis and mental retardation, may need neurosurgical treatment by lobectomy (Arzimanoglou et al. 2000, Buttler and Schulte 1975, Rosen and Salford 1984), hemispherectomy (Hoffman et al. 1979), corpus callosum section (Rappaport 1988) or lesionectomy (complete resection of the pial vascular malformation and underlying cortex). Lobectomy and hemispherectomy are the most commonly used surgical treatments. Surgical methods started to be used more than half a century ago (Polani 1952, Peterman et al. 1958). Lesionectomy (Fig. 13) has been found to be a good approach in cases of unilateral pial malformation and possibility of complete section (Arzimanoglou et al. 2000). Hemispherec-

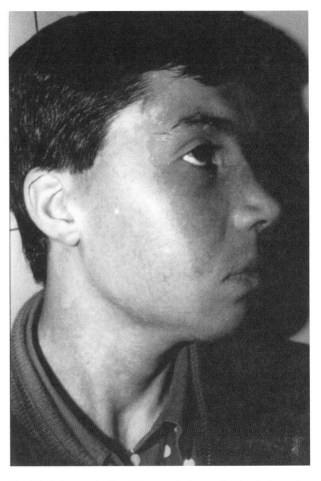

**Fig. 12.** A line marks the difference between the treated and the untreated areas of the facial nevus immediately after applying lasertherapy.

tomy gives gratifying results in a majority of patients who underwent surgery before 1 year of age (Ogunmekan et al. 1989). In some recent retrospective reviews, however, it was observed that the age at surgery does not have an adverse effect on either seizure or cognitive outcome, although children undergoing hemispherectomy at a younger age have frequent seizures for approximately 1 year but are later mostly seizure-free (Kossoff et al. 2002).

Asymmetry of lower extremities, scoliosis, and spasticity have been treated with physiotherapy, orthopaedic help or botulism toxin.

Problems at school that affect intellectual function and behaviour in most cases, may need special

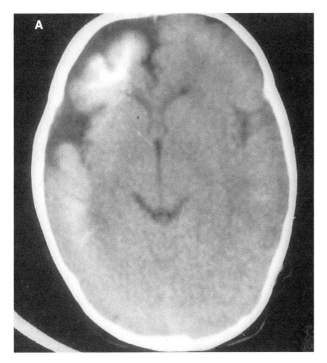
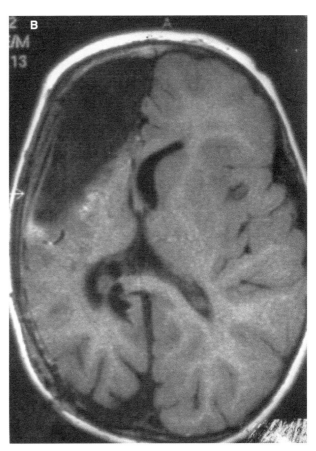

**Fig. 13.** SWS patient with a right frontal lesion and leptomeningeal capillary malformation at one year of age (**A**), and after lesionectomy at 7 years of age and complete control of the seizures (**B**).

help and stimulants drugs, such as methylphenidate, associated with antiepileptic treatment.

Glaucoma and buphthalmos must be treated and followed periodically by the ophthalmologist (Patrianakos et al. 2008).

## Psychomotor outcome

A comparison between data on adults and patients of all ages with SWS shows very similar prevalence figures of body asymmetry, seizures, neurologic deficits, and special educational requirements (Sujansky and Conradi 1995).

Abnormality of the cerebral parenchyma can be detected from birth in some patients and has a pro-

gressive character; occasionally it has been observed prenatally (Campistol et al. 1999, Portilla et al. 2002). The clinical disease follows a course parallel to the anatomic and physiologic changes. The patients who had extensive and severe lesions also had severe neurologic abnormalities, with hemiplegia, early onset of uncontrolled seizures, low intellectual level and, frequently, aggressive behaviour. A worse prognosis was observed in patients with bilateral cerebral lesions (only one fourth of patients with bilateral nevus flammeus develop bilateral cerebral lesions) (Pascual-Castroviejo et al. 1993), and in patients having unilateral lesions in whom there was severe involvement of the entire hemisphere (Pascual-Castroviejo et al. 1993).

No relationship exists between the size of the facial nevus flammeus or its unilateral or bilateral

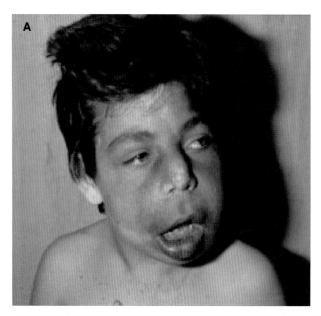

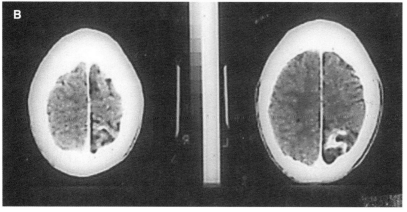

Fig. 14. (**A**) Patient with bilateral large facial nevus flammeus. (**B**) Enhanced MR with Gd-DTPA shows unilateral lesion in the left occipital region.

location (Fig. 14) and neurologic impairment. Conversely, a direct relationship exists between greater anatomic manifestations (i.e., atrophy, calcification) in the involved hemisphere when the lesion is unilateral (Fig. 15) as well as the presence of leptomeningeal vascular malformation in both cerebral hemispheres in patients with bilateral facial nevus flammeus, the presence of intractable seizures, the severity of clinical disorders and the white matter volume and loss (Juhasz et al. 2008). Keith et al. (1955) found that the incidence of mental retardation was 65% when onset of seizures occurred before age 6 months, 49% between 6 months and 2 years, and 34% between 2 and 4 years.

Mental retardation was present in 60% of a series of 40 children and young patients, and was severe in 32.5% (Pascual-Castroviejo et al. 1993). In a series of 52 adults, 65% had neurologic deficit (Sujansky and Conradi 1995), 55% were consider intellectually subnormal and 45% normal, with 43% with development delay, 85% with emotional and behavioural problems, 71% required special education, 46% obtained gainful employment, 39% were financially self-sufficient, and 55% were eligible or already married. In the series of 35 cases of Peterman et al. (1958), 54% had mental retardation. Bebin and Gomez (1988) reported a series of 102 patients of SWS who were seen at the Mayo Clinic between 1942 and 1986; they studied retrospectively the cases to determine the difference in prognosis between unihemispheric and bihemispheric involvement. Of

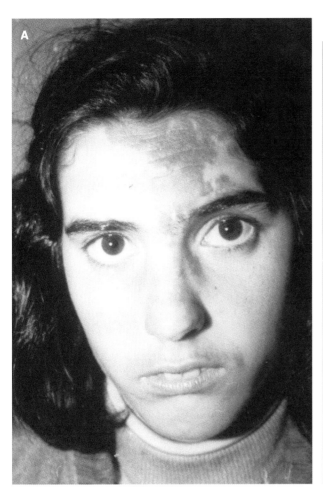
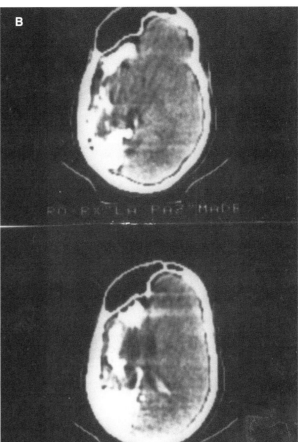

**Fig. 15.** (**A**) Patient with facial nevus flammeus located on a part of the territory of the left first sensory branch of the trigeminal nerve. (**B**) CT images of the same patient show severe left cerebral atrophy with calcification of almost the entire hemisphere and marked development of the left frontal sinus.

the patients with unihemispheric lesions, 19% were severely or moderately mentally retarded, 27% were mentally retarded but educable, and 45% had average intelligence. In the bihemispheric involvement group, 46% were severely or moderately mentally retarded, 38% were retarded but educable, and only 8% had average intelligence.

Most of the patients with SWS present with attention deficit and hyperactivity disorder (ADHD), predominating the combined subtype. The 22% of cases with ADHD reported by Chapiesky et al. (2000) may be lower than the true incidence observed personally by us. Eighty five per cent of patients with mental retardation have emotional or behavioural pro-

blems, such as violence towards others and self-abuse (Sujansky and Conradi 1995). No severe depression has been found in almost 50% of adults with normal intellectual functioning. Depression is related to the frustration of poor seizure control, headaches, or poor self-esteem due to the cosmetic consequences of facial nevus flammeus (Sujansky and Conradi 1995).

Adults show a higher prevalence of headaches than children and young patients with SWS: a proportion of 69% vs 48% was seen by Sujansky and Conradi (1995). Special educational requirements for adults, however, are similar as compared to younger people.

Only limited information about long-term outcome, including psychopathology, social integration or the possibility of working in regular employment of adult patients, is available in the literature (Lee 1990, Oakes 1992, Sujansky and Conradi 1995). Almost 50% of adults with SWS would be able to work in regular employment, but the presence of seizures, problems of intelligence or character, depression, motor or sensory handicaps, low self-esteem, and a low motivation to work, decrease the possibilities to live independently in society.

Neurologic deficits persist or may even increase as the child grows older. Motor and sensory functions do not change after they become permanent during childhood in most cases. Spastic hemiparesis or hemiplegia, cortical hemisensory deficit, or hemianopsia contralateral to the cerebral lesion persist for life. Either hemiparesis or hemiplegia has been reported in 18% of patients less than 14 years (Pascual-Castroviejo et al. 1978) and in 26% of patients of all ages (Peterman et al. 1958). Underdevelopment of the paretic hemibody is seen from the first years of age, and orthopaedic treatment does not improve motor function. At an early stage, a hemiparesis or hemiplegia may be only transient postictally and then, in the course of the disease, may become more permanent. The severity of the motor and sensory features is related to the degree of contralateral cerebral hemiatrophy or calcification.

# References

Adamsbaum C, Pinton F, Rolland Y, Chiron C, Dulac O, Kalifa G (1996) Accelerated myelination in early Sturge-Weber syndrome: RMI-SPECT correlations. Pediatr Radiol 26: 759–762.

Alonso A, Taboada D, Ceres L, Beltran J, Olave R, Nogués A (1979) Intracranial calcification in a neonate with the Sturge-Weber síndrome and additional problems. Pediatr Raiol 8: 39–41.

Arzimanoglou AA, Andermann F, Aicardi J, Sainte-Rose C, Beaulieu MA, Villemure JC et al. (2000) Sturge-Weber syndrome. Indications and results of surgery in 20 patients. Neurology 55: 1472–1479.

Barsky SH, Rosen S, Geer D, Noe JM (1980) The nature and evolution of port-wine staind. J Invest Dermatol 74: 154–157.

Baselga E (2004) Sturge-Weber syndrome. Semin Cut Med Surg 23: 87–98.

Bebin EM, Gomez MR (1988) Prognosis in Sturge-Weber disease: comparison of unihemispheric and bihemispheric involvement. J Child Neurol 3: 181–184.

Benedikt RA, Brown DC, Walker R, Ghaed UN, Mitchell M, Geyer CA (1993) Sturge-Weber syndrome: cranial MR imaging with Gd-DTPA. Am J Neuroradiol 14: 409–415.

Bentson JR, Wilson GH, Newton TH (1971) Cerebral venous drainage pattern of the Sturge-Weber syndrome. Radiology 101: 111–118.

Bodensteiner JB, Roach ES (1999) Sturge-Weber syndrome. Mt. Freedom: The Sturge Weber Foundation: 1–10.

Breugen CC, Alders M, Salieb-Beugelaar GB, Mannens MMAM, Van der Hosrts C, Hennekam RCM (2002) A locus for hereditary capillary malformations mapped on chromosome 5q. Hum Genet 110: 343–347.

Breuner RP, Sharbrough FW (1976) Electroencephalographic evaluation in Sturge-Weber syndrome. Neurology 26: 629–632.

Buttler G, Schulte FJ (1975) Zur operation behandbung des Sturge-Weber syndrome. Neuropediatrie 6: 135–141.

Cambon H, Truelle JL, Baron JC, Chiras J, Tran Dinh S, Chatel M (1987) Ischemiè chronique focale et migraine acompagné: forme atypique d'une angiomatose de Sturge-Weber. Rev Neurol (París) 143: 588–594.

Campistol J, Garcìa-Cazorla A, Gonzalez-Campo C (1999) Sturge-Weber disease with unusual cerebral atrophy and hydrocephalus. Eur J Paediatr Neurol 3: 227–229.

Chabriat H, Pappata S, Traykov L, Kurtz A, Bousser MG (1996) Angiomatose de Sturge-Weber responsible d'une hémiplégie sans infarctus cerebral en fin de grossesse. Rev Neurol (París) 152: 536–541.

Chamberlain MC, Press GA, Hesselink JR (1989) MR imaging and CT in three cases of Sturge-Weber syndrome: Prospective comparison. Am J Neuroradiol 10: 491–496.

Chapieski L, Friedman A, Lachar D (2000) Psychological functioning in children and adolescents with Sturge-Weber syndrome. J Child Neurol 15: 660–665.

Chiron C, Raynaud C, Tzourio N, Diebler C, Dulac O, Zilbovicius M et al. (1989) Regional cerebral blood flow by SPECT imaging in Sturge-Weber disease: an aid for diagnosis. J Neurol Neurosurg Psychiatr 52: 1402–1409.

Chugani HT, Mazziotta J, Pelps M (1989) Sturge-Weber syndrome. A study of cerebral glucose utilization with positron emission tomography. J Pediatr 114: 244–253.

Cohen MM Jr (2000) Klippel-Tranaunay syndrome: A critical analysis. Am J Med Genet 93: 171–175.

Cohen MM Jr, Neri G, Weksberg R (2002) Klippel-Trenaunay syndrome, Parkes Weber syndrome, and Sturge-Weber syndrome. In: Cohen MM Jr, Neri G, Weksberg R (eds.) Overgrowth Syndromes. New York: Oxford University Press, pp. 111–124.

Comati A, Beck H, Halliday W, Snipes GJ, Plate KH, Acker T (2007) Upregulation of hypoxia-inducible factor (HIF)-1alpha and HIF-2alpha in leptomeningeal vascular malformations of Sturge–Weber Syndrome. J. Neuropathol Exp Neurol 66: 86–97.

Comi AM (2003) Pathophysiology of Sturge-Weber syndrome. J Child Neurol 18: 509–516.

Comi AM (2006) Advancs in Sturge–Weber syndrome. Curr Opin Neural 19: 124–128.

Cushing H (1906) Cases of spontaneous intracranial hemorrhage associated with trigenimal nevi. JAMA 47: 178–183.

Debicka A, Adamczak P (1979) Przypadek dziedziczenia zespolu Sturge'a-Webera. Klin Oczna 81: 541–542.

Dimitri V (1923) Tumor cerebral congénito (Angioma cavernoso). Rev Assoc Med Argent 36: 1029–1037.

Di Rocco C, Tamburrini G (2006) Sturge–Weber syndrome. Childs Nerv Syst 22: 909–921.

Di Trapani G, Di Rocco C, Abbmonti AL, Calderelli M (1982) Light microscopy and ultrastructural studies of Sturge-Weber disease. Childs Brain 9: 23–26.

Eerola I, Boon L, Watanabe S, Grynberg H, Mulliken JB, Vikkula M (2002) Locus for susceptibility for familial capillary malformation ("port-wine stain") maps to 5q. Eur J Hum Genet 10: 375–380.

Eerola I, Boon L, Mulliken JB, Burrows PE, Dompmartin A, Watanabe S, Vanwijck R, Vikkula M (2003) Capillary malformation-arteriovenous malformation, a new clinical and genetic disorder caused by RASA1 mutations. Am J Hum Genet 73: 1240–1249.

Enjolras O, Riche MC, Merland JJ (1985) Facial port-wine stains and Sturge-Weber Syndrome. Pediatrics 76: 48–51.

Evans AL, Widjaja E, Connolly DJ, Griffiths PD (2006) Cerebral perfusion abnormalities in children with Sturge–Weber syndrome shown by dynamic contrast bolus magnetic resonance perfusion imaging. Pediatrics 117: 2119–2125.

Fukuyama Y, Tsuchiya S (1979) A study on Sturge-Weber syndrome. Eur Neurol 18: 194–202.

Garcìa JC, Roach ES, Mc Lean WT (1981) Recurrent thrombotic deterioration in the Sturge-Weber syndrome. Childs Brain 8: 427–433.

Gobbi G, Bouquet F, Greco L, Lambertini A, Tassinari CA, Ventura A et al. (1992) Coeliac disease, epilepsy, and cerebral calcifications. Lancet 340: 439–443.

Gobbi G (2005) Coeliac disease, epilepsy and cerebral calcifications. Brain Dev 27: 189–200.

Gomez MR, Bebin EM (1987) Sturge-Weber syndrome. In: Gomez MR (ed.) Neurocutaneous Diseases. A Practical Approach. Boston: Butterworths: 356–367.

Gorlin RJ, Cohen MM Jr, Hennekam RAC (2001) Klippel–Trenaunay syndrome, Parkes Weber syndrome, and Sturge–Weber syndrome. In: Gorlin RJ, Cohen MM Jr, Hennekam RAC (eds.) Syndromes of the Head and Neck, 4th ed, pp. 453–460.

Griffiths PD (1996) Sturge-Weber syndrome revisited: the role of neuroradiology. Neuropediatrics 27: 284–294.

Griffiths PD, Boodram MB, Blaser S, Altomare F, Buncic JR, Levin AV et al. (1996) Abnormal ocular enhancement in Sturge-Weber syndrome: Correlation of ocular MR and CT findings with clinical and intracranial imaging findings. Am J Neuroradiol 17: 749–754.

Guseo A (1975) Ultrastructure of calcification in Sturge-Weber. Virchows Arch Pathol Anat 366: 352–356.

Happle R (1987) Lethal genes surviving by mosaicism: a possible explanation for sporadic birth defects involving the. skin. J Am Acad Dermatol 16: 899–906.

Hatfield LA, Crone NE, Kossoff EH, Ewen JB, Pyzik PL, Lin DD, Kelley TM, Comi AM (2007) Quantitative EEG asymmetry correlates with clinical severity in unilateral Sturge–Weber Syndrome. Epilepsia 48: 191–195.

Hebold O (1913) Hemangiomen der weicjen Hirnhaut bei Naevus vasculosus des Gesischts. Arch Psychaitr Nervenkr 51: 445–456.

Hoffmann HJ, Hendrick EB, Dennis M, Amstrong D (1979) Hemispherectomy for Sturge-Weber syndrome. Childs Brain 5: 233–248.

Huq AHMM, Chugani DC, Hukku B, Sarajee FJ (2002) Evidence of somatic mosaicism in Sturge-Weber syndrome. Neurology 59: 780–782.

Iwach A, Hoskins HD, Heterington J, Shaffer R (1990) Analysis of surgical and medical management of glaucoma in Sturge-Weber syndrome. Ophthalmology 97: 904–909.

Jacoby CG, Yuh WTC, Afifi AK, Bell WE, Schelper RL, Sato Y (1987) Accelerated myelination in early Sturge-Weber syndrome demonstrated by MR imaging. J Comp Assist Tomogr 11: 226–231.

Jenning Milles W (1884) Naevus of the right temporal and orbital region: naevus of the choroid and detachment of the retina in the right eye. Trans Ophthalmol Soc 4: 168–171.

Juhasz C, Batista CE, Chugani DC, Muzik O, Chugani HT (2007) Evaluation of cortical metabolic abnormalities and their clinical correlates in Sturge–Weber syndrome. Eur J Ped Neurol 11: 277–284.

Juhasz C, Lai C, Behen ME, Muzik O, Helder EJ, Chugani DC, Chugani HT (2008) White matter volume as a major predictor of cognitive function in Sturge-Weber syndrome. Arch Neurol 64: 1169–1174.

Kalischer S (1897) Demonstration des Gehirns eines Kindes mit Telangiectasie der linkseitigen Gesichts. Kopfhatu und Hirnoberfläche. Berl Klin Wochenschr 34: 1059.

Kalischer S (1901) Ein Fall von Teleangiectasie (Angiom) des Gesichts und der weichen Hirnhaut. Arch Psychiatr 34: 169–180.

Keith HM, Ewert JC, Green MW, Gage RP (1955) Mental status of children with convulsive disorders. Neurology 5: 419–425.

Kelley TM, Hatfield LA, Lin DD, Comi AM (2005) Quantitative analysis of cerebral cortical atrophy and correlation with clinical severity in unilateral Sturge–Weber syndrome. J Child Neurol 20: 867–870.

Kiley MA, Oxburg JM, Coley SC (2002) Intracranial hypertension in Sturge-Weber/Klippel-Trenaunay-Weber overlap syndrome due to impairment of cerebral nevous outflow. J Clin Neurosci 9: 330–338.

Kitahara T, Maki Y (1978) A case of Sturge-Weber disease with epilepsy and intracranial calcification in the neonatal period. Eur Neurol 17: 8–12.

Kossoff EH, Buck C, Freeman JM (2002) Outcomes of 32 hemispherectomies for Sturge-Weber syndrome worldwide. Neurology 59: 1735–1738.

Krabbe KH (1934) Facial and meningeal angiomatosis associated with calcifications of brain cortex: clinical and anatomopathologic contribution. Arch Neurol Psychiatr 32: 737–755.

Lee S (1990) Psychopathology in Sturge-Weber syndrome. Can J Psychiatr 35: 674–678.

Lee JS, Asano E, Muzik O, Chugani DC, Juhász C, Pfund Z, Philip S, Behen M, Chugani HT (2001) Sturge-Weber syndrome. Correlation between clinical course and FDG PET findings. Neurology 57: 189–195.

Loevner L, Quint DJ (1992) Persistent trigeminal artery in a patient with Sturge-Weber syndrome. Am J Radiol 158: 872–874.

Lund M (1949) On epilepsy in Sturge-Weber disease. Acta Psychiatr Neurol 24: 569–586.

Maria BL, Neufeld JA, Rosainz LC, Ben-David K, Drane WE, Quisling RG, Hamed LM (1998a) High prevalence of bihemispheric structural and functional defects in Sturge–Weber syndrome. J Child Neurol 13: 595–605.

Maria BL, Neufeld JA, Rosainz LC, Drane WE, Quisling RG, Ben-David K, Hamed LM (1998b) Central nervous system structure and function in Sturge–Weber syndrome. Evidence of neurologic and radiologic progression. J Child Neurol 13: 606–618.

Nguyen CM, Yohn JJ, Huft C (1998) Facial port-wine stains in childhood: prediction of the rate of improvement as a function of the age of the patient size and location of the port-wine stain and the number of treatments with the pulsed dye (585 mm). Br J Dermatol 138: 821–825.

Oakes WJ (1992) The natural history of patients with Sturge-Weber syndrome. Pediatr Neurosurg 18: 287–290.

Ogunmekan AO, Hwang PA, Hoffmann HJ (1989) Sturge-Weber-Dimitri disease. Role of hemispherectomy in prognosis. Can J Neurol Sci 16: 78–80.

Parsa CF (2008) Sturge–Weber syndrome: a unified pathophysiologic mechanism. Curr Treat Options Neurol 10: 47–54.

Pascual-Castroviejo I (2004) Cutaneous hemangiomas: vascular anomaly complex. In: Roach ES, Miller VS (eds.) Neurocutaneous Disorders. Cambridge: Cambridge University Press, pp. 172–178.

Pascual-Castroviejo I, Roche Herrero MC, Lopez-Terradas JM, Lopez-Martìn V (1978) Sìndrome de Sturge-Weber. Hallazgos en 22 casos infantiles. An Pediatr (Spain) 11: 281–294.

Pascual-Castroviejo I, Dìaz-Gonzalez C, García-Melian RM, Gonzalez-Casado I, Muñoz-Hiraldo E (1993) Sturge-Weber sìndrome: Study of 40 patients. Pediatric Neurol 9: 283–288.

Pascual-Castroviejo I, Pascual-Pascual SI, Viaño J, Martinez V, Coya J (1995) Sturge-Weber syndrome without facial nevus. Neuropediatrics 26: 220–222.

Pascual-Castroviejo I, Viaño J, Moreno F, Palencia R, Martinez Fernandez V, Pascual-Pascual SI et al. (1996) Hemangiomas of the head, neck, and chest with associated vascular and brain anomalies: A complex neurocutaneous syndrome. Am J Neuroradiol 17: 461–471.

Patrianakos TD, Nagao K, Walton DS (2008) Surgical management of glaucoma with the Sturge–Weber syndrome. Int Ophthalmol Clin 48: 63–67.

Peterman AF, Hayles AB, Dockerty MB, Love JG (1958) Encephalotrigeminal angiomatosis (Sturge-Weber disease). Clinical study of thirty-five cases. JAMA 167: 2169–2176.

Pfund Z, Kagawa K, Juhász C, Shen C, Lee JS, Chugani DC, Muzik O, Chugani HT (2003) Quantitative analysis of gray – and white – matter volumes and glucose metabolism in Sturge-Weber syndrome. J Child Neurol 18: 119–126.

Polani PE (1952) Encephalotrigeminal angiomatosis (Sturge-Weber syndrome) treated by removal of affected cerebral hemisphere. Proc Roy Soc Med 45: 860–862.

Portilla P, Husson B, Lasjaunias P, Landrieu P (2002) Sturge-Weber disease with repercussion on the prenatal development of the cerebral hemisphere. Am J Neuroradiol 23: 490–492.

Ramli N, Sachet M, Bao C, Lasjaunias P (2003) Cerebrofacial venous metameric syndrome (CVMS) 3: Sturge-Weber syndrome with bilateral lymphatic/venous malformations of the mandible. Neuroradiology 45: 685–690.

Rappaport ZH (1988) Corpus callosum section in the treatment of intractable seizures in the Sturge-Weber syndrome. Childs Nerv Syst 4: 231–232.

Riela AR, Stump DA, Roach ES, Mc Lean WT, Garcìa JC (1985) Regional cerebral blood flow characteristics of the Sturge-Weber syndrome. Pediatr Neurol 1: 85–90.

Roach ES (1988) Diagnosis and management of neurocutaneous syndromes. Surg Neurol 8: 83–96.

Roach ES (1992) Neurocutaneous syndromes. Pediatr Clin N Amer 39: 591–621.

Rosen E (1950) Hemangioma of the choroid. Ophthalmologica 120: 127–148.

Rosen I, Salford L (1984) Sturge-Weber disease – neurophysiological evaluation of a case with secondary epileptogenesis, successfully treated with lobectomy. Neuropediatrics 15: 95–98.

Rosen S, Smoller BR (1987) Port-wine stains: a new hypothesis. K Am Acad Dermatol 17: 164–166.

Schirmer R (1860) Ein Fall von Telangiektasie. Von Graefes Arch Ophth 7: 119–121.

Schnyder UW (1957) Zur klinic and histology der angiome. 4. Mitteilung: Die planotuberösen angiome des Kleinkindes. Arch Klin Exp Dermatol 204: 457–471.

Shuper A, Merlob P, Garty B, Varsano I (1984) Familial multiple naevi flammei. J Med Genet 21: 112–113.

Simonati A, Colamaria V, Bricoo A, Dalla Bernardina B, Rizzuto N (1994) Microgyria associated with Sturge-Weber angiomatosis. Child Nerv Syst 10: 392–395.

Smoller BR, Rosen S (1986) Port-wine stains. A disease of altered neural modulation of blood vessels? Arch Dermatol 122: 177–179.

Sperner J, Schmauser I, Bittner R, Henkes H, Bassir C, Sprung C et al. (1990) MR imaging findings in children with Sturge-Weber syndrome. Neuropediatrics 21: 146–152.

Stevenson RF, Thomson HG, Morin JD (1974) Unrecognized ocular problems associated port-wine stain of the face in children. Can Med Assoc J 111: 953–954.

Sturge WA (1879) Case of partial epilepsia apparently due to lesion of one of vasomotor centres of brain. Trans Clin Soc London 12: 162–167.

Sugama S, Yoshimura H, Ashimine K, Eto Y, Maekawa K (1997) Enhanced magnetic resonance imaging of leptomeningeal angiomatosis. Pediatric Neurol 17: 262–265.

Sujansky E, Conradi S (1995) Outcome of Sturge-Weber syndrome in 52 adults. Am J Med Genet 57: 35–45.

Sullivan TJ, Clarke MP, Morin JD (1992) The ocular manifestations of Sturge-Weber syndrome. J Pediatr Opthalmol Strabismus 29: 349–356.

Tallman B, Tan OT, Morelli JG, Piepenbrink J, Stafford TJ, Trainor S et al. (1991). Location of port-wine stains and the likehood of ophthalmic and/or central nervous system complications. Pediatrics 87: 323–327.

Tan OT, Sherwood K, Gilchrest BA (1989) Treatment of children with port-wine stains using the plashlamppulsed tunable dye laser. N Engl J Med 320: 416–421.

Taybi H (1996) Sturge–Weber syndrome. In: Taybi H, Lachman RS (eds.) Radiology of syndromes, metabolic disorders, and skeletal dysplasias. 4th ed. St. Louis: Mosby, pp. 473–476.

Thomas-Sohl KA, Vaslow DF, Maria BL (2004) Sturge–Weber syndrome: a review. Pediatr Neurol 30: 303–310.

Tönnis W, Friedmann G (1964) Roentgenologic and clinical findings in 23 patients with Sturge-Weber disease. Zentralbl Neurochir 25: 1–10.

Van der Hoeve (1937) A fourth type of phakomatosis. Arch Ophthalmol 18: 679–682.

Van der Horst CMAM, van Eijk TGJ, de Borgie CAJM, Koster PHL, Struycken PM, Strackee SD (1999) Hereditary port-wine stains, do they exist? Lasers Med Sci 14: 238–243.

Vogl TJ, Stemmler J, Bergman C, Pfluger T, Egger E, Lissner J (1993) MR and MR angiography of Sturge-Weber syndrome. Am J Neuroradiol 14: 417–425.

Weber FP (1922) Right-sided hemi-hypotrophy resulting from right-sided congenital spastic hemiplegia, with morbid condition of left side of brain, revealed by radiograms. J Neurol Psychopath 2: 134–139.

Weber FP (1929) A note on the association of extensive haemangiomatous nevus of the skin with cerebral (meningeal) haemangioma, especially case of facial vascular naevus with contralateral hemiplegia. Proc Roy Soc Med 22: 431.

Whitschel H, Font RL (1976) Hemangioma of the choroids: A clinopathological study of 71 cases and review of the literature. Surv Ophthalmol 20: 415–431.

Yeakley JW, Woodside M, Fenstermacher MJ (1992) Bilateral neonatal Sturge-Weber-Dimitri disease: CT and MR findings. Am J Neuroradiol 13: 1179–1182.

Yu TW, Liu HM, Lee WT (2007) The correlation between motor impairment and cerebral blood flow on Sturge–Weber syndrome. Eur J Ped Neurol 11: 96–103.

# Chapter 11

# OSLER-WEBER-RENDU SYNDROME (HEREDITARY HEMORRHAGIC TELANGIECTASIA)

**Haneen Sadick, Maliha Sadick, and Karl Hörmann**

Department of Otorhinolaryngology, Head and Neck Surgery, University Hospital Mannheim, Mannheim, Germany (HS, KH);
Department of Clinical Radiology, University Hospital Mannheim, Mannheim, Germany (MS)

## Introduction and eponyms of the disease

Osler-Weber-Rendu syndrome, also known as "Rendu-Osler-Weber disease", "Osler's disease" or "hereditary hemorrhagic telangiectasia (HHT)", was first described more than a century ago as a rare condition producing minor discomfort for affected people. Nowadays, this disorder is considered to be more common than previously thought, and its association to brain, liver and pulmonary lesions are sources of substantial morbidity and mortality and represent even these days a continuing challenge for many sub-specialities (Guttmacher et al. 1995).

## Historical perspective

It is still discussed controversially whether it was Sutton in 1864 who was the first to report on HHT as a disorder of epistaxis and degeneration of the vascular system. One year later, Babington was said to have noted a possible familial relationship saying that the occurrence of nosebleeds could be inherited (Babington 1865). Over the years, recurrent epistaxis concurrent with "petits angiomes cutanes et muqueux" was again described by Rendu in 1896 (Rendu 1896) as well as in 1901 by Sir William Osler who reported on a family with recurrent epistaxis as well as skin and mucous membrane telangiectases (Osler 1901). In 1907, Weber followed with his description of multiple hereditary angiomata associated with recurrent haemorrhage (Weber 1907). The term hereditary hemorrhagic telangiectasia (HHT) was finally attributed to Hanes, who wrote on "multiple hereditary telangiectases causing haemorrhage" in 1909 (Hanes 1907). The typical clinical triad with characteristic multiple telangiectases, recurrent nosebleeds and familial occurrence have become firmly established as a medical entity.

## Incidence and prevalence

Hereditary hemorrhagic telangiectasia occurs with a wide geographic distribution among many ethnic and racial groups, but white patients are primarily affected. Men and women are affected equally. In previous studies, the incidence of the disease was estimated at 1–2 in 100.000 (Garland and Anning 1950). However, the HHT prevalence nowadays shows to be more frequent than formerly thought. Recent careful epidemiologic studies in France, Denmark and Japan reveal an incidence of 1 in 5–8000 (Bideau et al. 1989, Kjeldsen et al. 1999, Dakeishi et al. 2002).

## Clinical manifestations

### Nose

Spontaneous recurrent nose bleeds from telangiectasia of the nasal mucosa are the most common clinical manifestation of HHT. In more than 90% of cases they represent the first clinical symptom of the disease (Römer et al. 1992) (Fig. 1). However, while some patients experience significant nosebleeds on a daily basis leading to chronic anaemia, others will have only occasional nosebleeds (Aassar et al. 1991). Recurrent epistaxis begins in more than 50% before the age of 20 (Haitjema et al.

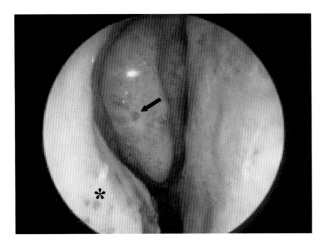

**Fig. 1.** Left nasal cavity with multiple telangiectasia on the head of the inferior turbinate (arrow) and the anterior part of the nasal septum (asterisk).

1995, 1996). The onset of clinical manifestation has been described in many cases by the age of 10, and in most cases by the age of 21, becoming more severe in later decades in about two thirds of affected individuals.

## Skin

Muco-/cutaneous telangiectases occur in about 50–80% of individuals. As already described by Rendu in 1896, they appear as "small purplish stains", of the size of a pinhead, the largest reaching the size of a lentil. In general, these lesions manifest later in life than epistaxis, but typically arise during youth, with most cases developing these lesions at the third or even forth decade of life, and increasing in size and number with age (Plauchu et al. 1989). They mostly occur on the face, lips, mouth, tongue and buccal mucosa, ears, hands, fingertips and chest in descending order of frequency and in any combination, but can also occur elsewhere (Figs. 2–5). They may bleed but this is rarely clinically significant and the main concern is rather cosmetic (Guttmacher et al. 1995).

## Lung

Pulmonary arteriovenous malformations consist of direct connections between a branch of a pulmonary

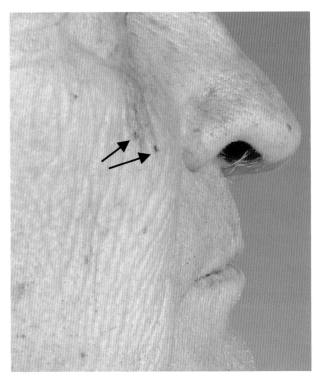

**Fig. 2.** Manifestation of cutaneous telangiectasia (→) on the face of an HHT patient.

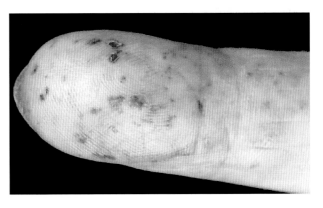

**Fig. 3.** Manifestation of cutaneous telangiectasia on the right forefinger of an HHT patient.

artery and a pulmonary vein through a thin-walled aneurysm. They are often multiple and appear in both lungs, with a predilection for the lower lobes. It is estimated that approximately 60–70% of pulmonary arteriovenous malformations (pAVM) occur in patients with HHT (Dines et al. 1974, Schneider et al. 2008). Therefore, their detection should

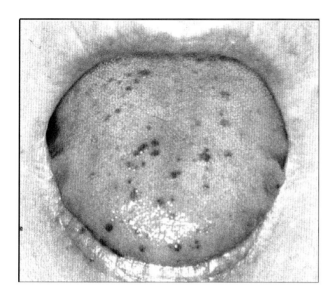

**Fig. 4.** Typical sight of an HHT patient with clinical manifestation of mucocutaneous telangiectases on the tongue.

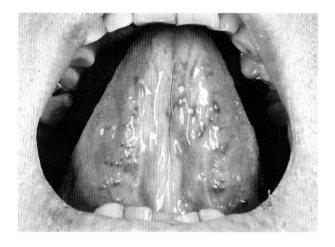

**Fig. 5.** Front view into the oral cavity with few mucocutaneous telangiectasia below the tongue.

prompt a thorough review of the patient and his or her family. The incidence of pAVM apparently varies according to the specific gene for the condition that is present (Kjeldsen et al. 2000). The HHT subgroup with endoglin mutations has a higher risk (40%) than HHT patients with ALK1 mutations (Mc Allister et al. 1994, Porteous et al. 1994). Pulmonary AVMs tend to increase in size, especially if multiple, and rarely regress spontaneously (Bosher

et al. 1959, Sluiter-Eringa et al. 1969, Vase et al. 1985). In female, pAVM have been reported more often than in males. During the course of pregnancy, pAVMs also increase in size and can cause severe complications (Shovlin et al. 1995). Therefore, female patients with HHT need a thorough screening for pAVMs before pregnancy or need to be categorized as patients with a "high risk pregnancy" who need strict follow-up examinations (Shovlin et al. 1995, Shovlin and Letarte 1999). The mortality rate in untreated but usually symptomatic patients with pAVMs range from 4 to 22% (Dines et al. 1974, Shovlin and Letarte 1999), in severe cases even up to 40% (Stringer et al. 1955). The abnormal vessels can bleed into the bronchus or the pleural cavity, sometimes with a fatal outcome (Muri 1955). The direct communication between the pulmonary and systemic circulation, bypassing the capillary bed, with their functional consequences are the most commonly caused problems. Such right-left-shunts cause hypoxaemia and the absence of a filtering capillary bed allows embolism which can reach the systemic arteries, inducing clinical sequelae especially in the cerebral circulation with brain abscesses and stroke. These processes account for the clinical features such as dyspnoea, fatigue, haemoptysis, cyanosis or polycythemia (Burke et al. 1986). Small pAVMs with shunting of less than 25% of pulmonary blood flow are asymptomatic in half of the cases. These patients show no cyanosis but demonstrate dyspnoea on exertion and easy fatigability. Additionally, a possible correlation of HHT with pulmonary hypertension is been discussed (Shovlin and Letarte 1999). The histological and pathophysiological features of HHT and primary pulmonary hypertension seem to be different. Pulmonary arteriovenous dilatation is the hallmark of lung involvement in hereditary hemorrhagic telangiectasia, leading to decreased pulmonary vascular resistance and increased cardiac output, with normal to low pulmonary arterial pressure. In contrast, primary pulmonary hypertension is characterized by obliteration of small pulmonary arteries, leading to increased pulmonary vascular resistance, marked elevation of pulmonary arterial pressure, and ultimately, a reduction in cardiac output.

## Brain

Cerebral vascular malformations (CVMs) as well as most of their complications are thought to affect up to 15% of patients with HHT. Neurologic symptoms can include migraine headache, brain abscess, transient ischemic attack, stroke, seizure, and intracerebral as well as subarachnoid haemorrhage (White et al. 1988, Robin et al. 1976), and affect particularly those HHT patients who have a personal or family history of pulmonary arteriovenous malformations (Burke et al. 1986, Porteous et al. 1992, Willinsky et al. 1990, Press and Ramsey 1984, Hewes et al. 1985). In two thirds of cases, in whom neurologic symptoms develop, pulmonary AVMs are the source of the symptoms. In the remaining third, cerebral or spinal arteriovenous malformations cause subarachnoid haemorrhage, seizure, or less common paraparesis (Matsubara et al. 2000). Brain or spinal abscess, transient ischemic attack, and ischemic stroke occur particularly in patients with pulmonary AVMs who have right-to-left shunting that facilitates the passage of septic and bland emboli into the cerebral circulation (Burke et al. 1986, Maldonado et al. 2007).

## GI-tract and liver

Recurrent haemorrhage of the upper or lower gastrointestinal (GI-) tract occurs in a minority of patients with hereditary hemorrhagic telangiectasia (Plauchu et al. 1989, Kjeldsen and Kjeldsen 2000). Usually, GI-bleedings do not start until the fifth or sixth decade. It often presents as an iron deficiency anaemia but occasionally as an acute gastrointestinal haemorrhage. In few cases, the coincidence of HHT with hereditary juvenile polyposis could be observed. A possible genetic association between these two disease is of major importance, as juvenile polyposis has a known high rate of possible malignancies (Reilly and Nostrant 1984).

Liver involvement with fistulas due to the presence of multiple arteriovenous malformations or atypical cirrhosis is a rare but important manifestation of hereditary hemorrhagic telangiectasia (Bernard et al. 1993, Garcia-Tsao et al. 2000). Though many patients are asymptomatic, a high cardiac output caused by left-to-right shunting within the liver can lead to heart failure. Cases with hepatomegaly, portal hypertension, biliary manifestation with pain in the right upper quadrant, jaundice as well as

**Table 1.** Clinical features and current diagnostic methods in HHT

| Organ | Incidence | Type of lesion | Clinical symptoms | Diagnostic methods |
|---|---|---|---|---|
| Nose | >90% | Telangiectasia | Epistaxis | Visual inspection |
| Skin | 50–80% | Telangiectasia | Bleeding (minor) | Visual inspection |
| Lung | >20% | Arteriovenous malformation | Cyanosis, Cerebral abscess, Embolic stroke, Migraine | Arterial-blood gas measurement, Pulse oximetry, Contrast echocardiography, High-resolution helical CT, Angiography |
| Central nervous system | 15% | (Arterio-)venous malformation, AV-Fistula => especially multiple, cortical | Headache, Subarachnoid hemorrhage | MRI, MR-angiography |
| GI-tract, Liver | 11–25% 8–16% | Angiodysplsia, Arteriovenous malformation, Telangiectasia | Bleeding, Ascites, Hyperdynamic circulation, Portosystemic shunts | Endoscopy, Ultrasound, CT |

abdominal angina from a mesenteric arterial "steal" have been described (Bernard et al. 1993). Patients with clinically significant liver lesions most often present with a hyperdynamic circulation due to a shunting from hepatic arteries to hepatic veins, portal veins to hepatic veins, or both. This condition often results in pseudocirrhosis, with nodular transformations of the parenchyma without fibrous septa.

On overview on the main clinical features and diagnostic measures is given in Table 1.

## Pathogenesis

The characteristic manifestations of HHT are all due to abnormalities of the vascular structure. The earliest morphologic change in the pathogenesis of HHT appears to be a focal dilatation of postcapillary venules, often surrounded by a mononuclear infiltrate. As the venules increase in size, both in luminal diameter and vascular wall thickness, they become convoluted and connect to enlarging arterioles through capillary segments. Eventually, these segments disappear, leading to the formation of a direct arteriovenous communication (Fig. 6a–c) (Braverman et al. 1990, Menefee et al. 1975). In fully developed telangiectases, most venules show excessive layers of smooth muscle cells without any elastic fibres or have an incomplete layer of smooth muscle cells. Additional defects in endothelial junctions have been described (Hashimoto and Pritzker 1972, Jahnke 1970). Whereas telangiectases appear nearly universal, arteriovenous malformations which represent the other prominent lesions of HHT, appear only at certain forms of the condition. Similar to telangiectases, these malformations lack capillaries and consist of direct connections between arteries and veins, but are much larger in size (Porteous et al. 1994). In general, HHT patients have a normal thrombocyte function and an unimpaired coagulation. However, rare cases of HHT associated with von Willebrand's disease have been described (Ahr et al. 1977).

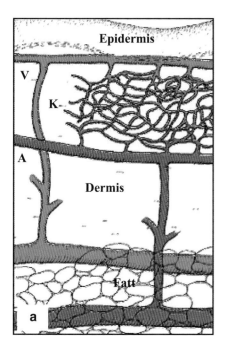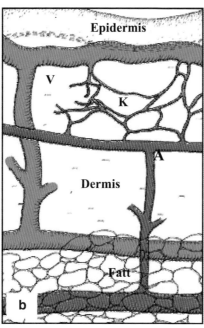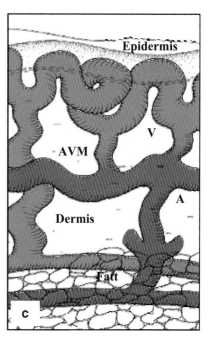

Fig. 6. (a–c) Development of telangiectasia in the region of the skin and mucosa. (a) Normally, arterioles (A) in the papillary dermis are connected to venules (V) through multiple capillaries (C). (b) In the early stage of telangiectases, the capillary bed (C) becomes more and more rare with the development of dilated venules which are still connected to arterioles through one or more capillaries. (c) In a fully developed telangiectasia, the venules and their braches become markedly dilated, elongated, and convoluted. The arterioles become also dilated and communicate directly with the venules without intervening capillaries.

## Molecular genetics

The mode of inheritance is autosomal dominant and affected individuals are heterozygous. Homozygous forms are considered to be lethal (Snyder and Doan 1944). In HHT patients the penetrance, which is estimated at 97–100%, is age-dependent (Porteous et al. 1992). In spite of the high HHT penetrance, evidence of disease may not be present until after the age of 30 (Plauchu et al. 1989, Porteous et al. 1992). Nevertheless, about 20% of patients can have a negative familial history, indicating the occurrence of spontaneous mutations, the differences in the individual clinical manifestations or an incomplete and insufficient screening examination of all family members and relatives (Römer et al. 1992).

Mutations which cause HHT have been identified in at least two different genes. The genetic linkage to both these genes has been established on chromosome 9q33–q34 (Shovlin et al. 1994, Mc Donald et al. 1994), and on chromosome 12q (Johnson et al. 1995). The gene for HHT at chromosome 9q3 has been identified by Mc Allister and co-workers as endoglin (ENG) (Mc Allister et al. 1994). The gene encoding for HHT at chromosome 12q has been identified as activin receptor-like kinase 1 (ALK1) (Johnson et al. 1996). In HHT type 1, chromosome 9q33–q34 mutations alter the coding sequence of endoglin, whereas in HHT type 2, chromosome 12q mutations alter the coding sequence of ALK1. Previous studies could demonstrate that subjects with known endoglin mutations have an incidence of pulmonary arteriovenous malformations of approximately 30%, but that the incidence is less than 5% in subjects in whom the endoglin locus had been excluded (Berg et al. 1996). Endoglin and ALK1 encode proteins which are expressed on vascular endothelial cells and are involved with signalling by the transforming growth factor beta (TGF-β) superfamily.

A possible correlation of HHT with familial juvenile polyposis (FJP) is discussed. Familial juvenile polyposis is characterized by the appearance of juvenile polyps in the gastrointestinal tract. Patients with this syndrome are at an increased risk for cancer of the colon, stomach, and pancreas. Similar to HHT, familial juvenile polyposis is an autosomal dominant disorder. It is caused by mutations in the MADH4 gene, encoding proteins which are also involved in the transforming growth factor-beta signalling pathway.

In addition, primary pulmonary hypertension (PPH) has also been reported in association with hereditary hemorrhagic telangiectasia type 2. PPH, an autosomal dominant progressive disease, is characterized by plexiform lesions of endothelial cells in pulmonary arterioles in which widespread occlusion of the smallest pulmonary arteries leads to increased pulmonary vascular resistance, and subsequently right ventricular failure. The gene for PPH encodes bone morphogenetic protein receptor II (*BMPR2*), located on human chromosome 2, which is also a member of the transforming growth factor superfamily of receptors.

## Diagnosis of HHT

Diagnosis of HHT is made clinically by the Curaçao criteria which were established in June 1999 by the Scientific Advisory Board of the "HHT Foundation International Inc." to standardize research and to improve the management of individuals with HHT (Shovlin et al. 2000). The criteria are based on four main clinical features, comprising:

1. spontaneous recurrent nosebleeds,
2. muco-cutaneous telangiectasia,
3. visceral involvement, and
4. an affected first degree relative.

These parameters define "definite HHT" where three criteria are present, "suspected HHT" with two criteria, most commonly family history and

**Table 2.** Curaçao criteria with the four main clinical symptoms

1. Epistaxis: spontaneous, recurrent nose bleeds
2. Multiple (muco-)cutaneous telangiectasia
3. Visceral lesions such as:
   – gastrointestinal telangiectasia (with or without bleeding)
   – pulmonary AVM (arteriovenous malformation)
   – hepatic AVM
   – cerebral AVM
4. Family history with an HHT-affected first degree relative

nosebleeds, or "unlikely HHT" with one criterion – for example, spontaneous nosebleeds without a family history, or a first degree relative of an HHT patient without any signs of the disease (Table 2).

## Management and follow-up

### Nose and skin

Diagnostic measures for nose and skin involvement are bases primarily on visual inspection. To enable a comparability of the severity of epistaxis with other studies, a standardize protocol was developed by Bergler et al. which helps to categorize the degree of epistaxis according to the frequency and intensity of bleeding (Bergler et al. 2002) Table 3.

**Table 3.** Intensity and frequency of epistaxis according to Bergler et al. (2002)

| Intensity of bleeding | Frequency of bleeding |
|---|---|
| Grade I: slight stains on the handkerchief | Grade 1: less than once a week |
| Grade II: soaked handkerchief | Grade 2: a few times a week |
| Grade III: bowl or similar utensil necessary | Grade 3: more than once a day |

### Lungs

A screening examination for PAVMs is strictly recommended due to the severe complications which can arise from PAVMs such as stroke or brain abscess. Supine and erect pulse oximetry, conventional chest radiography (Fig. 7) as well as arterial-blood gas analyse serve as important screening method to detect individuals with suspected PAVMs (Haitjema et al. 1995, Sluiter-Eringa et al. 1969, Shovlin and Letarte 1999, Robin et al. 1976). However, many pulmonary arteriovenous malformations appear below the diaphragm because of their posterior location in the lung (Haitjema et al. 1995, Sluiter-Eringa et al. 1969), making chest X-ray not sufficient enough. Contrast echocardiography has the ability to detect intracardiac shunts and has shown to detect pulmonary AVM when pulse oximetry examination or even pulmonary angiographic findings are negative. Agitated saline, with its small air bubbles – also called micro-bubbles – is injected intravenously and creates visible contrast that can be observed in the left atrium on echocardiography. The presence of contrast in the left ventricle indicate right-left-shunts (Ueki et al. 1994, Shub et al. 1976). The presence of shunts detected by contrast echocardiography, can be verified by high-resolution helical computed tomography scanning with three-dimensional reconstructions

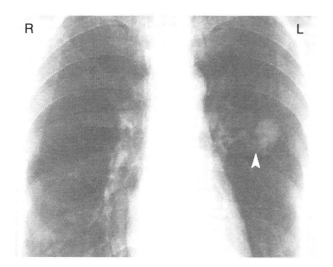

**Fig. 7.** Conventional chest X-ray showing a nodular lesion (arrow) in the upper lobe of the left lung.

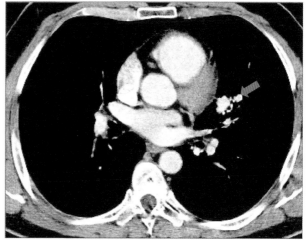

**Fig. 8.** Axial multi-slice CT scan after intravenous contrast confirms a hypervascularized pulmonary AVM in the left upper pulmonary lobe (→).

(Fig. 8). It conveniently identifies small, multiple lesions and effectively demonstrates the architecture of vessels in pulmonary arteriovenous malformations (Remy et al. 1994). Apart from the helical CT scan with contrast agent which also implicates an exposure to radiation and can be very cost-effective, pulmonary angiography has been advocated as an important screening method for pulmonary AVMs. It is required for therapeutic embolisation and is also mandatory to determine the position and structure of abnormal vascular lesions prior to surgical treatment. However, angiography is labour-, cost- and radiation-intensive, asks for a hand of an experienced radiologist and its use should be limited to individuals in whom non-invasive diagnostic tests strongly suggest the presence of PAVMs. According to recent studies, a prophylactic measure with antibiotics before any surgical intervention in HHT patients with known or assumed PAVMs is strongly recommended as complications arising from PAVM can be of septic event with severe cerebral involvement, such as brain abscess or hemiplegia due to a thrombembolic event (Kjeldsen et al. 1999).

### Brain

For diagnostic screening purposes, cerebral magnetic resonance imaging (MRI) is currently the most sensitive non-invasive method, though it can also fail to detect the presence of AVMs. Though recommended, the question of whether asymptomatic HHT patients should be screened for cerebral AVM still remains controversially discussed (Easey et al. 2003).

### GI-tract and liver

Telangiectasia occur throughout the GI-tract, and are more commonly situated in the stomach or duodenum, than in the colon. They are visualised by endoscopy and are similar in size and appearance to mucocutaneous telangiectasia, but may be surrounded by an anaemic halo. Arteriovenous malformations as well as aneurysms are less common (Reilly and Nostrant 1984). For possible liver involvement, ultrasound imaging as well as abdominal CT scan are in routine clinical use for detection of possible liver involvement.

## Differential diagnosis

The clinical triad of telangiectases, recurrent epistaxis and inheritance is typical for patients with HHT. Possible differential diagnosis are idiopathic telangiectasia with occurrence at an older age or CRST (calcinosis, Raynaud phenomenon, sclerodermia, telangiectasia) syndrome. This syndrome, a variation of sclerodermia, is defined by cutaneous calcinosis, Raynaud phenomenon, hypomobility of the oesophagus, sclerodermia and telangiectasia. Antibodies against centromeric structures are typical for the syndrome (Maire et al. 1986).

## Treatment

As curative treatments are not available for patients with HHT, all therapeutic effects remain symptomatic, or organ-directed.

Especially in the management of epistaxis with failure to medical treatment, a vast majority of different treatment options has been established, e.g. systemic hormone therapy, electrocautery, brachytherapy, embolisation or laser surgery using the Nd:YAG-, KTP- or $CO_2$ laser. In recent years, very encouraging and positive results could be gained with a new combined treatment approach consisting of "argon plasma coagulation" (APC) and topically applied estriol nose ointment (Bergler et al. 2002). In the treatment of skin lesions, the KTP laser has shown to be very effective.

Treatment of PAVM is based on the size, number and location of the lesions and the specific complications as well as the general condition of the patient. The therapy for symptomatic congenital PAVMs previously consisted of surgical resection entailing local excision, segmental resection, lobectomy or pneumonectomy. However nowadays, percutaneous transcatheter embolisation by coil or balloon is the treatment of choice in patients with PAVM (Fig. 9a–c) (Guttmacher et al. 1995, Kjeldsen et al. 1999).

## Future diagnostic developments

The understanding of HHT is expanding rapidly. However, many multi-centred research studies are still

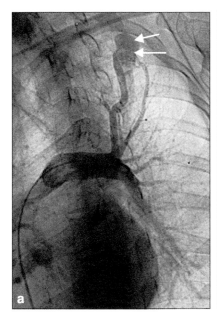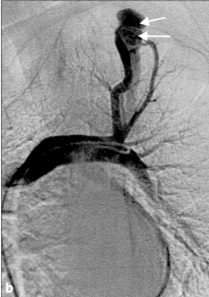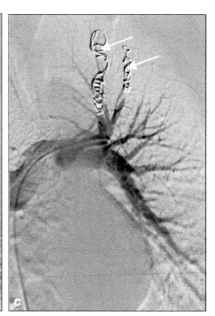

**Fig. 9. (a–c)** Pulmonary angiography confirms 2 AVMs arising from the upper segmental branches of the left pulmonary artery (→). Selective embolisation with platinum coils (**c**) results in successful occlusion of the pulmonary AVMs.

necessary to establish the needed correlations between genotype and phenotype. Currently, there are only a few specialised human genetic laboratory centres that offer diagnostic blood tests for HHT genotype identifications. However, these genetic tests are still very expensive and not in daily clinical use. At times, it is difficult to specify the genotype within members of the same family, as mutations within a family can vary immensely. Recently, different cytokines and pro-angiogenic factors such as the vascular endothelial growth factor (VEGF) have been identified, which have shown to be highly elevated in serum samples of HHT patients. These cytokines might serve as a potential plasma marker for HHT screening purposes (Sadick et al. 2005a,b). However, further studies are still necessary for a better understanding of HHT which may also bring critical insights into other diseases involving vascular damage and repair.

## References

Aassar OS, Friedman CM, White RI (1991) The natural history of epistaxis in hereditary hemorrhagic telangiectasia. Laryngoscope 101: 977–980.

Ahr DJFR, Rickles LW, Hoyer DS, O'Leary ME (1977) Conrad: von Willebrand's disease and hemorrhagic telangiectasia. Association of two complex disorders of hemostasis resulting in life-threatening hemorrhage. Am J Med 62: 452–456.

Babington BG (1865) Hereditary hemorrhagic telangiectasia. Lancet 2: 362–363.

Berg JN, Guttmacher AE, Marchuk DA, Porteous ME (1996) Clinical heterogeneity in hereditary haemorrhagic telangiectasia: are pulmonary arteriovenous malformations more common in families linked to endoglin? J Med Genet 33: 256–257.

Bergler W, Sadick H, Götte K, Riedel F, Hörmann K (2002) Topical estrogens combined with argon plasma coagulation in the management of epistaxis in hereditary hemorrhagic telangiectasia. Ann Otol Rhinol Laryngol 111: 222–228.

Bernard G, Mion F, Henry L, Plauchu H, Paliard P (1993) Hepatic involvement in hereditary haemorrhagic telangiectasia: clinical, radiological, and hemodynamic studies of 11 cases. Gastroenterology 105: 482–487.

Bideau A, Plauchu H, Brunet G, Robert J (1989) Epidemiological investigation of Rendu-Osler disease in France: its geographical distribution and prevalence. Population 1: 9–28.

Bosher LH, Blake A, Byrd BR (1959) An analysis of the pathologic anatomy of pulmonary arteriovenous aneurysms with particular reference to the applicability of local excision. Surgery 45: 91–104.

Braverman IM, Keh A, Jacobson BS (1990) Ultrastructure and three-dimensional organization of the telangiectasia of hereditary hemorrhagic telangiectasia. J Invest Dermatol 95: 442–447.

Burke CM, Safai C, Nelson DP, Raffin TA (1986) Pulmonary arteriovenous malformations: a critical update. Am Rev Respir Dis 134: 334–339.

Dakeishi M, Shioya T, Wada Y, Shindo T, Otaka K, Manabe M, Nozaki J, Inoue S, Koizumi A (2002) Genetic epidemiology of hereditary haemorrhagic telangiectasia in a local community in the northern part of Japan. Human Mutat 19: 140–148.

Dines DE, Arms RA, Bernatz PE, Gomes MR (1974) Pulmonary arteriovenous fistulas. Mayo Clinic Proc 49: 460–465.

Easey AJ, Wallace GMF, Hughes JMB, Jackson JE, Taylor WJ, Shovlin CL (2003) Should asymptomatic patients with hereditary haemorrhagic telangiectasia (HHT) be screened for cerebral vascular malformations? Data from 22061 years HHT patient life. J Neurol Neurosurg Psychiatry 74: 743–748.

Garcia-Tsao G, Korzenik JR, Young L, Henderson KJ, Jain D, Byrd B, Pollak JS, White RI Jr (2000) Liver disease in patients with hereditary hemorrhagic telangiectasia. N Engl J Med Sept 28; 343(13): 931–936.

Garland HG, Anning St (1950) Hereditary hemorrhagic telangiectasia: genetic and biographical study. Br J Dermatol 62: 289–310.

Guttmacher AE, Marchuk DA, White RI Jr (1995) Current concepts. Hereditary hemorrhagic telangiectasia. New Eng J Med 10: 918–924.

Haitjema T, Disch E, Overtoom TTC, Westermann TJJ, Lammers JWJ (1995) Screening of family members of patients with hereditary hemorrhagic telangiectasia. Am J Med 99: 519–524.

Haitjema T, Balder W, Disch FJM, Westermann CJJ (1996) Epistaxis in hereditary hemorrhagic telangiectasia. Rhinology 34: 176–178.

Hanes FM (1907) Multiple hereditary telangiectases causing hemorrhage (hereditary hemorrhagic telangiectasia). Bull Johns Hopkins Hosp 1909, 20: 63–73.

Hashimoto K, Pritzker M (1972) Hereditary hemorrhagic telangiectasia: an electron microscope study. Oral Surg Oral Med Oral Pathol Radiol Endod 34: 751–768.

Hewes RC, Auster M, White RI Jr (1985) Cerebral embolism – first manifestation of pulmonary arteriovenous malformation in patients with hereditary hemorrhagic telangiectasia. Cardiovasc Intervent Radiol 8: 151–155.

Jahnke V (1970) Ultrastructure of hereditary hemorrhagic telangiectasia. Arch Otolaryngol Head and Neck Surg 91: 262–265.

Johnson DW, Berg JN, Gallione CJ, Mc Allister KA, Warner JP, Helmbold EA, Markel DS, Jackson CE, Porteous ME, Marchuk DA (1995) A second locus for hereditary hemorrhagic telangiectasia maps to chromosome 12. Genome Res 5: 21–28.

Johnson DW, Berg JN, Baldwin MA, Gallione CJ, Marondel I, Yoon SJ, Stenzel TT, Speer M, Pericak-Vance MA, Diamond A, Guttmacher AE, Jackson CE, Attisano L, Kucherlapati R, Porteous ME, Marchuk DA (1996) Mutations in the activin receptor-like kinase 1 gene in hereditary haemorrhagic telangiectasia type 2. Nature Genet 13: 189–195.

Kjeldsen A, Kjeldsen J (2000) Gastrointestinal bleeding in patients with hereditary hemorrhagic telangiectasia. Am J Gastroenterol 95: 415–418.

Kjeldsen AD, Vase P, Green A (1999) Hereditary hemorrhagic telangiectasia (HHT): a population-based study of prevalence and mortality in Danish HHT patients. J Intern Med 245: 31–39.

Kjeldsen AD, Oxhoj A, Andersen PE, Elle B, Jacobsen JP, Vase P (1999) Pulmonary arteriovenous malformations: screening procedures and pulmonary angiography in patients with hereditary hemorrhagic telangiectasia. Chest 116: 432–439.

Kjeldsen AD, Oxhøj H, Andersen PE, Green A, Vase P (2000) Prevalence of pulmonary arteriovenous malformations (PAVMs) and occurrence of neurologic symptoms in patients with hereditary haemorrhagic telangiectasia (HHT). J Int Med 248: 255–262.

Maire R, Schnewlin G, Bollinger A (1986) Video-microscopic studies of telangiectases in Osler's disease and scleroderma. Schweiz Med Wochenschr 116: 335–339.

Maldonado LV, Soloaga ED, Veltri MA, Chertcoff FJ, Ubaldini JE (2007) Spinal abscess in a patient with hereditary hemorrhagic telangiectasia. Medicina (B Aires) 67: 714.

Matsubara S, Mandzia JL, ter Brugge K, Willinsky RA, Faughnan ME (2000) Angiographic and clinical characteristics of patients with cerebral arteriovenous malformations associated with hereditary hemorrhagic telangiectasia. AJNR Am J Neuroradiol 21(6): 1016–1020.

Mc Allister KA, Grogg KM, Johnson DW, Gallione CJ, Baldwin MA, Jackson CE, Helmbold EA, Markel DS, McKinnon WC, Murrell J, et al. (1994) Endoglin, a TGF-β binding protein of endothelial cell, is the gene for hereditary haemorrhagic telangiectasia type 1. Nat Genet 8: 345–351.

Mc Donald MT, Papenberg KA, Ghosh S, Glatfelter AA, Biesecker BB, Helmbold EA, Markel DS, Zolotor A, McKinnon WC, Vanderstoep JL, et al. (1994) A disease locus for hereditary haemorrhagic telangiectasia maps to chromosome 9q33–34. Nat Genet 6: 197–204.

Menefee MG, Flessa HC, Glueck HI, Hogg SP (1975) Hereditary hemorrhagic telangiectasia (Osler-Weber-Rendu disease): an electron microscopic study of the vascular lesions before and after therapy with hormones. Arch Otolaryngol Head Neck Surg 101: 791–792.

Muri JW (1955) Arteriovenous aneurysm of the lung. Am J Surg 89: 265–271.

Osler W (1901) On family form of recurring epistaxis, associated with multiple telangiectases of skin and mucous membranes. Bull Johns Hopkins Hosp 12: 333–337.

Plauchu H, de Chadarevian JP, Bideau A, Robert JM (1989) Age-related clinical profile of hereditary hemorrhagic telangiectasia in an epidemiologically recruited population. Am J Med Genet 32: 291–297.

Porteous ME, Burn J, Proctor SJ (1992) Hereditary hemorrhagic telangiectasia: a clinical analysis. J Med Genet 29: 527–530.

Porteous MEM, Curtis A, Williams O, Marchuk D, Bhattacharya SS, Burn J (1994) Genetic heterogeneity in hereditary haemorrhagic telangiectasia. J Med Genet 31: 925–926.

Press OW, Ramsey PG (1984) Central nervous system infections associated with hereditary hemorrhagic telangiectasia. Am J Med 77: 86–92.

Reilly PJ, Nostrant TT (1984) Clinical manifestations of hereditary hemorrhagic telangiectasia. Am J Gastroenterol 79: 363–367.

Remy J, Remy-Jardin M, Giraud F, Wattinne L (1994) Angioarchitecture of pulmonary arteriovenous malformations: clinical utility of three-dimensional helical CT. Radiology 191: 657–664.

Rendu HJLM (1896) Épistaxis répétées chez un sujet porteur de petits angiomes cutanés et muqueux. Bull Soc med Hop 13: 731–733.

Robin ED, Laman D, Horn BR, Theodore G (1976) Platypnea related to orthodeoxia caused by true vascular lung shunts. N Engl J Med 294: 941–943.

Römer W, Burk M, Schneider W (1992) Hereditäre hämorrhagische Teleangieltasie (Morbus Osler). Dtsch Med Wochenschr 117: 669–675.

Sadick H, Naim R Gössler U, Hörmann K, Riedel F (2005a) Angiogenesis in hereditary hemorrhagic telangiectasia: VEGF plasma concentration in correlation to the VEGF expression and microvessel density. Int J Mol Med 15(1): 15–19.

Sadick H, Riedel F, Naim R, Goessler U, Hörmann K, Hafner M, Lux A (2005b) Patients with hereditary hemorrhagic telangiectasia have increased plasma levels of vascular endothelial growth factor and transforming growth factor-beta1 as well as high ALK1 tissue expression. Haematologica 90(6): 818–828.

Schneider G, Uder M, Koehler M, Kirchin MA, Massmann A, Buecker A, Geisthoff U (2008) MR angiography for detection of pulmonary arteriovenous malformations in patients with hereditary hemorrhagic telangiectasia. Am J Roentgenol 190: 892–901.

Shovlin CL, Hughes JMB, Tuddenham EGD, Temperley I, Perembelon YF, Scott J, Seidman CE, Seidman JG (1994) A gene for hereditary haemorrhagic telangiectasia maps to chromosome 9q3. Nat Genet 6: 205–209.

Shovlin CL, Winstock AR, Peters AM, Jackson JE, Hughes JM (1995) Medical complications of pregnancy in hereditary hemorrhagic telangiectasia. Quart J Med 88: 879–887.

Shovlin CL, Letarte M (1999) Hereditary haemorrhagic telangiectasia and pulmonary arteriovenous malformations: issues in clinical management and review of pathogenic mechanisms. Thorax 54: 714–729.

Shovlin CL, Guttmacher AE, Buscarini E, Faughnan ME, Hyland RH, Westermann CJ, Kjeldsen AD, Plauchu H (2000) Diagnostic criteria for hereditary haemorrhagic telangiectasia (Rendu-Osler-Weber syndrome). Am J Med Genet 91: 66–67.

Shub C, Tajik AJ, Seward JB, Dines DE (1976) Detecting intrapulmonary right-to-left shunt with contrast echocardiography. Mayo Clin Proc 51: 81–84.

Sluiter-Eringa H, Orie NGM, Sluiter HJ (1969) Pulmonary arteriovenous fistula. Diagnosis and prognosis in non-complaint patients. Am Rev Respir Dis 100: 177–188.

Snyder LH, Doan CA (1944) Clinical and experimental studies in human inheritance. Is the homozygous form of multiple telangiectasia lethal? J Lab Clin Med 29: 1211–1367.

Stringer CJ, Stanley AL, Bates RC, Summers JE (1955) Pulmonary arteriovenous fistula. Am J Surg 89: 1054–1080.

Ueki J, Hughes JMB, Peters AM, Bellingan GJ, Mohammed MA, Dutton J, Ussov W, Knight D, Glass D (1994) Oxygen and $^{99m}$Tc-MAA shunt estimations in patients with pulmonary arteriovenous malformations: effects of changes in posture and lung volume. Thorax 49: 327–331.

Vase P, Holm M, Arendrup H (1985) Pulmonary arteriovenous fistulas in hereditary hemorrhagic telangiectasia. Acta Med Scand 218: 105–109.

Weber EP (1907) Multiple hereditary developmental angiomata (telangiectasia) of the skin and mucous membranes associated with recurring hemorrhages. Lancet 2: 160–162.

White RI Jr, Lynch-Nyhan A, Terry P, Buescher PC, Farmlett EJ, Charnas L, Shuman K, Kim W, Kinnison M, Mitchell SE (1988) Pulmonary arteriovenous malformations: techniques and long-term outcome of embolotherapy. Radiology 169: 663–669.

Willinsky RA, Lasjaunias P, Terbrugge K, Burrows P (1990) Multiple cerebral arteriovenous malformations (AVMs): review of our experience from 203 patients with cerebral vascular lesions. Neuroradiology 32: 207–210.

# Chapter 12

# MACROCEPHALY-CUTIS MARMORATA TELANGIECTATICA CONGENITA (MACROCEPHALY-CAPILLARY MALFORMATION)

**Pablo Lapunzina and Jill Clayton-Smith**

Department of Genetics, University Hospital La Paz, University of Madrid, Madrid, Spain (PL); Academic Department of Medical Genetics, St. Mary's Hospital, Manchester, United Kindom (JCS)

## Introduction

This recently recognised entity (OMIM # 602501) (OMIM 2006) is characterised by the association of macrocephaly (megalencephaly), capillary malformation of the cutis marmorata telangectatica congenita type, cavernous haemangioma, asymmetric growth pattern, central nervous system malformations, and neurological abnormalities (Clayton-Smith et al. 1997, Gerritsen et al. 2000, Moore et al. 1997, Lapunzina et al. 2004). Despite extensive investigation of many of affected cases, no specific cause for the condition has yet been identified (Lapunzina et al. 2004).

In this chapter, we discuss the clinical findings, natural history, diagnostic criteria, and possible mode of inheritance of M-CMTC.

Recently, this entity has been renamed macrocephaly-capillary malformation (M-CM) (Conway et al. 2007, Toriello and Mulliken 2007) in line with the current terminology for vascular anomalies, hemangiomas and malformations (Enjorlas et al. 2007, Mulliken et al. 2006).

We chose to retain the original name throughout the text as this is still used in the current medical literature (Katugampola et al. 2008).

## Historical perspective and eponyms

Although the association of macrocephaly, limb asymmetry, and capillary malformations was documented around 30 years ago, it was not until 1997 that Moore and co-workers (Moore et al. 1997) and Clayton-Smith and colleagues (Clayton-Smith et al. 1997) independently reported on 22 patients with common clinical findings and a similar facial gestalt. The main clinical features of these patients were overgrowth, macrocephaly and cutis marmorata telangiectatica congenita (M-CMTC) along with other associated anomalies. Subsequent communications pointed out that some patients reported by other authors might well have had this syndrome (Carcao et al. 1998, Stephan et al. 1975, Vogels et al. 1998, Wrobleski et al. 1988). A recent paper reported 6 additional cases, reviewed the literature and critically analysed the published evidence in order to further delineate the syndrome (Lapunzina et al. 2004). Since then, a further two patients have been described (Akcar et al. 2004, Dinleyici et al. 2004, Nyberg et al. 2005) bringing the total number of patients with M-CMTC described so far to 77 (Cohen et al. 2002).

## Incidence and prevalence

Seventy-seven patients so far reported (Akcar et al. 2004, Dinleyici et al. 2004, Lapunzina et al. 2004, Nyberg et al. 2005). There is a slight preponderance of males but this is not statistically significant (M:F = 42:34).

## Clinical manifestations

The main characteristics of M-CMTC are macrocephaly, pre and postnatal overgrowth, cutis marmorata, syndactyly, capillary malformation of the lip and/or philtrum, skin and joint laxity and develop-

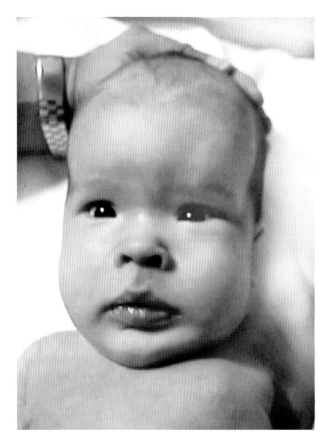

**Fig. 1.** Characteristic capillary malformation on the philtrum and the upper lips.

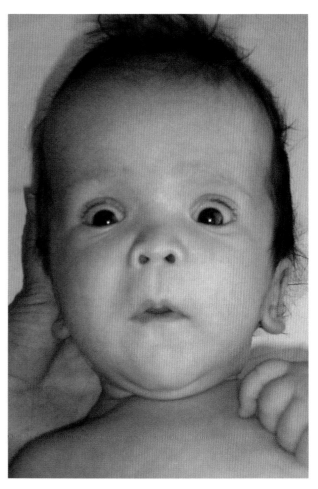

**Fig. 2.** Typical facial appearance of MCMTC demonstrating sunsetting" appearance of the eyes with frontal bossing, large forehead, and short nose, small chin and full lips.

mental delay (Figs. 1–6). In the following sections we discuss the clinical features by region.

## Skin and connective tissue

The skin is affected in almost all patients with M-CMTC. Most of them have a combination of CMTC, nevus flammeus and flat or cavernous hemangiomas, usually most conspicuous in the limbs (Fig. 5). The capillary malformation on the philtrum and/or the upper lip is perhaps the most characteristic (Fig. 1) but some children have had a capillary malformation also of the back or buttocks. The generalised cutis marmorata tends to fade with time. One patients developed a mastocytoma-like nodule in the face (Giuliano et al. 2004). Deep vein thrombosis was observed in 2 cases.

The majority of patients have demonstrable increased skin laxity with or without thickening of the

subcutaneous tissue. Pigmentary abnormalities (hyper or hypopigmentation, following the Blaschko lines) epidermal nevus and deep plantar and palmar creases have been observed in some patients (Baralle and Firth 2000). Hyperextensible joints, diastasis recti, umbilical hernia and inguinal hernia are additional findings suggesting a connective tissue component to the condition.

## Craniofacial anomalies

The facial features and craniofacial anomalies seen in these patients are striking and give rise to a dis-

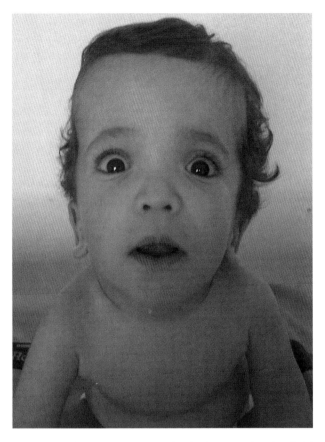

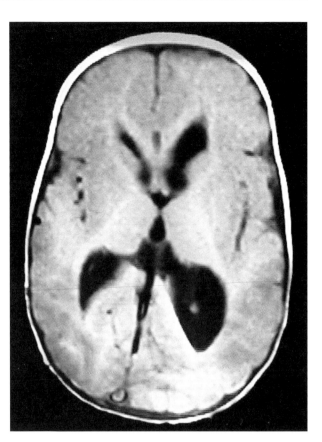

**Fig. 3.** Note the prominent supraorbital ridges associated to facial asymmetry.

**Fig. 4.** Axial T1-weighted MR image of the brain demonstrating left hemimegalencephaly with dilated ventricular horns.

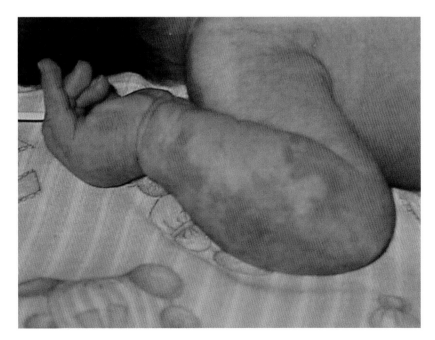

**Fig. 5.** Combination of CMTC, nevus flammeus and flat haemangioma in the right upper limb.

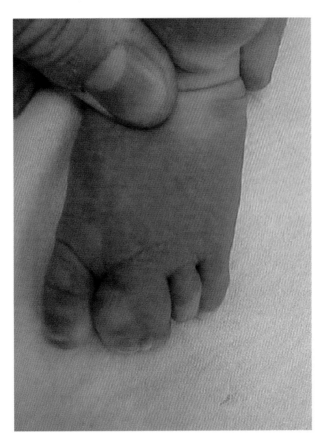

**Fig. 6.** Syndactyly of the 2nd–3rd toes.

tinctive facial *"gestalt"* (Figs. 1–3). Macrocephaly, present at birth and progressive in nature has been present in more than 95% of cases of M-CMTC (Lapunzina et al. 2004). The increased occipito-frontal circumference (OFC) is often independent of the presence of hydrocephalus and the head size may continue to increase in size disproportionately even after shunting. Frontal bossing, large forehead, short nose, small chin, full lips and thick gums are usually present. A characteristic finding is a mid-facial capillary malformation, found mostly on the philtrum and/or upper lip (Fig. 1). This finding is a useful diagnostic feature. The cheeks may be full and fleshy and sometimes with patchy reddish areas of skin. Most patients have deep-set eyes with prominent supraorbital ridges. A "sun-setting" appearance of the eyes may be present along with ptosis of the eyelids and facial asymmetry (Figs. 2 and 3). Along

with the latter there may also be asymmetric gingival hyperplasia. Macroglossia and craniosynostosis are infrequent findings (Moore et al. 2004, Vogels et al. 1998).

## Growth

More than 95% of the patients have had prenatal overgrowth with a high birth weight and increased OFC. Length was normal or just slightly increased in the majority of children. In view of the neonatal macrosomia this syndrome is included in the nosology of the overgrowth syndromes (Cohen et al. 2002). Postnatal overgrowth may occur but is less common and with age the weight and height tend to normalise or even fall below the normal centiles for age and sex (Moore et al. 1997). Postnatal failure to thrive was reported in a small number of cases (Moore et al. 2004, Reardon et al. 1996).

Asymmetric growth in the form of hemihyperplasia/hemihypertrophy or unilateral overgrowth of the face, thorax and/or limbs is commonly observed (Table 1).

## Central nervous system and performance

Brain imaging by MRI or CT scans demonstrated that hydrocephalus with or without hemimegalencephaly is very frequent in M-CMCT (Fig. 4). White matter anomalies demonstrated by MRI have been recorded in ~12% of children (consisting in white matter irregularities with increased signal on T2-weighted images) (Conway et al. 2008). Cortical dysgenesis, a thickened, hyposplastic or agenetic corpus callosum, enlarged cerebellum, Chiari type I malformation, loss of normal sulcation, pachygyria, polymycrogyria and abnormal myelinisation with prominent Virchow-Robin spaces have all been observed (Akcar et al. 2004, Carcao et al. 1998, Conway et al. 2008, Franceschini et al. 2000, Garavelli et al. 2005, Vogels et al. 1998, Reardon et al. 1996). A distinctive feature in more than 50% of patients in one study (Conway et al. 2008) was cerebellar tonsillar herniation (which was acquired in some cases) associated with rapid brain growth and progressive

**Table 1.** Summary of Findings in 77 cases[#] of Macrocephaly-Cutis Marmorata Telangiectatica Congenita (modified from Lapunzina 2005)

| Very frequent (>77%) | |
| --- | --- |
| Macrocephaly | 75/77 |
| Cutis marmorata telangiectatica | 72/77 |
| Asymmetry of the head, face or body | 66/77 |
| Overgrowth/high birth weight | 60/77 |
| Hemangioma of the lip and/or philtrum | 60/77 |

| Frequent (25–77%) | |
| --- | --- |
| Developmental delay[a] | 49/77 |
| Syndactyly of the 2nd–3rd toes | 48/77 |
| Hydrocephalus | 48/77 |
| High forehead/frontal bossing | 42/77 |
| Joint laxity/hypermobility | 42/77 |
| Hypotonia | 36/77 |
| Hemimegalencephaly | 28/77 |
| Hypereslatic skin | 25/77 |
| Thick subcutaneous tissue | 25/77 |

| Less frequent (<25%) | |
| --- | --- |
| Dolichocephaly | 15/77 |
| Polyhydramnios | 15/77 |
| Polydactyly | 16/77 |
| True hypertelorism | 12/77 |
| White matter anomalies | 11/77 |
| Syndactyly 3rd–4th fingers | 11/77 |
| Internal A-V malformation | 10/77 |
| Seizures | 8/77 |
| Pigmentary abnormalities | 8/77 |
| Venous aneurysms/thromboses | 7/77 |
| Gap between 1st and 2nd toes | 9/77 |
| Small palpebral fissures | 9/77 |
| Failure to thrive | 6/77 |
| Chiari-type malformation | 6/77 |
| Hypoglycaemia | 5/77 |
| Stridor | 5/77 |
| Thick gums | 5/77 |
| Arrhythmia/sudden death | 4/77 |
| Ptosis of eyelids | 4/77 |
| Tumours* | 4/77 |
| Cardiac malformation | 5/77 |
| Umbilical hernia | 3/77 |
| Deep plantar creases | 4/77 |
| Pectus carinatum | 2/77 |
| Intestinal lymphangiectasia | 2/77 |
| Epidermal nevus | 2/77 |
| Macroglossia | 2/77 |
| Hip dysplasia | 2/77 |
| Macrodactyly | 2/77 |
| Hip dysplasia | 2/77 |
| Single umbilical artery | 1/77 |
| Hydronephrosis | 1/77 |
| Mesenteric anomalies | 1/77 |
| Atrophic abdominal aorta | 1/77 |

Females 34 cases; Males 42 cases; 1 case gender not reported.

[#]Including the cases of Ringrose et al. (1965); 4 cases of Stephan et al. (1975); 1 case of Meyer (1979); 2 of López-Herce Cid et al. (1985); 1 of Wroblewski et al. (1988); 2 of Cristaldi et al. (1995); 1 of Barnicoat et al. (1996); 1 of Reardon et al. (1996); 9 of Clayton-Smith et al. (1997); 13 of Moore et al. (1997); 1 of Carcao et al. (1998); 4 of Vogels et al. (1998); 1 of Berbel Tornero et al. (1999); 1 of Moffit et al. (1999); 1 of Thong et al. (1999); 1 of Baralle and Firth (2000); 2 of Franceschini et al. (2000); 1 of Gerritsen et al. (2000); 5 of Robertson et al. (2000); 1 of Howells et al. (2000); 1 of Bottani et al. (2000); 3 of Yano and Watanabe (2001); 1 of Schwartz et al. (2002); 1 of Mégarbané et al. (2003); 1 of Stoll (2003), 7 cases of Giuliano et al. (2003), 6 of Lapunzina et al. (2004); 1 of Nyberg et al. (2005); and 1 of Dinleyici et al. (2004) and Akcar et al. (2004) (both the same case).

[a]Some patients did not reach the age for evaluation.

growing of the posterior fossa during infancy. Other findings have been ventriculomegaly, bifrontal extraaxial fluid collections, and cavum septi pellucidum and vergae. Focal CNS infarcts and ischaemic changes have occasionally been reported (Giuliano et al. 2004). Conway et al. (2008) postulated that this constellation of unusual brain features suggests a dynamic process of mechanical compromise in the posterior fossa, perhaps initiated by a rapidly growing cerebellum, which leads to congestion of the venous drainage, compromised cerebrospinal fluid reabsorption, increased posterior fossa pressure and acquired tonsillar herniation.

All degrees of developmental delay have been observed in M-CMTC, with a predominance of moderate to severe retardation (Robertson et al. 2000). This retardation seems to be related not only to brain anatomic anomalies (increased size of cerebral ventricles, hemimegalencephaly, white matter abnormalities, etc) but also to probable CNS cortical dysplasia as developmental delay may be present in the absence of significant structural malformations of the brain. Ventriculo-peritoneal shunts were inserted in about half of the patients but these had little influence on the macrocephaly, suggesting a true megalencephaly (Moore et al. 1997, Vogels et al. 1998). Hypotonia, anisocoria, esotropia, facial nerve palsy, optic atrophy and brain arteriovenous malformation were observed in several patients. Seizures have occurred in a few patients but are not a common finding (Lapunzina et al. 2004).

## Limbs

The hands are usually large and broad with a "fleshy" appearance. Some patients may have polydactyly (postaxial) and syndactyly of the fingers (Fig. 6) (Clayton-Smith et al. 1997, Franceschini et al. 2000, Moore et al. 1997). Macrodactyly was observed in one case.

Cutaneous syndactyly of the second and third toes, usually up to the distal phalanx is very frequent (Fig. 6). There is often a wide space between the first and second toes. One patient had bilateral oligodactyly with absent fifth toes (Giuliano et al. 2003). Hypoplastic toenails were observed sporadically. In some patients the nails are flattened and have an appearance similar to that seen when there has been oedema in utero.

A degree of body disproportion and asymmetry has been observed in a high percentage of cases, with or without vascular compromise of the involved region (Table 1). Joints may be hyperelastic with a tendency to subluxation in some occasions. Hip dysplasia was reported in a small number of cases.

## Thorax and abdomen

Complex cardiac malformations were described in two cases (Clayton-Smith et al. 1997, Giuliano et al. 2003), a ventricular septal defect (VSD) in another and a dilated aortic root in further children (Moore et al. 1997, Nyberg et al. 2005). Akcar et al. (2004), reported a child with an atrial septal defect and a giant atrial septal aneurysm, and Giuliano et al. (2003) reported a further patient with an atrial septal defect (ASD). Cardiac arrhythmias such as atrial flutter or supraventricular tachycardia have been observed and are often life-threatening situations requiring intervention. (Clayton-Smith et al. 1997, Giuliano et al. 2003, Yano and Watanabe 2001). Mesenteric angina was reported by Howells et al. (Howells et al. 2000), and intestinal lymphangiectasia and atrophic abdominal aorta by others (Megarbané et al. 2003, Thong et al. 1999). Unlike other overgrowth syndromes, enlargement of the liver, spleen or kidneys are not often seen.

## M-CMTC and Tumours

A total of four patients with M-CMTC have developed tumours (acute leukemia, meningioma, Wilms tumour and retinoblastoma) (Lapunzina et al. 2004, Moore et al. 1997, Schwartz et al. 2002). The boy with retinoblastoma reported by Schwartz et al. (2002) did not have the typical characteristics of M-CMTC however and might be an atypical case. One patient was found to have a frontal perifalcine mass resembling a meningioma at age 5 years in one study (Conway et al. 2008). Although the number of patients with M-CMTC currently reported is low and the types of neoplasia seen so far are heterogeneous, the putative 5–6% tumour risk appears to be similar to other overgrowth syndromes (Cohen 1989, Lapunzina 2005, Lapunzina et al. 1998). Thus it has been recommended that patients with this syndrome should have regular screening for tumours (Lapunzina 2005) and this will be discussed in more detail below.

## Pathogenesis and molecular genetics

The cause of M-CMTC is not known. All cases reported to date have been sporadic. There is a slight preponderance of males but this is not statistically significant (M:F = 42:34). No affected parents or siblings have been observed but increased paternal age has been noted in several cases. All these data would seem to support an autosomal dominant pattern of inheritance with the condition arising due to a new dominant mutation. The parents of patient 4 of Vogels et al. (1998) were consanguineous (second cousins) with otherwise unremarkable family history and the parents of the patient of Berbel Tornero et al. (1999) were first cousins of Gypsy ancestry (an ethnic group with a high degree of consanguinity). Clayton-Smith et al. (1997) suggested that some of the clinical findings of this disorder such as patchy vascular markings of the skin, asymmetry, and occasional pigmented skin lesions which follow Blaschko's lines might be due to somatic mosaicism. Chromosome anomalies have been observed in three patients with M-CMTC; mosaicism in skin fibroblasts (diploidy/tetraploidy; 92, XXXY [2]/46, XY [17]) in one patient was reported by Bottani et al. (2000). Skin fibroblast chromosomes from other patients failed to confirm any similar alteration (Lapunzina et al. 2004). The other chromosome abnormalities were a 16q deletion in a girl (Cristaldi et al. 1995) and recently, an apparently balanced translocation 2:17 (p11; p13) (Stoll 2003). Although the latter may be significant the t(2; 17) could be purely coincidental or due to culture artefact. Data of the 16q deletion in the report by Cristaldi et al. (1995) is scant and unfortunately no breakpoint on 16q is given and molecular studies were not done. Thus, a cryptic balanced translocation was not excluded and the significance of this finding remains unclear. The

cause of M-CMTC thus remains elusive but will probably be elucidated as further patients are described (Lapunzina et al. 2004).

## Diagnosis and diagnostic criteria

Diagnosis must be based on clinical findings as no molecular defect has been defined so far. The clinical findings observed in the majority of patients are listed in Table 1. Major and minor criteria of M-CMTC were set forth by Franceschini et al. (2000) who suggested that the diagnosis could be made in the presence of: a) macrocephaly and at least two other findings such as b) cutis marmorata, overgrowth, capillary malformation, syndactyly or asymmetry. Other groups have proposed similar criteria (Baralle and Firth 2000, Yano and Watanabe 2001), suggesting that the diagnosis should be sustained on the presence of macrocephaly and at least two of the following findings: overgrowth, cutis marmorata, capillary malformation, polydactyly/syndactyly and asymmetry. Robertson et al. (2000) have laid down more stringent criteria. They suggested as major criteria the presence of: congenital macrocephaly and CMTC and in addition at least 4 of the following findings: neonatal hypotonia, developmental delay, connective tissue defect, frontal bossing, midline facial nevus flammeus, cutaneous toe syndactyly, segmental overgrowth and hydrocephalus. With a condition such as M-CMTC where the spectrum of problems is broad, more stringent criteria might exclude milder cases which could provide useful clues to the aetiology of the condition. On the other hand, the less stringent criteria may not be restrictive enough. Only when the underlying genetic basis is identified will it be possible to validate the different sets of diagnostic criteria suggested.

Abnormalities have been identified prenatally in several patients when macrocephaly, macrosomia, limb asymmetry, hemimegalencephaly, polyhydramnios, ascitis and/or pleural effusions were observed (Moore et al. 1997, Nyberg et al. 2005, Robrtson et al. 2000, Vogels et al. 1998) Elevated maternal serum alpha fetoprotein was observed one one occasion (Robertson et al. 2000). It is difficult to make a firm diagnosis of M-CMTC prenatally, however, as the characteristic skin signs, one of the diagnostic hallmarks of the condition, cannot be visualised.

## Differential diagnosis

Differential diagnosis includes other disorders with overgrowth/macrocephaly (Barnicoat et al. 1996, Cohen et al. 2002, Lopez-Herce Cid et al. 1985, Meyer 1979, Mofitt et al. 1999, Ringrose et al. 1965) such as Beckwith Wiedemann syndrome, Simpson Golabi Behmel syndrome, Sotos syndrome, Perlman syndrome, Proteus syndrome, Costello syndrome and Bannayan–Zonana syndrome. Disorders with skin vascular malformations and asymmetry such as Klippel–Trenaunay, Parkes Weber must also be considered. M-CMTC may be easily diagnosed when the full phenotype, characteristic features and typical *gestalt* are present.

## Prognosis and follow-up

Long-term prognosis is usually determined by the neurological (Giuliano et al. 2003) and cardiac mani-

**Table 2.** Management Plan For A Child With M-CMTC

| Age | Problem | Health Check/Investigation |
|---|---|---|
| At Birth | Macrocephaly/overgrowth | Plot baseline growth parameters |
| | Structural heart defects | Echocardiogram |
| | Cardiac arrhythmia | ECG |
| | Internal vascular malformations | Abdominal ultrasound scan |
| | | Brain imaging |
| | Hip dysplasia | Ultrasound scan hips |
| 0–12 months Paediatric follow-up at monthly intervals for first three months, then three monthly | Ventriculomegaly | Plot OFC monthly |
| | | Monthly neuro examination |
| | | Refer neurosurgeon if excessive increase or signs of raised intracranial pressure |
| | Predisposition to malignancy | 3 monthly abdominal ultrasound examination |
| | Ophthalmological | Formal ophthalmological examination |
| | General | Monitor growth and development with physiotherapy/occupational therapy referral as appropriate |
| | | Regular vision and hearing checks |
| Early childhood | Predisposition to malignancy | 3 monthly abdominal ultrasound scans until age 5 |
| | General | Six monthly paediatric assessment with abdominal and neuro examinations |
| | | Offer genetic referral |
| | Developmental problems | Formal developmental assessment at 12 months. Early intervention programme |
| | Hemihypertrophy | Refer to orthopaedic surgeon if significant leg length discrepancy |
| 5–10 years | General | Monitor growth and development 6–12 monthly |
| | | Regular vision and hearing checks |
| | Developmental problems | Pre-school assessment of special educational needs |
| 10 years plus | General | Annual health check with general examination |
| | Developmental problems | Review educational needs on a regular basis |

festations. There is almost always some degree of mental impairment, ranging from mild to severe. About half of the patients need a ventricular shunt for treatment of hydrocephalus. Some children can attend normal school, but in general almost all of them will need support and a special educational program. An ECG, together with neurological and cardiac evaluations are recommended for all patients with M-CMTC due to the fact that some patients have had life-threatening arrhythmias. It is not clear whether or not these children need to enter a tumour surveillance program. It has been suggested recently that regular physical examination, abdominal and renal ultrasound and AFP analysis should be carried out (Lapunzina 2005). This recommendation is empirical and more patients need to be followed up for a longer period of time before it can be validated. Table 2 summarises the management plan for a child with M-CMTC.

It is clear from the patients reported so far that there is a great deal of variability between patients with M-CMTC. This should be borne in mind when discussing the diagnosis with the parents, emphasising that perhaps the best guide to determining the prognosis for an individual child, after ruling out any significant medical complications, is observation of the child's progress during the first years of life.

# References

Akcar N, Adapinar B, Dinleyici C, Durak B, Ozkan IR (2004) A case of macrocephaly-cutis marmorata telangiectatica congenita and review of neuroradiologic features. Ann Genet 47: 261–265.

Baralle D, Firth H (2000) A case of the new overgrowth syndrome-macrocephaly with cutis marmorata, haemangioma and syndactyly. Clin Dysmorphol 9: 209–211.

Barnicoat A, Salman M, Chitty L, Baraitser M (1996) A distinctive overgrowth syndrome with polysyndactyly. Clin Dysmorphol 5: 339–346.

Berbel Tornero O, Rometsch S, Ridaura Gastaldo S, Perez-Aytes A (1999) Macrocephaly-cutis marmorata telangectasica congenita: another case of a newly recognized entity. An Esp Pediatr 51: 399–401.

Bottani A, Chevallier I, Dahoun S, Cossali D, Pfister R (2000) Macrocephaly-cutis marmorata telangiectatica congenita (M-CMTC) syndrome can be caused by diploidy/tetraploidy skin mosaicism. Eur J Hum Genet (Suppl 1): 187 (abstract).

Carcao M, Blaser SI, Grant RM, Weksberg R, Siegel-Bartelt J (1998) MRI findings in macrocephaly-cutis marmorata telangiectatica congenita. Am J Med Genet 76: 165–167.

Clayton-Smith J, Kerr B, Brunner H, Tranebjaerg L, Magee A, Hennekam RC, Mueller RF, Brueton L, Super M, Steen-Johnsen J, Donnai D (1997) Macrocephaly with cutis marmorata, haemangioma and syndactyly – a distinctive overgrowth syndrome. Clin Dysmorphol 6: 291–302.

Cohen MM Jr (1989) A comprehensive and critical assesment of overgrowth and overgrowth syndromes. In: Harris H, Hirschhorn K (eds.) "Advances in Human Genetics". Vol. 18. New York: Plenum Press, pp. 181–303 and 373–376.

Cohen MM Jr, Neri G, Weksberg R (2002) Overgrowth syndromes. Oxford Monographs on Medical Genetics. Oxford University Press.

Conway RL, Pressman BD, Dobyns WB, Danielpour M, Lee J, Sanchez-Lara PA, Butler MG, Zackai E, Campbell L, Saitta SC, Clericuzio CL, Milunsky JM, Hoyme HE, Shieh J, Moeschler JB, Crandall B, Lauzon JL, Viskochil DH, Harding B, Graham JM Jr (2008) Neuroimaging findings in macrocephaly-capillary malformation: a longitudinal study of 17 patients. Am J Med Genet A 143: 2981–3008.

Cristaldi A, Vigevano F, Antoniazzi G (1995) Hemimegalencephaly, hemihypertrophy and vascular lesions. Eur J Pediatr 154: 134–137.

Dinleyici EC, Tekin N, Aksit MA, Kilic Z, Adapinar B, Bozan G (2004) Macrocephaly-Cutis marmorata telangiectatica congenita with atrial septal aneurysm and magnetic resonance imaging (MRI) findings. Pediatr Int 46: 366–367.

Enjorlas O, Wassef M, Chapot R (2007) Color atlas of vascular tumours and vascular malformations. New York: Cambridge University Press.

Franceschini P, Licata D, Di Cara G, Guala A, Franceschini D, Genitori L (2000) Macrocephaly-cutis marmorata telangiectatica congenita without cutis marmorata? Am J Med Genet 90: 265–269.

Garavelli L, Leask K, Zanacca C, Pedori S, Albertini G, Della Giustina E, Croci GF, Magnani C, Banchini G, Clayton-Smith J, Bocian M, Firth H, Gold JA, Hurst J (2005) MRI and neurological findings in macrocephaly-cutis marmorata telangiectatica congenita syndrome: report of ten cases and review of the literature. Genet Couns 16: 117–128.

Gerritsen MJ, Steijlen PM, Brunner HG, Rieu P (2000) Cutis marmorata telangiectatica congenita: report of 18 cases. Br J Dermatol 142: 366–369.

Giuliano F, Edery P, Bonneau D, Cormier-Daire V, Philip N (2004) Macrocephaly-cutis marmorata telangiectatica congenita: seven cases including two with unusual cerebral manifestations. Am J Med Genet published online 126: 99–103.

Howells R, Curran A, Jardine P, Newbury-Ecob R, Sandhu B (2000) Mesenteric angina complicating a mesodermal anomaly. Eur J Paediatr Neurol 4: 181–183.

Katugampola R, Moss C, Mills C (2008) Macrocephaly-cutis marmorata telangiectatica congenita: a case report and review of salient features. J Am Acad Dermatol 58: 697–702.

Lapunzina P, Badia I, Galoppo C, De Matteo E, Silberman P, Tello A, Grichener J, Hughes-Benzie R (1998) A patient with Simpson–Golabi–Behmel syndrome and hepatocellular carcinoma. J Med Genet 35: 153–156.

Lapunzina P, Gairi A, Delicado A, Mori MA, Torres ML, Goma A, Navia M, Pajares IL (2004) Macrocephaly-cutis marmorata telangiectatica congenita: report of six new patients and a review. Am J Med Genet A130: 45–51

Lapunzina P (2005) Risk of tumorigenesis in the overgrowth syndromes. Am J Med Genet C Semin Med Genet 137: 53–71.

López-Herce Cid J, Roche Herrero MC, Pascual-Castroviejo I (1985) Cutis marmorata telangiectática congénita. Anomalías asociadas. An Esp Pediatr 22: 575–580.

Mégarbané A, Haddad J, Lyonnet S, Clayton-Smith J (2003) Child with overgrowth, pigmentary streaks, polydactyly, and intestinal lymphangiectasia: macrocephaly-cutis marmorata telangiectatica congenita syndrome or new disorder? Am J Med Genet 116A: 184–187.

Meyer E (1979) Neurocutaneous syndrome with excessive macrohydrocephalus.(Sturge–Weber/Klippel–Trenaunay syndrome). Neuropädiatrie 10: 67–75.

Moffitt DL, Kennedy CT, Newbury-Ecob R (1999) What syndrome is this? Macrocephaly with cutis marmorata, hemangioma, and syndactyly syndrome. Pediatr Dermatol 16: 235–237.

Moore CA, Toriello HV, Abuelo DN, Bull MJ, Curry CJ, Hall BD, Higgins JV, Stevens CA, Twersky S, Weksberg R, Dobyns WB (1997) Macrocephaly-cutis marmorata telangiectatica congenita: a distinct disorder with developmental delay and connective tissue abnormalities. Am J Med Genet 70: 67–73.

Mulliken JB, Fishman SJ, Bunows PE (2006) Vascula anomalies, hemangiomas and malformations. Oxford: Oxford University Press.

Nyberg RH, Uotila J, Kirkinen P, Rosendahl H (2005) Macrocephaly-cutis marmorata telangiectatica congenita syndrome – prenatal signs in ultrasonography. Prenat Diagn 25: 129–132.

Reardon W, Harding B, Winter RM, Baraitser M (1996) Hemihypertrophy, hemimegalencephaly, and polydactyly. Am J Med Genet 66: 144–149.

Ringrose RE, Jabbour JT, Keele DK (1965) Hemihyperthrophy. Pediatrics 36: 434–448.

Robertson SP, Gattas M, Rogers M, Ades LC (2000) Macrocephaly – cutis marmorata telangiectatica congenita: report of five patients and a review of the literature. Clin Dysmorphol 9: 1–9.

Schwartz IV, Felix TM, Riegel M, Schuler-Faccini L (2002) Atypical macrocephaly-cutis marmorata telangiectatica congenita with retinoblastoma. Clin Dysmorphol 11: 199–202.

Stephan MJ, Hall BD, Smith DW, Cohen MM Jr (1975) Macrocephaly in association with unusual cutaneous angiomatosis. J Pediatr 87: 353–359.

Stoll C (2003) Macrocephaly-cutis marmorata telangiectatica congenita: report of a patient with a translocation. Genet Couns 14: 173–179.

Thong MK, Thompson E, Keenan R, Simmer K, Harbord M, Davidson G, Haan E (1999) A child with hemimegalencephaly, hemihypertrophy, macrocephaly, cutaneous vascular malformation, psychomotor retardation and intestinal lymphangiectasia – a diagnostic dilemma. Clin Dysmorphol 8: 283–286.

Toriello HV, Mulliken JB (2007) Accurately renaming macrocephaly-cutis marmorata telangiectatica congenita (M-CMTC) as macrocephaly-capillary malformation (M-CM). Am J Med Genet A 143: 300.

Vogels A, Devriendt K, Legius E, Decock P, Marien J, Hendrickx G, Fryns JP (1998) The macrocephaly-cutis marmorata telangiectatica congenita syndrome. Long-term follow-up data in 4 children and adolescents. Genet Couns 9: 245–253.

Wroblewski I, Joannard A, François P, Baudain P, Beani JC, Beaudoing A (1988) Cutis marmorata telangiectatica congenita avec asymétrie corporelle. Pédiatrie 43: 117–120.

Yano S, Watanabe Y (2001) Association of arrhythmia and sudden death in macrocephaly-cutis marmorata telangiectatica congenita syndrome. Am J Med Genet 102: 149–152.

# Chapter 13

# BLUE RUBBER BLEB NEVUS SYNDROME (BRBNS)

María del Carmen Boente and María Rosa Cordisco

Department of Dermatology, Hospital del Niño Jesús, Tucumàn, Argentina (MDCB);
Department of Dermatology, Hospital de Pediatria "Prof. Dr. J. P. Garrahan", Buenos Aires, Argentina (MRC)

## Introduction

Blue rubber bleb nevus syndrome (BRBNS) is a rare congenital disorder (OMIM # 112200) characterized by multifocal venous malformations mainly of the skin, soft tissue and gastrointestinal tract which may occur however in any tissue including the nervous system (Enjolras and Mulliken 1997, Fretzin and Potter 1965, Moodley and Ramdial 1993, Mulliken and Glowacki 1982, Munkvad 1983, Nahm et al. 2004, Paules et al. 1993).

BRBNS is characterised by distinctive cutaneous lesions, nocturnal pain and regional hyperhidrosis. Bleeding of the gastrointestinal tract is an important, and often fatal, complication but lesions of the brain and spinal cord occur (Andersen 2004, Deng et al. 2008, Edelstein et al. 2005, Garen and Sahn 1994, Shannon and Auld 2005, Wong et al. 1994).

Most BRBNS are sporadic and do not harbour mutations in the receptor tyrosine kinase/TEK-TIE2 (on chromosome 9p21) like in the so-called *"venous malformation multiple cutaneous and mucosal"* (VMCM) (OMIM # 600195) (Boon et al. 1994, Gallione et al. 1995, Tille and Pepper 2004). Until now there is no clear clinical-genetic differentiation between BRBNS and VMCM.

## Historical background and eponyms

In 1860 Gascoyen probably reported the first case of an association of cutaneous and intestinal lesions with gastrointestinal bleeding in a 44-year-old man with anaemia and numerous cavernous hemangiomas of the skin. Gascoyen or Gaskoyen, referred to by one author, is probably the English dermatologist George Gaskoin (1818?–1887).

Almost a century later, in 1958, the hepatologist William Bean described a condition with similar findings in two individuals and reviewed the features of six others; he also coined the term *"blue rubber bleb nevus syndrome"* (Andersen 2004, Bean 1958).

**William Bennett Bean** was born in the Philippine Islands, but not long after the family moved to New Orleans and a few years later to Charlottesville, Virginia. Following graduation from medical school in Virginia, he interned on the Osler Service at Johns Hopkins and the following year he moved to Boston. Dr. Bean began his clinical career at the University of Cincinnati College of Medicine (1936–1946) and at Cincinnati General Hospital (1941–1948). In 1948 he became professor of medicine and head of internal medicine at the University of Iowa College of Medicine. In 1974, he was appointed Director, Institute for Medical Humanities and Professor of Internal Medicine at the University of Texas Medical Branch, Galveston. In 1980, he retired from the Institute and returned to Iowa City. Between 1937 and 1974, Bean published over 600 works in such diverse fields as nutrition, respiratory disease, myocardial infarction, climatology, arterial "spiders," slum eradication and housing, liver disease, William Osler, Walter Reed, and the history of medicine (History of Medicine 2006, Who named it? 2006).

The inaccurate use of the term *"hemangioma"* for the malformations of BRBNS in general reflected the traditional use of the cavernous hemangiomas when referring to venous malformations. Mulliken and Glowacki (1982) helped to clarify our thinking regarding vascular anomalies by proposing that these would be categorized as either hemangiomas or malformations on the basis of their cellular features in relation to their clinical appearance and natural history. A modification of this classification system was accepted by the International Society for the Study of Vascular Anomalies (ISSVA) (Enjolras and Mulliken 1997). They proposed that *vascular anomalies* (VA) can be classified as *tumours* or *malformations* of diverse vascular origin. *Vascular malformations* (VM) result from errors of vascular morphogenesis and are named by their predominant vessel type: arterial, venous, capillary, lymphatic or different combinations of each of them. Venous malformations, often improperly termed "cavernous hemangiomas", are the most frequent vascular abnormality. They are present at birth, thought often they often become apparent afterward. In BRBN, the vascular lesions represent a peculiar type of venous malformations (Tille and Pepper 2004).

BRBNS is also known as Bean's dollar bill skin; Bean syndrome; Blaues Gummiblasen-Syndrom (in Germany); cutaneous-intestinal cavernous hemangioma; and naevus caoutchouc-bleu (in France).

## Incidence and prevalence

The syndrome is quite rare with approximately 200 cases reported in the world's literature but its precise incidence is unknown (Andersen 2004, Cherpelis and Fenske 2006, Edelstein et al. 2005). BRBNS has been reported in persons of all races, although whites appear to be most frequently affected. Males and females are equally affected.

## Clinical manifestations

### Skin manifestations

BRBNS is characterized by highly distinctive cutaneous lesions, as multiple, protuberant, dark blue, compressible blebs, a few millimetres to several centimetres in diameter and varied in hues and shapes.

They usually do not bleed and can be classified into 3 types (Bean 1958):

- Type 1 is a large disfiguring, cavernous lesion that may compress and/or obstruct vital structures (Fig. 1).
- Type 2 are the most classic cutaneous lesions: these are rubbery raised bluish-to-black lesions, soft and easily compressible, leaving an empty sack after pressure that refills slowly they are considered nipple like lesions (Fig. 2). Sometimes hyperhidrosis is seen on their overlying skin (Moodley and Ramdial 1993, Tunkvad 1983).
- Type 3 is an irregular blue-black macule or papule that rarely may blanch when pressure is applied (Fig. 3).

Skin lesions may be seen on any cutaneous surface, but the trunk, limbs and face are the most frequently involved sites and may appear immediately after birth, in infancy, or even later beyond midlife (Cherpelis and Fenske 2006, Mejia-Rodriguez et al. 2008). The number and size of lesions can increase with age (Fine et al. 1961, Fretzin and Potter 1965, Moodley and Ramdial 1993, Nahm et al. 2004, Romao et al. 1999). They usually do not bleed and are rarely painful. No malignant change of skin lesions has been reported so far (Moodley and Ramdial 1993, Munkvad 1983).

## Systemic involvement

### Gastrointestinal tract

In addition to the cutaneous involvement, vascular lesions are usually found in the gastrointestinal tract, anywhere from the oral to the anal mucosa, but predominantly in the small bowel (McKinlay et al. 1998, Moodley and Ramdial 1993, Paules et al. 1993) (Fig. 4). The most common mode of presentation of BRBNS is gastrointestinal bleeding. Lesions are typically discrete mucosal nodules with a central bluish nipple, although they may be flat, macular or polyploid. They vary in size and number but there is no correlation with extent of cutaneous involvement (Gallo and McClave 1992, Nahm et al. 2004, Sandhu et al. 1987).

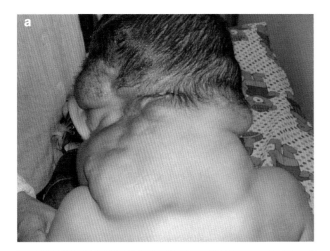

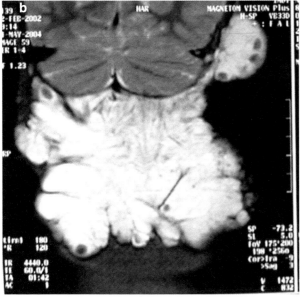

Fig. 1. (a) A large, complex, disfiguring, cavernous lesion of the neck and upper shoulders compressing vital structures in a child with BRBNS; (b) corenal T2-weighted MR image shows marked increased signal intensity of the venous component of a large tumour in the posterior fossa.

Gastrointestinal lesions may appear from infancy to adulthood, they are generally multiple and tend to bleed easily, often leading to iron deficiency anaemia, due to occult blood loss or acute haemorrhage, requiring iron supplementation or blood transfusions (Baker et al. 1971, Berlyne and Berlyne 1960, McIntosh and Harris 1970, Sandhu et al. 1987). Acute bleeding, presenting as hematemesis, melena or rectal bleeding may occur. Hemorrhage is

occasionally massive and life-threatening requiring blood transfusion or surgical intervention without any delay (Baker et al. 1971, Fishman et al. 2005, Romao et al. 1999, Shahed et al. 1990). Occasionally they cause other types of complications such as intussusception, volvulus, intestinal infarction, internal hemorrhage or rectal prolapse (Lee et al. 2008). Therefore, in a patient with BRBNS the presence of abdominal pain or signs of intestinal obstruction should always be evaluated carefully (Beluffi et al. 2004, Browne et al. 1983, Moodley and Ramdial 1993, Nahm et al. 2004).

## Other organs

Many other organs may be involved: liver, spleen, heart, lung, pleura, peritoneum, kidney, thyroid, pararotid, bladder, oronasopharyns, penis, vulva, cervix, eyes, skcletal muscle, bone and brain (Carvalho et al. 2003, Gascoyen 1860, Lichtig et al. 1971, Malhotra et al. 2008, Moodley and Ramdial 1993, Munkvad 1983, Paules et al. 1993, Radke et al. 1993, Starr et al. 2005, Tanaka et al. 2007) (Figs. 5 and 6). In addition to skin and gastrointestinal tract lesions orthopaedic abnormalities are often present. Skeletal anomalies may arise from pressure of adjacent venous malformations into bone structures (Fig. 6). Hypertrophy may occur as a result of hypervascularity. Skeletal bowing as well as pathologic fractures have also been reported (Manoury et al. 1990, Mckinlay et al. 1998, Tzoufi et al. 2007).

Sakurane et al. (1967) described cavernous hemangiomas characteristic of BRBNS over the entire surface of the body and in the mucosa of the oropharynx, oesophagus, distal ileum and anus. In addition the patient had multiple enchondromatosis (Sakurane et al. 1967).

## Central nervous system

Although central nervous system involvement is rarely described, there has been a number of reports of variable cerebral vascular and arteriovenous malformations in BRBNS (Fig. 1b) including dural arteriovenous fistula (Carvalho et al. 2003) vascular malformations

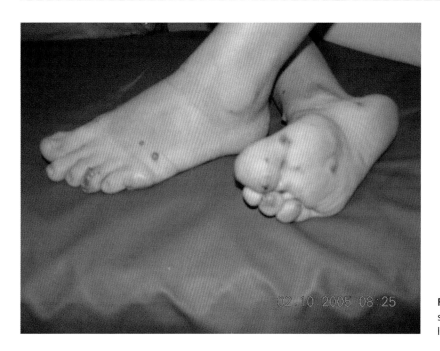

**Fig. 2.** Rubbery raised bluish-to black lesions, soft and easily compressible, nipple like lesions in the feet of a man with BRBNS.

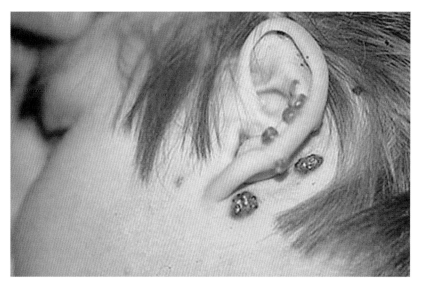

**Fig. 3.** Irregular blue-black papules in the auricular and sub auricular region in a child with BRBNS.

(Gil-Nunez et al. 1983, Hashimoto et al. 1989, Jaffe 1929, Kunishige et al. 1997, Satya-Murti et al. 1986, Wood et al. 1957), developmental venous anomalies including vein of Galen malformation (Waybright et al. 1978) and sinus periocranii (Gabikian et al. 2003) giant venous angioma (Sherry et al. 1984), vertebral hemangiomas (Garen and Sahn 1994), mixed vascular malformations (Rice and Fischer 1996, Rosenblum et al. 1978) and multiple cerebral and cerebellar vascular malformations with foci of haemorrhage in both occipital lobes (Shannon et al. 2005, Tzoufi et al. 2007).

Bleeding can occur in any affected site leading to different clinical pictures. If sufficiently severe, anaemia can cause additional neurological symptoms (Andersen 2004). Focal seizures seem to be the most common initial neurological problem (Bean 1958, Waybright et al. 1978, Kim 2000). Neurological

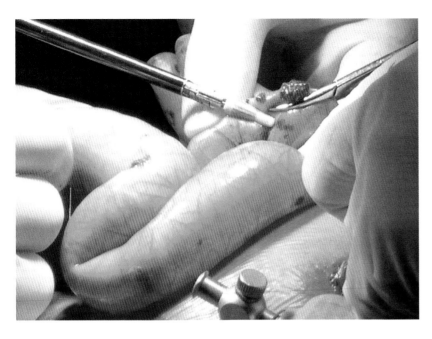

**Fig. 4.** Evidence of blue bleb lesions in a segment of gastrointestinal tract shown during resection of the involved segment of gut.

signs included so far weakness, ataxia, ophthalmoplegia, visual field defects and cortical blindness (Kim 2000, Satya-Murti et al. 1986, Shannon and Auld 2005, Wong et al. 1994). If the lesion is around the spinal cord, medullar compression requiring emergency surgery can occur (Garen and Sahn 1994, Wong et al. 1994) or progressive leg pain and weakness after minor back injury can ensue (Garen and Sahn 1994). Satya-Murti et al. (1986) described a young adult with central nervous system involvement: the patient presented with a slowly progressive ataxia and brain stem signs including palatal myoclonus. A large posterior fossa, and multiple smaller hemispheric vascular lesions were noted. Waybright et al. (1978) described another patient with severe headaches who had a thrombosed Galen's vein malformation.

## Imaging

Radiographic images may be useful in suspected bone or joint involvement to detect fractures, bony overgrowth, and articular derangement (Cherpelis and Fenske 2006). Radiographic contrast techniques may detect gastrointestinal lesions, but endoscopy is considered to be superior. Upper gastrointestinal endoscopy is more sensitive than an upper gastrointestinal series and colonscopy more useful than a barium enema. Endoscopy also provides the opportunity to treat and diagnose the lesion(s).

Multifocal intracranial calcifications (most often located in the caudate nucleus and posterior fossa) (Edelstein et al. 2005) are sometimes evident with computed cranial tomography (CT) (Waybright et al. 1978). These calcifications may stem from thrombosis within the vascular lesion (Andersen 2004). Contrast enhancing lobulated intraconal orbital lesions consistent with hemangiomas are demonstrated by computed tomography. Larger lesions of similar nature may be seen within the soft tissues of the neck, in association with partial thromboses and hyperdense phlebolyts (Edelstein et al. 2005).

CT scans show the extent of the lesions which are hypodense or heterogeneous before contrast and enhances peripherally and slowly after injection of contrast. Magnetic resonance imaging (MRI) is an excellent technique for defining the extent of the lesions and their relationship to adjacent structures. On T1-weighted images, venous malformations are hypointense or jointense compared to the muscle. They may present with an heterogeneous on intermediate signal secondary to

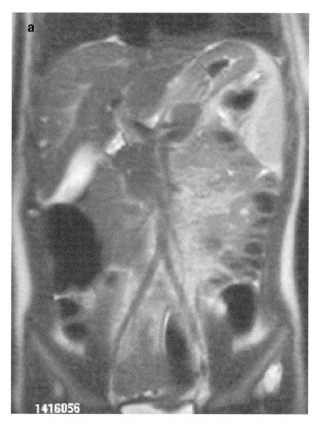

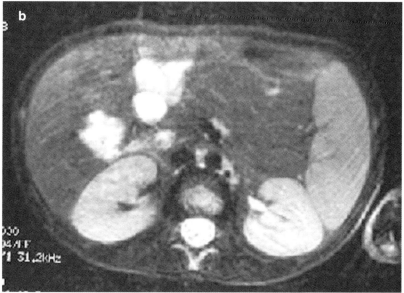

**Fig. 5.** MR (**a**) and CT (**b**) appearance of multiple cavernous lesions in the internal organs.

thrombosis or haemorrhage. Absence of flow voids is mandatory for the diagnosis of venous malformations.

MRI and/or MR angiography is a useful tool for detecting extracutaneous lesions and fro screening of asymptomatic members. Patients with brain involve-

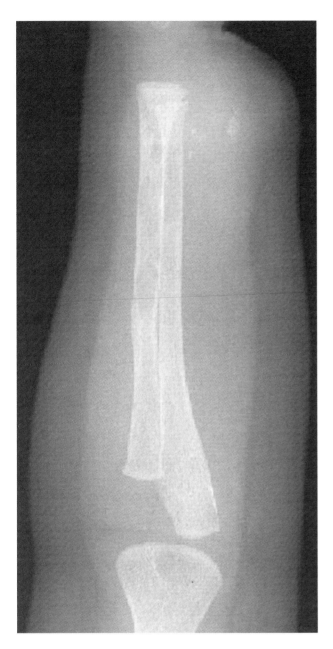

**Fig. 6.** X-ray demonstration of bone involvement.

ment show at MRI one or more lesions (Kim 2000). Flow voids and areas of moderate to marked contrast enhancement within the cerebellum, caudate nucleus, and cerebral cortex indicate vascular lesions of diverse size. These correlate angiographically with vascular malformations but are not true arterovenous malformations, since they show no definite arteri-

ovenous shunting (Edelstein et al. 2005). Larger lesions may be apparent in the late phases of cerebral angiography (Satya-Murti et al. 1986). MRI and MR angiography also display anomalous venous sinuses, thromboses of sinuses, and adjacent cerebral atrophy, presumably related to altered flow dynamics (Edelstein et al. 2005).

The vertebral bodies may show stippled "honey comb" lesions characteristic of vascular lesions and any associated epidural malformation within the spinal canal, as well as any concurrent epidural haematoma or spinal block (Edelstein et al. 2005).

## Natural history

The natural history and overall prognosis of BRBNS is unknown. However, systemic complications begin to appear after the age of 10–20 years (Oranje 1986), and sudden massive gastrointestinal hemorrhage remains the most frequent cause of death (Edelstein et al. 2005). Affected patients usually present to the dermatologist because of cosmetic concerns. Physical complaints or symptoms vary depending on the organ system involved. Venous malformations that occur intra or extra-articularly may lead to pain, decrease joint range of motion and occasionally deformity. Soft tissue involvement in or near a muscle bulk may adversely affect the surrounding or adjacent muscle function (Maunoury et al. 1990, Mckinlay et al. 1998).

Patients may present with blindness due to cerebral or cerebellar vascular lesions that may hemorrhage into the occipital lobes.

BRBNS has been also associated with several tumours: medulloblastoma, chronic lymphocytic leukaemia, hypernephroma, and squamous cell carcinoma (Hoffman et al. 1978, Lichtig et al. 1971, Rice and Fischer 1996).

Extensive venous malformations, mainly if located in the trunk or a limb, was associated with a lifelong, low-grade localized intravascular coagulopathy, characterized by low fibrinogen and high D-dimer levels. This could evolve to disseminated intravascular coagulopathy following trauma, surgery, or sclerotherapy (Hofhuis et al. 1990, Lichtig et al. 1971).

## Pathology

Histologically, the skin lesions consist of large, irregularly dilated, mature endothelial-lined channels with insufficient (or too thin) layer of connective tissue and surrounding smooth muscle. This abnormal mural structure allows the lesions to expand slowly over time. The first type of histopathology change has been observed in the superficial dermis, whereas in the deep dermis or in subcutaneous lesions, the second an third type of pathologic are generally described (Fine et al. 1961, Fretzin and Potter 1965, Rice and Fischer 1996, Walshe et al. 1966).

Little information is available about the brain pathology of BRBNS, but the brain lesions grossly and histologically resemble those of the skin (Waybright et al. 1978).

## Pathogenesis and molecular genetics

Although BRBNS usually occur sporadically, Berlyne and Berlyne (1960) demonstrated transmission through 5 generations; Walshe et al. (1966) reported on two families with affected persons in 3 and 5 successive generations; Munkvad (1983) reported a family with 7 affected persons (without visceral involvement) in 3 generations, including father-to-son transmission. Other families with autosomal dominant transmission have been reported by Moodley and Ramdial (1993) as well as families with only male to male transmission (Talbot and Wyatt 1970).

Knoell et al. (1998) described familial multiple blue nevi, histologically shown to be of the Jofassohn-Tieche type, occurring in a dominant inheritance pattern over 4 generations, without associated abnormalities (OMIM # 603670) (OMIM 2006). Additional families with several bluen nevi of the cellular type have been described by Blackford and Roberts (1991). Either families however appear to be distinct from the BRBNS (OMIM 2006).

Gallione et al. (1995) first postulated that BRBNS might be likely a variety of the so-called *"venous malformation multiple cutaneous and mucosal"* (VMCM), a phenotype first reported by Boon et al. (1994) in 15 members of 3 generations who had small cutaneous venous malformations associated to "slow-flow" venous malformations of soft tissues and bleeding of the gastrointestinal tract (OMIM # 600195) (OMIM 2006). The lesions in VMCM may present at birth but usually appear by puberty. Notably, histopathology examination of the affected blood vessels in this phenotype shows the same features as in BRBNS. Genetic linkage studies have implicated a region on chromosome 9p21 in two unrelated VMCM families (Boon et al. 1994, Gallione et al. 1995, Vikkula et al. 1996). The disease gene was subsequently identified as the receptor tyrosine kinase/TEK (TIE2) (Calvert et al. 1999, Gallione et al. 1995), a controller of endothelial cell assembling and remodelling which organises the vascular network hierarchically into large and small vessels and recruits perivascular cells that are necessary to stabilise vessel structures (Tille and Pepper 2004). It is important to note that some VMCM families do not show linkage to the TIE2 locus (Calvert et al. 1999) suggesting the existence of additional loci for inherited venous malformations (Tille and Pepper 2004). As we expressed earlier, the majority of true BRBNS are sporadic and do not carry the TIE2 mutation like in VMCM. Many reports in the literature of familial BRBNS are actually cases of glomangiomas and there is a potential for confusion because of the clinical similarities between both disorders (Lu et al. 2005). Autosomal dominant inheritance has also been reported in both diseases, although familial cases of multiple glomangiomas occur more frequently. For this reason, it is very important to perform a biopsy of all cutaneous lesions.

## Diagnosis

Diagnosis of BRBNS is initially based on clinical-cutaneous findings of the characteristic skin lesions, and confirm by imaging studies and endoscopic finding of the gastrointestinal lesions (Arguedas and Wilcox 1999, Baker et al. 1971, De Bona et al. 2005, Fish et al. 2004, Gallo and McClave 1992, Radke et al. 1993, Rosenblum et al. 1978).

Anaemia due to gastrointestinal bleeding is frequent and it is important to consider this syndrome in cases of unexplained anaemia to search for the characteristic skin lesions (Baker et al. 1971, Bean 1958, Berlyne and Berlyne 1960, Fretzin and Potter 1965).

Consumption coagulopathy associated with thrombosis is a different type of clinical presentation (Gonzalez et al. 2001, Hofhuis et al. 1990)

Careful examination of the patient, searching for other sites of involvement is helpful in supporting the diagnosis. Computed tomography (CT) and magnetic resonance imaging (MRI) also may be useful, non invasive methods, in evaluating internal lesions in these patients (Garen and Sahn 1994, Gascoyen 1860, Satya-Murti et al. 1986, Shannon and Auld 2005, Starr et al. 2005, Waybright et al. 1978).

For the gastrointestinal compromise, diagnosis can be established by upper endoscopies and colonoscopies if lesions involved oesophagus, stomach, duodenum and colon. For lesions in the small bowel several investigations can be employed: capsule endoscopies, intraoperative enteroscopy and push-enteroscopy (Fig. 4). Capsule endoscopy has recently been proposed as a new non-invasive endoscopic procedure for evaluating the small bowel (Arguedas and Wilcox 1999, Badran et al. 2007, De Bona et al. 2005, Fish et al. 2004, Kopacova et al. 2007, Maunoury et al. 1990, Radke et al. 1993).

For another unusual type of presentations such as acute abdominal pain due to intussusception, cortical blindness, spinal cord compression, other CNS symptoms, as well as, suffocation due to airway compromise, the syndrome should be suspected if the characteristic skin lesions are present or if there is an antecedent of gastrointestinal bleeding (Beluffi et al. 2004, Browne et al. 1983, Carvalho et al. 2003, Garen and Sahn 1994, Gascoyen 1860, Rice and Fischer 1996, Rosenblum et al. 1978, Shannon and Auld 2005, Starr et al. 2005, Waybright et al. 1978).

## Differential diagnosis

BRBN must be differentiate from hereditary hemorrhagic telangiectasia (Rendu Osler Weber Syndrome), where the skin lesions are red and pinpoint with noticeable telangiectasia (Moodley and Ramdial 1993).

Multiple glomangiomas have been confused with the lesions of BRBN, they never have gastrointestinal involvement (Lu et al. 2005).

Maffuci syndrome has widespread vascular low flow cutaneous and visceral involvement but its lesions are distinguishable by the bony abnormalities resulting from dyschondroplasia and defective ossification (Shepherd et al. 2005).

The dermal nodule of BRBN should be distinguished from a distinct type of vascular malformation named "venous nevus" or "nevus venous" (Zeitz et al. 2008) which consists in an extratruncal venous malformation of the skin or the neighbouring mucosa arranged in segmental patterns.

## Treatment

The most important clinical problem for these patients is the management of acute or chronic bleeding from the multiple gastrointestinal venous malformations. A conservative approach should be instituted whenever the clinical features and the bleeding episodes are mild. Another point in the surveillance and follow-up of BRBNS patients is iron deficiency anaemia due to acute of chronic gastrointestinal bleeding as was seen in almost all of the patients. Continuous oral iron are usually adequate to the management of most of the cases. Resection of the affected intestinal segment is recommended when there is significant bleeding and the lesions are confined to one segment of the gastrointestinal tract. Gastrointestinal lesions can be also treated by sclerosing agents (Baker et al. 1971, Berlyne and Berlyne 1960, Fishman et al. 2005, McKinlay et al. 1998, Moodley and Ramdial 1993, Munkvad 1983, Nahm et al. 2004, Paules et al. 1993).

Cutaneous lesions are seldom treated unless they are cosmetically or functionally troublesome. Recurrences or hypertrophic scars often result from surgical excision (Paules et al. 1993). Treatment of the skin lesions with $CO_2$ laser, whereas combined with oral steroids or not has been reported (Dieckermann et al. 1994, Fine et al. 1961).

A variety of therapeutic agents have been used for the management of GI bleeding in BRBNS including antiangiogenic agents such as corticosteroids and interferon alpha and endoscopic approaches (Boente et al. 1999, De Bona et al. 2005, Maunoury et al. 1990, Shahed et al. 1990).

Thrombocytopenia and chronic consumption coagulopathy have also seen described in this syndrome. Transfusions may occasionally be required (Hofhuis et al. 1990).

Octreotide a somatostatin analogue has been used to treat acute and chronic upper GI bleeding in adults and children (Bowers et al. 2000, Zellos and Schwarz 2000). Its role in long term treatment o chronic GI bleeding is unclear but is safe and affective for the management of chronic GI blood loss as a result of a variety of causes (Gonzalez et al. 2001, Siafakas et al. 1998, Zellos and Schwarz 2000).

The management of the GI lesions depends on the extent of involvement and the severity of GI bleeding. If the bleeding is significant and the vascular lesions are confined to a segment of gastrointestinal tract, resection of the involved segment of gut is indicated (Fishman et al. 2005).

## References

Andersen JM (2004) Blue rubber bleb nevus syndrome. In: Roach SE, Miller VS (eds.) Neurocutaneous Disorders. New York: Cambridge University Press, pp. 154–158.

Arguedas MR, Wilcox CM (1999) Blue rubber bleb nevus syndrome. Gastrointest Endosc 50: 544.

Badran AM, Vahedi K, Berrebi D, Catana D, De Lagausie P, Drouet L, Ferkadji F, Mougenot JF (2007) Pediatric ampullar and small bowel blue rubber bleb nevus syndrome diagnosed by wireless capsule endoscopy. J Pediatr Gastroenterol Nutr 44: 283–286.

Baker AL, Kahn PC, Binder SC, Patterson JF (1971) Gastrointestinal bleeding due to blue rubber bleb nevus syndrome. A case diagnosed by angiography. Gastroenterology 61: 530–534.

Bean WB (1958) Blue rubber-bleb nevi of skin and gastrointestinal tract. In: Bean WB (ed.) Vascular Spiders and Related Lesions of the skin. Springfield, IL: Charles Thomas Publishers, pp. 178–185.

Beluffi G, Romano P, Matteotti C, Minniti S, Ceffa F, Morbini P (2004) Jejunal intussusception in a 10-year-old boy with blue rubber bleb nevus syndrome. Pediatr Radiol 34: 742–745.

Berlyne GM, Berlyne N (1960) Anaemia due to blue rubber bleb nevus disease. Lancet 2: 1275–1277.

Blackford S, Roberts DL (1991) Familial multiple blue nevi. Clin Exp Dermatol 16: 308–309.

Boente MD, Cordisco MR, Frontini MD, Asial RA (1999) Blue rubber bleb nevus (Bean syndrome): evolution of four cases and clinical response to pharmacologic agents. Pediatr Dermatol 16: 222–227.

Boon LM, Mulliken JB, Vikkula M, Watkins H, Seidman J, Olsen BR, Warman ML (1994) Assignment of a locus for dominantly inherited venous malformations to chromosome 9p. Hum Mol Genet 3: 1583–1587.

Bowers M, McNulty O, Mayne E (2001) Octreotide in the treatment of gastrointestinal bleeding caused by angiodysplasia in two patients with von Willebrand's disease. Br J Haematol 108: 524–527.

Browne AF, Katz S, Miser J, Boles ET Jr (1983) Blue rubber bleb nevi as a cause of intussusception. J Pediatr Surg 18: 7–9.

Calvert JT, Riney TJ, Kontos CD, Cha EH, Prieto VG, Shea CR, Berg JN, Nevin NC, Simpson SA, Pasyk KA, Speer MC, Peters KG, Marchuk DA (1999) Allelic and locus heterogeneity in inherited venous malformations. Hum Mol Genet 7: 1279–1289.

Carvalho S, Barbosa V, Santos N, Machado E (2003) Blue rubber-bleb nevus syndrome: report of a familial case with a dural arteriovenous fistula. Am J Neuroradiol 24: 1916–1918.

Cherpelis BS, Fenske NA (2006) Blue rubber bleb nevus syndrome. E-medicine: http://www.emdeicine.com/derm/topic56.htm

De Bona M, Bellumat A, De Boni M (2005) Capsule endoscopy for the diagnosis and follow-up of blue rubber bleb nevus syndrome. Dig Liver Dis 37: 451–453.

Deng ZH, Xu CD, Chen SN (2008) Diagnosis and treatment of blue rubber bleb nevus syndrome in children. World J Pediatr 4: 70–73.

Dieckmann K, Maurage C, Faure N, Margulies A, Lorette G, Rudler J, Rolland JC (1994) Combined laser-steroid therapy in blue rubber bleb nevus syndrome: case report and review of the literature. Eur J Pediatr Surg 4: 372–374.

Edelstein S, Naidich TP, Newton TH (2005) The rare phakomatoses. In: Tortori-Donati P (ed.) Pediatric Neuroradiology. Brain. Berlin: Springer, pp. 819–854.

Enjolras O, Mulliken JB (1997) Vascular tumors and vascular malformations (new issues). Adv Dermatol 13: 375–423.

Fine ERM, Derbes VJ, Clatk WH Jr (1961) Blue rubber bleb nevus. Arch Dermatol 84: 802–805.

Fish L, Fireman Z, Kopelman Y, Sternberg A (2004) Blue rubber bleb nevus syndrome: small-bowel lesions diagnosed by capsule endoscopy. Endoscopy 36: 836.

Fishman SJ, Smithers CJ, Folkman J, Lund DP, Burrows PE, Mulliken JB, Fox VL (2005) Blue rubber bleb nevus syndrome: surgical eradication of gastrointestinal bleeding. Ann Surg 241: 523–528.

Fretzin DF, Potter B (1965) Blue rubber bleb nevus. Arch Intern Med 116: 924–929.

Gabikian P, Clatterbuck RE, Gailloud P, Rigamonti D (2003) Developmental venous anomalies and sinus pericranii in the blue rubber-bleb nevus syndrome. Case report. J Neurosurg 99: 409–411.

Gallione CJ, Pasyk KA, Boon LM, Lennon F, Johnson DW, Helmbold EA, Markel DS, Vikkula M, Mulliken JB, Warman ML, Perikac-Vance MA, Marchuk DA (1995) A gene for familial venous malformations maps to chromosome 9p in a second large kindred. J Med Genet 32: 197–199.

Gallo SH, McClave SA (1992) Blue rubber bleb nevus syndrome: gastrointestinal involvement and its endoscopic presentation. Gastrointest Endosc 38: 72–76.

Garen PD, Sahn EE (1994) Spinal cord compression in blue rubber bleb nevus syndrome. Arch Dermatol 130: 934–935.

Gascoyen M (1860) Case of naevus involving the parotid gland, and causing death from suffocation: naevi of the viscera. Trans Pathol Soc Lond 11: 267.

Gil-Nunez AC, Mateo D, Lazaro P, Gimenez-Roldan S (1983) Multiple calcified hemangiomas of the brain and the blue rubber bleb nevus syndrome. Arch Neurobiol (Madr) 46: 167–176.

Gonzalez D, Elizondo BJ, Haslag S, Buchanan G, Burdick JS, Guzzetta PC, Hicks BA, Andersen JM (2001) Chronic subcutaneous octreotide decreases gastrointestinal blood loss in blue rubber-bleb nevus syndrome. J Pediatr Gastroenterol Nutr 33: 183–188.

Hashimoto Y, Eto K, Uyama E, Uchino M, Araki S (1989) Blue rubber bleb nevus syndrome presented vascular dementia and chronic DIC: a case report. Rinsho Shinkeigaku 29: 202–208.

History of Medicine (2006) Website of the United States National Library of Medicine, National Institutes of health: http://www.nlm.nih.gov/hmd/manuscripts/ead/bean.html

Hoffman T, Chasko S, Safai B (1978) Association of blue rubber bleb nevus syndrome with chronic lymphocytic leukemia and hypernephroma. Johns Hopkins Med J 142: 91–94.

Hofhuis WJ, Oranje AP, Bouquet J, Sinaasappel M (1990) Blue rubber-bleb naevus syndrome: report of a case with consumption coagulopathy complicated by manifest thrombosis. Eur J Pediatr 149: 526–528.

Jaffe RH (1929) Multiple hemangiomas of the skin and of the internal organs. Arch Pathol 7: 44–54.

Kim SJ (2000) Blue rubber bleb nevus syndrome with central nervous system involvement. Pediatr Neurol 22: 410–412.

Kopacova M, Tacheci I, Koudelka J, Kralova M, Rejchrt S, Bures J (2007) A new approach to blue rubber bleb nevus syndrome: the role of capsule endoscopy and intraoperative enteroscopy. Pediatr Surg Int Jan 5 [Epub ahead of print].

Korpelainen EI, Karkainnen M, Gunji J, Vikkula M, Alitalo K (1999) Endothelial receptor tyrosine kinase activate the STAt signalling pathway: mutant Tie-2 causing venous malformations signals a distinct STAT activations. Oncogene 18: 1–8.

Kunishige M, Azuma H, Masuda K et al. (1997) Interferon alfa-2 for disseminated intravascular coagulation in a patient with blue rubber bleb nevus syndrome: a case report. Angiology 48: 273–277.

Lee C, Debnath D, Whitburn T, Farrugia M, Gonzalez F (2008) Synchronous multiple small bowel intussusceptions in an adult with blue rubber bleb naevus syndrome: report of a case and review of literature. World J Emerg Surg 3: 3.

Lichtig C, Alroy G, Gellei B, Valero A (1971) Multiple skin and gastro-intestinal haemangiomata blue rubber-bleb nevus. Report of case with thrombocytopenia, hypercalcemia and coinciding cystic cell carcinoma. Dermatologica 142: 356–362.

Lu R, Krathen RA, Sanchez RL, May NC, Hsu S (2005) Multiple glomangiomas: potential for confusion with blue rubber bleb nevus syndrome. J Am Acad Dermatol 52: 731–732.

Malhotra P, Menon MC, Anand SS, Narula A, Varma S (2008) Haemopericardium in blue rubber bleb naevus syndrome (Bean syndrome). Med J Aust 188: 416.

Maunoury V, Turck D, Brunetaud JM, Marti R, Cortot A, Farriaux JP, Paris JC (1990) Blue rubber bleb nevus syndrome. 3 Cases treated with a Nd:YAG laser and bipolar electrocoagulation. Gastroenterol Clin Biol 14: 593–595.

McCarthy JC, Goldberg MJ, Zimbler S (1982) Orthopaedic dysfunction in the blue rubber-bleb nevus syndrome. J Bone Joint Surg Am 64: 280–283.

McIntosh N, Harris J (1970) Multiple gastrointestinal haemangiomata. Br Med J 4: 600.

McKinlay JR, Kaiser J, Barrett TL, Graham B (1998) Blue rubber bleb nevus syndrome. Cutis 62: 97–98.

Mejía-Rodríguez S, Valencia-Herrera A, Escobar-Sánchez A, Mena-Cedillos C (2008) Dermoscopic features in Bean (blue rubber bleb nevus) syndrome. Pediatr Dermatol 25: 270–272.

Moodley M, Ramdial P (1993) Blue rubber bleb nevus syndrome: case report and review of the literature. Pediatrics 92: 160–162.

Mulliken JB, Glowacki J (1982) Hemangiomas and vascular malformations in infants and children: a classification based on endothelial characteristics. Plast Reconstr Surg 69: 412–422.

Munkvad M (1983) Blue rubber bleb nevus syndrome. Dermatologica 167: 307–309.

Nahm WK, Moise S, Eichenfield LF, Paller AS, Nathanson L, Malicki DM, Friedlander SF (2004) Venous malformations in blue rubber bleb nevus syndrome: variable onset of presentation. J Am Acad Dermatol 50: S101–S106.

Park J, Chung KY (2006) Blue rubber bleb nevus syndrome with central nervous system involvement. J Dermatol 33: 649–651.

Paules S, Baack B, Levisohn D (1993) Tender bluish papules on the trunk and extremities. Blue rubber-bleb nevus syndrome. Arch Dermatol 129: 1505–1506, 1508–1509.

Radke M, Waldschmidt J, Stolpe HJ, Mix M, Richter I (1993) Blue rubber-bleb-nevus syndrome with predominant urinary bladder hemangiomatosis. Eur J Pediatr Surg 3: 313–316.

Rice JS, Fischer DS (1996) Blue rubber-bleb nevus syndrome. Generalized cavernous hemangiomatosis or venous hamartoma with medulloblastoma of the cerebellum: case report and review of the literature. Arch Dermatol 186: 503–511.

Romao Z, Pontes J, Lopes H, Vasconcelos H, Portela F, Andrade P, Leitao MC, Donato A, Freitas D (1999) Endosonography in the diagnosis of "blue rubber bleb nevus syndrome": an uncommon cause of gastrointestinal tract bleeding. J Clin Gastroenterol 28: 262–265.

Rosenblum W, Nakoneczna I, Konerding H, Nochlin D, Ghatak N (1978) Multiple vascular malformations in the blue rubber bleb nevus syndrome: a case with aneurysm of veni of Galen and vascular lesions suggesting a link to the Weber-Osler-Rendu syndrome Histopathology 2: 301–311.

Sandhu KS, Cohen H, Radin R, Buck FS (1987) Blue rubber bleb nevus syndrome presenting with recurrences. Dig Dis Sci 32: 214–219.

Satya-Murti S, Navada S, Eames F (1986) Central nervous system involvement in blue-rubber-bleb-nevus syndrome. Arch Neurol 43: 1184–1186.

Shahed M, Hagenmuller F, Rosch T, Classen M, Encke A, Siewert JR, Ysawy MI, al Karawi M (1990) A 19-year-old female with blue rubber bleb nevus syndrome. Endoscopic laser photocoagulation and surgical resection of gastrointestinal angiomata. Endoscopy 22: 54–56.

Shannon J, Auld J (2005) Blue rubber bleb naevus syndrome associated with cortical blindness. Ausralas J Dermatol 46: 192–195.

Shepherd V, Godbolt A, Casey A (2005) Maffuci's syndrome with extensive gastrointestinal involvement. Australas J Dermatol 46: 33–37.

Sherry RG, Walker ML, Meredith VO (1984) Sinus pericranii and venous angioma in blue rubber bleb nevus syndrome. AJNR 5: 832–834.

Siafakas C, Fox VL, Nurko S (1998) Use of octreotide for the treatment of severe gastrointestinal bleeding in children. J Pediatr Gastroenterol Nutr 26: 356–359.

Starr BM, Katzenmeyer WK, Guinto F, Pou AM (2005) The blue rubber bleb nevus syndrome: a case with prominent head and neck findings. Am J Otolaryngol 26: 282–284.

Talbot S, Wyatt EH (1970) Blue rubber bleb naevi: report of a family in which only males were affected. Br J Dermatol 82: 37–39.

Tanaka N, Tsuda M, Samura O, Miyoshi H, Hara T, Kudo Y (2007) Blue rubber bleb nevus syndrome: report of a patient with hemangiomas of the vaginal portion of the cervix appearing during pregnancy. J Obstet Gynaecol Res 33: 546–548.

Tille JC, Pepper MS (2004) Hereditary vascular anomalies. New insights into their pathogenesis. Arterioscl Vasc Biol 24: 1578–1590.

Tzoufi MS, Sixlimiri P, Nakou I, Argyropoulou MI, Stefanidis CJ, Siamopoulou-Mavridou A (2007) Blue rubber bleb nevus syndrome with simultaneous neurological and skeletal involvement. Eur J Pediatr Oct 13 [Epub ahead of print].

Vikkula M, Boon LM, Carraway KL 3rd, Calvert JT, Diamonti AJ, Goumnerov B, Pasyk KA, Marchuk DA, Warman ML, Cantley LC, Mulliken JB, Olsen BR (1996) Vascular dysmorphogenesis caused by an activating mutation in the receptor tyrosine kinase TIE2. Cell 87: 1181–1190.

Vikkula M, Boon LM, Mulliken JB (2001) Molecular genetics of vascular malformations. Matrix Biol 20: 327–335.

Walshe MM, Evans CD, Warin RP (1966) Blue rubber bleb naevus. Br Med J 15: 931–932.

Waybright EA, Selhorst JB, Rosenblum WI, Suter CG (1978) Blue rubber bleb nevus syndrome with CNS involvement and thrombosis of a vein of galen malformation. Ann Neurol 3: 464–467.

Who Named it? 2006 An online catalogue of persons who named syndromes: http://www.whonamedit.com

Wong YC, Li YW, Chang MH (1994) Gastrointestinal bleeding and paraparesis in blue rubber bleb nevus syndrome. Pediatr Radiol 22: 600–601.

Wood MW, With RJ, Kermohan JW (1957) Cavernous hemangiomatosis involving the brain, spinal cord and kidney. Proc Mayo Clin 32: 249–254.

Zellos A, Schwarz KB (2000) Efficacy of octreotide in children with chronic gastrointestinal bleeding. J Pediatr Gastroenterol Nutr 30: 442–446.

Zietz S, Happle R, Hohenleutner U, Landthaler M (2008) The venous nevus: a distinct vascular malformation suggesting mosaicism. Dermatology 216: 31–36.

# Chapter 14

# WYBURN-MASON SYNDROME

Martino Ruggieri, Orhan Konez, and Concezio Di Rocco

Institute of Neurological Science, National Research Council, Catania, and Department of Paediatrics, University of Catania, Catania, Italy (MR); Department of Radiology, Vascular and Interventional Radiology, St. John West Shore Hospital, University Hospitals Case Medical Center, Westlake, OHIO, USA (OK); Section of Paediatric Neurosurgery, Department of Paediatrics, Catholic University of Sacred Heart, Rome, Italy (CDR)

## Introduction

Wyburn-Mason's syndrome is a rare neurocutaneous disorder characterised mainly by: (1) usually unilateral arteriovenous malformations of the (mid)brain; (2) vascular abnormalities of the retina, optic nerve, orbit, optic chiasm and tract; and (3) multiple cutaneous nevi consisting either of faint reddish-bluish discoloration or dilated enlarged superficial veins involving the trigeminal region (Younge 1987).

## Historical perspective and terminology

*Magnus* (1874) first described the retinal component of the malformation in 1874: however, that was regarded for many years as an ophthalmologic curiosity. A few patients with this retinal lesion developed signs suggesting more extensive vascular involvement of the head, and in 1930 *Yates* and *Paine* reported an extensive vascular malformation in the ipsilateral cerebral hemisphere, mid-brain, choroid plexus, sylvian veins and retina of a patient who died from an intracerebral haemorrhage.

The clinical association of retinal and cerebral arteriovenous malformation however was first reported in the French literature by the French ophthalmologist **Paul Bonnet** (1894–1959) along with the French neurosurgeons **Jean Dechaume** (1896–1968) and **Eugene Blanc** (1888–1961) (Bonnet et al. 1937). In the European literature this condition is still known as the *Bonnet-Dechaume-Blanc syndrome* (Younge 1987).

Northfield (1941) early in the era of angiography demonstrated the first retinocephalic arteriovenous malformation by this technique. However it was **Wyburn-Mason**, a British neurologist working at the National Hospital of Queen Square in London, who in 1943 described the association of retinal and intracranial vascular malformations in detail (Younge 1987). He reviewed the world literature on retinal arteriovenous malformations up untill 1943 and showed that of 27 cases, signs of intracranial arteriovenous malformations were present in 22 (Wyburn-Mason 1943). He surveyed 20 cases of midbrain arteriovenous malformations and found 14 instances of associated retinal arteriovenous malformations helping to initially categorise this condition which he regarded as a syndrome (Bidwell 2006, Brown et al. 1973, Rizzo et al. 2004). He described the "curious association of lesions, consisting of arteriovenous aneurysm of one or both sides of the mid-brain, arteriovenous aneurysm or some similar congenital vascular abnormality of the retina on the corresponding side and cutaneous naevi with physical changes" and stressed the fact that "sometimes the mid-brain or retinal lesions occurs alone, so that examples of arteriovenous aneurysms of the retina have been recorded without other abnormalities, but none of these cases have been followed for any length of time" (Wyburn-Mason 1943). Most of the reviewed cases however were not documented by contrast studies, operation, or autopsy and the diagnosis was made in the majority by clinical examination alone (Brown et al. 1973).

Shira and Guernsey (1965) first reported the extracranial vascular lesions and Archer et al. (1973) revealed by means of fluorescein the basic nature of the retinal lesion: one or more abnormal communications between arteries and veins, with a wide clinical spectrum. This has led to various descriptive names, but the primary defect is an arteriovenous communication (Younge 1987).

The entity is known also as mesencephalon-oculo-facial angiomatosis.

## Incidence and prevalence

Wyburn-Mason's syndrome is considered one of the rarest neurocutaneous syndromes (Taybi and Lachman, 1996, Younge 1897) with no calculated frequencies so far (Bidwell 2006) and no predilections of age and gender (Bidwell 2006, Edelstein et al. 2005). Approximately, 90 cases have been described so far in the literature.

## Clinical manifestations

Wyburn-Mason usually presents in childhood, occasionally at birth. Specific symptoms and signs vary with location and size of the arteriovenous malformation (Edelstein et al. 2005). Larger arteriovenous malformations causing visual or neurological impairment generally are diagnosed earlier in life, whereas smaller lesions may not be diagnosed until later in life (Bidwell 2006). Archer et al. (1973) subdivided the arteriovenous anastomoses of Wyburn-Mason's syndrome into three groups (Bidwell 2006, Edelstein et al. 2005, Younge 1987):

(1) *Group 1* is characterised by a (less severe type of) interposing arteriolar capillary bed between arteries and veins (small arteriole-venule anastomoses), which is usually localised to one sector or quadrant of the retina (often involving the macula) and may be subtle and difficult to detect clinically. It was their impression that these vascular retinal lesions were stable and not associated with cerebral anomalies;

(2) *Group 2* represents direct arteriovenous communications without intervening capillary or arteriolar elements. This group may represent an exaggerated form of the abnormalities included in group 1, and is likewise geographically seg-

mented within the fundus. There is the tendency to higher flow rates and pressures, and some decompensation of the involved vessel walls and surrounding tissues. Shunting of highly oxygenated blood past poorly perfused capillary beds may be evident. Haemorrhages, leakage of fluid with oedema, and exudates may cause decreased vision in some of these cases. With a few exceptions these, too, seem unassociated with cerebral lesions;

(3) *Group 3* includes malformations with more severe retinal involvement and a higher likelihood of intracranial and other site involvement. In these, the retinal vessels are very large communications; they are of large caliber and are interwined, convoluted, and highly arterialised in blood content. The abnormalities are extended throughout the entire fundus and there is a considerable retinal degeneration and generally poor vision. Varying amounts of exudation and pigmentary migration occur, and there are often ghost vessels and sheathed vessels in parts of the retina. This is the group that corresponds more closely to those reviewed by Wyburn-Mason in his original paper of 1943 (Wyburn-Mason 1943).

The expanded spectrum of Wyburn-Mason syndrome now includes variants with orbital arteriovenous malformations that spare the retina, bilateral orbital or retrolental arteriovenous malformations, and arteriovenous malformation of the cerebral hemisphere, basal ganglia, thalamus, optic nerves/chiasm, mandible and maxilla. At present, thus, unilateral and/or retinal arteriovenous malformation is not required for diagnosis.

## Skin abnormalities

Dermatological signs are subtle and detectable in less than 50% of cases. The facial naevi are generally present from birth and vary from faint reddish-bluish discoloration containing scattered punctate red spots to dilated enlarged superficial veins involving the trigeminal region (Fig. 1) or extensive angiomatous naevi. They are usually unilateral, infrequently bilateral. Cutaneous vascular nevus, port-

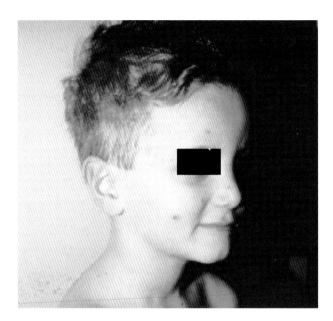

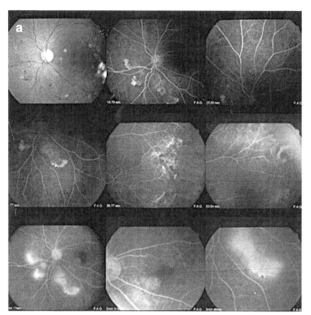

**Fig. 1.** Dilated enlarged superficial veins involving the trigeminal region of the right face in a child with Wyburn-Mason syndrome.

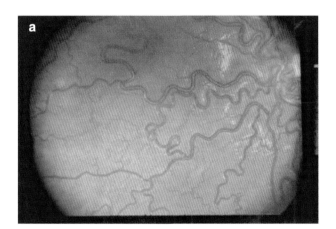

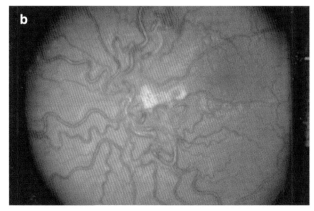

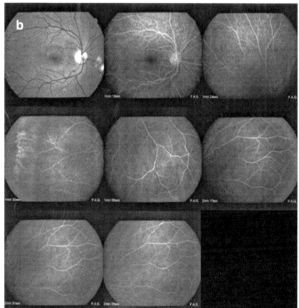

**Fig. 3.** Fluorescein angiographic examination of the eyes in a child with Wyburn-Mason's syndrome: the right eye (**a**) shows tortuos and dilated retinal vessels in a cirsoid pattern with spot haemorrhages (white dots); the left eye (**b**) shows only minimal spot haemorrhages (courtesy of Professor S. Li Volti, Department of Pediatrics, University of Catania, Italy).

**Fig. 2.** (**a**) and (**b**) Fundi examination showing mixed angiomatous/large masses of tortuous and dilated vessels covering almost the entire retina in a cirsoid/aneurismal pattern ("bag of worms") in a patient with Wyburn-Mason syndrome.

wine nevus, or dilated veins involving the eyelids have also been reported.

## Eye abnormalities

Ocular manifestations involving both the retina and orbits are diagnostic for the disease. An important sign is the presence of a vascular malformation in the bulbar conjunctiva as this can be easily detected at examination. The retinal lesions are usually unilateral and range from visible vascular malformations of the angiomatous type to large masses of tortuous and dilated vessels covering a substantial portion of the retina, a so-called (cirsoid) aneurismal pattern or "bag of worms" (Figs. 2 and 3) (Bidwell 2006). Normal acuity and normal disk do not exclude the presence of a malformation. In the original series of Wyburn-

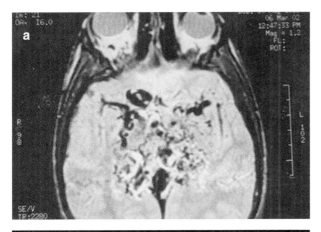

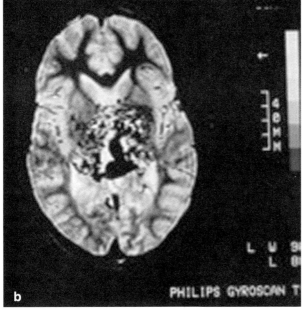

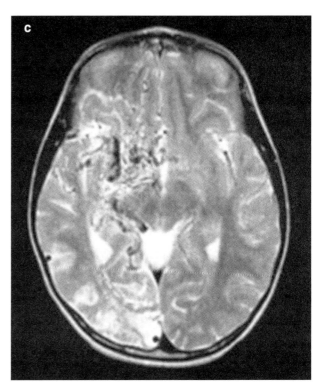

**Fig. 4.** Axial T1-weighted (**a–b**) and T2-weighted (**c**) magnetic resonance images of the brain showing typical vascular malformations: deeply located in the midbrain and brainstem (**a**) in a woman who had acute headache as presenting symptom at age 22 years; (**b**) deeply located in the entire thalami and basal ganglia regions in a 44-year-old woman who had hemiparesis at onset; (**c**) located in the entire right hemisphere with high signal areas in the posterior regions in a 6-year-old child (same child shown in Fig. 1) who had headache and later progressive cognitive deterioration (Figs. a and b are courtesy of Professor G. Pero, Institute of Neuroradiology, University of Catania, Italy).

Mason, six patients had normal fundi; visual impairment was reported in 50% of them (Wyburn-Mason 1943). Orbital manifestations include optic atrophy, involvement of the retrobulbar soft tissue by vascular malformations, or varying amounts of gliosis leading to mild, non-pulsating exophthalmos. The eye vascular malformations usually remain stable and generally do not demonstrate leakage on fluorescein angiography (Fig. 3) (Bidwell 2006). Rare associated ocular complications have been reported which include macular hole, central retinal vein occlusion, neovascular glaucoma, macroaneurysmal abnormalities, retinal haemorrhage and vitreous haemorrhage.

## Nervous system abnormalities

The vascular malformation of the central nervous system are deeply located (Figs. 4–6) and frequently related to the optic pathways, extending sometimes to the occipital lobe. Extension into the vermis is not frequent. Other sites of involvement are the hypothalamus, thalamus, basal ganglia, midbrain, temporo-occipital and fronto-temporo-parieto-occipital

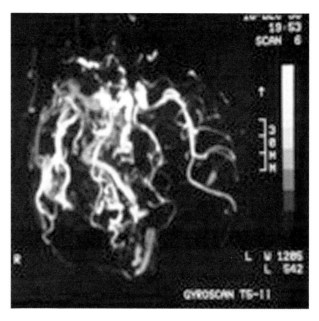

Fig. 6. Axial magnetic resonance angoiography showing the right arteriovenous malformation seen in Fig. 4c.

(Luo et al. 2006). The malformation is supplied either by the vertebral or the carotid system or both.

Arteriovenous malformations are dynamic structures that change over time. Substantial remodelling of an arteriovenous malformation has been observed in the retina and is evident on pathological analysis of intracranial lesions. Within the same lesion one can find atrophy of some vessels and dilatation of other vessels. These changes are most likely directed by vascular dynamic forces caused by spontaneous thrombosis and might account for the progression of neurological signs.

Clinically, the intracranial vascular malformation causes central nervous system signs in more than 80% of patients. The onset is generally sudden during puberty and adolescence. Affected individuals may present with acute headache, hemiplegia, and homonymous hemianopsia in 50% of cases. Seizures, cerebellar dysfunction, acute psychiatric signs, hallucinations and temporal/spatial disorientation are reported more rarely. Mental impairment is rarely present at onset but it becomes evident later in about 30% of cases. Arteriovenous shunting and steal may cause progressive neurological deficits and optic nerve atrophy.

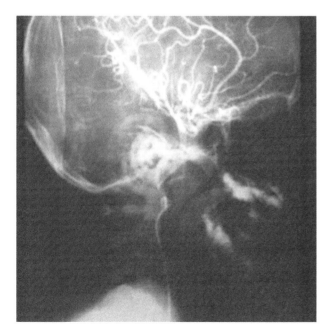

Fig. 5. Brain angiography showing the complex arteriovenous malformation in the left parieto-temporal region of a woman with Wyburn-Mason syndrome (courtesy of Professor G. Pero, Institute of Neuroradiology, University of Catania, Italy).

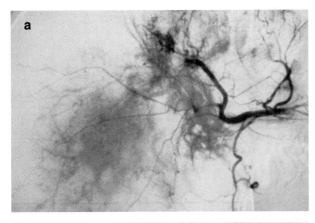

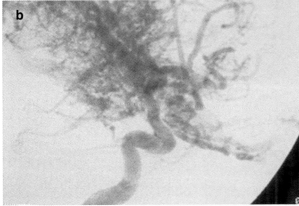

**Fig. 7.** Angiography (vein phase) (**a**) and (**b**) showing the arteriovenous malformation in the carotid and vertebral regions (courtesy of Professor G. Pero, Institute of Neuroradiology, University of Catania, Italy).

## Neuroimaging studies

The imaging findings reflect the primary vascular lesions and secondary complications (Edelstein et al. 2005). Thus, CT, MRI and angiography (Figs. 4–7) reveal arteriovenous malformations within the orbits, retro-orbital region, cerebral hemispheres and brainstem, any associated subarachnoid or intraparenchimal haemorrhage and any optic nerve atrophy that result from direct compression or chronic ischemia (Fig. 4c). The retinal arteriovenous malformation varies from tiny angiographically occult lesions to large, tortuous and dilated vessels covering much of the retina (Edelstein et al. 2005). Arterial supply to the arteriovenous malformations arises from the internal carotid artery more often than from the

vertebrobasilar arteries or the external carotid artery. Venous drainage is primarily via the cavernous sinus or the vein of Galen.

### Extracranial/systemic involvement

The intracranial and retinal vascular malformation in Wyburn-Mason's syndrome can (occasionally) extend to the jaw, nose and mouth and to the thyroid (Brown et al. 1973, Lee et al. 2007, Shira and Guernsey 1965). Severe bleeding from the gingiva and tonsils, following chewing hard foods or during dental extraction is frequently reported and recurrent bouts of nose bleeding has been also described. Lung and spinal involvement has also been recorded (Bidwell 2006).

## Pathology/pathophysiology

Arteriovenous anastomoses are characterised by variable alterations in capillary and arteriolar networks. Small anastomoses may have only minor alterations within the capillary system and can be subtle, whereas large, racemous aneurysms are characterised by direct artery-to-vein communication, without interposing capillary or arteriorial elements (Bidwell 2006). At pathology, most of the vascular malformations in Wyburn-Mason's syndrome are a grossly tangled mass of convoluted vessels that histologically are neither arteries nor veins, with direct continuity from the arterial side to venous side (Brock and Dyke 1932, Krug and Samuel 1932, Younge 1987). The vessel walls are ectatic and have a fibromuscular media of varying thickness with wide fibrohyaline adventitial coats showing hyaline degeneration, haemorrhage, and calcification; and may be of such size to occupy more than the entire thickness of the retina. Nearby tissues are often gliotica and have loss of neurons. This is evident in the retina (Cameron and Greer 1968, Younge 1987), presumably because of the great mechanical distortion and compression of the neurons, although optic atrophy can occur from compression elsewhere on the optic nerve or chiasm, even in the absence of the retinal lesion (Danis and Appen 1984). Thrombosis and organisation may be present to a variable degree.

## Natural history

The natural history of the syndrome is unpredictable, the long-term outcome largely depending on the extensiveness of the lesions (Rizzo et al. 2004, Younge 1987). The arteriovenous malformation could remain asymptomatic throughout the patient's life. In the literature, the presenting symptoms were reported at the mean age of 20 years. The risk of haemorrhage is not higher in children than in adults (Iizuka et al. 1992).

Bilateral involvement of the midbrain and early onset of symptoms are usually regarded as poor prognostic factors. However, a precise correlate between the size of the lesions and the haemorrhage does not exist. It seems that venous drainage is responsible for neurological and haemorrhagic symptoms. In our experience, slow, progressive cognitive impairment was evident in children whilst acute neurological symptoms (e.g., headache, focal neurological deficits) were the typical symptoms/sings at presentation. If the vascular malformation remains untreated, progressive deficits related to congested cerebral veins owing to ischaemic or to limited episodes of bleeding bring additional functional impairment.

## Diagnostic work-up

Imaging studies should include fluorescein angiography (Fig. 3), which may further demonstrate the abnormal retinal vascular communications; most arteriovenous aneurysms are stable nonleaking processes (Bidwell 2006). MRI studies of the brain (Fig. 4) (and the spine) and MR angiography (MRA) (Fig. 6) of the ipsilateral orbit and the brain may be considered. Additionally angiographic evaluation of the affected regions (Fig. 7) could be obtained.

## Pathogenesis and molecular genetics

The anomaly is considered to be the result of a persistent primordial stage of vascular development without separation of arteries from veins in that part of the circulation shared by the optic cup and prosencephalon. The various systems that are affected in the head likely represent the effect on the particular stage of differentiation at the time of the insult (Danis and Appen 1984, Younge 1987). No instance of familial transmission are known and no genetic mechanisms have been invoked so far to explain the syndrome.

## Treatment

The therapeutic strategies in Wyburn-Mason's syndrome are extremely challenging. In most cases, complete eradication of the arteriovenous malformation is not feasible. Partial or targeted surgical resection was undertaken to either decrease the symptoms or eradicate obvious dangerous portions of the lesions (Berenstein and Lasjaunias 1992, Lasjaunias et al. 1995). Endovascular management of arteriovenous malformations seems to be the best form of treatment (Lasjaunias et al. 1995). In a few cases, complementary radiosurgical treatment might follow the partial embolisation with bucrylate (Iizuka et al. 1992). Partial treatment performed with a permanent agent such as bucrylate is an acceptable therapeutic objective when complete eradication of the vascular lesion cannot be obtained due to the elevated risks. Partial removal of the most dangerous portions of the intracranial vascular anomaly might progressively minimise the deleterious affects to the adjacent brain (Lasjaunias et al. 1995).

Because of the stability of the retinal lesions, treatment from an ophthalmologist usually is not necessary beyond routine, periodic ophthalmic examination (Bidwell 2006).

## References

Archer DB, Deutman A, Ernest JT, Krill AE (1973) Arteriovenous communications of the retina. Am J Ophthalmol 66: 163–209.

Berenstein A, Lasjaunias P (1992) Surgical Neuroangography in Endovascular Treatment of Brain Lesions. Vol. 4. Berlin: Springer, pp. 10–20.

Bidwell AE (2006) Wyburn-Mason syndrome. http://www.emedicine.com/oph/topic357.htm

Bonnet BP, Dechauma J, Blanc E (1937) L'aneurisme cirsoide de la retine (Aneurysme racemeux). Ses relations avec l'aneurisme cirsoide de la face et avec l'aneurysme cirsoide du cerveaux. J Med (Lyon) 18: 165–178.

Brock S, Dyke CG (1932) Venous and arteriovenous angiomas of the brain: clinical and roentgenographic study of 8 cases. Bull Neurol Inst NY 2: 247–293.

Brown D, Hilal SK, Tenner SS (1973) Wyburn-Mason syndrome. Report of two cases without retinal involvement. Arch Neurol 28: 67–68.

Cameron ME, Greer CH (1968) Congenital arteriovenous aneurysm of the retina: a post mortem report. Br J Ophthalmol 52: 768–772.

Danis R, Appen RE (1984) Optic atrophy and the Wyburn-Mason syndrome. J Can Neuro Ophthalmol 4: 91–95.

Edelstein S, Naidich TP, Newton TH (2005) The rare phakomatoses. In: Tortori-Donati P (ed.) Pediatric Neuroradiology. Brain. Berlin New York: Springer, pp. 819–854.

Iizuka Y, Rodesch R, Garcia-Monaco R, Alvarez H, Burrows P, Hui F, Lasjaunias P (1992) Multiple cerebral arteriovenous shunts in children: report of 13 cases. Childs Nerv Syst 8: 437–444.

Krug EF, Samuels B (1932) Venous angioma of the retina, optic nerve, chiasm, and brain: a case report with postmortem observations. Arch Ophthalmol 8: 871–879.

Lasjaunias P, Hui F, Zerah M, Garcia-Monaco R, Malherbe V, Rodesch G, Tanaka A, Alvarez H (1995) Cerebral arteriovenous malformations in children. Management of 179 consecutive cases and review of the literature. Childs Nerv Syst 11: 66–79.

Lee AW, Chen CS, Gailloud P, Nyquist P (2007) Wyburn-Mason syndrome associated with thyroid arteriovenous malformation: a first case report. Am J Neuroradiol 28: 1153–1154.

Luo CB, Lasjaunias P, Bhattacharya J (2006) Craniofacial vascular malformations in Wyburn-Mason syndrome. J Chin Med Assoc 69: 575–580.

Magnus H (1874) Aneurisma arteriosovenosum retinale. Virchows Arch Pathol 60: 38–45.

Northfield DWC (1940–41) Angiomatous malformation of the brain. Guy's Hosp Rep 90: 149–170.

Rizzo R, Pavone L, Pero G, Curatolo P (2004) A neurocutaneous disorder with a severe course: Wyburn-Mason's syndrome. J Child Neurol 19: 908–911.

Shira RB, Guernsey LH (1965) Central caveronosu hemangoma of the mandible. J Oral Surg 23: 636–642.

Taybi H, Lachman RS (1996) Wyburn-Mason disease. In: Taybi H, Lachman RS (eds.) Radiology of syndromes, metabolic disorders, and skeletal dysplasia. 4th ed. St. Louis: Mosby, pp. 376–379.

Yates AG, Paine CG (1930) Case of arteriovenous aneurysm within brain. Brain 53: 38–46.

Younge BR (1987) Wyburn-Mason syndrome. In: Gomez (ed.) Neurocutaneous Disorders: a practical approach. Boston: Butterworths: 376–380.

Wyburn-Mason R (1943) Arteriovenous aneurysm of midbrain and retina, facial naevi and mental changes. Brain 66: 165–209.

# Chapter 15

# MAFFUCCI SYNDROME

Leida B. Rozeman, Yvonne M. Schrage, Judith V. M. G. Bovée, and Pancras C. W. Hogendoorn

Department of Pathology, Leiden University Medical Center, Leiden, The Netherlands

## Introduction

Maffucci syndrome is characterized by the presence of multiple enchondromas, referred to as enchondromatosis, combined with multiple haemangiomas and/or lymphangiomas, as described by Maffucci (1881). Both lesions tend to have an unilateral predominance (Albregts and Rapini 1995). Enchondromas are benign cartilaginous neoplasms and occur mainly in the tubular bones of hands and feet. Their presence in long bones can result in shortening and deformation of the limbs (Lewis and Ketcham 1973, Kaplan et al. 1993). Nowadays the World Health Organisation classifies the Maffucci syndrome as a subclass of enchondromatosis and defines it as a developmental disorder characterized by the presence of multiple cartilaginous masses and the presence of cutaneous, soft tissue or visceral haemangiomas (Mertens and Unni 2002).

Apart from Maffucci syndrome, other disorders can also be classified as "enchondromatosis". Of these the most frequent is Ollier disease, which is characterized by the presence of multiple enchondromas only, without accompanying vascular, or other tumours neither developmental abnormalities, aside the skeletal system. Both Maffucci syndrome and Ollier disease are non-hereditary, although some of the other rare subclasses of enchondromatosis, such as spondyloenchondromatosis, are autosomal dominant hereditary (Schorr et al. 1976, Bhargava et al. 2005).

## Historical perspective and terminology

The syndrome was first described by Maffucci (1881) **Angelo Maffucci** was born into a farming family at Calitri near Avellino. After graduating in medicine at Naples in 1872 he spent a few years in country practice. He then returned to Naples, where he commenced his scientific work in the institute of pathological anatomy under Otto von Schrön (1837–1917). At this time he earned his living as a vaccination physician to the city of Naples as well as surgeon at the Ospedale degli Incurabili. In 1882 he became head of general pathology at Messina University. In the following year he was called to the chair of anatomical pathology at Catania and in 1884 assumed the chair of pathological anatomy in Pisa, where he died in 1903. He worked in almost every field of pathological anatomy. He was a diligent researcher and a massive collection of his meticulous notes, which was found in his home after his death, is now in the Institute for the History of Medicine in Rome. He recorded details of classical chick experiments, in which he isolated the bacteria causing avian tuberculosis (B. gallinaceous) and determined that avian tuberculosis had a different aetiology from the bovine and human forms. He also recognised that chick embryos had defence mechanisms that could destroy bacteria. Despite the importance of his contributions, his work attracted little attention outside Italy. As a person he was described as sincere and genial.

In 1881 Maffucci reported the case of a 40-year-old woman died from complications following amputation (Maffucci 1881). The patient had frequent and severe hemorrhage from a vascular tumour for which she was admitted to the hospital. In view of the profuse bleeding, an amputation was performed and the patient died from infection. Maffucci reported a thorough autopsy that described all the main points of the syndrome named after him (Who named it? 2006).

Previously Chuveilheir in 1835 and Hanssen in 1863 reported similar cases. In 1889, possibly unaware of Maffucci's article, Alfred Kast and Fredrich Daniel von Recklinghausen (1833–1910) reported another example of the same disorder (Who named it? 2006). Thereafter the condition was known by a variety of descriptive titles and by the conjoined eponym, "Kast-Maffucci". However, Kast's name was soon abandoned and the syndrome finally received its name "Maffucci syndrome" in a report from Carleton et al. (1942).

## Incidence and prevalence

Maffucci syndrome is an extremely rare, non-hereditary disorder. Males and females are equally affected, and no particular ethnical distribution has been reported. No incidence figure is known. In literature, some 200 cases have been reported (Collins et al. 1992).

The incidence of solitary enchondroma is unknown as well, since most of these tumours cause no symptoms. Solitary conventional chondrosarcoma constitute about 17–24% of all primary bone tumours, which have an incidence of 1:100.000 (Huvos 1991, Mulder et al. 1993, Bertoni et al. 2002).

In children, solitary haemangiomas are common lesions, constituting 7% of all benign tumours (Weiss and Goldblum 2001).

## Clinical manifestations

### Skin abnormalities

In Maffucci syndrome skin abnormalities in the form of haemangiomas are present (Fig. 1 a–c). Haemangiomas are described as a benign overgrowth of normal blood vessels, clinically presenting with a bluish or reddish swollen-up appearance. The neoplastic-, or hamartomatous nature of this lesion is matter of debate: some speculate that there is a difference between congenital and non-congenital lesions, the former being regarded as malformations, whilst the latter are considered true neoplasms.

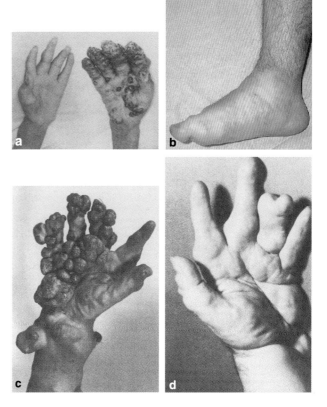

**Fig. 1.** Clinical aspects of the vascular malformations and enchondromatous involvement in the hand (**a**) (From Ma and Leung 1984) and in the foot (**b**) (courtesy of Dr. O. Konez, Cleveland, Ohio, USA); more severe involvement (**c**) (From Tisley and Buren 1985) and distortion from mutiple cartilagineous lesions (**d**) (From Bean 1955).

Haemangiomas occur as superficial skin lesions, often located in the face, but may occur in the internal organs as well (see below) and are clinically divided in two main groups: capillary haemangioma and cavernous haemangioma (Miller and Frieden 2005). In the non-Maffucci-syndrome patients, both groups are more frequently encountered in women and can fluctuate in size in pregnancy and menarche.

The most common form, the *capillary haemangioma*, varies in size from a few millimetres up to several centimetres. The colour of the lesions varies from bright red to blue. Capillary haemangiomas are histologically recognized by narrow, thin-walled capillaries and relatively thin epithelium, separated by connective tissue (Weiss and Goldblum 2001).

The *cavernous subtype* is less common in case of solitary lesions but in patients with Maffucci syndrome, the haemangiomas are mostly of the cavernous type (Fig. 1a–b). These haemangiomas involve deeper structures more often than the capillary subtype and form large, dilated, vascular channels. Histologically, the cavernous subtype is sharply defined though not encapsulated. The cavernous vascular spaces can be partly filled with blood. Intravascular thrombosis with associated dystrophic calcification is common. Those so-called phleboliths can be found in the soft tissue at X-ray screening of patients with enchondromatosis, and are diagnostic, together with the presence of enchondromas for Maffucci syndrome (Fig. 1) (Mertens and Unni 2002).

In addition, *spindle cell haemangiomas*, a lesion with cavernous haemangioma-like features together with Kaposi sarcoma-like features, are over-represented among patients with Maffucci syndrome (Fanburg et al. 1995, Perkins and Weiss 1996). These lesions have a high potential for recurrence, but not for metastasis.

The major clinico-pathological problem is lack of recognition of the benign entity and overdiagnosing it as either angiosarcoma or Kaposi sarcoma.

## Abnormalities of other systems and organs

Haemangiomas in the internal organs are mostly found by chance using computed tomography or magnetical resonance imaging (MRI). Nearly one third of the tumours occur in the liver.

Multiple enchondromas are an essential feature in Maffucci syndrome (Figs. 1–2). These are benign cartilaginous tumours growing in the medulla of bone (Mulder et al. 1993). Most often they can be found in the long bones, especially of hands (Fig. 1a, c, d) and feet (Fig. 1b). In about 25% of enchondromatosis patients malignant transformation of an enchondroma into a conventional central chondrosarcoma occurs compared to <1% in patients with a solitary enchondroma (Brien et al. 1997, Mertens and Unni 2002). Patient awareness, instructions for symptoms of malignant transformation and radiologic monitoring of deep-seated tumours are therefore essential. Signs for malignant transformation are sudden growth, fatigue and pain in the affected area (Collins et al. 1992). Pathologic fractures at the side of an enchondroma can occur, not necessarily pointing to malignant transformation.

Radiological screening may aid in the distinction between enchondroma and chondrosarcoma. On conventional radiographs (Fig. 2), ill-defined margins and lobulated contours are the only morphologic features seen on radiographs that help in discrimination. However, these do not improve the ability to differentiate between enchondromas and central grade I chondrosarcomas when compared to using rather aspecific features like size and location as markers for malignancy (Geirnaerdt et al. 1997). Fast contrast-enhanced MRI is a better tool to distinguish between benign lesions and chondrosarcomas since in contrast to benign tumours, chondrosarcomas have a highly vascularised pattern (Geirnaerdt et al. 2000). Analogously, at the histological level, enchondromas present radiologically as avascular cartilaginous matrix without overt induction of neo-

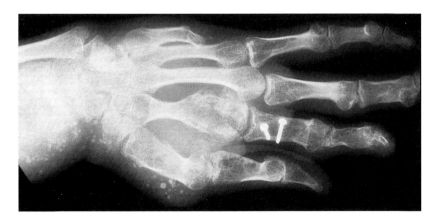

**Fig. 2.** Radiograph from hand of patient with Maffucci syndrome, containing enchondromas and calcified thrombi (phleboliths) in soft tissue haemangiomas (Source: The Netherlands Committee on Bone Tumours).

vascularisation. Low-grade chondrosarcomas have a fibrovascular stroma surrounding the avascular cartilaginous nodules (Ayala et al. 2000). These features thus form the basis for fast contrast-enhanced MRI (Geirnaerdt et al. 2000).

At the histological level, the distinction between enchondroma and low-grade central chondrosarcoma is mainly based on growth patterns and cytomorphological features. Host-bone entrapment (defined as the permeation of tumour around pre-existing lamellar host bone), tumour encasement (defined as new shells of reactive lamellar bone at the periphery of cartilage nodules), high cellularity, marked nuclear pleomorphism and irregular cell distribution are the main histological discriminators (Mirra et al. 1985, Eefting et al. 2001). The presence of mucoid matrix degeneration in 20% or more of the lesion, and the presence of host-bone entrapment, almost certainly indicates malignancy (Eefting et al. 2001).

Enchondromas in patients with enchondromatosis behave less aggressive, despite worrisome his-

**Table 1.** Additional neoplasms found in Maffucci syndrome (from 169 cases)

| Neoplasm | No. of cases | Refs. |
|---|---|---|
| Chondrosarcoma | 35 | Lewis and Ketcham (1973), Sun et al. (1985), Schwartz et al. (1987), Fanburg et al. (1995), Ramina et al. (1997), Retornaz et al. (1998), Ribeiro et al. (1998), Ahmed et al. (1999), Balcer et al. (1999), Tachibana et al. (2000), McDermott et al. (2001), Biber et al. (2004) |
| Glioma | 5 | Lewis and Ketcham (1973), Schwartz et al. (1987), Jirarattanaphochai et al. (1990), Balcer et al. (1999) |
| Angiosarcoma | 11 | Lewis and Ketcham (1973), Fanburg et al. (1995), Auyeung et al. (2003) |
| Brain tumour | 1 | Sun et al. (1985) |
| Olafactory neuroblastoma | 1 | Kurian et al. (2004) |
| Paraganglioma | I | Lamovec ct al. (1998) |
| Fibrosarcoma | 1 | Lewis and Ketcham (1973) |
| Malignant ovarium tumour | 2 | Lewis and Ketcham (1973) |
| Ovarium juvenile granulosa cell tumour | 3 | Tanaka et al. (1992) |
| Thyroid adenoma | 1 | Fanburg et al. (1995) |
| Pituitary adenoma | 2 | Lewis and Ketcham (1973), Marymont et al. (1987) |
| Adrenal adenoma | 2 | Lewis and Ketcham (1973) |
| Pancreatic adenocarcinoma | 3 | Lewis and Ketcham (1973), Sun et al. (1985), Schwartz et al. (1987) |
| Hepatic adenocarcinoma | 1 | Sun et al. (1985) |
| Biliairy adenocarcinoma | 1 | Schwartz et al. (1987) |
| Phyllodes tumour breast | 1 | Fernandez-Aguilar et al. (2004) |
| Fibroadenoma breast | 2 | Cheng et al. (1981) |
| Breast carcinoma | 1 | Marymont et al. (1987) |
| Squamous cell carcinoma | 1 | Yazidi et al. (1998) |
| Osteosarcoma | 1 | Schwartz et al. (1987) |
| Chordoma | 1 | Nakayama et al. (1994) |
| Giant thorax tumor (fibroadenoma and canalicular adenoma) | 1 | Strzalka et al. (2003) |
| Mixed abdominal tumour (fibroleioangioma and fibroangiosarcoma) | 1 | Koufos et al. (1998) |
| Acute myeloblastic leukemia | 1 | Fanburg et al. (1995) |

tological features, and slightly different criteria for malignancy are applied (Mertens and Unni 2002). As such, increased cellularity and more cytological atypia are allowed compared to solitary cases. The differential diagnosis between enchondroma and grade I chondrosarcoma in patients with Ollier disease or Maffucci syndrome is therefore difficult on histology and needs to be backed up by radiographic and clinical information.

In case of solitary chondrosarcomas, grade I tumours are histologically low in cellularity, and have a large amount of cartilaginous hyaline matrix. Binucleated cells are present. Grade II tumours are more cellular, in which the cells have atypical cell shapes and occasional mitoses are found. In grade III tumours the chondroid matrix has been replaced by mucomyxoid matrix, high cellularity is found and scatted mitotic activity is obvious (Evans et al. 1977).

Apart from haemangiomas and enchondromas/chondrosarcomas patients with Maffucci syndrome may suffer from various other tumours, both from mesenchymal as well as non-mesenchymal origin. In some reports it has even been suggested that all patients with Maffucci syndrome will develop a malignancy in time (Schwartz et al. 1987). The spectrum of tumours reported, is shown in Table 1.

### Nervous system abnormalities

Intracranial chondrosarcomas in patients with Maffucci syndrome may present with neuro-ophthalmologic symptoms like horizontal diplopia consistent with sixth (n. abducens) nerve palsy (Balcer et al. 1999). Primary brain tumours, especially gliomas, have been reported in patients with Maffucci syndrome (Lowell and Mathog 1979, Bender and Yunis 1979, Johnson et al. 1990, Jirarattanaphochai et al. 1990).

### Natural history

Vascular malformations, such as haemangioma, are often present at birth. These lesions do not enlarge out of proportion to body size and do not regress as is typical of congenital haemangiomas (Albregts and Rapini 1995).

Skeletal deformations become apparent after birth. Almost all patients with Maffucci syndrome have orthopaedic complications, of which short stature is the most prominent (Lewis and Ketcham 1973, Kaplan et al. 1993). Additionally, deformities of the tubular bones resulting in leg-length discrepancy are described (Lewis and Ketcham 1973, Kaplan et al. 1993). Both haemangiomas and enchondromas have a tendency to distribute with a unilateral predominance (Albregts and Rapini 1995) and can recur (Abdelmalek et al. 2008).

Unilateral, mosaic distributions of the typical skin and systemic lesions of Maffucci syndrome has been reported (Katz et al. 2008) including unilateral vascular malformations and atrophic overlying dermis and subcutis, enchondromas and multiple periosteal chondromas of the ipsilateral limb, congenital fibrosarcoma and thrombocytopenia.

Malignant transformation of enchondromas occurs in approximately 25% of patients with Maffucci syndrome (Mertens and Unni 2002). As described above, an increased incidence of other malignancies is reported (Table 1).

### Pathogenesis and molecular genetics

Few studies have been performed in which the pathogenesis or molecular genetics were investigated. Genetic analysis of tumours of patients with Maffucci syndrome is sparsely available in literature. Chromosomal aberrations were investigated in patients with Maffucci syndrome, but were usually not observed (Elmore and Cantrell 1966, Lewis and Ketcham 1973, Collins et al. 1992). However, one case with an inversion on chromosome 1 of p11 and q21 was reported (Matsumoto et al. 1986). Germ-line abnormalities are not found so far and not expected – given the non-hereditary character – to occur. Given the fact that unilateral predominance is found in some patients it suggests that the cause of this syndrome lies in early development and could be a result from mosaicism.

Mutational analysis of the *Parathyroid Hormone Receptor 1* (*PTHR1*) gene in enchondromas from 3 patients with Maffucci syndrome revealed no abnormalities (Rozeman et al. 2004). Also, expression studies of PTHR1 on enchondromas and chondrosarcomas of patients with Ollier disease and Maffucci syndrome revealed that they were similar to solitary enchondromas and chondrosarcomas (Rozeman et al. 2004).

Expression analyses of neuropeptides, using immunohistochemistry on sections with haemangiomas and enchondromas, as well as their surrounding tissues revealed that the nerve density in both solitary and Maffucci syndrome-related cases was similar. The only difference was observed for calcitonin gene-related peptide (CGRP) positive fibres, which covered significantly more surface area of the sections of Maffucci syndrome-related haemangiomas as compared to solitary ones (Robinson et al. 1994). The presence of nerve fibres was investigated in only one Maffucci syndrome-related enchondroma and identified nerves present in very close proximity to some of the cartilage cells (Robinson et al. 1994). However, this result was not compared to solitary enchondromas.

More research has been performed on solitary enchondromas and chondrosarcomas. Genomic analysis of enchondromas and central chondrosarcomas revealed that in benign and low-grade central chondrosarcomas few aberrations are present, whereas in high-grade central chondrosarcomas the number of aberrations increases (Sandberg and Bridge 2003, Rozeman et al., manuscript in submission). Possible targets have been identified, such as loss of chromosomal region 9p21 (Bovée et al. 2001). In this region the gene *CDKN2A/p16* is located and loss of p16 protein expression was associated with tumour progression (Asp et al. 2000, van Beerendonk et al. 2004). Loss of chromosome 6 and amplification of 12q12 were found to associate with tumour progression whereas loss of 4q13 and 4q34, chromosome 10 and gain of 9q34 correlated with adverse prognosis (Rozeman et al., manuscript in submission).

Also several molecular markers have been investigated (Rozeman et al. 2002). The signal transduction of the Indian Hedgehog (IHH)/Parathyroid Hormone Like Hormone (PTHLH) pathway plays an important role in the growth and differentiation of normal cartilage. It is also thought to be of importance in solitary chondrosarcomas (Rozeman et al. 2005).

For solitary haemangiomas no molecular changes are known.

## Diagnosis, follow-up and management

The diagnosis of Maffucci syndrome is based on the rontgenographic appearance, documenting the presence of multiple enchondromas as well as vascular lesions, and clinical features.

If superficial haemangiomas are present, evaluation for intestinally located haemangiomas is recommended, as these may form a potential risk of internal bleeding and obstruction of the organs. Magnetic resonance imaging is the best radiological option to assess the presence of internal haemangiomas.

The increased risk of malignant transformation of benign enchondromas makes close follow-up and surveillance mandatory for all patients with Maffucci syndrome. Signs for malignant transformation are sudden growth and pain. Radiological checks at regular interval of all deep-seated lesions are advisable. In addition, the high risk of development of other malignancies favours strict follow-up. Since brain, abdominopelvic organs and endocrine glands are commonly affected, periodic imaging of these locations has been suggested (Sun et al. 1985).

When progression to chondrosarcoma occurs, surgical treatment is required because of the risk of local spread and metastatic potential. This is the only therapeutic option, since chondrosarcomas are highly resistant to chemotherapy and radiotherapy. Enchondromas, mainly located in the hand, are usually expectatively followed, and only treated locally in case of fracture or cosmetic or functional complaints. Low-grade chondrosarcoma are often treated by curettage, possibly combined with cryosurgery or phenol treatment (Veth et al. 2005). Grades II and III lesions need to be resected with wide margins. For chondrosarcomas located in the phalanges, grading has not proven to be of prognostic value. Treatment of these lesions is predominantly prompted by the local destructive behaviour, since chondrosarcomas at this site are rarely reported to metastasize (Bovée et al. 1999).

Treatment of haemangiomas can be useful when traumatic ulceration and bleeding are causing complications. Haemangioma can be treated with injections of steroids or laser to reduce the size of the lesions (Chan and Giam 2005).

So far there is no option for patients with inoperable tumours or patients that present with metastatic disease.

## Differential diagnosis

The most important differential diagnosis of Maffucci syndrome is Ollier disease and Klippel-Trenaunay syndrome. Patients with Ollier disease, as well as other subclasses of enchondromatosis (Rozeman et al. 2004, Bhargava et al. 2005) have multiple enchondromas similar to patients with Maffucci syndrome, but lack vascular neoplasms. In some patients diagnosed with Ollier disease, the diagnosis needs to be adjusted after the finding of haemangiomas, even at later stages of life (Ahmed et al. 1999).

Klippel-Trenaunay syndrome is a combination of three symptoms: haemangioma, varicosis, and soft tissue and bony hypertrophy. Distinction between this syndrome and Maffucci can be made based on the limb deformities. Whereas patients with Maffucci syndrome have shortened or deformed limbs, patients with Klippel-Trenaunay syndrome usually display excessive growth of the affected limb (Ben Itzhak et al. 1988).

Another syndrome hallmarked by multiple cartilaginous lesions is Multiple Osteochondromas (MO), an autosomal dominant condition (Bovée and Hogendoorn 2002, Hameetman et al. 2004). Osteochondromas are cartilage capped bony protuberances arising on the external surface of bone, containing a marrow cavity that is continuous with that of the underlying bone (Khurana et al. 2002). These tumours can readily be separated from enchondromas at radiology in expert hands.

In addition to the differentiation from other rare syndromes, patients with Maffucci syndrome may be mistaken for patients having solitary tumours, since benign enchondroma and haemangioma can be asymptomatic. This confusion may be harmful, since the risk of malignant transformation increases drastically with the diagnosis of Maffucci syndrome.

## Genetic counselling

Referring to a clinical geneticist can be useful to ascertain the diagnosis of Maffucci syndrome. Although Maffucci syndrome is a congenital disease, there is no evidence for this syndrome to be considered hereditary, thus germ-line genetic screening is not valuable.

In contrast, multiple osteochondroma (MO) syndrome, which can be mistaken for Maffucci syndrome, is hereditary. In these patients mutations in the *Exostosis (EXT)* genes are found.

## References

Abdelmalek M, Stanko C (2008) Recurrent chondrosarcoma of the right skull base in a patient with Maffucci syndrome. Am J Clin Dermatol 9: 61–65.

Ahmed SK, Lee WC, Irving RM, Walsh AR (1999) Is Ollier's disease an understaging of Maffucci's syndrome? J Laryngol Otol 113: 861–864.

Albregts AE, Rapini RP (1995) Malignancy in Maffucci's syndrome. Dermatol Clin 13: 73–78.

Asp J, Sangiorgi L, Inerot SE, Lindahl A, Molendini L, Benassi MS, Picci P (2000) Changes of the p16 gene but not the p53 gene in human chondrosarcoma tissues. Int J Cancer 85: 782–786.

Auyeung J, Mohanty K, Tayton K (2003) Maffucci lymphangioma syndrome: an unusual variant of Ollier's. J Pediatr Orthop B 12: 147–150.

Ayala G, Liu C, Nicosia R, Horowitz S, Lackman R (2000) Microvasculature and VEGF expression in cartilaginous tumors. Hum Pathol 31: 341–346.

Balcer LJ, Galetta SL, Cornblath WT, Liu GT (1999) Neuroophthalmologic manifestations of Maffucci's syndrome and Ollier's disease. J Neuroophthalmol 19: 62–66.

Bean WB (1955) Dyschondroplasia with hemangiomata (maffucci's syndrome). Arch Intern Med 95: 767–778.

Ben Itzhak I, Denolf FA, Versfeld GA, Noll BJ (1988) The Maffucci syndrome. J Pediatr Orthop 8: 345–348.

Bender BL, Yunis E (1979) Fibrocartilaginous lesions of bone and hemangiomas and lipomas of soft tissue resembling Maffucci's syndrome. A case report. J Bone Joint Surg Am 61: 1104–1108.

Bertoni F, Bacchini P, Hogendoorn PCW (2002) Chondrosarcoma. In: Fletcher CDM, Unni KK, Mertens F (eds.) World Health Organisation classification of tumours. Pathology and genetics of tumours of soft tissue and bone. Lyon: IARC Press, pp. 247–251.

Bhargava R, Leonard NJ, Chan AK, Spranger J (2005) Autosomal dominant inheritance of spondyloenchondrodysplasia. Am J Med Genet A 135: 282–288.

Biber C, Ergun P, Turay UY, Erdogan Y, Hizel SB (2004) A case of Maffucci 's syndrome with pleural effusion: ten-year. Ann Acad Med Singapore 33: 347–350.

Bovée JVMG, Hogendoorn PCW (2002) Multiple osteochondromas. In: Fletcher CDM, Unni KK, Mertens F (eds.) World Health Organization classification of tumours. Pathology and genetics of tumours of soft tissue and bone. Lyon: IARC Press, pp. 360–362.

Bovée JVMG, Sciot R, Cin PD, Debiec-Rychter M, Zelderen-Bhola SL, Cornelisse CJ, Hogendoorn PCW (2001) Chromosome 9 alterations and trisomy 22 in central chondrosarcoma: a cytogenetic and DNA flow cytometric analysis of chondrosarcoma subtypes. Diagn Mol Pathol 10: 228–235.

Bovée JVMG, Van der Heul RO, Taminiau AHM, Hogendoorn PCW (1999) Chondrosarcoma of the Phalanx: a locally aggressive lesion with minimal metastatic potential. A report of 35 cases and a review of the literature. Cancer 86: 1724–1732.

Brien EW, Mirra JM, Kerr R (1997) Benign and malignant cartilage tumors of bone and joint: their anatomic and theoretical basis with an emphasis on radiology, pathology and clinical biology I. The intramedullary cartilage tumors. Skeletal Radiol 26: 325–353.

Carleton A, Elkington J, Greenfield J, Robb-Smith A (1942) Maffucci's syndrome (dyschondroplasia with haemangiomata). Q J Med 11: 203–228.

Chan YC, Giam YC (2005) Guidelines of care for cutaneous haemangiomas. Ann Acad Med Singapore 34: 117–123.

Cheng FC, Tsang PH, Shum JDOGB (1981) Maffucci's syndrome with fibroadenomas of the breast. J Roy Coll Surg Edinburgh 26: 181–183.

Collins PS, Han W, Williams LR, Rich N, Lee JF, Villavicencio JL (1992) Maffucci's syndrome (hemangiomatosis osteolytica): a report of four cases. J Vasc Surg 16: 364–371.

Eefting D, Geirnaerdt MJ, Le Cessie S, Taminiau AHM, Hogendoorn PCW (2001) Diagnostic impact of histologic parameters in dedifferentiating enchondroma from grade I central chondrosarcoma. Sarcoma 5 (Supplement 1), S29.

Elmore SM, Cantrell WC (1966) Maffucci's syndrome. Case report with a normal karyotype. J Bone Joint Surg Am 48: 1607–1613.

Evans HL, Ayala AG, Romsdahl MM (1977) Prognostic factors in chondrosarcoma of bone. A clinicopathologic analysis with emphasis on histologic grading. Cancer 40: 818–831.

Fanburg JC, Meis-Kindblom JM, Rosenberg AE (1995) Multiple enchondromas associated with spindle-cell hemangioendotheliomas. An overlooked variant of Maffucci's syndrome. Am J Surg Pathol. 19: 1029–1038.

Fernandez-Aguilar S, Buxant F, Noel JC (2004) Benign phyllodes tumor associated with Maffucci's syndrome. Breast 13: 247–249.

Geirnaerdt MJA, Hermans J, Bloem JL, Kroon HM, Pope TL, Taminiau AHM, Hogendoorn PCW (1997) Usefulness of radiography in differentiating enchondroma from central grade I chondrosarcoma. A J R 169: 1097–1104.

Geirnaerdt MJA, Hogendoorn PCW, Bloem JL, Taminiau AHM, Van der Woude HJ (2000) Cartilaginous tumors: Fast contrast-enhanced MR imaging of cartilaginous tumors. Radiology 214: 539–546.

Hameetman L, Bovée JVMG, Taminiau AHM, Kroon HM, Hogendoorn PCW (2004) Multiple osteochondromas: clinicopathological and genetic spectrum and suggestions for clinical management. Hereditary Cancer in Clinical Practice 2: 161–173.

Huvos AG (1991) Cartilage-forming tumors, benign and malignant. Bone tumors. Diagnosis, treatment, and prognosis. Philadelphia: W.B. Saunders Company, pp. 253–334.

Jirarattanaphochai K, Jitpimolmard S, Jirarattanaphochai K (1990) Maffucci's syndrome with frontal lobe astrocytoma. J Med Assoc Thai 73: 288–293.

Johnson TE, Nasr AM, Nalbandian RM, Cappelen-Smith J (1990) Enchondromatosis and hemangioma (Maffucci's syndrome) with orbital involvement. Am J Ophthalmol 110: 153–159.

Kaplan FS, Tabas JA, Gannon FH, Finkel G, Hahn GV, Zasloff MA (1993) The histopathology of fibrodysplasia ossificans progressiva. J Bone Joint Surg Am 75A: 220–230.

Katz P, Colbert R, Drolet B (2008) Unilateral mosaic cutaneous vascular lesions, enchondroma, multiple soft tissue chondromas and congenital fibrosarcoma – a variant of Maffucci syndrome? Pediatr Dermatol 25: 205–209.

Khurana J, Abdul-Karim F, Bovée JVMG (2002) Osteochondroma. In: Fletcher CDM, Unni KK, Mertens F (eds.) World Health Organization classification of tumours. Pathology and genetics of tumours of soft tissue and bone. Lyon: IARC Press, pp. 234–236.

Koufos C, Tsavaris N, Travlou A (1998) Unusual development of an abdominal neoplasm in a patient with. Panminerva Med 40: 338–342.

Kurian S, Ertan E, Ducatman B, Crowell EB, Rassekh C (2004) Esthesioneuroblastoma in Maffucci's syndrome. Skeletal Radiol 33: 609–612.

Lamovec J, Frkovic-Grazio S, Bracko M (1998) Nonsporadic cases and unusual morphological features in. Arch Pathol Lab Med 122: 63–68.

Lewis RJ, Ketcham AS (1973) Maffucci's syndrome: functional and neoplastic significance. Case report and review of the literature. J Bone Joint Surg Am 55: 1465–1479.

Lowell SH, Mathog RH (1979) Head and neck manifestations of Maffucci's syndrome. Arch Otolaryngol 105: 427–430.

Ma GFY, Leung PC (1984) The management of the soft tissue haemangiomatous manifestations of Maffucci's syndrome. Br J Plast Surg 37: 615–618.

Maffucci A (1881) Di un caso di encondroma ed angioma multiplo. Movimento medico-chirurgico. Napoli 3: 399–412: 565–575.

Marymont JV, Fisher RF, Emde GE, Limbird TJ (1987) Maffucci's syndrome complicated by carcinoma of the breast, pituitary adenoma, and mediastinal hemangioma. South Med J 80: 1429–1431.

Matsumoto N, Fukushima T, Tomonaga M, Imamura M (1986) Maffucci's syndrome with intracranial manifestation and chromosome abnormalities – a case report. No Shinkei Geka 14: 403–410.

McDermott AL, Dutt SN, Chavda SV, Morgan DW (2001) Maffucci's syndrome: clinical and radiological features of a rare condition. J Laryngol Otol 115: 845–847.

Mertens F, Unni KK (2002) Enchondromatosis: Ollier disease and Maffucci syndrome. In: Fletcher CDM, Unni KK, Mertens F (eds.) World Health Organization classification of tumours. Pathology and genetics of tumours of soft tissue and bone. Lyon: IARC Press, pp. 356–357.

Miller T, Frieden IJ (2005) Hemangiomas: new insights and classification. Pediatr Ann 34: 179–187.

Mirra JM, Gold R, Downs J, Eckardt JJ (1985) A new histologic approach to the differentiation of enchondroma and chondrosarcoma of the bones. A clinicopathologic analysis of 51 cases. Clin Orthop Relat Res 201: 214–237.

Mulder JD, Schütte HE, Kroon HM, Taconis WK (1993) Radiologic atlas of bone tumors, Amsterdam: Elsevier.

Nakayama Y, Takeno Y, Tsugu H, Tomonaga M (1994) Maffucci's syndrome associated with intracranial chordoma: case. Neurosurgery 34: 907–909.

Perkins P, Weiss SW (1996) Spindle cell hemangioendothelioma. An analysis of 78 cases with reassessment of its pathogenesis and biologic behavior. Am J Surg Pathol 20: 1196–1204.

Ramina R, Coelho NM, Meneses MS, Pedrozo AA (1997) Maffucci's syndrome associated with a cranial base chondrosarcoma. Neurosurgery 41: 269–272.

Retornaz F, Duffaud F, Baciuchka-Palmaro M, Nicoara A, Bordes G, Guidicelli R, Zanaret M, Favre R (1998) Chondrosarcoma in nasal fossae and Maffucci's syndrome. Rev Med Interne 19: 501–505.

Ribeiro C, Fernandes P, Reis FC (1998) The Maffucci syndrome with axial bone lesions. A rare cause of low. Acta Med Port 11: 559–562.

Robinson D, Tieder M, Halperin N, Burshtein D, Nevo Z (1994) Maffucci's syndrome – the result of neural abnormalities? Evidence of mitogenic neurotransmitters present in enchondromas and soft tissue hemangiomas. Cancer 74: 949–957.

Rozeman LB, Hameetman L, Cleton-Jansen AM, Taminiau AHM, Hogendoorn PCW, Bovée JVMG (2005) Absence of IHH and retention of PTHrP signalling in enchondromas and central chondrosarcomas. J Pathol 205: 476–482.

Rozeman LB, Hogendoorn PCW, Bovée JVMG (2002) Diagnosis and prognosis of chondrosarcoma of bone. Expert Rev Mol Diagn 2: 461–472.

Rozeman LB, Sangiorgi L, Briaire-de Bruijn IH, Mainil-Varlet P, Bertoni F, Cleton-Jansen A-M, Hogendoorn PCW, Bovée JVMG (2004) Enchondromatosis (Ollier disease, Maffucci syndrome) is not caused by the PTHR1 mutation p.R150C. Human Mutation 24: 466–473.

Sandberg AA, Bridge JA (2003) Updates on the cytogenetics and molecular genetics of bone and soft tissue tumors: osteosarcoma and related tumors. Cancer Genet Cytogenet 145: 1–30.

Schorr S, Legum C, Ochshorn M (1976) Spondyloenchondrodysplasia. Enchondromatomosis with severe platyspondyly in two brothers. Radiology 118: 133–139.

Schwartz HS, Zimmerman NB, Simon MA, Wroble RR, Millar EA, Bonfiglio M (1987) The malignant potential of enchondromatosis. J Bone Joint Surg Am 69: 269–274.

Strzalka M, Drozdz W, Kulawik J (2003) Maffucci's syndrome with giant tumor of the thoracic wall. Przegl Lek 60 (Suppl 7): 77–80.

Sun TS, Swee RG, Shives TC, Unni KK (1985) Chondrosarcoma in Maffucci's syndrome. J Bone Joint Surg 67A: 1214–1219.

Tachibana E, Saito K, Takahashi M, Fukuta K, Yoshida J (2000) Surgical treatment of a massive chondrosarcoma in the skull base associated with Maffucci's syndrome: a case report. Surg Neurol 54: 165–169.

Tanaka Y, Sasaki Y, Nishihira H, Izawa T, Nishi T (1992) Ovarian juvenile granulosa cell tumor associated with Maffucci's. Am J Clin Pathol 97: 523–527.

Tisley DA, Burden PW (1981) A case of Maffucci's syndrome. Br J Dermatol 105: 331–336.

van Beerendonk HM, Rozeman LB, Taminiau AHM, Sciot R, Bovée JVMG, Cleton-Jansen AM, Hogendoorn PCW (2004) Molecular analysis of the INK4A/INK4A-ARF gene locus in conventional (central) chondrosarcomas and enchondromas: indication of an important gene for tumour progression. J Pathol 202: 359–366.

Veth R, Schreuder B, van Beem H, Pruszczynski M, de Rooy J (2005) Cryosurgery in aggressive, benign, and low-grade malignant bone tumours. Lancet Oncol 6: 25–34.

Weiss SJ, Goldblum JR (2001) *Soft Tissue Tumors*, the C.V. Mosby Company, St. Louis.

Yazidi A, Benzekri L, Senouci K, Bennouna-Biaz F, Hassam B (1998) Maffucci syndrome associated with epidermoid carcinoma of the nasopharynx. Ann Dermatol Venereol 125: 50–51.

# Chapter 16

# HYPOMELANOSIS OF ITO AND RELATED DISORDERS (PIGMENTARY MOSAICISM)

Ignacio Pascual-Castroviejo and Martino Ruggieri

Paediatric Neurology Service, University Hospital La Paz, University of Madrid, Madrid, Spain (IPC); Institute of Neurological Science, National Research Council, Catania, and Department of Paediatrics, University of Catania, Catania, Italy (MR)

## Introduction

The term *hypomelanosis of Ito* (HI) (OMIM # 300337) encompasses a heterogeneous group of disorders characterised by hypopigmented whorls and streaks following the lines of Blaschko (Taibjee et al. 2004). Blaschko's lines represent a non-random developmental system of linear and/or whorled streaks first described in 1901 (Blaschko 1901) as a constant pattern of cutaneous markings characterising the distribution of various linear and segmental skin disorders (Bologna et al. 1994; Happle 1985, 1993).

HI still represents a challenging disorder for clinicians (Editorial 1992; Pascual-Castroviejo 1989; Pascual-Castroviejo et al. 1988, 1998; Ruggieri and Pavone 2000, 2007; Ruiz-Maldonado et al. 1992) and a controversial issue in the medical literature (Sybert 1994, Sybert et al. 1990, Taibjee et al. 2004). In fact, even though Ito's original report in 1952 described a purely cutaneous disease (Ito 1952), subsequent case reports and case series (Esquivel et al. 1991; Glover et al. 1989; Nehal et al. 1996; Pascual-Castroviejo 1989; Pascual-Castroviejo et al. 1988, 1998; Ruiz-Maldonado et al. 1992; Ruggieri and Pavone 2000; Ruggieri et al. 1996, 1998; Schwartz et al. 1977; Steiner et al. 1996; Zappella 1992) have reported a 33–94% association with multiple and sometimes severe extra-cutaneous manifestations including cognitive/behavioural deficits, epilepsy and/or asymmetric abnormalities in other organs leading to frequent characterisation as a neurocutaneous disorder (Editorial 1992; David 1981; Pascual-Castroviejo 1987, 1989, 2004; Pascual-Castroviejo et al. 1988, 1998; Ruggieri and Pavone 2000, 2007).

Initially designated "incontinentia pigmenti achromians" to differentiate it from classical *incontinentia pigmenti* (IP) (OMIM # 308300) in which the lines are hyperpigmented, HI also differs from classical IP in the absence of preceding inflammatory or verrucous lesions, and the occurrence of a much wider spectrum of associated abnormalities. Furthermore, HI occurs as a sporadic trait (Ruggieri 2000, Taibjee et al. 2004), whereas IP is X-linked and now known to be due to mutations of the IKBKG (NEMO) gene (Smahi et al. 2000).

More recently, conditions have been recognised which resemble HI in all but the arrangement of hypopigmentation or the colour of the skin markings (*HI related disorders*) (Moss and Savin 1995, Taibjee et al. 2004). In *linear and whorled naevoid hypermelanosis* (LWNH), the skin lesions are hyperpigmented, and in several patients both hypopigmented and hyperpigmented streaks are seen (Nehal et al. 1996, Taibjee et al. 2004). Other hyper- and hypopigmented cutaneous patterns include the phylloid (leaf-like), checkerboard, patchy pigmentation without midline separation (Happle 1993) and spiral patterns (Ruggieri 2000, Ruggieri et al. 2003) and the nevus depigmentosus (Bologna et al. 1994). In all these HI related disorders a wide spectrum of associated extracutaneous features has been recorded (Happle 2005).

For HI several models of inheritance have been proposed but not proved (Amon et al. 1990; Cram and Fukuyama 1974; David 1981; Griffihs and Payne 1975; Grosshans et al. 1971; Hara et al. 1987; Masumizu 1963; Moss and Burn 1988; Pascual-Castroviejo 1987; Pinol et al. 1969; Rubin 1972; Sacrez et al. 1970; Sybert 1990, 1994; Vormittag et al.

1992; reviewed in Ruggieri 2000) and a number of cytogenetic studies (which included HI related disorders) has revealed an enormous range of mosaic chromosomal abnormalities, including polyploidy, aneuploidy, chromosomal deletions, insertions and translocations (reviewed in Taibjee et al. 2004). Almost any chromosome has been affected, hence the wide heterogeneity of associated systemic features (Taibjee et al. 2004). Thus, it has been suggested that this group of conditions (i.e., HI and related disorders) are rather non-specific manifestations (i.e., phenotypes) reflecting genetic mosaicism which likely disrupts expression or function of pigmentary genes (Taibjee et al. 2004). Pigmentary mosaicism (PM) could be a useful term to encompass all these different phenotypes (Taibjee et al. 2004).

Hypopigmentation distributed along the lines of Blaschko seems to be the most common pattern in clinical practice (Nchal et al. 1996, Pascual-Castroviejo et al. 1988, Ruggieri and Pavone 2000). For this phenotype the term "*hypomelanosis of Ito*" is used for historical reasons (Jelinek et al. 1973). Of the other pigmentary mosaicism, only *nevus depigmentosus* and *LWNH* have been recently recognised as distinctive entities genetically related to HI (Happle 2004, 2006), and thus will be described in this chapter.

The so-called *phylloid hypomelanosis* (previously regarded as a HI related disorder) appears to be constantly associated to trisomy 13 mosaicism (Happle 2001) and therefore it will be treated in a separate chapter.

## Hypomelanosis of Ito

### Historical perspective and terminology

### Lines of Blaschko

**Alfred Blaschko** (1858–1922) was a private practitioner of dermatology in Berlin whose interests ranged from leprosy to occupational skin diseases (Bologna et al. 1994). In 1901 he presented his findings on the distribution patterns of linear skin disorders at the German Dermatological Society meeting in Breslau (Blaschko 1901, Jackson 1976). He examined more

than 140 patients with linear lesions such as epidermal nevi, sebaceous nevi, and nevus lipomatosus and carefully transposed the pattern in each patient onto dolls and statues (Blaschko 1901, Bologna et al. 1994, Jackson 1976). A composite diagram of these distribution patterns was then drawn that has subsequently been referred to as the lines of Blaschko. During the later years of his life, Dr. Blaschko focused on social hygiene and founded the "German Society for the Fight against Venereal Disease (Jackson 1977). In 1976, Jackson provided a detailed review of the 1901 publication and introduced the concept of the lines of Blaschko into the English-language literature, although it had been well known in the European community for decades (Bologna et al. 1994). In his original 1901 treatise (Blaschko 1901), Dr. Blaschko made a distinction between the distribution of herpes zoster and that of nevoid conditions. Happle (Happle 1990, 2006; Happle et al. 1984) added to the Blaschko's original definition lines to the posterior scalp (Bologna et al. 1994).

### Hypomelanosis of Ito

In 1952 **Minor Ito** (Ito 1952) described a 22-year-old Japanese girl with the skin of her upper half of the body looking as "if the normal pigment was brushed off". The depigmented skin lesions were widespread and symmetric, arranged in irregular shapes with "zigzag borders and splash-like spots" on the trunk and in a "linear pattern" down her arms ("*nevus depigmentosus systematicus bilateralis*"). No other physical abnormality was reported apart from asymmetry of breast size. At that time, Ito (Ito 1952) coined the term *incontinentia pigmenti achromians* (Pascual-Castroviejo 2004), because the pattern of colour loss was similar to that of the hyperpigmented changes seen in incontinentia pigmenti of the Bloch-Sulzberger type (OMIM # 308300) (Jones 2005, OMIM 2006). Subsequent observations expanded the phenotype and the name *hypomelanosis of Ito* was proposed (Jelinek et al. 1973) to avoid confusion with incontinentia pigmenti. However, this term was in itself incorrect as Ito's patient (Ito 1952) was described as having "depigmented", not hypopigmented lesions (Ruggieri and Pavone 2000; Sybert 1990,

1994). Ironically, the original patient by Ito (Ito 1952) may actually have had incontinentia pigmenti, as Ito himself believed (Ito 1952). Further changes to the term were *Ito's disease* (Sacrez et al. 1970), *Ito syndrome* (Happle et al. 1986, Ishikawa et al. 1985) and *Ito hypomelanosis* (Donnai 1985, Sybert 1994).

As the condition was no longer considered a syndrome (Donnai 1985; Editorial 1992; Sybert 1990, 1994) it was proposed to drop the term "*hypomelanosis of Ito*"[3]. Proposed changes in terminology, so far, include the terms *pigmentary dysplasia*, *mosaic dyspigmentation*, *pigmentary mosaicism*, *pigmentary mosaicism of the Ito type* or *hypopigmentation along the lines of Blaschko* to reflect the disease pathogenesis or recall the cutaneous patterns (Donnai 1985; Editorial 1992; Moss et al. 1993; Pascual-Castroviejo 1987, 2004; Ruggieri et al. 1996; Sybert 1990, 1994; Sybert et al. 1994).

## Incidence and prevalence

HI is the fourth most frequent neurocutaneous condition, exceeded only by "vascular anomaly complex or Pascual-Castroviejo type II syndrome", neurofibromatosis type 1 (NF1) and tuberous sclerosis (TS) thus surpassing Sturge–Weber disease (Pascual-Castroviejo et al. 1996, Pascual-Castroviejo 2004).

HI is underestimated by most medical colleagues. A frequency of 1 in every 7805 general paediatric outpatients, 1 in every 790 general paediatric dermatology outpatients, 1 in every 2983 general paediatric inpatients, and 1 in every 63 paediatric dermatology inpatients was reported by Ruiz-Maldonado et al. (1992), and a prevalence of about 1 per 600–700 new patients referred to a paediatric neurology service at a large National Children's Hospital was reported by Pascual-Castroviejo (1989). No data however were available from the general population in either study (Pascual-Castroviejo et al. 1989, Ruiz-Maldonado et al. 1992). Notably, pigmentation disorders in a recent study (Eul et al. 2008) were as frequent as 3.8%.

The calculated incidence and prevalence data in the area of Catania, Italy (800,000 inhabitants with approximately 13,000 births per year out of the 6 million inhabitants of Sicily) were 1 in 7540 births (or 0.013%) and 1 in 82,000 individuals in the general population (or 0.0012%) (Ruggieri and Pavone 2000).

While in the past series there was a predominance of women, with a female/male ratio of 1.7 (Donnai 1985, Editorial 1992), in our populations we recorded a ratio of 0.7, as confirmed by other studies (Pascual-Castroviejo et al. 1998, Ruiz-Maldonado et al. 1992, Ruggieri and Pavone 2000).

## Clinical manifestations

HI is a multisystem disease in which most organs of the body may show anomalies. However, the most frequent alterations are found in the skin and the central nervous system (CNS).

The main features that define HI are the cutaneous anomalies. In many instances, patients only present skin hypopigmentation following the lines of Blaschko without any other associated anomaly (Nehal et al. 1996). The frequency of cutaneous abnormalities in published reviews depends on the type of specialists who studied the series. Paediatric neurologists usually analyse patients with neurological problems, and paediatric dermatologists are closely associated with paediatric neurologists in the hospital for comprehensive medical evaluation. Although any part of the body of patients with HI may show some alteration, the most frequent and important are the neurological anomalies (Pascual-Castroviejo 1987, 2004; Pascual-Castroviejo 1989; Ruggieri and Pavone 2000). Metzker et al. (1982) did not find extracutaneous involvement in an analysis of 30 children with HI. Low frequencies of extracutaneous abnormalities (30%) were recorded by Nehal et al. (1996) and Ruggieri and Pavone (2000). However, Ruiz-Maldonado et al. (1992) reported nearly 100%, Pascual-Castroviejo et al. (1988) 94%, Glover et al. (1989) 79% and Zvulunov and Esterly (1995) 75%.

## Skin manifestations

The pigmentary lesions in HI are either recognizable at birth or become visible during childhood. The typical phenotype is characterized by hypopigmented areas consisting of bilateral or unilateral irregular borders, whorls, patches or linear white streaks or lines of the Blaschko type (Happle 1993, 1996, 1997, 2000). These pattern of lines that characterized the distribution of various linear and segmental skin disorders are those originally described by Blaschko in 1901. In HI the system of lines known now as Blaschko's lines, forms streaks displaying a V-shape or fountain-like pattern over the face or the spine (Fig. 1) and S-shape or whorled patterns over the anterior and lateral aspects of the trunk, and a linear arrangement over the extremities (Fig. 2) with a characteristic sharp midline cut-off (Blaschko 1901). The lines of Blaschko are always associated with mosaicism (Happle 1993, 1997a, b). Pigmentary anomalies associated with human mosaicism may show several patterns of distribution in the skin: (1) type 1 along the lines of Blaschko (either narrow band type 1a or broad band type 1b); (2) type 2 checkerboard pattern; (3) type 3 phylloid pattern; (4) type 4 patchy pattern without midline separation (Happle 1993); and (5) type 5 spiral pattern (Ruggieri 2000b, Ruggieri et al. 2003). Accordingly, other types of cutaneous pigmentary patterns such as a the checkerboard pattern or a zoosteriform or dermatome or plaque-like arrangement have likewise been observed in HI (Metzker et al. 1982). All of these cutaneous changes are associated with mosaicism, but not all are hypopigmented zones

and not all correspond to HI skin patterns other than those following Blaschko's lines in patients with different types of mosaicism reported and accepted in the group of HI (Ohashi et al. 1992). Some believe that skin changes like a systematized nevus depigmentosus (Fukai et al. 1993) should be included in the group of pigmentary mosaicism, although a chromosomal mosaic has not been shown in all of these cases (Küster and König 1999).

Skin changes in HI are observed within the first year of age in about 64% (Pascual-Castroviejo et al. 1998) to 70% of patients (Pascual-Castroviejo et al. 1988, Pascual-Castroviejo 1989). The hypopigmented zones can be seen localized to in any part of the body: head, face, neck, trunk or extremities (see Figs. 1 and 2). These also have been observed in the iris (Happle and Vakilzadeh 1982, Pascual-Castroviejo et al. 1998, Ruiz-Maldonado et al. 1992, Schwartz et al. 1977). Hyperpigmentation following the lines of Blaschko may also be seen, as a counterpart to the hypopigmentation. In many patients, determination that the lighter areas of skin were hypopigmented rather than the darker areas hyperpigmented has been arbitrary (Flannery 1990; Sybert 1994). The hypo- and hyperpigmented patterns reflect the presence of two cell lines with a different pigment production. It is a necessary prereq-

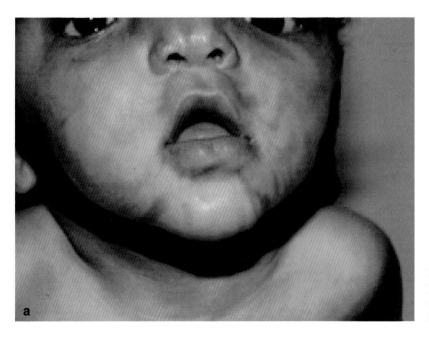

a

**Fig. 1.** Hypopigmented lesions showing a linear (**a**), "V-shape" (**b**) and "fountain-like" (**c**) pattern over the face (**a**) and spine (**b, c**) following the Blaschko lines.

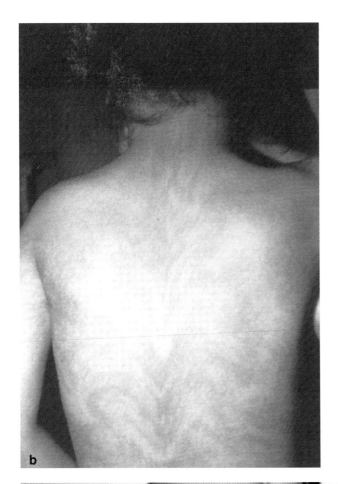

b

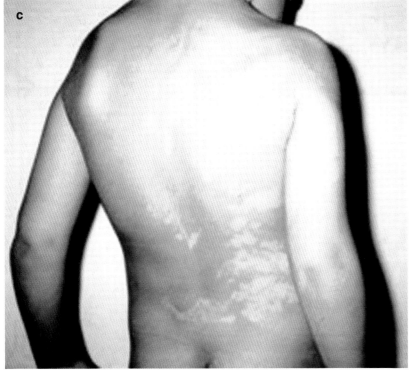

c

Fig. 1. (Continued)

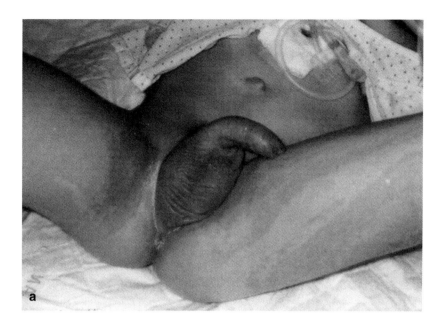

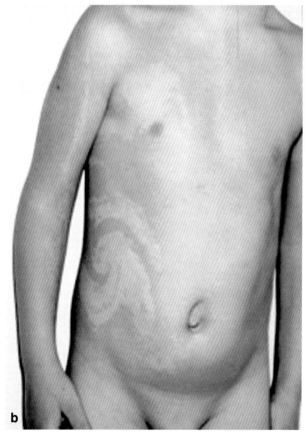

**Fig. 2.** Linear (**a**) and whorled (**b**) arrangements of the cutaneous hypomelanotic lesions in the lower extremities (**a**) and trunk (**b**).

uisite that hypopigmented skin is not preceded by vesicular or verrucous stages because cutaneous lesions in the IV stage of IP is indistinguishable from that of HI (Happle 1998) (see Chapter on IP). Areas of hypomelanosis are more easily detected in ethnic groups with increased skin pigmentation, such as Asians (David 1981), Hispanics (Rosenberg et al. 1984) or Africans (Schwartz et al. 1977). Inspection with a Wood (ultraviolet) lamp, however, could help in distinguishing hypochromic zones, especially in Caucasians with fair skin (Schwartz et al. 1977, Ardinger and Bell 1986).

The extent of the hypopigmented cutaneous lesion does not correlate either with the severity of neurological disease or with the neuroimaging or histological findings (Ruggieri et al. 1996). It appears related, however, to an early onset of symptoms (Editorial 1992, Pascual-Castroviejo et al. 1998). On the other hand, segmental nevus depigmentosus and cutaneous hypopigmented zones of HI show indistinguishable appearances. However, segmental nevus, even when distributed along Blaschko's lines, is commonly a benign lesion associated with systemic features only in a minority of cases (Di Lernia 1999), while HI is more frequently associated with extracutaneous (neurological) disorders.

Sweat glands and fingernails also may be abnormal (Marohashi et al. 1977, Pascual-Castroviejo et al. 1988, Ruiz-Maldonado et al. 1992). Decreased sweat production is known since Ito described HI in 1952. Hypohydrosis corresponds to hypopigmented areas, which may represent a pathological cell line. This feature has been found in about one third of patients with HI (Küster and König 1999). Absence of sweating with absence of glands in a skin biopsy has been also reported (Moss and Burn 1988), and this may be an argument in favour of the heterogeneity of HI.

Other types of cutaneous lesions associated with HI include café-au-lait spots, nevus marmoratus, angiomatous nevi, nevus fusceruleous of Ota and Mongolian blue spot.

## Scalp and hair

Scalp alterations mainly include changes in hair colour (Fig. 3), diffuse alopecia (Marohashi et al. 1977, Ardinger and Bell 1986, Lestringant et al. 1997, Pascual-Castroviejo et al. 1998) and hair with trichorrhexia and white-greyish colour (Fig. 4) (Pascual-Castroviejo 1989). Some patients show alopecia in some areas of the scalp until 3–5 years of age, at which time trichorrhexia and grey-white hair appear

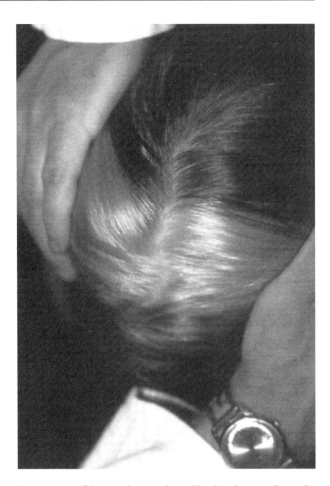

**Fig. 3.** Area of hypomelanotic skin with white hair on the scalp.

(Fig. 5) (Pascual-Castroviejo et al. 1988, 1998). Macrocephaly is a common complication of HI, particularly in cases with hair colour changes. In our series of more than two hundred cases, patients with hair anomalies, mostly consisting in colour changes, showed more anomalies elsewhere in the body than patients without hair changes: these anomalies most frequently consisted of macrocephaly, hemicranial and/or hemifacial hypertrophy, ocular, nasal, or oral abnormalities, cerebral malformations, asymmetry of the trunk or extremities, and others. Hypochromic hair may appear as areas of patches, streaks or extending over the entire scalp, associated with achromic or hypochromic skin. Focal hypertrichosis of the genital area without signs of precocious puberty has been observed by Ballmer-Weber et al. (1996). Macrocephaly was present in 16% of the patients in this series (Ballmer-

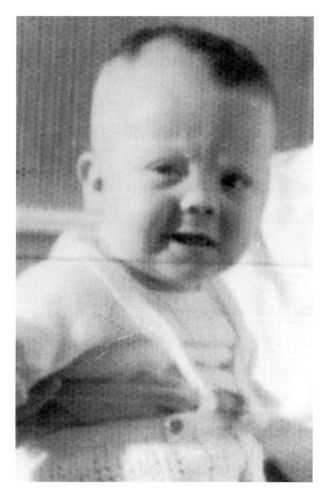

**Fig. 4.** Diffuse alopecia in the scalp of the midline and the right side of a 11 month-old child with HI.

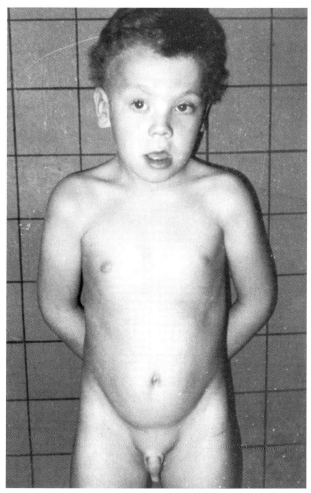

**Fig. 5.** The same patient as in Fig. 4 at age 5 years shows alopecia, trichorrhexia, and grey-white hair in the scalp along with the typical cutaneous lesions of HI also shows macrosomy and macrogenitosomy.

Weber et al. 1996) and usually is associated with coarse facies (Pascual-Castroviejo et al. 1998).

## Oral manifestations

Oral anomalies are of a wide variety and consist of defective dental implantation, partial anodontia, dental hypoplasia or dysplasia, conical teeth (Fig. 6), and defective enamel (Bartholomew et al. 1987, Happle and Vakilzadeh 1982, Maize et al. 1972, Pascual-Castroviejo et al. 1998). Hamartomatous cuspids protruding from the dental crowns of permanent teeth might be histologically reminiscent of odontoma (Happle and Vakilzadeh 1982, Maize et al. 1972). Bifid uvula and submucosal cleft palate are rarer anomalies.

## Eye manifestations

Non specific ocular alterations include strabismus, nystagmus, dacryostenosis, hypertelorism, ptosis, symblepharon, nonclosure of the upper lid, myopia, amblyopia, iridal heterocromia, scleral melanosis, cataracts, striated patchy hypopigmented fundi, atrophy of the choroid, corneal opacity, micro-ophthalmia, macro-ophthalmia, optic nerve hypoplasia and retinal degeneration (Jelinek et al. 1973, Peña et al. 1977, Schwartz et al. 1977, Pascual-Castroviejo et al. 1988, Ruiz-Maldonado et al. 1992, Pascual-Castroviejo et al. 1999). An important point in the

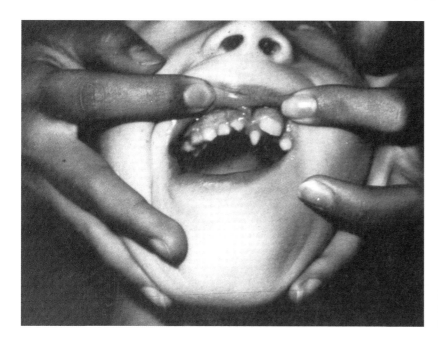

**Fig. 6.** Imperfect implantation of the teeth, which also show abnormalities in size and morphology.

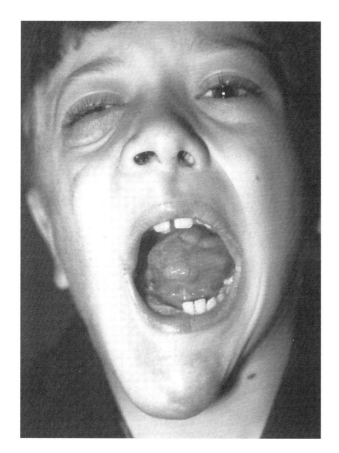

**Fig. 7.** Hypertrophy of the right hemiface and tongue.

differential diagnosis between HI and IP is the commonly severe ocular lesions in IP as sequelae of the neonatal pathology (Pascual-Castroviejo et al. 1994), while in HI, ocular lesions are usually very discrete or do not exist.

## Nervous system manifestations

Anomalies of the CNS may include mental and motor retardation, microcephaly or macrocephaly, seizures, unbalanced gait, hyperkinesias, and hypotonia (Jelinek et al. 1973; Pascual-Castroviejo et al. 1988, 1998; Ruiz-Maldonado et al. 1992). The most frequent and severe complications of HI are related to involvement of the CNS. There is a consistent discrepancy between clinical series reported by neurologists and child neurologists who record higher frequencies (94–100%) and wider spectrum of associated CNS alterations than do dermatologists or paediatric dermatologists (33–60%). This could be due to referral and reporting bias in previous studies. By literature review the incidence of neurological disease is reported to be as high as 100 percent (Hara et al. 1987), 94% (Pascual-Castroviejo et al. 1988) or 80% (Hamada et al. 1979) or as low as 61% (Rosenberg et al. 1984), 50%

(Hamada et al. 1967), 40% (Ortonne et al. 1979) or 30% (Nehal et al. 1996, Ruggieri and Pavone 2000).

**Cognitive/behavioural problems**. The most frequent neurological problem in individuals with HI who present with associated extracutaneous features is mental retardation. An intellectual quotient (IQ) below 70, that is to say below borderline, has been reported in 30% (Nehal et al. 1996, Ruggieri and Pavone 2000), 57% (Pascual-Castroviejo et al. 1998) or 70% (Ruiz-Maldonado et al. 1992) of cases likely depending to ascertainment bias in tertiary referral centres (reviewed in Ruggieri and Pavone 2000). Between 8 and 10% of the patients with mental retardation have been reported to exhibit autistic behaviour or autism spectrum disorders (Pascual-Castroviejo et al. 1989, Glover et al. 1989, Akefeldt and Gillberg 1991, Ruiz-Maldonado et al. 1992, Zappella 1993) but again this is likely due to a bias towards child neuropsychiatry referrals. Twenty-one (out of 100) patients seen in Madrid had borderline mental level (IQ between 70 and 85) (Pascual-Castroviejo et al. 1998). Most patients with mental retardation and/or autism spectrum disorders previously had suffered of infantile spasms or severe seizures (Pascual-Castroviejo 1989, Ruiz-Maldonado et al. 1992, Pascual-Castroviejo et al. 1998). The association of mental retardation with seizures is seen in 65% of cases (Ruiz-Maldonado et al. 1992, Pascual-Castroviejo et al. 1998).

**Epilepsy**. The second most frequent extracutaneous neurological manifestation of HI is epilepsy. Seizures may occur in 11% (Nehal et al. 1996) to about 50% (Pascual-Castroviejo et al. 1988, 1998) of cases depending on ascretainment bias. Seizures commonly appear early, within the first year of life, and usually are refractory to anticonvulsant drugs. Seizures are mostly associated with mental retardation. Both alterations, seizures and mental retardation, as well as electroencephalographic (EEG) changes, may be caused by underlying neuronal migration disorders (Hara et al. 1989), and may be accompanied by macrocephaly (Rubin 1972, Peña et al. 1977, Ross et al. 1982, Schwartz et al. 1977, Pascual-Castroviejo et al. 1988 and 1998, Pascual-Castroviejo 1989, Ruiz-Maldonado et al. 1992) or microcephaly (Ishikawa et al. 1985; Ardinger and

Bell 1986; Pascual-Castroviejo et al. 1988, 1998; Pascual-Castroviejo 1989; Ruiz-Maldonado et al. 1992). There is no consistent EEG pattern in HI (Esquivel et al. 1991, Ogino et al. 1996). The EEG can yield normal results or show a wide range of abnormalities in different combinations.

**Language abnormalities**. Speech delay in HI has been occasionally reported (Golden and Kaplan 1986, Ruggieri et al. 1996, Zappella 1992). Overall, these studies recorded higher scores on performance IQ (mean PIQ=90) than verbal IQ (mean VIQ=73) in HI patients of whom 20% had mental retardation. There was delay in the production of speech sound and in communication milestones, and specific expressive language disabilities according to the DSM-IV-R. In 80% of patients with language disabilities MRI revealed hyperintensities on T2-weighted images (Ruggieri et al. 1996). Language disturbances were not progressive in most children and improved after placement in special and early pre-schooling intervention programs (Ruggieri and Pavone 2000, Ruggieri et al. 1996, Zappella 1992).

**Other neurological manifestations**. There are other neurological alterations found in isolated cases including muscular hypotonia or hypertonia, hyperkinesias, nystagmus, ataxia and neurosensorial deafness (reviewed in Ruggieri and Pavone 2000). These alterations, however, could be simply related to the overall neurological (mosaic) phenotype or it may be a chance association due to bias in report.

**Imaging findings**. Most intracranial anomalies can be demonstrated by CT and MRI even though there are no constant findings in HI, as expected. Most HI cases (and likely almost all cases with no clinical neurological signs/symptoms) display normal neuroimaging studies (Barkovich 2005, Edelstein et al. 2005) or only show enlarged perivascular spaces (Ruggieri et al. 1996). In the remainder, abnormalities may be grouped into white matter alterations (Fig. 8) and structural malformations (Fig. 9) (Edelstein et al. 2005). More than 50% of HI patients with neurological involvement have MRI-demonstrable non progressive *white matter abnormalities* (Fig. 8), thought to be pathologically related to dilated Virchow-Robin spaces and/or altered/delayed myelination (Ardinger and Bell 1986, Battistella et al.

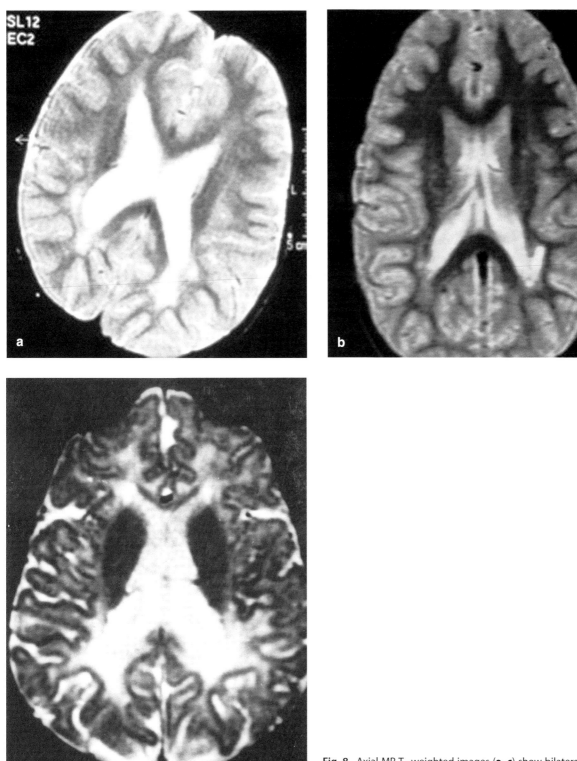

**Fig. 8.** Axial MR T$_2$-weighted images (**a–c**) show bilateral and symmetric changes in the perivenricular white mater in three children with hypomelanosis of Ito.

1990, Bhushan et al. 1989, Hara et al. 1989, Pascual-Castroviejo et al. 1998, Ruggieri et al. 1996, Steiner et al. 1996, Turleau et al. 1984, Williams and Elster 1990). These abnormalities appear as early as a few months of age (Ruggieri et al. 1996) and on T2-weighted and FLAIR sequences show multifocal, symmetric high signal foci in the periventricular (Fig. 8a, b) and subcortical (Fig. 8c) white matter particularly in the centrum semiovale (Edelstein et al. 2005, Ruggieri and Pavone 2000, Ruggieri et al. 1996). CT shows the same features as multiple low density areas in the deep white matter of the hemispheres, or as a

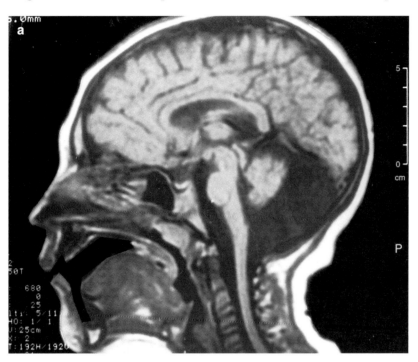

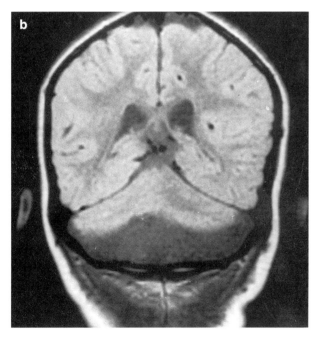

**Fig. 9.** MRI study in a girl with chromosomal alterations (46XX, 16qh+) and HI. Sagittal (**a**) and coronal (**b**) T$_1$-weighted views show neocerebellar hypoplasia which affects the brainstem and the posterior and inferior cerebellum.

diffuse low density in the white matter (when a large number of lesion is present) (Edelstein et al. 2005). White matter lesions are static over time (Fryburg et al. 1996), and show no correlation between the extent of the lesions and the patient age (Ruggieri et al. 1996). The most frequent *structural anomalies* are cerebellar hypoplasia (Fig. 9) or atrophy (Ross et al. 1982, Turleau et al. 1984, Golden and Kaplan 1986, Pini and Faulkner 1995, Pascual-Castroviejo et al. 1998d), focal cerebral atrophy (Golden and Kaplan 1986, Urgellés et al. 1996) or generalized cerebral atrophy (Hamada et al. 1979, Davis 1981, Ardinger and Bell 1986, Rufo and Sierra 1996, Pascual-Castroviejo et al. 1998), cerebral dysplasias and/or other migrational abnormalities often associated with hemimegalencephaly (Ross et al. 1982, Ardinger and Bell 1986, Peserico et al. 1988, Hara et al. 1989, Williams and Elister 1990, Batistella et al. 1990, Malherbe et al. 1993, Kimura et al. 1994, Tagawa et al. 1984, Steiner et al. 1996, Ono et al. 1997). Other anomalies include grey matter heterotopia, blurred grey/white matter junction, agiria, polymicrogyria, porencephaly, and periventricular cysts (reviewed in Barkovich 2005, Edelstein et al. 2005, Pascual-Castroviejo 2004, Ruggieri and Pavone 2000). Macroencephaly may be associated with generalized dilatation of the cerebral ventricles.

## Musculoskeletal manifestations

Musculoskeletal disturbances are commonly seen in HI when the phenotype is more severe and are exceeded only by the mental retardation, seizures and hypotonia (Ross et al. 1982, Rosenberg et al. 1984, Pascual-Castroviejo 1989, Ruiz-Maldonado et al. 1992, Pascual-Castroviejo et al. 1998). Skeletal defects include short stature, asymmetry showing hemihypertrophy or hemihypotrophy of a part or of an entire side of the body (Fig. 7) (Pascual-Castroviejo 2004, Riyaz et al. 2004), scoliosis, thoracic deformities (pectus carinatum or excavatum), and various finger and toe anomalies (clinodactyly, polydactyly, syndactyly, brachydactyly), (Jelinek et al. 1973; Stewart et al. 1979; Pascual-Castroviejo et al. 1988, 1989, 1998; Fryburg et al. 1996). Hypertrophic or hy-

potrophic areas are usually on the same side as the hypomelanotic skin. Bilateral hypertrophy is found in some cases with generalized hypomelanotic skin. The patients usually show coarse facies and macrocephaly (Schwartz et al. 1977; Pascual-Castroviejo et al. 1988, 1989, 1998). All these defects are likely related to the age dependent effect of the genetic mosaic abnormality (Ruggieri 2000, Ruggieri and Pavone 2000).

## Other system's anomalies

These include congenital cardiac disease (Pascual-Castroviejo et al. 1988, 1998; Ruiz-Maldonado et al. 1992), single kidney or ureteral duplication, cryptorchidism, micropenis or macrogenitosomy and glomerulo cystic kidney disease (Pascual-Castroviejo 1989; Pascual-Castroviejo et al. 1988, 1998; Ruiz-Maldonado et al. 1992, Vergine et al. 2008). Asymmetric breast development has been reported occasionally (Ito 1952; Pascual-Castroviejo et al. 1989, 1998) and, more rarely, gynecomastia may appear in boys or prepubertal girls (Pascual-Castroviejo 1989). HI occasionally is associated with vascular anomalies as Moya-Moya syndrome (Echenne et al. 1995), intracranial arteriovenous malformation (AVM) (Urgellés et al. 1996), or intestinal lymphangiectasia (Riyaz et al. 2004).

## Hypomelanosis of Ito and tumours

There is a limited number of HI cases occasionally associated with benign tumours (Browne and Byrd 1976, Happle and Vakilzadeh 1982, Ishikawa et al. 1985, Oguma et al. 1986, Steichen-Gersdorf et al. 1993, Steiner et al. 1996, Tateno et al. 1981, Turleau et al. 1986, Zajac et al. 1997), including cystic teratoma in association with diploic epidermoid cyst (Ishikawa et al. 1985), complex mature sacrocoxygeal dysembryonal tumour (Turleau et al. 1986), choroid plexus papilloma (Steichen-Gersdorf et al. 1993, Zajac et al. 1997) and dental hamartomatous tumour (complex composite odontome-like) (Happle and Vakilzadeh 1982, Browne and Byrd 1976). Rarely, malignant tumours such as acute lymphoblastic leukemia (Tateno et al. 1981), medulloblastoma (Steiner et al. 1996), and neuroblastoma (Oguma et al. 1986) have been reported.

One explanation to such phenomenon could be that tumours are often associated with chromosomal abnormalities or this may well be just a coincidental occurrence of rare features due to report bias (Ruggieri et al. 2001). Notably, in some of these cases (Ishikawa et al. 1985, Steichen-Gersdorf et al. 1993, Tateno et al. 1981, Zajac et al. 1997) mosaic chromosomal abnormalities were found while no chromosomal mosaic could be found in the blood and tumour karyotypes as occurred in the medulloblastoma reported by Steiner et al. (1996). No genetic data were reported in the remaining cases (Browne and Byrd 1976, Happle and Vakilzadeh 1982, Oguma et al. 1986, Turleau et al. 1986).

## Pathology

Histological abnormalities of HI are not specific. Rounded melanocytes with reduced or absent dendrites visible on DOPA stain or by electron microscopic studies have been described (Stoebner and Grosshans 1970, Grosshans et al. 1971, Meinecke et al. 1985, Sáxena et al. 1989). These histopathological findings, however, are not characteristic changes. The hypopigmented lesions may be the result of a decrease in the number of melanocytes, as well as of the number of premelanosomes and melanosomes (Stoebner and Grosshans 1970, Hamada et al. 1979). These results also do not represent a specific characteristic criterion and are of limited diagnostic value (Küster and Köning 1999, Hamada et al. 1967, Stoebner and Grosshans 1970). The pathogenesis of these disorders in still incompletely understood and microscopic examination of the lesions reveals only non-specific findings. Ultrastructural studies disclose fewer than normal melanosomes and incomplete melanisation (Cram and Fukuyama 1974).

The neuropathologic findings have consisted of abnormal cortical morphogenesis with disarray of cortical lamination, heterotopic areas, laminar or band heterotopia, pachygyria, cerebral or cerebellar micropolygyria, focal or generalised brain atrophy, brainstem and cerebellum hypoplasia with demyelinization of the corticospinal tracts, existence of abnormal neurons in the white matter and periventricular areas and impressive astrocytes reaction, resulting from the coexistence of neural cells undergoing a normal migration and cells exhibiting *arête en route* or even complete absence of migration (reviewed in Pascual-Castroviejo 2004 and Ruggieri and Pavone 2000).

## Nevus depigmentosus

Naevus depigmentosus (ND) (also known as *achromic nevus*) is a congenital, nonfamilial, well circumscribed, uniformly hypopigmented macule or patch, the relative size and distribution of which is stable throughout life. ND is usually present at birth (35% of case in one study) (Xu et al. 2008), but may also appear during the first 3 years of life (Kim et al. 2006, Xu et al. 2008). Its frequency has been calculated as about 0.4% in the general population (Shih et al. 2007). The trunk and the proximal extremities are the most commonly affected sites, and the lesions usually have serrated, irregular borders. Under Wood's lamp, the lesions have an off-white accentuation without fluorescence.

Three patterns of distribution of lesions have been described so far including: (1) the classical *isolated* (circumscribed, irregular oval to round lesion) form; and (2) the *segmental* form (Di Lernia 1999) which are the most common types; and (3) the less common *systematised* form (Kandpur and Sumanth 2005). The segmental and systematised forms more often consist in multiple macules or patches in a segmental or widespread distribution (Di Lernia 1999, Kim et al. 2006) bet may also present as unilateral broad bands or streaks with a blocklike configuration or arranged along one or more Blaschko lines (type 2 pattern along the lines of Blashko) (Bologna et al. 1994, Di Lernia 1999, Happle 1993). According to our experience and by literature review (unreported data), when the ND is reportedly as arranged in streaks or bands is indistinguishable from HI (Di Lernia 1999, Fuermann and Wolf 1982) and likely the reports describe the same entity (i.e., HI; see later under "misdiagnosis of HI").

Immunohistochemistry studies show that the melanin content of ND lesions is decreased compared with perilesional normal skin (Kim et al. 2006, Xu et al. 2008) with decreased (Kim et al. 2006) or normal (Xu et al. 2008) number of melanocytes. Ultrastructural studies (Jimbow et al. 1975, Xu et al. 2008) showed that some aggregated melanosomes were present in the affected keratinocytes.

Occasionally, superimposed or distant areas of congenital (Alkemade and Juhlin 2000, Baba et al. 2002, Bardazzi et al. 2008, Shim et al. 2002, Taniguchi et al. 1995) and acquired (In and Kang 2008) lentiginosis have been reported in the context of ND as a possible example of twin spotting. Further examples of twin spotting phenomena in this context – associated (Baba et al. 2002, Chen and Liao 2004, Jagia et al. 2004) or not (Afsar et al. 2007, Dippel et al. 2003) with partial lentiginosis – include the coexistence of ND along with ipsilateral Becker's naevus (Afsar et al. 2007), capillary malformations (Nevi flammei) (Dippel et al. 2003), ipsilateral breast hypoplasia (Jagia et al. 2004), inflammatory linear verrucous epidermal nevus (Ogunbiji and Ogunbiji 1998) and congenital linear punctate keratoderma (Chen and Liao 2004).

Occasionally, associated extra-cutaneous features have been reported (likely reflecting more generalised mosaicism expressed throughout the body) including musculoskeletal abnormalities (cranial and thoracic asymmetry, scoliosis, leg length discrepancy) (Dawn et al. 1995, Di Luria 1999), eye abnormalities (iris and lens colobomas, and drusen) (Sharma et al. 2008), and neurological deficits (psychomotor retardation, seizures behavioural disturbances and language impairment) (Di Luria 1999) associated or not to nervous system anomalies (corpusa callosum agenesis, cerebral asymmetry).

Successful results have been obtained in the treatment of ND by autologous in vitro epidermal grafts (Raskovic et al. 2006). However cases of recurrence of ND after autologous epidermal graft have been recored (Kim do et al. 2008).

# Linear and whorled naevoid hypermelanosis

Linear and whorled nevoid hypermelanosis (LWNH) is a sporadic disorder first described by Kalter et al. in 1988. Clinically, is characterised by: (1) asymmetrically distributed linear and whorled hyperpigmentation following Blaschko's lines as well as reticulated hyper-

pigmentation; (2) coexistence (in some cases) of hyper- and hypopigmented lesions in the same patient; (3) skin lesions noted at birth or within the first two years of life; (4) no preceding inflammatory event or palpable lesion; (5) gradual increase (spread) of involvement during the first two years of life and subsequent stabilisation or gradual fading; (6) sparing of mucous membranes, palms, and soles; (7) sporadic male and female (equal) incidence; (8) increased pigmentation of the basal layer and prominence or vacuolation of melanocytes, with no pigment incontinence or dermal melanophages on histological examination; and (9) in approximately 30% of cases (Bolognia et al. 1994, Di Lermia 2007, Nehal et al. 1996, Pinheiro et al. 2007), associated systemic anomalies consisting in atrial septal defects, dextrocardia, mild hypereosinophilia, cerebral palsy, psychomotor delay, seizures and deafness.

Previous eponyms have been reticulate hyperpigmentation with zoosteriform patter, reticulated hyperpigmentation of Ijima, Naito and Uyeno, zebra-like hyperpigmentation and zoosteriform lentiginous nevus which have been currently unified under the umbrella term of LWNH (Bologna et al. 1994, Quecedo et al. 1997).

Under the term LWNH two different clinical presentations may be included corresponding to the same spectrum: (a) the classical generalised pattern with onset within the first two weeks of life; and (b) unilateral cases involving only one quadrant of the body, with a later onset at about the 2nd decade of life.

Recently (Hong et al. 2008) LWNH has been associated with chromosomal abnormality inv (9)

## Pathogenesis and molecular genetics

### Mendelian transmission

There have been a number of single case reports claiming familial occurrence and supporting single gene inheritance (Amon et al. 1990; Cram and Fukuyama 1974; David 1981; Griffiths and Payne 1975; Grosshans et al. 1971; Hara et al. 1987; Masumizu 1963; Moss and Burn 1988; Pascual-Castroviejo 1987; Pinol et al. 1969; Rubin 1972; Ruggieri 2000; Sacrez et al. 1970; Sybert 1990, 1994; Vormittag et al. 1992). None, however, has been proved. Nonetheless, there is still an entry for HI in the *McKusick catalogue* under the autosomal dominant disorders (OMIM # 146150) (Jones 2005, OMIM 2006).

A number of pedigrees (reviewed in Sybert 1994, Ruggieri 2000b) have been used to support *X-linked dominant inheritance* despite: 1) the findings in these families are now recognised as classic for incontinentia pigmenti; 2) there is no history of recurrent pregnancy losses of presumed affected male foetuses in HI; and 3) an only moderately distorted male:female ratio was reported in HI (Editorial 1992; Sybert 1990, 1994).

The same applies to the pedigrees inferring *autosomal dominant inheritance* where in none of the family members, besides the probands, were the skin changes described typical for HI. The only exception is still considered (Various Authors 1999) the family reported by Patrizi et al. (1987) and Montagna et al. (1991), where two sibs – a man and a woman in their twenties – were described as having the typical skin changes of HI associated with psychomotor delay and cerebellar disturbances; their fifty-year-old mother had the same pigmentary abnormalities without neurological defects while the maternal grandfather (who died prior to the family referral) was said to have been affected with similar neurological disturbances. However, the pigmentary abnormalities in the sibs and the mother were "bilateral, irregular, dyschromic regions at the level of the flanks or the iliac crest" which faded in the daughter. The natural history of the disease in the sibs was that of a complex neurodegenerative (autosomal dominant?) disorder with neuroimaging evidence of cerebellar vermian atrophy associated to patchy dyspigmentation of the skin. Moreover, no cytogenetic analysis was performed in the skin biopsies in this family (see also Ruggieri 2000).

The argument for *autosomal recessive inheritance* of HI has been based on classical reports (reviewed in Ruggieri 2000b) on affected probands with consanguineous parents. However, not all of the affected individuals in these families had skin and/or systemic abnormalities, all of these cases were isolated and there were no recurrences among siblings.

Two families were reported (Amon et al. 1990, Vormittag et al. 1992) both with a mother and her daughter affected by HI. A diploid/tetraploid mosaicism was found in the mother reported by Vormittag et al. (1992) (while the daughter was not investigated) and "a suspect" (sic !) chromosome mosaic was found in both family members in the case of Amon et al. (1990). Members of the same family having HI have been mentioned in other series (Pascual-Castroviejo et al. 1998) but a description of the cutaneous markings was not available in all the affected family members and genetic analysis was not carried out. We personally observed a brother and a sister with typical HI skin lesions and unaffected consanguineous parents (Ruggieri et al. 1996). Both the children, their father and paternal grandmother had a balanced autosome translocation t(5;17) (q35;q11).

## Chromosome studies

The recognition of chromosomal mosaicism as the pathogenic basis of many cases of HI and related disorders was a clue to explain the protean clinical manifestations of this condition and their often asymmetrical expression. Chromosomal abnormalities of several types, however, have been documented in only 30–60% of the reported cases and in a recent literature survey (Taibjee et al. 2004) the mosaicism could be classified, in the cases identified, as follows:

1) Mosaicism with two or more different karyotypes involving structural abnormalities of chromosomes ($n=70$);
2) Mosaicism involving structural abnormalities of chromosomes, where the chromosome was undetermined ($n=2$);
3) Chromosomal abnormality apparently affecting all cells, but where undetected mosaicism remains a possibility ($n=5$);
4) Balanced X; autosome translocations affecting all cells, with functional mosaicism due to lyonisation ($n=19$);
5) Polyploidy mosaicism, i.e., cells having different multiples of 23 chromosomes ($n=7$). One case was also mosaic for trisomy 18;
6) Chimerism ($n=6$).

The primary question addressed is how such disparate genotypes could produce the common cutaneous phenotype of patchy pigmentation. By cross-comparing karyotype abnormalities in HI and related disorders (pigmentary mosaicism) with 76 pigmentary and candidate pigmentary gene loci, either in humans or animals, Taibjee et al. (2004) tried to answer to this question. In their study (Taibjee et al. 2004) they showed extensive (88%) overlaps between cytogenetic abnormalities and one or more pigmentary genes as well as significant (74%) overlaps between pigmentary genes and one or more karyotype abnormalities supporting the hypothesis of a pathogenic role for the individual chromosomal abnormalities in causing the hypo- and hyperpigmented whorls and patches (besides chance occurrence). In pigmentary mosaicism therefore the pigmentary phenotype could arise through karyotype abnormalities specifically disrupting either expression or function of pigmentary genes. Likely mechanisms to explain the disruption are (reviewed in Taibjee et al. 2004): (a) parallel co-migration of genetically different but not necessarily abnormal, cell clones; (b) X-chromosome functional disomy; (c) "spreading" of X inactivation to autosomes; (d) transposons (transposable elements of retroviral origin) regulating gene activation and silencing and modulating the activity of pigmentary genes; (e) genetic imprinting; and (f) phenotype reversion. The various processes controlled by the (disrupted) pigmentary genes are: (a) melanoblast migration from the neural crest in foetal life; (b) melanocytes function including synthesis, transport and degradation of melanosomes; (c) physiology of the surrounding melanocytes milieu which include keratinocytes, intercellular matrix, growth factors, etc.

In light of the above explanations, demonstrated chromosomal abnormalities found in parents of children with HI or running in families with multiple affected members, might be the only plausible explanation for *recurrence* in *HI*.

## Natural history and outcome

Approximately one third (or less) of patients with HI and related disorders (depending on the reported series) may have psychomotor delay in infancy and present with cognitive/behavioural deficits later in childhood and adult life. Approximately the same percent-age of individuals present some type of seizure with complete control by antiepileptic drugs in less than a 50%. Seizures in these disorders often are refractory (Hara et al. 1989, Pascual-Castroviejo 1989), especially because of disordered neuronal migration (Hara et al. 1989, Esquivel et al. 1991). However, control of seizures in a 70% of patients with HI has been reported in the series of Pascual-Castroviejo et al. (1998).

Severe mental retardation is almost always present in patients with a severe and complex phenotype (usually associated to other system's involvement) who had infantile spasms (i.e., about a 10% of the overall HI population) (Pascual-Castroviejo et al. 1988, Pascual-Castroviejo 1989). The high frequency of hypotonia also contributes to the motor sequelae. Autistic spectrum disorders in isolated cases must be taken into consideration (Pascual-Castroviejo et al. 1989, 1998; Ruiz-Maldonado et al. 1992).

## Differential diagnosis

HI may be confused with other pigmentary disorders, but the differential diagnosis usually is not difficult for expert specialists in neurocutaneous disorders. HI presents many similarities with other diseases with hypopigmented spots on the skin. These diseases are incontinentia pigmenti (IP) of Bloch and Sulzberger, vitiligo, and skin fungal infections. Identical to HI, IP shows the streaky pigmentary changes and the frequent occurrence of extracutaneous abnormalities. However, IP is characterized by affecting almost only females, and by a dynamic course of distinct cutaneous lesions that appear successively soon after birth (see also chapter on IP): 1) linear dermatitis with vesicles and erythema; 2) linear verrucous anomalies; 3) hyperpigmented streaks; and 4) hypochromic or achromic lesions very similar to those of HI. In contrast to IP, the hypopigmentation in patients with HI is either recognized at birth or during the neonatal period or in early childhood, and remains unchanged during many years or during the entire life. Vitiligo and skin fungal lesions are local problems of the skin that do not involve the CNS and they can disappear after a variable period of time, while cutaneous lesions of HI do not disappear.

## Misdiagnosis of HI

In the absence of a recognised diagnosis, the label of HI has been often used for individuals having diffuse or patchy, generalised or limited, linear or spotty skin depigmentation or hypopigmentation distributed along the lines of Blaschko but also in many other patchy or streaky configuration. This has caused a great confusion and has expanded the phenotype of HI, melting under the same rubric several conditions of different aetiologies because of the solely presence of hypopigmented skin lesions. Often, in such cases, the presumptive diagnosis of a child having CNS or musculoskeletal abnormalities associated to cutaneous anomalies has been based only upon a single or a pair of pigmentary skin lesions which could ultimately have been merely a presenting symptom of other diseases (see Ruggieri 2000b, Ruggieri and Pavone 2000). Notably, in the *London Dysmorphology Database* (Winter and Baraitser 2006) there are >70 different syndromes (including HI) under the same entry "*patchy depigmentation of skin*". Thus, we would favour the use of the term HI (and related disorders) only in cases with "*overt*" and "*widely distributed*" pigmentary abnormalities, with or without associated extra-cutaneous manifestations.

## Follow-up and management issues

Patients who exhibit pigmentary anomalies (hypopigmentation or depigmentation or hyperpigmentation) along the lines of Blaschko, in a patchy or linear distribution, unilaterally or bilaterally, should be fully evaluated for structural systemic abnormalities. Laboratory or imaging tests, including EEG and neuroimaging, should be only oriented by the abnormal findings on clinical examination. Karyotyping of peripheral blood, and if this is normal, skin fibroblasts or better keratinocytes or melanocytes, obtained from biopsies taken from affected and unaffected areas, should be performed in affected individuals to support the diagnosis.

The recommended *follow-up protocol* calls for an annual clinical review. However, each case should be examined individually and further evaluated to the extent that the history, careful clinical examination and investigations dictate with more frequent re-evalua-

tions in children with unusual symptoms or complications requiring special care. The assumption of a high risk of associated abnormal features in these individuals is without basis. Parents should be reassured that serious complications, if present, are congenital and thus typically evident clinically early in infancy. The chance occurrence of a tumour in an affected patient should be almost the same as in the general population.

The routine or screening use of brain MRI does not improve HI prognosis because the majority of CNS abnormalities are either unspecific or not treatable and overall do not predict a poor outcome. Conversely, it is warranted a full brain MRI study if and when seizures ensues because a minority of such patients could have underlying neuronal migration anomalies.

No special *treatment* is indicated for the *skin lesions* and no precaution has to be taken with regard to sun exposure or cream applications. Malignant transformation of a hypomelanotic zone of the skin (the so-called "nevus of Ito") has occasionally been reported (Van Krieken et al. 1988) but this was never recorded in the skin lesions in the largest series so far reported, including ours. There are no data available in the literature about pregnant mothers with pigmentary mosaicism who suffered complications or about children who suffered complications during gestation or delivery.

Convulsive episodes should be treated similar to seizures of other aetiologies, using anticonvulsant drugs in doses appropriate for the age and weight of the patient. Motor disturbances may be minimized with good physiotherapy and orthopaedic care.

Mental retardation is approached educationally rather than medically and special vocational training should be appropriate to each patient's individual capabilities.

Ocular, oral, urogenital, and other disturbances must receive appropriate individual treatment.

## Genetic counselling

Affected parents should be fully reassured that the risk of the same condition in his/her offspring is low. Peripheral blood Karyotyping is warranted however in the affected child and his/her parents before considering further pregnancies.

Even though the majority of daughters from mothers with balanced X; autosome translocations with breakpoint above the juxtacentromeric X region are likely to be phenotypically normal, an "unfortunate" X inactivation may occur resulting in a severe phenotype. Conversely, reassurance can be given to a phenotypically normal mother, with a balanced X; autosome translocation, having a male offspring with the same translocation that the son will be phenotypically normal although male infertility would be expected (Hatchwell et al. 1996, Ruggieri 2000b).

# References

Afsar FS, Aktas S, Ortac R (2007) Becker's naevus and segmental naevus depigmentosus: an example of twin spotting? Australas J Dermatol 48: 224–246.

Akefeldt A, Gillberg C (1991) Hypomelanosis of Ito in three cases with autism and autistic-like conditions. Develop Med Child Neurol 33: 737–743.

Alkemade H, Juhlin L (2000) Unilateral lentiginosis with nevus depigmentosus on the other side. J Am Acad Dermatol 43: 361–363.

Amon M, Menapace R, Kirnbauer R (1990) Ocular symptomatology in familial hypomelanosis of Ito. Ophthalmologica 200: 1–6.

Ardinger HH, Bell WE (1986) Hypomelanosis of Ito. Wood's light and magnetic resonance imaging as diagnostic measures. Arch Neurol 43: 848–850.

Baba M, Akcali C, Seçkin D, Happle R (2002) Segmental lentiginosis with ipsilateral nevus depigmentosus: another example of twin spotting? Eur J Dermatol 12: 319–321.

Ballmer-Weber BK, Inaebnit D, Brand CU, Baathen LR (1996) Sporadic hypomelanosis of Ito with focal hypertrichosis in a 16-months-old girl. Dermatology 193: 63–64.

Bardazzi F, Balestri R, Antonucci A, Spadola G (2008) Lentigines within nevus depigmentosus: a rare collateral effect of UVB therapy? Pediatr Dermatol 25: 272–274.

Barkovich AJ (2005) The Phakomatoses. In: Barkovich AJ (ed.) Pediatric Neuroimaging. 4th ed. Philadelphia: Lippincott Williams & Wilkins, pp. 440–505.

Bartholomew DW, Jabs EW, Levin LS, Ribovich R (1987) Single maxillary central incisor and coloboma in hypomelanosis of Ito. Clin Genet 31: 370–373.

Battistella PA, Peserico A, Bertoli P, Drigo P, Laverda AM, Casara GL (1990) Hypomelanosis of Ito and hemimegalencephaly. Childs Nerv Syst 6: 421–423.

Bhushan V, Gupta RR, Weinreb J, Kairam R (1989) Unusual brain MRI findings in a patient with hypomelanosis of Ito. Pediatr Radiol 20: 104–104.

Blaschko A (1901) Der Nervenverteilung in der Haut ihrer Bezielung zu den Erkrankungen der Haut. Wien: Wilhelm Braumuller.

Bologna JL, Orlow SJ, Glick SA (1994) Lines of Blaschko. J Am Acad Dermatol 31: 157–190.

Browne RM, Byrne JPH (1976) Dental dysplasia in incontinentia pigmenti achromians (Ito). An unusual form. Br Dent J 140: 211–214.

Chen HH, Liao YH (2004) Coexistence of congenital linear punctate keratoderma and nevus depigmentosus with lentigines: a case of twin spotting? Acta Derm Venereol 84: 408–410.

Cram DL, Fukuyama K (1974) Unilateral systemised hypochromic nevus. Arch Dermatol 109: 416.

David TJ (1981) Hypomelanosis of Ito: a neurocutaneous syndrome. Arch Dis Child 56: 798–800.

Dawn G, Dhar S, Handa S, Kanwar AJ (1995) Nevus depigmentosus associated with hemihypertrophy of the limbs. Pediatr Dermatol 12: 286–287.

Di Lernia V (1999) Segmental nevus depigmentosus: analysis of 20 patients. Pediatr Dermatol 16: 349–353.

Di Lernia V (2007) Linear and whorled hypermelanosis. Pediatr Dermatol 24: 205–210.

Dippel E, Utikal J, Feller G, Fackel N, Klemke CD, Happle R, Goerdt S (2003) Nevi flammei affecting two contralateral quadrants and nevus depigmentosus: a new type of phacomatosis pigmentovascularis? Am J Med Genet A 119: 228–230.

Donnai D, McKeown C, Andrews T, Read AP (1986) Diploid/triploid mixoploidy and hypomelanosis of Ito. Lancet 21: 1443–1444.

Donnai D, Read AP, McKeown C, Andrews T (1988) Hypomelanosis of Ito: a manifestation of mosaicism or chimaerism. J Med Genet 25: 809–818.

Echenne BP, Leboucq N, Humbertclaude V (1995) Ito hypomelanosis and moya-moya disease. Pediatr Neurol 13: 179–181.

Edelstein S, Naidich TP, Newton TH (2005) The rare phakomatoses. In: Tortori-Donati P (ed.) Pediatric Neuroradiology. Brain. Berlin: Springer, pp. 819–854.

Esquivel EE, Pitt MC, Boyd SG (1991) EEG findings in hypomelanosis of Ito. Neuropediatrics 22: 216–219.

Feuerman EJ, Wolf R (1982) Incontinentia pigmenti achromians (systematized depigmented nevus). Hautarzt 33: 159–161.

Flannery DB (1990) Pigmentary dysplasias, hypomelanosis of Ito and genetic mosaicism. Am J Med Genet 35: 18–21.

Flannery DB, Byrd JR, Freeman WE, Perlman SA (1985) A cutaneous marker of chromosomal mosaicism. Am J Hum Genet 37: A93.

Fritz B, Küster W, Orstavik KH, Naumova A, Spranger J, Rehder H (1998) Pigmentary mosaicism in hypomelanosis of Ito. Further evidence for functional disomy of Xp. Hum Genet 103: 441–449.

Fryburg JS, Lin KY, Matsumoto J (1996) Abnormal head MRI in a neurologically normal boy with hypomelanosis of Ito. Am J Med Genet 66: 200–203.

Fukai K, Ishii M, Kadoya A, Hamada T, Wakamatsu K, Ito S (1993) Nevus depigmentosus systematicus with partial yellow scalp hair due to selective suppression of eumelanogenosis. Pediatr Dermatol 10: 205–208.

Glover MT, Brett EM, Atherton DJ (1989) Hypomelanosis of Ito: spectrum of the disease. J Pediatr 115: 75–80.

Golden SE, Kaplan AM (1986) Hypomelanosis of Ito: neurologic complications. Pediatr Neurol 2: 170–174.

Griffihs A, Payne C (1975) Incontinentia pigmenti achromians. Arch Dermatol 111: 751–752.

Grosshans EM, Stoebner P, Bergoend H, Stoll C (1971) Incontinentia pigmenti achromians (Ito): etude clinique et histopathologique. Dermatologica 142: 65–78.

Gül U, Cakmak SK, Gönül M, Kiliç A, Bilgili S (2008) Pediatric skin disorders encountered in a dermatology outpatient clinic in Turkey. Pediatr Dermatol 25: 277–278.

Hamada K, Tanaka T, Ohdo S, Hayakawa K, Kikuchi I, Katsuya H (1979) Incontinentia pigmenti achromians as part of a neurocutaneous syndrome: a case report. Brain Dev 1: 313–317.

Hamada T, Saito T, Sugai T, Morita Y (1967) Incontinentia pigmenti achromians (Ito). Arch Dermatol 96: 673–676.

Happle R (1985) Lyonization and the lines of Blaschko. Hum Genet 70: 200–206.

Happle R (1986) Lyonization and the lines of Blaschko. Hum Genet 70: 200–206.

Happle R (1990) Absence de bipolarité dans les lignes de Blaschko. Ann Dermatol Venereol 117: 397.

Happle R (1993) Mosaicism in human skin. Understanding the patterns and mechanisms. Arch Dermatol 129: 1460–1470.

Happle R (1997a) Segmental forms of autosomal dominant skin disorders: different types of severity reflect different states of zygosity. Am J Med Genet 66: 241–242.

Happle R (1997b) A rule concerning the segmental manifestations of autosomal dominant skin disorders: review of clinical examples providing evidence for dichotomous types of severity. Arch Dermatol 133: 1505–1509.

Happle R (1998) Incontinentia pigmenti versus hypomelanosis of Ito: The whys and wherefores of a confusing issue. Am J Med Genet 79: 64–65 (letter).

Happle R (2001) Phylloid hypomelanosis and mosaic trisomy 13: a new etiologically defined neurocutaneous syndrome Hautarzt 52: 3–5.

Happle R (2004) Patterns on the skin. New aspects of their embryologic and genetic causes Hautarzt 55: 960-961, 964–968.

Happle R (2005) Principles of genetics, mosaicism and molecular biology. In: Harper J, Oranje A, Prose N (eds.). Textbook of Pediatric Dermatology. 2nd ed. Oxford: Blackwell Science, pp. 1221–1246.

Happle R (2006) X-chromosome inactivation: role in skin disease expression. Acta Paediatr Suppl 95: 16–23.

Happle R, Vakilzadeh F (1982) Harmatomatous dental cusps in hypomelanosis of Ito. Clin Genet 21: 65–68.

Happle R, Fuhrmann-Rieger A, Fuhrmann W (1984) Wie verlaufen die Blaschko-Lienen am behaarten Kopf? Hautarzt 35: 366–369.

Hara M, Kozasa M, Mituisi Y, Yajima K, Saito K, Fukuyama Y (1989) Ito syndrome (Hypomelanosis of Ito) as a cause of intractable epilepsy. In: Pascual-Castroviejo I (ed.) Trastornos Neuroectodérmicos. Barcelona. JR Prous, pp. 221–225.

Hatchwell E (1996) Hypomelanosis of Ito and X;autosome translocations: a unifying hypothesis. J Med Genet 33: 177–183.

Hatchwell E, Robinson D, Crolla JA, Cockwell AE (1996) X inactivation analysis in a female with hypomelanosis of Ito associated with a balanced X; 17 translocation: evidence for functional disomy of Xp. J M Genet 33: 216–220.

Hodgson SV, Neville B, Jones RWA, Fear C, Bobrow M (1985) Two cases of X/autosome translocation in females with incontinentia pigmenti. Hum Genet 71: 231–234.

Hong SP, Ahn SY, Lee WS (2008) Linear and whorled nevoid hypermelanosis: unique clinical presentations and their possible association with chromosomal abnormality inv(9). Arch Dermatol 144: 415–416.

Horn D, Happle R, Neitzel H, Kunze J (2002) Pigmentary mosaicism of the hyperpigmented type in two half brothers. Am J Med Genet 112: 65–69.

In SI, Kang HY (2008) Partial unilateral lentiginosis colocalized with naevus depigmentosus. Clin Exp Dermatol 33: 337–339.

Ishikawa T, Kanayama M, Sugiyama K, Katoh T, Wada Y (1985) Hypomelanosis of Ito associated with benign tumors and chromosomal abnormalities: a neurocutaneous syndrome. Brain Dev 7: 45–49.

Ito M (1952) Studies of melanin XI. Incontinentia pigmenti achromians: a singular case of nevus depigmentosus systematicus bilateralis. Tohoku Exper Med 55 (suppl): 57–59.

Jackson R (1976) Blaschko's lines: a review and reconsideration of observations on the cause of certain unusual linear conditions of the skin. Bt J Dermatol 95: 349–360.

Jackson R (1977) Correspondence. Br J Dermatol 97: 341–342.

Jagia R, Mendiratt V, Koranne RV, Sardana K, Bhushan P, Solanki RS (2004) Colocalized nevus depigmentosus and lentigines with underlying breast hypoplasia: a case of reverse mutation? Dermatol Online J 10: 12.

Jelinek JE, Bart RS, Shiff GM (1973) Hypomelanosis of Ito "Incontinentia pigmenti achromians" Arch Dermatol 107: 596–601.

Jimbow K, Fitzpatrick TB, Szabo G, Hori Y (1975) Congenital circumscribed hypomelanosis: a characterization based on electron microscopic study of tuberous sclerosis, nevus depigmentosus, and piebaldism. J Invest Dermatol 64: 50–62.

Jones KL (2005) Smith's RecognizabÚe Patterns of Human Malformation. Philadelphia: Saunders.

Kalter DC, Griffiths WA, Atherton DJ (1988) Linear and whorled nevoid hypermelanosis. J Am Acad Dermatol 19: 1037–1044.

Kim SK, Kang HY, Lee ES, Kim YC (2006) Clinical and histopathologic characteristics of nevus depigmentosus. J Am Acad Dermatol 55: 423–428.

Kim do Y, Park YK, Hann SK (2008) Recurrence of nevus depigmentosus after an autologous epidermal graft. J Am Acad Dermatol 58: 527–529.

Kimura M, Yoshino K, Maeoka Y, Suzuki N (1994) Hypomelanosis of Ito: MR findings. Pediatr Radiol 24: 68–69.

Khandpur S, Sumanth MK (2005) Systematized nevus depigmentosus. Indian Pediatr 42: 1046–1047.

Koiffmann CP, de Souza DH, Diament A, Ventura HB, Alves RS, Kihara S, Wajntal A (1993) Incontinentia pigmenti achromians (Hypomelanosis of Ito, MIM 146 150): Further evidence of localization at Xp11. Am J Med Genet 46: 529–533.

Küster W, König A (1999) Hypomelanosis of Ito: no entity, but a cutaneous sign of mosaicism. Am J Med Genet 85: 346–350.

Lancet (1992) Hypomelanosis of Ito. Editorial. Lancet 339: 651–652.

Lestringant GG, Topley J, Sztriha L, Frossard PM (1977) Hypomelanosis of Ito may or may not involve hair growth. Dermatology 195: 71–72.

Lungarotti MS, Martello C, Calabro A, Baldari F, Mariotti G (1991) Hypomelanosis of Ito associated with chromosomal translocation involving Xq11. Am J Med Genet 40: 447–448.

Maize JC, Headington JT, Lynch PJ (1972) Systematized hypochromic nevus. Incontinentia pigmenti achromians of Ito. Arch Dermatol 106: 884–885.

Malherbe V, Pariente D, Tardieu M, Lacroix C, Venencie PY, Hibon D, Vedrenne J, Landrieu P (1993) Central nervous system lesions in hypomelanosis of Ito: an MRI and pathological study. J Neurol 240: 302–304.

Marohashi M, Hashimoto K, Gooman TF, Newton DE, Rist T (1977) Ultrastructural studies of vitiligo. Vogt-Koyanagi syndrome, and incontinentia pigmenti achromians. Arch Dermatol 113: 755–766.

Masumizu T (1963) Incontinentia pigmenti achromians. Jpn J Dermatol 73: 303.

Meinecke P, Müller EP, Happle R (1985) Das Ito-syndrom (Hypomelanosis of Ito). "Incontinentia pigmenti achromians". Pädiatr Praxis 32: 129–137.

Metzker A, Morag C, Weitz R (1982) Segmental pigmentation disorder. Acta Derm Venereol (Stockh) 63: 1276–1269.

Montagna P, Procaccianti G, Galli G, Ripamonti, Patrizi A, Baruzzi A (1991) Familial hypomelanosis of Ito. Eur Neurol 31: 345–347.

Moss C (1999) Cytogenetic and molecular evidence for cutaneous mosaicism: the ectodermal origin of Blaschko lines. Am J Med Genet 85: 330–333.

Moss C, Burn J (1988) Genetic counseling in hypomelanosis of Ito: case report and review. Clin Genet 4: 109–115.

Moss C, Savin J (1995) Dermatology and the new genetics. Oxford, Blackwell Science.

Moss C, Larkins S, Stacy M, Blight A, Ferndon PA, Davison EV (1993) Epidermal mosaicism and Blaschko's lines. J Med Genet 30: 752–755.

Nehal KS, Pe Benito R, Orlow SJ (1996) Analysis of 54 cases of hypopigmentation and hyperpigmentation along the lines of Blaschko. Arch Dermatol 132: 1167–1170.

Ogino T, Hata H, Minakuchi E, Iyoda K, Narahara K, Ohtahara S (1994) Neurophysiologic dysfunction in hypomelanosis of Ito: EEG and evoked potential studies. Brain Dev 16: 407–412.

Oguma E, Aihara T, Shimanuki Y, Moritani T, Kikuchi A, Imaizumi S, Ogawa Y, Fukushima Y, Samejima T (1996) Hypomelanosis of Ito associated with neuroblastoma. Pediatr Radiol 26: 273–275.

Ogunbiyi AO, Ogunbiyi JO (1998) Nevus depigmentosus and inflammatory linear epidermal nevus – an unusual combination with a note on histology. Int J Dermatol 37: 600–602.

Ohashi H, Tsukahara M, Murano I, Naritomi K, Nishioka K, Miyake S, Kajii T (1992) Pigmentary dysplasias and chromosomal mosaicism: report of nine cases. Am J Med Genet 43: 716–721.

Ono J, Harada K, Kodaka R, Ishida M, Okada S (1997) Regional cortical dysplasia associated with suspected hypomelanosis of Ito. Pediatr Neurol 17: 252–254.

Ortonne JP, Coiffet J, Floret D (1979) Hypomelanosis of Ito: report of one case (author's transl) Ann Dermatol Venereol 106: 47–50.

Pascual-Castroviejo I (1989) Hipomelanosis de Ito. Alteraciones neurológicas en una serie de 48 casos. In Trastornos neuroectodermicos. Pascual-Castroviejo I (ed.) Barcelona. JR Prous: 127–137.

Pascual-Castroviejo I (2004) Hypomelonosis of Ito. In: Roach ES, Miller VS (eds.) "Neurocutaneous Disorders". Cambridge: Cambridge University Press, pp. 123–130.

Pascual-Castroviejo I, Lopez Martin V, Tendero A, Martinez Bermejo A, Lopez-Terradas JM, Roche C (1989a) Epidemiología y experiencia personal de los trastornos neuroectodérmicos. Barcelona. JR Prous, In: Pascual-Castroviejo I (ed.) Trastornos Neuroectodérmicos. Barcelona JR Prous: 1–71.

Pascual-Castroviejo I, Lopez Rodriguez L, de la Cruz Medina M, Salamanca Maesso C, Roche Herrero C (1988) Hypomelanosis of Ito. Neurological complications in 34 cases. Can J Neurol Sc 15: 124–129.

Pascual-Castroviejo I, Roche MC, Martinez Fernandez V, Pérez-Romero M, Escudero RM, Garcia-Peñas JJ et al. (1994) Incontinentia pigmenti: MR demonstration of brain changes. Am J Neuroradiol 15: 1521–1527.

Pascual-Castroviejo I, Roche C, Martinez-Bermejo A, Arcas J, Lopez-Martin V, Tendero A et al. (1998) Hypomelanosis of Ito. A study of 76 infantile cases. Brain Dev 20: 36–43.

Patrizi A, Masina M, Varrotti C (1987) Familial hypomelanosis of Ito. Pediatr Dermatol News 6: 302–305.

Peña L, Ruiz-Maldonado R, Tamayo L, Astengo OC, Gonzalez-Mendoza A (1977) Incontinentia pigmenti achromians (Ito's hypomelanosis). Int J Dermatol 16: 194–202.

Peserico A, Battistella PA, Bertoli P, Drigo P (1988) Unilateral hypomelanosis of Ito with hemimegalencephaly. Acta Paediatr Scand 77: 446–447.

Pinheiro A, Mathew MC, Thomas M, Jacob M, Srivastava VM, Cherian R, Raju R, George R (2007) The clinical profile of children in India with pigmentary anomalies along the lines of Blaschko and central nervous system manifestations Pediatr Dermatol 24: 11–17.

Pini G, Faulkner LB (1995) Cerebellar involvement in hypomelanosis of Ito. Neuropediatrics 26: 208–210.

Pinol J, Mascaró JM, Romaguera C, Asprer J (1969) Considèrations sur l'incontinentia pigmenti achromians de Ito: a propos de deux nouveaux cas. Bull Soc Fr Dermatol Syphiligr 76: 533–535.

POSSUM (2006) Pictures of Standard Syndromes and Undiagnosed Malformations. Version 7.0. Melbourne: Murdoch Institute for Research into Birth Defects.

Quecedo E, Febrer I, Aliaga A (1997) Linear and whorled naevoid hypermelanosis. A spectrum of pigmentary disorders. Pediatr Dermatol 14: 247–248.

Raskovic D, Bondanza S, Gobello T, Luci A, Zambruno G, Happle R, Guerra L (2006) Autologous in vitro reconstituted epidermis in the treatment of a large nevus depigmentosus. J Am Acad Dermatol 54(5 Suppl): S238–S240.

Ritter CL, Steele MW, Wenger SL, Cohen BA (1990) Chromosome mosaicism in hypomelanosis of Ito. Am J Med Genet 35: 14–17.

Riyaz A, Riyaz N, Anoop P, Chansni B, Noushad K (2004) Hemihypertrophy and primary small intestinal lymphangiectasia in incontinentia pigmenti achromians. Ind J Pediatr 71: 947.

Rosenberg S, Artia FN, Campos C, Alonso F (1984) Hypomelanosis of Ito. Case report with involvement of the central nervous system and review of the literature. Neuropediatrics 15: 52–55.

Ross DL, Liwnicz BH, Chun RWM, Gilbert E (1982) Hypomelanosis of Ito (incontinentia pigmenti achromians) – a clinicopathologic study: Macrocephaly and gray matter heterotopias. Neurology 32: 1013–1016.

Rubin MB (1972) Incontinentia pigmenti achromians. Multiple cases within a family. Arch Dermatol 105: 424–425.

Rufo M, Sierra J (1996). Facomatosis con discromias extensas: incontientia pigmenti, nevus acrómico. Rev Neurol 24: 1060–1067.

Ruggieri M (2000) "Cutis tricolor": congenital hyper- and hypopigmented lesions in a background of normal skin, with and without associated systemic features: further expansion of the phenotype. Eur J Pediatr 159: 745–749.

Ruggieri M (2000) Familial hypomelanosis of Ito: implications for genetic counseling. Am J Med Genet 95: 82–84.

Ruggieri M, Pavone L (2000) Hypomelanosis of Ito: clinical syndrome or just phenotype? J Child Neurol 15: 635–644.

Ruggieri M, Pavone L (2007) Hypomelanosis of Ito. San Diego: MedLink Neurology Database. http://www.medlink.com

Ruggieri M, Tigano G, Mazzone D, Tiné A, Pavone L (1996) Involvement of the white matter in hypomelanosis of Ito (incontinentia pigmenti achromiens). Neurology 46: 485–492.

Ruggieri M, Polizzi A, Franzò A, Tiné A, Pavone L (1996) Speech and language disabilities in association with parietotemporal white matter anomalies in hypomelanosis of Ito: an anatomical substrate for a behavioural phenotype? Ann Neurol 40: 312–313 (Abstract).

Ruggieri M, Magro G, Polizzi A (2001) Tumours and hypomelanosis of Ito. Arch Pathol Lab Med 125: 599–601.

Ruggieri M, Iannetti P, Pavone L (2003) Delineation of a newly recognised neurocutaneous malformation syndrome with "cutis tricolor". Am J Med Genet 120A: 110–116.

Ruggieri V, Granana N, Palacios C (1998) Nervous system involvement in 38 children with hypomelanosis of Ito. Brain Dev 20: 372 (Abstract).

Ruiz-Maldonado R, Toussaint S, Tamayo L, Laterza A, del Castillo V (1992) Hypomelanosis of Ito: Diagnostic criteria and report of 41 cases. Pediat Dermatol 9: 1–10.

Sacrez R, Gigonnet JM, Stoll C (1970) Quatre cas de maladie d'Ito familiale (encephalopathia congenitale et dyschromie). Rev Intern Pediatr 7: 5–23.

Sáxena U, Ramesh V, Iyengar B, Misra RS (1989) Hypomelanosis of Ito. Histochemical and ultrastructural observations. Austral J Dermatol 30: 45–47.

Schwartz MF, Esterly NB, Fretzin DF, Pergament E, Rozenfeld IH (1977) Hypomelanosis of Ito (incontinentia pigmenti achromians): A neurocutaneous syndrome. J Pediatr 90: 236–240.

Sharma P, Pai HS, Kamath MM (2008) Nevus depigmentosus affecting the iris and skin: a case report. J Eur Acad Dermatol Venereol 22: 634–635.

Shih IH, Lin JY, Chen CH, Hong HS (2007) A birthmark survey in 500 newborns: clinical observation in two northern Taiwan medical center nurseries. Chang Gung Med J 30: 220–225.

Shim JH, Seo SJ, Song KY, Hong CK (2002) Development of multiple pigmented nevi within segmental nevus depigmentosus. J Korean Med Sci 17: 133–136.

Smahi A, Courtois G, Vabres P, Yamaoka S, Heuertz S, Munnich A, Israel A, Heiss NS, Klauck SM, Kioschis P, Wiemann S, Poustka A, Esposito T, Bardaro T, Gianfrancesco F, Ciccodicola A, D'Urso M, Woffendin H, Jakins T, Donnai D, Stewart H, Kenwrick SJ, Aradhya S, Yamagata T, Levy M, Lewis RA, Nelson DL (2000) Genomic rearrangement in NEMO impairs NF-kappaB activation and is a cause of incontinentia pigmenti. The International Incontinentia Pigmenti (IP) Consortium. Nature 405: 466–472.

Steichen-Gersdorf E, Tragower R, Duba HC, Mayr U, Felber S, Utermann G (1993) Hypomelanosis of Ito in a girl with plexus papilloma and translocation (X; 17). Hum Genet 90: 611–613.

Steiner J, Adamsbaum C, Desguerres I, Lalande G, Raynaud F, Ponsot G (1996) Hypomelanosis of Ito and brain abnormalities: MRI findings and literature review. Pediatr Radiol 26: 763–768.

Stewart RE, Funderburk S, Setoguchi Y (1979) A malformation complex of ectrodactyly, clefting and hypomelanisis of Ito (incontinentia pigmenti achromians). Cleft Palat J 16: 358–362.

Stoebner P, Grosshans EM (1970) Incontinentia pigmenti achromians (Ito): Etude ultrastructurale. Arch Klin Exper Dermatol 239: 227–240.

Sybert VP (1994) Hypomelanosis of Ito: A description, not a diagnosis. J Invest Dermatol 103: 141S–143S.

Sybert VP, Pagon RA (1994) Hypomelanosis of Ito in a girl with plexus papilloma and translocation (X;17) Hum Genet 93: 227.

Sybert VP, Pagon RA, Donlan M, Bradley CM (1990) Pigmentary abnormalities and mosaicism for chromosomal aberration: association with clinical features similar to hypomelanosis of Ito. J Pediatr 116: 581–586.

Tagawa T, Otani K, Futagi Y, Arai H, Mushiake S, Nakayama M, Morita Y (1984) Hypomelanosis of Ito associated with hemimegalencephaly. No To Hattatus 26: 518–521.

Taibjee SM, Bennett DC, Moss C (2004) Abnormal pigmentation in hypomelanosis of Ito and pigmentary

mosaicism: the role of pigmentary genes. B J Dermatol 151: 269–282.

Taniguchi S, Tsuruta D, Higashi J, Hamada T (1995) Coexistence of generalized milia and naevus depigmentosus. Br J Dermatol 132: 317–318.

Tateno A, Sasaki S, Tsukimoto I, Mizuno K (1981) A case of incontinentia pigmenti achromians with acute lymphatic leukemia. Shonika Rinsho 34: 831–835.

Thomas T, Frias JL, Cantu ES, Lafer CZ, Flannery DB, Graham JG (1989) Association of pigmentary anomalies with chromosomal and genetic mosaicism and chimerism. Am J Hum Genet 45: 193–205.

Turleau C, Taillard F, Doussau de Bezignan M, Delépine N, Desbois JC, de Grouchy J (1984) Hypomelanosis of Ito (incontinentia pigmenti achromians) and mosaicism for a microdeletion of 15q1. Hum Genet 74: 185–187.

Urgellés E, Pascual-Castroviejo I, Roche C, Hernandez Moneo JL, Martinez MA, Vega A (1996) Arteriovenous malformation in hypomelanosis of Ito. Brain Dev 18: 78–80.

Van Krieken JHJM, Boom BW, Scheffer E (1988) Malignant transformation in a nevus of Ito. A case report. Histopathology 12: 100–102.

Various Authors (1998) Mosaicism in human skin. Proceedings of a symposium in honour of Rudolf Happle. Marburg, Germany. Am J Med Genet 1999; 85: 323–364.

Vergine G, Mencarelli F, Diomedi-Camassei F, Caridi G, El Hachem M, Ghiggeri GM, Emma F (2008) Glomerulocystic kidney disease in hypomelanosis of Ito. Pediatr Nephrol Apr 5 [Epub ahead of print].

Vormittag W, Ensinger C, Raff M (1992) Cytogenetic and dermatoglyphic findings in a familial case of hypomelanosis of Ito (incontinentia pigmenti achromians). Clin Genet 41: 309–314.

Williams DW, Elster AD (1990) Cranial MR imaging in hypomelanosis of Ito. J Comp Assist Tomogr 14: 981–983.

Winter RM, Baraitser M (2006) Winter-Baraitser Dysmorphology Database. Oxford, Oxford University Press.

Xu AE, Huang B, Li YW, Wang P, Shen H (2008) Clinical, histopathological and ultrastructural characteristics of naevus depigmentosus. Clin Exp Dermatol Mar 18 [Epub ahead of print].

Zajac V, Kirchhoff T, Levy ER, Horsley SW, Miller A, Steichen-Gersdorf E, Monaco AP (1997) Characterisation of X;17(q12q13) translocation breakpoints in a female patient with hypomelanosis of Ito and choroid plexus papilloma. Eur J Hum Genet 5: 61–68.

Zappella M (1993) Autism and hypomelanosis of Ito in twins. Develop Med Child Neurol 35: 826–832.

Zvulunov A, Esterly NB (1995) Neurocutaneous syndromes associated with pigmentary skin lesions. J Am Acad Dermat 32: 915–935.

# Chapter 17

# PHYLLOID HYPOMELANOSIS

**Carmelo Schepis**

Unit of Dermatology, I.R.C.C.S. OASI Maria Santissima, Troina, Italy

## Introduction

Phylloid hypomelanosis is a peculiar pigmentary disorder related to the mosaicism on the human skin resembling a leaf-like or a floral ornament. This pattern of mosaicism is strongly related to mosaic trisomy involving chromosome 13 (Happle 2000). A severe mental retardation and various dysmorphic features are the extra-cutaneous manifestations more frequently associated with it (Horn et al. 1997, Ribeiro Noce et al. 2001, Schepis et al. 2001).

## Historical perspective and terminology

The term phylloid was coined and introduced in the international literature by Happle (1993) to describe the patterns of mosaicism in human skin: Type 1 follows the lines of Blaschko on narrow or broad bands; Type 2, called "checkerboard", consists of alternate squares of hyperpigmentation with a midline separation; Type 3 or "phylloid" pattern presents with hypo- or hyperchromic maculae which look like a floral ornament with a midline separation (Fig. 1); Type 4 consists of a large patchy pattern without separation on the midline.

The Greek term of "*phylloid*" means similar to a leaf.

## Incidence and prevalence

Phylloid hypomelanosis is a very rare condition and less than 10 cases have been documented until now in the literature (Hansen et al. 2003). In a recent review of 1,188 cases of nevi of various shapes and patterns no cases of phylloid shape have been observed (Torrelo et al. 2005). The sex ratio calculated on the cases published until now is 8 females/0 males.

## Clinical manifestation

### Skin abnormalities

The maculae are already recognizable in infancy (Happle 1993, Horn et al. 1997, Schepis et al. 2001) but probably are present since the first year of life (Ribero Noce et al. 2001) or at birth (Pillay et al. 1998). The trunk is the region of the body more affected but macules are also present over limbs. The lesions present with a shape of a begonia leaves (Fig. 1), or more irregularly, or like a pear. The majority of these are hypochromic, this justifies the name of phylloid hypomelanosis (Figs. 2, 3), but in some reports surrounding hyperchromic maculae have also been described (Ribero Noce et al. 2001, Schepis et al. 2001) (Fig. 2). Recently, a case of phylloid hyperpigmentation has been described in association with tetrasomy of chromosome 5p (Hansen et al. 2003).

In addition, linear hypopigmented streaks, which look like the pattern of Hypomelanosis of Ito, have been inconstantly detected over the leg (Horn et al. 1997, Schepis et al. 2001).

### Nervous system abnormalities

Since the first well documented cases (Ohashi et al. 1992) the central nervous system (CNS) defects appeared to be part of the spectrum of the disease. All the subjects reported until now showed various degrees of mental retardation or epileptic seizures

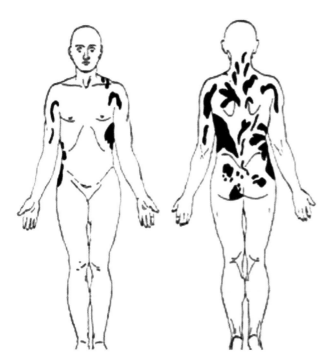

**Fig. 1.** Leaf-shaped or phylloid pattern of mosaicism.

(Happle 2000, Schepis et al. 2001, Ribero Noce et al. 2001, Hansen et al. 2003).

## Abnormalities of other systems and organs

Several facial dysmorphic features have been reported. Microcephaly is frequently detected (Horn et al. 1997, Pillay et al. 1998, Schepis et al. 2001, Ribero Noce et al. 2001) but other different dysmorphic features seem to be often present in the cases described in the literature.

## Pathology

Only one biopsy study of hypochromic maculae is available with histopathological and electron microscopy examination (Pillay et al. 1998) and the histopathological features resembled those of lesions of hypomelanosis of Ito with hypopigmentation due to local loss of functioning melanocytes (Cavallari et al. 1996). Normally, pigmented keratinocytes can

be observed in proximity of preserved melanocytes, whereas no melanocytes or single elements are found in the hypochromic areas of hypomelanosis of Ito.

## Molecular genetics and pathogenesis

### Familial occurrence

The totality of cases reported so far have been observed in females (Happle 2000, Schepis et al. 2001, Ribero Noce et al. 2001, Hansen et al. 2003) but parental transmission has never been described. The risk of recurrence for the parents of the affected patients is calculated to be low (Hansen et al. 2003).

### Pathogenesis

Phylloid Hypomelanosis is interpreted as a peculiar pattern of human genomic mosaicism (Happle 1993). Noteably, the totality of the cases reported are young females, whereas no males have been reported so far.

## Natural history

The Phylloid macular mosaicism has been described in an age range from 8 months to 6 years but we can suppose it to be present since the first infancy. We have no report on the evolution of the cutaneous features, although similar macular forms of mosaicism, such as *"Hypomelanosis of Ito"* and the so-called *"Linear and Whorled Hypermelanosis"*, observed in the clinical practice, undergo spontaneously improvement or fading with age.

## Differential diagnosis

The differential diagnosis of phylloid hypomelanosis is prevalently with linear and whorled dyschromic maculae which follow the "Blaschko lines" (Harre and Millikan 1994, Bolognia et al. 1994).

The first dilemma regards the *"Hypomelanosis of Ito"*. The diagnosis of Hypomelanosis of Ito was

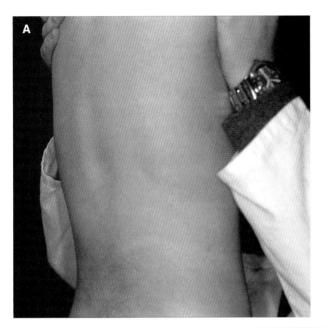

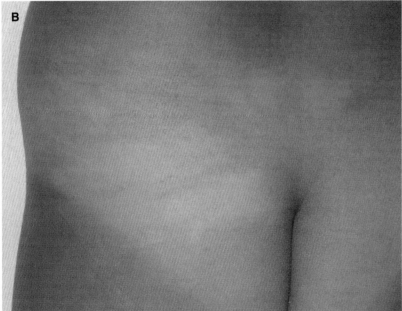

**Fig. 2. (A)** Leaf-shaped hyperpigmentation on the right side, **(B)** phylloid hypopigmentation present with a shape of a begonia leaves on the left buttock.

stressed by Mexican authors (Maldonado et al. 1992) when they described 41 cases from personal series and proposed the guidelines for its diagnosis. The authors invoked the presence of the congenital or early macular hypopigmentations in linear streaks or whorls as a "*sine qua non* criterion" and involving at least two body segments, with one or more major symptoms consistent with CNS or musculoskeletal involvement. More rarely, the pattern of distribution is patchy.

The diagnosis of "*Nevus Depigmentosus*" is used to define a hypomelanotic congenital or an early onset macula in patches or along the Blaschko lines, without systemic involvement. This condition might be considered as a "mild" expression of mosaicism, as opposed to Hypomelanosis of Ito that is a severe condition.

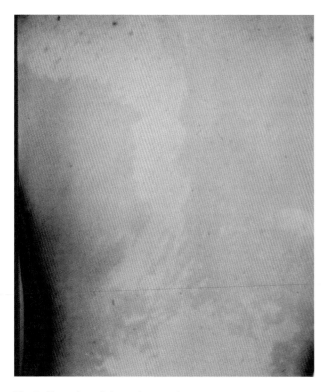

**Fig. 3.** Hypochromic irregular maculae.

*"Linear and Whorled Nevoid Hyperpigmentation"* is a rare well defined condition (Kalter et al. 1988) that appears as the reverse feature of the "Hypomelanosis of Ito", if associated with neurological involvement; it can be considered as the opposite of the *"Nevus Depigmentosus"* if it lacks systemic involvement. This entity has been differently named in the literature; as examples, *"Reticulate Hyperpigmentation* or *Progressive Cribiform and zosteriform Hyperpigmentation"* (Romano et al. 1999). To date many eponyms exist for a single disease with a large spectrum of severity. These conditions do not overlap with phylloid mosaicism because their pattern of distribution is along the lines of Blaschko and because of their lack of association with a specific chromosomal pattern.

Cytogenetic analysis is recommended in the case of cutaneous mosaicism in association with systemic abnormalities, such as mental retardation or birth defects. Recently, a case of Hypomelanosis of Ito has been described in association with Trisomy 13 mosaicism (Ronger et al. 2003) by a group of au-

thors who were revising the few cases reported so far. In our opinion, every patient showing pigmentary dysplasia needs to be investigated by karyotyping. It is likely that the Phylloid Pigmentary Dysplasia is strongly associated with trisomy 13 but such a trisomy might be also detected, occasionally, in association with other forms of human mosaicism.

## Management and follow-up

When Phylloid Mosaicism is suspected, karyotyping of blood and skin biopsy fibroblasts is necessary. The presence of eventual CNS pathology must be assessed and it is recommended to analyze eventual dysmorphic features. Other laboratory and imaging investigations can be performed, according to previous clinical suggestions.

## Treatment

No treatment is available for the cutaneous pigmentary dysplasia.

Neurologic impairment, e.g., seizures and mental retardation, requires treatment and appropriate rehabilitation.

## Genetic counseling

Phylloid Macular Mosaicism is a very infrequent entity. The risk of transmission to affected subjects is considered rather low or absent unless a chromosomal abnormality is detected in parents.

## References

Bolognia JL, Orlow SJ, Glick SA (1994) Lines of Blaschko. J Am Acad Dermatol 31(2-1): 157–190.

Cavallari V, Ussia AF, Siragusa M, Schepis C (1996). Hypomelanosis of Ito: electron microscopical observations on two new cases. J Dermatol Sci 13: 87–92.

Hansen LK, Brandrup F, Rasmussen K (2003) Pigmentary mosaicism with mosaic chromosome 5p tetrasomy. Br J Dermatol 149: 414–416.

Happle R (1993) Mosaicism in human skin: understanding the patterns and mechanism. Arch Dermatol 129: 1460–1470.

Happle R (2000) Phylloid hypomelanosis is closely related to mosaic trisomy 13. Eur J Dermatol 10: 511–512.

Harre J, Millikan LE (1994) Linear and whorled pigmentation. Int J Dermatol 33: 529–537.

Horn D, Rommeck M, Sommer D, Körner H (1997) Phylloid pigmentary pattern with mosaic trisomy 13. Pediatr Dermatol 14: 278–280.

Kalter DC, Griffiths WA, Atherton DJ (1988) Linear and whorled nevoid hypermelanosis. J Am Acad Dermatol 19: 1037–1044.

Ohashi H, Tsukahara M, Murano I, Naritomi K, Nishioka K, Miyake K, Kajii T (1992) Pigmentary dysplasias and chromosomal mosaicism: report of 9 cases. Am J Med Genet 43: 716–721.

Pillay T, Winship WS, Ramdial PK (1998) Pigmentary abnormalities in trisomy of chromosome 13. Clin Dysmorphol 7: 191–194.

Ribeiro Noce T, Montero de Pina-Neto J, Happle R (2001) Phylloid pattern of pigmentary disturbance in a case of complex mosaicism. Am J Med Genet 98: 145–147.

Romano C, Pirrone P, Siragusa M, Schepis C, Cavallari V (1999) An additional case of Linear and Whorled Nevoid Hypermelanosis associated with birth defects and mental retardation. Pediatr Dermatol 16: 71–73.

Ronger S, Till M, Kanitakis J, Balme B, Thomas L (2003) Ètude cytogènètique d'une hypomèlanose de Ito chez une malade atteinte d'une trisomie 13 en mosaïque. Ann Dermatol, Venereol 130: 1033–1038.

Ruiz-Maldonado R, Toussaint S, Tamayo L, Laterza A, del Castillo V (1992) Hypomelanosis of Ito: diagnostic criteria and report of 41 cases. Pediatr Dermatol 9: 1–10.

Schepis C, Failla P, Siragusa M, Romano C (2001) An additional case of macular phylloid mosaicism. Dermatology 202: 73.

Torrelo A, Baselga E, Nagore E, Zambrano A, Happle R (2005) Delineation of the various shapes and patterns of nevi. Eur J Dermatol 15: 439–450.

# Chapter 18

# INCONTINENTIA PIGMENTI

Ignacio Pascual-Castroviejo and Martino Ruggieri

Paediatric Neurology Service, University Hospital La Paz, University of Madrid, Madrid, Spain (IPC); Institute of Neurological Science, National Research Council, Catania, and Department of Paediatrics, University of Catania, Catania, Italy (MR)

## Introduction

Incontinentia pigmenti (IP) or *Bloch–Sulzberger syndrome* (OMIM # 308310), is a rare ectodermal dysplasia that segregates as an X-linked dominant disorder and is usually lethal to affected males in utero. In affected females it causes highly variable congenital abnormalities of the skin, hair, nails, teeth, and eyes associated to non progressive, chronic central nervous system (CNS) involvement (Bruckner 2004). Other anatomical regions are less frequently affected. Development of benign subungual tumors involving distal phalanges in adult age is not rare.

The prominent skin signs occur in 4 classic cutaneous stages: (1) perinatal inflammation with erythematous and vesicular rash; (2) verrucous patches; (3) a distinctive pattern of hyperpigmentation; and (4) dermal scarring. Cells expressing the mutated X chromosome are eliminated selectively around the time of birth, so females with IP exhibit extremely skewed X-inactivation (OMIM™ 2006).

The gene responsible for IP has been mapped to the locus Xq28 (Sefani et al. 1998, Smahi et al. 1994), a region known to encode the nuclear *factor κB essential modulator* (NEMO) (Jin and Jeang 1999). Also known as the *γ-subunit of the inhibitor κB kinase* (IKKγ), NEMO is involved in regulating the *nuclear factor κB* (NF-κB) pathway. NF-κB is a transcription factor that regulates the expression of genes involved in the immune and stress response, ectodermal development, inflammatory reactions, cell adhesion and protection against apoptosis (Bruckner 2004, Smith et al. 2002). Significant mutations in the NEMO gene result in the IP phenotype, with a single deletion in exons 4 through 10 being the culprit in over 80% of cases (The International Incontinentia Pigmenti (IP) Consortium 2000).

## Historical perspective and terminology

The first description of this disorder was by *Garrod* (1906) who in 1905 briefly described a 2$^1$/$_2$-year-old girl who presented with "peculiar pigmentation of the skin" and "scvere neurodevelopment deficits". She reportedly had always been very backward, had never sat or talked, had a brachycephalic head and spastic legs, and was said to have shown "some of the characteristics of the *Mongolian* variety of idiocy" (Garrod 1906). The most remarkable feature of the case was a peculiar pigmentation of the skin, of gray–brown tint, which had a linear distribution and in places was arranged in whorls. A photograph of the child accompanied the report which appeared in *Transaction of the Clinical Society of London* in 1906 (Garrod 1906, Rosman 1987). The second case description was by *Adamson* (1908) who reported on a 19-year-old girl, small and of feeble intellect, whose skin showed a generalized retiform red–brown pigmentation with areas of scarring. The girl laso had absent earlobes, facial asymmetry, patchy alopecia, absence of two fingers on one hand, only four toes on each foot, and two nipples on the right breast (Adamson 1908, Rosman 1987). The next report was by *Bardach* who reported in 1925 on the disorder in identical twins said to have systematized naevi.

The disease, however, is known as IP of Bloch-Sulzberger syndrome (OMIM™ 2006) because of the publications of Bloch (1926) (which represented the fifth case in the literature) who studied a 1$^1$/$_2$-year-old girl with "splashed pigmented skin lesions" and first introduced the term *"incontinentia pigmenti"*, and Sulzberger (1928) who observed the association of other features in the same patient reported two years earlier by Bloch. Though Bloch's original patient was said to have been neurologically intact, one of her eyes had been surgically removed at 1 month of age because of glioma or pseudoglioma (Rosman 1987).

**Bruno Bloch** was a Swiss dermatologist, born January 19, 1878, in Endingen, Canton Aargau and died in 1933 (Obituary 1933, Who named it? 2006) He attended the University of Basel, where he graduated in 1900 obtaining his doctorate in 1902. Bloch received further education at the medical and dermatological clinic in Basel, as well as in Vienna under Gustav Riehl (1855–1943), Berlin, Paris, and in Bern under Josef Jadassohn. In 1908, he was appointed as head of dermatology at the University of Basel. In 1916, he was called to the newly established chair of dermatology at the University of Zurich, where he remained until his death in 1933 (Obituary 1933). Bloch was influenced by Jadassohn in applying laboratory techniques in the study of skin disorders. He made important contributions in the field of allergy and he was an expert on disorders of pigmentation (Who named it? 2006, Sulzberger 1980).

**Marion Baldur Sulzberger** was an American dermatologist, born on March 12, 1895, in New York City and died November 23, 1983 (Who named it? 2006). He was the son of Ferdinand Sulzberger, the owner of one of the largest international meat packing firms in the world. Marion's mother was Stella, his father's third wife. He was a brilliant scholar during his school years, but in his teens he indulged in a rather uninhibited lifestyle, before traveling the world, working as a kitchen hand in Switzerland, a docker in England and a shepherd in Australia (Hunter and Holubar 1984, MacKee 1955). His father died while he was overseas. During World War I Sulzberger was an aviator and eventually achieved the rank of flying instructor. He began his medical studies in Geneva, Switzerland, in 1920, but later changed to the University of Zurich. During this period he came into contact with Josef Jadassohn (1863–1936), professor of dermatology in Bern, and Bruno Bloch (1878–1933), who had been appointed to the chair of dermatology at Zurich. Sulzberger was thus well trained in European dermatology when he returned to America. He entered private practice with Fred Wise (1881–1950), who became his friend and

mentor (Who named it? 2006). During World War II Sulzberger served with the Naval Reserve as a lieutenant commander. He was decorated by the United States and France for his outstanding contributions to the understanding and treatment of the dermatoses caused by poison gases, burns and tropical skin diseases. In 1949, Sulzberger became professor of dermatology and syphilology of the New York University-Bellevue Medical Center. He retired from the chair of dermatology in 1961, but three years later he accepted an appointment as professor of clinical dermatology at the University of California in San Francisco. He retired from his tenure in 1970 (Hunter and Hoular 1984, MacKee 1955, Who named it? 2006).

Notably, the same patient of Bloch (1926) and Sulzberger (1928) was reported once again, in adult life, by Franceschetti and Jadassohn (1954), showing at this age that the skin lesions had completely cleared (Rosman 1987).

The syndrome has also been known as: Asboe-Hansen disease from **Gustav Asboe-Hansen** a Danish physician, born in 1917 who reported on the initial phase of the Bloch–Sulzberger syndrome; and Bloch–Siemens syndrome and Siemens–Bloch pigmented dermatosis from the German dermatologist **Hermann Werner Siemens**, born on August 20, 1891, in Charlottenburg and died in 1969 (Who named it? 2006) who worked for a brief period of time under Josef Jadassohn (1863–1936) in Breslau. Other eponyms are Bloch–Sulzberger melanoblastoma; incontinentia pigmenti 1; melanoblastosis cutis linearis sive systematisata; melanosis corii degenerativa; and nevus pigmentosus systematicus.

## Prevalence and incidence

While over than 700 cases have been reported in the world literature (Berlin et al. 2002, Bruckner 2004, Carney 1976), there are likely many additional cases not diagnosed or reported (Bruckner 2004, Berlin et al. 2002, Morgan 1971) and thus the exact prevalence of IP in so far unknown. The reported series on IP still present only isolated or very few cases, and relatively few series describe eight or more patients (Goldberg and Custis 1993, O'Brien and Feingold 1985, Pascual-Castroviejo et al. 1994, 2006). IP affects individuals of all races. Over 97% of affected individuals are female (Carney 1976). This high female to male sex ratio, coupled with the female to female transmission and a high rate of early spontaneous miscarriages in female carriers supported the X-linked dominant transmission with lethality in males as the mode of inheritance. Surviving males with the classic phenotype are explained by a 47, XXY karyotype (Klinefelter syndrome) or somatic mosaicism (Kenwrick et al. 2001). The most common abnormalities are dental, which are present in 65%, disorders of the eye in 35%, and CNS involvement in 30% (Carney 1976) of cases.

## Clinical manifestations

Dermatological, ocular and CNS are the prevalent and more severe manifestations of IP. Skin, hair and eyes must be studied in the suspect of IP and clinical and imaging studies of the CNS, skeleton, teeth and nails (this, especially in adult age) must be obtained. The only hematological abnormality is the presence of eosinophils, with more than 65% during the stages 1 and 2.

### Skin and appendages

#### Cutaneous manifestations

Skin lesions are the first manifestation of the disease and the hallmark of IP. They usually pass through four distinctive but somewhat overlapping stages. The onset, and duration of each stage vary among patients. Skin lesions usually occur along Blaschko lines, which correspond to migration or growth pathways of skin cells.

The evolution of the disorder is divided into the following stages (Bruckner 2004):

**Stage 1** (*inflammatory stage*): the characteristic lesions are erythematous, macular, popular, vesicular, bullous and, finally, pustular in most cases (Fig. 1).

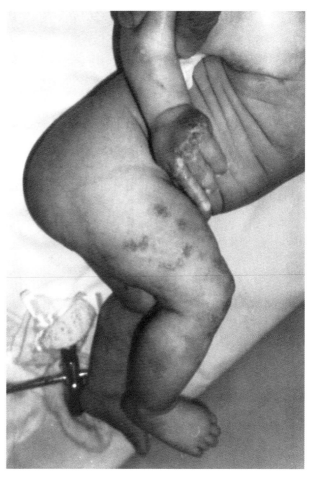

**Fig. 1.** Cutaneous pustular lesions in stage 1.

These can appear anywhere in the body. Lesions in the scalp are often associated with underlying cerebral pathology. They appear within the first 2 weeks in 90% of cases, but in half of these, the lesions are present at birth. Only 10% of cases show the first manifestations of skin abnormalities between the second week and the second month of age. On the limbs, the lesions are linear in distribution and affect proximal, middle and distal areas. Vesicular and bullous skin lesions and the underlying dermis contain eosinophils, and most infants present with eosinophilia. Lesions during the first phase can last from some days to several months. Histological studies of skin biopsies in our patients during the neonatal period when the lesions were in the first stage, demonstrated the presence of free pigment, melanophages, and eosinophils over the superficial dermis (Pascual-Castroviejo et al. 1994). The epidermis showed mild papillomatous lesions with subjacent perivascular inflammation. The basal layer was irregularly pigmented.

**Stage 2** (*verrucous stage*): This is a pustular-verrucous stage. The peak age for this stage is between the second and the sixth weeks, but it can be prolonged during many months or several years. The

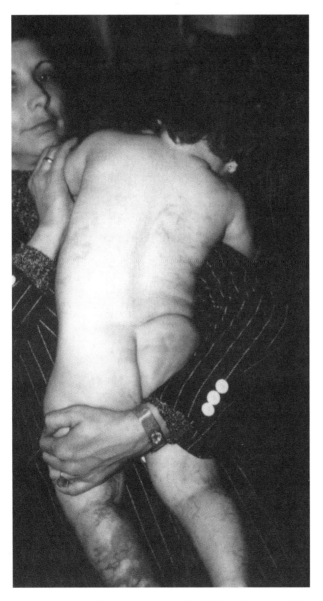

**Fig. 2.** Cutaneous lesions in stage 2. The left leg shows pustular-verrucous lesions and the right leg shows pigmentary lesions.

lesions are variously pustular, lichenoid, verrucous, keratotic, and dyskeratotic (Fig. 2). During this period one can start to notice the changes in the lids, eyelids, eye, nails and hair that follow the cutaneous lesions of the first stage, and abnormalities of teeth eruption are also observed. The lesions are most prominent over the limbs, most frequently on the distal parts of the legs and arms: these may disappear without sequelae, but often are followed by hypopigmentation or atrophy of the skin and, in many cases, of the underlying conjunctival and muscular tissues.

**Stage 3** (*hyperpigmented*): This is the hyperpigmentation (Fig. 3) period. It occurs during months or (few) years, and is the most characteristic stage of IP. The discoloration can show many different configurations, such as streaks, whorls, stellate macules, and flecks of slate gray, chocolate brown, or tan. The pigmentation is most prominent as a circumferential lesion on the trunk and linear is streaks on the limbs, mostly following a pattern along Blaschko's lines. Skin lesions of the second and third stages often overlap in the same patient. The pigmentation commonly persists for many years, and usually begins to fade in the second or third decade of life. Severe lesions in the second stage, particularly in the extremities, usually last many years and the affected skin shows atrophy or violaceus pigmentation.

**Stage 4** (*atrophic stage*): This is a sequelar hypopigmentation (Fig. 4) stage that may persist for the entire life. The skin that showed hyperpigmentation or violaceous scarring appearance changes to hypopigmented color following Blaschko lines. This occurs after the second decade and can most frequently be observed in limbs. Streaked hypomelanotic areas of the calves may be the only dermatological sign of IP in adult life (Wiley and Frias 1974). Hypopigmented skin in adulthood shows the same aspect of the skin lesions of Hypomelanosis of Ito (HI) but the lack of an X-linked pattern of transmission, the static skin lesions and some other characteristics of HI (see chapter on HI and related disorders) can facilitate the differential diagnosis. It is thought than not all patients with IP show the hypopigmented lesions in adulthood, but we could find these after a carefully inspection of the skin in all affected women.

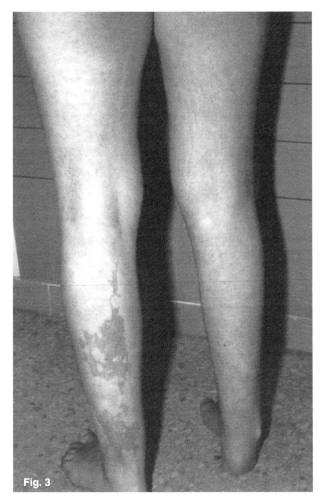
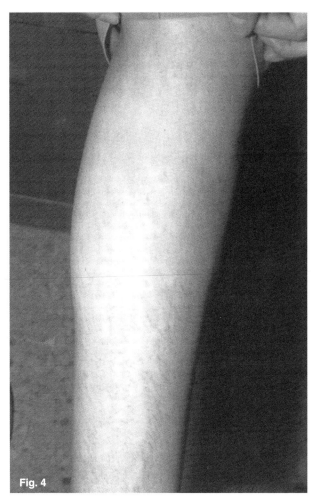

**Figs. 3 and 4.** Same case as Fig. 2. showing lesions in stage 3 (hyperpigmentation of the left leg), and in stage 4 (hypopigmentation) respectively.

## Hair

An additional dermatological finding in IP is alopecia of the scalp, that has been described in more than a third of patients (Carney 1976). It is mostly seen in the stage 4 and not only is there alopecia, but also loss of epidermal glands. Alopecia occurs most frequently in the scalp, especially at the vertex, but it can be found in the trunk and extremities, particularly in areas of skin hypopigmentation where lesions were present during the stages 1, 2 and 3. The hair surrounding the areas of alopecia is coarse, depigmented and wiry (Fig. 5). Similar alterations to the scalp hair can be seen in the eyebrows.

## Nails

Dystrophic changes in nails appear early, commonly during stage 2. Nails may appear streaked, ridging, pitting or brittle. Lesions can become recurrent. During adult life, patients with IP can present sub-ungual tumors (Simmons et al. 1986). They are painful keratotic tumors which must be radically removed despite their histologic benignity (Mascaró et al. 1985). This complication may present in more than one finger of the same hand (Fig. 6), although not all at the same time. These tumors frequently recur and it is necessary to remove again the distal phalanx and seldom the middle phalanx.

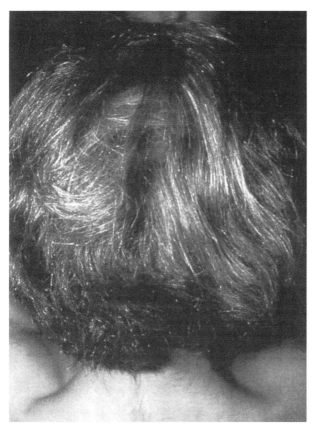

**Fig. 5.** Area of alopecia in the scalp surrounded by coarse and depigmented hair.

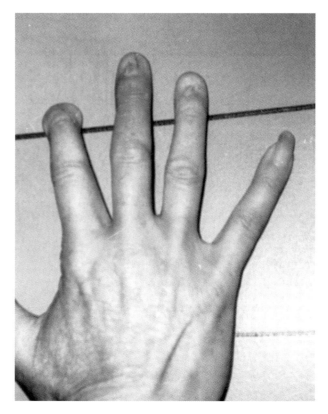

**Fig. 6.** Hand of an adult woman with IP with nails anomalies in the three middle fingers. It lacks the nail and distal phalanx of the second finger which have been removed because of a subungual tumor.

## Non dermatological features

Between 50 and 80% of patients with IP present extracutaneous manifestations. The most important affected organs are the CNS and the eyes, but teeth, skeleton, breast, and other organs or systems may also present changes. Besides eye, teeth, breas, skeletal and CNS abnormalities the other associated findings in IP have reported sporadically and thus they likely appear to be coincidental manifestations not part of the syndrome. The onset of these manifestations is different in every patient.

## Eyes

Ophthalmologic manifestations are present in 35% of cases, and more than half are severe. They may be divided into retinal and non retinal findings. Non retinal associations include microphthalmos (Fig. 7), ptosis, strabismus, cataracts, conjunctival and iris changes of pigmentation, uveitis, myopia, blue sclera, changes of the pupile size, ciliary body atrophy, persistence of the hyaloid artery, absence of the anterior chamber, nystagmus, and optic atrophy. Retinal abnormalities can be subdivided into those in the periphery, which are the most frequent, and those in the posterior pole (Goldberg and Custis 1993). Peripheral abnormalities are: peripheral avascular zone, tortuous and irregular vessels, aneurysmal-like dilatation and neovascular changes, exudates, vitreous hemorrhage, preretinal fibrovascular proliferation, retinal detachment, retinal pigment epithelium mottling/granularity, or with hypopigmentation/coloboma. Posterior pole

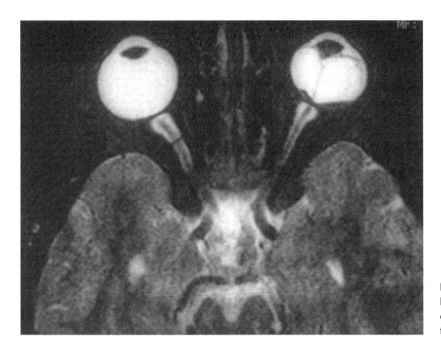

**Fig. 7.** Axial view of the MR study shows the left microphthalmic eye with corpus vitreous and retinal lesions (see right part of the figure).

abnormalities consist of foveal hypoplasia, paramacular vascular dilatations and aneurysms, neovascularization, vitreous hemorrhage, preretinal fibrosis, retinal detachment, retinal pigment epithelium mottling/granularity with hypopigmentation/coloboma. Although all types of ocular lesions can be found, the most typical abnormality is a retrolental mass with detachment of a dysplastic retina; this mass has been called a pseudoglioma, retrolental fibroplasia, or persistent hyperplastic primary vitreous (François 1984). The cause of these abnormalities and other lesions in IP remains uncertain (Bell et al. 2008).

## Teeth

Between 35 and 90% of patients present with teeth abnormalities (Fig. 8), that include delayed dentition, lack of some teeth (the most frequently lacking are both lateral incisors), conical crown deformities, microdontia, or malpositioning. Both deciduous and permanent teeth can be affected. In contrast to the skin manifestations of IP, the dental manifestations are permanent, making them an

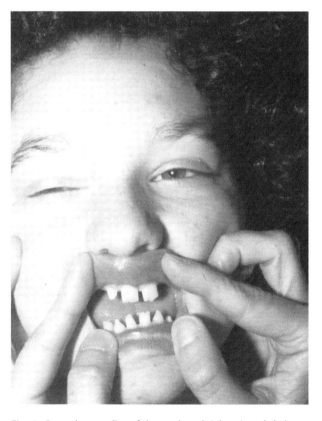

**Fig. 8.** Several anomalies of the teeth and right microphthalmus.

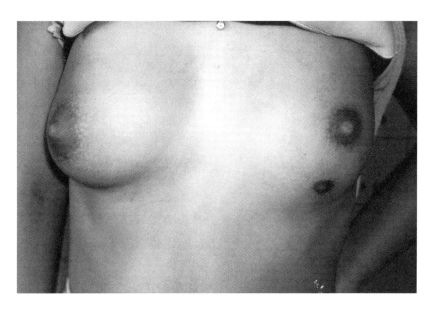

**Fig. 9.** Asymmetry between both breasts and supernumerary nipple on the left breast.

excellent late marker for the disorder (Bruckner 2004).

## Breast

Manifestations usually include abnormalities of the size and the number. Aplasia of one breast, asymmetry between both breasts, and supernumerary nipples may be found (Fig. 9).

## Skeletal system

More than 20% of patients with IP have some bony abnormality (François 1984, Taybi 1996). Skeletal manifestations usually include skull deformities, extra ribs, hemivertebrae, hip dislocation, spina bifida, syndactyly, shortening of the legs and arms and chondrodystrophy. The presence of club foot and bone hemihypotrophy of the ipsilateral limb and scoliosis are usually present in patients with contralateral cerebral hemiatrophy.

## Other somatic abnormalities

These include alterations which appear occasionally, but they have been described in some patients, such

as ear deformities, cleft lip and palate, genitourinary and cardiovascular anomalies (Morgan 1971). Facial asymmetry in neurological normal adults with IP is often observed.

## Neurological abnormalities

The CNS is affected in 30–50% of patients (Carney 1976), causing mental retardation, seizures, spastic paralysis, microcephaly, somatic malformations – club foot, hemihypotrophy or scoliosis – and cerebellar ataxia. Between 13.3 (O'Brien and Feingold 1985) and 16.4% (Carney 1976) of patients with IP have mental retardation. Generalized or focal seizures are present in 15% (O'Brien and Feingold 1985) and 25% (Pascual-Castroviejo et al. 1994) of patients. Spastic hemiparesis in cases with unilateral lesions of the brain, or bilateral pyramidal disease in patients with lesions in both hemispheres are usually found. The overlap of mental retardation, seizures and ocular abnormalities is often seen. Bilaterality of the brain lesions and seizures in the first week of life may indicate a poor prognosis with subsequent developmental delay, which may be profound in some patients. However, the evolution can be favorable if the brain lesions are not severe despite the bilaterality (Pörksen et al. 2004). Unilateral cerebral lesions, even associated with focal seizures controlled with antiepileptic medication, may develop with hemiparesis and hypotrophic hemibody, but with normal intelligence. Attention deficit and hyperactivity are frequently associated with IP. Brain damage may occur in the prenatal (O'Doherty and Norman 1968, Mangano and Barbagallo 1993), perinatal (Siemes et al. 1978, Frontera Izquierdo et al. 1981, Shuper et al. 1990, Triki et al. 1992), and postnatal (Brunquell 1987) periods.

Magnetic resonance imaging (MRI) does not reveal abnormalities in IP patients without neurologic disease. MRI shows brain changes (developmental and acquired lesions) in most patients with neurologic disease associated with the cutaneous lesions of IP (Edelstein et al. 2005, Loh et al. 2008, Lou et al. 2008, Maingay-de Groof et al. 2007, Pascual-Castroviejo et al. 1994). Abnormalities are located in the cerebral hemisphere contralateral to the most severely affected side of the body and the most

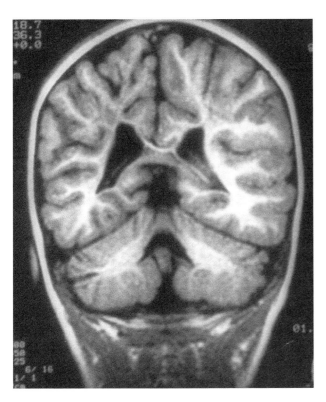

**Fig. 10.** Coronal T$_1$-weighted image shows corticosubcortial atrophy of the right cerebral hemisphere and atrophy of the corpus callosum.

severe MRI changes are subjacent to the scalp areas where the most severe cutaneous lesions appear located in the neonatal period. Hypoplasia of the corpus callosum, probably secondary to atrophy of one or both cerebral hemispheres, may be seen as well (Fig. 10). Abnormal signal and atrophy of the lateral regions of one of the cerebellar hemispheres also are found. Although the changes can be seen in both T$_1$- and T$_2$-weighted images, they are most evident in the latter. Cerebral areas that show MRI signal changes seem to correspond to areas where there is neuronal loss by histological observation and appear as minor dysplasias (O'Doherty and Norman 1968). However, not all of the IP patients have histological findings of this type. In some cases, generally coinciding with an infectious or vaccination process, an encephalitis develops (Siemes et al. 1978, Frontera Izquierdo et al. 1981, Avrahami et al. 1985, Mangano and Barbagallo 1993) that results in cerebral lesions with necrotic cavitation in the grey matter (Siemes et al. 1978, Frontera Izquierdo et al. 1981); in other reports these have been interpreted as originating from a postnatal insult (Hauw et al. 1977). In some of these cases, humoral or cellular immunologic deficiencies have been found (Siemes et al. 1978, Brunquell 1987). A mutant protein with variable expression, capable of causing malformations and encephaloclastic processes in the CNS also has been suggested as origin of the destructive process (Shuper et al. 1990). The pathogenesis of cerebral lesions in IP has been attributed to a microangiopathic process with secondary ischemia at a time of particular vulnerability of the neonatal brain (Hennel et al. 2003).

The dominant pathology in the cerebral white matter, despite involvement of a major vessel, which supplies both white matter and cortex (Hennel et al. 2003), has been related to the particular vulnerability of the neonatal white matter to ischemic insults (Volpe 2001). However, MRI of our patients demonstrated that the lesions extended radially through cortical and subcortical zones, involving cortex, subcortical and deep white matter, ependymal and subependymal zones of one or both cerebral hemispheres (Fig. 11), as well as cortical and subcortical zones of the cerebellar hemispheres (Fig. 12) the most severe lesions located mainly in the subcortical

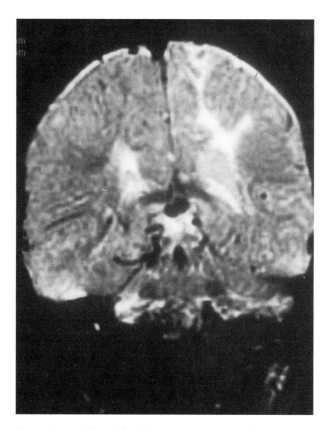

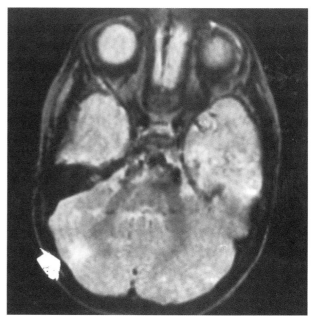

**Fig. 12.** Axial T$_2$-weighted (2000/100) image reveals hyperintense signal in cortico-subcortical zones of the cerebellum with marked predominance in the right side (arrow).

**Fig. 11.** Coronal T$_2$-weighted (2000/100) image reveals asymmetric increased signal in the deep white mater of both cerebral hemispheres, more extensively involving the left side, which also reveals cortical and ependymal involvement.

white matter (Pascual-Castroviejo 1994, 2006). This pathologic finding and the location of the lesions following a radial direction from the cortex to the deep zones of the white matter not always reaching the ependymal or subependymal zones, and the higher frequency of these lesions in cerebral or cerebellar areas subjacent to the scalp lesions of IP in the neonatal period, suggest a relationship between the pathogenesis of the skin and the cerebral lesions. This could be a non-specific inflammatory disease which would include locally arterial vessels as well, as occurs in many cases of Landau–Kleffner syndrome (Pascual-Castroviejo et al. 1992). The inflammatory disease can be of autoimmune origin. Moreover, histologic studies of biopsies from affected skin obtained during the neonatal period show perivascular inflammation. We believe that cutaneous and subjacent

cerebral lesions during the neonatal period have the same pathogenesis. Although both external and internal inflammatory processes commonly present combined in the same patients, there are patients that only show cutaneous or cerebral lesions, but this is not frequently seen.

## Pathology

The histopathological findings of IP vary based on the stage of disease that is biopsied. The findings of the *inflammatory stage* are the most specific for the disease (see above). The combination of eosinophilic spongiosis with dyskeratotic keratinocytes is considered pathognomonic for IP (Machado-Pinto et al. 1996). The epidermal hyperplasia and hyperkeratosis of the *verrucous lesions in the second stage* are also highly suggestive of IP. Edema and intraepidermal eosinophils may persist in this stage but are mild. Scattered melanophages are seen in the papillary dermis (Bruckner 2004). In the *hyperpigmented stage*, prominent dermal melanophages (including incontinence of pigment) are the main histological finding (Bruckner 2004). In this stage, a specific diagnosis of IP cannot be made based on the histology alone as postinflammatory hyperpigmentation appears identical. Stage 4 lesions demonstrate an atrophic epidermis with effacement of the rete ridges. Adnexal structures such as dermal sweat duct coils and pilosebaceous units are reduced or absent as well (Bruckner 2004, Nazzaro et al. 1990, Zillikens et al. 1991).

There have been few postmortem studies of the CNS in IP (O'Doherty and Norman 1968, Hauw et al. 1977, Siemes et al. 1978). Neuropathologic lesions usually consisted of necrotic foci in the white matter and cortex in the affected cerebral hemispheres, probably developing at or around the time of birth , and some cortical areas of polymicrogyria; the cerebellar cortex showed multiple demarcated areas of neuronal loss, resembling minor dysplasias (O'Doherty and Norman 1961). Hauw et al. (1977) reported destructive encephalopathy, apparently of perinatal onset, with cerebral ulegyria, white matter cavitation, scarring of cerebellar cortex, diffuse inflammatory cell infiltration of the pia-arachnoid and brain parenchyma. The case of Siemes et al. (1978) was complicated by a post vaccinal encephalitis and the patient showed evidence of a perivenous encephalitis.

## Pathogenesis and molecular genetics

IP is an X-linked dominant disorder that is usually lethal prenatally in males (OMIM 2006). Cells expressing the mutated X-chromosome are eliminated selectively around the time at birth, and females with IP exhibit extremely skewed X-inactivation (Parrish et al. 1996).

The gene responsible for IP has been mapped to the locus Xq28 (Sefani et al. 1989, Smahi et al. 1994), a region known to encode the nuclear *factor κB essential modulator* (NEMO) (Jin and Jeang 1999). Significant mutations in the NEMO gene result in the IP phenotype, with a single deletion in exons 4 through 10 being the culprit in over 80% of cases (The International Incontinentia Pigmenti (IP) Consortium 2000). Also known as the γ-*subunit of*

*the inhibitor κB kinase* (IKKγ), NEMO is required for activation of the *nuclear factor κB* (NF-κB) a transcription factor that regulates the expression of genes involved in the immune and stress response, inflammatory reactions, cell adhesion and protection against apoptosis (Rothwarf et al. 1998, Smith et al. 2002, Yamaoka et al. 1998). NF-κB factor is composed of homo- and heterodimers of 5 proteins belonging to the *Rel* family and is sequestered in the cytoplasm by inhibitory proteins of the IκB family. In response to various stimuli such as tumor necrosis factor (TNF), interleukin-1 (IL-1), and lipopolysaccharide, the inhibitory molecule is phosphorylated and then degraded, allowing NF-κB to enter the nucleus and activate transcription of targeted genes. The kinase phosphorylating IκB (IKK) is a complex of three molecules IKK1/IKKα, IKK2/IKKβ, and NEMO. IKK1 and IKK2 act as catalytic subunits, while NEMO is a structural and regulatory subunit vital to the function of the unit as a whole (Fig. 13). The absence of NEMO results in no NF-κB activity in response to stimuli (Bruckner 2004).

The phenotype of IP is the result of genetic mosaicism. Due to lyonization of the X-chromosome in early embryogenesis, individuals with IP are born with two populations of cells: those that do (IKKγ[+]) and do not (IKKγ[−]) express NEMO/IKKγ. Leukocytes in affected females with IP demonstrate skewed X-inactivation towards the affected chromosome (Parrish et al. 1996). The normal function of the remaining X chromosome explains the survival and progressive improvement in both affected females and males with Klinefelter syndrome and IP. In the skin, mosaicism presents along the lines of Blaschko (Happle 1985). Although less well understood, extracutaneous examples of mosaicism are found in the eye, teeth, bones and possibly brain (Rott 1999).

Several studies have shed light on how abnormalities in the NF-κB pathway produce IP (reviewed in Bruckner 2004 and Fusco et al. 2008). The activation of NF-κB is critical in preventing apoptosis induced by TNF-α (Beg and Baltimore 1996, Van Antwerp et al. 1998). Male NEMO knockout mice die early in utero and often demonstrate massive liver apoptosis (Makris et al. 2000, Rudolph et al. 2000, Schmid-Supprian et al. 2000).

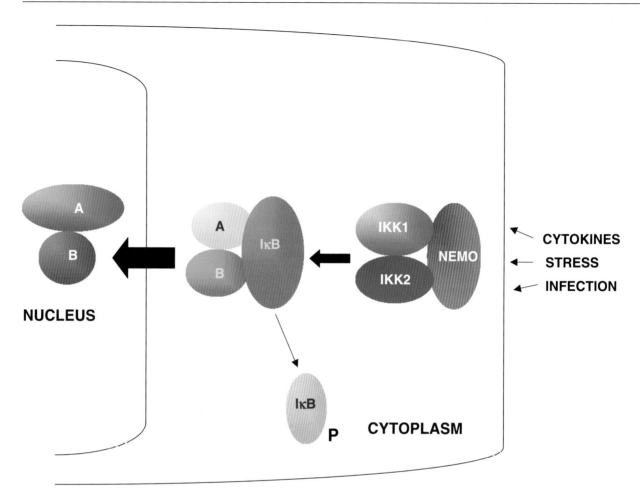

**Fig. 13.** Normal activation of the NF-κB pathway (see text for explanation). A, B = representative proteins of the Rel family (adapted from Bruckner 2004).

On the other hand, female mice heterozygous for NEMO deficiency (IKKγ±) develop transitory skin changes that are phenotypically and histologically similar to those of IP (Makris et al. 2000, Schmid-Supprian et al. 2000). The skin of these mice contains elevated levels of several cytokines and chemokines such as TNF-α (Makris et al. 2000). *Stage 1 IP lesions* of human skin strongly express eotaxin, an eosinophil-selective chemokine that is activated by NF-κb (Jean-Baptiste et al. 2002). These findings suggest that in the vesicular stage of IP, IKK-γ⁻ cells undergo apoptosis, while IKK-γ⁺ cells in turn upregulate the production of TNF-α, IL-1, eotaxin and other cytokines and chemokines. This further drives apoptosis of IKK-γ⁻ cells and also produces an influx

of eosinophils into the skin. As the population of IKK-γ⁻ cells declines, inflammation subsides, heralding the end of the 1st stage of disease. Residual IKK-γ⁻ cells that undergo apoptosis in response to circulating cytokines explain the recurrence of vesicular lesions with febrile illnesses (Brucker 2004).

The mechanism producing subsequent skin changes, as well as other findings associated with IP, are poorly understood. The skin of NEMO knockout mice over expresses cytokeratins 6 and 17 which are markers of an inflammatory response, in part explaining the hyperkeratotic lesions (Makris et al. 2000). The pathogenesis of the hyperpigmented lesions is unclear, as these areas often do not correspond to preceding inflammation, making purely post inflammatory hyperpigmentation unlikely. Atrophic skin changes may represent residual scarring but may also be due to developmental malformation of the affected areas.

It is known that certain proteins of the Rel family are critical in the generation of mature osteoclasts (Iotsova et al. 2000, Franzoso et al. 1997), which are essential for the degradation of alveolar bone leading to tooth eruption, providing some insight into the dental anomalies seen with IP (Bruckner 2004).

Initially, IP was considered a lethal factor in males. However, some males may survive, showing symptoms of IP or presenting with a phenotype of *anhydrotic/hypohydrotic ectodermal dysplasia (HED)* and features of *immunodeficiency (ID)* and/or *osteopetrosis and lymphoedema (OL)* (Zonana et al. 2000, Mansour et al. 2001, Aradhya et al. 2001, Chang et al. 2008, Fusco et al. 2008). The ectodermal dysplasia (ED) are an uncommon, heterogeneous group of disorders with varying modes of inheritance characterized by the abnormal development of cutaneous appendages, such as teeth, hair, nails and sweat glands (Pinheiro and Freire-Maia 1994). In the HED-ID forms, individuals demonstrate characteristic facies, sparse hair, dry skin, eczema, decreased to absent sweating and dental abnormalities. The X-linked form is most common and is caused by mutations in the *ectodysplasia gene* (EDA1), a member of the TNF cytokine super family; autosomal forms are either caused by mutations in the genes encoding EDAR (the receptor for EDA) or EDARADD (EDAR-associated death domain (Smahi et al. 2002). EDA activates EDAR which uses EDARADD as a bridge to trigger NF-κB activation, a process that is dependent on NEMO. Alterations in this pathway lead to abnormal ectodermal morphogenesis (Bruckner 2004). Males with HED-ID offspring of mothers with IP harbor missense mutations or minor deletions in the coding region of NEMO, while those with OL-HED-ID have mutations in the stop codon of NEMO (Zonana et al. 2000, Mansour et al. 2001, Aradhya et al. 2001). While the NEMO deletion of IP results in no activation of the NF-κB, these hypomorphic mutations lead to decreased or altered function of the NF-κB pathway (Bruckner 2004).

# Differential diagnosis

All neurocutaneous diseases that affect brain, eye and skin overlap some features, but each one has some particular characteristics that help to make the differential diagnosis. These characteristics are: age at onset of the symptoms, sex and type of transmission, distribution of the lesions and their evolution, and imaging features. The highest difficulty to make a correct diagnosis is the limited experience of most dermatologists, pediatric neurologists and ophthalmologists because of the low incidence of IP and the other syndromes with overlapping features. However, only IP has an evolution of four stages of the cutaneous lesions, that show focal cerebral lesions of the acquired type (Pascual-Castroviejo et al. 1994). Cutaneous lesions in stage 1 may be the most difficult to classify because these show many similarities with those of staphylococcal or streptococcal bullous impetigo, severe cases of epidermolysis bullosa, varicella, or congenital herpes simplex, but the particular associated features with each disease and the cutaneous lesions along the lines of Blaschko in IP facilitate the diagnosis. During the neonatal period, Naegeli syndrome, an autosomal dominant disorder that presents with hyperhydrosis and punctate hyperkeratosis of the palms and soles, may cause to hesitate on the identity of the disease, but the lack of abnormalities in eyes, brain and the lines of Blaschko discard the possibility of IP. The highest difficulty for a differential diagnosis and the most confusing diagnosis is hypomelanosis of Ito (HI) in adults, but not in children. Skin lesions of IP in stage 4 are hypopigmented areas that before had shown hyperpigmentation, and they present almost the same aspect as skin lesions of HI. However, the lesions of both entities present some differences, apart from the previous history. Skin lesions of HI show patches or lines of hyperpigmentation besides the hypopigmented areas, while lesions of IP in stage 4 are more similar to the cicatrisation of this area after a rubbing of the skin.

# Management

Treatment of IP is most often symptomatic. Cutaneous lesions usually do not need treatment unless secondary infection of the skin lesions develops in stage 1 during the neonatal period. Ocular lesions may or may not need treatment, but intervention depends on the kind eye abnormality. Spastic disorders, pyramidal disease, club foot, scoliosis, and other features need specific treatment for each alteration, such as physiotherapy, specific surgery for scoliosis or other orthopedic problems, botulinum toxin administration, antiepileptic drugs substances for epilepsy, etc. Learning problems required educational evaluation and remediation.

Following molecular genetic findings recently reported (Jin and Jeang 1999, The International Incontinentia Pigmenti (IP) Consortium 2000), intrauterine investigations in pregnant women with IP may be able to confirm the presence of IP in the fetus.

## References

Adamson HG (1908) Congenital pigmentation with atrophic scarring associated with other congenital abnormalities. Proc R Soc Med 1: 9–10.

Aradhya S, Courtois G, Raikovic A, Lewis RA, Levy M, Israël A, Nelson DL (2001) Atypical forms of incontinentia pigmenti in male individuals result from mutations of a cytosine tract in exon 10 of NEMO (IKK-γ). Am J Hum Genet 68: 765–771.

Avrahami E, Harel S, Jurgenson U, Cohn DF (1985) Computed tomographic demonstration of brain changes in incontinentia pigmenti. Am J Dis Child 139: 372–374.

Bardach M (1925) Systematisierte Navusbildungen bei einem eineiigen Zwillingspaar. Ein Beitrag zur Navusatiolgie. Z Kinderheilkd 39: 542–550.

Beg AA, Baltimore D (1996) An essential role for NF-kappaβ in preventing TNF-induced cell death. Science 274: 782–784.

Bell WR, Green WR, Goldberg MF (2008) Histopathologic and trypsin digestion studies of the retina in incontinentia pigmenti. Ophthalmology 115: 893–897.

Berlin AL, Paller AS, Chan LS (2002) Incontinentia pigmenti: a review and update on the molecular basis of pathophysiology. J Am Acad Dermatol 47: 169–187.

Bloch B (1926) Eigentumliche, bisher nicht beschriebene Pigmentafektion (incontinentia pigmenti). Schweiz Med Wochen 7: 404–405.

Bruckner AL (2004) Incontinentia pigmenti: a window to the role of NF-κB function. Semin Cut Med Surg 23: 116–124.

Brunquell PJ (1987) Recurrent encephalomyelitis associated with incontinentia pigmenti. Pediatr Neurol 3: 174–177.

Carney RG (1976) Incontinentia pigmenti: a world statistical analysis. Arch Dermatol 112: 535–542.

Chang TT, Behshad R, Brodell RT, Gilliam AC (2008) A male infant with anhidrotic ectodermal dysplasia/immunodeficiency accompanied by incontinentia pigmenti and a mutation in the NEMO pathway. J Am Acad Dermatol 58: 316–320.

Edelstein S, Naidich TP, Newton TH (2005) The rare phakomatoses: In: Tortori-Donati P (ed.) Pediatric Neuroradiology. Brain. Berlin: Springer, pp. 818–854.

Franceschetti A, Jadassohn W (1954) A propos de l'incontinentia pigmenti: délimitation de deux síndromes différents figurant sous le même teme. Dermatologica 108: 1–28.

François J (1984) Incontinentia pigmenti (Bloch-Sulzberger syndrome). Br J Ophthalmol 68: 19–25.

Franzoso G, Carslon L, Xing L, Poljak L, Shores EW, Brown KD, Leonardi A, Tran T, Boyce BF, Siebenlist U (1997) Requirement for NF-κβ on osteoclasts and B-cell development. Genes Dev 11: 3482–3496.

Frontera Izquierdo P, Cabezuelo Huerta G, Mulas F, Monfort Marti A (1981) Afectación neurológica en la incontinentia pigmenti (síndrome de Bloch–Sulzberger). Estudio de tres casos. An Esp Pediatr 14: 272–278.

Fusco F, Fimiani G, Tadini G, Michele D, Ursini MV (2007) Clinical diagnosis of incontinentia pigmenti in a cohort of male patients. J Am Acad Dermatol 56: 264–267.

Fusco F, Pescatore A, Bal E, Ghoul A, Paciolla M, Lioi MB, D'Urso M, Rabia SH, Bodemer C, Bonnefont JP, Munnich A, Miano MG, Smahi A, Ursini MV (2008) Alterations of the IKBKG locus and diseases: an update and a report of 13 novel mutations. Hum Mutat 29: 595–604.

Garrod AE (1906) Peculiar skin pigmentation of the skin in an infant. Trans Clin Soc Lond 39: 216–217.

Goldberg MF, Custis PH (1993) Retinal and other manifestations of incontinentia pigmenti (Bloch–Sulzberger syndrome). Ophthalmology 100: 1645–1654.

Happle R (1985) Lyonisation and the lines of Blaschko. Hum Genet 70: 200–206.

Hauw JJ, Perié G, Bonette J, Escourelle R (1997) Les lesions cerebrales de l'incontinentia pigmenti (a propos d'un cas anatomique). Acta Neuropathol 38: 159–162.

Hennel SJ, Ekert PG, Volpe JJ, Inder TE (2003) Insights into the pathogenesis of cerebral lesions in incontinentia pigmenti. Pediatr Neurol 29: 148–150.

Hunter JAA, Holubar K (1984) Sulzberger! Biography, Autobiography, Iconography. A posthumous festschrift. Am J Dermatopathol 6: 345–370.

Iotsova V, Caamaño J, Loy J, Yang Y, Lewin A, Bravo R (2000) Osteopetrosis in mice lacking NF-kappa-b1 and kappa-b2. Nature Med 3: 1285–1289.

Jean-Baptiste S, O'Toole EA, Chen M, Guitart J, Paller A, Chan LS (2002) Expression of eotaxin, an eosinophil-selective chemokine, parallels eosinophil accumulation in the vesiculobullous stage of incontinentia pigmenti. Clin Exp Immunol 127: 470–478.

Jin DY, Jeang KT (1999) Isolation of full-length cDNA and chromosomal localization of human NF-Kappa B modulator NEMO to Xq28. J Biomed Sci 6: 115–120.

Kenwrick S, Woffendin H, Jakins T, Shuttleworth SG, Mayer E, Greenhalgh L, Whittaker J, Rugolotto S, Bardaro T, Esposito T, D'Urso M, Soli F, Turco A, Smahi A, Hamel-Teillac D, Lyonnet S, Bonnefont JP, Munnich A, Aradhya S, Kashork CD, Shaffer LG, Nelson DL, Levy M, Lewis RA; International IP Consortium (2001) Survival of male patients with incontinentia pigmenti carrying a lethal mutation can be explained by somatic mosaicism. Am J Hum Genet 69: 1210–1217.

Loh NR, Jadresic LP, Whitelaw A (2008) A genetic cause for neonatal encephalopathy: incontinentia pigmenti with NEMO mutation. Acta Paediatr 97: 379–381.

Lou H, Zhang L, Xiao W, Zhang J, Zhang M (2008) Nearly completely reversible brain abnormalities in a patient with incontinentia pigmenti. Am J Neuroradiol 29: 431–433.

Machado-Pinto J, McCalmon TH, Golitz LE (1996) Eosinophilic and neutrophilic spongiosis: clues to diagnosis of immunobullous diseases and other inflammatory disorders. Semin Cutan Med Surg 15: 308–316.

MacKee GM (1955) Dr Marion B Sulzberger. J Invest Dermatol 24: 141–154.

Maingay-de Groof F, Lequin MH, Roofthooft DW, Oranje AP, de Coo IF, Bok LA, van der Spek PJ, Mancini GM, Govaert PP (2007) Extensive cerebral infarction in the newborn due to incontinentia pigmenti. Eur J Paediatr Neurol Oct 18 [Epub ahead of print].

Makris C, Godfrey VL, Krahn-Senftleben G, Takahashi T, Roberts JL, Schwarz T, Feng L, Johnson RS, Karin M (2000) Female male heterozygous for IKK gamma/NEMO deficiencies develop a dermatopathy similar to the human X-linked disorder incontinentia pigmenti. Mol Cell 5: 969–979.

Mangano S, Barbagallo A (1993) Incontinentia pigmenti: clinical and neuroradiological features. Brain Dev 15: 362–366.

Mansour S, Woffendin H, Mitton S, Jeffery I, Jakins T, Kenwrick E, Murday VA (2001) Incontinentia pig-

menti in a surviving male is accompanied by hypohydrotic ectodermal dysplasia and recurrent infection. Am J Med Genet 99: 172–177.

Mascaró JM, Palou J, Vives P (1985) Painful subungueal keratotic tumors in incontienentia pigmenti. J Am Acad Dermatol 13: 913–918.

Morgan JD (1971) Incontinentia pigmenti (Bloch–Sulzberger syndrome): report of four additional cases. Am J Dis Child 122: 294–300.

Nazzaro V, Brusasco A, Gelemetti C, Ermacora E, Caputo R (1990) Hypochromic reticulated streaks in incontinentia pigmenti: an immunohistochemical and ultrastructural study. Pediatr Dermatol 7: 174–178.

Obituary (1933) Br J Dermatol 45: 269–271.

O'Brien JE, Feingold M (1985) Incontinentia pigmenti: A longitudinal study. Am J Dis Child 139: 711–712.

O'Doherty NY, Norman RM (1968) Incontinentia pigmenty (Bloch–Sulzberger syndrome) with cerebral malformation. Dev Med Child Neurol 10: 168–174.

OMIM™ (2006) Online Mendelian Inheritance in Man. Baltimore: The Johns Hopkins University Press: http://www.ncbi.nlm.nih.gov/omim

Parrish JE, Scheuerle AE, Lewis RA, Levy ML, Nelson DL (1996) Selection against mutant alleles in blood leukocytes is a consistent feature in incontinentia pigmenti type 2. Hum Mol Genet 5: 1777–1783.

Pascual-Castroviejo I, Lopez Martin V, Martinez Bermejo A, Perez Higueras A (1992) Is cerebral arteritis the cause of the Landau–Kleffner syndrome? Four cases in childhood with angiographic study. Can J Neurol Sci 19: 46–52.

Pascual-Castroviejo I, Roche MC, Martínez-Fernandez V, Perez-Romero M, Escudero MR, García-Peñas JJ et al. (1994) Incontinentia pigmenti: MR demonstration of brain changes. Am J Neuroradiol 15: 1521–1527.

Pascual-Castroviejo I, Pascual-Pascual SI, Velazquez-Fragua R, Martinez Z (2006) Incontinentia pigmenti. Hallazgos clinicos y radiologicos en una serie de 12 pacientes. Neurologia 21: 239–248.

Pörksen G, Pfeiffer C, Hahn G, Poppe M, Friebel D, Kreuz F, Gahr M (2004) Neonatal seizures in two sisters with incontinentia pigmenti. Neuropediatrics 35: 139–142.

Pinheiro and Freire-Maria (1994)

Rosman NP (1987) Incontinentia pigmenti. In: Gomez MR (ed.) Neurocutaneous diseases. A practical approach. Boston: Butterworths, pp. 293–300.

Rothwarf DM, Zandi E, Natoli G, Karin M (1998) IKK-γ is an essential regulatori subunit of the I κB kinase complex. Nature 395: 297–300.

Rott HD (1999) Extracutaneous analogies of Blaschko lines. Am J Med Genet 85: 338–341.

Rudolph D, Yeh WC, Wakeham A, Rudolph B, Nallainathan D, Potter J, Elia AJ, Mak TW (2000) Severe liver degeneration and lack of NF-kappaβ activation in NEMO/IKKgamma deficient mice. Genes Dev 14: 854–862.

Schmidt-Supprian M, Bloch W, Courtois G, Addicks K, Israel A, Rajewsky K, Pasparakis M (2000) NEMO/IKK gamma-deficient mice model incontinentia pigmenti. Mol Cell 5: 981–992.

Sefani A, Abel L, Heuertz S et al. (1998) The gene for incontinentia pigmenti is assigned to Xq28. Genomics 4: 427–429.

Shuper A, Bryan RN, Singer HS (1990) Destructive encephalopathy in incontinentia pigmenti: a primary disorder? Pediatr Neurol 6: 137–140.

Siemes H, Sneider H, Dening D, Hanefeld F (1978) Encephalitis in two members of a family with incontinentia pigmenty (Bloch–Sulzberger syndrome): the possible role of the inflammation in the pathogenesis of CNS involvement. Eur J Pediatr 129: 103–115.

Simmons DA, Kegel MF, Scher RK, Hines YC (1986) Subungueal tumors in incontinentia pigmenti. Arch Dermatol 122: 1431–1434.

Smahi A, Hyden-Granskog C, Peterlin B, Vabres P, Heuertz S, Fulchignoni-Letaud MC (1994) The gene for the familial form of incontinentia pigmenti (IP2) maps to the distal part of Xq28. Hum Mol Genet 3: 273–278.

Smith C, Andreakos E, Crawley JB, Brennan FM, Feldmann M, Foxwell BM (2001) NF-kappaB-inducing kinase is dispensable for activation of NF-kappaB in inflammatory settings but essential for lymphotoxin beta receptor activation of NF-kappaB in primary human fibroblasts. J Immunol 15: 5895–5903.

Sulzberger MB (1928) Über eine bisher nicht beschriebene congenitale Pigmentonomalie (incontinenetia pigmenti). Arch Derm Syph (Berlín) 154: 19–32.

Sulzberger MB (1980) Three lessons learned in Bloch's clinic. Am J Dermatopathol 2: 321–325.

Taiby H (1996) Incontinentia pigmenti. In: Taiby H, Lachman RS (eds.) Radiology of syndromes, metabolic disorders, and skeletal dysplasias. 4th ed. St. Louis, Mosby, pp. 251–252.

The International Incontinentia Pigmenti (IP) Consortium (2000) Genomic rearrangement in NEMO impairs NF-κB activation and is a cause of incontinentia pigmenti. Nature 405: 466–472.

Triki C, Devictor D, Kah S, Roge-Wolter M, Lacroix C, Venencie PY, Landrieu P (1992) Complications cérébrales de l'incontinentia pigmenti. Etude clinique et pathologique d'un cas. Rev Neurol (Paris) 148: 773–776.

Van Antwerp DJ, Martin SJ, Verma IM, Green DR (1998) Inhibition of TNF-induced apoptosis by NF-kappaβ. Trends Cell Biol 8: 107–111.

Volpe JJ (2001) Neurobiology of periventricular leukomalacia in the premature infant. Pediatr Res 50: 553–562.

Who named it? (2006) An online catalog of eponyms in medical literature. http://www.whonamedit.com

Wiley HE, Frias JL (1974) Depigmented lesions in incontinentia pigmenti: a useful diagnostic sign. Am J Dis Child 128: 546–547.

Yamaoka S, Courtois G, Bessia C, Whiteside ST, Weil R, Agou F, Kirk HE, Kay RJ, Israel A (1998) Complementation cloning of NEMO, a component of the IkappaB kinase complex essential for NF-kappaB activation. Cell 26: 1231–1240.

Zillikens D, Mehringer A, Lechner W, Burg G (1991) Hypo- and hyperpigmented areas in incontinentia pigmenti: light and electronic microscopic studies. Am J Dermatopathol 13: 57–62.

Zonana J, Elder ME, Schneider LC, Orlow SJ, Moss C, Golabi M, Shapira SK, Farndon PA, Wara DW, Emmal SA, Ferguson BM (2000) A novel X-linked disorder of immune deficiency and hypohydrotic ectodermal dysplasia is allelic to incontinentia pigmenti and due to mutation in IKK-gamma (NEMO). Am J Hum Genet 67: 1555–1562.

# Chapter 19

# SILVER HAIR SYNDROMES: CHEDIAK-HIGASHI SYNDROME (CHS) AND GRISCELLI SYNDROMES (GS)

Marimar Saez-De-Ocariz, Luz Orozco-Covarrubias, Carola Duràn-McKinster, and Ramòn Ruiz-Maldonado

Department of Dermatology, National Institute of Paediatrics, Mexico City, Mexico

Normal pigmentation is a complex biological process and in the human, at least 127 different genes have been identified (Bennett and Lamoreaux 2003). Colour loci are the genetic loci in which mutations can affect pigmentation of the hair, skin, and/or eyes.

Differences in skin and hair colour are basically genetically determined and depend on the uniform distribution of melanin polymers produced by melanocytes and secreted into keratinocytes. The movement of melanosomes from post-Golgi compartments to the periphery of melanocytes is known to be regulated by motor proteins, e.g. myosin -V and Rab27, interacting with each other and functioning by means of vesicle trafficking. Motor proteins play a critical role in transporting melanosomes within melanocytes as well as neurosecretory vesicles within neurons. Therefore, mutations in these proteins can produce a dilute or silvery hair colour and various neurologic defects (Lambert et al. 1998).

The so-called *silver hair syndromes* have misleading been referred to as partial albinism syndromes. Oculocutaneous albinism comprises a group of congenital hypopigmentation disorders related to mutations in genes interacting in melanin formation pathway, resulting from aberrant processing of tyrosinase, the enzyme critical to pigment production in mammals. In contrast, the phenotype of patients with silver hair syndrome is characterized by a silver-grey sheen hair (Fig. 1) and hypopig-

mented skin at birth followed by a prolonged bronzed skin after sun exposure (Fig. 2a and b). This phenotype is associated to the following clinical conditions:

- **Chediak-Higashi syndrome (CHS):** associated to defective chemotaxis secondary to impaired synthesis and/or maintenance of storage/secretory granules;
- **Griscelli syndromes (GS):** (1) with primary and severe neurological disorder (**GS1** also known as *Griscelli/Elejalde syndrome*); (2) with severe disturbed B-cell and T-cell immunity (**GS2**, as originally described by Griscelli); and (3) without extracutaneous abnormalities (**GS3** or *GS restricted to hypopigmentation/pigment dilution*).

Skin/hair hyperpigmentation is the result of a failure to transfer melanine to keratinocytes which provokes a hyperpigmented epidermal basal layer. Light microscopic examination of a skin biopsy shows the same characteristics in the four conditions, making it difficult to distinguish between each other. An accumulation of melanin in basal melanocytes contrasting with an extremely scant pigment in adjacent keratinocytes is observed, especially with Fontana-Masson stain. Electron microscopy examination reveals accumulation of mature melanosomes in the cytoplasm around the nucleus of a melanocytes or melanocytes with different stages of melanosomes formation.

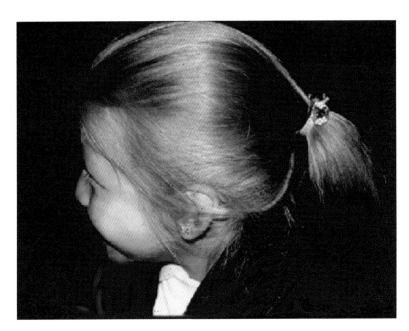

**Fig. 1.** Silver shine of hair and bronzed skin characteristic of silver hair syndromes.

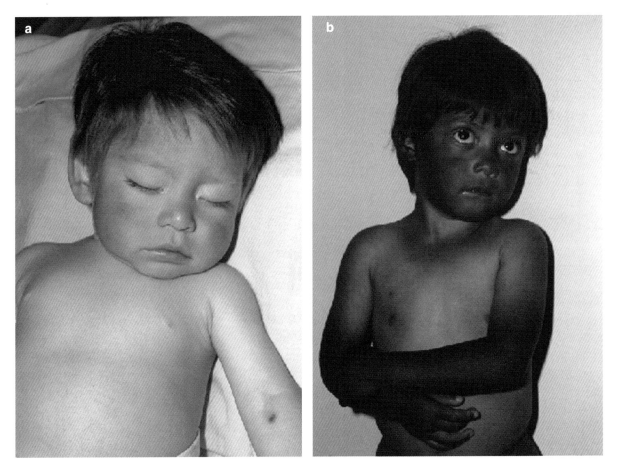

**Fig. 2.** (**a**) and (**b**) Chediak-Higashi syndrome. Characteristic hypo and hyperpigmented skin after sun exposure.

The silver-grey sheen (Fig. 1) of the scalp and body hair, eyebrows and eyelashes is the result of an abnormal distribution of pigment in clumps in the hair shaft leaving spaces free of melanin that impairs the refraction and absorption of light.

The natural course of the diseases and outcome is dictated by the site of involvement and the type of genetic mutation.

## References

Bennett DC, Lamoreaux ML (2003) The colour loci of mice-a genetic century. Pigment Cell Res 16: 333–344.

Lambert J, Onderwater J, Vander Haeghen Y, Vancoillie G, Koerten HK, Mommaas AM, Naeyaert JM (1998) Myosins V-colocalized with melanosomes and subcortical actin bundles not associated with stress fibers in human epidermal melanocytes. J Invest Dermatol 111: 835–840.

# CHEDIAK-HIGASHI SYNDROME (CHS)

**Marimar Saez-De-Ocariz, Luz Orozco-Covarrubias, Carola Duràn-McKinster, and Ramòn Ruiz-Maldonado**

Department of Dermatology, National Institute of Paediatrics, Mexico City, Mexico

## Introduction

This is a rare autosomal recessive immunodeficiency disorder (OMIM # 214500) where silvery hair was first recognized as a pathological feature (Beguez-Cesar 1943, Chediak 1952, Higashi 1954, Steinbrinck 1948). The hallmark of the disorder are the pathognomonic giant inclusion bodies seen in all granule-containing cells, including granulocytes, lymphocytes, melanocytes, mast cells and neurons (see below). CHS is a special lysosomal disorder in that it is not due to a specific enzyme deficiency but to a fusion defect of primary lysosomes.

The features of CHS are decreased pigmentation of hair and eyes, photophobia, nystagmus, large eosinophilic, peroxidase-positive inclusion bodies in the myeloblasts and promyelocytes of the bone marrow, neutropenia, abnormal susceptibility to infection, enterocolitis, and peculiar malignant lymphoma. Various neurological abnormalities have been described including clumsiness, abnormal gait, peripheral neuropathy, cranial nerve palsies and a variable degree of cognitive impairment with imaging evidence of diffuse atrophy of the brain, cerebellum and spinal cord (Ballard et al. 1994, Farah and Rogers 2004, Misra et al. 1991, Pettit and Ballard 1984, Tardieu et al. 2005, Uyama et al. 1994).

Most patients eventually enter a usually fatal *"accelerated phase"* of accelerated reaction manifested by fever, pancytopenia and non malignant lympho-histiocytic lymphoma-like organ infiltrates (Farah and Rogers 2004, Nowicki and Szarmach 2006). This lymphoma-like stage is precipitated by viruses, particularly by infection by the Epstein-Barr virus. It is associated to anaemia, bleeding episodes, and overwhelming infections (mostly of the skin, lungs, and respiratory tracts) often leading to early death without appropriate treatment (i.e., bone marrow transplantation).

The CHS locus has been mapped to chromosome 1q42.1–42.2 (Barrat et al. 1996, Fukai et al. 1996). The defective gene is the lysosomal trafficking regulator gene (**LYST**) currently termed **CHS1** gene which encodes a clue protein to regulate the secretory processes of intracellular lysosomal vesicles and melanosomes. An increased susceptibility to recurrent infections secondary to an impaired phagocytosis and a lack of natural killer cell function is characteristic.

## Historical perspective and eponyms

This syndrome was first described in 1943 by a Cuban pediatrician in three siblings (Beguez-Cesar 1943). Steinbrink reported 1 case in 1948. In 1952, **Alexander Moisés Chédiak**, a Cuban physician and serologist, born in 1903, reported 4 cases in 13 Cuban siblings, and in 1954 **Otokata Higashi**, a Japanese pediatrician, graduated from Tohoku University, Sendai, Japan, who later was Professor of pediatrics at Akita University, described 4 cases in 7 Japanese siblings. In these cases the parents were related; however, subsequent cases have not necessarily involved related parents (Van Hale 1987). Sato (1955) recognized the similarity between Chediak and Higashi's cases (Chediak 1952, Higashi 1954) reporting the probable identity of a "new leucocyte anomaly" (Chediak) and "congenital gigantism of peroxidase granules" (Higashi) and first named the disease Chediak-Higashi syndrome along with Donohue and Bain (1957) (Farah and Rogers 2004).

## Incidence and prevalence

CSH has been described in all ethnic groups and is usually rare except for a cluster of cases that has been described in an isolated area of the Venezuelan-Andes (Ramirez-Duque et al. 1983). A similar syndrome has been described in numerous animal species including the Aleutian mink, partial albino Hereford cattle, blue foxes, albino whales and the beige mouse (the latter used as an animal model for the disease) (Farah and Rogers 2004, Windhorst and Padgett 1973).

## Clinical manifestations

CHS commonly affects the skin, eyes, and central nervous system. The age at diagnosis ranges from 1 month to 39 years (median age, 5.6 years). The disease is usually first suspected either because of coexistent hypopigmentation (Fig. 2) (infants born with CHS have non pigmented skin – similar to albinos but in a patchy distribution – blonde hair, and blue eyes) and a history of recurrent pyogenic infections, or on the basis of a sibling in whom the diagnosis has been previously made, or after incidental observation of giant peroxidase-positive intracellular granules on a peripheral blood smear (Fig. 3) or bone

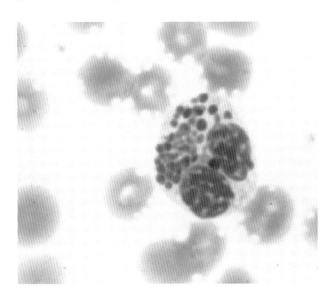

**Fig. 3.** Giant cytoplasmic granules in neutrophils pathognomonic of Chediak-Higashi syndrome.

marrow examination. Signs and symptoms that usually appear soon after birth include adenopathy, aphthae, gingivitis, hyperhidrosis, malaria, jaundice, severe and extensive pyoderma, recurrent sinopulmonary infections and fever usually unrelated to recognizable infections (Nowicki and Szarmach 2006).

## Skin manifestations

Most patients with CHS exhibit oculocutaneous albinism in at least one of three sites: the skin, the hair, or the eyes. Hair are sparse and colour varies from blonde to dark brown, bur always has a silvery tint that is particularly noticeable in strong light. CHS patients also have less skin pigmentation that their siblings and are susceptible to sunburns. This lack of pigmentation is also noticeable in the areolas and genitals. The pigmentary disturbance is not due to absence of melanin, but to its abnormal aggregation into giant melanosomes (Farah and Rogers 2004, Zhao et al. 1994).

## Eye involvement

The albinism in CHS is often more evident in the eyes than in the skin. Ocular alterations include a lack of pigmentation in the iris and the retina, pigmentary degeneration of the peripheral retina with progressive visual loss (Sayanagi et al. 2003). Overall, in CHS the skin is fair, the retinae are pale, and the irides are translucent. Ocular involvement can also be manifested clinically by photophobia, rotatory nystagmus, and an increased red reflex. Abnormal giant melanosomes have been found in the optic cup and neural crest derived melanocytes (Farah and Rogers 2004): therefore the ocular hypopigmentation in patients with CHS is related to an ultrastructural melanosomal defect.

## Recurrent infections

Recurrent infections affect mainly the skin, respiratory tract and mucous membranes. The most commonly involved organisms are Staphylococcus aureus, beta-haemolytic streptococci, Streptococcus pneuomniae, and other bacteria, fungi, and viruses. Recurrent skin infections range from superficial pyoderma to deep subcutaneous abscesses and ulcers that heal slowly and result in atrophic scars. Deep ulcerations resembling pyoderma gangrenosum have been also described.

This increased susceptibility has been attributed to the various immunologic defects observed in CHS including cellular immune deficiency, absent natural killer (NK) cytotoxic activity, altered neutrophils and monocytes numbers, diminished chemotactic responses, and delayed degranulation and intracellular killing of microorganisms (Farah and Rogers 2004, Gallin et al. 1975, Merino et al. 1983, Root et al. 1972).

## Neurological abnormalities

CHS may present with neurological dysfunction and should be considered in the differential diagnosis of children and young adults first seen with symptoms of spinocerebellar degeneration or movement disorders. In many persons with CHS, neurological changes appear in the lymphoproliferative phase. Progressive neurological deterioration is common in patients who survive early childhood. The adult form of CHS manifests during late childhood to young adulthood and is marked by various neurological sequelae (see below).

The various neurological abnormalities of CHS have been mainly described in young adult patients (Ballard et al. 1994, De Freitas et al. 1999, Farah and Rogers 2004, Fukuda et al. 2000, Hauser et al. 2000, Jacobi et al. 2005, Lockman et al. 1967, Misra et al. 1991, Pettit and Berdal 1984, Sheramata et al. 1974, Tardieu et al. 2005, Uyama et al. 1994, Van Hale 1987). Among the most common are signs of spinocerebellar degeneration such as clumsiness and abnormal gait, progressive parkinsonian syndrome (e.g., bradykinesia, resting tremor and oculogyric crises), dystonia, and peripheral neuropathy which is manifested by dysesthesias and paresthesias, transitory pareses (including cranial nerve palsies), and sensory deficit of the glove-stocking type (Van Hale 1987). The sensorineural neuropathy may begin early in childhood and progress to complete loss of muscle stretch reflexes, weakness, atrophy, and sensory deficits. Ataxia, with broad-based gait and dysdiadochokinesia, seizures, and behavioural abnor-

malities also occur. Headaches or emotional lability may occur occasionally in a setting of cognitive deterioration. The patient may become bedridden and totally incapacitated. Mental retardation or progressive intellectual decline have been also associated with CHS and appear to be independent of other neurological signs. The intellectual limitation may progress even after cure of the haematological manifestations with bone marrow transplantation (Uyama et al. 1994). Tardieu et al. (2005) reported on 3 CHS patients who underwent successful allogenic bone marrow transplantation in childhood with sustained mixed chimerism and no subsequent recurrent infections or haemophagocytic syndrome. At the age of 22–24 years, each patient developed a neurological syndrome combining difficulty walking, loss of balance and tremor. Examination revealed cerebellar ataxia and signs of peripheral neuropathy. Electrophysiology studies showed motor-sensory axonal neuropathy, there was moderate axon loss and rarefaction of large demyelinated fibres on peripheral nerve biopsy, and cerebellar atrophy was detected on brain MRI in two patients. Tardieu et al. (2005) reviewed also the neurological status of other 8 patients with CHS who had survived the initial bone marrow post transplantation period: 2 manifested neurological lesions immediately after transplantation; 1, aged 24 years, began having gait abnormality, falls when walking, and decreased cognitive abilities at the age of 21; 3 other patients, aged 2, 14 and 17 years, had borderline IQ scores but normal neurological examination. Tardieu et al. (2005) noted that the neurological signs/symptoms observed were identical to those in adults with mild CHS who did not undergo bone marrow transplantation, and concluded that the neurological syndrome including the low cognitive abilities most likely resulted from steady long-term progression, despite bone marrow transplantation, of the lysosomal defect in neurons and glial cells.

## Coagulation defects

There is usually a mild bleeding diathesis associated with CHS (Farah and Rogers 2004). Coagulation studies usually show a prolonged bleeding time, a normal platelet count, and impaired platelet aggregation with epinephrine and collagen (Buchanan and Handin 1976). This results form a platelet storage pool dense granule deficiency (Apitz-Castro et al. 1985). Patients usually experience increased cutaneous bruising during the chronic phase, even though thrombocytopenia and severe hemorrhage can occur during the accelerated phase.

## Imaging

Nonspecific radiological manifestations are hilar and mediastinal lymphadenopathy, hepatosplenomegaly; lymphangiography with a reticular pattern of enlarged inguinal and para-aortic lymph nodules. Oral radiographs reveal extensive loss of alveolar bone, leading to tooth exfoliation in most cases (Taiby 1996).

CT and/or MRI may show marked temporal dominant (or diffuse) brain atrophy and diffuse spinal cord atrophy (Uyama et al. 1991, 1994); periventricular decreased density (CT); increased signal intensity on T2-weighted images and lack of enhancement on T1-weighted images in periventricular and coronal radiated regions (Ballard et al. 1994). The overall pattern is quite similar to that seen in other lysosomal disorders (e.g., GM2 gangliosidosis) with extensive, diffuse white matter disease (probably a combination of hypomyelination and demyelination), showing an antero-posterior gradient and abnormalities in the deep cerebral grey matter (Patay 2005).

## Pathology

The hallmark of CHS is the occurrence of giant lysosomal inclusion bodies and organelles in all granule-containing cells (Fig. 3), including granulocytes, lymphocytes, monocytes, erythroid precursors, histiocytes, mast cells, platelets, melanocytes, Schwann cells, neurons and fibroblasts (Farah and Rogers 2004, Windhorst et al. 1966). Electron microscopy and histochemical staining have demonstrated that these are abnormal giant lysosomes. These contain lipoidal material in varying stages of

degradation (Barak and Nir 1987). Ultrastructural studies by means of immunogold electron microscopy have suggested that the giant granules are derived from azurophilic granules containing myeloperoxidase and CD63 and not from specific and gelatinase granules (Kjeldsen et al. 1998).

Histological studies support the association between peripheral neuropathy and the cellular infiltrates of the accelerated phase of the disease. Giant lysosomes are present in the cytoplasm of the Schwann cells of myelinated peripheral nerve axons.

## Pathogenesis and molecular genetics

Chediak-Higashi syndrome is inherited as autosomal recessive and is caused by mutation in the lysosomal trafficking regulator gene (**LYST**), currently named **CHS1** gene, located on chromosome 1q42.1–42.2 (Barrat et al. 1996, Fukai et al. 1996). The defective gene encodes a clue protein to regulate the secretory processes of intracellular lysosomal vesicles and melanosomes. The CHS protein is expressed in the cytoplasm of cells of a variety of tissues and may represent an abnormality of organelles protein trafficking. The CHS gene affects the synthesis and/or maintenance of storage/secretory granules in various types of cells: lysosomes of leukocytes and fibroblasts, dense bodies of platelets, azurophilic granules of neutrophils, and melanosomes and melanocytes which are generally larger in size and irregular in morphology, indicating that a common pathway in the synthesis of organelles responsible for storage is affected in patients with CHS. In the early stages of neutrophils maturation, normal azurophilic granules fuse to form megagranules, whereas in the later stage (i.e., during myelocyte stage), normal granules are formed. The mature neutrophils contain both populations. A similar phenomenon occurs in monocytes. The impaired function in the polymorphonuclear leukocytes may be related to abnormal microtubular assembly (Nowicki and Szarmach 2006). The mechanism of peripheral nervous system damage in CHS has not completely elucidated: both the axonal and demyelinating types of peripheral neuropathy associated to CHS have been reported. Defective melanisation of melanosomes occurs in hypopigmentation associated to CHS: in melanocytes autophagocytosis of melanosomes occurs. The increased susceptibility to recurrent infections is likely secondary to an impaired phagocytosis and a lack of natural killer cell function.

The pathophysiology of the so-called accelerated phase (see above and below) seems related to an immune dysregulation (similar to what occurs in the haemophagocytic lymphohistiocytosis syndromes) (Rubin et al. 1985, Kinugawa 1990) with uncontrolled activation of lymphocytes and macrophages, possibly secondary to the lack of NK cell function.

Karim et al. (2002) performed mutation analysis of 21 unrelated patients with the childhood, adolescent, and adult forms of CHS: in patients with severe childhood CHS, they found only functionally null mutant CHS1 alleles, whereas in patients with the adolescent and adult forms of CHS they also found missense mutant alleles that likely encode CHS1 polypeptides with partial function.

## Animal model

Disorders similar to CHS occur in many mammalian species besides man, including mouse, cattle, mink, and killer whale. Kahraman and Prieur (1990) stated that this disorder has been identified in at least 10 species including humans. They succeeded in prenatal diagnosis of CHS in cats by demonstrating abnormally large lysosomes (stained for acid phosphatase) in cultured amniotic fluid cells. In mink and cattle the disorder is autosomal recessive (Padgett et al. 1964).

The beige mouse has been used as an animal model for the disease (Windhorst and Padgett 1973). The mouse *beige (bg)* locus consists of a s series of seven mutant alleles of a gene located on chromosome 13. The human CSH1 (LYST) gene was mapped to a chromosome region (1q42.1–42.2) homologous to the position of the mouse *beige* gene (Barrat et al. 1996). When the mouse *beige* gene was positionally cloned (Barbosa et al. 1996; Perou et al. 1996a, b) cDNAs were used to isolate the human gene (Nagle et al. 1996) and to demonstrate the homology between mouse beige and humans (Barbosa

et al. 1997). Thus far the pathologic mutations identified all resulted in lack of expression of the normal CHS protein (Spritz 1998, Farah and Rogers 2004).

Kunieda et al. (2000), by using a bovine/murine somatic cell hybrid panel, demonstrated linkage between the CHS locus and marker loci on the proximal end of bovine chromosome 28. CHS in Japanese black cattle is a hereditary disease with prolonged bleeding time and partial albinism.

## Natural history

The disease typically proceeds along with an indolent course, with relapsing febrile episodes and infections, usually of the upper respiratory tract and skin. Intercellular vesicle formation is deficient, resulting in giant granules in many cells with deposition of lymphohistiocytes in the liver, spleen, lymph nodes and bone marrow, resulting in hepatosplenomegaly, bone marrow infiltration, bleeding tendency and haemophagocytosis. Most patients develop progressive neurologic deterioration, as a secondary event with a heterogeneous clinical picture (Silveira-Moriyama et al. 2004).

## Accelerated phase

Viral infection, particularly due to Epstein-Barr virus, has been associated to the so-called "accelerated phase". Spritz (1998) stated that about 85–90% of CHS patients eventually develop this strange *lymphoproliferative syndrome* which is characterized by generalized lymphohistiocytic infiltrates, fever, jaundice, hepatosplenomegaly, lymphadenopathy, pancytopenia, and bleeding. This in turn leads to worsening of the neutropenia and increases the risk of infections (Farah and Rogers 2004). Thrombocytopenia ensues which intensifies the bleeding disorder. Onset of this phase may occur shortly after birth or may be delayed of years. It usually leads to death from infection or hemorrhage. This phase can resemble some lymphoma but it is not a true malignancy.

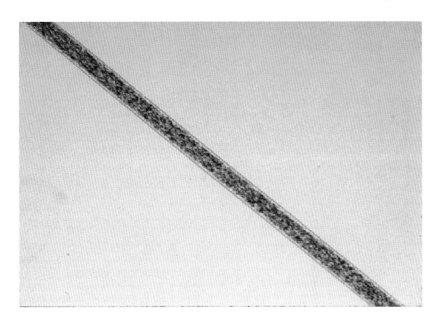

**Fig. 4.** Light microscopy of hair in Chediak-Higashi syndrome. Small granules regularly distributed are pathognomonic.

## Diagnosis

With simple methods, light microscopy of the hair and a peripheral blood smear the diagnosis of CHS can be confirmed based on the presence of pathognomonic anomalous giant cytoplasmic granules in neutrophils (Fig. 3) or in leukocyte precursor cells (bone marrow smears) and multiple small clumps of melanine along the hair shaft distributed in a regular pattern (Fig. 4). Fluorescent cytometric analysis reveals the characteristic leukocyte dysfunction, the cellular granularity and surface molecules.

Light and electron microscopy examinations of biopsy specimens of periodontal tissues reveal massive bacterial invasion of epithelial tissue, epithelial cells and connective tissue.

Prenatal diagnosis can be made by examination of the hair from foetal scalp biopsy and from leukocytes from foetal blood samples.

## Differential diagnosis

It should include albinism, bacterial mouth infections, cutaneous T-cell lymphoma, Griscelli syndrome (see below) and pyoderma gangrenosum.

## Treatment and prognosis

The prognosis of CHS is generally poor: early death occurs without treatment from infections, hemorrhage, or complications of the accelerated phase. However, there is significant clinical heterogeneity among patients with CHS, and some patients may survive into adulthood with few or even no severe infections, although they may develop progressive neurological deterioration (Tardieu et al. 2005, Uyama et al. 1994).

Current treatment protocols for CHS include prophylactic trimethoprim-sulphamethoxazole and aggressive parenteral antibiotic treatment of infections. Ascorbic acid (vitamin C) at doses of 20 mg/Kg or 0.2–6 grams per day has been shown to improve neutrophils function in vitro, although there is no proof that this provides clinical benefit (Malech and Nauseef 1997).

High dose of methylprednisolone and splenectomy in the accelerated phase may improve significantly the clinical, radiological and haematological findings (Aslan et al. 1996).

Allogeneic bone marrow transplantation from an HLA-matched sibling is the therapy of choice and should be performed early. In absence of a family donor, an unrelated donor or a placental blood graft is a good alternative (Mottonen et al.

2003): cure of the accelerated phase can be achieved even when transplantation results only in mixed chimerism, suggesting that even a small fraction of donor cells are sufficient to suppress this phase. Conversely, ocular and skin pigmentary disturbances are not corrected by the bone marrow transplantation and neurological complications can still develop or progress after the transplant (Haddad et al. 1995, Tardieu et al. 2005, Uyama et al. 1994).

## References

Apitz-Castro R, Cruz MR, Ledezma E, Merino F, Ramirez-Duque P, Dangelmeier C, Holmsen H (1985) The storage pool deficiency in platelets from humans with the Chediak-Higashi syndrome: study of six patients. Br J Haematol 59: 471–483.

Aslan Y, Erduran E, Gedik Y, Mocan H, Yildiran A (1996) The role of high dose methylprednisolone and splenectomy in the accelerated phase of Chediak-Higashi syndrome. Acta Haematol 96: 105–107.

Ballard R, Tien RD, Nohria V, Juel V (1994) The Chediak-Higashi syndrome: CT and MRI findings. Pediatr Radiol 24: 266.

Barak Y, Nir E (1987) Chediak-Higashi syndrome. Am J Pediatr Hematol Oncol 9: 42–55.

Barbosa MDFS, Nguyen QA, Tchernev VT, Ashley JA, Detter JC, Blaydes SM, Brandt SJ, Chotai D, Hodgman C, Solari RC, Lovett M, Kingsmore SF (1996) Identification of the homologous beige and Chediak-Higashi syndrome. Nature 382: 262–265.

Barbosa MDFS, Barrat FJ, Tchernev VT, Nguyen QA, Mishra VS, Colman SD, Pastural E, Dufourq-Lagelouse R, Fisher A, Holcombe RF, Wallace MR, Brandt SJ, de Saint Basile G, Kingsmore SF (1997) Identification of mutations in two major mRNA isoforms of the Chediak-Higashi syndrome gene in human and mouse. Hum Molec Genet 6: 1091–1098.

Barrat FJ, Auloge L, Pastural E, Lagelous RD, Vilmer E, Cant AJ, Weissenbach J, Le Paslier D, Fischer A, de Saint Basile G (1996) Genetic and physical mapping of the Chediak-Higashi syndrome on chromosome 1q42–43. Am J Hum Genet 59: 625–632.

Beguez-Cesar A (1943) Neutropenia crónica maligna familiar con granulaciones atípicas de los leucocitos. Bol Soc Cubana Pediatr 15: 900–922

Buchanan GR, Handin RI (1976) Platelet function in the Chediak-Higashi syndrome. Blood 47: 941–948.

Chediak MM (1952) Nouvelle anomalie leucocytaire de caractere constitutionnel et familial. Rev Hematol 7: 362–367.

De Freitas GR, de Oliveira CP, Reis RS, Sarmento MR, Gaspar NK, Fialho M, Praxedes H (1999) Seizures in Chediak-Higashi syndrome. Arq Neuropsiquiatr 57: 495–497.

Farah RA, Rogers R (2004) Chediak-Higashi syndrome. In: Roach ES, Allen VS (eds.) Neurocutaneous Disorders. New York: Cambridge University Press, pp. 296–300.

Fukai K, Oh J, Karim MA, Moore KJ, Kandil HH, Ito H, Burger J, Spritz RA (1996) Homozygosity mapping of the gene for Chediak-Higashi syndrome to chromosome 1q42–44 in a segment of conserved synteny that includes the mouse beige locus (bg). Am J Hum Genet 59: 620–624.

Fukuda M, Morimoto T, Ishida Y, Suzuki Y, Murakami Y, Kida K, Ohnishi A (2003) Improvement of peripheral neuropathy with oral prednisone in Chediak-Higashi syndrome. Eur J Pediatr 31: 87–90.

Gallin JL, Klinerman JA, Padgett GA, Wolff SM (1975) Defective mononuclear leukocyte chemotaxis in the Chediak-Higashi syndrome of humans, mink and cattle. Blood 45: 863–870.

Haddad E, Le Diest F, Blanche S, Benkerrou M, Rohrlich P, Vilmer E, Griscelli C, Fischer A (1995) Treatment of Chediak-Higashi syndrome by allogeneic bone marrow transplantation: report of 10 cases. Blood 85: 3328–3333.

Hauser RA, Friedlander J, Baker MJ, Thomas J, Zuckerman KS (2000) Adult Chediak-Higashi parkinsonian syndrome with dystonia. Mov Disord 15: 705–708.

Higashi O (1954) Congenital gigantism of peroxidase granules: the first case ever reported of qualitative abnormality of peroxidase. Tokai J Exp Clin Med 59: 315–332.

Jacobi C, Koerner C, Fruehauf S, Rottenburger C, Storch-Hagenlocher B, Grau AJ (2005) Presynaptic dopaminergic pathology in Chediak-Higashi syndrome with parkinsonian syndrome. Neurology 24: 1814–1815.

Kahraman MM, Prieur DJ (1990) Chediak-Higashi syndrome in the cat: prenatal diagnosis by evaluation of amniotic fluid cells. Am J Med Genet 36: 321–327.

Karim MA, Suzuki K, Fukai K, Oh J, Nagle D, Moore KJ, Barbosa E, Falik-Borenstein T, Filipovich A, Ishida Y, Kivrikko S, Klein C, Kreuz F, Levin A, Miyajima H, Regueiro J, Russo C, Uyama E, Vierimaa O, Spritz RA (2002) Apparent genotype-phenotype correlation in childhood, adolescent, and adult Chediak-Higashi syndrome. Am J Med Genet 108: 16–22.

Kinugawa N (1990) Epstein-Barr virus infection in Chediak-Higashi syndrome mimicking acute lymphocytic leukemia. Am J Pediatr Hematol Oncol 12: 182–186.

Kjeldsen L, Calafat J, Borregaard N (1998) Giant granules of neutrophils in Chediak-Higashi syndrome are derived from azurophil granules but not from specific and gelatinase granules. J Leukoc Biol 64: 72–77.

Kunieda T, Ide H, Nakagiri M, Yoneda K, Konfortov B, Ogawa H (2000) Localization of the locus responsible for Chediak-Higashi in cattle to bovine chromosome 28. Anim Genet 31: 87–90.

Lockman LA, Kennedy WR, White JG (1967) The Chediak-Higashi syndrome electrophysiological and electron microscopic observations on the peripheral neuropathy. J Pediatr 70: 924–951.

Malech HL, Nauseef WM (1997) Primary inherited defects in neutrophil function: etiology and treatment. Semin Hematol 34: 279–290.

Merino E, Klein GO, Henle W, Ramirez-Duque P, Forsgren M, Amesty C (1983) Elevated antibody titers to Epstein-Barr virus and low natural killer cell activity in patients with Chediak-Higashi syndrome. Clin Ummunol Immunopathol 27: 326–339.

Misra VP, King RH, Harding AE, Muddle JR, Thomas PK (1991) Peripheral neuropathy in the Chediak-Higashi syndrome. Acta Neuropathol (Berl) 81: 354–358.

Mottonen M, Lanning M, Baumann P, Saarinen-Pihkala UM (2003) Chediak-Higashi syndrome: four cases from Northern Finland. Acta Pediatr 92: 1047–1051.

Nagle DL, Karim MA, Woolf EA, Holmgren L, Bork P, Misumi DJ, McGrail SH, Dussault BJ Jr, Perou CM, Boissy RE, Duyk GM, Spritz RA, Moore KJ (1996) Identification and mutation analysis of the complete gene for Chediak-Higashi syndrome. Nat Genet 14: 307–311.

Nowicki R, Szarmach H (2006) Chediak-Higashi syndrome. E-medicine from webMD: http://emedicine.com/derm/topic704.htm

Padgett GA, Leader RW, Gorham JR, O'Mary CC (1964) The familial occurrence of Chediak-Higashi syndrome in mink and cattle. Genetics 49: 505–512.

Patay Z (2005) Metabolic disorders. In: Tortori-Donati P (ed.) Pediatric Neuroradiology. Brain. Berlin: Springer, pp. 543–721.

Perou CM, Moore KJ, Nagle DL, Misumi DJ, Woolf EA, McGrail SH, Holmgren L, Brody TH, Dussault BJ Jr, Monroe CA, Duyk GM, Pryor RJ, Li L, Justice MJ, Kaplan J (1996a) Identification of the murine beige gene by YAC complementation and positional cloning. Nature Genet 13: 303–308.

Perou CM, Justice MJ, Pryor RJ, Kaplan J (1996b) Complementation of the beige mutation in cultured cells by episomally replicating murine yeast chromosomes. Proc Nat Acad Sci USA 93: 5905–5909.

Pettit RE, Berdal KG (1984) Chediak-Higashi syndrome. Neurologic appearance. Arch Neurol 41: 1001–1002.

Roder JC, Haliotis T, Laing L, Kozbor D, Rubin P, Pross H, Boxer LA, White JG, Fauci AS, Mostowski H, Matheson DS (1982) Further studies of natural killer cell function in Chediak-Higashi patients. Immunology 46: 555–560.

Root RK, Rosenthal AS, Balestra DJ (1972) Abnormal bacterial, metabolic and lysosomal function of Chdeiak-Higashi syndrome leukocytes. J Clin Invest 51: 649–665.

Rubin CM, Burke BA, McKenna RW, McClain KL, White JG, Nesbit ME Jr, Filipovich AH (1985) The accelerated phase of Chediak-Higashi syndrome. An expression of the virus associated haemophagocytic syndrome? Cancer 56: 524–530.

Sayanagi K, Fujikado T, Onodera T, Tano Y (2003) Chediak-Higashi syndrome with progressive visual loss. Jpn J Ophthalmol 47: 304–306.

Sheramata W, Kott SK, Cyr DP (1974) The Chediak-Higashi-Steinbrinck syndrome. Presentation of three cases with features resembling spinocerebellar degeneration. Arch Neurol 25: 289–294.

Silveira-Moriyama L, Moriyama TS, Gabbi TV, Ranvaud R, Barbosa ER (2004) Chediak-Higashi syndrome with parkinsonism. Mov Disord 19: 472–475.

Spritz RA (1998) Genetic defects in Chediak-Higashi syndrome and the beige mouse. J Clin Immunol 18: 97–105.

Stato A (1955) Chediak and Higashi's disease. Probable identity of "new leukocytal anomaly (Chediak)" and "congenital gigantism of peroxidase granules (Higashi)". Tohoku J Exp Med 61: 201–210.

Steinbrinck W (1948) Uber eine neue Granulationsanomalie der Leurkocyten. Dtsch Arch Klin Med 193: 577–581.

Taiby H (1996) Chediak-higashi syndrome. In: Taiby H, Lachman RS (eds.) Radiology of Syndromes, Metabolic Disorders, and Skeletal Dysplasia. St-Louis: Mosby, pp. 81–82.

Tardieu M, Lacroix C, Neven B, Bordigoni P, de Saint Basile G, Blanche S, Fisher A (2005) Progressive neurologic dysfunctions 20 years after allogeneic bone marrow transplantation for Chediak-Higashi syndrome. Blood 106: 40–42.

Uyama E, Hirano T, Yoshida A, Doi O, Maruoka S, Araki S (1991) An adult case of Chediak-Higashi syndrome with parkinsonism and marked atrophy of the central nervous system. Rinsho Shinkeigaku 31: 24–31.

Uyama E, Hirano T, Ito K, Nakashima H, Sugimoto M, Naito M, Uchino M, Ando M (1994) Adult Chediak-Higashi syndrome presenting as parkinsonism and dementia. Acta Neurol Scand 89: 175–183.

Van Hale P (1987) Chediak-Higashi syndrome. In: Gomez MR (ed.) Neurocutaneous Diseases. A Practical Approach. Boston: Butterworths, pp. 209–213.

Windhorst DB, Padgett G (1973) The Chediak-Higashi syndrome and the homologous trait in animals. J Invest Dermatol 60: 529–537.

Zhao H, Boissy YL, Abdel-Malek Z, King RA, Nordlund JJ, Boissy RE (1994) On the analysis of the pathophysiology of Chediak-Higashi syndrome. Defects expressed by cultured melanocytes. Lab Invest 71: 25–34.

# GRISCELLI SYNDROMES (GS)

Marimar Saez-De-Ocariz, Luz Orozco-Covarrubias, Carola Duràn-McKinster, and Ramòn Ruiz-Maldonado

Department of Dermatology, National Institute of Paediatrics, Mexico City, Mexico

## Introduction

Griscelli syndrome (GS) is a rare autosomal recessive disorder (OMIM # 214450, 607624 and 609227) characterized by pigmentary dilution of the skin, due to abnormal melanosomal transport which result in abnormal accumulation of end-stage melanosomes in the centre of melanocytes, and by silvery grey hair, due to pigment clumping in hair shafts. While most patients also develop an *haemophagocytic syndrome*, characterized by uncontrolled activation of T lymphocytes and macrophages leading to death if not treated by bone marrow transplantation (OMIM # 607624) (Menasche et al. 2000), some show *severe primary neurological impairment* early in life without apparent immune abnormalities (OMIM #214450) (Anikster et al. 2002) and other have *hypomelanosis only with no immunologic or neurological manifestations* (Menasche et al. 2003) (OMIM # 609227). Recently, all these phenotypes (see Figs. 5–8) have been grouped under the same umbrella name (i.e., Griscelli syndrome/GS) because of shared biological mechanisms, but divided into three different subtypes (GS1–GS3), as they result from defects in three separate genes, located on chromosome 15q21 and 2q37 (Anikster et al. 2002; Menasche et al. 2000, 2002, 2003; Pastural et al, 1997, 2000):

- Myosin VA (MYO5A) gene, located on chromosome 15q21 (OMIM # 160777), causing GS with neurological impairment without haemophagocytic syndrome or **GS1** (OMIM # 214450);
- Ras-associated protein RAB27A gene, located on chromosome 15q21 (OMIM # 603868), causing GS with haemophagocytic syndrome or **GS2** (OMIM # 60764);

- Slac2-a/melanophilin (SLAC2A/MLPH) gene, located on chromosome 2q37 (OMIM # 606526), causing GS with no immunologic or neurological involvement or **GS3** (OMIM # 609227).

The protein products of the three genes are functionally closely linked one to each other as interacts in the same molecular pathways, resulting in melanosome transport of actin filaments to dock at the plasma membrane (i.e., in melanosome movement): defects in each gene result in pigmentary dilution because of defective release of melanosome content to neighbouring cells, such as keratinocytes in the skin (Menasche et al. 2002). In some body and cellular sites, however, MYO5A and RAB27A are expressed differently: for example, MYO5A is expressed in the brain, whereas RAB27A is not. Defects in MYO5A cause primary neurological dysfunction, whereas defects in RAB27A do not cause neurological abnormalities (unless as secondary effects of lymphocyte infiltration of central nervous system) (see GS2). Unlike myosin Va (the protein product of MYOVA), the GTP-binding protein (the protein product of RAB27A) appears to be involved in the control of the immune system thus causing the haemophagocytic syndrome. Melanophilin (Mlph) links the function of myosin Va and the GTP-Rab27a protein in the melanosome without additional functions: this explains why expression is restricted to the characteristic hypopigmentation in the third form of GS. In the protein complex *Rab27a-Mlph-MyoVa*, Mlph interacts with Rab27a through its N-terminal part (SHD) and with MyoVa through its C-terminal part (F-exon) (Fig. 9).

It is now accepted that the GS form caused by mutations in the MYOVA gene (GS1) and the so-called **Elejalde syndrome** (OMIM # 256710) (see below) are allelic or better represent the same entity. The GS form caused by mutations in the Slac2-a/melanophilin (SLAC2A/MLPH) gene (GS restricted to hypopigmentation) represents the so-called "**silvery hair syndrome restricted to pigment dilution**" (OMIM # 609227) (see below).

## Historical perspective and eponyms

Historically, Griscelli and co-workers (Griscelli et al. 1978), who worked at the Hospital Necker pour les enfants maladies in Paris, France, and his colleague Siccardi first described a condition characterized by partial albinism, frequent pyogenic infections and acute episodes of fever, neutropenia and thrombocytopenia. The pigmentary dilution was characterized by large clumps of pigment in the hair shafts and an accumulation of melanosomes in melanocytes. Despite an adequate number of T and B lymphocytes, the patients were hypogammaglobulinemic, deficient in antibody production, and incapable of delayed skin hypersensitivity and skin graft reaction. Their leukocytes did not stimulate normal leukocytes. A defect of helper T-cells was postulated. One patients was an 11-year-old North African girl with unrelated parents with a brother and sister with silvery hair who had died at 30 and 18 months of age, respectively. The morphological normality of polymorphonuclear leukocytes and lack of giant granules distinguished the disorder form Chediak-Higashi syndrome. The morphologic characteristics of hypopigmentation also distinguished the disorder from Chediak-Higashi syndrome, as well as from other pigmentary anomalies. These original cases (Griscelli et al. 1978) fit with the GS2 phenotype.

In 1977, Elejalde and co-workers described a new pigment mutation in two males and one female each from a consanguineous marriage in an inbred Columbian kindred. Elejalde et al. (1979) described this condition as neuroectodermal melanolysosomal disease (NEMLD). Dr. Elejalde (Elejalde et al. 1977, 1979) is credited for having first recognized a (primary) neurological impairment in patients with a silver hair syndrome. His original observation (Elejalde et al. 1977) credited to him the name of his own syndrome and an entry in the McKusick catalogue (OMIM # 256710) (OMIM 2006). This syndrome however is currently regarded as the same entity of GS1 (because both entities are caused by mutations in the MYOVA gene, see also above) and some authors continue to use only the eponym Griscelli syndrome type 1 (GS1) to characterize the Elejalde syndrome (Menanche et al. 2002). According to other authors (Duran-McKinster et al. 1999, Huizing et al. 2002, Ivanovich et al. 2001) the absence of immunological defects allows Elejalde syndrome to be distinguished from GS (at least from GS1). We believe that perhaps Dr. Griscelli should be (at least) credited for the accuracy of his ascertainment in recognizing a primary neurological involvement in the GS spectrum and the term *Griscelli/Elejalde syndrome* could be used as an alternative eponym for GS1.

## Incidence and prevalence

GS is a rare disease in all populations. Male and female are equally affected. Most reported cases are from Turkish and Mediterranean populations; however, in 2004, Manglani et al. (2004) and Rath et al. (2004) reported several cases from India. In the US is rare with fewer than 10 cases reported (Scheinfeld and Johnson 2006). The largest series of patients with GS1 (Griscelli/Elejalde syndrome) have been reported in Mexico (Duran-McKinster et al. 1999).

## Clinical manifestations

Often the first manifestation of GS that is noted is silvery hair. Not long after the immunologic effects of GS caused by mutations in the Rab27A gene (GS2) are noted. These immunologic defects resemble those of the haemophagocytic lymphohistiocytosis (HLH) and the X-linked lymphoproliferative syndrome. The neurological effects of GS caused by defects in MYOVA gene usually manifest early in life closer to birth.

Mutations in both MYO5A and RAB27A genes cause pigmentary dilution and other internal organ abnormalities. Skin manifestations of both GS12 and

GS2 include granulomatous skin lesions, partial albinism, and generalized lymphadenopathy. The skin is usually pale, but the hypopigmentation is not complete. Liver manifestations include hepatosplenomegaly and jaundice as a result of hepatitis. Patients can present with pallor as a result of pancytopenia. Partial ocular hypopigmentation has been observed in some patents but retinal degeneration has not been reported.

We will describe the main clinical features, the pathogenesis and molecular genetic aspects and the natural history of GS according to the three different subtypes.

## Griscelli syndrome type 1 (GS1) or Griscelli/Elejalde syndrome [GS with neurological involvement]

GS1 (OMIM # 214450) represents hypomelanosis with a primary neurological deficit and without immunologic impairment or manifestations of haemophagocytic syndrome (Menasche et al. 2002). Neuromuscular disorders are the hallmark of the disease. Psychomotor impairment may have two forms of presentation: congenital or infantile, first developing during childhood (Fig. 6). The sudden presentation of central nervous system dysfunction can be compared with the "accelerated phase" described in CHS and GS2 (see below). A severe regressive psychomotor process develops rapidly with loss of normal skills until patients die. A triggering factor for this sudden dysfunction has not yet been identified. Severe migraine status followed by hemiparesis has also been described. In general, normal humoral and cellular immunity is observed and recurrent infections are not the rule as in CHS and GS3. Ocular abnormalities are quite frequent. Patients may present congenital amaurosis or progressive loss of vision, nystagmus, diplopia as well as hypopigmented retina.

The natural history in GS1 is characterized by initial referred because of hypotonia, marked motor developmental delay, and mental retardation, with

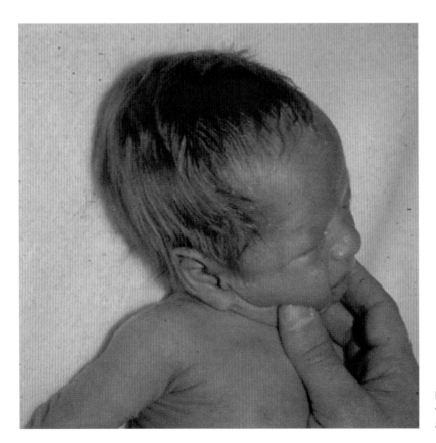

**Fig. 5.** Patient with Griscelli syndrome. Silvery hair is evident in hair scalp, eyelashes and eyebrows.

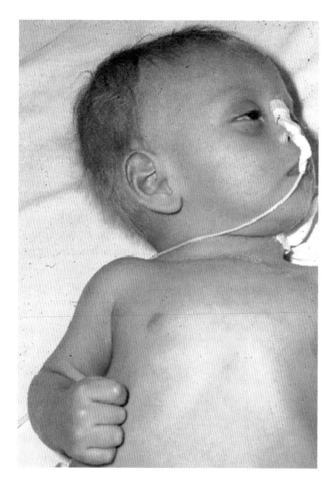

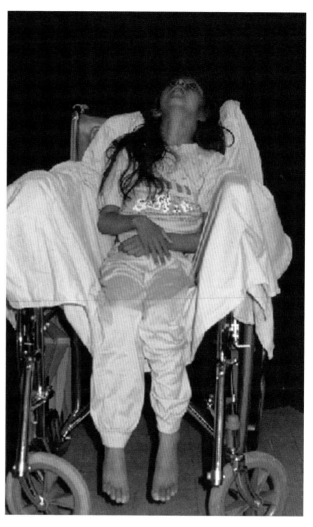

**Fig. 6.** Characteristic silvery hair in scalp in a patient with Elejalde syndrome with spastic quadriplegia.

**Fig. 7.** Flaccid quadriparesis in a 6-year old patient with Elejalde syndrome.

no history of infections or "accelerated phase". Psychomotor development may be normal early in life but suddenly the patients present with a regressive neurological process. One typical manifestation at onset include recurrent vomiting, acute febrile illness and/or lethargy after which patients typically deteriorate neurologically as indicated by regression of cognitive and motor function. Central nervous system disorder is stable and never regresses with time. The age of onset of neurological signs ranges from 1 month to 11 years. Clinical features include also periodic episodes of ocular alterations (e.g., exotropia and nystagmus), ataxia, brainstem signs, hemiparesis, peripheral facial palsy, spasticity, and seizures (Fig. 7). In addition to the silver-leaden hair, bronze skin with diffuse freckling may develop after sun

exposure. Large granules of melanin unevenly distributed in the hair shaft are observed. Usually, the long-lasting bronzed skin in patients with ES is not as darker as in patients with CHS or GS2. Death usually occur within the first decade of life when the patients are not treated.

Electroencephalogram usually reveals a diffuse and severe encephalopathy. Magnetic resonance imaging and computed tomography have demonstrate abnormal non-specific findings. Isolated congenital cerebellar atrophy was observed in a patient with the MYO5A defect. No evidence of infiltration of lymphocytes is present in these patients. MRI can reveal areas of increased T2 signal intensity and focal areas of abnormal enhancement in the subcortical white matter.

GS1 is caused by mutations in the gene encoding myosin Va (or myosin 5a) (MYO5A) located on chromosome 15q21 (Pastural et al. 1997). MYO5A is a motor molecule, one of the large family of unconventional class myosin V, involved in melanosome movement as well as neurosecretory vesicles. Mutation in MYO5A has been found in synaptic terminals in the retina and brain. It is required for normal photoreceptor signalling, suggesting that it might function in central nervous system synapses in general, with aberrant synaptic activity. Bahadoran et al. (2003a, b) characterized GS1 as comprising hypomelanosis and severe central nervous system dysfunction, corresponding to the "dilute" phenotype in the mouse.

Anikster et al. (2002), Huizing et al. (2002), Menasche et al. (2002) and Bahadoran et al. (2003a, b) suggested that *Elejalde syndrome* and GS1 may represent allelic conditions or (at least) in some patients the same entity (see below). Sanal et al. (2000) suggested that ashen is a mouse model of Elejalde syndrome: however, in 2000 Wilson et al. showed that a mutated Rab27a gene, not the MYOVA gene, causes the pathology of Mouse. Anikster et al. (2002) suggested also that neurological involvement in some patients with GS occurred secondarily to the haemophagocytic syndrome and that patient with primary central nervous system complications and MYOVA mutations (i.e., with the GS1 form) have Elejalde syndrome. Several other reports established that neurological manifestations in patients with GS caused by RAB27A (i.e., the GS2 form) were related to lymphocyte infiltration of the central nervous system (De Saint Basil and Fisher 2001, Menasche et al. 2000, Pastural et al. 2000), whereas patients with GS caused by MYO5A mutations (i.e., the GS1 form) exhibited a primary neurological disease, potentially described as Elejalde syndrome.

## Griscelli syndrome type 2 (GS2) [GS with haemophagocytic syndrome]

GS2 (OMIM # 607624) is characterized by hypomelanosis with immunologic abnormalities with or without neurological impairment. The GS2 phenotype currently corresponds to the original patients reported by Griscelli et al. (1978) (see above "historical perspective and eponyms"). GS2 patients exhibit various degrees of skin hypopigmentation and a silvery-gray sheen of the hair with large pigment aggregates in hair shafts. In most patients at least one episode of haemophagocytic syndrome (HS) or haemophagocytic lymphohistiocytosis (HLH) (the so-called "accelerated phase"), which is a lymphohistiocytic proliferation of unknown origin consisting of multivisceral infiltration, haemophagocytosis, pancytopenia, hypertriglyceridaemia, hypofibrinogenaemia, and hypoproteinaemia (Fig. 5) occurs. It is triggered by infectious episodes (usually viral but also bacterial) and is associated with a poor prognosis. When a remission is obtained, recurrent, accelerated phases with increasing severity are seen. The immunodeficiency is characterized by absent delayed-type cutaneous hypersensitivity and impaired natural killer cell function. No abnormal cytoplasmic granules are present in leukocytes. Patients with GS2 have immunologic abnormalities during the course of the haemophagocytic syndrome leading to leukocyte brain infiltration that sometimes result in secondary neurological involvement with diffuse white matter abnormalities seen at MRI (Anikster et al. 2002, Aksu et al. 2003): main signs include hyperreflexia, seizures, signs of intracranial hypertension, (e.g., vomiting or altered consciousness), strabismus, dysartrhia, ataxia, or regression of developmental milestones. The primary clinical differentiation between GS2 and GS1 is that the former has no primary neurological features. Occasionally, neurological problems may be the first sign of the accelerated phase.

CT and MRI findings are usually normal at birth. When the disease manifests, imaging findings are abnormal: CT can shoe areas of coarse calcification in the globus pallidus bilaterally, left parietal white matter, periventricular and left brachium pontis. Patients with GS2 can manifest unilateral hypodense signals in the genu and posterior limb of the internal capsulae (compatible with inflammatory changes), as well as posterior aspects of both thalami, together with minimal generalized atrophy. CT scanning can also suggest cell infiltration of the brain. The subcortical white matter can be affected as occurs in the GS1 variant.

GS2 is caused by mutations in the RAB27A gene which encodes a GTP-binding protein (rab27) that functions in the targeting and re fusion of transport vesicles with their appropriate acceptor membranes (Mamishi et al. 2008). Like other rab proteins, rab27 requires geranylgenarylation of two consensus C-terminal cysteine residues in order to be anchored to membranes. Truncation of the carboxy-terminal part of rab27 would render it inactive (Westbroek et al. 2008). To date all patients with GS and mutations in RAB27A have developed the haemophagocytic syndrome.

Mutations in Munc 13-4 cause *familial haemophagocytic lymphohistiocytosis subtype 3* (FHL3), a syndrome that resembles GS2. Neeft et al. (2005) have shown that Munc 13-4 intimately interacts with the Rab27 protein: both proteins are intensely expressed in cytolytic T lymphocytes and mast cells and co-localize on secretory lysosomes.

## Griscelli syndrome type 3 (GS3) [GS restricted to hypopigmentation]

The third form of GS, GS3, is characterized by the fair skin at birth of CHH and the other forms of GS followed by bronzed skin after sun exposure. Children can be referred because of unspecific complaints of failure to gain weight or recurrent tonsillitis and then noticed to have silver-gray hair, eyebrows, and eyelashes. Clinically, GS3-associate albinism is indistinguishable from that described in the other forms of GS. Skin biopsy and light microscopic examination reveals the same pattern as GS1 and GS2. Microscopic analysis of hair shafts show the characteristic features of GS, i.e., the presence of large clumps of pigment in the hair shaft. Most importantly, longitudinal follow-up reveals that phenotypic presentation is restricted to hypopigmentation, without any immune or neurological manifestation.

GS3 is caused by mutations in the gene that encodes melanophilin (Mlph) (SLAC2A/MLPH gene), the orthologue of the gene mutated in leaden mice. It has also been shown that an identical phenotype can result from the deletion of the MYOVA F-exon, an exon with a tissue-restricted expression pattern. The protein Mlph links the function of myosin Va and the GTP-Rab27a protein in the melanosome without additional functions: this explains why expression in GS3 is restricted to the characteristic hypopigmentation. In GS3 the Mlph is unable to associate with Rab27a, either transiently over expressed or endogenously expressed in melanocytes.

## Diagnosis

As silver hair syndrome present four different clinical and genetic patterns, in view of the restricted or failure of current therapeutic measures, a correct diagnosis is mandatory to offer a correct genetic counseling to the families with affected children. Skin biopsy and light microscopic examination in all the three forms of GS reveals the same pattern (Fig. 8). Light microscopy of the hair reveals a different distribution of melanin in small and large clumps irregularly arranged along the hair shaft. MYOVA and RAB27A interact in the same molecular pathway, resulting in melanosome transport. Menasche et al. (2002) suggested that patients with partial (albinos-like) hypopigmentation and manifestations of haemophagocytic syndrome, with or without neurological involvement, should be screened for mutation in RAB27A, and patients with partial (albinos-like) hypopigmentation and primary neurological disease without haemophagocytic syndrome should be screened for MYO5A mutations.

Characteristic laboratory features in GS2 include pancytopenia, hypofibrinogenaemia, and hypoproteinaemia.

## Treatment and prognosis

Medical treatment for patients with GS is difficult. For patients with defects in RAB27A (GS2), antibiotics and antiviral agents are used with mixed effects. Similarly medications may not control the neurological signs/symptoms of the disease. In GS related to MYO5A mutations (GS1), no specific treatment exists because the defect is in the brain rather than in the blood cells as in cases caused by

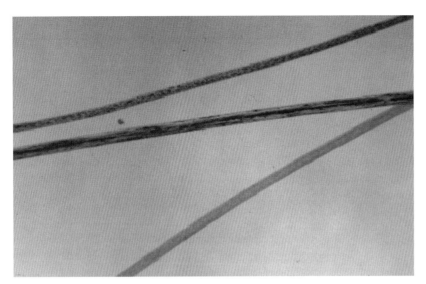

**Fig. 8.** Light microscopy of hair showing clumped pigment in small granules regularly distributed in CH syndrome (above) and small and large granules irregularly distributed characteristic of GS1 and GS2 patients without abnormalities, restricted to pigment dilution (middle) contrasting with normal hair (below).

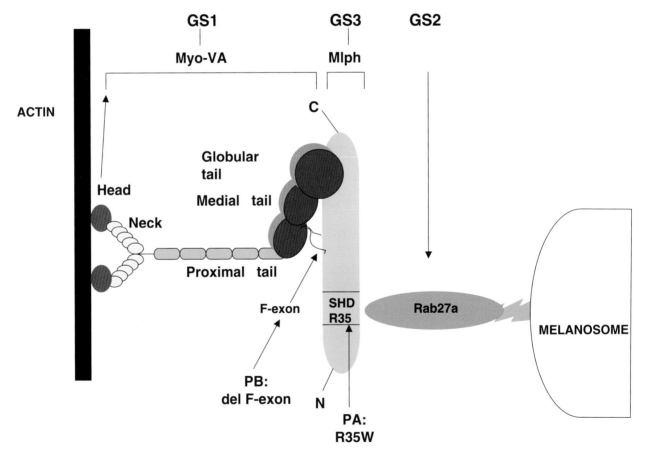

**Fig. 9.** Scheme of the heterotrimeric protein complex involved in human melanosome transport. A defect in any of the proteins, MyoVa, Rab27a, or Mlph, leads to identical pigmentary dilution, found in the three forms of GS (see text for further explanation). The F-exon of MyoVa is required for MyoVa-Mlph interaction and the SHD of Mlph for Mlph-Rab27a interaction (adapted from Menasche et al. 2000).

mutations in the RAB27A mutations (GS2). The severe neurological impairment and retarded psychomotor development do not improve with time.

Only allogeneic bone marrow transplantation is the treatment of choice in the early period of the disease (Arico et al. 2002). In preparation for a transplant, particularly in patients with GS caused by mutations in RAB27A (GS2), various immunosuppressive regimens have been used to attenuate the accelerated phase. Even a low number of donor cells in the patient's bone marrow can be sufficient to control symptoms of GS in cases caused by mutations of the RAB27A gene (GS2).

# References

Aksu G, Kutekculer N, Genel F, Vergin C, Omowaire B (2003) Griscelli syndrome without hemophagocytosis in an eleven-year-old girl: expanding the phenotypic spectrum of Rab27A mutations in humans. Am J Med Genet A 116: 329–333.

Anikster Y, Huizing M, Anderson PD, Fitzpatrick DL, Klar A, Gross-Kieselstein E, Berkun Y, Shazberg G, Gahl WA, Hurvitz H (2002) Evidence that Griscelli syndrome with neurological involvement is caused by mutations in Rab27A, not Myo5a. Am J Hum Genet 71: 407–414.

Arico M, Zecca M, Santoro N, Caselli D, Maccario R, Danesino C, de Saint Basile G, Locatelli F (2002) Successful treatment of Griscelli syndrome with unrelated donor allogenic hematopoietic stem cell transplantation. Bone Marrow Transplant 29: 995–998.

Bahadoran P, Ballotti R, Ortonne JP (2003a) hypomelanosis, immunity, central nervous system: no more "and", not the end. Am J Med Genet 116A: 334–337.

Bahadoran P, Ortonne JP, Ballotti R, de Saint-Basile G (2003b) Comment on Elejalde syndrome and relationship with Griscelli syndrome. Am J Med Genet 166A: 408–409.

De Saint Basile G, Fisher A (2001) The role of cytotoxicity in lymphocyte homeostasis. Curr Opin Immunol 13: 549–554.

Duran-McKinster C, Rodríguez-Jurado R, Ridaura C, Orozco-Covarrubias ML, Tamayo L, Ruiz-Maldonado R (1999) Elejalde syndrome – A melanolysosomal neurocutaneous syndrome. Clinical and Morphological findings in 7 patients. Arch Dermatol 135: 182–186.

Elejalde BR, Valencia A, Gilbert EF, Marin G, Molina J, Holguin J (1977) Neuro-ectodermal melanolysosomal disease: an autosomal recessive pigment mutation in man. Am J Hum Genet 29: 39A (abstract).

Elejalde BR, Holguin J, Valencia A, Gilbert EF, Molina J, Marin G, Arango LA (1979) Mutations affecting pigmentation in man: I. Neuroectodermal melanosomal disease. Am J Med Genet 3: 65–80.

Fukuda M (2005) Versatile role of Rab27 in membrane trafficking: focus on the Rab27 effector families. J Biochem 137: 9–16.

Griscelli C, Durandy A, Guy-Grand D, Daguillard F, Herzog C, Pruneiras M (1978) A syndrome associating partial albinism and immunodeficiency. Am J Med 65: 691–702.

Huizing M, Anikster Y, Gahl WA (2002) Reply to Menasche et al. Am J Hum Genet 71: 1238.

Hume AN, Collinson LM, Hopkins CR, Strom M, Burral DC, Bossi G, Griffiths GM, Seabra MC (2002) The leaden gene product is required with Rab27a to recruit myosin Va to melanosomes in melanocytes. Traffic 3: 193–202.

Ivanovich J, Mallory S, Storer T, Ciske D, Ciske D, Hing A (2001) 12-year-old male with Elejalde syndrome (neuroectodermal melanolysosomal disease). Am J Med Genet 98: 313–316.

Libby RT, Lillo C, Kitamoto J, Williams DS, Steel KP (2004) Myosin Va is required for normal photoreceptor synaptic activity. J Cell Sci 117: 4509–4515.

Mamishi S, Modarressi MH, Pourakbari B, Tamizifar B, Mahjoub F, Fahimzad A, Alyasin S, Bemanian MH, Hamidiyeh AA, Fazlollahi MR, Ashrafi MR, Isaeian A, Khotaei G, Yeganeh M, Parvaneh N (2008) Analysis of RAB27A Gene in Griscelli Syndrome type 2: Novel Mutations Including a Deletion Hotspot. J Clin Immunol Mar 19 [Epub ahead of print].

Mancini AJ, Chan LS, Paller AS (1998) Partial albinism with immunodeficiency: Griscelli syndrome. Report of a case and review of the literature. J Am Acad Dermatol 38: 295–300.

Manglani M, Adhvaryu K, Seth B (2004) Griscelli syndrome – a case report. Indian Pediatr 41: 734–737.

Marks MS, Seabra MC (2001) The melanosome: membrane dynamics in black and white. Nat Rev Mol Cell Biol 2: 738–748.

Menasche G, Pastural E, Feldman J, Certain S, Ersoy F, Dupuis S, Wulfraat N, Bianci D, Fisher A, Le Deist F, de Saint Basile G (2000) Mutations in RAB27A cause Griscelli syndrome associated with haemophagocytic syndrome. Nat Genet 25: 173–176.

Menasche G, Fisher A, de Saint Basile G (2002) Griscelli syndrome types 1 and 2. Am J Hum Genet 71: 1237–1238.

Menasche G, HoCh, Sanal O, Feldmann J, Tezcan I, Ersoy F, Houdusse A, Fischer A, de Saint Basile G (2003) Griscelli syndrome restricted to hypopigmentation results from a melanophilin defect (GS3) or a

MYO5A F-exon deletion (GS1). J Clin Invest 112: 450–456.

Neeft M, Wieffer M, de Jong AS, Negroiu G, Metz CH, van Loon A, Griffith J, Krijgsveld J, Wulffraat N, Koch H, Heck AJ, Brose N, Kleijmeer M, van der Sluijs P (2005) Munc13-4 is an effector of rab27a and controls secretion of lysosomes in hematopoietic cells. Mol Biol Cell 16: 731–741.

OMIM™ (2006) Online Mendelian Inheritance in Men. Baltimore: Johns Hopkins University Press, http://www.ncbi.nlm.nih.gov/omim

Pastural E, Barrat JF, Dufourcq-Lagelouse R, Certain S, Sanal O, Jabado N, Sager R, Griscelli C, Fisher A, de Saint Basile G (1997) Griscelli disease maps to chromosome 15q21 and is associated to mutations in myosin Va. Nat Genet 116: 289–292.

Pastural E, Ersoy F, Yalamn N, Wulffrat N, Grillo E, Ozkinay F, Tezcan I, Gedikoglu G, Philippe N, Fisher A, de Saint Basile G (2000) Two genes are responsible for Griscelli syndrome at the same 15q21 locus. Genomics 63: 299–306.

Provance DW, James TL, Mercer JA (2002) Melanophilinn, the product of the leaden locus is required for targeting of myosin-Va to melanosomes. Traffic 3: 124–132.

Rath S, Jain V, Marwaha RK, Trehan A, Rajesh LS, Kumar V (2004) Griscelli syndrome. Indian J Pediatr 71: 173–175.

Seabra MC, Mules EH, Hume AN (2002) Rab GTPase, intracellular traffic and disease. Trends Mil Med 8: 23–30.

Sanal O, Yel L, Kucukali T, Gilbert-Barnes E, Tardieu M, Texcan I, Ersoy F, Metin A, de Saint Basile G (2000) An allelic variant of Griscelli disease: presentation with severe hypotonia, mental-motor retardation, and hypopigmentation consistent with Elejalde syndrome (neuroectodermal melanolysosomal disorder). J Neurol 247: 570–572.

Scheinfeld NS (2003) Syndromic albinism: a review of genetics and phenotypes. Dermatol Online 9: 5–14.

Scheinfeld NS, Johnson AM (2006) Griscelli syndrome. E-medicine from webMD. http://www.emedicine.com/derm/topic926.htm

Westbroek W, Tuchman M, Tinloy B, De Wever O, Vilboux T, Hertz JM, Hasle H, Heilmann C, Helip-Wooley A, Kleta R, Gahl WA (2008) A novel missense mutation (G43S) in the switch I region of Rab27A causing Griscelli syndrome. Mol Genet Metab Apr 6 [Epub ahead of print].

Wilson SM, Yip R, Swing DA, O'Sullivan TN, Zhang Y, Novak EK, Swank RT, Russel LB, Copeland NG, Jenkins NA (2000) A mutation in Rab27a causes the vesicle transport defects observed in ashen mice. Proc Nat Acad Sci 97: 7933–7938.

# Chapter 20

# LEOPARD SYNDROME

**Sergiusz Jóźwiak**

Department of Neurology and Epileptology, Children's Memorial Health Institute, Warsaw, Poland

## Introduction

LEOPARD syndrome is a complex dysmorphogenetic disorder transmitted as an autosomal dominant trait with variable penetrance and expressivity. In recent years this multifaceted syndrome has attracted the interest of dermatologists, pediatricians, neurologists, cardiologists, endocrinologists, orthopedists, and radiologists.

Lentiginosis is a hallmark of this familial syndrome, which is regarded as a neuroectodermal defect. Gorlin et al. (1969) introduced the acronym LEOPARD as the name of the syndrome to recall the main features of the disorder:

- Lentigines (multiple)
- Electrocardiographic conduction abnormalities
- Ocular hypertelorism
- Pulmonary stenosis
- Abnormalities of genitalia
- Retardation of growth
- Deafness

## Historical perspective and terminology

Progressive generalized lentigines were reported in 1936 by Zeisler and Becker in a 24-year-old woman with hypertelorism, pectus carinatum, and prognatism (Zeisler and Becker 1936). The first familial cases were reported in twins by Rosen in 1942 and subsequently Pipkin and Pipkin (1950) described 8 members of a large 3-generation family. The possible association of abnormal skin pigmentation with some cardiovascular defects in a series of 1188 cases was stressed in Lamy et al. paper (Lamy et al. 1957), however, the associated syndrome with cardiac abnormalities and short stature was first reported by Moynahan in 1962. Soon afterwards, descriptions of patients with other features of LEOPARD syndrome appeared in the literature. The description of the full spectrum of the syndrome and the name LEOPARD syndrome was given by *Gorlin* in 1969 (Gorlin et al. 1969).

The syndrome is known by a number of names: cardiocutaneous lentiginosis syndrome, multiple lentigines syndrome, generalized lentiginosis, centrofacial lentiginosis, lentiginosis profusa syndrome, lentiginosis-deafness-cardiopathy syndrome, cardiocutaneous syndrome, progressive cardiomyopathic lentiginosis, Moynahan syndrome. However, the most widely accepted term is LEOPARD syndrome.

## Incidence and prevalence

There are no reliable epidemiological data. The syndrome seems to be rare, with no racial predilection. So far more than 100 patients have been reported and only few review have been published (Sarkozy et al. 2004, Voron et al. 1976). In a large collection from the literature of 77 patients, a slight preponderance of men has been documented (47:30) (Voron et al. 1976). Due to unpredictable variability of clinical manifestations most patients may lead a normal life. Some cardiac pathologic findings, as dysrhythmias and obstructive cardiomyopathy may be a cause of death in selected patients (Limongelli et al. 2006).

## Clinical manifestations

Not all of the findings are present in any given patient.

### Lentigines

Typically, lentigines are very characteristic in this syndrome, making the diagnosis relatively easy. They

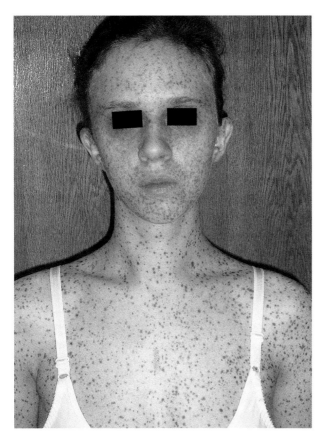

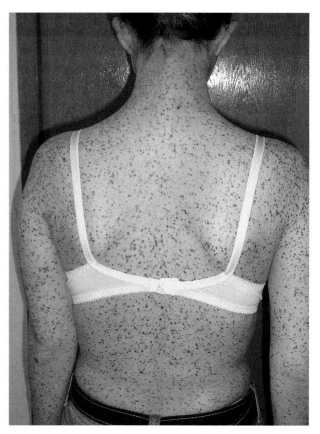

**Fig. 1.** Multiple lentigines on the face and trunk of the patient with LEOPARD syndrome.

**Fig. 2.** Multiple lentigines on the trunk of the same patient, posterior view.

were reported in 74 of 80 patients collected by Voron et al. (1976). However, according to recent observations they are not seen in every single patient. There are several descriptions of patients with features of the LEOPARD syndrome, but without lentigines (Watson 1967). We reported a male with full spectrum of LEOPARD syndrome, whose one sister had multiple lentigines, short stature, mental retardation and cardiac dysrhythmia, but another sister only cardiac myxoma without concomitant skin lesions (Jóźwiak et al. 1998).

Lentigines are often small, dark brown, irregularly shaped, usually from pinpoint to 5 mm in diameter, but sometimes larger, even up to 1–1.5 cm. Usually they are located on the upper part of the trunk and neck, but also often present on the face, palms, soles, genitalia, and even on the sclerae. With age they become darker and more numerous.

On histological examination, an increased number of melanocytes per unit skin area and prominent rete ridges are seen. Electron microscopic examination reveals large accumulation of melanosomes within the Langerhans cells and giant melanosomes. The giant melanosomes were revealed in normal and pigmented skin of patients with the LEOPARD syndrome, but they are not specific and also found in neurofibromatosis and nevus spilus (Slater et al. 1986).

On careful skin examination, other cutaneous abnormalities may be detected: axillary freckling, café-au-lait spots, hypopigmentations, onychodystrophy or hyperelastic skin. In some cases, patches of hair loss on the scalp can be observed (Shamsadidni et al. 1999).

Some isolated lentigines may be successfully treated with intense pulsed light and cryosurgery (Kontoes et al. 2003). However, such treatment modalities are less effective in respect to multiple lentigines. For some patients, treatment with tretinoin cream and hydroquinone cream may be helpful.

## Cardiac and vascular abnormalities

Voron et al. (1976) reported that about 40% of patients with LEOPARD syndrome have pulmonary stenosis, either valvular or infundibular type. Frequently, an obstruction of left or right ventricular outflow tracts was related to obstructive hypertrophic cardiomyopathy with clinical manifestations even in infancy (Cetinkaya et al. 2004, Hagspiel et al. 2005). According to Sarkozy et al. (2004) hypertrophic cardiomyopathy should be considered an important hint in the search of LEOPARD syndrome related to *PTPN11* mutations in the absence of multiple lentigines. The authors stress that hypertrophic cardiomyopathy should be regarded as more common and specific for LEOPARD syndrome than pulmonary stenosis, as according to their observations the incidences are 47% vs 10%, respectively.

Several other types of cardiac or vascular structural defects were revealed, including atrial myxomas, atrial insufficiency or aneurysms of large vessels (Limongelli et al. 2008). Yagubyan et al. (2004) reported a patient with recurrent upper extremity aneurysms requiring multiple operations. Another unusual vascular finding in LEOPARD syndrome was congenital intrahepatic portosystemic venous shunt (Digilio et al. 2005).

Electrocardiograms usually reflect the underlying structural anomalies. The most common electrocardiographic abnormality seen in patients with LEOPARD syndrome is left axis deviation which has been reported in one third of the patients with performed electrocardiographic studies (Voron et al. 1976). Other types of rhythm or conduction abnormalities include premature ventricular contractions, paroxysmal atrial tachycardia, prolonged PR intervals, left anterior or left posterior hemiblock, bundle branch block or combination of these with a complete heart block.

Despite frequent cardiac involvement, most patients are asymptomatic, and routine physical examination may be negative. Normal electrocardio-

gram does not exclude a risk of sudden death. The conduction impairment tends to occur gradually and progressively.

In patients with cardiac structural abnormalities beta-adrenergic receptor or calcium channel blocking agents are applied to reduce outflow tract obstruction and adrenergic responsiveness. Antiarrhythmic treatment may be given in selected patients with ventricular rhythm abnormalities.

## Neurologic abnormalities

Mental retardation, the most frequent neurologic abnormality among patients with the LEOPARD syndrome, was documented in 30% of subjects reviewed by Voron et al. (1976), and 27% those reported by Sarkozy et al. (2004). Mental retardation is usually of mild degree.

Sensorineural hearing loss appears in 20–25% of affected persons (Sarkozy et al. 2004, Voron et al. 1976). As melanocyte participates in the formation of the inner ear, some postulate, that this kind of deafness may be due to a primary abnormality in neural crest development (Polani and Moynahan 1972).

Other uncommon neurological manifestations of LEOPARD syndrome include nystagmus, hyposmia, seizures and abnormalities in electroencephalograms (Garty et al. 1989, Voron et al. 1976). In few patients, mild cerebral atrophy (Garty et al. 1989) or corpus callosum agenesis (Bonioli et al. 1999) can be found in neuroimaging examinations.

Recently, an association of LEOPARD syndrome with neuroblastoma development was postulated (Merks et al. 2005). Further studies are needed to assess the risk of neuroblastoma in these patients, however, in case of neurological symptoms appearance neuroimaging examination should be performed.

There is no specific treatment for neurological abnormalities in LEOPARD syndrome. If seizures occur, EEG and antiepileptic therapy is recommended.

## Genitourinary abnormalities

The most common abnormalities of genitourinary system in LEOPARD syndrome comprise cryptorchidism, either unilateral or, more likely, bilateral, hypospadius and delayed puberty (Ruiz-Maldonado et al. 1983, Voron et al. 1976). All of these features are distinctly more frequently seen in males, but this predominance can reflect the involvement of visible genitalia and resulting easier diagnosis. In few patients, other disturbances, as absent ovary, cystic hyperplastic ovary, agenesia of the kidney and ureter with contralateral hydroureter, double ureter or small penis attached to anterior abdominal wall, were reported (Voron et al. 1976). Taken together, genitourinary abnormalities affect 26% of LEOPARD syndrome patients (Voron et al. 1976).

There is no established method to treat genitourinary abnormalities in LEOPARD syndrome. In some cases, hormonal therapy to bring testes into scrotum can be effective (Gorlin et al. 1971). Surgical treatment is required in hypospodias and hormone-resistant cryptorchidism.

## Endocrine abnormalities

As retardation of growth and genitourinary disturbances including delayed puberty are pivotal symptoms of LEOPARD syndrome, endocrine abnormalities are apparently very much involved in the pathogenesis of the disease. Unfortunately, systematic hormonal examinations of LEOPARD syndrome patients are lacking. In some patients, hypogonadotropic hypogonadism or hypothyroidism were described. Laboratory studies performed in few patients revealed low level of follicle stimulating hormone (FSH), and luteinizing hormone (LH), low levels of T3 or T4, elevated urinary concentration of 17-hydroxy- and 19-ketosteroids in some cases (Swanson et al. 1971, Carney et al. 1986, Danoff et al. 1987, Wilsher et al. 1986). Interestingly, despite retardation of growth seen in many patients with LEOPARD syndrome, growth hormone levels were reported to be normal (Nordlund et al. 1973, Polani and Moynahan 1972).

## Dysmorphic features

Retardation of growth is one of key LEOPARD syndrome features. One third of patients demon-strate short stature and 20% of cases are below 3rd percentile (Voron et al. 1976). In majority of patients birth weight is normal (Polani and Moynahan 1972), suggesting that postnatal factors are involved in this symptom pathogenesis.

The detailed background of growth retardation in LEOPARD syndrome is not known. Although in few cases it seemed to be related to puberty delay, there are no reliable data supporting the association of growth retardation with other coexisting features or low level of growth hormone (Nordlund et al. 1973, Polani and Moynahan 1972). Therefore, defects in skeletal growth center response to physiological levels of various growth factors as well as mesodermal disorder manifestation are taken into consideration.

Ocular hypertelorism is the most common cephalofacial abnormality, seen in 25% of patients with LEOPARD syndrome (Voron et al. 1976). Other features include: mandibular prognatism, low-set large auricles, ptosis, high palatal arch, epicanthic fold and broad nasal root (Voron et al. 1976, Sarkozy et al. 2005). Different craniofacial dysmorphic features can be noticed in as much as 90% of patients with LEOPARD syndrome (Sarkozy et al. 2005).

## Skeletal abnormalities

Skeletal anomalies are relatively frequently found in LEOPARD syndrome patients (Voron et al. 1976, Sarkozy et al. 2005). Most are minor and do not require special treatment. Chest deformity (either pector excavatum or carinatum) is the most common anomaly. Others include kyphoscoliosis, retarded bone age, winging scapulae, rib anomalies, cervical spine fusion, syndactyly and supernumerary teeth (Voron et al. 1976, Ho et al. 1989, David 1973, Sarkozy et al. 2005). In some cases, surgical treatment can be beneficial.

## Other findings

LEOPARD syndrome was randomly reported to be associated with coeliac disease (Sarkozy et al. 2005), myelodysplasia (Sarkozy et al. 2005), bilateral congenital corneal tumor – choristoma (Choi et al.

2004) and severe caries of primary teeth (Sheehy et al. 2000). The detailed relation of these findings to LEOPARD syndrome pathogenesis requires further studies.

## Natural history

Although short stature is observed in one third of the patients, most newborns are of normal weight.

Lentigines may be present at birth or develop during childhood. They become more numerous and darker with age. Other skin lesions, such as nevocellular nevi and malignant melanomas, reported sporadically in the LEOPARD patients, may undergo depigmentation.

Cardiac pathologic findings, especially obstructive cardiomyopathy, are often progressive and responsible for morbidity, and in some cases, death. Progressive cardiac dysrhythmias may be a cause of sudden death.

## Pathogenesis/molecular genetics

The LEOPARD syndrome is an autosomal dominant condition that shares several clinical features with Noonan syndrome. About 40% of patients with Noonan syndrome have missense mutations in the *PTPN11* gene, which encodes for the protein tyrosine phosphatase SHP2.

The recent developments in molecular genetics demonstrate that the LEOPARD syndrome is allelic to Noonan syndrome, with two recurrent *PTPN11* mutations in exons 7 (Tyr279Cys) and 12 (THr468Met) (Legius et al. 2002). These two mutations are detected in about 80% of the patients with LEOPARD syndrome. Other patients have 5 additional mutations (Conti et al. 2003, Digilio et al. 2004, Kalidas et al. 2005, Limongelli et al. 2008, Pacheco et al. 2004, Sarkozy et al. 2005).

The revealed mutations suggest that distinct molecular and pathogenetic mechanisms cause the peculiar cutaneous manifestations of the syndromes (Digilio et al. 2002, 2006b). Clinical variability seen in patients with the same mutation likely reflects the effect of modifier genes or environmental factors, or both, which influences the phenotypes associated with *PTPN11* mutations.

## Diagnosis

The diagnosis of the syndrome may be difficult, especially in sporadic patients, due to the absence of any pathognomonic morphologic or biochemical markers and its highly variable expressivity. As seventy percent of cases are familial, careful examination of the first degree relatives may be an useful diagnostic tool (Digilio et al. 2006a).

In the majority of patients, we cannot confirm presence of all of the features included in 1969 by Gorlin at al. in the acronym LEOPARD. Although this classification has the advantage of being easily remembered, most patients have only three to five of these criteria (Pennelli et al. 1988).

Based on a clinical analysis of a large series of patients collected from the literature Voron et al. proposed in 1976 their own criteria for the diagnosis. Apart from lentigines, they grouped the features of the syndrome into nine categories: other cutaneous abnormalities, cardiac structural lesions, electrocardiographic abnormalities, genitourinary abnormalities, endocrine abnormalities, neurological defects, cephalofacial dysmorphism, shortness of stature and skeletal abnormalities.

They proposed the following "minimum" criteria for diagnosis:

- if the patient has multiple lentigines, features in at least two other categories must be present;
- if lentigines are absent, a diagnosis of LEOPARD syndrome may be established if the patient has features in at least 3 above-mentioned categories and has an immediate relative with the defined multiple lentigines syndrome.

## Differential diagnosis

First distinction should be made between lentigines and freckles. Lentigines occur at an earlier age than freckles and, unlike the latter, do not increase in number upon solar exposure.

There is also a clinical overlap between LEOPARD syndrome and neurofibromatosis 1. Café-au-lait spots and multiple lentigines are skin lesions common to both disorders. However a differential diagnosis in children may be difficult, as café-au-lait spots increase in number with age in both conditions, whereas the lentigines characteristic of LEOPARD syndrome are not present at younger age and develop during childhood. In adolescents and adult patients the lentigines of LEOPARD syndrome are distinguishable from those found in neurofibromatosis 1, being generalized and dark in color.

Patients with Noonan syndrome have café-au-lait spots similar to those found in neurofibromatosis 1 and frequently pulmonary stenosis.

Watson syndrome, an autosomal dominant disorder characterized by pulmonary stenosis, café-au-lait spots, short stature and limited intelligence should also be differentiated with LEOPARD syndrome.

## Follow up

Most patients are capable of leading a normal life.

All patients with the LEOPARD syndrome should be studied for the possible presence of serious dysrhythmia such as ventricular ectopy or supraventricular tachycardia, which may be responsible for sudden death in patients with hypertrophic obstructive cardiomyopathy. As the heart conduction impairment tends to occur gradually but progressively the patients should undergo periodic cardiac assessment with echocardiography, twenty-four hour ambulatory electrocardiogram and exercise stress testing (Chong et al. 2004). Outflow tract obstruction and significant cardiac dysrhythmias should exclude patients from performing strenuous physical exercises.

Periodic skin evaluation is also recommended due to an increased risk of malignant melanomas.

## Management

Cryosurgery and laser therapy may be beneficial for isolated lentigines, however, due to the large number of the lesions this type of treatment may last very long. Treatment with tretinoin cream and hydroquinone cream may be helpful in some patients.

To reduce outflow tract obstruction and adrenergic responsiveness, therapeutic regimens including betaadrenergic receptor or calcium channels blocking agents are recommended. Amiodarone treatment may be applied in cases of life-threatening ventricular ectopy (McKenna et al. 1985). Surgery may be necessary in cases with severe outflow tract obstruction.

Surgery may also be necessary in patients with cryptorchidism, hypospadias, or severe skeletal deformity. Other supportive measures may be applied for the management of psychomotor retardation and sensorineural deafness.

## Genetic counseling

Sarkozy et al. (2005) suggest that *PTPN11* screening should be carried out at first in children with café-au-lait spots associated with facial anomalies or congenital heart disease, or both, although in the absence of multiple lentigines.

In addition, *PTPN11* analysis should be considered in patients with café-au-lait spots or multiple lentigines when neurofibromas or Lisch nodules are not detectable and molecular analysis for mutations of *NF1* is negative.

Conversely, screening of the *NF1* gene should be performed in patients with skin manifestations of LEOPARD syndrome without a detectable *PTPN11* mutation.

## References

Bonioli E, Di Stefano A, Costabel S, Bellini C (1999) Partial agnesis of corpus callosum in LEOPARD syndrome. Int J Dermatol 38: 855–862.

Carney JA, Headington JT, Su WPD (1986) Cutaneous myxomas. A major component of the complex of myxomas, spotty pigmentation, and endocrine overactivity. Arch Dermatol 122: 790–798.

Cetinkaya E, Günal N, Sönmez N, Aycan Z, Vidinlisan S, Kahramanyol O, Paşaoğlu I (2004) LEOPARD syndrome and hypertrophic obstructive cardiomyopathy: a case report. Turk J Pediatr 46(4): 373–376.

Choi WW, Yoo JY, Park KC, Kim KH (2004) Leopard syndrome with a new association of congenital corneal tumor, choristoma. Pediatr Dermatol 20(2): 158–160.

Chong WS, Klanwarin W, Giam YC (2004) Generalized lentiginosis in two children lacking systemic associations: case report and review of the literature. Pediatr Dermatol 21(2): 139–145.

Conti E, Dottorini T, Sarkozy A, Tiller GE, Esposito G, Pizzuti A, Dallapiccola B (2003) A novel PTPN11 mutation in LEOPARD syndrome. Hum Mutat 21(6): 654.

Danoff A, Jormak S, Lorber D, Fleischer N (1987) Adrenocortical micronodular dysplasia, cardiac myxomas, lentigines and spindle cell tumors. Arch Intern Med 147: 443–448.

David LM (1973) Multiple lentigines syndrome. Arch Dermatol 108: 590.

Digilio MC, Conti E, Sarkozy A, Mingarelli R, Dottorini T, Marino B, Pizzuti A, Dallapiccola B (2002) Grouping of multiple-lentigines/LEOPARD and Noonan syndromes on the PTPN11 gene. Am J Hum Genet 71(2): 389–394.

Digilio MC, Pacileo G, Sarkozy A, Limongelli G, Conti E, Cerrato F, Marino B, Pizzuti A, Calabro R, Dallapiccola B (2004) Familial aggregation of genetically heterogeneous hypertrophic cardiomyopathy: a boy with LEOPARD syndrome due to PTPN11 mutation and his nonsyndromic father lacking PTPN11 mutations. Birth Defects Res Part A Clin Mol Teratol 70(2): 95–98.

Digilio MC, Capolino R, Marino B, Sarkozy A, Dallapiccola B (2005) Congenital intrahepatic portosystemic venous shunt: an unusual feature in LEOPARD syndrome and in neurofibromatosis type 1. Am J Med Genet A 134(4): 457–458.

Digilio MC, Sarkozy A, de Zorzi A, Pacileo G, Limongelli G, Mingarelli R, Calabro R, Marino B, Dallapiccola B. (2006a) LEOPARD syndrome: clinical diagnosis in the first year of life. Am J Med Genet A 140: 740–746.

Digilio MC, Sarkozy A, Pacileo G, Limongelli G, Marino B, Dallapiccola B (2006b) PTPN11 gene mutations: linking the Gln510Glu mutation to the "LEOPARD syndrome phenotype". Eur J Pediatr 165: 803–805.

Garty BZ, Waisman Y, Weitz R (1989) Gertsmann tetrad in leopard syndrome. Pediatr Neurol 5: 391–392.

Gorlin RJ, Anderson RC, Blaw M (1969) Multiple lentigines syndrome. Am J Dis Child 117: 652–662.

Gorlin RJ, Anderson RC, Moller JH (1971) The Leopard (multiple lentigines) syndrome revisited. Birth Defects Orig Artic Ser 7: 110–115.

Hagspiel KD, Candinas RC, Hagspiel HJ, Amann FW (2005) LEOPARD syndrome: cardiac imaging findings. Am J Roentgenol 184(3 Suppl.): S21–S24.

Ho IC, O'Donnell D, Rodrigo C (1989) The occurrence of supranumerary teeth with isolated, non-familial Leopard (multiple lentigines) syndrome: report of case. Spec Care Dentist 9: 200–202.

Jóźwiak S, Schwartz RA, Krysicka-Janniger C, Zaremba J (1998) Familial occurrence of the LEOPARD syndrome. Int J Dermatol 37: 48–51.

Kalidas K, Shaw AC, Crosby AH, Newbury-Ecob R, Greenhalgh L, Temple IK, Law C, Patel A, Patton MA, Jeffery S (2005) Genetic heterogeneity in LEOPARD syndrome: two families with no mutations in PTPN11. J Hum Genet 50(1): 21–25.

Kontoes PP, Vlachos SP, Marayiannis KV (2003) Intense pulsed light for the treatment of lentigines in LEOPARD syndrome. Br J Plast Surg 56(6): 607–610.

Lamy M, De Grouchy J, Schneisguth O (1957) Genetic and non-genetic factors in the etiology of congenital heart disease: a study of 1,188 cases. Am J Hum Genet 9: 17–41.

Legius E, Schrander-Stumpel C, Schollen E, Pulles-Heintzberger C, Gewillig M, Fryns JP (2002) PTP11 mutations in LEOPARD syndrome. J Med Genet 39(8): 571–574.

Limongelli G, Pacileo G, Calabro R (2006) Is sudden cardiac death predictable in LEOPARD syndrome? Cardiol Young 16(6): 599–601.

Limongelli G, Sarkozy A, Pacileo G, Calabrò P, Digilio MC, Maddaloni V, Gagliardi G, Di Salvo G, Iacomino M, Marino B, Dallapiccola B, Calabrò R (2008) Genotype-phenotype analysis and natural history of left ventricular hypertrophy in LEOPARD syndrome. Am J Med Genet A 146: 620–628.

McKenna WJ, Oakley CM, Krikler DM, Goodwin JF (1985) Improved survival with amiodarone in patients with hypertrophic cardiomyopathy and ventricular tachycardia. Br Heart J 53: 412–416.

Merks JH, Caron HN, Hennekam RC (2005) High incidence of malformation syndromes in a series of 1,073 children with cancer. Am J Med Genet A 134(2): 132–143.

Moynahan EJ (1962) Multiple symmetrical moles, with psychic and somatic infantilism and genital hypoplasia: first male case of a new syndrome. Proc R Soc Med 55: 959–960.

Nordlund JJ, Lerner AB, Braverman IM, Mc Guire JS (1973) The multiple lentigines syndrome. Arch Dermatol 107: 259.

Pacheco TR, Oreskovich N, Fain P (2004) Genetic heterogeneity in the multiple lentigines/LEOPARD/Noonan syndromes. Am J Med Genet 127A(3): 324–326.

Pennelli GM, Guolo S, Pavoncello S, Ferraris AM (1988) La syndrome della lentigginosi multipla o syndrome

"Leopard". Presentazione di un caso clinico. Minerva Med 79: 575–578.

Pipkin AC, Pipkin SB (1950) A pedigree of a generalized lentigo. J Hered 41: 79–83.

Polani PE, Moynahan EJ (1972) Progressive cardiomyopathic lentiginosis. Quart J Ed 41: 205–225.

Rosen I (1942) Society transactions. Manhattan Dermatologic Society. Generalized lentigo. Arch Dermatol Syphilol 45: 979–980.

Ruiz-Maldonado R, Trevizo L, Tamayo L, de los Rios MF, Skurovich M, Carrillo J, Dominguez D, del Castillo V (1983) Progressive cardiomyopathic lentignosis. Report of six cases and one autopsy. Pediatr Dermatol 1: 146–153.

Sarkozy A, Conti E, Cristina Digilio MC, Marino B, Morini E, Pacileo G, Wilson M, Calabro R, Pizzuti A, Dallapiccola B (2004) Clinical and molecular analysis of 30 patients with multiple lentigines LEOPARD syndrome. J Med Genet 41: e68.

Shamsadidni S, Abazardi H, Shamsadini F (1999) Leopard syndrome. Lancet 354: 1530.

Sheehy EC, Soneji B, Longhurst P (2000) The dental management of a child with LEOPARD syndrome. Int J Paediatr Dent 10(2): 158–160.

Slater C, Hayes M, Saxe N, Temple-Camp C, Beighton P (1986) Macromelanosomes in the early diagnosis of neurofibromatosis. Am J Dermatopathol 8: 284–289.

Swanson SL, Santen RJ, Smith DW (1971) Multiple lentigines syndrome. New findings of hypogonadotropism, hyposmia and unilateral renal agenesis. J Pediatr 78: 1032–1042.

Voron DA, Hatfield HH, Kalkhoff RK (1976) Multiple lentigines syndrome. Case report and review of the literature. Am J Med 60: 447–456.

Watson GH (1967) Pulmonary stenosis, café-au-lait spots and dull intelligence. Arch Dis Child 42: 303–307.

Wilsher ML, Rohe AHG, Neutze JM, Synek BJ, Holdaway IM, Nicholson GI (1986) A familial syndrome of cardiac myxomas, myxoid neurofibromata, cutaneous pigmented lesions and endocrine abnormalities. Aust NZ J Med 16: 393–396.

Yagubyan M, Panneton JM, Lindor NM, Conti E, Sarkozy A, Pizzuti A (2004) LEOPARD syndrome: a new polyaneurysm association and an update on the molecular genetics of the disease. J Vasc Surg 39(4): 897–900.

Zeisler EP, Becker SW (1936) Generalized lentigo: its relation to systemic nonelevated nevi. Arch Dermatol Syphilol 33: 109–125.

# Chapter 21

# NEVUS OF OTA

Ignacio Pascual-Castroviejo and Martino Ruggieri

Paediatric Neurology Service, University Hospital La Paz, University of Madrid, Madrid, Spain (IPC); Institute of Neurological Science, National Research Council, Catania, and Department of Paediatrics, University of Catania, Catania, Italy (MR)

## Introduction

The "nevus of Ota" is a hypermelanotic melanocytic phacomatosis, characterised by: (1) a (usually unilateral) area of non-hairy, macular or slightly raised hamartomatous hyperpigmentation (usually blue or grey in colour) involving the skin and mucous membranes at the forehead, temple, or eyelids over the distribution of the 1st and 2nd division of the trigeminal nerve; commonly associated with (2) ocular melanosis (involving the conjunctiva, iris, choroid, sclera, and optic disk) and (3) intracranial melanosis (involving the skull, periostium, dura, cerebral hemispheres, Meckel's cave, pineal gland, and optic chiasm) (Edelstein et al. 2005).

The blue nevus, the nevus of Ota and Ito, and the Mongolian spot are all classified as benign dermal dendritic melanocytoses (blue naevi) (Newton Bishop 2005). Histologically are characterised by the presence of increased numbers of dermal melanocytes deep in the dermis, scattered between collagen bundles differing in size, depth, anatomic location, and concentration and arrays of dendritic melanocytes (Lui and Zhou 2006, Newton Bishop 2005). The colour of these lesions is blue because of the optical effects of light reflecting off melanin deep in the dermis (Newton Bishop 2005).

## Historical background and terminology

The disorder was first described by *Hulke* in 1861 in a patient who presented with unilateral cutaneous hyperpigmentation associated with malignant melanoma of the sclera. In 1939, **Ota** described 26 patients in a Japanese population.

Specific variants of the nevus of Ota have been described in the literature under the names of "nevus fusca-caeruleus-ophthalmomaxillaris" (Ota 1939), "scleral melanocytosis", "oculodermal melanocytosis", "plaque-type variant of blue nevus", and "Hori's nevus" (Fitzpatrick et al. 1956). Some clinicians consider Hori nevus to be a distinct entity that is separate from nevus of Ota. Differential features of these conditions are related to location of patch or macules, extent of involvement, age of onset, tendency to occur as familial cases, and presence of a papular component (Lui and Zhou 2006).

## Prevalence and incidence

The nevus of Ota is most often described in Asian populations, especially the Japanese (Leung 1999, Leung et al. 2000), and is rare in Caucasians (Terheyden et al. 2001). In Japan, 0.4 (Yoshida 1952) to 1.1% (Tanino 1940) of all patients seen in dermatological clinics showed scleral melanocytosis.

The age at presentation has a bimodal distribution with one peak at birth-infancy and a second at adolescence (Hidano et al. 1967, Sekar et al. 2008). The characteristic cutaneous pigmentation is noted at birth or perinatally in approximately 50% of patients. In the other 50%, the dermal pigmentation becomes evident later, most frequently at puberty (Leung 1999, Leung et al. 2000). Isolated cases of delayed-onset nevi of Ota that first appear in adults, including in older patients, have been reported (Lui and Zhou 2006). Women are more commonly affected than men, in a ratio ranging from 5:1 to 7:3 (Patel et al. 1998). Leung et al. (2000) found scleral melanocytosis in 4.9% of boys and 4.1% of girls in

Chinese children under the age of 1 year, but oculo-dermal melanocytosis occurred only in one patient.

## Clinical manifestations

### Scleral and cutaneous features

The hallmark lesion is a congenital melanocytic hyperpigmentation of the sclera, which is usually black or grey-blue in colour (but it has also been described as brown, purple, blue/black, or slate grey) and it is a common characteristic of Asian and Africans subjects (Leung 1999). The condition is most often unilateral (95%) and infrequently bilateral (5%) (Leung et al. 2000). Scleral melanocytosis may occur as an isolated finding or in association with oculodermal melanocytosis (nevus of Ota). The nevus of Ota is

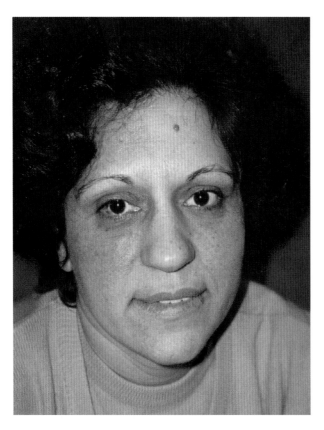

**Fig. 1.** A woman shows scleral and periorbital soft tissue nevus of Ota on the right side.

typically characterized by scleral melanocytosis and melanocytic hyperpigmentation of the skin and mucous membranes in the areas innervated by the 1st and 2nd sensory branches of the trigeminal nerve. According to our experience, the skin pigmentation in the nevus of Ota is usually unilateral and commonly affects the forehead, temple, eyelids or periorbital soft tissue (Fig. 1) (Pascual-Castroviejo et al. 2003). Up to 10% of affected patients may suffer of glaucoma (Teekhasaenee et al. 1990).

Associated melanosis of the mucous membranes may also be seen in the nasal mucosa, palate, pharynx, or tympanum. Half of the cases show ocular lesions, particularly hyperpigmentation of the sclera, conjunctiva, iris, choroids, or optic disc.

The colour (or perception of the colour) of the affected skin may fluctuate in extent and coloration (according to the personal and environmental conditions such as fatigue, menstruation, insomnia, and cloudy, cold or hot weather conditions) varying from light brown to dark brown, blue black or slate grey, but does not undergo spontaneous regression.

The nevus of Ota may be associated with or be encountered in the setting of other neurocutaneous disorders most often of vascular origin, such as Sturge-Weber or Klippel-Trenaunay syndromes (Furukawa et al. 1970, Noriega-Sanchez et al. 1972). Pascual-Castroviejo et al. (2003) reported a patient with cutaneous and intracranial hemangiomas (Pascual-Castroviejo type II syndrome) whose mother had nevus of Ota.

### Intracranial involvement

The nevus of Ota may also be associated with intracranial lesions consisting in diffuse (or circumscribed) melanosis (melanocytosis) involving the skull, periostium, dura, cerebral hemispheres, Meckel's cave, pineal gland, and optic chiasm (Edelstein et al. 2005). Diffuse leptomeningeal melanosis (or diffuse melanocytosis) is seen in addition to true melanocytomas (see below). Early neurological symptoms usually are mild or non-specific. Neurological manifestations of diffuse melanosis/melanocytosis include seizures, psychiatric disturbances, and signs of raised intracranial pressure due to hydrocephalus (Jellinger et al. 2005). Adult asymptomatic patients have been described as well as cases with probable only peripheral nervous system involvement (Wassima et al. 2007). Melanocytomas and malignant melanomas present with signs of raised intracranial pressure or compression of the spinal cord by an external mass, with local neurological signs, depending on the location. CSF cytology may be positive for malignant cells in some patients.

Imaging studies of diffuse melanocytosis show diffuse thickening and enhancement of the leptomeninges. MRI typically reveals prominent signal increase on T1-weighted images and signal decrease on T2-weighted images in the periostium and/or meninges caused by the inherent paramagnetic effects of melanin, which shortens T1 and T2 relaxation times. On non-contrast T1-weighted images, the melanin-containing periostium and meninges are displayed as high signal structures juxtaposed to the dark border formed by the cortical bone of the adjacent inner table. If a malignant melanocytic transformation occurs this bleeds frequently and thus can be detected as haemorrhage within the lesion that appears less homogeneous as compared to the surrounding tissue (Edelstein et al. 2005).

## Nevus of Ota and melanoma

The nevus of Ota rarely gives rise to cutaneous melanoma, but it is occasionally associated with melanomas of the optic tract, iris, choroids, orbits, and brain (Balmaceda et al. 1993, Dorsey and Montgomery 1954, Hartman et al. 1989, Horsey et al. 1980, Sagar et al. 1983, Piercecchi-Marti et al. 2002). Balmaceda et al. reviewed 12 published cases (including two of their own) of nevus of Ota with intracranial melanoma until 1993. All patients were adults, most of them whites. Intracranial melanomas mostly developed ipsilaterally in the tissues underlying the nevus. Exceptionally, the nevus of Ota has been reported with contralateral cerebral melanoma (Sang et al. 1977, Balmaceda et al. 1993).

Central nervous system melanomas associated with nevus of Ota primarily involve the meninges, and, in some cases, they are intraparenchymal

(Balmaceda et al. 1993). The typical intracranial lesions consist of diffuse (or circumscribed) leptomeningeal melanosis (or melanocytosis), and, in others, leptomeningeal melanosis/melanocytosis is seen in addition to the melanoma. Intracranial melanocytic tumours (as all melanocytic lesions) are quite variable in their malignant potential (Balmaceda et al. 1993).

## Pathology

The histological findings of the nevus of Ota are characterised by: 1) normal overlying dermis; 2) papillary and reticular dermis with increased number of pigmented dendritic melanocytes oriented parallel to the epidermis without disturbing the normal architecture of the skin and surrounding fibrosis and melanophages (Lui and Zhou 2006). The histological pattern of scleral melanocytosis, the Mongolian spots, the blue nevus and the nevus of Ota is similar, but the changes are more superficial in the nevus of Ota; in addition, in the Mongolian spot there is no surrounding fibrosis and in the blue nevus the dermal proliferation is nodular with heavily pigmented spindle cells.

Nevi of Ota have been classified histologically into 5 types based on the location of the dermal melanocytes, which are: (1) superficial; (2) superficial-dominant; (3) diffuse; (4) deep dominant; (5) deep. The histological classification correlates clinically with the observation that the more superficial lesions tend to be localised on the cheeks, while deep lesions occur on periorbital areas, the temple and forehead (Lui and Zhou 2006).

Malignant transformation of the skin lesion itself or a separate melanoma may be seen, especially in whites (Dorsey and Montgomery 1954).

Grossly, diffuse melanocytic lesions of the central nervous system may appear as dense black replacement of the subarachnoid space or as a dusky clouding of the meninges. Melanocytoma and malignant melanoma are single, often encapsulated lesions that may appear black, red-brown, blue or macroscopically non-pigmented (Jellinger et al. 2005). Neuropathology differentiates (1) diffuse melanocytosis (diffuse or multifocal proliferation of uniform nevoid polygonal cells in the leptomeninges which may spread into the Virchow-Robin spaces or frankly invade the brain); (2) melanocytoma (composed of monomorphic, spindle, fusiform, epithelioid or polyhedral cells, with round vescicular nuclei, prominent nucleoli, and a cytoplasm usually rich in melanin and arranged in whorls, sheets, nests, and interlacing bundles with a focal storiform configuration); (3) malignant melanoma (showing considerable pleomorphism, with large and bizarre tumour cells, and variable amount of melanin pigment associated to high mitotic rate, necroses, haemorrhage and invasion of brain and spinal cord parenchyma).

## Pathogenesis and molecular genetics

The aetiology and pathogenesis of nevi of Ota are not known. Hyperpigmentation is believed to result from mal development and abnormal migration of neural crest cells, particularly melanocytes. We know that melanoblasts arise from the neural crest and normally migrate to the skin, leptomeninges, ocular structures, and the internal ear (Maize and Ackerman 1987). The Mongolian spot, blue nevus, and nevus of Ota (although unconfirmed) are thought to represent arrested melanocytes in the migration (melanocytes that have not migrated completely) which remained in the dermis during the embryonic stages (while other cells arrived to the dermoepidermal junction to become branched melanocytes that produce melanin throughout life).

The variable prevalence among different populations suggests genetic influence – although typically sporadic, the nevus of Ota may occur in successive generations (reviewed in Trese et al. 1981). Incidental nevus of Ota has been reported in an autosomal dominant form of familial cerebellar degeneration with slow eye-movements and progressive mental deterioration (Whyte and Dekaban 1976). Nevus of Ota has been recorded also in a mother and her daughter (Agero et al. 2008). No specific genetic defect however has been identified so far.

Mutations in several genes may underlie susceptibility to uveal melanoma (UVM). Susceptibility loci have been mapped to chromosome 3q24-q26 (UVM1)

(OMIM # 606660) and chromosome 3p25.2-p25.1 (UVM2) (OMIM # 606661) (OMIM 2006).

## Management

Management is symptomatic. Skin and scleral lesions have no particular treatment however cosmetic camouflage makeup can minimise the disfiguring facial pigmentation resulting from the nevus. Pulsed Q-switched laser surgery (Q-switched ruby, Q-switched alexandrite, Q-switched Nd:YAG lasers) is unquestionably the current treatment of choice and it works via selective photothermal and photomechanical destruction of dermal melanocytes and melanophages (Kouba et al. 2008). After 4–8 treatments skin pigmentation is reduced dramatically or removed up to 90–100% of cases, with less than 1% risk of scarring.

Meningeal, cerebral and ocular tumours are usually removed.

Further follow-up care should require periodic ophthalmologic examination for the scleral nevus of Ota for the development of glaucoma (calculated risk of 10%). Skin biopsies are warranted if clinical changes are suspected of malignant transformation (e.g., ulceration, new papular lesions, variegations in colour) within the involved skin, ocular, or mucosal tissues.

## References

Agero AL, Lahmar JJ, Holzborn RM, Martin LK, Freckmann ML, Murrell DF (2008) Naevus of Ota presenting in two generations: a mother and daughter. J Eur Acad Dermatol Venereol Apr 14 [Epub ahead of print].

Balmaceda CM, Fetell MR, Powers J, O'Brien JL, Housepian EH (1993) Nevus of Ota and leptomeningeal melanocytic lesions. Neurology 43: 381–386.

Dorsey CS, Montgomery H (1954) Blue nevus and its distinction from Mongolian spot and the nevus of Ota. J Invest Dermatol 22: 225–236.

Edelstein S, Naidich TP, Newton TH (2005) The rare phakomatoses. In: Tortori-Donati P (ed.) Pediatric Neuroradiology. Brain Berlin: Springer, pp. 818–854.

Fitzpatrick TB, Zeller R, Kukita A, Kitamura H (1956) Ocular and dermal melanocytosis. Arch Ophthalmol 56: 830–832.

Furukawa T, Igata A, Toyokura Y, Ikeda S (1970) Sturge-Weber and Klippel-Trenaunay syndrome with nevus of Ota and Ito. Arch Dermatol 102: 640–645.

Hartmann LC, Oliver F, Winkelmann RK, Colby TV, Sundt TM, O'Neill BP (1989) Blue nevus and nevus of Ota associated with dural melanoma. Cancer 64: 182–186.

Hidano A, Kajima H, Ikeda M, Miyasato H, Númura M (1967) Natural history of nevus of Ota. Arch Dermatol 95: 187–195.

Horsey WJ, Bilbao JM, Nethercott J, Myers R, Hoffman HJ (1980) Oculodermal melanosis (naevus of Ota) complicated by multiple intracranial tumors. Can J Neurol Sci 7: 101–107.

Hulke JW (1861) A series of cases of carcinoma of the eyeball. Ophthalmic Hosp Rep 3: 279–286.

Jellinger K, Chou P, Paulus W (2005) Melanocytic lesions. In: Kleihues P, Cavenee K (eds.) Pathology and Genetics: Tumours of the Nervous System. Lyon: IARC Press, pp. 193–195.

Kouba DJ, Fincher EF, Moy RL (2008) Nevus of Ota successfully treated by fractional photothermolysis using a fractionated 1440-nm Nd:YAG laser. Arch Dermatol 144: 156.

Leung AKC (1999) Scleral melanocytosis. Am Fam Physician 59: 163–164.

Leung AKC, Kao CP, Cho EYH, Siu MPM, Choi MCK, Sauve RS (2000) Scleral melanocytosis and oculodermal melanocytosis (nevus of Ota) in Chinese Children. J Pediatr 137: 581–584.

Lui H, Zhou Y (2006) Nevi of Ota and Ito. E-medicine: Instant access to the minds of Medicine. http://www.emedicine.com/DERM/topic290.htm

Maize JC, Ackerman BA (1987) Pigmented lesions of the skin. Philadelphia: Bernard, Lea and Febiger, pp. 73–162.

Newton Bishop JA (2005) Melanocytic naevi and melanoma. In: Harper J, Oranje A, Prose N (eds.) Textbook of Pediatric Dermatology. 2nd edn. Oxford: Blackwell Science, pp. 937–951.

Noriega-Sanchez A, Markand ON, Herndon JH (1972) Oculocutaneous melanosis associated with the Sturge-Weber syndrome. Neurology 22: 256–262.

Ota M (1939) Naevus fusco-caeruleus-ophthalmomaxillaris. Jpn J Dermatol 46: 369–372.

Pascual-Castroviejo I, Pascual-Pascual SI, Moreno F, Viaño J, Martínez V (2003) Anomalías vasculares extracraneales e intracraneales y nevus de Ota en la misma familia. Neurología 18: 102–106.

Piercecchi-Marti MD, Mohamed H, Liprandi A, Gambarelli D, Grisoli F, Pellissier JF (2002) Intracranial meningeal melanocytoma associated with ipsilateral nevus of Ota. Case report. J Neurosurg 96: 619–623.

Sagar HJ, Ilgren EB, Adams CBT (1983) Nevus of Ota associated with meningeal melanosis intracranial melanoma. J Neurosurg 58: 280–283.

Sang DN, Albert DM, Sober AJ, McMeekin TO (1977) Nevus of Ota with contralateral cerebral melanoma. Arch Ophthalmol 95: 1820–1824.

Sekar S, Kuruvila M, Pai HS (2008) Nevus of Ota: a series of 15 cases. Indian J Dermatol Venereol Leprol 74: 125–127.

Tanino H (1940) Über eine in Japan haüfig vorkommende nävusform: "Naevus fusco-caeruleous ophthalmo-maxillais Ota". Jpn J Dermatol Urol 47: 51–53.

Teekhasaenee C, Ritch R, Rutnin U, Leelawongs N (1990) Glaucoma in oculodermal melanocytosis. Ophthalmology 97: 562–570.

Terheyden P, Rickert S, Kampgen E, Munnich S, Hofmann UB, Brocker EB, Becker JC (2001) Nevus of Ota and choroid melanoma. Hautarzt 52: 803–806.

Trese MT, Pettit TH, Foos RY, Hofbauer J Links (1981) Familial Nevus of Ota. Ann Ophthalmol 13: 855–857.

Wassima Z, Laissaoui K, Amal S, Sbai K, Kissani N (2007) Naevus of Ota and idiopathic facial neuralgia: association or coincidence? Ann Dermatol Venereol 134: 77–78.

Whyte MP, Dekaban AS (1976) Familial cerebellar degeneration with slow eye-movements, mental deterioration and incidental nevus of ota (oculo-dermal melanocytosis). Dev Med Child Neurol 18: 373–380.

Yoshida K (1952) Nevus fusco-caeruleus ophthalmo-maxillaris Ota. Tohok J Exp Med 55 (Suppl 1): 34–43.

# Chapter 22

# PHACOMATOSIS PIGMENTOKERATOTICA

María del Carmen Boente and Rudolf Happle

Department of Dermatology, Hospital del Niño Jesús, Tucumán, Argentina (MCB); Department of Dermatology, Philipp University of Marburg, Germany (RH)

## Introduction

Epidermal nevi are mosaic lesions reflecting an abnormal ectodermal embryonic development of the epidermis or its appendages, with excess or deficiency or structural changes of tissue elements being either present at birth or developing in postnatal life (Boente et al. 2000, Happle and Rogers 2002, Mehregan and Pinkus 1965, Rogers 1992, Solomon and Esterly 1975). The group of *epidermal nevus syndromes* denotes the association of an epidermal nevus with other cutaneous or extracutaneous anomalies (Boente et al. 2000, Happle 1995) each type being associated with specific additional defects (Happle 1991).

Among the epidermal nevus syndromes Happle delineated a separate clinical entity characterized by the presence of: (1) an organoid epidermal nevus usually showing sebaceous differentiation; and (2) a speckled lentiginous nevus (SLN) of the papular type; sometimes associated with (3) extracutaneous anomalies including neurological, ophthalmological, and skeletal abnormalities. The organoid nevus follows the lines of Blaschko whereas the SLN is arranged in a checkerboard pattern.

## Historical background and eponyms

Happle et al. (1996) first coined the term Phacomatosis Pigmentokeratotica (PPK) after reviewing a series of eight patients previously reported in the literature (Brufau et al. 1986, Goldberg et al. 1987, Happle 1993, Happle et al. 1996, Kopf and Bart 1980, Misago et al. 1994, Stein et al. 1972, Tadini et al. 1995, Wauschkuhn and Rohde 1972). Since then the condition has been documented in at least further 10 cases.

## Prevalence and incidence

PPK is a rare entity more frequently reported in men with a proportion male/female of 12:5 (Martinez-Menchòn et al. 2005).

## Clinical manifestations

The epidermal nevus associated with PPK constantly follows the lines of Blaschko (Fig. 1). If it involves the head, histopathological examination always shows hyperplasia of sebaceous glands consistent with a sebaceous nevus. In other parts of the body, however, the sebaceous component may be minimal or even absent, as generally noted in cases of systematized nevus sebaceus, including Schimmelpenning syndrome. Remarkably, however, Tadini et al. (1995) reported a diffuse ichthyosis-like hyperkeratosis involving the entire body. A similar finding was reported in one of the cases of Boente et al. (2000). Such unusual cases may be best explained by the concept of loss of heterozygosity for a mutation that in the homozygous state gives rise to a nonorganoid epidermal nevus (Happle 1999). Such diffuse ichthyosis-like hyperkeratosis has so far never been described in cases of simple nevus sebaceus or isolated Schimmelpenning syndrome. Does that mean that the epidermal nevus associated with PPK may sometimes be of a non-organoid type, thus differing from nevus sebaceus? Future research may address and hopefully answer this question.

The extracutaneous anomalies to be considered as part of this epidermal "half" of the didymosis (twin spotting) (Happle et al. 1996) include: mental retardation, seizures, coloboma, lipodermoid of con-

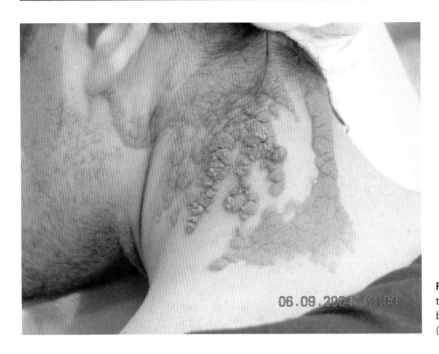

**Fig. 1.** Epidermal nevus of the sebaceous type, arranged along Blaschko's lines, in a boy with phacomatosis pigmentokeratotica (Figs. 2–5 show the same patient).

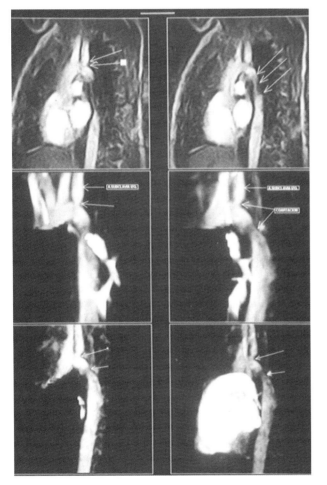

**Fig. 2.** Angiography showing pronounced coarctation of the aorta.

junctiva, skeletal defects, vascular abnormalities, and arterial hypertension (Gorlin et al. 2001, Marden and Venters 1966, Happle 2004). We want to highlight the vascular defects that appear to be present in PPK more frequently than in the Schimmelpenning syndrome (Boente et al. 2008), in the form of arterial hypertension (Aizawa et al. 2000, Boente et al. 2008, Ratzenhofer et al. 1981), changes in bone structure that originated from a vascular dysplasia with arterio-venous shunt involving the left iliac artery, resulting in increased length of the affected limb (Ratzenhofer et al. 1981), paradoxical pulse due to coarctation of the aorta (Fig. 2) (Boente et al. 2008), or hypertension with elevated plasma renin activity due to stenosis of a renal artery (Aizawa et al. 2000). In another case, juvenile hypertension was found to be due to compression of renal arteries by tumors (Okada et al. 2004).

On the other hand, the associated speckled lentiginous nevus (SLN) constituting the other "half" of the didymosis (Happle et al. 1996) consists of a café-au-lait macule superimposed by multiple dark papules that represent melanocytic nevi (Vidaurri-

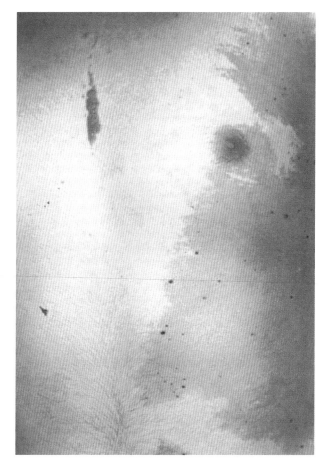

**Fig. 3.** Speckled lentiginous nevus of the papular type, arranged in a checkerboard pattern.

de la Cruz and Happle 2006). The SLN does not follow the lines of Blaschko but is arranged in a checkerboard pattern (Fig. 3) (Boente et al. 2000; Happle 1993, 2002a; Tadini et al. 1995, 1998). The spectrum of systemic involvement considered as part of the newly described SLN syndrome includes sensory and motor neuropathy, nerve palsy with thinning of the nerve, spinal muscular atrophy with fasciculations, muscular hypertrophy, and hyperhidrosis (Fig. 4) (Happle 2002a, Vente et al. 2004). Hemiatrophy is a frequent finding in PPK. This anomaly could be regarded as part of the SLN component if we assume it as a sequela of neurological defects rather than a genuine hypoplasia (Boente et al. 2008).

Other anomalies as noted in cases of PPK are so far difficult to assign to one of the twinned components, e. g., pinhead-sized vascular lesions superimposing the SLN (Boente et al. 2000, Tadini et al. 1995), linear connective tissue nevus of the collagen type (Fig. 5) (Boente et al. 2000, 2008) or suprasellar dermoid cyst (Majmudar et al. 2007).

Because many of the systemic complications appeared during follow-up of the reported patients it is important to bear in mind all of the possible cutaneous and extracutaneous anomalies of this syndrome, in order to ascertain a correct diagnosis at an early age.

**Fig. 4.** Circumscribed area of hyperhidrosis on the trunk.

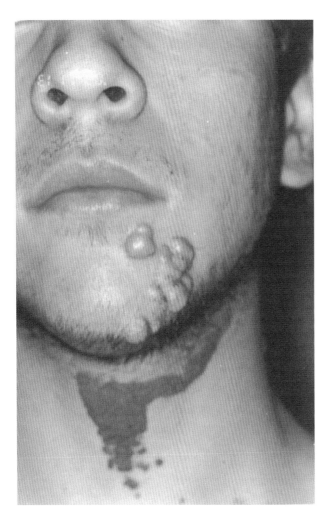

**Fig. 5.** Collagen nevus arranged along Blaschko's lines involving the chin. In addition, lesions of the epidermal nevus are seen on the neck.

## Pathogenesis and molecular genetics

The temporal and spatial relationship between the sebaceous nevus and the SLN of the papular type (Boente et al. 2000, Happle et al. 1996, Vidaurri-de la Cruz and Happle 2006) has been tentatively explained by the genetic mechanism of twin spotting (Happle 1999, Happle et al. 1990, Hermes et al. 1997, Tadini et al. 1995). Twin spotting or didymosis is a well-recognized mechanism extensively studied in plants and animals and used to test the mutagenic or recombinogenic activity of chemicals (Graf et al. 1989, Harrison and Carpenter 1977,

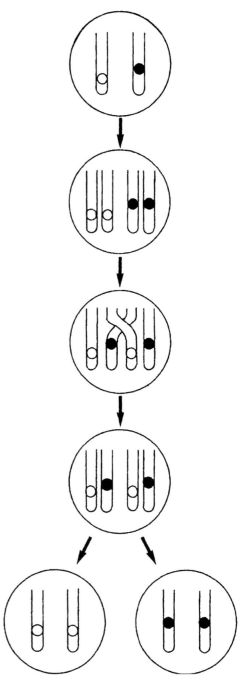

**Fig. 6.** Origin of non-allelic didymosis from a doubly heterozygous cell. The mutations of SLN and sebaceous nevus would be located in different regions on either of a pair of homologous chromosomes. After semiconservative replication, postzygotic crossing-over would give rise to homologous chromosomes that either contains a different chromatid. This mechanism may result in two different homozygous daughter cells, representing the stem cells of two different clones.

Patterson 1929, Vig and Paddock 1970), and proposed to likewise occur in human skin (Happle 1993, 1999; Happle and Steijlen 1989, Koopman 1999). The phenomenon of non-allelic twin-spotting requires an organism heterozygous for two different recessive mutations that would be located at different regions on either of a pair of homologous chromosomes. The segments bearing these loci are exchanged by somatic recombination at an early stage of the embryogenesis, giving rise to two homozygous daughter cells, representing the stem cells of two different cell populations that generate two different mosaic patches (Fig. 6) (Happle 1999, Happle et al. 1996, Happle and König 1999, Tadini et al. 1995). Hence, twin spots can be defined as paired patches of mutant tissues that differ from each other and from the background tissue. These two distinct mosaic spots are, by the nature of the process, usually in close proximity to each other and are therefore called twin spots or didymosis (Happle 2002b).

Proposed examples of didymosis in human skin so far include vascular twin nevi, cutis tricolor, lesions of overgrowth and deficient growth in Proteus syndrome, paired patches of excessive involvement or uninvolved skin in epidermolytic hyperkeratosis of Brocq, as well as phacomatosis pigmentovascularis and phacomatosis pigmentokeratotica (Happle 2002b).

Within the spectrum of anomalies noted in PPK, one "half" should be regarded as representing Schimmelpenning syndrome (Happle 1991, Schimmelpenning 1957, Feuerstein and Mims 1962). According to the concept of didymosis, this "half" of PPK does not reflect a heterozygous but rather a homozygous state of the underlying genetic defect (Happle et al. 1996). This assumption is further supported by the presence of a diffuse ichthyosis-like hyperkeratosis as noted in some PPK patients (Tadini et al. 1995). The other "half" of the twin-spot phenotype would be SLN syndrome (Happle 2002a) resulting in a melanocytic-epidermal didymosis (Happle 2002b; Happle et al. 1996; Misago et al. 1994; Tadini et al. 1995, 1998). The number of mutated cells, the time of the mutational event during embryogenesis, and the cellular type can modify the pattern and the degree of the cutaneous and systemic involvement. The time and location of the post-zygotic mutation can also explain why in some cases the two types of nevi are located on either side of the body, whereas in other cases they are located ipsilaterally (Boente et al. 2000, Happle et al. 1996).

All of the cases of PPK described so far have been sporadic and, therefore, at least one of the underlying genes might represent a lethal mutation surviving by mosaicism (Happle 1987, 1993; Happle et al. 1996; Tadini et al. 1995). The action of a lethal gene that survives by mosaicism may be suspected in a disorder that always occurs sporadically and is arranged in a mosaic pattern. The degree of severity is rather variable but the involvement is never diffuse or complete, and the sex ratio is 1:1. If the mutation is present in a zygote, the embryo dies at an early developmental stage. The cells carrying the mutations can only survive in close contact with normal cells, in a mosaic state. This mosaic may arise either from an early postzygotic mutation, or from a half chromatid mutation that has occurred before fertilization in one of the two gametes forming the zygote (Happle 1987).

## Diagnosis

If we consider PPK as a melanocytic-epidermal twin nevus syndrome (Happle et al. 1996) we should note, in a given case, both cutaneous components of this syndrome in order to establish the diagnosis. The SLN and the epidermal nevus of an organoid type are usually found either in adjacent areas on one side of the body or in corresponding regions of either side of the body, suggesting a common origin from a post-zygotic mutational event.

Either "half" of the syndrome, however, may occur as a separate entity. The epidermal component is so far considered to be identical with Schimmelpenning syndrome (Happle et al. 1996) including the full spectrum of its extracutaneous anomalies. The other "half" is SLN syndrome that can also occur as an isolated entity as delineated recently by Happle (2002a). Besides the cutaneous speckled lentiginous melanocytic nevus of the papular type, it is characterized by several neurological abnormalities, such as hyperhidrosis, muscular weakness and dysesthesia. In both isolated SLN syndrome and PPK, these neurological defects tend to be ipsilateral to the SLN (Tadini et al. 1995, 1998; Vente et al. 2004).

## Differential diagnosis

For differential diagnosis of the SLN component of PPK, partial unilateral lentiginosis and segmental neurofibromatosis may be considered. Other separate entities are multiple agminated Spitz nevi (Martínez-Menchón et al. 2005) and cases of linear arrangement of multiple congenital melanocytic nevi (Effendy and Happle 1992). The epidermal nevus present in PPK should be distinguished from other types of epidermal nevi and their corresponding extracutaneous anomalies (Happle 1991, 1995; Happle and Rogers 2002, Rogers 1992).

In several cases of PPK, an association with vitamin D-resistant rickets has been reported (Aschinberg et al. 1977, Goldblum and Headington 1993, Happle et al. 1996, Sugarman and Reed 1969). It is unlikely that such cases represent a distinct entity because hypophosphatemic rickets appears to belong to the clinical spectrum of Schimmelpenning syndrome (Zutt et al. 2003).

## Follow-up and management

The number of PPK cases so far reported is rather small. Moreover, several complications were noted only during the follow-up of such cases. Hence, the full spectrum of cutaneous and extracutaneous features of PPK has not been delineated yet. For this reason it is necessary, after the diagnosis of PPK, to inform the patient or the parents of the importance of a careful follow-up in order to notice any of the previously reported features or any other possible associations that are so far unknown. These patients should be managed by a team of specialists who are aware of the possible complications of PPK within their areas of expertise.

## References

Aizawa K, Nakamura T, Ohyama Y, Saito Y, Hoshino J, Kanda T, Sumino H, Nagai R (2000) Renal artery stenosis associated with epidermal nevus syndrome. Nephron 84: 67–70.

Aschinberg LC, Solomon LM, Zeis PM, Justice P, Rosenthal IM (1977) Vitamin D-resistant rickets associated with epidermal nevus syndrome: demonstration of a phosphaturic substance in the dermal lesions. J Pediatr 91: 56–60.

Boente M, Asial R, Happle R (2008) Phacomatosis pigmentokeratotica: a follow-up report documenting additional cutaneous and extracutaneous anomalies. Pediatr Dermatol 25: 76–80.

Boente M, Pizzi de Parra N, Larralde de Luna M, Bibas-Bonet H, Sanchez-Muñoz A, Parra V, Gramajo P, Moreno S, Asial RA (2000) Phacomatosis pigmentokeratotica: another epidermal nevus syndrome and a distinct type of twin spotting. Eur J Dermatol 10: 190–194.

Effendy I, Happle R (1992) Linear arrangement of multiple congenital melanocytic nevi. J Am Acad Dermatol 27: 853–854.

Feuerstein RC, Mims LC (1962) Linear nevus sebaceus with convulsions and mental retardation. Am J Dis Child 104: 675–679.

Goldblum JR, Headington JT (1993) Hypophosphatemic vitamin D-resistant rickets and multiple spindle and epithelioid nevi associated with linear nevus sebaceus syndrome. J Am Acad Dermatol 29: 109–111.

Gorlin RJ, Cohen MM Jr, Hennekam RCM (2001) Syndromes of the Head and Neck. 4th ed. Oxford: Oxford University Press.

Graf U, Frei H, Kägi A, Katz AJ, Würgler FE (1989) Thirty compounds tested in the Drosophila wing spot test. Mutat Res 222: 359–373.

Happle R (1987) Lethal genes surviving by mosaicism: a possible explanation for sporadic birth defects involving the skin. J Am Acad Dermatol 16: 899–906.

Happle R (1991) How many epidermal nevus syndromes exist? A clinicogenetic classification. J Am Acad Dermatol 25: 550–556.

Happle R (1993) Mosaicism in human skin: understanding the patterns and mechanisms. Arch Dermatol 129: 1460–1470.

Happle R (1995) Epidermal nevus syndromes. Sem Dermatol 14: 111–121.

Happle R (1999) Loss of heterozygosity in human skin. J Am Acad Dermatol 41: 143–161.

Happle R (2002a) Speckled lentiginous nevus syndrome: delineation of a new distinct neurocutaneous phenotype. Eur J Dermatol 12: 133–135.

Happle R (2002b) Dohi memorial lecture: new aspects of cutaneous mosaicism. J Dermatol 29: 681–692.

Happle R (2004) Gustav Schimmelpenning and the syndrome bearing his name. Dermatology 209: 84–87

Happle R, Hoffmann R, Restano L, Caputo R, Tadini G (1996) Phacomatosis pigmentokeratotica: a melanocytic-epidermal twin nevus syndrome. Am J Med Genet 65: 363–365.

Happle R, König A (1999) Dominant traits may give rise to paired patches of either excessive or absent involvement. Am J Med Genet 84: 176–177.

Happle R, Koopman R, Mier PD (1990) Hypothesis: vascular twin naevi and somatic recombination in man. Lancet 335: 376–378.

Happle R, Rogers M (2002) Epidermal nevi. Adv Dermatol 18: 175–201.

Happle R, Steijlen PM (1989) Phacomatosis pigmentovascularis gedeutet als ein Phänomen der Zwillingsflecken. Hautarzt 40: 721–724.

Harrison BJ, Carpenter R (1977) Somatic crossing-over in *Antirrhinum majus*. Heredity 38: 169–189.

Hermes B, Cremer B, Happle R, Henz BM (1997) Phacomatosis pigmentokeratotica: a patient with the rare melanocytic-epidermal twin nevus syndrome. Dermatology 194: 77–79.

Koopman RJJ (1999) Concept of twin spotting. Am J Med Genet 85: 355–358.

Marden PM, Venters HD (1996) A new neurocutaneous syndrome. Am J Dis Child 112: 79–81.

Majmudar V, Loffeld A, Happle R, Salim A (2007) Phacomatosis pigmentokeratotica associated with a suprasellar dermoid cyst and leg hypertrophy. Clin Exp Dermatol 32: 690–692.

Martínez-Menchón T, Mahiques Santos L, Vilata Corell JJ, Febrer Bosch I, Fortea Baixauli JM (2005) Phacomatosis pigmentokeratotica: a 20-year follow-up with malignant degeneration of both nevus components. Pediatr Dermatol 22: 44–47.

Mehregan A, Pinkus H (1965) Life history of organoid nevi. Arch Dermatol 91: 574–588.

Misago N, Narisawa Y, Nishi T, Kohda H (1994) Association of nevus sebaceus with an unusual type of combined nevus. J Cutan Pathol 21: 76–81.

Okada E, Tamura A, Ishikawa O (2004) Phacomatosis pigmentokeratotica complicated with juvenile on-set hypertension. Acta Derm Venereol 84: 397–398. 58.

Patterson JT (1929) The production of mutations in somatic cells of Drosophila melanogaster by means of X-rays. J Exp Zool 53: 327–372.

Ratzenhofer E, Hohlbrugger H, Gebhart W, Lubec G (1981) Linearer epidermaler Naevus mit multiplen Mißbildungen ("epidermal nevus syndrome" Solomon). Klin Pädiatr 117: 117–119.

Rogers M (1992) Epidermal nevi and epidermal nevus syndromes: a review of 233 cases. Pediatr Dermatol 9: 342–344.

Schimmelpenning GW (1957) Klinischer Beitrag zur Symptomatologie der Phakomatosen. Fortschr Röntgenstr 87: 716–720.

Solomon LM, Esterly NB (1975) Epidermal and other congenital organoid nevi. Curr Probl Pediatr 6: 1–56.

Sugarman GI, Reed WB (1969) Two unusual neurocutaneous disorders with facial cutaneous signs. Arch Neurol 21: 242–247.

Tadini G, Ermacora E, Carminati G, Gelmetti C, Cambiaghi S, Brusasco A, Caputo R, Happle R (1995) Unilateral specked lentiginous naevus, contralateral verrucous epidermal naevus, and diffuse ichthyosis-like hyperkeratosis: an unusual example of twin spotting? Eur J Dermatol 5: 659–663.

Tadini G, Restano L, Gonzales-Perez R, Gonzales-Enseñat A, Vincente-Villa MA, Cambiaghi S, Marchettini P, Mastrangelo M, Happle R (1998) Phacomatosis pigmentokeratotica: report of new cases and further delineation of the syndrome. Arch Dermatol 134: 333–342.

Vente C, Neumann C, Bertsch H, Rupprecht R, Happle R (2004) Speckled lentiginous nevus syndrome: report of a further case. Dermatology 209: 228–229.

Vidaurri-de la Cruz H, Happle R (2006) Two distinct types of speckled lentiginous nevi characterized by macular versus papular speckles. Dermatology 212: 53–58.

Vig BK, Paddock EF (1970) Studies on the expression of somatic crossing over in Glycine max L. Theoret Applied Genet 40: 316–321.

Zutt M, Strutz F, Happle R, Habenicht EM, Emmert S, Haenssle HA, Kretschmer L, Neumann C (2003) Schimmelpenning-Feuerstein-Mims syndrome with hypophosphatemic rickets. Dermatology 207: 72–76.

# Chapter 23

# PHAKOMATOSIS PIGMENTOVASCULARIS

Ramón Ruiz-Maldonado, Carola Duràn-McKinster, Luz Orozco-Covarrubias, and Marimar Saez-De-Ocariz

Department of Dermatology, National Institute of Paediatrics, Mexico City, Mexico

## Introduction

Phakomatosis pigmentovascularis (PPV) is defined as the coexistence of a widespread *vascular* (usually capillary) *nevus* (nevus flammeus) and an extensive *pigmentary nevus* (usually of the Mongolian spot type or blue/slate/grey oculo-cutaneous melanocytosis) associated to a variety of other cutaneous nevus (e.g., anaemicus, epidermal nevus, telangiectatic nevus, nevus spilus or cutis marmorata telangiectatica) and/or extracutaneous alterations (Happle 2005, Ruiz-Maldonado et al. 1987, Vidaurri-de la Cruz et al. 2003). All types of PPV so far described have been best explained as examples of twin spotting (Happle 1999, 2005).

## Historical perspective and eponyms

Ota, Kawamura and Ito first described PPV in 1944 (Ota et al. 1947). PPV derives its name from the Greek words *phakos*, which means spot (as referred to the retinal abnormalities originally seen in neurocutaneous disorders such as von Hippel-Lindau disease, Sturge-Weber syndrome or tuberous sclerosis) (Gomez 1987), *oma* that means tumour and *osis*, which means condition. The term phakomatosis (spelled with "k" instead of "c") was originally used and still is synonymous with neurocutaneous syndromes whilst the term phacomatosis (spelled with "c" instead of "k") has been mainly applied to genetically determined diseases characterised by the presence of 2 or more different naevi, such as "phacomatosis pigmentovascularis" or "phacomatosis pigmentokeratotica" (Happle 2005). The term *"pigmento"* refers to the pigmentary nevus while the term *"vascularis"* refers to the red spots due to dermal capillary malformations.

According to Happle (2005) the spelling "phacomatosis" would be preferable to "phakomatosis" when the term is followed by a Latin adjective. We propose that in order to avoid unnecessary accumulation of meaningless and confusing terminology, only the original name "Phakomatosis pigmento vascularis" should be re-adopted.

## Incidence and prevalence

Over 200 cases of PPV have been so far reported, mainly in Asian or Asian related populations, as are the Latin Americans. Isolated cases have been reported worldwide. All cases have been sporadic (Vidaurri-de la Cruz et al. 2003).

At the National Institute of Pediatrics in Mexico City, over a 35- years period 35 cases of PPV have been diagnosed, one every year with a calculated incidence of 7.9 per 100,000 paediatric patients and 88 per 100,000 paediatric dermatology patients. Fifteen were males and 20 females (Vidaurri-de la Cruz et al. 2003). After Mexico, the country with the highest number of reported cases of PPV is Argentina (Ruiz-Maldonado et al. 1987, Vidaurri-de la Cruz et al. 2003).

## Clinical manifestations

### Major skin manifestations

In 1985, Hasegawa and Yasuhara proposed a classification of PPV into four types. Enjolras and Mulliken (2000) described a fifth type.

**Type I:** Nevus flammeus (capillary malformation) and epidermal nevus.

**Type II:** Nevus flammeus and Mongolian spot (Dermal melanocytosis) with or without nevus anaemicus.
**Type III:** Nevus flammeus and nevus spilus with or without nevus anaemicus.
**Type IV:** Nevus flammeus and Mongolian spot and nevus spilus with or without nevus anaemicus.
**Type V:** Mongolian spot and cutis marmorata telangiectatica congenita.

Each type was subdivided into:

A. With oculocutaneous involvement.
B. With extra-oculocutaneous involvement.

While in Caucasians the dermal melanocytosis is an unusual finding, in native Americans, Mestizo, and Asian populations, "classic" or ectopic dermal melanocytosis (Mongolian spot), is present in over 90% of newborns (Bleehen 1998), therefore its association with cutaneous and extracutaneous alterations may be fortuitous. This could explain why phakomatosis pigmentovascularis is sometimes reported "in association" with known vascular syndromes with nevus flammeus as for example the Sturge-Weber syndrome (SWS) (Al Robaee et al. 2004): in these cases the "true" phenotype could be that of the complex vascular malformation (in this case the SWS) whilst the pigmentary nevus (in this case the Mongolian spot) would be coincidentally associated. An extensive pigmentary ne-

vus however should orient towards a "true" PPV (see also below).

On the basis of the observation of 35 cases of PPV over 35 years at the National Institute of Pediatrics in Mexico City (the largest series so far), we propose to consider PPV as a single clinical-pathological entity with variable expression. All of our cases, and the vast majority of those published, correspond to the original description by Ota et al. (1947) and to the type 2 PPV according to the Hasegawa and Yasuhara classification (Hasegawa and Yasuhara 1985). Under the diagnostic term PPV only patients with nevus flammeus (cutaneous capillary malformations) and classic or ectopic Mongolian spots (dermal melanocytosis) should be considered (Fig. 1). Associated cutaneous and extra-cutaneous abnormalities should be recorded and their frequency and characteristics reported as part of the syndromic spectrum, not as new types (Figs. 2–4).

In a recent paper Happle (2005) proposed a new classification based on three types only and insisted to use the term phacomatosis instead of phakomatosis:

(a) *Phacomatosis cesioflammea* (blue spots [*caesius* = blue grey used as equivalent of *fuscocoeruleus* to describe an aberrant Mongolian spot] and nevus flammeus) which is identical with the traditional types IIa and IIb (Castori et al. 2008);

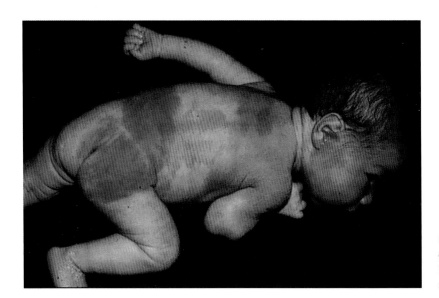

**Fig. 1.** Typical dermal melanocytosis or Mongolian spots (Grey spots) and capillary vascular malformations or nevus flammeus (Red spots) in phakomatosis pigmentovascularis.

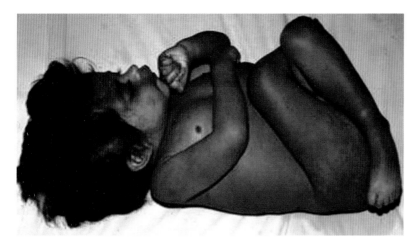

**Fig. 2.** Phakomatosis pigmentovascularis with extensive Mongolian spot and profound mental retardation.

(b) *Phacomatosis spilorosea* (Nevus spilus coexisting with a pale-pink telangiectatic nevus) corresponding to types IIIa and IIIb (Karabudak et al. 2007);

(c) *Phacomatosis cesiomarmorata* (blue spots and cutis marmorata telangiectatica congenita), which is a descriptive term for type V (Torrelo et al. 2006).

In this classification phacomatosis spilorosea lacks Mongolian spots and phacomatosis cesiomarmorata lacks nevus flammeus.

## Associated skin and systemic manifestations

Associated alterations in our patients and in the cases reported in the literature (Cho et al. 2001, Du et al. 1998, Fernández-Guarino et al. 2008, Guiglia and Prendeville 1991, Happle 2005, Happle and Staijlen 1989, Hall et al. 2007, Hasegawa and Yasuhara 1985, Kikuchi and Okasaki 1982, Kim et al. 2002, Ota et al. 1947, Ruiz-Maldonado et al. 1987, Tsuruta et al. 1991, Vidaurri-de la Cruz et al. 2003) were as follows:

### Cutaneous

In our series we recorded café-au-lait spots, nevus anaemicus, hypochromic nevus, pre-auricular tags, plexiform neurofibroma and linear morfea. Associated cutaneous alterations in the literature not present in our patients included vitiligo (Kim et al. 2002), congenital patches of alopecia (Kikuchi and Okasaki 1982), multiple granular-cell tumours (Guiglia and

Prendeville 1991), hypoplastic nails (Guiglia and Prendeville 1991) and unilateral lymphoedema (Happle and Steijlen 1989).

### Ocular

In our patients we found melanosis bulbi, glaucoma, iris mammillations, megalocornea and buphthalmos. Associated ocular abnormalities in the literature not present in our patients were Goniodysgenesis with iris abnormalities (Kono et al. 2003).

### Musculoskeletal

Musculoskeletal alterations in our patients included limb hypertrophy, Klippel-Trenaunay type abnormalities, hemifacial hypertrophy, hemicorporal hypertrophy, macrocephaly and scoliosis. We did not record additional musculoskeletal alterations in the literature besides unilateral lipohyplasia (Castori et al. 2008).

## Central nervous system manifestations

The central nervous system (CNS) abnormalities recorded in our patients included seizures, Sturge-Weber syndrome manifestations, cerebral atrophy, mental retardation, hydrocephalus, abnormal electroencephalogram, sensorineural deafness and intracranial hypertension (Al Robaee et al. 2004, Cho et al. 2001, Hagiwara et al. 1998, Onsun et al. 2007,

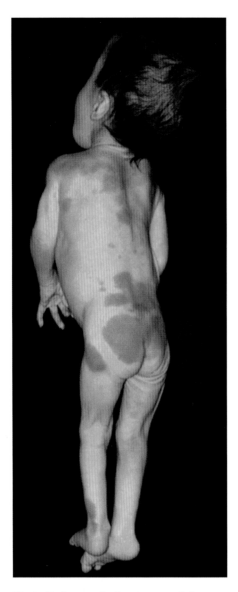

**Fig. 3.** Phakomatosis pigmentovascularis macrocephaly and mental retardation.

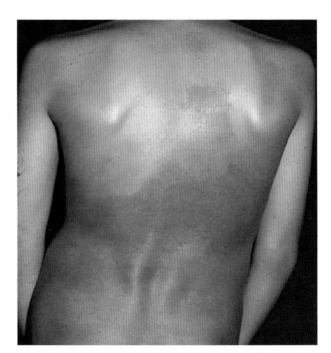

**Fig. 4.** Phakomatosis pigmentovascularis and scoliosis.

Saricaoglu et al. 2002, Uysal et al. 2000). CNS findings in the literature not present in our patients were hemiplegia or hemiparesis (Cho et al. 2001), Chiari 1 malformation (Du et al. 1998), meningeal capillary malformations (Ruiz-Maldonado 1987) and Moyamoya disease (Tsuruta et al. 1991). In our series we found a positive correlation between extracutaneous alterations and extension of the body surface area involved by the capillary vascular malformation (nevus flammeus).

## Pathology

Seldom is it necessary to biopsy for histopathological analysis to make the diagnosis of PPV, which is essentially a clinical one. The pathology of Mongolian spots or dermal melanocytosis consists in the presence of more or less abundant melanocytes in the middle and deep dermis that can be seen with the routine haematoxylin eosin staining or become evident with silver stains or by means of immunohistochemistry (S-100 reactant). The capillary (nevus flammeus) component consists in increased numbers of dilated capillaries in the papillary and superficial dermis.

## Pathogenesis

PPV is currently explained as an example of twin spotting phenomenon as proposed by Happle (1999, 2005) and Happle and Steijlen (1989): loss of heterozygosity in an embryo that is heterozygous for two different mutations, during somatic recombination, gives origin to three different cell lines, two homozygous for different mutations (hence, the coexistence of different naevi) and the third heterozygous not expressing any mutation (Happle 1999).

## Diagnosis

The clinical diagnosis is easily made by the presence of Mongolian spots (Dermal melanocytosis) with their typical slate-grey colour located in any body area, usually extensive and sometimes coexisting in the same area with a nevus flammeus that may be more difficult to identify. The capillary malformation (nevus flammeus) may also be extensive involving several body segments, of dark- red or pink colour that fades under pressure. With time both, the Mongolian spots and the nevus flammeus may partially or totally spontaneously disappear. The diagnosis of FPV is further supported by the presence of associated cutaneous or extra-cutaneous alterations, more frequently neurological or musculoskeletal.

## Differential diagnosis

The main differential diagnosis should be made with the Sturge-Weber Syndrome (SWS) which shares with PPV the presence of a nevus flammeus, usually hemi-facial, seldom bilateral or involving other body areas. Buphthalmos, seizures and meningeal calcifications are frequent findings in SWS and can also be found in PPV (Al Robaee et al. 2004, Cho et al. 2001, Diociaiuti et al. 2005, Hagiwara et al. 1998, Lee et al. 2005, Saricaoglu et al. 2002, Uysal et al. 2000). In contrast to PPV, however, SWS is characterised by a typical capillary malformation of the cerebral leptomeninges, which is almost always ipsilateral to the facial vascular malformation and is often associated to a capillary malformation of the retina (eventually leading to glaucoma) and/or the conjunctiva. It could be that the overlapping phenotypes between PPV and SWS could represent phenotypic variability. Therefore, the definite diagnosis of PPV is made on the presence of usually extensive Mongolian spots (Figs. 1–4). In patients with facial naevus flammeus not involving the ocular branch of the trigeminal nerve, there are usually no underlying brain abnormalities and no as-

sociated neurological component and the diagnosis of SWS cannot be easily made.

In patients with extensive nevus flammeus involving the limbs and causing hypertrophy, but without involvement of the trigeminal area the diagnosis of Klippel-Trenaunay Syndrome (KTS) should be made. In patients with KTS and arteriovenous fistula the corresponding diagnosis is that of Parkes Weber syndrome.

The coexistence of clinical and/or imaging features of PPV, SWS and KTS in the same patient is not an exceptional event. The loci of the responsible genes for these three conditions might be probably close neighbours.

In presence of classic, ectopic, small or extensive Mongolian spot, associated to cutaneous or systemic alterations but in the absence of nevus flammeus the diagnosis of PPV should not be made.

## Treatment

The vascular capillary malformation (nevus flammeus) of the PPV when involving the face represents an aesthetic nuisance and may be successfully treated with the laser of anilines (580 nanometres) or with multiple lasers (Kono et al. 2003). Factors that should be taken into consideration before deciding to treat are: (a) the neurological manifestations and the status of the patient; (b) the extent of the cutaneous lesion; (c) the skin complexion (dark skins respond poorly to laser treatment); and (d) the high cost of treatment.

Mongolian spots representing an aesthetic problem and not showing signs of spontaneous regression may also be treated with laser (Q-switch ruby or similar).

Cutaneous or systemic associated anomalies should be referred to and treated by the corresponding specialist.

## Prognosis

Prognosis depends of the type and severity of associated abnormalities, in particular neurological (mental retardation may be profound and seizures refractory to therapy).

# References

Al Robaee A, Banka N, Alfadley A (2004) Phakomatosis pigmentovascularis type IIb associated with Sturge-Weber syndrome. Pediatr Dermatol 21: 642–645.

Bleehen SS (1998) Disorders of skin colour. In: Champion RH, Burton JL, Burns DA, Breathnach SM (eds.) Rook/Wilkinson/Ebling Textbook of Dermatology. 6th ed. Oxford: Blackwell Science, pp. 1791–1792.

Castori M, Rinaldi R, Angelo C, Zambruno G, Grammatico P, Happle R (2008) Phacomatosis cesioflammea with unilateral lipohypoplasia. Am J Med Genet A 146: 492–495.

Cho S, Choi JH, Sung KJ, Moon KC, Koh JK (2001) Phakomatosis pigmentovascularis type IIb with neurologic abnormalities. Pediatr Dermatol 18: 263.

Diociaiuti A, Guidi B, Aguilar Sanchez JA, Feliciani C, Capizzi R, Amerio P (2005) Phakomatosis pigmentovascularis type IIb: a case associated with Sturge-Weber and klippel-Trenaunay syndrome. J Am Acad Dermatol 53: 536–539.

Du LC, Delaporte E, Catteau B, Destee A, Piette F (1998) Phakomatosis pigmentovascularis Type II. Eur J Dermatol 8: 569–572.

Enjolras O, Mulliken JB (2000) Vascular malformations. In: Harper J, Oranje A, Prose N (eds.) Textbook of Dermatology. Oxford: Blackwell Science, pp. 975–976.

Fernández-Guarino M, Boixeda P, de Las Heras E, Aboin S, García-Millán C, Olasolo PJ (2008) Phakomatosis pigmentovascularis: clinical findings in 15 patients and review of the literature. J Am Acad Dermatol 58: 88–93.

Gomez MR (1987) Neurocutaneous diseases. A Practical Approach. Boston: Butterworths.

Guiglia MC, Prendeville JS (1991) Multiple granular-cell tumors associated with giant speckled lentiginous nevus and nevus flammeus in a child. J Am Acad Dermatol 24: 359–363.

Hagiwara K, Uezato H, Nonaka S (1998) Phacomatosis pigmentovascularis type IIb associated with Sturge-Weber syndrome and pyogenic granulom. J Dermatol 25: 721–729.

Hall BD, Cadle RG, Morrill-Cornelius SM, Bay CA (2007) Phakomatosis pigmentovascularis: implications for severity with special reference to Mongolian spots associated with Sturge-Weber and Klippel-Trenaunay syndromes. Am J Med Genet A 143: 3047–3053.

Happle R (1999) Loss of heterozygosity in human skin. J Am Acad Dermatol 14: 143–161.

Happle R (2005) Phacomatosis pigmentovascularis revisited and reclassified. Arch Dermatol 141: 385–388.

Happle R, Steijlen PM (1989) Phacomatosis pigmentovascularis gedeuted als ein Phänomen der Zwillingsflecken. Hautarzt 40: 721–724.

Hasegawa Y, Yasuhara M (1985) Phakomatosis pigmentovascularis type Iva. Arch Dermatol 121: 651–655.

Karabudak O, Dogan B, Basekim C, Harmanyeri Y (2007) Phacomatosis spilorosea (phacomatosis pigmentovascularis type IIIb). Australas J Dermatol 48: 256–258.

Kikuchi I, Okasaki M (1982) Congenital temporal alopecia in Phakomatosis pigmentovascularis. J Dermatol 9: 485–487.

Kim YC, Park HJ, Cinn YW (2002) Phakomatosis pigmento vascularis type IIa with generalized vitiligo. Br J Dermatol 147: 1028–1029.

Kono T, Ercöcen AR, Chan HH, Kikuchi Y, Hori H, Uezono S, Nozaki M (2003) Treatment of phakomatosis pigmento-vascularis: A combined multiple laser approach. Dermatol Surg 29: 642–646.

Lee CW, Choi DY, Oh YG, Yoon HS, Kim JD (2005) An infantile case of Sturge-Weber syndrome in association with Klippel-Trenaunay-Weber syndrome and phakomatosis pigmentovascularis. J Korean Med Sci 20: 1082–1084.

Onsun N, Inandirici A, Kural Y, Teker C, Atilganoglu U (2007) Phakomatosis pigmentovascularis type II b with bilateral hearing impairment. J Eur Acad Dermatol Venereol 21: 402.

Ota M, Kawamura T, Ito N (1947) Phakomatosis pigmentovascularis. Jpn J Dermatol 57: 1–3.

Ruiz-Maldonado R, Tamayo L, Laterza AM, Brawn G, Lopez A (1987) Phakomatosis pigmentovascularis: A new syndrome? Report of four cases. Pediatr Dermatol 4: 189–196.

Saricaoglu MS, Guven D, Karakurt A, Sengun A, Ziraman I (2002) An unusual case of Sturge-Webers syndrome in association with phakomatosis pigmentovascularis and klippel-Trenaunay-Weber syndrome. Retina 22: 368–371.

Tsuruta D, Fukai K, Seto M, Fujitani K, Shindo K, Hamada T, Ishii M (1991) Phakomatosis pigmentovascularis (TypeIIIa) associated with Moyamoya disease. Pediatr Dermatol 16: 35–38.

Torrelo A, Zambrano A, Happle R (2006) Large aberrant Mongolian spots coexisting with cutis marmorata telangiectatica congenita (phacomatosis pigmentovascularis type V or phacomatosis cesiomarmorata). J Eur Acad Dermatol Venereol 20: 308–310.

Uysal G, Guven A, Ozhan B, Ozturk MH, Mutluay AH, Tulunay O (2000) Phakomatosis pigmentovascularis with Sturge-Weber syndrome. J Dermatol 27: 467–470.

Vidaurri-de la Cruz H, Tamayo-Sanchez l, Duran-McKinster C, Orozco-Covarrubias Mde L, Ruiz-Maldonado R (2003) Phakomatosis Pigmentovascularis II and II B: Clinical findings in 24 patients. J Dermatol 30: 381–388.

# Chapter 24

# SPECKLED LENTIGINOUS NEVUS SYNDROME

**Martino Ruggieri**

Institute of Neurological Science, National Research Council, Catania, and Department of Paediatrics, University of Catania, Catania, Italy

## Introduction

*Speckled lentiginous nevus syndrome* has recently been recognized as a neurocutaneous phenotype characterised by: (a) a papular speckled lentiginous nevus consisting in a light brown macule (usually of rather limited dimensions but sometimes involving large areas of the body) superimposed by multiple melanocytic nevi in the form of papules or nodules that show a more uneven distribution reminiscent of a "star map"; and (b) ipsilateral neurological abnormalities such as hyperhidrosis, muscular weakness and dysesthaesia (Happle 2002). This postulated new mosaic phenotype has been tentatively categorized as a paradominant trait (Happle 2002, Vente et al. 2004).

## Historical perspective and terminology

The *papular* speckled lentiginous nevus (recently separated from its counterpart the *macular* speckled lentiginous nevus) (Vidaurri-de La Cruz and Happle 2006) can be observed either alone or in association with the nevus sebaceous (which is the hallmark of Schimmelpenning-Feuerstein-Mims/nevus sebaceous syndrome) to form the so-called phakomatosis pigmentokeratotica a further example of twin spot phenomenon (Vente et al. 2004, Vidaurri-de La Cruz and Happle 2006). Some authors use the term "nevus spilus" as a synonym for speckled lentiginous nevus, and French dermatologists describe this lesion as "naevus sur naevus"; other authors hace confusingly and interchangeably used the terms "speckled lentiginous nevus", "zoosteriform lentiginous nevus",

and "partial unilateral lentiginosis" (Happle 2002, Viadauuri-de La Cruz and Happle 2006).

For the association of speckled lentiginous nevus with ipsilateral neurological abnormalities Happle (2002) first introduced the term of "speckled lentiginous nevus syndrome".

## Incidence and prevalence

The full-blown syndromic phenotype is rare with 5 cases (4 men, 1 woman) so far reported in the medical literature (Brufau et al. 1986, Hofman et al. 1998, Holder et al. 1994, Piqué et al. 1995, Vente et al. 2004, reviewed in Happle 2002 and Vidaurri-de La Cruz and Happle 2006). No racial or sexual predilection has been noted for the isolated speckled lentiginous nevus in the general population (Lazova 2006). Low prevalence rates of up to 0.2% in newborns and 1.3–2.1% in school-aged children and adults have been reported for the isolated nevus (Lazova 2006).

## Clinical manifestations

### Skin abnormalities

The hallmark of the syndrome is the speckled lentiginous nevus of the papular type (Fig. 1) as likewise found in phakomatosis pigmentokeratotica (Vente et al. 2004). This nevus is characterised by a light brown macule superimposed by multiple melanocytic nevi in the form of papules or nodules that show a more uneven distribution reminiscent of

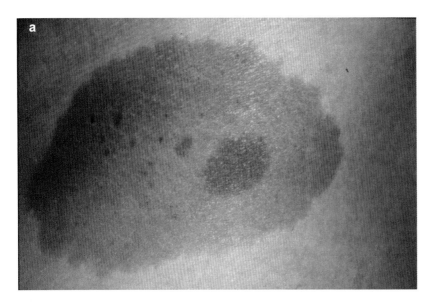

**Fig. 1.** The typical nevus spilus lesion in two women (**a**, **b**) who had in addition hyperhidrosis and dysesthaesia in the ipsilateral region.

a star map (Vidaurri-de La Cruz and Happle 2006). Small dark macules may likewise be present. The superimposed melanocytic aggregations are mandatory for the diagnosis (Vente et al. 2004) and may also be present in the form of blue naevi (Happle et al. 1996, Kinoshita et al. 2003). Some of the darker papules are covered with pigmented scales that can be scratched off making the lesion lighter in colour (Vente et al. 2004). The brownish-blue papules (and macules) are usually arranged in a segmental pattern superimposed on a darker background pigmentation (in the form of a large café-au-lait spot or a hyperpigmented nevus) which reflects the limits of distribution of spots in the involved area (Fig. 2). The affected area can be as small as a quadrant of the body or more widespread to involve an entire hemibody with a sharp midline and clear-cut borders (Fig. 1) (Happle 2002, Vente et al. 2004). The skin lesions are usually present at birth or noted during the first year of life (Lazova 2006). The darker background as well as the spots within tend to fade with age (Vente et al. 2004).

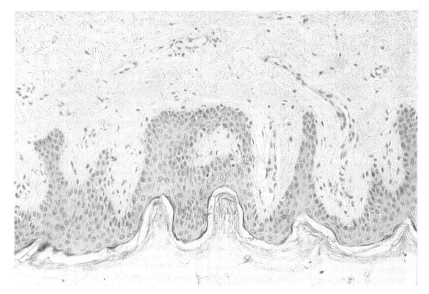

**Fig. 2.** Histopathological examination of the melanocytic nevi shows lentigines and dermal or compound nevi that in part produce epidermal extension of pigment.

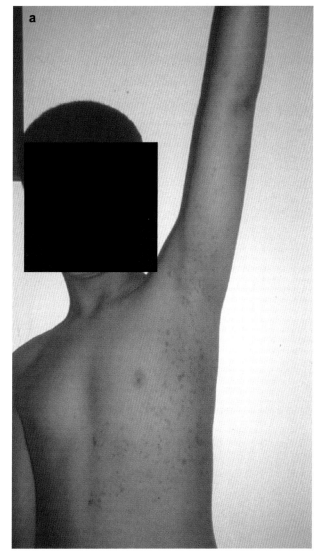

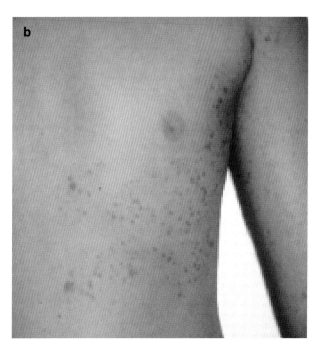

**Fig. 3.** Comparison with similar (flat) lesions in mosaic/localised (segmental) (**a, b**) neurofibromatosis type 1 (reprinted with permission from Ruggieri and Huson, 2001).

**Table 1.** Neurological abnormalities associated with speckled lentiginous nevus syndrome

| | |
|---|---|
| Sensory neuropathy | |
|   Hyperalgesia/paresthesia | Piqué et al. (1995), Vente et al. (2004) |
| Motor neuropathy | Piqué et al. (1995) |
| Nerve palsy with thinning of nerve | Holder et al. (1994) |
| Spinal muscular atrophy with fasciculation | Hofmann et al. (1998) |
| Hyperhidrosis | Happle (2002), Vente et al. (2004) |

## Neurological abnormalities

The associated neurological abnormalities reported so far are listed in Table 1.

Typically, the neurological abnormalities are confined to the involved body area with the nevus. In some cases with sensory neuropathy just touching the skin in the darker background macule of the nevus was felt as uncomfortable (Vente et al. 2004). The hyperhidrosis may be ipsilateral to the entire area involved with the nevus. In an affected 43-year-old woman (Holder et al. 1994) electrocardiography showed a right bundle branch block while in a 27-year-old man (Brufau et al. 1986) in addition to the nevus there was hypertrophy of the underlying pectoralis muscle.

## Pathology

Histopathological examination of the melanocytic nevi shows lentigines and dermal or compound nevi that in part produce epidermal extension of pigment (Fig. 3) (Vente et al. 2004). Sometimes these nevi are diagnosed as dysplastic nevi and therefore it seems reasonable to assume that this nevus harbours an increased risk of developing malignant melanoma (Bolognia 1991, Kurban et al. 1992).

## Diagnosis and differential diagnosis

The papular speckled lentiginous nevus must be distinguished firstly from its macular counterpart,

which is characterised clinically by a tannish-brown background with darker flat speckles (Vidaurri-de La Cruz and Happle 2006). The distribution of speckles in the macular form is rather even and resembles a polka-dot pattern. Histopathologically, the macular speckled lentiginous nevus is characterised by what has been called a "jentigo" pattern in the darker speckles and by some nests of melanocytes at the dermoepidermal junction at the tips of the papillae whereas the background pigmentation shows the microscopical features of a lentigo.

Speckled lentiginous nevus syndrome should be distinguished form *phakomatosis pigmentokeratotica* that represents a combination of the nevus sebaceous typically seen in Schimmelpenning-Feuerstein-Mims syndrome and the papular speckled lentiginous nevus.

In the *LEOPARD syndrome* the lentiginosis is usually diffuse without melanocytic papules.

*Phakomatosis pigmentovascularis* may be associated with a speckled lentiginous nevus (Libow 1993), but this particular type of nevus is quite flat and does never show melanocytic papules (Vente et al. 2004, Vidaurri-de La Cruz and Happle 2006).

*Partial unilateral lentiginosis* can be confused sometimes with speckled lentiginous nevus but the former is never superimposed by melanocytic macules (Hofmann et al. 1998, Piqué et al. 1995, Vente et al. 2004). *Partial unilateral lentiginosis* is presently taken as a mosaic manifestation of neurofibromatosis type 1 (NF1): in most cases of *segmental NF1* however additional typical cafè-au-lait spots are recorded within the involved area with the nevus (see Fig. 2) (Ruggieri and Huson 2001).

## Pathogenesis and molecular genetics

Speckled lentiginous nevus may represent a localised defect in neural crest melanoblasts that populate a particular area of the skin. Environmental and genetic factors may also play a role. Mosaicism however is currently regarded as the best explanation for the development of this segmentally distributed nevus. Likewise, all of the neurological manifestations have been reported in the ipsilateral area of the nevus (Brufau et al. 1986, Hofman et al. 1998, Holder et al. 1994, Piqué et al. 1995, Vente et al. 2004).

In analogy to its syndromic complex counterpart, phakomatosis pigmentokeratotica, speckled lentiginous nevus syndrome occurs as a sporadic trait and has been clinically categorised as a possible example of paradominant trait (Happle 2002, Vente et al. 2004). The hitherto unknown mutation would give rise to a normal phenotype when present in a heterozygous state (Happle 2002). Speckled lentiginous nevus syndrome would only become manifest when postzygotic loss of heterozygosity results in a cell clone in which the corresponding wild type allele is present (Happle 1999, Vente et al. 2004).

## Management and follow-up

There are no particular management or follow-up issues for the syndromic complex. One important issue however is represented by the potentially increased risk of developing malignant melanoma in one or more melanocytic papules (Vente et al. 2004). Predictors of the risk of malignant transformation of a speckled lentiginous nevus have yet to be determined. The surface area, the number of nevi within the speckled nevus, and/or the presence of cytological atypia may be factors that affect the potential for transformation. Regular visits to a dermatologist and careful examination with the use of photography should be used for early recognition of atypical features within the nevus (Lazova 2006). Biopsy is necessary to rule out cytological atypia eventually developing within the nevus.

## References

Brufau C, Moran M, Armijo M (1986) Nevus on nevus. Apropos of 7 case reports, 3 of them associated with other dysplasias, and 1 with an invasive malignant melanoma. Ann Dermatol Venereol 113: 409–411.

Happle R (1999) Loss of heterozygosity in human skin. J Am Acad Dermatol 41: 143–161.

Happle R (2002) Speckled lentiginous nevus syndrome: delineation of a new distinct neurocutaneous phenotype. Eur J Dermatol 12: 133–135.

Happle R, Hoffmann R, Restano L, Caputo R, Tadini G (1996) Phacomatosis pigmentokeratotica: a melanocytic-epidermal twi nevus syndrome. Am J Med Genet 65: 363–365.

Hofmann UB, Ogilivie P, Mullges W, Bröcker EB, Hamm H (1998) Congenital unilateral speckled lentiginous blue naevi with asymmetric spinal muscular atrophy. J Am Acad Dermatol 39: 326–329.

Holder JE, Graham-Brown RAC, Camp RDR (1994) Partial unilateral lentiginosis associated with blue naevi. Br J Dermatol 130: 390–393.

Kinoshita K, Shinkai H, Utani A (2003) Phacomatosis pigmentokeratotica without extracutaneous abnormalities. Dermatology 207: 415–416.

Lazova R (2006) Speckled lentiginous nevus. http://www.emedicine.com/derm/topic902/htm

Piqué E, Aguilar A, Farina MC, Gallego MA, Escalonilla P, Requena L (1995) Partial unilateral lentiginosis: report of seven cases and review of the literature. Clin Exp Dermatol 20: 319–322.

Ruggieri M, Huson SM (2001) The clinical and diagnostic implications of mosaicism in the neurofibromatoses. Neurology 56: 1434–1443.

Vente C, Neumann C, Bertsch H, Rupprecth H, Happle R (2004) Speckled lentiginous nevus syndrome: report of a further case. Dermatology 209: 228–229.

Vidauuri-de La Cruz H, Happle R (2006) Two distinct types of speckled lentiginous nevi characterised by macular versus popular speckles. Dermatology 212: 53–58.

# Chapter 25

# CUTIS TRICOLOR (RUGGIERI–HAPPLE SYNDROME)

**Martino Ruggieri, Mario Roggini, Ingo Kennerknecht, Carmelo Schepis, and Paola Iannetti**

Institute of Neurological Science, National Research Council, Catania, and Department of Paediatrics, University of Catania, Catania, Italy (MR); Paediatric Radiology Unit, Department of Paediatrics, University "La Sapienza", Rome, Italy (MR); Institute of Human Genetics, Westfallische Wilhelms – University of Munster, Munster, Germany (IK); Unit of Dermatology, IRCCS OASI Maria Santissima, Troina, Italy (CS); 2nd Chair of Paediatrics, Division of Paediatric Neurology, Department of Paediatrics, University "La Sapienza", Rome, Italy (PI)

## Introduction

The term cutis tricolor describes the combination of congenital hyper- and hypopigmented lesions (in the form of macules, patches or streaks), in close proximity to each other, in a background of normal skin (Baba et al. 2003; Happle 2006; Happle et al. 1997; Khumalo et al. 2001; Ruggieri 2000; Ruggieri et al. 2003, 2008; Seraslan and Atik 2005). This phenomenon has been reported either as an isolated skin disorder (Baba et al. 2003, Khumalo et al. 2001, Ruggieri 2000, Seraslan and Atik 2005) or as a part of a neurocutaneous malformation syndrome (Cutis tricolor syndrome or Ruggieri–Happle syndrome) (POSSUM 2006) in association with multiple congenital anomalies, including facial anomalies, cortical cataract (Ruggieri et al. 2008) neurological (mild hypotonia, mild to moderate mental retardation, epilepsy and EEG abnormalities) and behavioural abnormalities and specific skeletal defects consisting in skull, vertebral and long bones dysplasia (Happle et al. 1997; Ruggieri 2000; Ruggieri et al. 2003, 2008).

Cutis tricolor has been postulated to represent a twin-spotting phenomenon (Happle 2006, Koopman 1999, Ruggieri et al. 2003). Paradominant inheritance has been postulated as a possible mechanism (Happle 2006) to explain familial occurrence as in the case of Baba et al. (2003) who reported an isolated skin phenotype of the "cutis tricolor" type in two sisters.

Recently, Larralde and Happle (2005) distinguished a possible subtype of *cutis tricolor parvimaculata* with smaller hyperpigmented and hypopigmented skin spots in close proximity to each other, in a background of normal skin.

## Historical perspective and terminology

In 1997 Happle and co-workers coined the term "*cutis tricolor*" for the unusual combination of three degrees of skin pigmentation in close proximity to each other. In their 17-year-old boy they described congenital hyper- and hypopigmented macules confined to circumscribed body segments on a background of normal intermediate skin complexion in association with multiple birth defects (Happle et al. 1997). Ruggieri (2000) and Ruggieri et al. (2003, 2008) subsequently expanded the cutaneous phenotype by including cases with abnormal pigmentation in the form of large patches or streaks diffusely involving the body associated (case 2, Ruggieri 2000, Ruggieri et al. 2003) or not (case 1, Ruggieri 2000) to systemic defects. Variant forms have been also reported (Larralde and Happle 2005). The suggested explanation to this phenomenon was allelic twin spotting [Happle et al. 1997, Koopman 1999, Ruggieri 2000, Ruggieri et al. 2003].

Suggested eponyms for the complex malformation syndrome with cutis tricolor are Cutis tricolor syndrome or Ruggieri-Happle syndrome (POSSUM 2006).

## Incidence and prevalence

By literature review (Baba et al. 2003, Happle et al. 1997, Khumalo et al. 2001, Ruggieri 2000, Ruggieri et al. 2003, Seraslan and Atik 2005) and personal observations we have recorded 13 cases of cutis tricolor so far with no sex and race differences (Ruggieri et al. 2008, Ruggieri, unreported cases).

**Table 1.** Clinical findings in 8 cases with cutis tricolor syndrome

| Main features (*) | 1 | 2 | 3 | 4 | 5 | 6 | 7 | 8 |
|---|---|---|---|---|---|---|---|---|
| Sex | M | F | F | M | M | F | F | M |
| Age | 8 | 10 | 14 | 14 | 18 | 15 | 22 | 28 |
| *Clinical manifestations* | | | | | | | | |
| Height | 25th | 50th | 95th | 50th | 50th | 75th | 50th | <3rd |
| Weight | 50th | 50th | 97th | 90th | 50th | 97th | 50th | <3rd |
| OFC | 25th | 50th | 98th | 25th | 50th | 25th | 50th | <3rd |
| Cutis tricolor (pattern) | L, P | P | L, P | P | Spiral | L, P | M | M |
|    Face | + | − | − | + | ± | − | − | ± |
|    Trunk | + | + | + | + | + | + | + | − |
|    Upper limbs | − | + | + | − | − | + | − | R |
|    Lower limbs | + | + | + | + | − | − | − | − |
| Coarse face | + | − | + | + | − | + | − | + |
| Facial asymmetry | + | − | + | + | − | + | − | − |
| Dolichocephalism | + | − | + | + | − | + | − | − |
| Frontal bossing | + | − | + | + | − | + | − | − |
| Orbital bossing | + | − | + | + | − | + | − | + |
| Brushy eyebrows | + | + | + | + | + | + | + | + |
| Hypertelorism | + | − | + | + | − | + | − | − |
| Epicanthus | + | − | − | + | − | + | − | + |
| Deep nasal bridge | + | − | + | + | − | + | − | + |
| Large/bulbous nose | + | − | + | + | − | + | − | + |
| Large/anteverted nostrils | + | − | − | + | − | + | − | + |
| Low set ears | + | − | − | + | − | + | − | + |
| Posteriorly angulated ears | + | − | − | + | − | + | − | + |
| Wide philtrum | + | − | + | + | − | + | − | + |
| Prominent/thick lips | + | − | − | + | − | + | + | − |
| Prominent chin | + | + | + | + | − | + | + | + |
| Clinodactyly | + | + | + | − | − | + | − | − |
| Short neck | + | + | + | + | − | + | − | + |
| Pectus excavatum | + | + | + | + | + | + | + | + |
| Developmental milestones | D | N | D | D | N | D | N | D |
| Hypotonia | + | − | ± | + | − | + | − | − |
| Poor co-ordination | + | − | − | − | − | + | − | − |
| Language | D | N | D | D | N | D | N | D |
| Epilepsy | − | − | − | + | − | + | − | + |
|    Onset | NA | NA | NA | 6 y | NA | 2 y | NA | 8 y |
|    Seizure type | NA | NA | NA | GTCS | NA | GTCS | NA | GTCS |
|    Outcome/age ceased | NA | NA | NA | 9 y | NA | 11 y | NA | 19 y |
| Behavioural anomalies | + | − | − | − | − | + | − | − |
| Mental retardation | Mo | − | Mi | Mo | − | Mo | − | Se |
| Other | cataract(*) | − | − | cataract(*) | − | cataract(*) | − | VSD |

*Present cases are as follows: cases 1–3 = unreported cases; case 4 = case 2 (Ruggieri 2000); case 5 = case 1 (Ruggieri 2000); case 6 = case from Ruggieri et al. (2003); case 7 = unreported; case 8 = case from Happle et al. (1997).

M = male; F = female; L = linear; P = patches; M = multiple maculae; N = normal; D = delayed; NA = not applicable; y = years; GTCS = generalised tonic clonic seizures; Mi = mild; Mo = moderate; Se = severe; VSD = ventricular septal defect.

(*) = as reported in Ruggieri et al. (2008).

## Clinical manifestations

The main clinical, laboratory and imaging features in the syndromic cases so far recorded are summarised in Tables 1 and 2.

## Skin manifestations

These consist in the combination of hypopigmented and hyperpigmented lesions in close proximity one to each other in a background of normal

**Table 2.** Laboratory and imaging findings in 8 cases with cutis tricolor syndrome

| Main features (*) | 1 | 2 | 3 | 4 | 5 | 6 | 7 | 8 |
|---|---|---|---|---|---|---|---|---|
| Sex | M | F | F | M | M | F | F | M |
| Age | 8 | 10 | 14 | 14 | 18 | 15 | 22 | 28 |
| *Radiographic features* | | | | | | | | |
| Small skull | + | − | − | + | − | + | − | + |
| Prognathism | + | − | + | − | − | + | − | |
| Obtuse angle of mandible | + | − | + | + | − | + | − | + |
| Absent posterior arch atlas | + | − | − | − | − | + | − | + |
| Scoliosis | + | + | + | + | + | + | − | + |
|   Cervical | + | − | − | − | − | + | − | + |
|   Thoracic | + | + | + | + | + | + | + | + |
|   Lumbar | − | − | + | + | + | + | + | + |
| Kyphosis | + | − | + | + | − | + | + | + |
| Lordosis | + | + | + | + | + | + | + | + |
| Vertebral scalloping | + | − | + | + | + | + | + | + |
| Increased distance pedicles | + | − | + | + | − | + | − | + |
| Altered pedicles | + | − | + | + | − | + | − | + |
| Metaphyseal osteosclerosis | − | − | − | + | − | + | − | + |
| Rib abnormalities | + | − | + | + | − | + | + | + |
| Bowing of long bones | + | − | + | + | − | + | + | + |
|   Upper limbs | − | − | − | − | − | − | − | + |
|   Lower limbs | + | − | + | + | − | + | + | + |
| Leg length discrepancy | + | − | + | + | − | + | + | + |
| *Neuroimaging features* | | | | | | | | |
| Asymmetric ventricles | + | − | + | − | − | − | − | − |
| White matter anomalies | + | − | − | + | − | − | − | − |
| Corpus callosum anomalies | − | − | − | − | − | + | − | − |
| *Laboratory findings* | | | | | | | | |
| EEG abnormalities | + | − | + | − | − | + | − | + |
| *Cytogenetic analysis* | | | | | | | | |
| Karyotype (anomalies) | | | | | | | | |
|   Lymphocyte | − | − | − | − | − | − | − | − |
|   Fibroblasts | − | − | − | − | − | − | − | − |
| ZFHX1B gene (FISH) | − | − | − | NP | − | − | − | NP |
| *DNA analysis* | | | | | | | | |
| ZFHX1B gene | − | − | − | NP | − | − | − | NP |

*Present cases are as follows: cases 1–3 = unreported cases; case 4 = case 2 (Ruggieri 2000); case 5 = case 1 (Ruggieri 2000); case 6 = case from Ruggieri et al. (2003); case 7 = unreported; case 8 = case from Happle et al. (1997).
M = male; F = female; NP = not performed.

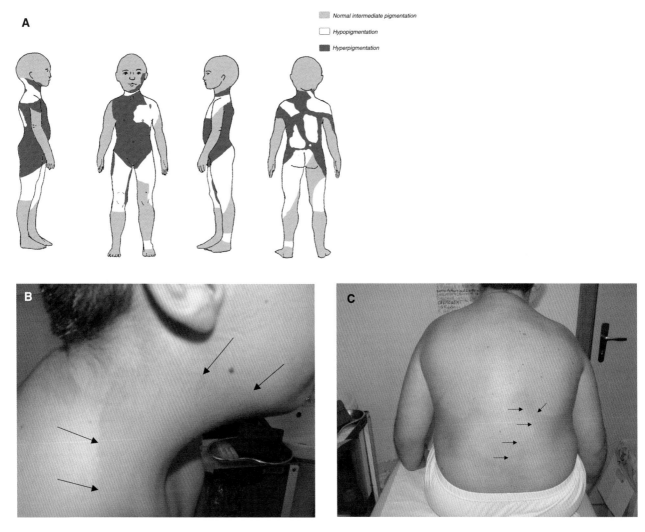

**Fig. 1. (A)** Ideogram showing the arrangement of the three different degrees of pigmentation in a child with cutis tricolor syndrome; **(B, C)** Different degrees of pigmentation (of the cutis tricolor type) observed at follow-up (case 2 of Ruggieri 2000 seen at age 11): **(A)** face and **(B)** trunk in the same child shown in the ideogram presenting hyperpigmented patches in close proximity to hypopigmented patches (black arrows) and a normal complexion (A reprinted with permission from Ruggieri 2000).

complexion (Figs. 1–3). There are a wide variety of juxtaposed cutaneous lesions including macules, patches, and streaks, arranged in different patterns (i.e., patchy, linear, spiral, diffuse) over confined or large body areas (Figs. 1–3). The hallmark of the condition is the close spatial proximity of the two different birthmarks (Fig. 2A) and the coexistence of three different complexions (Figs. 2A–B), which reflect the twin-spotting phenomenon (see below). Lesions usually manifest at birth or in the first months of life. The degree and (more rarely) the extent of pigmentary dysplasia can increase in the

first years of life: then they stabilise and could also fade and/or revert to normal in some areas.

## Facial phenotype

In the most severely affected cases the face (Fig. 4) is coarse and mildly asymmetric with dolichocephaly and prominent metopic suture; there is orbital bossing, thick and brushy eyebrows, hypertelorism, mild epichantus, deep nasal bridge with large, bulbous nose and anteverted nostrils; low set and anteriorly

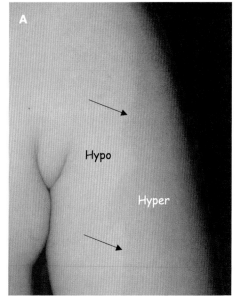

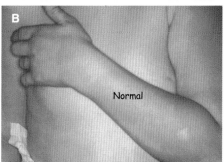

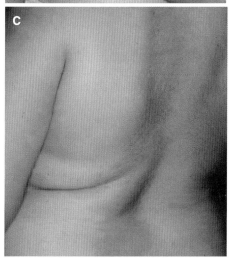

Fig. 2. (A–C) Different degrees of pigmentation observed in a girl with cutis tricolor syndrome: note (A) the hypopigmented lesions (hypo) in close proximity (black arrows) to the hyperpigmented patches (hyper) in a background of normal complexion (B); (C) shows the moderate kyphoscoliosis (reprinted in colour from Ruggieri et al. 2003).

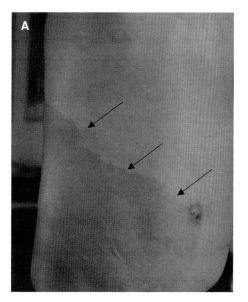

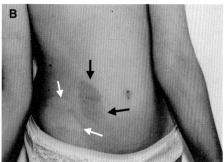

Fig. 3. (A, B) Different arrangements of the skin lesions: (A) spiral arrangement in the trunk showing the hyper- and hypopigmented skin lesions in close proximity to each other (black arrows); (B) macular arrangement in the abdomen of a girl with skin lesions only showing an hyperpigmented spot (black arrow) in close proximity to an hypopigmented macula (white arrow) in the context of a normal complexion (A reprinted with permission from Ruggieri 2000).

rotated ears; large phyltrum and thick lips; the palate is narrow with small and spaced teeth; the chin is prominent (see also Table 1). There is also clinodactyly of the fifth fingers.

## Nervous system involvement

It consists in mild hypotonia, urinary and faecal incontinence, mental retardation, epilepsy, EEG abnormalities, altered behaviour and hypoplasia of the corpus callosum (Fig. 5).

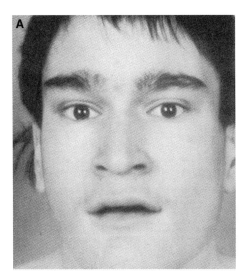
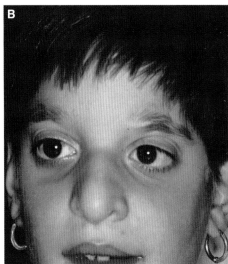

**Fig. 4.** Facial phenotype in two syndromic cases of cutis tricolor: (**A**) from Happle et al. (1997) and (**B**) from Ruggieri et al. (2003). Note the coarse and mildly asymmetric face with dolichocephaly, orbital bossing, thick and brushy eyebrows, hypertelorism, mild epichantus, deep nasal bridge with large, bulbous nose and anteverted nostrils, anteriorly rotated ears, large philtrum and thick lips and prominent chin.

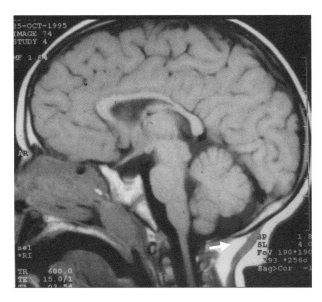

**Fig. 5.** Sagittal T1-weighted (TR 450, TE 50) MRI image of the head showing mild corpus callosum hypogenesis in a irl with cutis tricolor syndrome (reprinted from Ruggieri et al. 2003).

### Skeletal abnormalities

The radiographic features in the patients so far analyse include a small skull (not micro cephalic) (Fig. 6A) with prognathism (Fig. 6B); absent posterior arch of the atlas (Fig. 6C); obtuse angle of the mandible; scoliosis of different degrees and location [with additional lordosis and kyphosis: the abnormal curvature of the spine can be dystrophic in appearance, right-sided lower thoracic (T10–12) and upper lumbar (L1–3) with asymmetric peduncles and sloping ribs ($n = 6$) or left- and right-sided upper thoracic (T4–T7) and lower lumbar (L1–L4)] (Fig. 7); metaphyseal osteosclerosis of the femurs; mild to moderate bowing of long bones (Fig. 8); and increased bone age.

### Pathology

Punch biopsies collected from the involved areas showed histologically (Ruggieri 2000) an increase in melanin content of the basal layer, but no dermal melanin or melanophages in the hyperpigmented areas and a decrease in the melanin content and in the number of melanocytes in the hypopigmented lesions. A normal epidermal and dermal architecture was present in the normally intermediate pigmented areas. Electron microscopy showed (C. Schepis, unreported data): (1) in the hypopigmented area basal keratinocytes containing isolate melanosomes, some

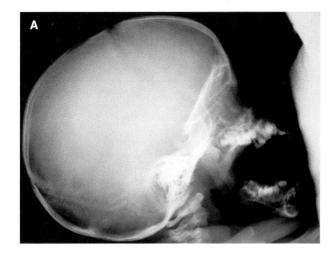

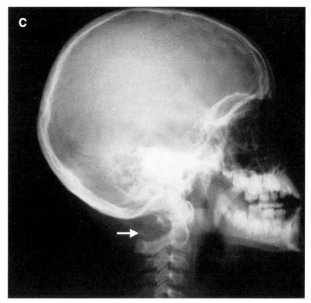

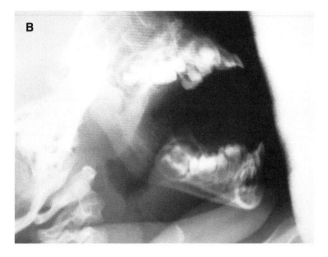

Fig. 6. Lateral (**A**) X-ray study of the skull with close up view of the mandible (**B**) showing small skull (**A**) with prognathism and (**A, B**) obtuse angle of mandible; lateral view of the skull at age 18 years (**A**) showing small skull and absent posterior arch of the atlas (white arrow).

of them displaying an incomplete maturation; and (2) in the hyperpigmented area basal keratinocytes filled of mature melanosomes (Fig. 9).

## Molecular genetics and pathogenesis

A tentative genetic explanation of this postulated new phenotype could be a post zygotic somatic mutation: loss of heterozygosity for the underlying mutation at an early developmental stage would give rise to one single mosaic skin disorder (e.g., generalised skin manifestations of the cutis tricolor type in association to extracutaneous anomalies) as in the original case of Happle et al. (1997) and in the subsequent reports (Ruggieri 2000, Ruggieri et al. 2003); post zygotic recombina-

tion occurring later during embryo genesis would give rise to isolated forms (e.g., manifestations confined to the skin only) (Khumalo et al. 2001, Case 1, Ruggieri 2000, Seraslan and Atik 2005). Paradominant inheritance has been postulated as a possible mechanism to explain familial occurrence as in the case of Baba et al. (2003) who reported an isolated skin phenotype of the "cutis tricolor" type in two sisters.

## Differential diagnosis

Similar dysmorphic, neurological and behavioural features have been observed in the *inv dup(15) syndrome* (Battaglia et al. 1997, Winter and Baraitser 2001) which is caused by an extra inv dup(15) marker

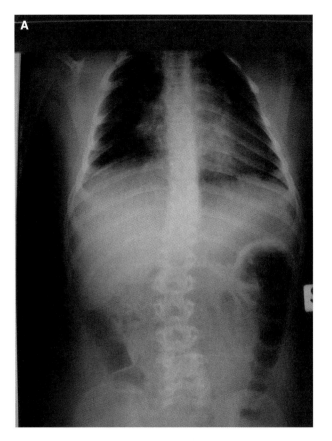

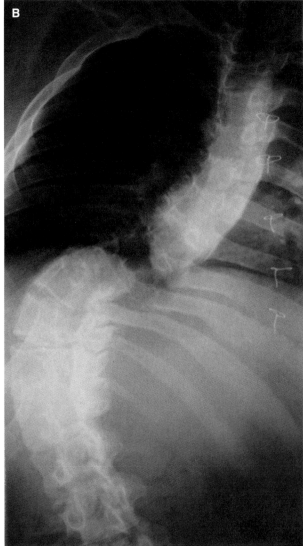

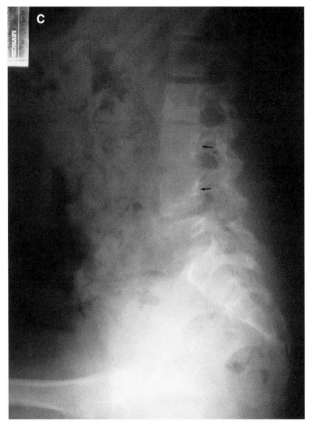

**Fig. 7.** Anteroposterior X-rays of the spine showing mild (**A**) to severe (**B**) dystrophic scoliosis; lateral X-rays of the lumbar and sacral spine (**C**, **D**) reveals scalloping of the posterior aspect of the lumbar vertebrae (black and white arrows).

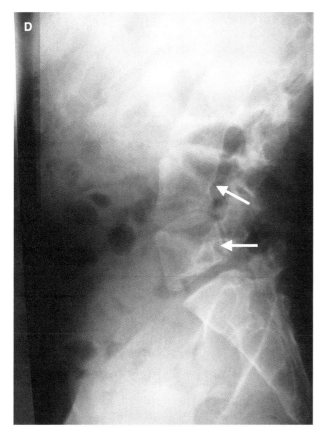

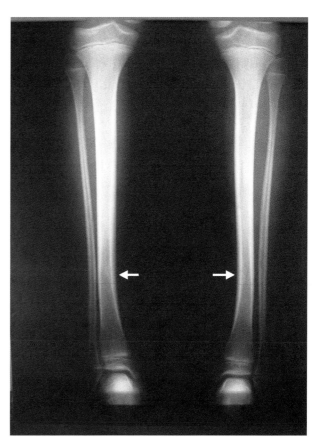

**Fig. 7.** (Continued)

**Fig. 8.** Anteroposterior view of the lower limbs at age 12 years reveal moderate bowing of the tibial bones (white arrows).

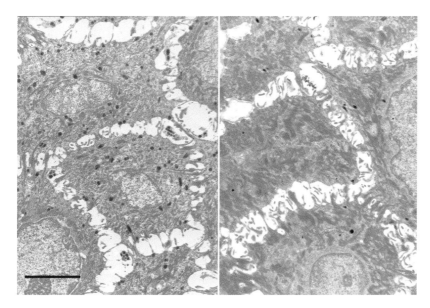

**Fig. 9.** Electron microscopy study of an hyperpigmented (left) and hypopigmented (right) area taken from a patchy skin lesions in a girl with cutis tricolor syndrome: the hyperpigmented area reveals features of abundant mature (type IV) melanosomes; the hypopigmented area shows decreased melanosomes in the basal keratinocytes; in addition some of them are of type III. Uranyl acetate and lead citrate. Bar = 4 μm.

chromosome cytogenetically defined as inv dup(15) (pter → q12–13:q12–13 → pter). The most consistent clinical findings are developmental delay, severe epilepsy, moderate to severe mental retardation, diffuse hypotonia, peculiar behavioural pattern consisting in lack of social interaction, stereotypies, non functional use of objects, primordial type of exploration, absent or very poor echolalic language and very limited comprehension (Battaglia et al. 1997). The associated dysmorphic and cutaneous signs consist of coarse face, hypertelorism, downslanting palpebral fissures with mild epichantus, low set ears and multiple hypo pigmented whorled areas in the skin of the arms, trunk and legs (Battaglia et al. 1997). One can exclude such syndrome on cytogenetic grounds by means of FISH analysis in peripheral leukocytes and fibroblasts. Notably, the neurological and behavioural abnormalities in the inv dup (15) syndrome are more severe (Battaglia et al. 1997). In addition, the pigmentary changes consists only of hypopigmented patches (Battaglia et al. 1997, Winter and Baraitser 2001); by contrast, the pigmentary changes in cutis tricolour consists of three different degrees of pigmentation adjacent to each other.

The cutaneous patterns in cutis tricolor are unlike any known type of human mosaicism proposed so far.

Some features in a few of the present cases were reminiscent of those seen in the so-called *Mowat-Wilson syndrome* (MWS) (OMIM # 235730), a multiple congenital anomaly characterised by typical facial dimorphic features in association with (postnatal) microcephaly and short stature, eye abnormalities (e.g., microphthalmia), variable malformations (e.g., Hirschprung disease, heart and genitourinary defects), severe intellectual disability, seizures and behavioural disturbances (Adam et al. 2006, Mowat and Wilson 2003). This phenotype is caused by defects of the transcriptional repressor ZFHX1B (Dastot-Le Moral et al. 2007, Cerruti-Mainardi et al. 2004, Zweier et al. 2005). Notably, some patients with MWS have been disclosed to have "patchy" or "drop-like" pigmentary anomalies of the hyperpigmented or hypopigmented type. However, many pathognomonic features of the MWS lack in cases with cutis tricolor (e.g., microcephalyand associated

systemic abnormalities) and the pigmentary changes are different in that hyper- and hypopigmented patches in the present cases were in close proximity to each other. Extensive cytogenetic and molecular analyses could rule out this diagnosis (see also Table 2).

The pigmentary changes seen in cutis tricolor are dissimilar to the skin anomalies seen in the *hypomelanosis of Ito* phenotype (Ruggieri and Pavone 2000) or in *incontinentia pigmenti* of the Bloch-Sulzberger type (OMIM # 308310) (Bruckner 2004). The lesion patterns in these conditions are typically distributed along the lines of Blaschko in rather narrow bands (Happle 1993a, b) forming whorls, streaks, "V" or "S" shaped and linear arrangements. In addition, in this case there were three degrees of pigmentation and clinically there were no preceding eruptive phases (Donnai 2006). This case was also dissimilar from the *McCune Albright* syndrome in that there were no associated polyostotic fibrous dysplasia or endocrine abnormalities (Sybert 1997, Winter and Baraitser 2000). It is also dissimilar from the *whorled hyperpigmented nevus* because of the coexistence of three different complexions (Moss and Savin 1995, Sybert 1997). *Acquired Blaschkolinear dermatoses* can also be ruled out because the skin abnormalities in cutis tricolour are congenital and not preceded by erithematous and/or eruptive phases (Grosshans 1999, Moss and Savin 1995).

## Management

There is no specific management issue. Due to the lens opacities recorded in some affected patients (see Table 1) annual slit-lamp examination is warranted at follow-up.

## References

Adam MP, Schelley S, Gallagher R, Brady AN, Barr K, Blumberg B, Shieh JT, Graham J, Slavotinek A, Martin M, Keppler-Noreuil K, Storm AL, Hudgins L (2006) Clinical features and management issues in Mowat-Wilson syndrome. Am J Med Genet A 140: 2730–2741.

Baba M, Seckin D, Akcali C, Happle R (2003) Familial cutis tricolor: a possible example of paradominant inheritance. Eur J Dermatol 13: 343–345.

Battaglia A, Gurrieri F, Bertini E, Bellacosa A, Pomponi MG, Paravatou-Petsotas M, Mazza S, Neri G (1997) The inv dup(15) syndrome: a clinically recognizable syndrome with altered behaviour, mental retardation, and epilepsy. Neurology 48: 1081–1086.

Bruckner AL (2004) Incontinentia pigmenti: a window to the role of NF-κB function. Semin Cut Med Surg 23: 116–124.

Cerruti-Mainardi P, Pastore G, Zweier C, Rauch A (2004) Mowat-Wilson syndrome and mutation in the zinc finger homeobox 1B gene; a well defined clinical entity. J Med Genet 41: e16

Dastot-Le Moal F, Wilson M, Mowat D, Collot N, Niel F, Goossens M (2007) ZFHX1B mutations in patients with Mowat-Wilson syndrome. Hum Mutat 28: 313–321.

Donnai D (2006) Incontinentia pigmenti and pigmentary mosaicism. In: Harper J, Oranje A, Prose N (eds.) Textbook of Pediatric Dermatology. 2nd ed. Oxford: Blackwell Science, pp. 1237–1247.

Grosshans EM (1999) Acquired Blaschkolinear dermatoses. Am J Med Genet 85: 334–337.

Happle R (1993a) Mosaicism in human skin. Understanding the patterns and mechanisms. Arch Dermatol 129: 1460–1470.

Happle R (1993b) Pigmentary patterns associated with human mosaicism: a proposed classification. Eur J Dermatol 3: 170–174.

Happle R (1997a) Segmental forms of autosomal dominant skin disorders: different types of severity reflect different states of zygosity. Am J Med Genet 66: 241–242.

Happle R (1997b) A rule concerning the segmental manifestations of autosomal dominant skin disorders: review of clinical examples providing evidence for dichotomous types of severity. Arch Dermatol 133: 1505–1509.

Happle R (2006) Principles of genetics, mosaicism and molecular biology. In: Harper J, Oranje A, Prose N (eds.) Textbook of Pediatric Dermatology. 2nd ed. Oxford: Blackwell Science, pp. 1221–1246.

Happle R, Barbi G, Eckert D, Kennerknecht I (1997) "Cutis tricolor": congenital hyper- and hypopigmented macules associated with a sporadic multisystem birth defect: an unusual example of twin spotting? J Med Genet 34: 676–678.

Khumalo NP, Joss DV, Huson SM, Burge S (2001) Pigmentary anomalies in ataxia-telangiectasia: a clue to diagnosis and an example of twin spotting. Br J Dermatol 1444: 369–371.

Koopman RJJ (1999) Concept of twin spotting. Am J Med Genet 85: 355–358.

Larralde M, Happle R (2005) Cutis tricolor parvimaculata: a distinct neurocutaneous phenotype? Dermatology 211: 149–151.

Moss C, Savin J (1995) Dermatology and the new genetics. Oxford: Blackwell Science.

Mowat DR, Wilson MJ, Goosens M (2003) Mowat-Wilson syndrome. J Med Genet 40: 305–310.

POSSUM (2006) Pictures of standard syndromes and undiagnosed malformations. Version 7.0. Melbourne: Murdoch Institute for Research into Birth Defects.

Ruggieri M (2000) "Cutis tricolor": congenital hyper- and hypopigmented lesions in a background of normal skin, with and without associated systemic features: further expansion of the phenotype. Eur J Pediatr 159: 745–749.

Ruggieri M, Pavone L (2000) Hypomelanosis of Ito: clinical syndrome or just phenotype? J Child Neurol 15: 635–644.

Ruggieri M, Iannetti P, Pavone L (2003) Delineation of a newly recognised neurocutaneous malformation syndrome with "cutis tricolor". Am J Med Genet 120A: 110–116.

Ruggieri M, Iannetti F, Polizzi A, Puzo L, Iannetti L, Di Pietro M, Caltabiano R, Magro G, Iannetti P (2008) Congenital cataract in a newly recognised neurocutaneous malformation syndrome with "cutis tricolor". Br J Ophthalmol (in press).

Seraslan G, Atik E (2005) Cutis tricolor: two case reports. Case Rep Clin Pract Rev 6: 317–319.

Spitz JL (2005) Genodermatoses. A full-color clinical guide to genetic skin disorders. 2nd ed. Baltimore: Williams & Wilkins.

Sybert VP (1997) Genetic Skin Disorders. New York: Oxford University Press.

Taybi H, Lachman RS (1996) Radiology of Syndromes, Metabolic Disorders and Skeletal Dysplasia. 4th ed. St. Louis: Mosby.

Zweier C, Thile CT, Dufke A, Crow YJ, Meinicke P, Suri M, Ala-Mello S, Beemer F, Bernasconi S, Bianchi P, Bier A, Devriendt K, Dimitrov B, Firth H, Gallagher RC, Garavelli L, Gillesen-Kaesbach G, Hudgins L, Kaariainen H, Karstens S, Krantz I, Mannhardt A, Medne L, Mucke J, Kibaek M, Krogh LN, Peippo M, Rittinger O, Schulz S, Schelley SL, Temple IK, Dennis NR, van der Knaap MS, Wheeler P, Yerushalmi B, Zenker M, Seidel H, Lachmeijer A, Prescott T, Kraus C, Lowry RB, Rauch A (2005) Clinical and mutational spectrum of Mowat-Wilson disease. Eur J Med Genet 48: 97–111.

# Chapter 26

# NEUROCUTANEOUS MELANOSIS

**Sergiusz Józwiak and Julita Borkowska**

Department of Neurology and Epileptology, Children's Memorial Health Institute, Warsaw, Poland

## Introduction

Neurocutaneous melanosis (NCM) is a rare congenital, dysmorphogenetic disorder characterized by the large or multiple congenital intradermal melanotic nevi and benign/malignant proliferation of melanocytes in the central nervous system, with the infiltration of leptomeninges.

## Historical perspective and terminology

The first report of this phacomatosis was presented by Rokitansky in 1861 (Rokitansky 1861). He reported a 14-year-old girl with mental retardation, hydrocephalus and multiple large pigmented skin nevi. On postmortem examination she was found to have leptomeningeal infiltration with melanocytes. This disease has been described by different names: giant melanotic nevus, melanose neurocutanee, dark hairy nevus syndrome, congenital melanotic hairy nevi, giant hairy nevus, garment hairy pigmented nevus, nevus pigmentosus at pillosus, nevomelanotic nevus, melanotic nevus, Becker hairy nevus, heredofamiliar melanosis or van Bogaert syndrome (Miller 2004). In 1948 van Bogaert described a heredofamiliar disorder and used the name neurocutaneous melanosis (Van Bogaert 1948). In 1949 Touraine reported 23 patients with proliferation of melanocytes in the skin and in the CNS and he classified them as NCM (Touraine 1949).

In 1972 Fox first proposed three criteria of NCM: 1) large or numerous pigmented nevi in association with leptomeningeal melanosis or melanoma, 2) no evidence of malignant change in any cutaneous lesion, 3) no evidence of melanoma in any location other then the meninges (Fox 1972).

In 1991 Kadonaga and Frieden revised aforementioned criteria and suggested the new ones:

1. large (in adults at least 20 cm largest diameter, 9 cm on the head and 6 cm in body region for newborns and infants) or multiple (3 or more) congenital melanotic nevi
2. no evidence of cutaneous melanoma, except patients with benign meningeal lesion proven by histology
3. no evidence of meningeal melanoma, except patients with benign cutaneous lesion proven by histology (Kadonaga and Frieden 1991).

## Incidence and prevalence

Neurocutaneous melanosis is a rare syndrome. This disease affects males and females with the same frequency. It occurs more often in white race, sporadically in blacks. (DeDavid et al. 1996, Acosta et al. 2005). However it's true epidemiology is not established.

## Clinical manifestations

### Cutaneous findings

The cutaneous lesions in NCM are present at birth. These lesions – single or numerous – are giant melanotic nevi with abundant hair. The color of the skin and hair is similar, it may be very dark and light brown, darker in the blacks (Pascual-Castroviejo 1987). According to the current criteria of NCM the large congenital melanotic nevi (LCMN) is defined as equal to or greater than 20 cm in adult, 9 cm on the scalp in infant or 6 cm in the body in infant (Miller 2004).

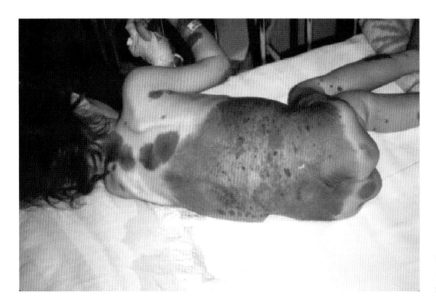

**Fig. 1.** Extensive, giant, black-brown pigmented nevus in lumbosacral area. Note also satellite nevi on the neck and extremities.

LCMN is usually located on the lower trunk, in gluteal-perineal-genital region (64%) or over the shoulders, upper arms and lover neck (32%) (Figs. 1, 2 and 3). It may be localized also on the head, it may cover the extremities giving the appearance of stockings or long gloves (Makkar and Frieden 2004, Sasaki et al. 1996) In some cases the multiple (three

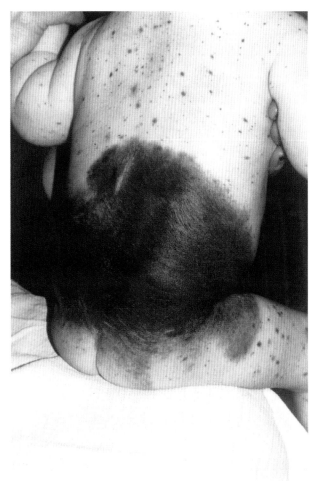

**Fig. 2.** Giant hairy pigmented nevus in bathing-trunks distribution. Small satellite nevi are not hairy.

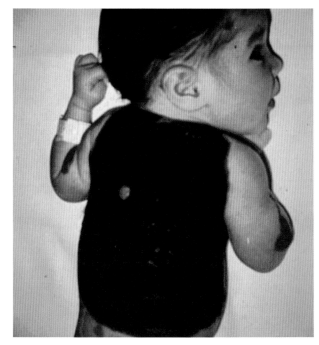

**Fig. 3.** Very large melanocytic nevus in upper trunk distribution.

or more) congenital pigmented nevi in the absence of a single large congenital melanotic nevus were found. New small satellite nevi may appear during the first years of life.

In NCM the melanocytes were found in the subcutis, muscles, peritoneum, lymphatic vessels and fascies (Kadonaga et al. 1991).

Histopathological findings of the NCM lesions are the nevus cells extending into the dermis or into the deep dermis or even the subcutis, surrounding nerves and blood vessels (Miller 2004).

## Neurological findings

Patients with NCM may be symptomatic – when the neurological manifestations occur or asymptomatic with or without the typical changes in MRI of the central nervous system.

Neurological manifestations of NCM are caused by leptomeningeal melanosis (see Fig. 4), intracranial melanoma, intracerebral or subarachnoid hemorrhage. Leptomeningeal melanosis tends to occur in the inferior surface of cerebellum, the frontal, temporal and occipital lobes, the ventral surface of the pons, medulla, cerebral peduncles, the upper cervical cord and the ventral surface of the lumbosacral cord. It is probably the most common cause of neurological symptoms in patients with NCM (Makkar and Frieden 2004).

Neurological symptoms usually occur before the age of 2 years. Fifty percent of patients with CNS involvement demonstrate the symptoms during the first 12 months of life. In infants the neurological symptoms have acute course. Sporadically the neurological manifestations occur in the 2nd or 3rd decade of life (Makkar and Frieden 2004). The symptoms appearing later in life are chronic and may be associated with neuropsychiatric manifestations like depression or psychosis (Azzoni et al. 2001).

The most frequent manifestations are caused by increased intracranial pressure – headache, vomiting, generalized seizures, increased head circumference, cranial nerve palsies, papilledema, meningeal signs, ataxic gait. Spinal involvement occurs in about 20% of patients. They demonstrate bowel and bladder dysfunction, myelopathy and radiculopathy. Motor

deficit and acute hemiparesis may also occur. Khera et al. (2005) reported an 11-year-old child with quadriparesis, who had had difficulties in walking since the age of two and a half years. In about 10% of patients the developmental delay was diagnosed (Berker et al. 2000, Burstein et al. 2005, Makkar and Frieden 2004).

The most frequent neurological symptom, hydrocephalus, is reported in two thirds of symptomatic patients. It's mechanism is probably related to reduced cerebrospinal fluid flow due to melanocyte infiltration of the arachnoid villi, cerebral aqueduct or cerebellar foramina (Dunin-Wasowicz et al. 1996).

In patients with the later onset of presentation – first neurological manifestation at average age of 8.5 year – the presence of discrete intracranial masses was reported. In this group of patients focal seizure activity, localized sensorimotor deficits and difficulties in speech are more often (de Andrade et al. 2004, Makkar and Frieden 2004).

Neurological symptoms in patients with NMC may be also related to the development of leptomeningeal melanoma with extremely poor prognosis. It occurs in 40–64% of symptomatic cases of NMC (Arunkumar et al. 2001, Makkar and Frieden 2004, Hayashi et al. 2004).

Histological material from meningeal biopsy or CSF analysis reveal cytoplasmic reactivity to melanoma-specific antigen HMB-45, neuron specific enolase (NSE) and protein S-100 (Sasaki et al. 1996, Peretti-Viton et al. 2002).

There is one report of a patient with NCM and intracranial amelanotic melanoma (Vanzieleghem et al. 1999).

## Other abnormalities

In some symptomatic NCM cases structural CNS anomalies are also reported, especially the Dandy-Walker complex (DWC), arachnoid cyst and occult spinal dysraphism. Association has also been reported with the syringomyelia, intraspinal subdural melanotic arachnoid cyst, spinal lipoma and orbital tumor (Acosta et al. 2005, Berker et al. 2000).

The Dandy-Walker complex has been frequently reported (Arai et al. 2004, Berker et al.

2000, Caceres and Trejos 2006, Mena-Cedillos et al. 2002). The pathogenesis of the association DWC and NCM is unknown. There are some hypothesis. The obstruction by melanocytes in the outgoing foramen of the fourth ventricle may result in the DWC. Maybe the leptomeningeal anomalies affect the development of the cerebellum and fourth ventricle. The most accepted hypothesis is that leptomeningeal melanosis interferes with the normal inductive effects of primitive meningeal cells resulting in vermian hypogenesis and retrocerebellar cyst formation.

NCM has been rarely reported with other neurocutaneous syndromes like neurofibromatosis type 1, Sturge-Weber syndrome, encephalocraniocutaneous lipomatosis and multiple hamartoma syndrome (Acosta et al. 2005, Ahmed et al. 2002).

Urinary tract anomalies including renal pelvis and urethral malformations, duodenal atresia, neoplasm including unilateral renal cyst and rhabdomyosarcoma have been also reported (Köksal et al. 2003).

In the literature there is a single report of NCM associated with Hirschprung's disease and the other associated with transposition of the great arteries and renal agenesis (Iwabuchi et al. 2005, Köksal et al. 2003).

Except for melanoma in individuals with NCM other malignancies may also occur. Embryonic rhabdomyosarcoma, melanoblastoma, malignant schwannoma and neuroectodermal neoplasm have been reported (Dunin-Wasowicz et al. 1996, Makkar and Frieden 2004).

## Natural history

The characteristic skin lesion – LCMN or multiple melanotic nevi are present at birth. During the first years of life the small satellite nevi may appear. The risk of development of symptomatic NCM in a patient with a LCMN is 2.5–11%, especially if the patient has the LCMN in a posterior axial location with satellite melanotic nevi (Acosta et al. 2005, DeDavid et al. 1996). In about 0.7–15% patients the malignant melanoma may develop in the setting of LCMN (Bittencourt et al. 2000, Hale et al. 2005,

Mena-Cedillos et al. 2002, Krengel et al. 2006). The melanoma risk strongly depends on the size of LCMN (Krengel et al. 2006).

The prognosis in symptomatic NCM is poor, even in the absence of malignant melanoma (Chu et al. 2003, Gondo et al. 2000, Miranda et al. 2005, Zhang et al. 2008). The prognosis for asymptomatic patients is more difficult to predict (Foster et al. 2001). The neurological manifestations of NCM usually appear in the first 2 years of life. Median survival time is 6.5 months after onset of symptoms, with more than 50% of deaths within the first 3 years of onset of neurological manifestations (Acosta et al. 2005, Makin et al. 1999, Schaffer et al. 2001).

Patients with NCM and Dandy-Walker complex experience rapid neurological deterioration and usually die by the age of 4 years (Berker et al. 2000).

Patients with leptomeningeal involvement have a potential for malignant degeneration with prevalence of 40–64% according to different reports (Hayashi et al. 2004, Makkar and Frieden 2004).

## Pathogenesis and molecular genetics

The precise pathogenesis of NCM is not clear. The syndrome seems to be a result of an error in morphogenesis of neural ectoderm in developing embryo. Cutaneous melanocytes derive from the pluripotent precursor cells of the neural crest. There are suggestions that the aberrancy in migration of melanocytes from the neural crest to skin may lead to leptomeningeal infiltration by pigmented cells. Another hypothesis suggests that the abnormality during the critical stage between 11th and 17th week, when the pia matter and basal leptomeninges originate from the neural crest, may result in the proliferation of melanocytes in the leptomeninges (Berker et al. 2000, Makkar and Frieden 2004).

The recent data suggest that alteration in hepatocyte growth factor (HGF)/scatter factor (SF) signaling though the *MET* receptor during embryogenesis might play the most important role in the development of NCM. HGF/SF signaling through the *MET* receptor in melanocytes derived from the neural crest promotes the proliferation, motility and melanin synthesis in vivo. Transgenic mice over-expressing HGF/SF develop pigmented nevi and leptomeningeal melanocytosis (Makkar and Frieden 2004). The abnormal expression of the *MET* receptor has been immunohistochemically detected also in a congenital nevus of the infant with NCM. (Acosta et al. 2005, Takayama et al. 2001).

## Diagnosis

Diagnosis of the disease is based on the clinical examination and MRI of the CNS. The characteristic skin lesions found at birth usually are the first symptoms of NCM (Paprocka et al. 2004). On clinical examination Ruiz-Maldonado et al. (1997) found neurological abnormalities, such as mild or minimal motor deficits,

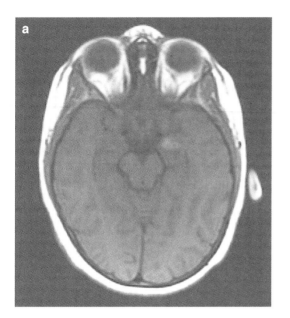
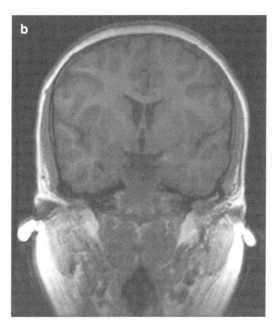
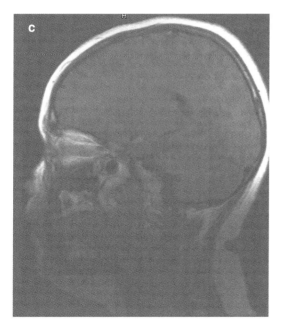

**Fig. 4.** Axial (**a**), coronal (**b**) and sagittal (**c**) T1-weighted magnetic resonance images of the brain in a child with a giant melanocytic nevus of the skin showing high signal lesion (likely melanocyte infiltration) in the paraippocampal region.

nerve dysfunction and impaired mental status in patients thought to be asymptomatic. In brain MRI studies there is an increased signal intensity on T1-weighted images without contrast and decreased signal intensity on T2-weighted sequences of MRI (diffuse or localized in the leptomeninges; the cortical and subcortical plaque and nodular lesions) as a reflection of the paramagnetic properties of melanin (Byrd et al. 1995, Dermici et al. 1995, Gondo et al. 2000).

Since 1991 the MRI has been recognized as a useful screening for neurocutaneous melanosis in asymptomatic patients with LCMN (Frieden et al. 1994). In 25% of asymptomatic infants with NCM the MRI allows to detect the CNS melanosis (Fig. 4). The most common finding in this group was the T1-signal shortening compatible with melanin deposits in the infratentorial structures (Acosta et al. 2005, Caceres and Trejos 2006, Chu et al. 2003). The FLAIR findings – leptomeningeal hyperintensity has been also described (Hayashi et al. 2004). Neuroimaging is also useful in diagnosis of associated malformations in the central nervous system like Dandy – Walker complex and others.

Results of CSF examination were reported in few cases. Increased intracranial pressure of CSF, elevated protein, aseptic leukocytosis and normal glucose were found. The presence of melanin-containing cells may be helpful in the diagnosis. (Akinwunmi et al. 2001, Makkar and Frieden 2004).

Electroencephalographic studies may be useful both in diagnosis of epilepsy, both in localization of the CNS tumor. Especially when seizures appear focal or generalized abnormalities may be detected (Pascual-Castroviejo 1987).

## Differential diagnosis

Differential diagnosis may require a cooperation between dermatologists, neurologists and neuroradiologists.

Differential diagnosis of NCM should be carried out with respect to:

1. heredofamiliar melanosis – a benign melanosis affecting the skin and leptomeninges with autosomal dominant inheritance
2. primary malignant melanoma of the leptomeninges
3. metastatic melanoma or intracranial dissemination of malignant melanoma of the skin – found at any age
4. progonoma – benign tumor with different tissue components in addition to melanotic cells, appears in cranial bones and in neighboring areas of the meninges, without infiltration of the brain
5. melanotic nerve sheath tumor – solitary, melanin-bearing slow growing plexiform neurofibroma with no metastasis (Pascual-Castroviejo 1987, Peters et al. 2000).
6. SCALP syndrome, a newly described entity consisting of sebaceous nevus syndrome, CNS malformations, aplasia cutis congenita (of the membranous type), limbal dermoid of the eye, and pigmented nevus (of the giant congenital melanocytic type) (Lam et al. 2008).

## Follow up

The melanotic nevi should be examined by parents at home once a month and by physician every 6 months with making photos for later comparison.

The asymptomatic patients should be followed with repeated neurological examination. The routine MRI examination in these patients is debated. Schaffer et al. (2001) report a case of an infant with asymptomatic NCM, an increased signal in the right temporal lobe on T1-weighted images and with a long-term outcome after the surgical intervention. The sensitivity of MR imaging has permitted detection of melanosis in about 25% asymptomatic infants. (Frieden et al. 1994). Some authors recommend the MRI in the first 4 months of life, as due to the poor mielinisation of CNS the signal of melanin is easier to detect (Agero et al. 2005).

When the clinical signs of increased intracranial pressure occur or the new neurological symptoms appear the neuroimaging should be performed for exclusion of the hydrocephalus and the malignant transformation in CNS.

## Management

There is no one established opinion about the excision the LCMN (Heffel and Thaller 2005). Removing of the nevi reduces the potential for malignant transformation and improves cosmetic outcome. However due to large diameters of the nevi patients after excision are left with large wounds that are difficult to close. Traditionally these defects have been repaired with split-thickness skin grafts, full-thickness skingrafts, the use of tissue expanders and a variety of flaps. But the complete excision of giant nevus involves multiple surgical procedures beginning in infancy and completing in adolescence (Arneja and Gosain 2005). This surgical excision causes scarring which creates other problems. Dermabrasion is probably less effective in reducing the risk of malignancy. The removal of cutaneous lesion does not reduce the risk of malignant melanoma of CNS. Some authors do not recommend the surgical procedures in symptomatic patients because of poor prognosis (Miller 2004).

Recently, new methods have been developed for the closure of large skin defects in pediatric patients with the use of artificial skin substitutes. Advantages include coverage of large wounds, decrease or elimination of donor site pain and morbidity, and decreased scarring and wound contractures (Earle and Marshall 2005).

Neurosurgical treatment (ventriculoperitoneal shunt) may be recommended in patients with hydrocephalus. A shunt filter may limit the spread of malignant cells (Pascual-Castroviejo 1987).

If the syringomyelia is associated with NCM the syrinx drainage should be considered.

Children with epilepsy should be treated with anticonvulsant medication. The radicular pain secondary to infiltration of the roots should be treated with analgetics (Pascual-Castroviejo 1987).

Treatment options for symptomatic NCM are unsatisfactory. There is a little experience in chemo- and radiotherapy, with relatively little effects on the symptoms and no effects on survival (Acosta et al. 2005, Di Rocco et al. 2004, Peters et al. 2000). In these cases due to the extremely poor prognosis the psychological support of the family is very important.

## Genetic counseling

NCM is non familial, very rare neuroectodermal dysplasia. The genetic background of this disorder is not known therefore genetic counseling is not applicable.

## References

Acosta FL Jr, Binder DK, Barkovich AJ, Frieden IJ, Gupta N (2005) Neurocutaneous melanosis presenting with hydrocephalus. J Neurosurg 102(1 Suppl): 96–100.

Agero ALC, Benvenuto-Andrade C, Dusza SW, Halpern AC, Marghoob AA (2005) Asymptomatic neurocutaneous melanocytosis in patients with large congenital melanocytic nevi: a study of cases from an internet-based registry. J Am Acad Dermatol 53(6): 959–965.

Ahmed I, Tope WD, Young TL, Miller DM, Bloom KE (2002) Neurocutaneous melanosis in association with the encephalocraniocutaneous lipomatosis. J Am Acad Dermatol 47(2): 196–200.

Akinwunmi J, Sgouros S, Moss C, Grundy R, Green S (2001) Neurocutaneous melanosis with leptomeningeal melanoma. Pediatr Neurosurg 35: 277–279.

Arai M, Nosaka K, Kashihara K, Kaizaki Y (2004) Neurocutaneous melanosis associated with Dandy – Walker malformation and a meningohydroencephalocele. Case report. J Neurosurg 100(5): 501–505.

Arneja JS, Gosain AK (2005) Giant congenital melanocytic nevi of the trunk and an algorithm for treatment. J Craniofac Surg 16(5): 886–893.

Arunkumar MJ, Ranjan A, Jacob M, Rajshekhar V (2001) Neurocutaneous melanosis: a case of primary intracranial melanoma with metastasis. Clin Oncol 13(1): 52–54.

Azzoni A, Argentieri R, Raja M (2001) Neurocutaneous melanosis and psychosis: a case report. Psychiatry Clin Neurosci 55(2): 93–95.

Berker M, Oruckaptan HH, Oge KH, Benli K (2000) Neurocutaneous melanosis associated with Dandy – Walker malformation. Pediatr Neurosurg 33: 270–273.

Bittencourt FV, Marghoob AA, Kopf AW, Koenig KL, Bart RS (2000) Large congenital melanocytic nevi and the risk for development of malignant melanoma and neurocutaneous melanocytosis. Pediatrics 106: 736–741.

Burstein F, Seier H, Hudgins PA, Zapiach L (2005) Neurocutaneous melanosis. J Craniofac Surg 16(5): 874–876.

Byrd SE, Reyes-Mugica M, Darling CF, Chou P, de Leon GA, Radkowski MA (1995) MR of leptomeningeal melanosis in children. Eur J Radiol 20: 93–99.

Caldarelli M, Tamburrini G, Di Rocco F (2005) Neurocutaneous melanosis. J Neurosurg 103(4 Suppl): 382

Caceres A, Trejos H (2006) Neurocutaneous melanosis with associated Dandy-Walker complex. Child's Nerv Syst 22(1): 67–72.

Chu WCW, Lee V, Chan YL, Shing MM, Chik KW, Li CK, Ma KC (2003) Neurocutaneous melanomatosis with a rapidly deteriorating course. Am J Neuroradiol 24: 287–290.

De Andrade DO, Dravet C, Raybaud C, Broglin D, Laguitton V, Girard N (2004) An unusual case of neurocutaneous melanosis. Epileptic Disord 6(3): 145–152.

DeDavid M, Orlow SJ, Provost N, Marghoob AA, Rao BK, Wasti Q, Huang CL, Kopf AW, Bart RS (1996) Neurocutaneous melanosis: clinical features of large congenital melanocytic nevi in patients with manifest central nervous system melanosis. J Am Acad Dermatol 35: 529–538.

Dermici A, Kawamura Y, Sze G, Duncan C (1995) MR of parenchymal neurocutaneous melanosis. Am J Neuroradiol 16(3): 603–606.

Di Rocco F, Sabatino G, Koiutzoglou M, Battaglia D, Caldarelli M, Tamburrini G (2004) Neurocutaneous melanosis. Childs Nerv Syst 20(1): 23–28.

Dunin-Wasowicz D, Józwiak S, Chrzanowska K, Dabrowski D (1996) Neurocutaneous melanosis-report of cases. Neur Dziec 5(10): 95–100.

Earle SA, Marshall DM (2005) Management of giant congenital nevi with artificial skin substitutes in children. J Craniofac Surg 16(5): 904–907.

Foster RD, Williams ML, Barkovich AJ, Hoffman WY, Mathes SJ, Frieden IJ (2001) Giant congenital melanocytic nevi: the significance of neurocutaneous melanosis in neurologically asymptomatic children. Plast Reconstr Surg 107(4): 933–941.

Fox H (1972) Neurocutaneous melanosis. In: Vinken PJ, Bruyn GW (eds.) The phacomatoses. Handbook of clinical neurology, Amsterdam: North Holland, vol. 14: 414–428.

Frieden IJ, Williams ML, Barkovich AJ (1994) Giant congenital melanocytic nevi: brain magnetic resonance findings in neurologically asymptomatic children. J Am Acad Dermatol 31: 423–429.

Gondo K, Kira R, Tokunaga Y, Hara T (2000) Age-related changes of the MR appearance of CNS involvement in neurocutaneous melanosis complex. Pediatr Radiol 30: 866–868.

Hale EK, Stein J, Ben-Porat L, Panageas KS, Eichenbaum MS, Marghoob AA, Osman I, Kopf AW, Polsky D (2005) Association of melanoma and neurocutaneous melanocytosis with large congenital melanocytic naevi – results from the NYU – LCMN registry. Br J Dermatol 152: 512–517.

Hayashi M, Maeda M, Maji T, Matsubara T, Tsukahara H, Takeda K (2004) Diffuse leptomeningeal hyperintensity on fluid-attenuated inversion recovery MR images in neurocutaneous melanosis. Am J Neuroradiol 25: 138–141.

Heffel DF, Thaller S (2005) Congenital melanosis: an update. J Craniofac Surg 16(5): 940–944.

Iwabuchi T, Shimotake T, Furukawa T (2005) Neurocutaneous melanosis associated with Hirschsprung's disease in male neonate. J Pediatr Surg 40: 11–13.

Kadonaga JN, Frieden IJ (1991) Neurocutaneous melanosis. Definition and review of the literature. J Am Acad Dermatol 24: 747–755.

Khera S, Sarkar R, Jain RK, Saxena AK (2005) Neurocutaneous melanosis: an atypical presentation. J Dermatol 32(7): 602–605.

Köksal N, Bayram Y, Murat I, Dogru M, Bostan O, Sevinir B, Yazici Z (2003) Neurocutaneous melanosis with transposition of the great arteries and renal agenesis. Pediatr Dermatol 20(4): 332–334.

Krengel S, Hauschild A, Schafer T (2006) Melanoma risk in congenital melanocytic naevi: a systematic review. Br J Dermatol 155: 1–8.

Lam J, Dohil MA, Eichenfield LF, Cunningham BB (2008) SCALP syndrome: sebaceous nevus syndrome, CNS malformations, aplasia cutis congenita, limbal dermoid, and pigmented nevus (giant congenital melanocytic nevus) with neurocutaneous melanosis: a distinct syndromic entity. J Am Acad Dermatol 58: 884–888.

Makin GW, Eden OB, Lashford LS, Moppett J, Gerrard MP, Davies HA, Powell CV, Campbell AN, Frances H (1999) Leptomeningeal melanoma in childhood. Cancer 86(5): 878–886.

Makkar HS, Frieden IJ (2004) Neurocutaneous melanosis. Semin Cutan Med Surg 23(2): 138–144.

Mena-Cedillos CA, Valencia-Herrera AM, Arrovo-Pineda AL, Salgado-Jimenez MA, Espinoza-Montero R, Martinez-Avalos AB, Perales-Arroyo A (2002) Neurocutaneous melanosis in association with the Dandy – Walker complex, complicated by melanoma: report of a case and literature review. Pediatr Dermatol 19(3): 237–242.

Miller VS (2004) Neurocutaneous melanosis. In: Roach ES, Miller VS (eds.) Neurocutaneous disorders, Cambridge: Cambridge University Press, pp. 71–76.

Miranda P, Esparza J, Hinojosa J, Munoz A (2005) Neurocutaneous melanosis and congenital melanocytic nevus in the head. Pediatr Neurosurg 41: 109–111.

Paprocka J, Jamroz E, Kajor M, Marszal E (2004) Neurocutaneous melanosis – case report. Wiad Lek 57(9–10): 520–523.

Pascual-Castroviejo I, Neurocutaneous melanosis (1987) In: Gomez MR, Adams RD (eds.) Neurocutaneous Diseases. A practical approach. Boston: Butterworths, pp. 329–334.

Peretti-Viton P, Gorincour G, Feuillet L, Lambot K, Brunel H, Raybaud C, Pellissier JF, Cherif AA (2002) Neurocutaneous melanosis: radiological – pathological correlation. Eur Radiol 12(6): 1349–1353.

Peters R, Jansen G, Engelbrecht V (2000) Neurocutaneous melanosis with hydrocephalus, intraspinal arachnoid collections and syringomyelia: case report and literature review. Pediatr Radiol 30(4): 284–288.

Rokitansky J (1861) Ein ausgezeineter Fall von Pigment-Mal mit ausgebreiteter Pigmentierung der inneren Hirn und Rückenmarkshaute. Allg Wien Med Z 6: 113–116.

Ruiz-Maldonado R, del Rosario Barona-Mazuera M, Hidalgo-Galvan LR (1997) Giant congenital melanocytic nevi, neurocutaneous melanosis and neurological alterations. Dermatology 195: 125–128.

Sasaki Y, Kobayashi S, Shimizu H, Nishikawa T (1996) Multiple nodular lesions seen in a patient with neurocutaneous melanosis. J Dermatol 23(11): 828–831.

Schaffer JV, McNiff JM, Bolognia JL (2001) Cerebral mass due to neurocutaneous melanosis: eight years later. Pediatr Dermatol 18(5): 369–377.

Takayama H, Nagashima Y, Hara M, Takagi H, Mori M, Merlino G, Nakazato Y (2001) Immunohistochemical detection of the c-met proto-oncogene product in the congenital melanocytic nevus of an infant with neurocutaneous melanosis. J Am Acad Dermatol 44(3): 538–540.

Touraine PA (1949) Les mélanoses neuro-cutanee. Ann Derm Syph 9: 489–523.

Van Bogaert LC (1948) La mélanose neurocutanée diffuse hérédofamiliale. Bull Acad R Med Belg 3: 397–427.

Vanzieleghem BD, Lemmerling MM, Van Coster RN (1999) Neurocutaneous melanosis presenting with intracranial amelanotic melanoma. Am J Neuroradiol 20(3): 457–460.

Zhang W, Miao J, Li Q, Liu R, Li Z (2008) Neurocutaneous melanosis in an adult patient with diffuse leptomeningeal melanosis and a rapidly deteriorating course: case report and review of the literature. Clin Neurol Neurosurg Apr 11 [Epub ahead of print].

# Chapter 27

# GENETICS OF PTEN HAMARTOMA TUMOR SYNDROME (PHTS)

**Corrado Romano**

Unit of Paediatrics and Medical Genetics, IRCCS OASI Maria Santissima, Troina, Italy

## Introduction

PTEN hamartoma tumor syndrome (PHTS) (Marsh et al. 1999) can be defined as a syndromic condition including one or more hamartomas which has its biological basis in a germline mutation of the Phosphatase and Tensin Homolog deleted on Chromosome 10 (PTEN) gene. Following such assumption, PHTS includes patients with the previous diagnosis of Cowden syndrome (CS) (Weary et al. 1972), Bannayan-Riley-Ruvalcaba syndrome (BRRS) (Cohen 1990), Proteus syndrome (PS) (Wiedemann et al. 1983), Proteus-like syndrome (PLS) (Zhou et al. 2000) and Lhermitte–Duclos syndrome (LDS) (Dastur et al. 1975). Conversely, those conditions not including hamartomas within their phenotype but presenting with a PTEN mutation (Butler et al. 2005) cannot be considered as part of the PHTS spectrum. Currently, failure to detect a PTEN mutation doesn't imply the ruling out of a clinical diagnosis of CS, BRRS, PS, PLS or LDS in patients who fulfill the clinical diagnostic criteria for these conditions; however, the term PHTS should be avoided in this case.

## The PHTS

CS, BRRS, PS, PLS and LDS are extensively addressed in other chapters of this book. The aim of this paragraph is to make the reader aware of how the discovery of PTEN gene has changed the understanding of the above mentioned conditions and has prompted the need of using the new definition of PHTS.

The International Cowden Consortium proposed in 1995 a set of operational criteria for the diagnosis of CS cases and families aimed at the search for the CS gene (Nelen et al. 1996, Liaw et al. 1997). The importance and robustness of these criteria are highlighted by the PTEN mutation rate, which is 80% (Liaw et al. 1997, Marsh et al. 1998b), when they are administered strictly, whereas is 10–50% (Tsou et al. 1997, Lynch et al. 1997, Nelen et al. 1997), when they are not used. A study has been performed in 1998 on CS-like families (Marsh et al. 1998a), in order to increase the knowledge about the PTEN mutation clinical spectrum. One of the 64 CS-like cases was found to have a germline PTEN mutation. Bilateral breast cancer, follicular thyroid carcinoma, and endometrial adenocarcinoma were running in that family. Five out of 103 (5%) women with multiple primary cancers were found to have PTEN germline missense mutations, with proven resulting loss of function (De Vivo et al. 2000). Two of these five cases had endometrial cancer. Consequently, PTEN germline mutations can be found in hamartomatous conditions not fulfilling the diagnostic criteria of CS, and endometrial carcinoma might be an important part of CS, increasing the probability of finding a PTEN mutation in CS-like cases. The International Cowden Consortium has included, in the version released during year 2000, endometrial carcinoma in the operational criteria for the diagnosis of CS.

The PLS is an effect of the use of PTEN analysis in borderline cases. Indeed, Zhou et al. (2000) reported a germline R335X PTEN mutation and a R130X somatic mutation in three separate tissues on a simplex case (e.g., a patient of unknown family history) showing PLS with hemihypertrophy, microcephaly, lipomas, connective tissue nevi, and multiple arteriovenous malformations.

PHTS has been coined as the best definition for hamartomatous conditions sharing PTEN germline mutations for the following reasons. CS, BRRS, PS, PLS and LDS appear now to be five conditions caused by the same genetic anomaly. Consequently, following the definition of a syndrome, they cannot be five syndromes, but one syndrome which can appear in at least five different ways. This assumption can be considered the lumper's view. However, some data may strengthen this position. First of all, CS and BRRS have been shown to be allelic, because 50–60% of patients with BRRS have PTEN germline mutations and the highest PTEN mutation frequencies (>92%) have been found in CS-BRRS overlap families (Marsh et al. 1999). Secondly, germline PTEN promoter mutations have been found only in CS patients (Zhou et al. 2003a). Thirdly, large deletions or rearrangements involving PTEN gene have been found only in BRRS or CS/BRRS overlap cases (Marsh et al. 1999, Zhou et al. 2003b, Ahmed et al. 1999). These results appear as the first cornerstone of genotype-phenotype correlations in PHTS. However, further data are needed to better clarify the whole picture.

## The PTEN gene

The PTEN gene is one of the most important tumor-suppressor genes, being second only to p53 as mutation frequency in human cancer. The involvement of its alteration in tumorigenesis has been first suspected and subsequently proven in 1997 (Li et al. 1997), when high frequency of loss of heterozygosity (LOH) at 10q23 chromosome band was observed in several human tumors. Furthermore, the suppression of tumorigenesis in glioblastoma murine cells by the wild type chromosome 10 led to envision a tumor suppressor gene mapping in 10q23 (Fig. 1). Such gene was eventually isolated by the above-mentioned authors and called PTEN (Fig. 2). They detected homozygous deletions, frame shift, or nonsense mutations in PTEN in 63% (5/8) of glioblastoma cell lines, 100% (4/4) of prostate cancer cell lines, and 10% (2/20) of breast cancer cell lines. Steck et al. (1997) independently isolated the same gene and called it Mutated in Multiple Advanced Cancers-1 (MMAC-1). Indeed, a common feature of PTEN somatic mutations, already presented in 10q LOH, is the association with advanced stage tumors (mainly glial and prostate cancers),

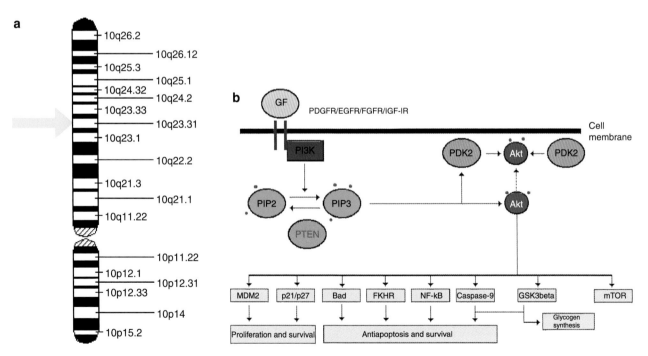

**Fig. 1.  a, b** Chromosomal mapping of PTEN gene (from http://ghr.nlm.nih.gov/gene=pten).

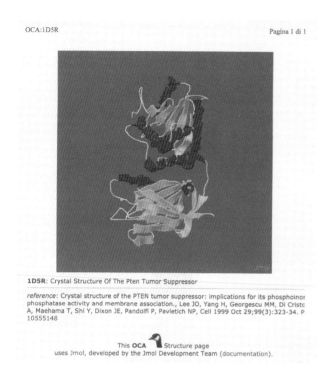

**1D5R:** Crystal Structure Of The Pten Tumor Suppressor

*reference:* Crystal structure of the PTEN tumor suppressor: implications for its phosphoinos phosphatase activity and membrane association., Lee JO, Yang H, Georgescu MM, Di Cristo A, Maehama T, Shi Y, Dixon JE, Pandolfi P, Pavletich NP, Cell 1999 Oct 29;99(3):323-34. P 10555148

This **OCA** Structure page uses Jmol, developed by the Jmol Development Team (documentation).

**Fig. 2.** Crystal structure of PTEN gene.

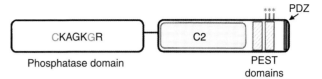

**Fig. 3.** Catalytic domains of the PTN gene.

whereas this is not true for endometrial cancer, being affected equally all the stages. This has led to the suggestion that the activation of PTEN is at an early stage in endometrial carcinogenesis, but later on in glial and prostatic carcinogenesis.

In the same year (Liaw et al. 1997) germline mutations of PTEN gene were found in families with CS, showing the function of tumor suppressor gene also in the germline. Furthermore germline PTEN mutations lead to increased breast cancer incidence, but do not cause frequently familial breast cancer (Chen et al. 1998), notwithstanding 10% of breast cancer cell lines have inactivated PTEN (Li et al. 1997, Steck et al. 1997).

Li et al. (1997) have shown that PTEN gene is an human cdc14 homolog, like CDC14A and CDC14B. The cdc 14 gene is a key point for the progression of cell cycle in Saccharomyces cerevisiae: its protein acts in late nuclear division preparing for subsequent DNA replication. The human PTEN gene spans 103,207 bases, is made up of 9 exons and codes for a 1212-bp transcript and a 403-amino acid protein.

The PTEN product has the kinetic properties of dual-specific phosphatases (Myers et al. 1997) and acts on G1 cell cycle progression through negative regulation of the PI3-kinase/Akt signaling pathway (Li and Sun 1998). PTEN is a member of the Protein-Tyrosine Phosphatase (PTP) gene superfamily (Li et al. 1997, Steck et al. 1997). These are genes consisting of conserved catalytic domains, flanked by noncatalytic regulatory sequences (Denu et al. 1996). The PTP catalytic domains show a "signature motif", which is the canonical sequence HCXXGXXRS/T. Among the PTP superfamily genes a further split is made in "classic" PTP (acting only towards phosphotyrosine residues) and dual-specificity phosphatase families (desphosphorylating phosphotyrosine, phosphoserine and/or phosphothreonine). PTEN is a dual-specificity phosphatase. The catalytic domain of PTEN has been proven to be essential for its function, which is lost following any mutation within the signature motif (Fig. 3) (Myers et al. 1997).

PTEN gene in glioblastoma-derived cell lines regulates hypoxia- and IGF-1-induced angiogenic gene expression by regulating Akt activation of HIF-1 activity (Zundel et al. 2000). Restoration of wild-type PTEN to glioblastoma cell lines lacking functional PTEN ablates hypoxia and IGF-1 induction of HIF-1-regulated genes. In addition, Akt activation leads to HIF-1α stabilization, whereas PTEN attenuates hypoxia-mediated HIF-1α stabilization. Loss of PTEN during malignant progression contributes to tumor expansion through the deregulation of Akt activity and HIF-1-regulated gene expression. PTEN abnormalities have been found also in primary acute leukemias and non-Hodgkin lymphomas (Dahia et al. 1999).

PTEN and phosphorylated Akt levels are inversely correlated in the large majority of the examined samples, suggesting that PTEN regulates phosphatidylinositol 3,4,5-triphosphates and may play a role in apoptosis. Over expression of PTEN inhibits cell migration, whereas antisense PTEN enhances migration (Tamura et al. 1998). The phosphatase domain of PTEN is essential because its inactivation does not allow the down regulation of integrin-mediated cell spreading and formation of focal adhesions, peculiar of wild type PTEN. Over expression of focal adhesion kinase (FAK) partially antagonizes the effects of PTEN. Thus, the negative regulation of cell interactions with the extra cellular matrix could be the way PTEN phosphatase acts as a tumor suppressor.

PTEN gene plays an essential role in human development. Indeed, the additional effect of three homozygotic mutations produce together early embryonic lethality in mice, whereas heterozygosis increases tumor incidence (Di Cristofano et al. 1998, Suzuki et al. 1998, Podsypanina et al. 1999). Furthermore, PTEN antagonizes growth factor-induced Shc phosphorylation and inhibits the MAP kinase (MAPK) signaling pathway (Fig. 4a) (Weng et al.

2001). The way this inhibition is accomplished is currently understood as a suppression by the PTEN protein phosphatase activity (Weng et al. 2002).

## The PI3K/Akt/mTOR signaling pathway

The function of PTEN gene and the way its mutation can cause a disease can barely be understood if one do not see the PTEN protein inside the PI3K/Akt/mTOR signaling pathway (Fig. 4b) (Newton 2004). The activation of Phosphoinositide 3' Kinase (PI3K) is the primary event in this pathway (Vivanco and Sawyers 2002). This can occur from several growth factor receptors (GFRs), such as PDGFR, EGFR, FGFR, IGF-1R, VEGFR, IL-R, interferon receptors (IF-Rs), integrin receptors and the Ras pathway (Martin and Blenis 2002, Wymann and Pirola 1998, Rameh and Cantley 1999). The major role of PI3K is the phosphorylation of phosphatidylinositol (4,5) P (PIP2) to phosphatidylinositol (3,4,5) P (PIP3). PIP3 binds and translocates Akt near the cell membrane where it can be phosphorylated and activated by phosphatidylinositol (3,4,5) P dependent kinase 1 (PDK1) and phosphatidylinositol (3,4,5) P dependent kinase 2 (PDK2). Akt has several downstream effectors which mediate its ability to promote cell survival and growth. Then, activation of PI3K/Akt pathway is observed in several human cancers. PTEN is the antagonist of PI3K because dephosphorylates PIP3 to PIP2. The PI3K/PTEN imbalance, caused for instance by a mutation of PTEN, is then responsible for the progression to human cancer.

## Diagnosis of PHTS

The diagnosis of PHTS can be made only when in a person usually showing the CS phenotype, or the BRRS phenotype, or the PS phenotype, or the PLS syndrome phenotype, or the LDS phenotype, a PTEN mutation is recognized.

## Genetic counseling in PHTS

PHTS has an autosomal dominant mode of inheritance. Consequently, it is paramount to know if a

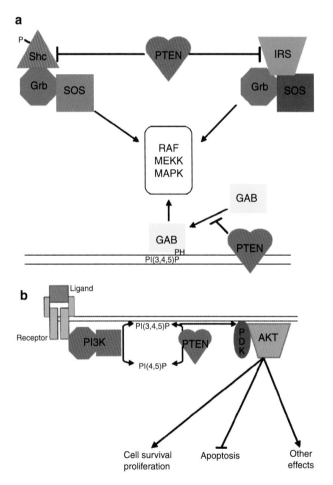

**Fig. 4.** The (**a**) MAP kinase (MAPK) signalling pathway and (**b**) PI3K/Akt pathway.

parent of the proband is affected. If the answer is affirmative, a 50% recurrence risk can be offered to the couple. The same risk is counseled for each pregnancy of the proband. If the parents are not affected, the recurrence risk would be negligible, because gonadal mosaicism has never been reported in PHTS. Prenatal diagnosis is feasible when the proband's mutation is known.

## Molecular genetic testing

The clinical uses of molecular genetic testing of PTEN gene in PHTS are essentially three: confirmation of diagnosis, predictive testing, and prenatal diagnosis. The sequence analysis of PTEN gene is currently available on a clinical basis. The Human Gene Mutation Database in Cardiff lists 156 different mutations on July 29, 2005 (Table 1).

The mutation detection rate for patients fulfilling clinical diagnostic criteria is currently 85–90% (Pilarski and Eng 2004) for CS, 83% for LDS (Zhou et al. 2003a), 65% for BRRS (Pilarski and Eng 2004), up to 50% for PLS (Zhou et al. 2001) and up to 22% for PS (Zhou et al. 2001). Heterozygous germline mutations in the PTEN promoter have been found in 10% of patients with CS who are negative for mutations in the coding sequence (Zhou et al. 2003b). Furthermore, sequence analysis cannot exclude a PTEN deletion: 11% of PTEN mutation-negative BRRS patients have been recently found affected by a PTEN deletion (Zhou et al. 2003b). Unfortunately, the PTEN deletion analysis, performed by southern blot or monochromosomal hybrid analysis or real-time PCR or semiquantitative multiplex PCR, is currently available only on a research basis. A few data were available by June 2005 on germline mutations in putative splice-sites: only 23 mutations have been published with limited resulting downstream data. On July 13, 2005, Agrawal et al. have published electronically in the Human Molecular Genetics journal website a study on splicing defects within the PTEN gene in 40 germline PTEN mutation positive and 33 mutation negative cases with classic CS, BRRS and CS- or BRRS-like features. They have found altered splicing in 4/40 mutation positive patients and 2/33 mutation negative patients. This latter result highlights furthermore the chance that a PTEN alteration can escape the usual mutation detection screening and a search for splicing defects should be done in all mutation screening negative cases showing the clinical features of PHTS.

## Genotype–phenotype relationship

Currently available data show that families with CS and germline PTEN mutations have an increased risk of malignant breast disease versus those families with clinical CS without a PTEN mutation (Marsh et al. 1998b). Missense mutations and mutations 5′ to or within the phosphatase core motif resulted to be associated with involvement of five or more organs (Marsh et al. 1998b). The overlap of BRRS and CS mutational range suggests that CS and BRRS are allelic (Marsh et al. 1999). A comparison between sporadic and familial cases of BRRS doesn't allow to find any difference in mutation frequencies. Patients with overlapping CS-BRRS phenotype had PTEN mutations identified in over 90% of cases. Zhou et al. (2000) reported a germline R335X PTEN mutation and a R130X somatic mutation in three separate tissues on a simplex case (e.g., a patient of unknown family history) showing PLS with hemihypertrophy, microcephaly, lipomas, connective tissue nevi, and multiple arteriovenous malformations. Both mutations are known in CS and BRRS patients.

**Table 1.** Mutations in the PTEN gene reported by HGMD, Cardiff on July 29, 2005

| Mutation type | Total No. of mutations |
|---|---|
| Nucleotide substitutions (missense/nonsense) | 66 |
| Nucleotide substitutions (splicing) | 19 |
| Nucleotide substitutions (regulatory) | 11 |
| Small deletions | 26 |
| Small insertions | 22 |
| Small indels | 3 |
| Gross deletions | 8 |
| Complex rearrangements (including inversions) | 1 |
| **Total** | **156** |

# References

Agrawal S, Pilarski R, Eng C (2005) Different splicing defects lead to differential effects downstream of the lipid and protein phosphatase activities of PTEN. Hum Mol Genet 2005 Jul 13 [Epub ahead of print].

Ahmed SF, Marsh DJ, Weremowicz S, Morton CC, Williams DM, Eng C (1999) Balanced translocation of 10q and 13q, including the PTEN gene, in a boy with an HCG-secreting tumor and the Bannayan–Riley–Ruvalcaba syndrome. J Clin Endocrinol Metab 84: 4665–4670.

Butler MG, Dasouki MJ, Zhou XP, Talebizadeh Z, Brown M, Takahashi TN, Miles JH, Wang CH, Stratton R, Pilarski R, Eng C (2005) Subset of individuals with autism spectrum disorders and extreme microcephaly associated with germline PTEN tumour suppressor gene mutations. J Med Genet 42: 318–321.

Chen J, Lindblom P, Lindblom A (1998) A study of the PTEN/MMAC1 gene in 136 breast cancer families. Hum Genet 102: 124–125.

Cohen MM Jr (1990) Bannayan–Riley–Ruvalcaba syndrome: renaming three formerly recognized syndromes as one etiologic entity. Am J Med Genet 35: 291–292.

Dahia PLM, Aguiar RCT, Alberta J, Kum JB, Caron S, Sill H, Marsh DJ, Ritz J, Freedman A, Stiles C, Eng C (1999) PTEN is inversely correlated with the cell survival factor Akt/PKB and is inactivated via multiple mechanisms in haematological malignancies. Hum Molec Genet 8: 185–193.

Dastur HM, Pandya SK, Deshpande DH (1975) Diffuse cerebellar hypertrophy Lhermitte-Duclos disease. Neurol India 23: 53–56.

Denu JM, Stuckey JA, Saper MA, Dixon JE (1996) Form and function in protein dephosphorylation. Cell 87: 361–364.

De Vivo I, Gertig DM, Nagase S, Hankinson SE, O'Brien R, Speizer FE, Parsons R, Hunter DJ (2000) Novel germline mutations in the PTEN tumour suppressor gene found in women with multiple cancers. J Med Genet 37: 336–341.

Di Cristofano A, Pesce B, Cordon-Cardo C, Pandolfi PP (1998) Pten is essential for embryonic development and tumour suppression. Nat Genet 19: 348–355.

Li DM, Sun H (1998) PTEN/MMAC1/TEP1 suppresses the tumorigenicity and induces G1 cell cycle arrest in human glioblastoma cells. Proc Nat Acad Sci USA 95: 15406–15411.

Li J, Yen C, Liaw D, Podsypanina K, Bose S, Wang SI, Puc J, Miliaresis C, Rodgers L, McCombie R, Bigner SH, Giovanella BC, Ittmann M, Tycko B, Hibshoosh H, Wigler MH, Parsons R (1997) PTEN, a putative protein tyrosine phosphatase gene mutated in human brain, breast, and prostate cancer. Science 275: 1943–1946.

Liaw D, Marsh DJ, Li J, Dahia PL, Wang SI, Zheng Z, Bose S, Call KM, Tsou HC, Peacocke M, Eng C, Parsons R (1997) Germline mutations of the PTEN gene in Cowden disease, an inherited breast and thyroid cancer syndrome. Nat Genet 16: 64–67.

Lynch ED, Ostermeyer EA, Lee MK, Arena JF, Ji H, Dann J, Swisshelm K, Suchard D, MacLeod PM, Kvinnsland S, Gjertsen BT, Heimdal K, Lubs H, Moller P, King MC (1997) Inherited mutations in PTEN that are associated with breast cancer, Cowden syndrome and juvenile polyposis. Am J Hum Genet 61: 1254–1260.

Marsh DJ, Dahia PL, Caron S, Kum JB, Frayling IM, Tomlinson IP, Hughes KS, Eeles RA, Hodgson SV, Murday VA, Houlston R, Eng C (1998a) Germline PTEN mutations in Cowden syndrome-like families. J Med Genet 35: 881–885.

Marsh DJ, Coulon V, Lunetta KL, Rocca-Serra P, Dahia PL, Zheng Z, Liaw D, Caron S, Duboue B, Lin AY, Richardson AL, Bonnetblanc JM, Bressieux JM, Cabarrot-Moreau A, Chompret A, Demange L, Eeles RA, Yahanda AM, Fearon ER, Fricker JP, Gorlin RJ, Hodgson SV, Huson S, Lacombe D, Eng C (1998b) Mutation spectrum and genotype-phenotype analyses in Cowden disease and Bannayan–Zonana syndrome, two hamartoma syndromes with germline PTEN mutation. Hum Mol Genet 7: 507–515.

Marsh DJ, Kum JB, Lunetta KL, Bennett MJ, Gorlin RJ, Ahmed SF, Bodurtha J, Crowe C, Curtis MA, Dasouki M, Dunn T, Feit H, Geraghty MT, Graham JM Jr, Hodgson SV, Hunter A, Korf BR, Manchester D, Miesfeldt S, Murday VA, Nathanson KL, Parisi M, Pober B, Romano C, Eng C (1999) PTEN mutation spectrum and genotype-phenotype correlations in Bannayan–Riley–Ruvalcaba syndrome suggests a single entity with Cowden syndrome. Hum Mol Genet 8: 1461–1472.

Myers MP, Stolarov JP, Eng C, Li J, Wang SI, Wigler MH, Parsons R, Tonks NK (1997) P-TEN, the tumor suppressor from human chromosome 10q23, is a dual-specificity phosphatase. Proc Nat Acad Sci USA 94: 9052–9057.

Nelen MR, Padberg GW, Peeters EAJ, Lin AY, van den Helm B, Frants RR, Coulon V, Goldstein AM, van Reen MMM, Easton DF, Eeles RA, Hodgson S, Mulvihill JJ, Murday VA, Tucker MA, Mariman ECM, Starink TM, Ponder BAJ, Ropers HH, Kremer H, Longy M, Eng C (1996) Localization of the gene for Cowden disease to 10q22-23. Nat Genet 13: 114–116.

Nelen MR, van Staveren CG, Peeters EAJ, Ben Hassel M, Gorlin RJ, Hamm H, Lindboe CF, Fryns JP, Sijmons RH, Woods DG, Mariman ECM, Padberg GW,

Kremer H (1997) Germline mutations in the PTEN/MMAC1 gene in patients with Cowden disease. Hum Mol Genet 6: 1383–1387.

Newton HB (2004) Molecular neuro-oncology and development of targeted therapeutic strategies for brain tumors. Part 2: PI3K/Akt/PTEN, mTOR, SHH/PTCH and angiogenesis. Expert Rev Anticancer Ther 4(1): 105–128.

Pilarski R, Eng C (2004) Will the real Cowden syndrome please stand up (again)? Expanding mutational and clinical spectra of the PTEN hamartoma tumour syndrome. J Med Genet 41: 323–326.

Podsypanina K, Ellenson LH, Nemes A, Gu J, Tamura M, Yamada KM, Cordon-Cardo C, Catoretti G, Fisher PE, Parsons R (1999) Mutation of Pten/Mmac1 in mice causes neoplasia in multiple organ systems. Proc Natl Acad Sci USA 96: 1563–1568.

Steck PA, Pershouse MA, Jasser SA, Yung WKA, Lin H, Ligon AH, Langford LA, Baumgard ML, Hattier T, Davis T, Frye C, Hu R, Swedlund B, Teng DHF, Tavtigian SV (1997) Identification of a candidate tumour suppressor gene, MMAC1, at chromosome 10q23.3 that is mutated in multiple advanced cancers. Nat Genet 15: 356–362.

Suzuki A, de la Pompa JL, Stambolic V, Elia AJ, Sasaki T, del Barco Barrantes I, Ho A, Wakeham A, Itie A, Khoo W, Fukumoto M, Mak TW (1998) High cancer susceptibility and embryonic lethality associated with mutation of the PTEN tumor suppressor gene in mice. Curr Biol 8: 1169–1178.

Tamura M, Gu J, Matsumoto K, Aota S, Parsons R, Yamada KM (1998) Inhibition of cell migration, spreading, and focal adhesions by tumor suppressor PTEN. Science 280: 1614–1617.

Tsou HC, Teng DH, Ping XL, Brancolini V, Davis T, Hu R, Xic XX, Gruener AC, Schrager CA, Christiano AM, Eng C, Steck P, Ott J, Tavtigian SV, Peacocke M (1997) The role of MMAC1 mutations in early-onset breast cancer: causative in association with Cowden syndrome and excluded in BRCA1-negative cases. Am J Hum Genet 61: 1036–1043.

Vivanco I, Sawyers CL (2002) The phosphatidylinositol 3-kinase-Akt pathway in human cancer. Nature Rev Cancer 2: 489–501.

Weary PE, Gorlin RJ, Gentry WC Jr, Comer JE, Greer KE (1972) Multiple hamartoma syndrome (Cowden's disease). Arch Dermatol 106: 682–690.

Weng LP, Smith WM, Brown JL, Eng C (2001) PTEN inhibits insulin-stimulated MEK/MAPK activation and cell growth by blocking IRS-1 phosphorylation and IRS-1/Grb-2/Sos complex formation in a breast cancer model. Hum Mol Genet 10: 605–616.

Weng LP, Brown JL, Baker KM, Ostrowski MC, Eng C (2002) PTEN blocks insulin-mediated ETS-2 phosphorylation through MAP kinase, independently of the phosphoinositide 3-kinase pathway. Hum Mol Genet 11: 1687–1696.

Wiedemann HR, Burgio GR, Aldenhoff P, Kunze J, Kaufmann HJ, Schirg E (1983) The proteus syndrome. Partial gigantism of the hands and/or feet, nevi, hemihypertrophy, subcutaneous tumors, microcephaly and other skull anomalies and possible accelerated growth and visceral affections. Eur J Pediatr 140: 5–12.

Zhou X, Hampel H, Thiele H, Gorlin RJ, Hennekam RC, Parisi M, Winter RM, Eng C (2001) Association of germline mutation in the PTEN tumour suppressor gene and Proteus and Proteus-like syndromes. Lancet 358: 210–211.

Zhou XP, Marsh DJ, Hampel H, Mulliken JB, Gimm O, Eng C (2000) Germline and germline mosaic PTEN mutations associated with a Proteous-like syndrome of hemihypertrophy, lower limb asymmetry, arteriovenous malformations and lipomatosis. Hum Mol Genet 9: 765–768.

Zhou XP, Marsh DJ, Morrison CD, Chaudhury AR, Maxwell M, Reifenberger G, Eng C (2003a) Germline inactivation of PTEN and Dysregulation of the Phosphoinositol-3-Kinase/Akt pathway cause human Lhermitte-Duclos disease in adults. Am J Hum Genet 73: 1191–1198.

Zhou XP, Waite KA, Pilarski R, Hampel H, Fernandez MJ, Bos C, Dasouki M, Feldman GL, Greenberg LA, Ivanovich J, Matloff E, Patterson A, Pierpont ME, Russo D, Nassif NT, Eng C (2003b) Germline PTEN promoter mutations and deletions in Cowden/Bannayan-Riley-Ruvalcaba syndrome result in aberrant PTEN protein and dysregulation of the phosphoinositol-3-kinase/Akt pathway. Am J Hum Genet 73: 404–411.

Zundel W, Schindler C, Haas-Kogan D, Koong A, Kaper F, Chen E, Gottschalk AR, Ryan HE, Johnson RS, Jefferson AB, Stokoe D, Giaccia AJ (2000) Loss of PTEN facilitates HIF-1-mediated gene expression. Genes Dev 14: 391–396.

# Chapter 28

# LHERMITTE–DUCLOS AND COWDEN DISEASE COMPLEX

**Dennis A. Nowak**

Department of Neurology, University of Cologne, Germany

## Introduction

*Lhermitte–Duclos disease* is a highly unusual and controversial condition, characterised by a space-occupying lesion within the posterior fossa of the skull arising from the cerebellar cortex (*dysplastic gangliocytoma of the cerebellum*). Clinically, the disease is characterised by a slowly progressive neurological deterioration associated with headaches, cerebellar ataxia and unsteadiness of gait, visual disturbances, other cranial nerve lesions and signs of increased intracranial pressure due to non-communicating hydrocephalus.

Today, the fundamental nature of this apparently benign entity remains unknown. The debate on whether it represents a neoplastic, malformative or hamartomatous lesion is still in progress (Nowak and Trost 2002). Lhermitte–Duclos disease was recently recognised to be part of a multiple hamartoma/neoplasia complex called Cowden disease (Koch et al. 1999, Murata et al. 1999, Padberg et al. 1995, Vinchon et al. 1994, Williams et al. 1992, Prabhu et al. 2004).

*Cowden disease* is an autosomal dominant hereditary condition with variable expression that results from a mutation in the PTEN gene, a tumour suppressor gene, localised on chromosome 10q22–23 (see also Chapter 28) (Gustafson et al. 2007, Hanssen and Fryns 1995, Liaw et al. 1997, Longy and Lacombe 1996, Marsh et al. 1998, Nelen et al. 1996, Zori et al. 1998). Patients with Cowden disease are prone to multiple neoplasms of the skin and mucosa, gastrointestinal tract, bones, central nervous system, eyes, and genitourinary tract. Skin is involved in 90–100% of affected cases (Lloyd and Dennis 1963, Mallory 1995, Starink et al. 1986, Tsao 2000). Morbidity and mortality from Cowden disease primarily is associated with an increased frequency of malignant tumours. Benign tumours that develop in Cowden disease patients also can cause significant morbidity.

The association between Lhermitte–Duclos disease and Cowden syndrome probably represents a single true *neurocutaneous syndrome* caused by abnormalities in the PTEN tumour suppressor gene (Delatycki et al. 2003, Eng et al. 1994, Murata et al. 1999, Zhou et al. 2003). At the present time more than 40 clinical observations document an association between Lhermitte–Duclos disease and the Cowden disease complex (for recent literature reviews see Derrey et al. 2004, Prabhu et al. 2004, Perez-Nunez et al. 2004). Based on these data, the association between both disorders was recently considered to represent a new phakomatosis, named *Cowden and Lhermitte–Duclos Disease Complex* (COLD), with Lhermitte–Duclos disease being the neurological manifestation of the genetically determined disease complex (Robinson and Cohen 2000). Today, Lhermitte–Duclos disease is regarded as a benign, treatable and even curable condition. Nevertheless, it is the apparently frequent, but under-recognised association with the Cowden disease complex that should prompt an extensive diagnostic work-up in any individual case of Lhermitte–Duclos disease in order to detect or disclose concomitant malignancies.

## Historical perspective and terminology

Lhermitte and Duclos described the disorder in 1920. Although Lhermitte and Duclos were credited with eponymic recognition of this entity, Spiegel (1920) described a similar case in the same year.

Lhermitte and Duclos were two French physicians (Who named it? 2006).

***Jacques Jean Lhermitte*** was a neurologist and neuropsychiatrist born in 1877 in Mont-Saint-Pére son of an artist. Following early education at St. Etienne he studied in Paris, graduating in medicine in 1907. He specialised in neurology and became Chef-de-clinique for nervous diseases in 1908, 1910 Chef de laboratoire, and professeur agrégé for psychiatry 1922. He later became Médecin at the Hospice Paul Brousse, head of the Fondation Dejerine, and clinical director at the Salpêtrière. During World War I he studied spinal injuries and became interested in neuropsychiatry. This led to publications on visual hallucinations of the self. A deeply religious man, he explored the common territory between theology and medicine, and this led to interesting studies on demoniacal possession and stigmatisation. Lhermitte was a great clinical neurologists whose enthusiasm infected his younger contemporaries and led to many discoveries and syndromic descriptions (Jean Lhermitte 1959, Who named it? 2006).

Lhermitte and Duclos originally described the lesion under the name of "ganglioneurome myélinique diffus de l' écore cérébelleuse". Subsequently, this entity was referred to by a variety of synonymous descriptions, such as *diffuse ganglioneuroma of the cerebellar cortex* (Bielschowsky and Simons 1930), *(benign) hypertrophy of the cerebellum* (Duncan and Snodgrass 1943, Oppenheimer 1955), *Purkinjoma* (Christensen 1937), *hamartoma of the cerebellum* (Hallervorden 1959), *gangliocytoma myelinicum diffusum of the cerebellar cortex* (Foerster and Gagel 1933), *dysplastic gangliocytoma of the cerebellum* (Roski et al. 1981, Roessmann and Wongmongkolrit 1984, Pritchett and King 1978, Leech et al. 1977, Rainov et al. 1995, Riliett and Mori 1979, Nowak et al. 2001), *granule cell hypertrophy of the cerebellum* (Ambler et al. 1969, Bellamy et al. 1963, Cessaga 1980) or simply *Lhermitte–Duclos disease* (Reznik and Schoenen 1983, Marano et al. 1988, Lobo et al. 1999, Tuli et al. 1997). At present, the disorder is usually referred to by the names of the first describers or by the term *dysplastic gangliocytoma of the cerebellum*. In this chapter the terms Lhermitte–Duclos disease

and dysplastic gangliocytoma of the cerebellum are used synonymous.

Regarding the nature of the disease, the original opinion expressed by Lhermitte and Duclos (1920) was that the tumour was a combination of a congenital malformation and a neoplasm arising from ganglion cells. Other early observers of this entity considered the lesion to represent a *neurocystic blastoma* (Bielschowsky and Simons 1930), a *hamartoma* (Roski et al. 1981) or a *hyperplasia* (Duncan and Snodgrass 1943, Oppenheim 1955, Ambler et al. 1961, Spiegel 1920). In 1930, Bielschowsky and Simons used the somewhat contradictory terms "hamartoma" and "hamartomablastoma" regarding their final conclusion that the lesion seems to be neoplastic in nature. Foerster and Gagel (1933) agreed with this opinion. Duncan and Snodgrass (1940) pointed out that the tumour originates from a pure hypertrophy of granule cells, suggesting the lesion to be of benign nature. Ambler et al. (1969) considered the tumour to originate from an ontogenetic developmental dysfunction of cell growth. Until now, the debate of whether Lhermitte–Duclos disease represents a malformation, hamartoma or neoplasm is still not settled (Nowak and Trost 2002, Demaerel et al. 2003). However, there is growing evidence to assume a benign hamartomatous character of the tumour.

Padberg et al. (1991) are credited for the first recognition of the coexistence of Lhermitte–Duclos disease and a multiple hamartoma-neoplasia complex, also called Cowden syndrome.

The syndrome of multiple hamartomas and carcinoma (Cowden disease) was originally described in detail by Lloyd and Dennis (1963) and has its name derived from an affected individual in the family of *Rachel Cowden* (Gorlin et al. 2001). However, Costello in 1941 had already reported the skin lesions in a patient who Brownstein et al. (1979) later documented with the disorder. Another early example is that of Witten and Kopf (1957). The syndrome is characterized by multiple mucocutaneous lesions and other systemic hamartomas associated with a high incidence of breast, thyroid, gastrointestinal and genitourinary malignancies (Hanssen and Fryns

1995, Mallory 1995, Longy et al. 1996, Starink et al. 1986).

Recent thorough clinical observations support the contention that Lhermitte–Duclos disease and Cowden syndrome are part of a single spectrum best classified as a single phakomatosis (Padberg et al. 1991, Koch et al. 1999, Murata et al. 1999, Robinson and Cohen 2000, Vantomme et al. 2001, Derrey et al. 2004, Prabhu et al. 2004). The term *Cowden and Lhermitte–Duclos disease complex* (COLD) has been proposed to refer to this new phakomatosis (Robinson and Cohen 2000).

## Incidence and prevalence

Lhermitte–Duclos disease is a very rare disorder. At present, more than 100 cases have been reported. Lhermitte–Duclos disease was associated with a very poor prognosis before the advances of neuroimaging within the last two decades. About one third of reported cases died from the mass effects directly resulting from the tumour's spread within the posterior fossa of the skull (Vinchon et al. 1994, Derrey et al. 2004, Prabhu et al. 2004). Reliable data about the incidence and prevalence of Lhermitte–Duclos disease do not exist. A high level of clinical suspicion is of particular importance when confronted with this entity as the frequent, but clearly under-reported association with the Cowden syndrome should prompt thorough clinical and apparative investigation to exclude concomitant malignancies or detect them at an early stage.

Cowden disease, also termed multiple hamartoma syndrome, is an autosomal dominant condition with variable expression that results from a mutation in the PTEN gene on chromosome arm 10q (Liaw et al. 1997, Nelen et al. 1996, Zori et al. 1998). Males and females inherit the mutated gene in equal numbers. The incidence of muco-cutaneous manifestations is similar in both genders. The incidence of concomitant malignancies appears to vary in between both sexes. For example, males are more likely to develop thyroid cancer, while females are at greater risk for breast cancer (Hanssen and Fryns 1995, Liaw et al. 1997, Longy and Lacombe 1996, Marsh

et al. 1998). Internationally, over 200 cases have been published. Similar to Lhermitte–Duclos disease reliable data about its incidence and prevalence among the population do not exist. Nelen et al. (1999) estimated that the prevalence of Cowden disease is 1 in 200.000 to 250.000 in the Dutch population.

## Clinical manifestation

### Lhermitte–Duclos disease

Lhermitte–Duclos disease is a cerebellar tumour and initial clinical symptoms result from tumour spread to the surrounding nervous structures located within the posterior fossa. Most common clinical signs and symptoms are headaches, nausea and vomiting, gait disturbance, upper limb ataxia and dysmetria, blurred vision and lower cranial nerve palsies (Derrey et al. 2004, Milbouw et al. 1988, Nowak and Trost 2002, Perez-Nunez et al. 2004, Tuli et al. 1997). Table 1 summarises the common clinical spectrum of Lhermitte–Duclos disease. More unusual symptoms associated with dysplastic gangliocytoma of the cerebellum are isolated orthostatic hypotension (Ruchoux et al. 1986) and tinnitus (Lobo et al. 1999). Occa-

**Table 1.** Presenting signs and symptoms of dysplastic gangliocytoma of the cerebellum and their frequency of occurrence among affected cases. [adapted from Nowak and Trost (2002)]

| Frequent signs and symptoms | |
| --- | --- |
| Headache | 70% |
| Nausea and vomiting | 60% |
| Papilloedema | 60% |
| Unsteadiness of gait | 50% |
| Upper limb ataxia and dsysmetria | 40% |
| Visual disturbances | 40% |
| Cranial nerve palsies | 30% |

| Less frequent signs and symptoms | |
| --- | --- |
| Sensory and motor deficits | 20% |
| Vertigo | 20% |
| Neuropsychological deficits | 15% |

sionally patients present with paroxysmal neurological deterioration, either spontaneously or following surgical intervention, presumably as a result of acute or subacutely decompensated chronic occlusive hydrocephalus (Ambler et al. 1969, Marano et al. 1988, Milbouw et al. 1988, Nowak et al. 2001).

In 1969, Ambler et al. first reported a familial cluster of Lhermitte–Duclos disease. The index case was a young man who died from dysplastic gangliocytoma of the cerebellum. His mother died from other reasons, but was found post-mortem to have had a dysplastic cerebellar gangliocytoma. Before her death she stated that a large head circumference was quite frequent within her family. The authors emphasised that some members of this patient's family were apparently asymptomatic carriers of the tumour, recognisable only by their megalocephaly (Ambler et al. 1969). Various concomitant abnormalities have been described in association with Lhermitte–Duclos disease (Oppenheimer 1955, Ambler et al. 1969, Padberg et al. 1991, Derrey et al. 2004). These include megalocephaly in about 50% of cases (Roski et al. 1981, Oppenheimer 1955, Pritchett and King 1978, Ambler et al. 1969, Marano et al. 1988, Robinson and Cohen 2000, Cessaga 1980, Reeder et al. 1988, Perez-Nunez et al. 2004), megalencephaly (Oppenheimer 1955, Leech et al. 1977, Ambler et al. 1969, Smith et al. 1989, Brown et al. 1980), syringomyelia (Bielschowsky and Simons 1930, Marcus et al. 1996, Wolansky et al. 1996), skeletal anomalies, such as polydactylia (Bielschowsky and Simons 1930, Delatycki et al. 2003) and cranial asymmetry (Pritchett and King 1978, Leech et al. 1977, Nowak et al. 2001, Spiegel 1930, Cessaga 1980), multiple hemangiomas (Ducan and Snodgrass 1943, Oppenheimer 1955) and muco-cutaneous lesions (Delatycki et al. 2003, Roski et al. 1981, Marano et al. 1988, Murata et al. 1999, Robinson and Cohen 2000). Table 2 gives an overview of malformations previously found to be associated with Lhermitte–Duclos disease.

The duration of symptoms ranges from a few months to more than 10 years (Leech et al. 1977, Ambler et al. 1969, Nowak and Trost 2002). Symptoms of increased intracranial pressure, such as headaches, nausea and vomiting, papilloedema,

**Table 2.** Concomitant malformations associated with dysplastic gangliocytoma of the cerebellum. [Adapted from Nowak and Trost (2002)]

**Frequent malformations**

Megalocephaly
Megalencephaly
Hydrocephalus
Syringomyelia

*Skeletal abnormalities*
Polydactylia
Syndactylia
Facial asymmetry
Small yaw
High arched palatae

**Less frequent malformations**

*Cutaneous and mucosal lesions*
Acral keratoses
Lipomas
Neurofibromas
Haemangiomas
Tongue plaques
Gingival papules and hyperplasia

*Benign lesions*
Thyroid (goitre, adenoma, thyreoglossal duct cyst)
Breast (fibroadenoma, fibrocystic disease)
Gastrointestinal (polyps)
Gynaecological (overian cyst, leiomyoma)

*Malignant lesions*
Genitourinary (prostate cancer, adenocarcinoma of urethra, renal cell carcinoma)
Breast (carcinoma)
Thyroid (adenocarcinoma)
Endometrial (adenocarcinoma, transitional carcinoma)
Ovarian (carcinoma, teratoma)

mental disturbances and loss of consciousness were frequently encountered features in the early cases and arose from the progressive mass effect of the growing tumour within the posterior fossa (Lhermitte and Duclos 1920, Bielschowsky and Simons 1930, Christensen 1937, Foerster and Gagel 1933, Oppenheimer 1955). Until 1955 most of the affected cases were diagnosed at autopsy. Today, patients are diagnosed in the early stage of the disease due to the advances of imaging techniques. Death directly related to dysplastic gangliocytoma of the cerebellum is now a rather rare occasion. Dysplastic gangliocytoma of the cerebellum most frequently presents in the third and forth decades of life (Derrey et al. 2004, Rainov et al. 1995, Nowak et al. 2001, Oppenheimer 1955, Perez-Nunez et al. 2004, Prabhu et al. 2004, Vinchon et al. 1994), however, the age at presentation varies from birth (Roessmann and Wongmongkolrit 1984) to the sixth decade (Cessaga 1980). There is no obvious sex preponderance.

From the very early cases until the end of the 1970s, the spectrum of preoperative imaging modalities targeting to evaluate indirectly the mass effect of dysplastic cerebellar gangliocytoma consisted of plain skull radiograms, conventional vertebral angiography and ventriculography (Hallervorden 1959, Duncan and Snodgrass 1943, Oppenheimer 1955, Foerster and Gagel 1933, Christensen 1937, Bielschowsky and Simons 1930, Pritchett and King 1978, Leech et al. 1977). Later computed tomography (CT) became the diagnostic radiographic tool to directly demonstrate the tumour, its distribution within the posterior fossa and its interference with the cerebellar parenchyma, brainstem, cranial nerves and cerebrospinal fluid (CSF) compartments (Roski et al. 1981, Ambler et al. 1969, Cessaga 1980, Brown et al. 1980). During the last decade magnetic resonance imaging (MRI) achieved major importance in the diagnosis of Lhermitte–Duclos disease (Ashley et al. 1990, Lobo et al. 1999, Marcus et al. 1996, Nowak et al. 2001, Reeder et al. 1988, Smith et al. 1989, Tuli et al. 1997, Wolasnky et al. 1996). Because of inherent Houndsfield artefacts in the posterior fossa with CT, MRI is the imaging modality of choice today. MRI typically reveals the characteristic non-enhancing gyriform patterns corresponding to the enlargement of cerebellar cortical folia (Carter et al. 1989, Nowak et al. 2001, Smith et al. 1989). The enlarged folia loose their secondary foldings and asymmetrically widen the affected cerebellar hemisphere. In particular, Lhermitte–Duclos tumours are hypointense on T1-weighted images and show a mild or none enhancement following Gadolinium-DTPA administration. The characteristic MRI features of Lhermitte–Duclos disease are shown in Fig. 1.

The lack of contrast enhancement suggests insignificant disturbances of the blood-brain barrier and/or missing of extracellular oedema. On T2-weighted images the lesion presents as a well circumscribed high signal intensity mass with an unique *striated pattern* with isointense bands within the area of hyperintensity corresponding to the widened gyri and displaced sulci of the cerebellar cortex (Fig. 2). The uniqueness of these MRI findings make it possible to diagnose Lhermitte–Duclos disease pre-operatively (Carter et al. 1989, Meltzer et al. 1995, Smith et al. 1989, Wolansky et al. 1996) obviating the necessity for an obligatory biopsy of the lesion in asymptomatic patients.

Functional imaging methods, such as positron emission tomography (PET), single photon emission CT (SPECT) and MR spectroscopy may give additional information about the pathophysiology and nature of the disorder (Klisch et al. 2001, Nagaraja et al. 2004, Ogasawara et al. 2001). In future, these imaging modalities may be helpful to predict the natural course of the disease and therefore may influence the indication for surgery in an individual case.

Dysplastic cerebellar gangliocytoma is histopathologically described as a non-neoplastic mass composed of cerebellar folia expanding by hypertrophic neurones of the internal granular layer (Burger and Scheithauer 1994, Kleihues and Cavenee 2000). Today, the lesion is graded a WHO grade 1 tumour. Grossly, the cerebellar hemispheres are markedly thickened and enlarged (Bellamy et al. 1963, Bielschowsky and Simons 1930, Burger and Scheithauer 1994, Cessaga 1980, Lhermitte and Duclos 1920, Oppenheimer 1955). Cross-section shows a fairly enlargement of the cerebellar cortex, sometimes extending into the vermis (Oppenheimer 1955), with gross reduction or even absence of the central white matter (Pritchett and King 1978, Ambler et al. 1969, Nowak and Trost 2002). The principal microscopic abnormality is massive replacement and expansion of the internal granular cell layer by large neurones with vesicular nuclei and prominent nucleoli (Bellamy et al. 1963, Cessaga 1980, Nowak and Trost 2002). These cells are smaller than the normal Purkinje cells and definitely larger than normal granule cells. The molecular layer is broadened by abundant, enlarged and irregularly myelinated axons. The axons belong to the abnormal hypertrophied neurones, composing the internal granular layer. Most authors agree that light and electron microscopy demonstrate that these neurones are hypertrophied granule cells (Ambler et al. 1969, Pritchett and King 1978, Reznik and Schoenen 1983, Roski et al. 1981). Fig. 3 illustrates the characteristic two-layered lamellar pattern of the cerebellar cortex and the abnormal granule cells to be found in dysplastic cerebellar gangliocytoma (compare it with Fig. 2).

The lack of a sharp border between the tumour and normal cerebellar tissue is limiting the accuracy

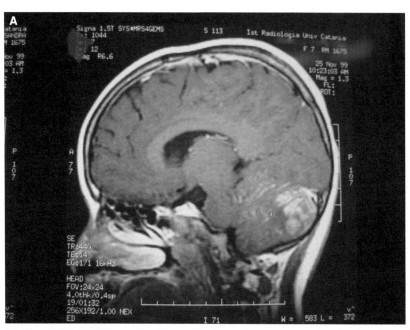

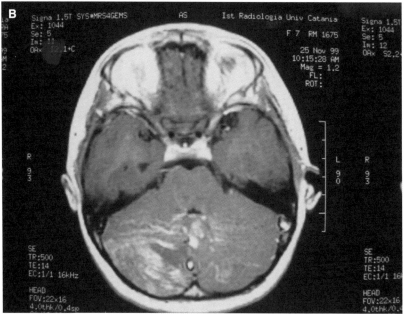

**Fig. 1.** Typical MRI findings of Lhermitte–Duclos disease: sagittal (**A**), axial (**B**) and coronal (**C**) T1-weighted images following intravenous administration of Gadolinium-DTPA show an enhancing lesion of the right cerebellar cortex; axial (**D**) T2-weighted images of the same patient show the right cerebellar lesion to be hyperintense with the typical widening of the cerebellar folia affected by the tumour lesion. The infratentorial midline structures are slightly displaced to the left (courtesy of P. Milone, Institute of Radiology, University of Catania, Italy).

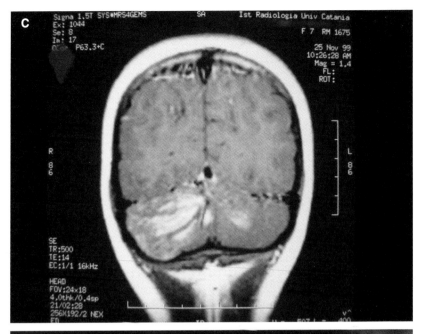

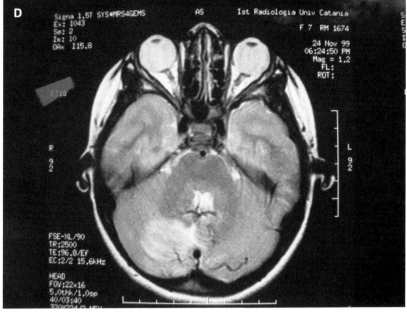

**Fig. 1.** (Continued)

of surgical excision. Mitoses have not been reported (Cessaga 1980, Ruchoux et al. 1986, Milbouw et al. 1988, Brown et al. 1980, Reeder et al. 1988, Nowak and Trost 2002). Recently, stainings with monoclonal antibodies to cell nuclear antigens and measurements of desoxyribonucleic acid proliferation indices gave new evidence to the suggestion, that

Lhermitte–Duclos lesions exhibit no proliferative activity (Hair et al. 1992). Long symptomatic periods over many years before severe clinical deterioration and a long-term survival over many years after surgical excision, support the notion that Lhermitte–Duclos tumours have a slow or even negligible growth potential (Christensen 1937, Brown et al.

HISTOLOGY                                      NEUROIMAGING

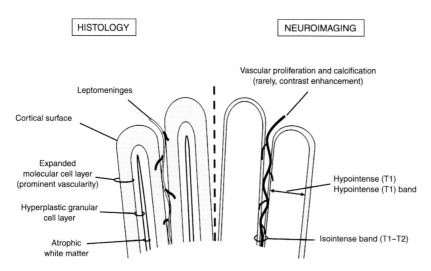

**Fig. 2.** The repeating/alternating bilaminar cortical patter evident on CT and MRI studies (right, *neuroimaging*) is compared with the histological alterations (left, *histology*), which characterise the Lhermitte–Duclos Cowden disease complex. The thicker inner portion of the folia consisting of the white matter layer, the abnormal granular cell layer, and deep molecular layer is hypodense on CT and hypointense on T1 and hyperintense on T2 MR images. The thinner outer portion of the folia consisting of the outer molecular layer and leptomeninges within affected sulci is isodense/isointense on CT and MRI studies. Vascular proliferation in the pial meninges and adjacent outer cortex may be occasionally associated with calcifications or (more rarely) with contrast enhancement within the isodencse/isointense bands. Adapted and modified from Kulkantrakorn et al. (1997).

1980, Reznik and Schoenen 1983, Robinson and Cohen 2000, Roski et al. 1981). The histopathological differential diagnosis includes glioma and ganglion cell tumour (Burger and Scheithauer 1994).

## Association between Lhermitte–Duclos disease and the Cowden disease complex

Recently, careful clinical reviews of reported cases added new evidence to the suggestion that there should be an apparently genetic association between Lhermitte–Duclos disease and the Cowden disease complex (Padberg et al. 1991, Robinson and Cohen 2000). Cowden syndrome is an autosomal dominant hereditary multiple hamartoma-neoplasia complex, presenting with systemic hamartomas and neoplasms affecting the skin, mucosa, skeletal system, breast, thyroid, genitourinary tract gastroinestinal tract and endometrium (Figs. 4 and 5) (Lloyd and Dennis 1963, Mallory 1995, Starink et al. 1986, Tsao 2000). Indeed, several genetic studies strongly support such an association based on the aberration of the PTEN

gene common to both disorders (Longy and Lacombe 1996, Marsh et al. 1998, Nelen et al. 1996, Zori et al. 1998, Delatycki et al. 2003, Eng et al. 1994, Murata et al. 1999, Zhou et al. 2003). Thus, Lhermitte Duclos disease is considered to represent the neurological manifestation of the Cowden disease complex and both disorders together are thought to form a single phakomatosis (Eng et al. 1994, Padberg et al. 1991, Robinson and Cohen 2000).

Recognition of the association between both disorders has direct clinical relevance given the high incidence of cancer among patients affected by the Cowden syndrome. Consequently, detection of Lhermitte–Duclos disease should prompt a careful search for signs and symptoms suggestive of the Cowden syndrome. Mucocutaneous features are present in 90–100% of Cowden disease cases (Lindor and Greene 1998, Mallory 1995, Requena et al. 1992, Tsao 2000). Benign or malignant disorders of the thyroid are present in about 70% of cases. In individuals suspected of having Cowden disease a careful family history should be obtained with regard to a familial cluster of malformations and

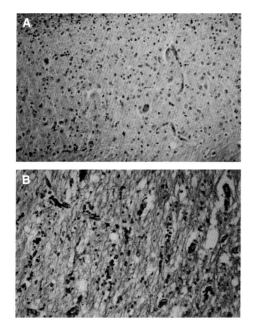

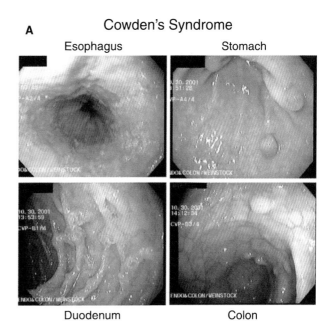

Cowden's Syndrome

**Fig. 3.** Photomicrograph of a surgically available specimen of Lhermitte–Duclos tumour (Nowak et al. 2001, 2002). (**A**) Haematoxylin and eosin staining, original magnification ×160. The cerebellar cortex reveals two clearly distinct layers. The outer molecular layer consists of myelinated axons (left upper border) and extends to an inner granular cell layer. In the inner layer atypical neurones are present, which are considerably larger than normal granule cells. (**B**) Periodic acid Schiff reaction, original magnification ×160. The neutropil shows spongiomatous transformation. Calcifications characterised by concentrically laminated deposits associated with capillary formations are frequent within the molecular layer of the cerebellar cortex. Calcareous deposits along small and very small vessels within the molecular layer of the cerebellar cortex were numerously described (Cessaga 1980, Marano et al. 1988, Nowak et al. 2001, Oppenheimer 1955, Pritchett and King 1978).

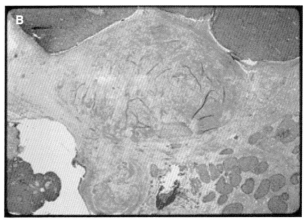

**Fig. 4.** (**A**) Gastrointestinal endoscopy showing small peduncolate lesions (hamartomatous polyps) in the oesophagus, stomach, duodenum and large intestine (colon); (**B**) histopathological examination shows an hamartomatous/hyperplastic gastric polyps.

malignancies, in particular breast and thyroid cancer, cutaneous and mucosal lesions, developmental and neurological abnormalities. Although the mutant gene is inherited, the onset of clinical manifestations of Cowden disease varies in age, ranging from birth to the fifth decade of life (Ferran et al. 2008, Hanssen and Fryns 1995, Liaw et al. 1997, Longy and Lacombe 1996, Marsh et al. 1998). Patients usually consult the physician because of cutaneous manifestations. A careful physical examination and additional apparative investigations, especially concerning the breast and thyroid, should be performed in affected cases with one-year follow up exams to detect malignancies at an early stage. Table 3 summarises physical signs and symptoms suggestive the Cowden disease complex.

Cowden disease is associated with the development of several types of malignancy. Gastrointestinal abnormalities are present in as many as 70% of patients (Liaw et al. 1997, Longy and Lacombe 1996, Marsh et al. 1998). Polyps can occur (Fig. 4A) in the oesophagus, stomach, small or large intestine,

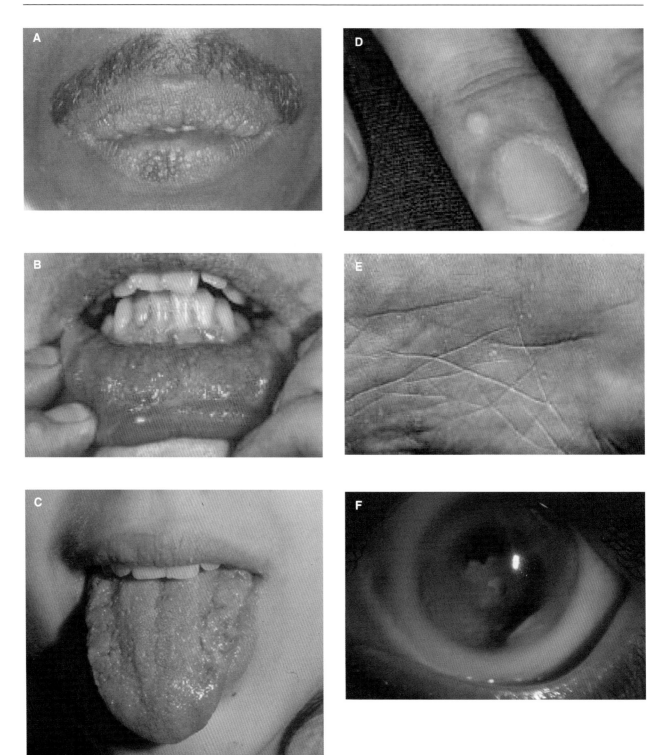

**Fig. 5.** Typical mucocutaneous lesions in the mouth (**A**, **B**), tongue (**C**), fingers (**D**), back (**E**) and eye (**F**) (see text for explanation).

**Table 3.** Physical signs suggestive of the Cowden disease complex

### Mucocutaneous lesions

*Cutaneous facial papules:* flesh colored, flat lichenoid or verrucoid papules; typically arranged in large numbers with a predisposition for the perioral region; commonly trichilemmomas

*Oral lesions:* whitish papules with a smooth surface present in the gingival, labial and palatal surfaces; lesions often form a confluent cobblestone like pattern; usually benign fibromas

*Acral keratoses:* Smooth or verrucoid papules on the dorsal surfaces of the hands and feet

*Palmoplantar keratoses:* translucent punctate leratoses on the palms and soles

*Other:* lipomas, neurofibromas, haemangiomas

### Head, face and throat

*Macrocephaly*
*Small yaw*
*High arched palate*
*Adenoid facies*

### Skeletal abnormalities

*Bone cysts*
*Kyphosis and kyphoskloliosis*

### Thyroid lesions

*Goitre*
*Benign adenomas*
*Follicular adenocarcinomas*

### Breast disease

*Fibrocystic disease*
*Fibroadenomas*
*Carcinoma*

### Gastrointestinal tract

*Polyps of the oesophagus, stomach, small and large intestine*
*Adenocarcinoma of the colon*

### Genitourinary tract

*Ovarian cysts*
*Leiomyomas*
*Teratomas*
*Adenocarcinoma of the urethra and cervix*
*Renal cell carcinoma*

or anus and are most common in the colon. These have been described as oesophageal squamous papilloma, hamartomatous and hyperplastic gastric polyps (Fig. 4B), adenoma, hamartoma and ganglioneuroma of colon. Although a few cases of adenocarcinoma of the colon in Cowden disease patients have been reported (Chen et al. 1987), the malignant potential of polyps is still uncertain.

Thyroid manifestations include goitre, benign adenomas, and follicular adenocarcinoma (Longy and Lacombe 1996, Starink et al. 1986). Thyroid cancer is diagnosed in about 5% of patients with a preponderance in men. Carcinoma of the breast occurs in 20–40% of female patients and is one of the most serious consequences of the syndrome. Fibrocystic disease and fibroadenomas of the breast are present in approximately 75% of patients. Breast screening should be initiated early in women with affected family members (possibly as soon as puberty is complete).

The international Cowden Syndrome Consortium has proposed operational criteria for the diagnosis

**Table 4.** Operational criteria for the diagnosis of Cowden disease (NCCN 1999)

### Pathognomonic criteria

Mucocutaneous lesions
Facial trichilemmomas
Akral keratoses
Papillomatous lesions
Mucosal lesions

### Major criteria

Breast cancer
Thyroid cancer (in particular follicular thyroid cancer)
Macrocephaly
Lhermitte–Duclos disease
Endometrial carcinomas

### Minor criteria

Other thyroid disease (adenoma, multinodular goitre)
Mental retardation
Gastrointestinal hamartomas
Fibrocsystic breast disease
Lipomas and fibromas

of the disease (NCCN 1999, Pilarski and Eng 2004), which are summarised in Table 4. In an individual the operational diagnosis of Cowden disease can be established based on the presence of mucocutaneous lesions (Fig. 5) alone if (a) 6 or more facial papules are present of which 3 or more are trichilemmomas, (b) cutaneous facial papules and oral mucosal papules are present, (c) oral papules and akral keratoses are present, (d) 6 ore more palmoplantar keratoses are present. The operational diagnosis in an individual can also be established if (a) two or more major criteria are met, but one must include either macrocephaly or Lhermitte–Duclos disease, (b) one major and 3 minor criteria are met and (c) four minor criteria are met.

## Natural history

The natural course of the early cases of Lhermitte–Duclos disease was associated with a very poor prognosis due to the progressive mass effect resulting from the tumour's spread within the posterior fossa of the skull (Bielschowsky and Simons 1930, Ducan and Snodgrass 1943, Foerster and Gagel 1933, Hallervorden 1959, Lhermitte–Duclos 1920, Oppenheimer 1955).

*In 1920, Lhermitte and Duclos, described the case of a 36-year old man, who suffered from a 10-month episode of left-sided hearing loss and occipital headaches. A few weeks prior to admission the man experienced episodes of paroxysmal vertigo with recurrent falls, unsteadiness of gait and cognitive symptoms, such as disorientation and memory deficits. On admission, the authors saw a confused, disoriented man with dysathria, nystagmus and ataxia of the upper and lower limbs. The spinal tap revealed an elevated cerebrospinal fluid protein level. One week after admission the neurological status deteriorated rapidly and the patient died in a coma.*

Surgery is the treatment of choice for Lhermitte–Duclos disease. However, surgical treatment produced very unsatisfactory results until 1955 with only three patients surviving from the intervention (Christensen 1937, Oppenheimer 1955).

*In 1930, Bielschowsky and Simons described the case of a 20-year old woman presenting with a 2-year history of gait unsteadiness, paroxysmal vertigo and paraesthesia of all four limbs. The patient complained about occasional headaches that were never severe. On admission clinical examination revealed bilateral papilloedema, nystagmus, cerebellar signs of both upper and lower extremities more dominant on the right and ataxia of gait. The spinal tap and radiographs of the skull revealed no indirect hints for increased intracranial pressure. The patient was scheduled for surgery of a right-sided cerebellar mass, but died following craniectomy before the dura mater was opened. This was the first time a surgical intervention was attempted in Lhermitte–Duclos disease.*

*In 1937, Christensen reported the first patient with Lhermitte–Duclos disease who underwent surgery and was discharged from hospital free of complains. This 34-year old man suffered from a 6-year period of paroxysmal "pressure feelings" of the head associated with a severe neck pain, "flickering" in both temporal visual fields, nausea and vomiting. Occasionally, the attacks led to unconsciousness. He was free of complains in between each episode. Clinical examination on admission revealed bilateral papilloedema, left trigeminal nerve dysfunction and mild facial nerve palsy on the right. There were no obvious cerebellar signs. Ventriculography showed a shift of the fourth ventricle and aqueduct to the left. During surgical exploration of the posterior fossa, the folia of the right cerebellar hemisphere appeared markedly thickened, but no circumscribed tumour could be detected. The lateral third of the right cerebellar hemisphere was resected and 18 months following the intervention the patients returned to work free of complains.*

Today, progress in anaesthesiology and surgical techniques have significantly improved the therapeutic management of the disease and survival over many years after successful tumour resection is no longer a rarity (Leech et al. 1977, Nowak et al. 2001, Robinson and Cohen 2000). In addition, the developments in neuroimaging allow preoperative diagnosis of the disorder (Carter et al. 1989, Meltzer et al. 1995, Smith et al. 1989, Wolansky et al. 1996). MRI is a useful tool to demonstrate the extension of tumour spread preoperatively (Kulkantrakorn et al.

1997, Meltzer et al. 1995, Nowak et al. 2001, Smith et al. 1989, Wolansky et al. 1996). The slow rate of growth permits survival over several years despite none or only partial tumour resection (Leech et al. 1977, Rilliet and Mori 1979, Ambler et al. 1969, Robinson and Cohen 2000). Long symptomatic periods over several years (Bielschowsky and Simons 1930, Nowak et al. 2001) and the continued incidental autopsy findings of Lhermitte–Duclos disease attribute to this assumption (Rilliet and Mori 1979, Cessaga 1980). Nowadays, the main threat of Lhermitte–Duclos disease is its frequent association with the Cowden disease complex, which is why recognition of individuals with the syndrome is of major importance.

## Pathogenesis and molecular genetics

Lhermitte and Duclos (1920) noted enlarged cerebellar folia containing circumscribed regions of abnormal ganglion cells. They regarded the lesion as a combination of a ganglion cell neoplasm and a malformation originating from precursors of Purkinje cells. Bielschowsky and Simons (1930) suggested the lesion to be *an experiment of nature* derived from a local agenesis of the superficial cerebellar cortex, which resulted in a tumour composed of neuroblasts. These authors related the lesion to other congenital malformations apparent in the described patients (see Table 2). They concluded that the clinical and histopathological appearance of dysplastic gangliocytoma unite the features of both a malformation and an infiltrating blastoma. The idea of a developmental abnormality of the cerebellar cortex was derived from the absence of normal cellular elements and the presence of abnormal cells in a more or less regular arrangement within the laminar pattern of the cerebellar cortex. Evidence for the existence of a neoplasm lies in the clinical picture of a progressive space occupying mass in adults and the appearance of immature cells similar to blastomatous cell types.

Duncan and Snodgrass (1943) regarded the tumour to be composed of hypertrophied granule cells. They did neither support nor reject the neoplasm and malformation theories. Later electron micro-

scopic studies confirmed that the abnormal cells to be found in dysplastic cerebellar gangliocytoma are granule cells (Pritchett and King 1978, Marano et al. 1988). Light microscopy revealed a perpendicular orientation of axons originating from the abnormal cells in relation to the pia (Roski et al. 1981, Pritchett and King 1978, Leech et al. 1977). Such an arrangement of the cell axons is characteristic for normal granule cells (Bellamy et al. 1963). It would be almost impossible to conceive dysplastic gangliocytoma as a true neoplasm, when its composing abnormal cells are under such strict neurobiotic control mimicking exactly the orientation of the granule cells they are replacing. So the objections to the view that Lhermitte–Duclos tumour is of neoplastic nature are very serious. The two-dimensional spread of tumour cells and the emission of axons which all follow a similar course in the molecular layer, are indicators for the well differentiated behaviour of the tumour. The absence of mitotic figures and the lack of proliferation activity (Hair et al. 1992). The theory favoured by Duncan and Snodgrass 60 years ago (1943) that the abnormal cells composing the lesion are hypertrophied granule cells is thus very attractive.

The fact that many of the patients described featured additional congenital abnormalities in other parts of the body to be attributed in part to the Cowden disease complex underline a genetic determination of the disease. The coexistence of Lhermitte–Duclos disease and Cowden disease was recognised by Padberg et al. (1991), highlighted by Eng et al. (1994) and was proved when mutations in the *PTEN* gene were recognised as the underlying cause (Liaw et al. 1997, Nelen et al. 1997). Germline mutations in the *PTEN* gene on chromosome subband 10q23 have been described in a family with Cowden syndrome with one member affected by Lhermitte–Duclos disease (Eng et al. 1994), in several individuals suffering from both disorders (Perez-Nunez et al. 2004) and in individuals with Lhermitte–Duclos disease alone (Sutphen et al. 1999, Zhou et al. 2003). However, it remains unclear why not all cases of Lhermitte–Duclos disease coexist with the Cowden disease complex. The protein product of the gene is a 3'-specific phosphatidylinositol-3,4,5-triphosphate phosphatase that regulates the function of other proteins by removing phosphate groups from those molecules. The *PTEN* protein product negatively controls the phosphoinositide 3-kinase-signaling pathway for regulating cell growth and survival by dephosphorylating the 3 position of phosphoinositide. The *PTEN* protein is believed to promote cell death. A mutation that causes loss of the protein's function may result in over-proliferation of cells, resulting in hamartomatous growths. Diseases resulting from germline *PTEN* mutations are grouped as the *PTEN* hamartoma-tumour syndrome (see also Chapter 14) (Waite and Eng 2002).

## Diagnosis, management and follow-up

Although a Lhermitte–Duclos tumour is obviously a hamartoma of benign behaviour and its incidence is extremely rare, the disease should be considered when confronted with a young adult in the third to fourth decade of life presenting with clinical signs and symptoms of a progressive posterior fossa mass. Characteristic symptoms include cranial nerve palsies, unsteadiness of gait, ataxia and sudden neurological deterioration because of acute or chronic hydrocephalus. MRI is sufficient to demonstrate the typical *striated pattern* of hyperintensity on T2-weighted images and corresponding hypointensity on T1-weighted images (Meltzner et al. 1995). Enhancement following Gadolinium-DTPA administration is typically mild or missing. Recognition of the disease should prompt radical surgical excision and warrants thorough investigation for concomitant hamartomas and/or neoplasms of other parts of the body associated with Cowden syndrome. In a few instances patients with Lhermitte–Duclos disease underwent radiation therapy, but the effect of posterior fossa irradiation was reported contradictory either with several years free of symptoms or progressive neurological deterioration (Marano et al. 1988). Suggesting the benign nature of dysplastic gangliocytoma with a very small growth potential, radiation therapy should not be considered when in toto excision of the tumour and thus, complete remission may be achieved. At the time, the role of gamma knife irradiation in the treatment of Lhermitte–Duclos dis-

ease was not yet intensively investigated to give appropriate conclusions about its therapeutic value.

Given the frequent coexistence of Lhermitte–Duclos disease with the Cowden disease complex, surveillance for the component tumours associated with the Cowden disease complex in accordance with the United States National Comprehensive Cancer Centre High Risk/Genetics Panel guidelines, which are similar to those of the International Cowden Consortium (Eng 2000), is recommended in any case of Lhermitte–Duclos disease. Annual history taking, physical exams, appropriate laboratory tests and imaging studies should be performed to check for malignancies. As mucocutaneous lesions are the most common abnormality in Cowden disease (even considered to be pathognomonic by some authors) a dermatological consultation (including skin biopsy if necessary) should be considered as a first step towards the diagnosis of Cowden disease. At least 40% of Cowden disease patients have a minimum of one malignant primary tumour, although with long-term follow-up care, this number may be higher. Many of the cancers are curable if detected early. Anaemia can be a sign of malignancy. Annual thyroid function tests should be performed to screen for thyroid disease (goitre, Hashimoto thyreoiditis, adenoma). Minimally, a single baseline thyroid ultrasound followed by careful physical examination of the neck is necessary. It is thought that clear cell renal cell carcinoma may be a component in male patients and so an annual urine dipstick for occult blood and/or abdominal ultrasound may be considered. The second is particularly important in families with a known history of renal cell carcinoma. A thorough screening for breast carcinoma in female patients with monthly breast self-examination and annual clinical breast examination is obligatory. Screening should be initiated early in women (possibly as soon as puberty is complete). Even men are thought to be at higher risk for breast cancer if affected by the Cowden syndrome (Fackenthal et al. 2001).

Annual or biannual mammography should be considered when there is strong suspicion on physical exams, a positive family history or in case the diagnosis of Cowden disease has been established.

Women with Cowden syndrome should receive endometrial cancer screening consisting of annual blind suction biopsies in pre-menopausal women beginning at age 30 (5 years before the youngest endometrial cancer diagnosis in the family) and annual transvaginal ultrasound examination with biopsy of suspicious areas in post-menopausal women. Stool analysis for occult blood and if positive upper and lower gastrointestinal endoscopy may be employed to rule out hamartomas or carcinoma. Other malignancies that have rarely been reported to occur in Cowden disease are lung cancer, ovarian cancer, acute myelogenous leukaemia, transitional cell carcinoma of the bladder, cervix carcinoma, non-Hodgkin lymphoma and osteosarcoma. On the other hand, individuals affected by the Cowden disease complex are presumably at increased risk of a cerebellar gangliocytoma. Given that Lhermitte–Duclos disease can present in childhood (Ambler et al. 1969, Heitkamp and Rose 1981, Marano et al. 1988) annual neurological examinations and a first MRI at 10 years of age and three yearly thereafter, if asymptomatic, may be recommended in individuals with Cowden disease.

## Differential diagnosis

The differential diagnosis of Lhermitte–Duclos disease includes any space occupying infratentorial mass lesion. The clinical signs of a posterior fossa mass are indistinguishable in between individual aetiologies. MRI is useful to demonstrate the cortical origin of dysplastic cerebellar gangliocytoma and the preservation of a gyral pattern within the cerebellar hemispheric lesion (*striated cerebellum*) (Carter et al. 1989, Meltzer et al. 1995, Smith et al. 1989, Wolansky et al. 1996). These MRI criteria are unique and may suggest the diagnosis preoperatively. There is no contrast enhancement and the lesion may be partially calcified (Marano et al. 1988, Milbouw et al. 1988, Roski et al. 1981). Ogasawara et al. (2001) investigated two patients with PET and SPECT. Hyperperfusion was found in both cases, suggesting that the lesion may have a retention mechanism for technetium-99m-ECD equivalent to that of normal neural tissue. Definitive diagnosis is established by histological examination of the tumour specimen obtained by surgery.

## Genetic counselling

Nelen et al. (1997) confirmed that the *PTEN* gene is the gene for Cowden disease by a refined localisation of the gene on chromosome 10q22–23 and by mutation analysis in 8 unrelated familial and 11 sporadic patients with Cowden disease. They detected 8 different mutations in various regions of the *PTEN* gene. Cowden disease is inherited in an autosomal dominant mode. When a *PTEN* mutation has been identified in an individual, testing of asymptomatic relatives can identify those who also have the mutation and are at risk of having Cowden disease. These individuals should be included in the ongoing management as specified above. Relatives who have not inherited the *PTEN* mutation found in an affected relative do not have the disease and the associated high risk of cancer. The actual proportion of non-familial cases of Cowden disease and familial cases (defined as two or more affected relatives) cannot be defined. Probably, the majority of Cowden disease cases are non-familial. Approximately 10–50% of individuals with Cowden disease have an affected parent (Marsh et al. 1999).

If a *PTEN* mutation is identified in an individual, his/her parents should be asked if they wish genetic testing to determine if one of them has the disease. If no mutation is identified in the affected individual, both parents should undergo a thorough clinical screening if they have signs of Cowden disease. Although some affected cases diagnosed with Cowden disease have an affected parent, the family history may seem to be negative due to under-recognition of the clinical signs in family members, early death of parents prior to clinical manifestation or late onset of the disease in the affected individual. The risk to the siblings of the affected individual depends on the genetic status of the parents. If one parent of the affected individual has Cowden disease, the risk to siblings is 50%. In case neither parent has the *PTEN* mutation found in the affected individual, the risk to the siblings is negligible. If no mutation of the *PTEN* gene is found in the affected individual, the disorder can be ruled out in family members based on clinical examination. In this case, unremarkable clinical exams in parents (aged ≥30 years) reduces the risk to siblings of the affected individual to minimal, since about 99% of affected individuals would have clinical manifestations of the disease by that age.

Each child of an affected individual has a 50% risk to inherit the gene mutation and develop the disorder. The risk to other family members of the affected individual depends on the genetic status of his/her parents. If one of the parents is carrier of the mutation his/her family members are at risk. When the gene mutation is found in an affected person, asymptomatic direct line relatives should be tested to identify those who also have the mutation. These individuals should undergo the clinical management as specified in detail above. If none of the parents of an affected individual has the same mutation, a de-novo mutation of the *PTEN* gene must be considered. However, alternative causes, such as undisclosed adoption, should be taken into account. Prenatal diagnosis is possible for at risk pregnancies. The genetic link between Lhermitte–Duclos disease and the Cowden disease complex appears not to be a fixed one (Eng et al. 1999, Liaw et al. 1997, Nelen et al. 1997) and there is clear evidence that Lhermitte–Duclos tumours frequently occur sporadically (Delatycki et al. 2003). However, in case the *PTEN* mutation is found in an affected individual the mode of inheritance and the risk for direct-line relatives appear to be similar to those of the Cowden syndrome as specified above.

## References

Ambler M, Pogacar S, Sidman R (1969) Lhermitte–Duclos disease (granule cell hypertrophy of the cerebellum). Pathological analysis of the first familial cases. J Neuropathol Exp Neurol 28: 622–647.

Ashley DG, Zee CS, Chandrasoma PT, Segall HD (1990) Lhermitte–Duclos disease. CT and MR findings. J Comput Assist Tomogr 14: 984–987.

Backman SA, Stambolic V, Suzuki A, Haight J, Ella A, Pretorius J, Tsao MS, Shannon P, Bolon B, Ivy GO,

Mak TW (2001) Deletion of PTEN in mouse brain causes seizures, ataxia and defects in soma size resembling Lhermitte–Duclos disease. Nat Gen 29: 396–403.

Bellamy JC, D'Aamato NA, Szakaks JE (1963) Diffuse cerebellar hypertrophy. Am J Clin Path 40: 395–404.

Bielschowsky M, Simons A (1930) Über diffuse Hamartome (Ganglioneurome) des Kleinhirns und ihrer Genese. J Psychol Neurol 41: 50–75.

Brown WR, Angelo JN, Kelly DL (1980) Lhermitte–Duclos disease: case report with computerized tomographic scan. Neurosurgery 6: 189–191.

Burger PC, Scheithauer BW (1994) Tumours of the central nervous system. In: Rosai J (ed.) Atlas of tumour pathology. 3rd ed. Washington, DC: Armed Forces Institute of Pathology, pp. 176–178.

Carter JE, Merren MD, Swann KW (1989) Preoperative diagnosis of Lhermitte–Duclos disease by magnetic resonance imaging, case report. J Neurosurg 70: 135–137.

Cessaga (1980) Lhermitte–Duclos disease (diffuse hypertrophy of the cerebellum). Report of two cases. Neurosurgery 3: 151–158.

Chen YM, Ott DJ, Wu WC, Gelfand DW (1987) Cowden's disease: a case report and literature review. Gastrointest Radiol 12: 325–239.

Christensen E (1937) Über die Ganglienzellgeschwülste im Gehirn. Virchows Arch (Pathol Anat) 300: 567–581.

Costello MJ (1941) A case for diagnosis (keratosis follicularis?) Arch Dermatol Syphil 44: 109–110.

Delatycki MB, Danks A, Churchyard A, Zhou XP, Eng C (2003) De novo germline PTEN mutation in a man with Lhermitte–Duclos disease which arose on the paternal chromosome and was transmitted to his child with polydactyly and Wormian bones. J Med Genet 40:e92 (http://www.jmedgenet.com/cgi/content/full/40/8/e92)

Demaerel P, Van Calenbergh F, Wilms G (2003) Lhermitte–Duclos disease: a tumor or not a tumor? Acta Neurol Scand 108: 294–295.

Derrey S, Proust F, Debono B, Langlois O, Layet A, Layet V, Longy M, Freger P, Laquerriere A (2004) Association between Cowden syndrome and Lhermitte–Duclos disease: report of two cases and review of the literature. Surg Neurol 61: 447–454.

Duncan D, Snodgrass SR (1943) Diffuse hypertrophy of the cerebellar cortex (Myelinated Neurocytoma). Arch Neurol Psychiatr 50: 677–684.

Eng C (2000) Will the real Cowden syndrome please stand up: revised diagnostic criteria. J Med Genet 37: 828–830.

Eng C, Murday V, Seal S, Mohammed S, Hodgson SV, Chaudary MA, Fentiman IS, Ponder BA, Eales RA (1994) Cowden syndrome and Lhermitte–Duclos disease in a family: a single genetic syndrome with pleiotropy? J Med Genet 31: 458–61.

Fackenthal JD, Marsh DJ, Richardson AL (2001) Male breast cancer in Cowden syndrome patients with germline PTEN mutations. J Med Genet 38: 159–164.

Ferran M, Bussaglia E, Lazaro C, Matias-Guiu X, Pujol RM (2008) Acral papular neuromatosis: an early manifestation of Cowden syndrome. Br J Dermatol 158: 174–176.

Foerster O, Gagel O (1933) Ein Fall von Gangliocytoma dysplasticum des Kleinhirns. Dtsch Z Nervenheilk 146: 792–803.

Gorlin RJ, Cohen MM Jr, Hennekam RCM (2001) Cowden syndrome (multiple hamartoma and carcinoma syndrome, Lhermitte–Duclos syndrome) In: Gorlin RJ, Cohen MM Jr, Hennekam RCM (eds.) Syndromes of the Head and Neck. 4th ed. Oxford: Oxford University Press, pp. 432–437.

Gustafson S, Zbuk KM, Scacheri C, Eng C (2007) Cowden syndrome. Semin Oncol 34: 428–434.

Hair LS, Symmans F, Powers JM, Carmel P (1992) Immunohistochemistry and proliferative activity in Lhermitte–Duclos disease. Acta Neuropathol (Berl) 84: 570–573.

Hallervorden J (1959) Über die Hamartome (Ganglioneurome) des Kleinhirns. Deutsch Z Nervenheilk 179: 531–563.

Hanssen AM, Fryns JP (1995) Cowden syndrome. J Med Genet 32: 117–119.

Kleihues P, Cavenee WK (2000) Pathology and genetics of tumours of the nervous system. WHO classification of tumours. Lyon: IARC Press, pp. 235–237.

Klisch J, Juengling F, Spreer J (2001) Lhermitte–Duclos disease. Assessment with MR imaging, positron emission tomography, single-photon emission CT, and MR spectroscopy. AJNR 22: 824–830.

Koch R, Scholz M, Nelen MR, Schwechheimer K, Epplen JT, Harders AG (1999) Lhermitte–Duclos disease as a component of Cowden's syndrome, case report and review of the literature. J Neurosurg 90: 776–779.

Kulkantrakorn K, Awward EE, Levy B, Selhorst JB, Cole HO, Leake D, Gussler JR, Epstein AD, Malik MM (1997) MRI in Lhermitte–Duclos disease. Neurology 48: 725–731.

Leech RW, Christoferson LA, Gilbertson RL (1977) Dysplastic gangliocytoma (Lhermitte–Duclos disease) of the cerebellum. J Neurosurg 47: 609–612.

Lhermitte J, Duclos P (1920) Sur un ganglioneuroma diffus du cortex du cervelet. Bull Assoc Franc Cancer 9: 99–107.

Liaw D, Marsh DJ, Li J, Dahia PL, Wang SI, Zheng Z, Bose S, Call KM, Tsou HC, Peacocke M, Eng C, Parsons R (1997) Germline mutations of the PTEN gene in Cowden disease, an inherited breast and thyroid cancer syndrome. Nat Genet 16: 64–67.

Lindboe CF, Helseth E, Myhr G (1995) Lhermitte–Duclos disease and giant meningioma as manifestations of Cowden's disease. Clin Neuropathol 14: 327–330.

Lindor NM, Greene MH (1998) The concise handbook of family cancer syndromes. Mayo Familial Cancer Program. J Natl Cancer Inst 90: 1039–1071.

Lloyd KM, Dennis M (1963) Cowden's disease. A possible new symptom complex with multiple system involvement. Ann Intern Med 58: 136–142.

Lobo CJ, Mehan R, Murugasu E, Laitt RD (1999) Tinnitus as the presenting symptom in a case of Lhermitte–Duclos disease. J Laryngol Otol 113: 464–465.

Longy KM, Lacombe D (1996) Cowden disease. Report of a family and a review. Ann Genet 39: 35–42.

Longy M, Lacombe D (1996) Cowden disease. Report of a family and review. Ann Genet 39: 35–42.

Mallory SB (1995) Cowden syndrome (multiple hamartoma syndrome). Dermatol Clin 13: 27–31.

Marano R, Johnson PC, Spetzler RF (1988) Recurrent Lhermitte–Duclos disease in a child. Case report. J Neurosurg 69: 599–603.

Marcus CD, Galeon M, Peruzzi P, Bazin A, Bernard HH, Pluot M, Menanteau B (1996) Lhermitte–Duclos disease associated with syringomyelia. Neuroradiology 38: 539–541.

Marsh DJ, Coulon V, Lunetta KL, Rocca-Serra P, Dahia PL, Zheng Z, Liaw D, Caron S, Duboue B, Lin AY, Richardson AL, Bonnetblanc JM, Bressieux JM, Cabarrot-Moreau A, Chompret A, Demange L, Eeles RA, Yahanda AM, Fearon ER, Fricker JP, Gorlin RJ, Hodgson SV, Huson S, Lacombe D, Eng C (1998) Mutation spectrum and genotype-phenotype analyses in Cowden disease and Bannayan-Zonana syndrome, two hamartoma syndromes with germline PTEN mutation. Hum Mol Genet 7: 507–515.

Meltzner CC, Smirniotopoulos JG, Jones RV (1995) The striated cerebellum: an MR imaging sign in Lhermitte–Duclos disease (dysplasic gangliocytoma). Radiology 194: 699–703.

Milbouw G, Born JD, Martin D, Collignon J, Hans P, Reznik M, Bonnal J (1988) Clinical and radiological aspects of dysplastic gangliocytoma (Lhermitte–Duclos disease): A report of two cases with review of the literature. Neurosurgery 22: 124–128.

Murata J, Tada M, Sawamura Y, Mitsumori K, Abe H, Nagashima K (1999) Dysplastic gangliocytoma (Lhermitte–Duclos disease) associated with Cowden disease. Report of a case and review of the literature for the genetic relationship between the two diseases. J Neurooncol 41: 129–136.

Nagaraja S, Powell T, Griffiths PD, Wilkinson ID (2004) MR imaging and spectroscopy in Lhermitte Duclos disease. Neuroradiology 46: 355–358.

NCCN (1999) NCCN practice guidelines: genetics/familial high risk cancer. Oncology 13: 161–186.

Nelen MR, van Staveren WC, Peeters EA, Hassel MB, Gorlin RJ, Hamm H, Lindboe CF, Fryns JP, Sijmons RH, Woods DG, Mariman EC, Padberg GW, Kremer H (1997) Germline mutations in the PTEN/MMAC1 gene in patients with Cowden disease. Hum Mol Genet 6: 1383–1387.

Nelen MR, Kremer H, Konings IBM, Schoute F, van Essen AJ, Koch R, Woods CG, Fryns J-P, Hamel B, Hoefsloot LH, Peeters EAJ, Padberg GW (1999) Novel PTEN mutations in patients with Cowden disease: absence of clear genotype-phenotype correlations. Europ J Hum Genet 7: 267–273.

Nowak DA, Trost HA (2002) Lhermitte–Duclos disease (dysplastic cerebellar gangliocytoma): a malformation, hamartoma or neoplasm? Acta Neurol Scand 105: 137–145.

Nowak DA, Trost HA, Porr A, Stölzle A, Lumenta CB (2001) Lhermitte–Duclos disease (dysplastic gangliocytoma of the cerebellum). Clin Neurol Neurosurg 103: 105–110.

Ogasawara K, Yasuda S, Beppu T, Kobayashi M, Doi M, Kuroda K, Ogawa A (2001) Brain PET and technetium-99m-ECD SPECT imaging in Lhermitte–Duclos disease. Neuroradiology 43: 993–996.

OMIM™ (2006) Online Mendelina Inheritance in Man. Baltimore: Johns Hopkins University Press. http://www.ncbi.nlm.nih.gov/omim

Oppenheimer DR (1955) A benign 'tumour' of the cerebellum. Report on two cases of diffuse hypertrophy of the cerebellar cortex with a review of nine previously reported cases. J Neurol Neurosurg Psychiatry 18: 199–213.

Padberg GW, Schot JD, Vielvoye GJ, Bots GT, de Beer FC (1991) Lhermitte–Duclos disease and Cowden disease: a single phakomatosis. Ann Neurol 29: 517–523.

Perez-Nunez A, Lagares A, Benitez J, Urioste M, Lobato RD, Ricoy JR, Ramos A, Gonzalez P (2004) Lhermitte–Duclos disease and Cowden disease: clinical and genetic study in five patients with Lhermitte–Duclos disease and literature review Acta Neurochir 146: 679–690.

Pilarski R, Eng C (2004) Will the real Cowden syndrome please stand up (again)? Expanding mutational and clinical spectra of the PTEN hamartoma tumour syndrome (Commentary). J Med Genet 41: 323–326.

Prabhu SS, Aldape KD, Bruner JM, Weinberg JS (2004) Cowden disease with Lhermitte–Duclos disease: case report. Can J Neurol Sci 31: 542–549.

Pritchett PS, King TI (1978) Dysplastic gangliocytoma of the cerebellum: an ultrastructural study. Acta Neuropathol 42: 1–5.

Rainov NG, Holzhausen HJ, Burkert W (1995) Dysplastic gangliocytoma of the cerebellum (Lhermitte–Duclos disease). Clin Neurol Neurosurg 97: 175–180.

Reeder RF, Sauders RL, Roberts DW, Fratkin JD, Cromwell LD (1988) Magnetic resonance imaging in the diagnosis and treatment of Lhermitte–Duclos disease (dysplastic gangliocytoma of the cerebellum). Neurosurgery 23: 240–245.

Requena L, Gutierrez J, Sanchez Yus E (1992) Multiple sclerotic fibromas of the skin. A cutaneous marker of Cowden's disease. J Cutan Pathol 19: 346–351.

Reznik M, Schoenen J (1983) Lhermitte–Duclos disease. Acta Neuropathol (Berl) 53: 88–94.

Riliett B, Mori Y (1979) Gangliocytome dysplasique du cervelet. Schweiz Arch Neurol Neurochir Psychiatr 124: 13–27.

Robinson S, Cohen AR (2000) Cowden disease and Lhermitte–Duclos disease: Characterization of a new phakomatosis. Neurosurgery 46: 371–383.

Roessmann U, Wongmongkolrit T (1984) Dysplastic gangliocytoma of cerebellum in a newborn. Case report. J Neurosurg 60: 845–847.

Roski RA, Roessmann U, Spetzler RF, Kaufman B, Nulsen FE (1981) Clinical and pathological study of dysplastic gangliocytoma. J Neurosurg 55: 318–321.

Ruchoux MM, Gray F, Gherardi R, Schaeffer A, Comoy J, Poirier J (1986) Orthostatic hypotension from a cerebellar gangliocytoma (Lhermitte–Duclos disease). J Neurosurg 65: 245–252.

Siegel E (1920) Hyperplasie des Kleinhirns. Beitr Pathol Anat 67: 539–548.

Smith R, Grossman R, Goldberg H, Hacjney D, Bilaniuk L, Zimmerman R (1989) MR imaging of Lhermitte–Duclos disease: a case report. Am J Neuroradiol 10: 187–189.

Spaargaren L, Cras P, Bomhof MAM, Lie ST, de Barsy AM, Croese PH, Teepen JLJM, Duwel VHJM, Van Goethem JW, Ozsarlak O, van den Hauwe L, De Schepper LM, Parizel PM (2003) Contrast enhancement in Lhermitte–Duclos disease of the cerebellum: correlation of imaging with neuropathology in two cases. Neuroradiology 45: 381–385.

Stapleton SR, Wilkins PR, Bell BA (1992) Recurrent dysplastic cerebellar gangliocytoma (Lhermitte–Duclos disease) presenting with subarachnoid haemorrhage. Br J Neurosurg 6: 153–156.

Starink TM, van der Veen JPW, Arwert F, de Waal LP, de Lange GG, Gille JJP, Eriksson AW (1986) The Cowden syndrome: a clinical and genetic study in 21 patients. Clin Genet 29: 222–233.

Sutphen R, Diamond TM, Minton SE, Peacocke M, Tsou HC, Root AW (1999) Severe Lhermitte–Duclos disease with unique germline mutation of PTEN. Am J Med Genet 82: 290–293.

Tsao H (2000) Update on familial cancer syndromes and the skin. J Am Acad Dermatol 42: 939–969.

Tuli S, Provias JP, Bernstein M (1997) Lhermitte–Duclos disease. Literature review and novel treatment strategy. Can J Neurol Sci 24: 155–160.

Vantomme N, van Calenbergh F, Goffin J, Sciot R, Demaerel P, Plets C (2001) Lhermitte–Duclos disease is a clinical manifestation of Cowden's syndrome. Surg Neurol 56: 201–205.

Vinchon M, Blond S, Lejeune JP (1994) Association of Lhermitte–Duclos and Cowden disease: report of a new case and review of the literature. J Neurol Neurosurg Psychiatry 57: 699–704.

Waite KA, Eng C (2002) Protean PTEN: form and function. Am J Hum Genet 70: 829–844.

Wells GB, Lasner TM, Yousem DM, Zager EL (1994) Lhermitte–Duclos disease and Cowden's syndrome in an adolescent patient. Case report. J Neurosurg 81: 133–136.

Who Named it? (2006) A biographical dictionary of medical eponyms, medical conditions and techniques and the people for whom they are named. http://www.whonamedit.com

Williams DW, Elster AD, Ginsberg LE, Stanton C (1992) Recurrent Lhermitte–Duclos disease. Report of two cases and association with Cowden's disease. Am J Neuroradiol 3: 287–290.

Witten VH, Kopf AW (1957) Case for diagnosis: Verrucae planae? Adenoma sebaceum? Epidermodysplasia verruciformis? Arch Dermatol 76: 799–800.

Wolansky LJ, Malantic GP, Heary R (1996) Preoperative MRI diagnosis of Lhermitte–Duclos disease: case report with associated enlarged vessels and syrinx. Surg Neurol 45: 470–475.

Zhou XP, Marsh DJ, Morrison CD, Chaudhury AR, Maxwell M, Reifenberger G, Eng C (2003) Germline inactivation of PTEN and dysregulation of the phosphoinositol-3-kinase/Akt pathway cause human Lhermitte–Duclos disease in adults. Am J Hum Genet 73: 1191–1198.

Zori RT, Marsh DJ, Graham GE, Marliss EB, Eng C (1998) Germline PTEN mutation in a family with Cowden syndrome and Bannayan-Riley-Ruvalcaba syndrome. Am J Med Genet 80: 399–402.

# Chapter 29

# BANNAYAN-RILEY-RUVALCABA SYNDROME

**Corrado Romano**

Unit of Paediatrics and Medical Genetics, IRCCS OASI Maria Santissima, Troina, Italy

## Definition

The term of Bannayan-Riley-Ruvalcaba syndrome (BRRS) has been suggested first by M. Michael Cohen Jr. in a letter to the American Journal of Medical Genetics (Cohen 1990). He lumped three already recognized syndromes combining the names of their first authors. For the sake of historical truth, Riley and Smith (1960) were the first ones to report on the association of macrocephaly, pseudopapilledema and multiple hemangiomata. Subsequently, Bannayan (1971) published on the combination of multiple lipomas, angiomas and macrocephaly, which was reported afterwards by Zonana et al. (1976). Ruvalcaba et al. (1980) described two males with macrocephaly, intestinal poliposis, and pigmentary spotting of the penis. Further reports (Halal 1982, 1983) confirmed the existence of this condition, which was considered distinct from Sotos syndrome by Cohen (1982) and called Ruvalcaba-Myhre syndrome. Additional reports from DiLiberti et al. (1982, 1983) were published naming it Ruvalcaba-Myhre-Smith syndrome. DiLiberti (1990) maintained that this lumping was a little bit premature, because it was based only on clinical judgment and not on sound research data. Subsequently, the same author (DiLiberti 1992) agreed on the suggestion that Ruvalcaba-Myhre-Smith (Ruvalcaba et al. 1980), Riley-Smith (Riley and Smith 1960) and Bannayan-Zonana (Bannayan 1971, Zonana et al. 1976) phenotypes may represent phenotypic variability at a single genetic locus on the basis of the presence of lipid storage myopathy in 14 evaluated children showing these phenotypes.

## The Bannayan-Riley-Ruvalcaba syndrome before the discovery of PTEN gene

The first careful review of the BRRS phenotype has been made by Gorlin et al. (1992). They reported on a family with 12 affected members, showing a pedigree which gave clinical evidence of the overlap between Ruvalcaba-Myhre-Smith, Riley-Smith and Bannayan-Zonana syndromes. Craniofacial manifestations, somatic, motor and intellectual development, skin, gastrointestinal system, neoplasms, skeletal system and other abnormalities were considered by these authors the thumbnail index of BRRS phenotype, which they reviewed as follows.

"The head circumference is at least 2.5 SD above the mean, with normal ventricular size. Downslanting palpebral fissures appear in 60% of cases. Prominent Schwalbe lines and clearly visible corneal nerves were reported (DiLiberti et al. 1983, Grezula et al. 1988) in 35% of these patients examined by ophthalmologists under slit lamp. Strabismus or amblyopia are observed in 15% of cases. Delayed closure of the anterior fontanel, ocular hypertelorism, and pseudopapilledema have been reported in some instances (Riley and Smith 1960, Dvir et al. 1988).

Birth weight is above 4,000 g, and birth length over the 97th centile. The postnatal growth decelerates with a resulting height and weight within the normal range by older childhood (Ruvalcaba et al. 1980; DiLiberti et al. 1983, 1984).

Approximately 50% of cases shows hypotonia, gross motor delay, speech delay, and mild-to-severe mental deficiency (Higginbottom and Schultz 1982, Saul et al. 1982, DiLiberti et al. 1983, Halal 1983, Miles et al. 1984, Moretti-Ferreira et al. 1989).

Seizures have been reported in 25% of patients (DiLiberti et al. 1984). A transient and improving with age asymmetric motor development has been described in 5 cases (DiLiberti and Budden 1988).

A myopathy in proximal muscles has been recognized in 60% of patients (DiLiberti et al. 1984, Christian et al. 1991) and muscle biopsy has confirmed a lipid storage myopathy, mainly in enlarged type I skeletal muscle fibers, in 13 out of 14 cases (DiLiberti 1992). Conversely, type II fibers are smaller than normal and their lipid content is intermediate between normal type II fibers and BRRS type I fibers. Christian et al. (1991) have reported on a response of such myopathy to carnitine treatment.

The peculiar feature in the skin is represented by pigmented macules on the penile glans and shaft (DiLiberti 1992), which may be subtle and recognizable only when searched for. Above 50% of patients show cutaneous angiolipomas, others suffer from lymphangiomyomas or angiokeratomas (Klein and Barr 1990, DiLiberti et al. 1983). Café-au-lait spots on the trunk and lower limbs have been reported in some instances, whereas acanthosis nigricans-like facial lesions and accessory nipples (Ruvalcaba et al. 1980) only in single cases.

Forty-five percent of cases shows hamartomatous polyps, which are usually multiple and confined to the distal ileum and colon, and appear in childhood or middle age. They may complicate with intussusception and rectal bleeding (DiLiberti et al. 1984, Foster and Kilkoyne 1986).

Lipomas have been found in 75% of patients, whereas hemangiomas in less than 10%. Mixed tumors are reported in 20% of cases. Usually the hamartomas are subcutaneous, rarely are intracranial (20%) or osseous (10%). In some cases the lipomas can be aggressive, causing severe complications (Miles et al. 1984).

About 50% of patients shows joint hyperextensibility, pectus excavatum, and scoliosis (DiLiberti et al. 1984, Moretti-Ferreira et al. 1989). Accelerated growth of the first metacarpal bone and first and second middle phalanges have been documented by metacarpophalangeal profile (Halal 1982).

Enlarged testes have been reported in 2 adults (DiLiberti et al. 1984).

The review of the BRRS phenotype started the search for its explanation. First, lipid storage myopathy was addressed by the report of Fryburg et al. (1994) on a boy with BRRS and long-chain-L-3-hydroxyacyl-CoA dehydrogenase (L-CHAD) deficiency. The authors postulated that L-CHAD deficiency may be the cause of lipid storage myopathy in BRRS. Secondly, the histologic findings of the facial lesions and pigmented macules of the penis were analyzed by Fargnoli et al. (1996). They studied two families with BRRS and observed verrucous changes in both lips of one patient, which resulted as epidermal hyperplasia with papillomatosis and hyperkeratosis on histologic examination. Facial papules showed the histology of syringomas and trichilemmomas. The penile macules unfolded epidermal lentiginous hyperplasia, hyperpigmentation of the basal layer and a slight increase in the number of melanocytes. Furthermore, the authors raised the possibility of a common genetic pathogenesis of BRRS and Cowden syndrome (CS), on the ground of their clinical similarities.

## The discovery of PTEN gene and its impact in Bannayan-Riley-Ruvalcaba syndrome

The above mentioned suggestion was reinforced when Arch et al. (1997) reported on a 18-month-old boy with an interstitial deletion at 10q23.2–q24.1 and the clinical features of BRRS. In the meantime, the gene for CS had been first mapped to 10q22–q23 (Nelen et al. 1996) and subsequently cloned (Li et al. 1997, Liaw et al. 1997). Arch et al. (1997) confirmed in their patient the absence of PTEN gene (see in the PHTS chapter of this book for a wider knowledge) by fluorescence in situ hybridization (FISH). The authors speculated on the fact that BRRS is a condition presenting in childhood, whereas CS is a disease of adulthood, on the overlap between BRRS and CS features in their boy, and on the previous report (Fargnoli et al. 1996) of BRRS patients, who later developed skin lesions pathognomonic of CS and showed malignancies uncommon in BRRS. These clinical considerations, added up to the documented PTEN deletion in their boy, suggested that both conditions are allelic and caused by loss of function of the PTEN gene.

Similar results were obtained by Zigman et al. (1997), who defined a maximal distance of 1.0 cM commonly deleted in 2 patients with juvenile intestinal poliposis and karyotypic abnormalities involving chromosome 10q. They concluded maintaining that BRRS, juvenile polyposis and CS may share the same genetic defect on chromosome 10q23.

Marsh et al. (1998) performed PTEN sequencing in 37 CD families and 7 BRRS families. PTEN mutations were found in 81% of CD families and 57% of BRRS families, respectively. A "hot spot" for PTEN mutations (43% of all mutations) was identified through CD families in exon 5, where the PTPase core motif is located. Interestingly enough, BRRS families didn't show any mutation in such position. A single nonsense point mutation, R233X, was observed in the germline DNA from two unrelated CD families and one BRRS family.

The chance that sporadic BRRS cases don't harbor PTEN mutations was raised by Carethers et al. (1998).

The availability of PTEN gene sequencing gave light to the issue of a possible role of L-CHAD deficiency in BRRS myopathy. Otto et al. (1999) studied the L-CHAD enzyme activity in cultured skin fibroblasts from a family showing dominant inheritance of BRRS through three generations. All the enzyme activities were normal, whereas the germline PTEN missense mutation P246L segregated with BRRS. The authors had the opportunity to test for PTEN mutations the original patient with BRRS and L-CHAD deficiency (Fryburg et al. 1994) and didn't find anything. The obvious conclusion of these results was that the case reported with BRRS and L-CHAD deficiency either is a coincidence of two rare genetic events or a gene different from PTEN is related to L-CHAD deficiency and BRRS.

In the meantime, the amount of new PTEN mutations in patients with BRRS was piling up (Boccone et al. 2008, Longy et al. 1998). Striking evidence of the clinical overlap between CS and BRRS was provided by Zori et al. (1998), who re-ported on a mother with CS and a son with BRRS sharing the same heterozygous nonsense mutation R130X of PTEN gene. These clinical findings were subsequently confirmed in other families (Marsh et al. 1999, Perriard et al. 2000).

Marsh et al. (1999) screened for PTEN mutations 43 BRRS individuals comprising 16 sporadic and 27 familial cases, 11 of which were families with both CS and BRRS. Mutations were identified in 26 of 43 (60%) BRRS cases. In contrast to Carethers et al. (1998), no significant difference in mutation status was found in familial versus sporadic cases of BRRS. The authors found similar mutation spectra among CS, BRRS and BRRS/CS overlap families that were PTEN mutation positive. Their consequent conclusion was that PTEN mutation-positive CS and BRRS may be different presentations of a single syndrome and, hence, both should receive equal attention with respect to cancer surveillance.

## The Bannayan-Riley-Ruvalcaba syndrome after the discovery of PTEN gene

Parisi et al. (2001) were the first to report on the spectrum and evolution of phenotypic findings in PTEN mutation positive cases of BRRS, exactly like the title of their letter to the Journal of Medical Genetics. Ten subjects in three families with BRRS and PTEN mutations were the basis for their considerations. Macrocephaly, mental retardation or developmental delay, and high arched palate were the features present in all the subjects. Overgrowth was shown by 89%, joint hypermobility by 88%, and penile macules by 67% of the patients. About the natural history of the BRRS, the authors confirmed that the distinctive finding of penile macules in males may not appear until mid childhood. Postnatal overgrowth during childhood may be common, and other features such as high arched palate and joint hypermobility may aid in diagnosis.

Subsequently, the term PTEN hamartoma tumor syndrome (PHTS) (Marsh et al. 1999) should be the best definition, but this doesn't explain the pathogenesis of patients with phenotypes compatible with BRRS not showing mutations in the PTEN gene. However, the definition of a syndrome implies the knowledge of its pathogenesis, and then the diagnosis of BRRS should be now limited only to patients with PTEN mutation.

## References

Arch EM, Goodman BK, Van Wesep RA, Liaw D, Clarke K, Parsons R, McKusick VA, Geraghty MT (1997) Deletion of PTEN in a patient with Bannayan-Riley-Ruvalcaba syndrome suggests allelism with Cowden disease. Am J Med Genet 71: 489–493.

Bannayan GA (1971) Lipomatosis, angiomatosis, and macrocephaly: A previously undescribed congenital syndrome. Arch Patol 92: 1–5.

Boccone L, Dessì V, Serra G, Zibordi F, Loudianos G (2008) Bannayan-Riley-Ruvalcaba syndrome with posterior subcapsular congenital cataract and a consensus sequence splicing PTEN mutation. Am J Med Genet A 146: 257–260.

Carethers JM, Furnari FB, Zigman AF, Lavine JE, Jones MC, Graham GE, Teebi AS, Huang HJ, Ha HT, Chauhan DP, Chang CL, Cavenee WK, Boland CR (1998) Absence of PTEN/MMAC1 germ-line mutations in sporadic Bannayan-Rilet-Ruvalcaba syndrome. Cancer Res 58: 2724–2726.

Christian CL, Fleisher DR, Feldman EJ, Pepkowitz SH, Jafolla AK, DiLiberti JH, Graham JM Jr (1991) Lipid storage myopathy associated with Ruvalcaba-Myhre-Smith syndrome: Treatment with carnitine. Clin Res 39: 64A.

Cohen MM Jr (1982) The large-for-gestational-age infant in dysmorphic perspective. In: Willey AM, Carter TP, Kelly S, Porter IM (eds.) Clinical Genetics: Problems in Diagnosis and Counselling. New York: Academic Press, pp. 153–169.

Cohen MM Jr (1990) Bannayan-Riley-Ruvalcaba syndrome: Renaming three formerly recognized syndromes as one etiologic entity. Am J Med Genet 35: 291.

DiLiberti JH, Weleber RG, Budden S (1983) Ruvalcaba-Myhre-Smith syndrome: A case report with probably autosomal dominant inheritance and additional manifestations. Am J Med Genet 15: 491–495.

DiLiberti JH, D'Agostino AN, Ruvalcaba RHA, Schimschock JR (1984) A new lipid storage myopathy observed in individuals with the Ruvalcaba-Myhre-Smith syndrome. Am J Med Genet 18: 163–168.

DiLiberti JH, Budden S (1988) Transient motor asymmetry in young children with the Ruvalcaba-Myhre-Smith syndrome. Ninth Annual David W. Smith Workshop on Malformations and Morphogenesis, Oakland, CA, August 3–7.

DiLiberti JH (1990) Comments on Dr. Cohen's Letter. Am J Med Genet 35: 292.

DiLiberti JH (1992) Correlation of skeletal muscle biopsy with phenotype in the familial macrocephaly syndromes. J Med Genet 29: 46–49.

Dvir M, Beer S, Aladjem M (1988) Heredofamilial syndrome of mesodermal hamartomas, macrocephaly and pseudopapilledema. Pediatrics 81: 287–290.

Fargnoli MC, Orlow SJ, Semel-Concepcion J, Bolognia JL (1996) Clinicopathologic findings in the Bannayan-Riley-Ruvalcaba syndrome. Arch Dermatol 132: 1214–1218.

Foster MA, Kilkoyne RF (1986) Ruvalcaba-Myhre-Smith syndrome: A new consideration in the differential diagnosis of intestinal poliposis. Gastrointest Radiol 11: 349–350.

Fryburg JS, Pelegano JP, Bennett MJ, Bebin EM (1994) Long-chain-L-3-hydroxyacyl-CoA dehydrogenase (L-CHAD) deficiency in a patient with the Bannayan-Riley-Ruvalcaba syndrome. Am J Med Genet 52: 97–102.

Gorlin RJ, Cohen MM Jr, Condon LM, Burke BA (1992) Bannayan-Riley-Ruvalcaba syndrome. Am J Med Genet 44: 307–314.

Grezula JC, Hevia O, Schachner LS, DiLiberti JH, Ruvalcaba RHA, Schimschock JR, Weleber RG, Halal F, Lipson MH, Blumberg B, Weber PJ (1988) Ruvalcaba-Myhre-Smith syndrome. Pediatr Dermatol 5: 28–32.

Halal F (1982) Male-to-male transmission of cerebral gigantism. Am J Med Genet 12: 411–419.

Halal F (1983) Cerebral gigantism, intestinal poliposis and pigmentary spotting of the genitalia. Am J Med Genet 15: 161.

Higginbottom MC, Schultz P (1982) The Bannayan syndrome: An autosomal dominant disorder consisting of macrocephaly, lipomas, hemangiomas, and a risk for intracranial tumors. Pediatrics 69: 632–634.

Klein JA, Barr RJ (1990) Bannayan-Zonana syndrome associated with lymphangiomyomatous lesions. Pediatr Dermatol 7: 48–53.

Li J, Yen C, Liaw D, Podsypanina K, Bose S, Wang SI, Puc J, Miliaresis C, Rodgers L, McCombie R, Bigner SH, Giovanella BC, Ittmann M, Tycko B, Hibshoosh H, Wigler MH, Parsons R (1997) PTEN, a putative protein tyrosine phosphatase gene mutated in human brain, breast, and prostate cancer. Science 275: 1943–1946.

Liaw D, Marsh DJ, Li J, Dahia PL, Wang SI, Zheng Z, Bose S, Call KM, Tsou HC, Peacocke M, Eng C, Parsons R (1997) Germline mutations of the PTEN gene in Cowden disease, an inherited breast and thyroid cancer syndrome. Nat Genet 16: 64–67.

Longy M, Coulon V, Duboue B, David A, Larregue M, Eng C, Amati P, Kraimps JL, Bottani A, Lacombe D, Bonneau D (1998) Mutations of PTEN in patients with Bannayan-Riley-Ruvalcaba phenotype. J Med Genet 35: 886–889.

Marsh DJ, Coulon V, Lunetta KL, Rocca-Serra P, Dahia PL, Zheng Z, Liaw D, Caron S, Duboue B, Lin AY, Richardson AL, Bonnetblanc JM, Bressieux JM, Cabarrot-Moreau A, Chompret A, Demange L, Eeles RA, Yahanda AM, Fearon ER, Fricker JP, Gorlin RJ, Hodgson SV, Huson S, Lacombe D, Eng C (1998) Mutation spectrum and genotype-phenotype analyses in Cowden disease and Bannayan-Zonana syndrome, two hamartoma syndromes with germline PTEN mutation. Hum Mol Genet 7: 507–515.

Marsh DJ, Kum JB, Lunetta KL, Bennett MJ, Gorlin RJ, Ahmed SF, Bodurtha J, Crowe C, Curtis MA, Dasouki M, Dunn T, Feit H, Geraghty MT, Graham JM Jr, Hodgson SV, Hunter A, Korf BR, Manchester D, Miesfeldt S, Murday VA, Nathanson KL, Parisi M, Pober B, Romano C, Eng C (1999) PTEN mutation spectrum and genotype-phenotype correlations in Bannayan-Riley-Ruvalcaba syndrome suggest a single entity with Cowden syndrome. Hum Mol Genet 8: 1461 1472.

Miles JH, Zonana J, McFarlane J, Aleck KA, Bawle E (1984) Macrocephaly with hamartomas: Bannayan-Zonana syndrome. Am J Med Genet 19: 225–234.

Moretti-Ferreira D, Koiffmann CP, Souza DH, Diament AJ, Wajntal A (1989) Macrocephaly, multiple lipomas, and hemangiomata (Bannayan-Zonana syndrome): Genetic heterogeneity or autosomal dominant locus with at least two different allelic forms? Am J Med Genet 34: 548–551.

Nelen MR, Padberg GW, Peeters EAJ, Lin AY, van den Helm B, Frants RR, Coulon V, Goldstein AM, van Reen MMM, Easton DF, Eeles RA, Hodgson S, Mulvihill JJ, Murday VA, Tucker MA, Mariman ECM, Starink TM, Ponder BAJ, Ropers HH, Kremer H, Longy M, Eng C (1996) Localization of the gene for Cowden disease to 10q22–23. Nat Genet 13: 114–116.

Otto LR, Boriack RL, Marsh DJ, Kum JB, Eng C, Burlina AB, Bennett MJ (1999) Long-chain L 3-hydroxyacyl-CoA dehydrogenase (LCHAD) deficiency does not appear to be the primary cause of lipid myopathy in patients with Bannayan-Riley-Ruvalcaba syndrome (BRRS). Am J Med Genet 83: 3–5.

Parisi MA, Dinulos MB, Leppig KA, Sybert VP, Eng C, Hudgins L (2001) The spectrum and evolution of phenotypic findings in PTEN mutation positive cases of Bannayan-Riley-Ruvalcaba syndrome. J Med Genet 38: 52–58.

Perriard J, Saurat JH, Harms M (2000) An overlap of Cowden's disease and Bannayan-Riley-Ruvalcaba syndrome in the same family. J Am Acad Dermatol 42: 348–50.

Riley HD, Smith WR (1960) Macrocephaly, pseudopapilledema and multiple hemangiomata. Pediatrics 26: 293–300.

Ruvalcaba RHA, Myhre S, Smith DW (1980) Sotos syndrome with intestinal poliposis and pigmentary changes of the genitalia. Clin Genet 18: 413–416.

Saul RA, Stevenson RE, Bley R (1982) Mental retardation in the Bannayan syndrome. Pediatrics 69: 642–644.

Zigman AF, Lavine JE, Jones MC, Boland CR, Carethers JM (1997) Localization of the Bannayan-Riley-Ruvalcaba syndrome gene to chromosome 10q23. Gastroenterology 113: 1433–1437.

Zonana J, Rimoin DL, Davis DC (1976) Macrocephaly with multiple lipomas and hemangiomas. J Pediatr 89: 600–603.

Zori RT, Marsh DJ, Graham GE, Marliss EB, Eng C (1998) Germline PTEN mutation in a family with Cowden syndrome and Bannayan-Riley-Ruvalcaba syndrome. Am J Med Genet 80: 399–402.

# Chapter 30

# ENCEPHALOCRANIOCUTANEOUS LIPOMATOSIS (HABERLAND SYNDROME)

Sergiusz Jóźwiak and Ignacio Pascual-Castroviejo

Department of Neurology and Epileptology, Children's Memorial Health Institute, Warsaw, Poland (SJ);
Paediatric Neurology Service, University Hospital La Paz, University of Madrid, Madrid, Spain (IPC)

## Introduction

Encephalocraniocutaneous lipomatosis (ECCL) or Haberland syndrome is a rare, congenital, neurocutaneous disorder. It is characterized by unilateral lipomatous hamartomata of the scalp, eyelid, and outer globe of the eye and ipsilateral neurologic malformations. Mental retardation and epilepsy may compromise the clinical status.

## Historical perspective and terminology

Haberland and Perou first described the disorder in 1970 in the clinical and necropsy findings of a 5-year-old boy who had epilepsy and mental retardation (Haberland and Perou 1970). They suggested that the child had a previously unreported neurocutaneous syndrome, which they termed encephalocraniocutaneous lipomatosis. Subsequently, Fishman et al. (1978) and Fishman (1987) reported three additional patients. All had epilepsy but their psychomotor skills were not so impaired as in the patient described by Haberland and Perou (1970). All had unilateral soft tissue tumours of the scalp with overlying alopecia, ipsilateral tumours of the sclera and skin tags of the face and eyelids. Their neuroimaging studies demonstrated ipsilateral cerebral hemiatrophy, porencephaly and defective opercularization. Two of the three patients had parenchymal calcifications and calcified vascular lesions.

In a patient reported by Sanchez et al. (1981) the cutaneous lesions were mostly unilateral, limited to the face, eyes and scalp. However, some soft tissue papules were present bilaterally, around both eyes and bulbar conjunctiva. Brain imaging revealed hydrocephalus, fatty tissue tumour and a porencephalic cyst ipsilaterally to a smooth patch of scalp alopecia. Such association of unilateral, or predominantly unilateral, cutaneous lesions on the face and scalp and ipsilateral cerebral malformations has been subsequently reported by other authors (Lasierra et al. 2003, Miyao et al. 1984, Parazzini et al. 1999).

In recent reports, the reporting authors termed the syndrome – Haberland syndrome, from the name of one of the original authors (Gawel et al. 2003). Recently, ECCL has also become known under the term of Fishman syndrome (Amor et al. 2000, Brumback and Leech 1987).

## Incidence and prevalence

Approximately, 40 patients are reported in the literature. No epidemiological data on the frequency of the disorder are available. There is no clear racial or gender predilection (Romiti et al. 1999).

Many patients with Haberland syndrome lead normal lives. Complications related to intracerebral malformations may be a cause of increased morbidity and mortality.

## Clinical manifestations

The clinical picture of Haberland syndrome may vary from patient to patient; however, a set of clinical features is regarded as characteristic for the disorder.

## Cutaneous lesions

The characteristic cutaneous neoplasm, named nevus psiloliparus (from Greek *psilos* – fat, fatty) is a
cutaneous hallmark of the ECCL syndrome. The
term was introduced by Happle and Kuster (1998)
to describe a distinct type of mesodermal nevus
characterized by the absence or paucity of scalp hair
and presence of an excessive amount of fatty tissue, giving rise to flat, smooth patch of hairlessness
(Figs. 1–3). Alopecia is a constant finding (Fig. 2).
These cutaneous soft tumours, often lipomas are skin
coloured and located on one side of the scalp, but bilateral involvement also has been reported (Grimalt et al.
1993, Rubegni et al. 2003, Sant'Anna et al. 1999).

Characteristic histopathologic features include
the absence or paucity of hair follicles, isolated peri-
follicular muscles mostly arranged at a single level
running parallel to the skin surface, and increased
lipomatous or fibrolipomatous tissue extending into
the upper reticular dermis (Happle and Kuster 1998,
Jóźwiak et al. 2001).

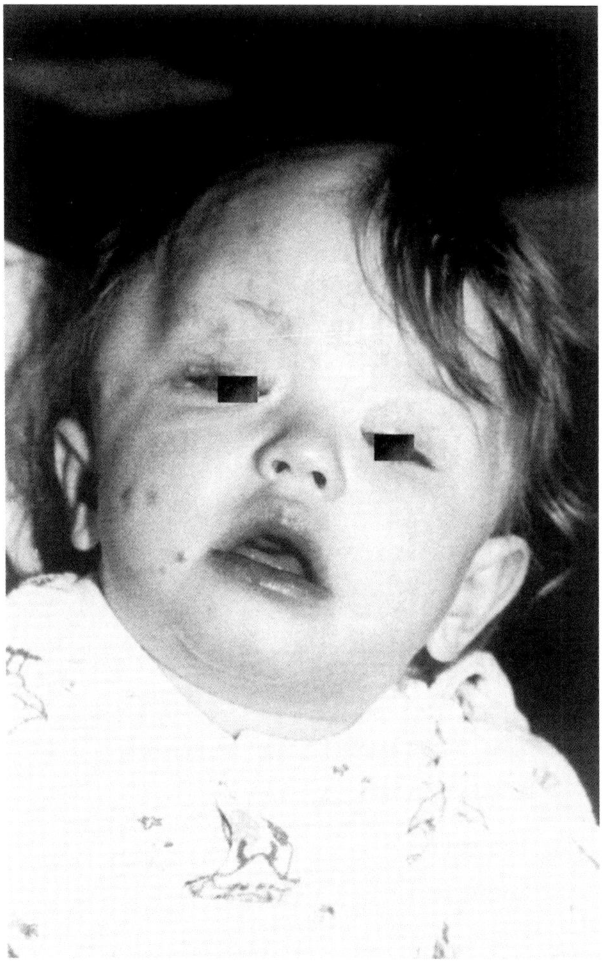

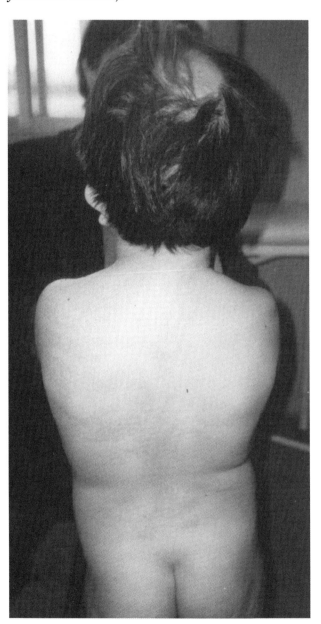

**Fig. 1.** Small cutaneous soft lipomas on the face and eyelid in a
patient with Haberland syndrome.

**Fig. 2.** Prominent alopecia in a child with Haberland syndrome.

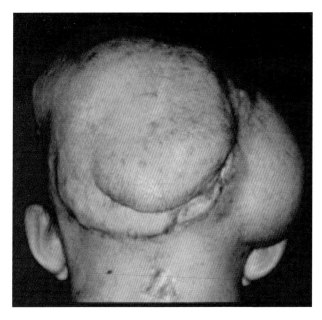

**Fig. 3.** Multiple bulky masses of the posterior aspect of the head that, at histology, were lipomatous-like (courtesy of professor G. Micali, Catania).

In 2004, Happle and Horster reported nevus psiloliparus in 2 otherwise healthy girls, suggesting that the skin lesion may be a nonsyndromic skin disorder (Happle and Horster 2004, Stieler et al. 2008).

Cutaneous abnormalities usually involve only the head and face. Some patients have ill-defined bony protuberances on the skull (associated with the scalp). Skin-coloured papular or polypoid cutaneous nodules may be observed on the face and eyelid in a unilateral distribution on the same side as the scalp lesions (Brown et al. 2003, Torrelo et al. 2005) (Figs. 1 and 3). These may represent small angiolipomas (Fig. 3), fibrolipomas, connective tissue nevi, or mixed hamartomas of cartilage, fat, and connective tissue (Fig. 1). A patient with unilateral odontomas was recently reported (Hauber 2003). Pigmented melanocytic nevi are another skin abnormality found in some patients with ECCL.

## CNS involvement

Mental status of the reported cases varies from totally normal to severe mental retardation. In most patients, testing of intellectual function revealed IQ scores ranging from 65 to 75.

Seizures are very frequent but not a constant feature and may become evident in some patients in the first year of life, leading to mental retardation. They are usually focal, contralateral to the skin and eye lesions. In most patients the seizures were well controlled with antiepileptic drugs.

Some patients with ECCL develop spasticity of contralateral limbs, hemiplegia, facial paresis and sensorineural hearing loss. One patient, delineated by Fishman in 1987, manifested a subarachnoid hemorrhage, presumably related to leakage of blood from an aneurysmal-type vascular malformation (Fishman 1987).

Neuroimaging studies are important part of the diagnosis (Fig. 4) (Moog et al. 2007). A hemiatrophy of the involved hemisphere with a porencephalic cysts communicating with the enlarged lateral ventricle ipsilateral to the cutaneous lipomatous hamartomas are among the most common findings (Nowaczyk et al. 2000). Some authors recognized a presence of porencephalic cysts as a typical feature of Haberland syndrome. Others have suggested different hypothesis: the areas of porencephaly in the temporal and parietooccipital regions associated with a dilatation of the ipsilateral ventricle could have been arachnoid cysts of the middle cranial fossa. They do not manifest mass effect because they are often associated with a primary hypogenesis of the temporal lobe or are part of a large dilatation of the lateral ventricle (see Fig. 4a). The histologic examination of the brain performed in a case reported by Haberland and Perou (1970) revealed a defective lamination of the cerebrum, polymicrogyria, and calcification in the outer cerebral cortex overlying the porencephalic cyst.

Other alterations, including pontocerebellar atrophy, endocranial hypertension, intracranial (Fig. 4b) and/or perimedullary (Fig. 4d) lipomas, and partial agenesis of the corpus callosum, also have been reported.

In some patients cortical calcifications and areas of cortical dysplasia (lissencephaly or polygyria) or hydrocephalus have been documented (Chittenden et al. 2002, Lasierra et al. 2003, Nosti-Martinez et al. 1995, Parazzini et al. 1999).

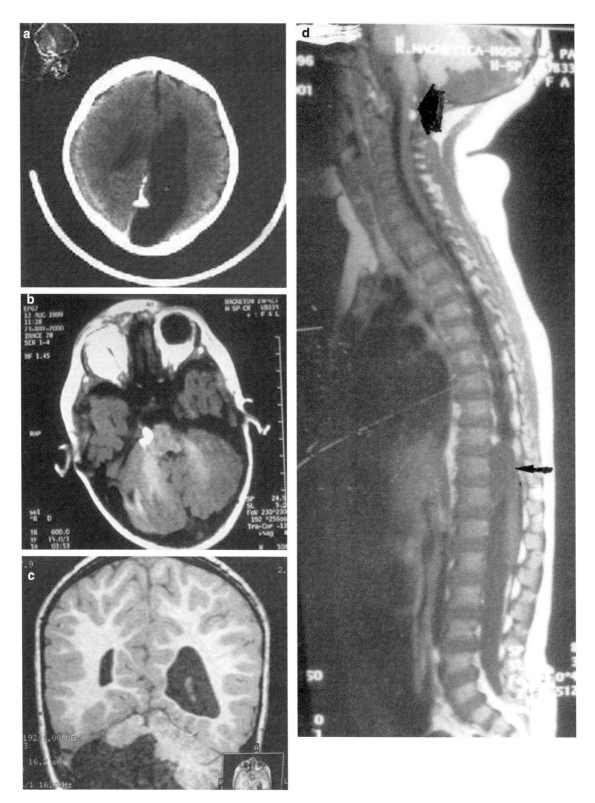

**Fig. 4.** Axial CT (**a**) and axial (**b**), coronal (**c**) and sagittal (**d**) T1-weighted images in patients with Haberland syndrome showing: (**a**) unilateral (left) ventricular dilatation with left calpocephaly and right cerebral hemiotrophy; (**b**) an intracranial lipoma in the right adjacent region of the brainstem; (**c**) ventricular asymmetry with unilateral (right) cerebellar hypoplasia; (**d**) multiple intradural lipomas of the cord (black arrows).

Neurologic symptoms do not appear to be related to the extent of neuroradiologic abnormalities. Most patients had extremely extensive cerebral abnormalities with only minimal symptomatology.

Donaire et al. (2005) reported a neurophysiological findings in a woman evaluated for epilepsy surgery. On functional magnetic resonance imaging the authors revealed transfer of memory and language functions to the nonaffected hemisphere, which may evidence the functional reorganization and restoration of cognitive functions in Haberland syndrome.

### Ocular findings

Ocular involvements appear to be a uniform feature of Haberland syndrome (see Fig. 2). The most common ocular lesions include epibulbar choristomas, small papules around the eyelids, and desmoid tumours of the scleral limb. Persistent hyaloid vessels, dislocation of the lens capsule, clouding of the cornea, iris dysplasia, colobomas, microphthalmia, ocular calcifications, and optic nerve pallor also have been reported (Fishman 2004).

In 2003, Almer et al. reported a case of ECCL with bilateral aniridia (Almer et al. 2003).

### Bone abnormalities

There are various skeletal abnormalities reported in patients with ECCL. They include vertebral abnormalities, extradural spinal cord lipomatous lesions, mandibular tumours, leg, arm, or chest asymmetry and multiple bone cysts (Andreadis et al. 2004, Moog et al. 2007, Savage et al. 1985, Zielinska-Kazimierska et al. 2005).

### Natural history

There are few studies on natural history of ECCL syndrome (Parazzini et al. 1999, Sofiatti et al. 2006). Skin manifestations are usually present at birth and do not seem to evolve with age. Seizures are usually well controlled and no decline in mental status is observed on follow up.

In some patients the serial neuroimaging studies demonstrated the development of progressive vasculopathy. Serial angiograms revealed the development of a sacular aneurysm in one patient (Fishman 1987). The lesions increased in size over time and were partially thrombosed.

## Pathogenesis/molecular genetics

The pathogenesis of the syndrome remains unknown. There is no evidence as yet of genetic transmission or chromosomal abnormality. However, the Happle hypothesis of somatic mosaicism may be an explanation for a number of hamartomatous syndromes. The survival of a lethal mutation by mosaicism may be important with this syndrome. We believe that somatic mosaicism will be proven to be the underlying pathophysiology in ECCL. In favor of Happle theory of a lethal mutation surviving only in the mosaic state could be the specific linear pattern of distribution of skin lesions with sharp midline delineation and marked clinical variability of cutaneous and tissue involvement (Hamm 1999).

Dysgenesia of the cephalic neural crest and the anterior neural tube is a most widely accepted explanation of this syndrome's pathogenesis. Haberland and Perou (1970) speculated as to whether the ectodermal malformations are caused by the same basic defect responsible for the mesenchymal malformations or whether they were secondary to the mesodermal dysgenesis.

The progression of the disease after birth is related to abnormalities in tissues derived from the mesenchyme, i.e., blood vessels and adipose tissue. One may therefore speculate that defects in the formation of the hemisphere are secondary to arterial circulatory impairment and that the whole syndrome is related to a primary defect in mesenchymal formation (Fishman 1987).

In 2004, Cultrera et al. described a female infant that showed significant overlap of ECCL with oculocerebrocutaneous Delleman syndrome. According to these authors, such overlap may support the theory of somatic mosaicism (Cultrera et al. 2004).

Legius et al. reported a unique case of a child having clinical findings of Haberland syndrome and features of neurofibromatosis type 1 (NF-1), in whom a de novo mutation of the *NF-1* gene was detected (Legius et al. 1995). However, due to the relatively high incidence of NF-1 in the general population, a coincidental occurrence of both disorders in the same patient cannot be excluded.

## Diagnosis

The diagnosis of the syndrome may be difficult, due to the absence of any pathognomonic morphologic or biochemical markers and its highly variable expressivity. Minimal diagnostic criteria for ECCL have been proposed by MacLaren et al. (1995). They include 1/unilateral skull hamartoma, 2/ocular choristoma, 3/skull asymmetry due to an increase in angiolipomatous tissue in the diploic space, and 4/intracranial anomalies.

## Differential diagnosis

The clinical features of ECCL overlap with other neurocutaneous syndromes: Delleman syndrome (oculocerebrocutaneous syndrome), nevus sebaceous syndrome, Proteus syndrome, Sturge-Weber syndrome, Goldenhar syndrome, Goltz syndrome, neurofibromatosis type 1.

Some have speculated that ECCL might represent a circumscribed form of the Proteus syndrome (McCall et al. 1992, Rizzo et al. 1993, Wiedemann and Burgio 1986). However, while the Proteus syndrome is an overgrowth syndrome which progresses from childhood to puberty, the lesions in ECCL syndrome remain usually static. Presence of porencephalic cysts has not been reported in the Proteus syndrome. ECCL affects one side of the face and brain, whereas the Proteus syndrome is usually characterized by bilateral lesions. Macrodactyly of the hands or feet, frequently observed in the Proteus syndrome, has also been reported in one patient with ECCL (Al-Mefty et al. 1987).

Choristomas, epilepsy and mental retardation may also be seen in the sebaceous nevus syndrome, with the cutaneous epidermal nevus affecting the face and upper part of the trunk, frequently located in the midline. Sebaceous lesions are composed of hyperplastic sebaceous glands, atypical apocrine glands and immature hair follicles. Neuroimaging may reveal unilateral ventricular enlargement, hemimegalencephaly, arachnoid cysts and porencephaly. Ocular findings are reported in approximately one-third of the patients with sebaceous nevus syndrome. Eyelid involvement by the sebaceous nevus and epibulbar choristomas are the most common ocular manifestations. Other developmental anomalies, as ventricular septal defects or tooth agenesis have been reported in sebaceous nevus syndrome but are very rare in ECCL syndrome. Some authors believe that ECCL and sebaceous nevus syndrome may represent a continuum of phenotypic expression. There are at least 2 reported cases of ECCL that demonstrated sebaceous nevi (Bamforth et al. 1989, Schlack and Skopnik 1985).

Delemann syndrome or oculocerebrocutaneous (OCC) syndrome and ECCL share many clinical features, such as skin, ocular and orbital defects, developmental delay, epilepsy and lack of progression (Narbay et al. 1996). In Delemann syndrome, the presence of orbital cysts, aplastic skin defects, as the absence of facial lipomas and scalp alopecia, are helpful in the diagnosis. Additionally, CNS malformations are rare in the syndrome and limited to intracranial cysts and agenesis of corpus callosum. Psychomotor retardation and seizures are reported in the majority of patients with OCC syndrome (Moog et al. 1997). Application of diagnostic criteria suggests that OCC syndrome and ECCL are distinct disorders (Hunter 2006).

The differential diagnosis of ECCL and Sturge-Weber syndrome (SWS) seems to be much easier. Cutaneous lesions in SWS are vascular, which is not characteristic for Haberland syndrome. Although both conditions have a gyriform pattern of intracranial calcifications, but the double line of calcifications seen in SWS has not been described in patients with ECCL. Contrary, a porencephaly and intracranial lipomatosis characteristic for ECCL is not reported in SWS patients.

Goldenhar syndrome, also known as facioauriculovertebral syndrome manifests with epibulbar choristomas as a prominent feature. Since first Goldenhar's report many additional features have been recognized. Ocular manifestations include eyelid colobomas, epibulbar dermolipomas, blepharoptosis and lacrimal drainage system abnormalities. Systemic anomalies include microsomia, cleft lip, vertebral and digital abnormalities, congenital urogenital or heart defects. There are reports in the literature of patients sharing some features of ECCL and Goldenhar syndromes, including the epibulbar choristoma and hemifacial microsomia (Kodsi et al. 1994).

Hypoplastic cutaneous plaques may resemble the skin findings in Goltz syndrome or congenital varicella zoster infection and may produce diagnostic difficulties. Tooth defects, scoliosis, syndactyly and polydactyly may support Goltz syndrome diagnosis (Hardman et al. 1998).

Rarely, pigmented skin nevi and neurofibromas can be seen in ECCL patients requiring the differentiation with neurofibromatosis type 1 (Fishman 2004).

## Follow up

The prognosis appears to correlate with the progression of neurologic lesions, either directly or secondary to complications from drug and surgical therapies. Many patients with ECCL syndrome may conduct normal life despite neurocutaneous lesions.

Due to the possible presence of extradural spinal cord lipomatous lesions, some authors suggest screening for spinal abnormalities in asymptomatic patients (Alfonso et al. 1986). Patients followed into early adulthood showed no evidence of progressive intellectual decline, however progressive hydrocephalus observed in some patients with ECCL syndrome may require a ventriculoperitoneal shunt justifying the necessity of brain CT follow up studies (Loggers et al. 1992, Parazzini et al. 1999).

In the 2005 study by Donaire et al. functional MRI revealed transfer of memory and language functions to the nonaffected hemisphere, providing evidence that functional reorganization and restoration

of cognitive function may occur in persons with ECCL (Donaire et al. 2005).

Periodic cardiologic assessment with echocardiography and electrocardiography may be indicated because of an anticipated progressive course.

## Management

Surgical treatment of cutaneous and subcutaneous lesions, especially on the face and cranium may be necessary. Antiepileptic treatment is administered in patients with clinical epileptic fits. Antiarrhythmic treatment may be required in patients with cardiac rhythm abnormalities due to lipomatous infiltration in the atrial myocardium.

Selected patients with drug-resistant epilepsy may benefit from neurosurgical intervention, as reported by Roszkowski and Dabrowski (1997).

Consultation with a neurosurgeon, neurologist, ophthalmologist, and cardiologist is warranted as determined by history and physical examination findings. No special activity limitations are required for most patients.

## Genetic counseling

All reported cases of ECCL were sporadic. A nonhereditary, autosomal mutation that may survive only in a mosaic state may be a cause of the clinical picture of ECCL.

## References

Alfonso I, Lopez PF, Cullen RF Jr, Martin-Jimenez R, Bejar RL (1986) Spinal cord involvement in encephalocraniocutaneous lipomatosis. Pediatr Neurol 2(6): 380–384.

Al-Mefty O, Fox JL, Sakati N, Bashir R, Probst F (1987) The multiple manifestations of the encephalocraniocutaneous lipomatosis syndrome. Childs Nerv Syst 3(2): 132–134.

Almer Z, Vishnevskia-Dai V, Zadok D (2003) Encephalocraniocutaneous lipomatosis: case report and review of the literature. Cornea 22: 389–390.

Amor DJ, Kornberg AJ, Smith LJ (2000) Encephalocraniocu-taneous lipomatosis (Fishman syndrome): a rare neurocu-taneous syndrome. J Paediatr Child Health 36: 603–605.

Andreadis DA, Rizos CB, Belazi M, Peneva M, Antoniades DZ (2004) Encephalocraniocutaneous lipomatosis ac-companied by maxillary compound odontoma and ju-venile angiofibroma: report of a case. Birth Defects Res A Clin Mol Teratol 70(11): 889–891.

Bamforth JS, Riccardi VM, Thisen P, Chitayat D, Friedman JM, Caruthers J, Hall JG (1989) Encephalocranio-cutaneous lipomatosis. Report of two cases and a review of the literature. Neurofibromatosis 2(3): 166–173.

Brown KE, Goldstein SM, Douglas RS, Katowitz JA (2003) Encephalocraniocutaneous lipomatosis: a neurocuta-neous syndrome. J AAPOS 7(2): 148–149.

Brumback RA, Leech RW (1987) Fishman's syndrome (en-cephalocraniocutaneous lipomatosis): a field defect of ectomesoderm. J Child Neurol 2(3): 168–169.

Chittenden HB, Harman KE, Robinson F, Higgins EM (2002) A case of encephalocraniocutaneous lipomato-sis. Br J Ophthalmol 86: 934–935.

Cultrera F, Guarnera F, Giardina MC (2004) Overlap among neurocutaneous syndromes. Observations on encephalo-craniocutaneous lipomatosis. Minerva Pediatr 56(2): 219–222.

Donaire A, Carreno M, Bargallo N, Setoain X, Agudo R, Martin G, Boget T, Raspall T, Pintor L, Rumia J (2005) Presurgical evaluation and cognitive functional reorganization in Fishman syndrome. Epilepsy Behav 6(3): 440–443.

Fishman MA (1987) Encephalocraniocutaneous lipomato-sis. J Child Neurol 2(3): 186–193.

Fishman MA, Chang CS, Miller JE (1978) Encephalocran-iocutaneous lipomatosis. Pediatrics 61(4): 580–582.

Fishman MA, Encephalocraniocutaneous lipomatosis (2004) In: Roach ES, Van S Miller (eds.) Neurocutaneous dis-orders, Cambridge University Press, Cambridge, pp. 301–305.

Gawel J, Schwartz RA, Jóźwiak S (2003) Encephalocranio-cutaneous lipomatosis. J Cutan Med Surg 7(1): 61–67.

Grimalt R, Ermacora E, Mistura L, Russo G, Tadini GL, Triulzi F, Cavicchini S, Rondanini GF, Caputo R (1993) Encephalocraniocutaneous lipomatosis: case re-port and review of the literature. Pediatr Dermatol 10(2): 164–168.

Haberland C, Perou M (1970) Encephalocraniocutaneous lipomatosis. A new example of ectomesodermal dysgen-esis. Arch Neurol 22(2): 144–155.

Hamm H (1999) Cutaneous mosaicism of lethal mutations. Am J Med Genet 85(4): 342–345.

Happle R, Kuster W (1998) Negus psiloliparus: a distinct fatty tissue nevus. Dermatology 197: 6–10.

Happle R, Horster S (2004) Nevus psiloliparus: report of two nonsyndromic cases. Eur J Dermatol 14(5): 314–316.

Hardman CM, Garioch JJ, Eady RA, Fry L (1998) Focal der-mal hypoplasia: report of a case with cutaneous and skeletal manifestations. Clin Exp Dermatol 23: 281–285.

Hauber K, Warmuth-Metz M, Rose C, Brocker EB, Hamm H (2003) Encephalocraniocutaneous lipomatosis: a case with unilateral odontomas and review of the literature. Eur J Pediatr 162: 589–593.

Hunter AG (2006) Oculocerebrocutaneous and encephalo-craniocutaneous lipomatosis syndromes: blind men and an elephant or separate syndromes? Am J Med Genet A 140: 709–726.

Jóźwiak S, Gawel J, Kasprzyk-Obara J (2001) En-cephalocraniocutaneous lipomatosis – case report. Pe-diatr Pol 76: 53–56.

Kodsi SR, Bloom KE, Egbert JE, Holland EJ, Cameron JD (1994) Ocular and systemic manifestations of en-cephalocraniocutaneous lipomatosis. Am J Ophthalmol 118(1): 77–82.

Lasierra R, Valencia I, Carapeto FJ, Ventura P, Samper MP, Rodriguez G, Perez-Gonzalez JM, Legido A (2003) Encephalocraniocutaneous lipomatosis: neurologic man-ifestations. J Child Neurol 18: 725–729.

Legius E, Wu R, Eyssen M, Marynen P, Fryns JP, Cassi-man JJ (1995) Encephalocraniocutaneous lipomatosis with a mutation in the NF1 gene. J Med Genet 32(4): 316–319.

Loggers HE, Oosterwijk JC, Overweg-Plandosen WCG, van Wilsem A, Bleeker-Wagemakers EM, Bijlsma JB (1992) Encephalocraniocutaneous lipomatosis and oculocerebro-cutaneous syndrome. Ophthalmic Genet 13: 171–177.

MacLaren MJ, Kluijt I, Koole FD (1995) Ophthalmologic abnormalities in encephalocraniocutaneous lipomato-sis. Doc Ophthalmol 90: 87–98.

McCall S, Ramzy MI, Cure JK, Pai GS (1992) En-cephalocraniocutaneous lipomatosis and the Proteus syndrome: distinct entities with overlapping manifesta-tions. Am J Med Genet 43(4): 662–668.

Miyao M, Saito T, Yamamoto Y, Kamoshita S (1984) En-cephalocraniocutaneous lipomatosis: a recently described neurocutaneous syndrome. Child's Brain 11: 280–284.

Moog U, de Die-Smulders C, Systermans JM, Cobben JM (1997) Oculocerebrocutaneous syndrome: report of three additional cases and aetiological considerations. Clin Genet 52: 219–225.

Moog U, Jones MC, Viskochil DH, Verloes A, Van Allen MI, Dobyns WB (2007) Brain anomalies in encephalocran-iocutaneous lipomatosis. Am J Med Genet A 143: 2963–2972

Moog U, Roelens F, Mortier GR, Sijstermans H, Kelly M, Cox GF, Robson CD, Kimonis VE (2007) Encephalocraniocutaneous lipomatosis accompanied by the formation of bone cysts: Harboring clues to pathogenesis? Am J Med Genet A 143: 2973–2980.

Narbay G, Meire F, Verloes A, Casteels I, Devos E (1996) Ocular manifestations in Delleman syndrome (Oculocerebrocutaneous syndrome, OCC-syndrome) and encephalocranio-cutaneous lipomatosis (ECCL). Report of three cases. Bull Soc Belge Ophtalmol 261: 65–70.

Nosti-Martinez D, del Castillo V, Duran-Mckinster C (1995) Encephalocraniocutaneous lipomatosis: an uncommon neurocutaneous syndrome. J Am Acad Dermatol 32: 387–389.

Nowaczyk MJ, Mernagh JR, Bourgeois JM, Thompson PJ, Jurriaans E (2000) Antenatal and postnatal findings in encephalocraniocutaneous lipomatosis. Am J Med Genet 91(4): 261–266.

Parazzini C, Triulzi F, Russo G, Mastrangelo M, Scotti G (1999) Encephalocraniocutaneous lipomatosis: complete neuroradiologic evaluation and follow up of two cases. Am J Neuroradiol 20: 173–176.

Rizzo R, Pavone L, Micali G, Nigro F, Cohen MM Jr (1993) Encephalocraniocutaneous lipomatosis, Proteus syndrome, and somatic mosaicism. Am J Med Genet 47(5): 653–655.

Romiti R, Rengifo JA, Arnone M, Sotto MN, Valente NY, Jansen T (1999) Encephalocraniocutaneous lipomatosis: a new case report and review of the literature. J Dermatol 26(12): 808–812.

Roszkowski M, Dabrowski D (1997) Encephalo-cranio-cutaneous lipomatosis (ECCL) – Haberland syndrome. A case report with review of the literature. Neurol Neurochir Pol 31(3): 607–613.

Rubegni P, Risulo M, Sbano P, Buonocore G, Perrone S, Fimiani M (2003) Encephalocraniocutaneous lipomatosis (Haberland syndrome) with bilateral cutaneous and visceral involvement. Clin Exp Dermatol 28: 387–390.

Sanchez NP, Rhodes AR, Mandell F, Mihm MC (1981) Encephalocraniocutaneous lipomatosis: a new neurocutaneous syndrome. Br J Dermatol 104(1): 89–96.

Sant'Anna GD, Saffer M, Mauri M, Facco S, Raupp S (1999) Encephalocraniocutaneous lipomatosis with otolaryngologic manifestations: a rare neurocutaneous syndrome. Int J Pediatr Otorhinolaryngol 49(3): 231–235.

Savage MG, Heldt L, Dann JJ, Bump RL (1985) Encephalocraniocutaneous lipomatosis and mixed odontogenic tumors. J Oral Maxillofac Surg 43(8): 617–620.

Schlack HG, Skopnik H (1985) Encephalocraniocutaneous lipomatosis and linear naevus sebaceus. Monatsschr Kinderheilkd 133(4): 235–237.

Sofiatti A, Cirto AG, Arnone M, Romiti R, Santi C, Leite C, Sotto M (2006) Encephalocraniocutaneous lipomatosis: clinical spectrum of systemic involvement. Pediatr Dermatol 23: 27–30.

Stieler KM, Astner S, Bohner G, Bartels NG, Proquitté H, Sterry W, Haas N, Blume-Peytavi U (2008) Encephalocraniocutaneous lipomatosis with didymosis aplasticopsilolipara. Arch Dermatol 144: 266–268.

Torrelo A, del C Boente M, Nieto O, Facco S, Raupp S (2005) Nevus psiloliparus and aplasia cutis: a further possible explanation of didymosis. Pediatr Dermatol 22: 206–209.

Wiedemann HR, Burgio GR (1986) Encephalocraniocutaneous lipomatosis and Proteus syndrome. Am J Med Genet 25(2): 403–404.

Zielinska-Kazmierska B, Grodecka J, Jablonska-Polakowska L, Arkuszewski P (2005) Mandibular osteoma in the encephalocraniocutaneous lipomatosis. J Craniomaxillofac Surg 33(4): 286–289.

# Chapter 31

# PROTEUS SYNDROME

**Martino Ruggieri and Ignacio Pascual-Castroviejo**

Institute of Neurological Science, National Research Council, Catania, and Department of Paediatrics, University of Catania, Catania, Italy (MR); Paediatric Neurology Service, University Hospital La Paz, University of Madrid, Madrid, Spain (IPC)

## Introduction

*Proteus syndrome* (OMIM # 176920) (OMIM™ 2005), a rare and highly variable congenital hamartomatous disorder (Gorlin et al. 2001), is a member of a group designated as local *"overgrowth diseases"* (Cohen et al. 2002). It consists of asymmetric (mosaic), disproportionate and progressive overgrowth of body parts, connective tissue nevi, epidermal nevi, dysregulated adipose tissue, vascular and lymphatic malformations, and visceral abnormalities (Cohen 2005; Biesecker 2001, 2006). Although the cause of Proteus syndrome is as yet unknown (Barker et al. 2001, Biesecker et al. 2001), it is thought to arise from a sporadic postzygotic mutation (Cohen et al. 2002, Gorlin et al. 2001, Turner et al. 2004).

Some authors in the dermatology literature (Happle 1991, 1995a, b, 2004; Sugarman and Frieden 2004; Vujevich and Mancini 2004) have suggested that this condition along with other complex malformation syndromes associated with epidermal nevi (e.g., Nevus comedonicus syndrome, (Becker's) pigmented hairy epidermal nevus syndrome, CHILD syndrome and Schimmelpenning-Feuerstein-Mims syndrome) should be comprised into the umbrella spectrum of the "epidermal nevus syndromes" (see also chapter on the epidermal nevus syndromes and Sugarman 2004).

## Historical perspective and terminology

Although first reported in contemporary medical literature by Cohen and Hayden (1979), who distinguished it from neurofibromatosis and Klippel-Trenaunay syndrome (Cohen et al. 2002, OMIM™ 2005), individual case reports of patients with Proteus syndrome can be traced as early as 1907 (Wieland 1907). The condition was not widely appreciated, however, until Wiedemann et al. (1983) reported four cases in the paediatric literature and delineated this condition with the name of *Proteus* ("The polymorphous"), because of the polymorphic and hamartoplastic nature of its features.

Proteus was a legendary ancient Greek hero, transformed by the gods into an immortal demon of the sea ("the old man of the sea") with prophetic powers (Child et al. 1998). He knew everything in the past, present and future but hated to divulge the information and therefore to evade capture was given the power to change his shape at will (Child et al. 1998, Clark 1994). His impressive ability of transfiguration was lyrically described in Homer's Odyssey. While engaged in a fight with Menelaus and his companions, Proteus appeared variously as a lion, a dragon, a tree, and even as water (Goodship et al. 1991, Bouzas et al. 1993). In order to obtain information from Proteus he had to be caught and bound during his noon-day slumber.

Wiedeman et al. (1983) suggested that the patient reported by Temtany and Rogers (1976) and probably also the case of Graetz (1928) may have had this disorder.

There is currently a body of evidence that supports the Proteus syndrome (rather than neurofibromatosis) as a diagnosis for Joseph Merrick, also known as the *"Elephant Man"*, (Cohen 1986, 1988a, b; Cohen et al. 2002; OMIM™ 2005; Seward 1994; Tibbles and Cohen 1986). Joseph Carey Merrick was born in 1862 in Leicester, UK with an apparently normal familial, obstetric and neonatal history. Typically, overgrowth began to develop at about 18 months of age and progressed to adulthood. When he was 22 years of age, his case was fully described by Sir Frederick Treves (Unsigned Comment 1884, 1886; Treves 1885a, b, 1923) who saw Merrick earning a living by exhibiting himself as a freak under the showman Tom Norton (Howard and Ford 1980). Treves negotiated to take Merrick (aged 24 years) to his room at the London Hospital Medical College. Following a continental tour under an Austrian manager (Howard and Hughes 1980, Treves 1923), Merrick returned to England and was housed in two rooms of the east Wing of the London Hospital where he died on April 1890 (Unsigned report 1890). Merrick had the following features of Proteus syndrome (Cohen 1986, 1988a, b; Tibbles and Cohen 1986): macrocephaly, hyperostoses of the skull, asymmetric long-bone overgrowth, macrodactyly, thickened skin and subcutaneous tissues particularly of the hands and feet (including moccasin-type plantar hyperplasia) and other unspecified subcutaneous masses (Clark 1994, Cohen et al. 2002). Besides NF1 other diagnoses have been entertained including Maffucci syndrome, Paget's disease of the bone, pyarthrosis, and fibrous dysplasia (Clark 1994, Cohen et al. 2002, Seward 1994). In the case of Joseph Merrick, there was no evidence of café-au-lait spots or neurofibromas in adulthood and whilst normal at birth he went on developing more severe manifestations than those usually encountered with NF1 (Cohen et al. 2002) (see also chapter 3 for discussion).

## Incidence and prevalence

Relatively few cases – approximately 100 meeting the revised diagnostic criteria (see Table 1) – have been reported so far (Cohen 1993, Cohen et al. 2002, Turner et al. 2004) with a male/female ratio of 1:9 (Turner et al. 2004). Similar figures have been recorded by Biesecker (Turner et al. 2004) at the NIH Proteus syndrome clinic (males vs. females ratio of 1:75). The parental age at the time of birth is usually within the normal reproductive age range.

Severe cases of Proteus syndrome may be diagnosed prenatally by ultrasonographic findings of cranial and extremity hemihypertrophy (Sigaudy et al. 1998). However even though birth weight may be increased

in Proteus syndromes with some newborns weighing 4000 g or more, normal birth weight and even small-for-gestational-age infants have been observed.

One issue in the literature has been the number of publications bearing the name "Proteus syndrome" in the title and in fact describing patients who can be demonstrated not to have the syndrome. Cohen et al. (2002) and Turner et al. (2004) critically reassessed the 250 cases published under the name of Proteus syndrome in the literature by applying the existing diagnostic criteria (Biesecker et al. 1999; Table 1) and found that only 47% could be truly diagnosed as having the condition while at least 39% clearly did not meet the criteria and a remaining 14% had features suggestive of Proteus syndrome but lacked sufficient clinical data to make this diagnosis. Several problems were apparent in these cases (Cohen et al. 2002, Turner et al. 2004): 1) misdiagnoses with other well known syndromes (e.g., Klippel-Trenaunay syndrome, hemihyperplasia/lipomatosis syndrome, etc.); 2) provisional, intriguing unique pattern syndromes similar but not fitting into the category of Proteus syndrome (see for example Dean et al. 1990, Ho et al. 1999, McMullin et al. 1993, Okumura et al. 1986, Raman et al. 1989, Reardon et al. 1996, Zhou et al. 2000); 3) misdiagnosis in cases of "congenital" hyperplastic overgrowth of limbs (patients with Proteus syndrome are usually normal at birth or may present with mild to moderate hyperplasia); 4) poor or little documentation in many reports to establish a diagnosis with certainty; 5) mismatch with lists/synopses of abnormalities not related to Proteus syndrome; and 6) reverse diagnostic situations with the so-called "Thanos syndrome" (Thanos et al. 1977) which in fact no longer exists (Cohen 1999).

## Clinical manifestations

The hallmarks of the disorder are asymmetrical, disproportionate overgrowth of the trunk, head, extremities or digits, bulky lipomatous or mixed tissue hamartomas (lipo/lymph/haemangiomas), linear epidermal nevi, prominent veins, exostoses (hyperostosis) of the skull and partial lypodystrophy (Table 1). Gyriform hyperplasia of the soles, and occasionally of the

**Table 1.** Revised* diagnostic criteria for Proteus syndrome

| For diagnosis | General criteria (all mandatory) + specific criteria (category signs) | |
|---|---|---|
| | Mosaic distribution of lesions | Either category A or |
| | Sporadic occurrence | 2 from category B or |
| | Progressive course | 3 from category C |
| Category signs | Manifestations | |
| A | 1. Cerebriform connective tissue nevi[a] | |
| B | 1. Linear epidermal nevus | |
| | 2. Asymmetric, disproportionate overgrowth[b] | |
| |    (one or more): | |
| |      Limbs | |
| |         Arms/legs | |
| |         Hands/feet/digits | |
| |         Extremities | |
| |      Hyperostoses of the skull | |
| |      External auditory meatus | |
| |      Megaspondylodysplasia | |
| |      Viscera | |
| |         Spleen/thymus | |
| | 3. Specific tumours before 2nd decade | |
| |    (one of the following): | |
| |      Ovarian cyst adenoma | |
| |      Parotid monomorphic adenoma | |
| | 4. Lung cysts | |
| C | 1. Dysregulate adipose tissue (either one): | |
| |      Lipomas | |
| |      Regional absence of fat | |
| | 2. Vascular malformations (one or more): | |
| |      Capillary malformations | |
| |      Venous malformations | |
| |      Lymphatic malformation | |
| | 3. Facial phenotype[c] (all): | |
| |      Dolichocephalism | |
| |      Long face | |
| |      Down slanting palpebral fissures and/or | |
| |         minor ptosis | |
| |      Low nasal bridge | |
| |      Wide or anteverted nostrils | |
| |      Open mouth at rest | |

[a]Cerebriform connective tissue nevi are skin lesions characterised by deep grooves and gyrations as seen in the surface of the brain.

[b]Asymmetric, disproportionate overgrowth should be carefully distinguished from asymmetric, proportionate overgrowth (see text).

[c]The facial phenotype has been found, so far, only in Proteus syndrome patients who have mental deficiency, and (in some cases) seizures and/or brain malformations.

*Adapted from Biesecker (2006), Biesecker et al. (1999), Cohen (2005), Cohen et al. (2002) and Turner et al. (2004).

palms is pathognomonic for Proteus syndrome (see also below).

## Skin abnormalities

The cutaneous lesions of Proteus syndrome are varied, distinctive and of diagnostic significance (Sampaio et al. 2006).

*Cerebriform connective tissue nevi* (which has replaced the terms connective tissue naevi, collagenoma, plantar hyperplasia and moccasin lesion) (Turner et al. 2004) are common, but not obligatory. They can be recorded anywhere in the body, but most frequently on the sole of the foot (Cohen and Haydn 1979), palm of the hands (Biesecker et al. 1998, Cohen et al. 2002), and more rarely on the chest and abdomen, dorsal aspects of the fingers, eyelid and nasal tissues (Cohen et al. 2002). Overgrowth of cutaneous-subcutaneous connective tissue of palms and soles gives them the appearance of cerebriform surface (Fig. 1a–e), but these aspects can also be seen in the skin of other regions of the body (Fig. 2). The typical cerebriform connective tissue naevi of Proteus syndrome are progressive, firm and nodular or cobblestone-like in structure and develop deep grooves and gyrations (hence the term cerebriform), a consistency that is firmer than the normal tissue (Cohen 1995, Cohen and Hayden 1979, Turner et al. 2004). Conversely, in non-Proteus patients (Turner et al. 2004) such overgrowth has only mildly exaggerated creases and is either softer or not different from the consistency of normal sole tissue. Areas of the body with these connective tissue anomalies usually present disproportionate overgrowth, commonly asymmetric in nature (Fig. 2) that can involve digits, hands, feet (Fig. 3), arms, legs, trunk (Fig. 4), head (Fig. 5) or facial regions (Fig. 6).

Histologically, connective tissue nevi are composed of highly collagenised fibrous connective tissue (Biesecker et al. 1999, Hoey et al. 2008) and a collagenoma has been defined as an abnormality of the extra-cellular dermal matrix, in which collagen is found in excess. Although cerebriform connective tissue naevi are collagenomas, the reverse is not always true.

Other skin lesions consist of flat, *non-organoid (epidermal) nevi* and are variable among the patients, most frequently evident in early life and located in the ipsilateral back (Fig. 7) or lateral zones of the trunk or extremities. The typical epidermal nevi of Proteus syndrome have a slightly raised and rough texture. The colour is most frequently brown/brown black or blue/grey and the consistency is soft rather than hard with faint lines coursing throughout; it is not waxy, yellow, or scaly. Histological characteristics

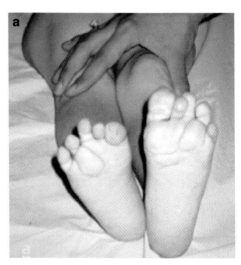

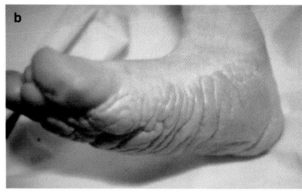

**Fig. 1.** Natural history of the cerebriform connective tissue nevus (of the feet) in Proteus syndrome: (**a**) early stages (age three years) of patchy hypertrophy of the upper region of the soles in both feet in a child with Proteus syndrome (same child shown in Figs. 3a–b, 4 and 6b); (**b**) and (**c**) further hypertrophy of the soles which have a "moccasin-like" aspect; (**d**) the soles of the feet show a cerebriform surface that extends partially in the right foot and totally in the hypertrophic left foot; (**e**) the left foot shows hypertrophy of the subcutaneous connective tissue and veins and gigantism of the toe and the second finger [(d) and (e) same child shown in Fig. 2] (Clinical and photographic follow-up of the case in Fig. 1b has been published by Schepis et al. 2008) [Fig. 1a, by courtesy of professor T. Mattina (Catania) and Fig. 1c, by courtesy of professor R. Ruiz-Maldonado (Mexico City)].

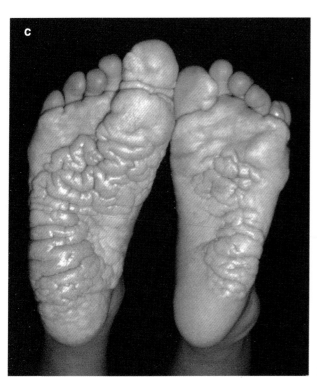

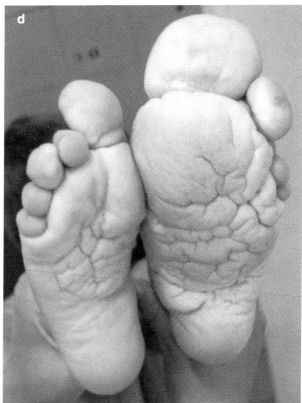

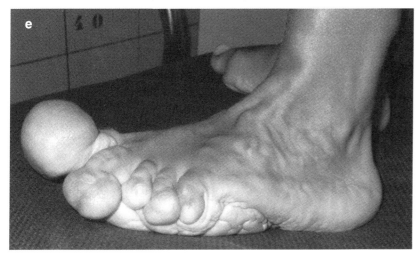

Fig. 1. (Continued)

have been seldom reported (Nazzaro et al. 1991), with lesions showing hyperorthokeratosis, acanthosis, and papillomatosis.

Infrequently, a single or few *café-au-lait spot* may be observed. Areas of patchy *dermal hypoplasia* (Fig. 8) with prominent veins in the allegedly unaffected areas of skin (explained as examples of twin spotting: see below "*Elattoproteus syndrome*") (Happle et al. 1997) and of *hypopigmentation* have also been noted.

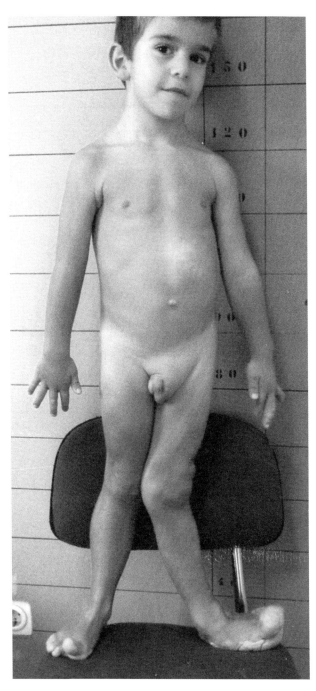

**Fig. 2.** This child with Proteus syndrome shows generalized asymmetric organs with overgrowth of the left structures, and large cutaneous nevus in the left side of the trunk.

## Vascular abnormalities

These may be of the capillary, venous, or lymphatic type, or may occur as combined channel anomalies

(Hoeger et al. 2004). The most commonly reported vascular abnormalities (70–100% of cases) in one series (Hoeger et al. 2004) were vascular tumours predominantly of the haemangioma or lymphangioma types or mixed lipo-/lympho-/heamangioma (the latter probably representing either lipomas with a vascular stroma and combined lymphatic-capillary malformations), port-wine stains, venous abnormalities including varicosities or prominent veins and other miscellaneous vascular malformations. Histologically these are developmental anomalies lined by flat endothelium which grow proportionately with the patient: they never regress but they can expand. Varicose veins have been reported in the abdomen and legs (Cohen et al. 2002).

## Tumours

The bulky and disfiguring subcutaneous masses, typically on the chest, back and abdomen (Fig. 4), are usually histologically benign *hamartomas* of mixed tissue origin. Often designated as lipomas, they are better described as lipomatous tumours because they usually lack the discrete encapsulated form required for the diagnosis of a true lipoma.

True *lipomas* composed mainly of mature adipocytes are occasionally present in Proteus syndrome, and these may be either confined or infiltrative. Decreased and increased fat in the same patient at different sites in the body have been reported (Cohen 1993, Happle 1995b, Shovby et al. 1993). Histologically, lipomas are benign tumours, and superficial lesions which tend to be confined, but the location is important as well due to the invasive behaviour of intrathoracic and intra-abdominal lipomas, despite benign histological appearance (Biesecker et al. 1999).

Several *unusual types of tumours*, such as ovarian cyst adenoma, testicular tumours, intracranial or spinal meningiomas, adenoma of the parotid gland, have been occasionally reported (Costa et al. 1985, Cohen 1993, Gordon et al. 1995). Unusual tumours are listed in Table 1 and reviewed by Cohen et al. (2002). Multiple tumours are found in some cases (Table 2). Malignant transformation is rare, although it has been documented.

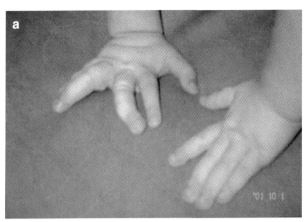

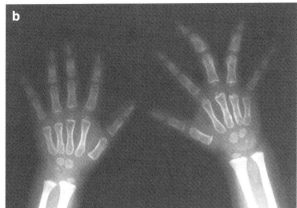

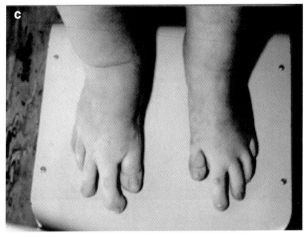

**Fig. 3.** Asymmetric growth of fingers as shown at clinical (**a**) and X-ray examination (**b**) of both hands in a child with Proteus syndrome as compared to symmetric overgrowth (**c**) in a child with non-Proteus syndrome.

## Abnormalities of other organs and systems

*Skeletal abnormalities.* Disproportionate overgrowth can also involve skeletal structures, such as hemicranium, hemivertebrae, bones of one limbs (or all extremities) (Fig. 3b), causing scoliosis, Kyphoscoliosis, genu valga, heel valgus, facial and/or cranial asymmetry (Fig. 5) involving teeth and nerves as well (Becktor et al. 2002) with associated instability of pelvic bones and pubic fracture (Fig. 9) (Velazquez Fraguas and Pascual-Castroviejo 2003). Even though external overgrowth is most common, any internal organ may be involved (Biesecker et al. 1998). An important issue (which delineates a specific diagnostic criteria) (Biesecker 2001, Turner et al. 2004) is the disproportionate bony overgrowth (often associated with invasion of the joints) which is typical of Pro-

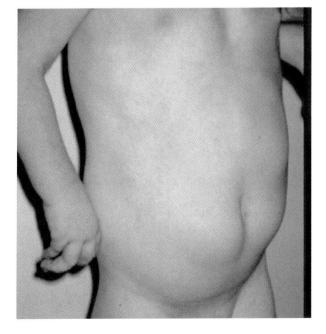

**Fig. 4.** Mutiple subcutaneous, bulky masses (lipoma-lke) in a child with Proteus syndrome.

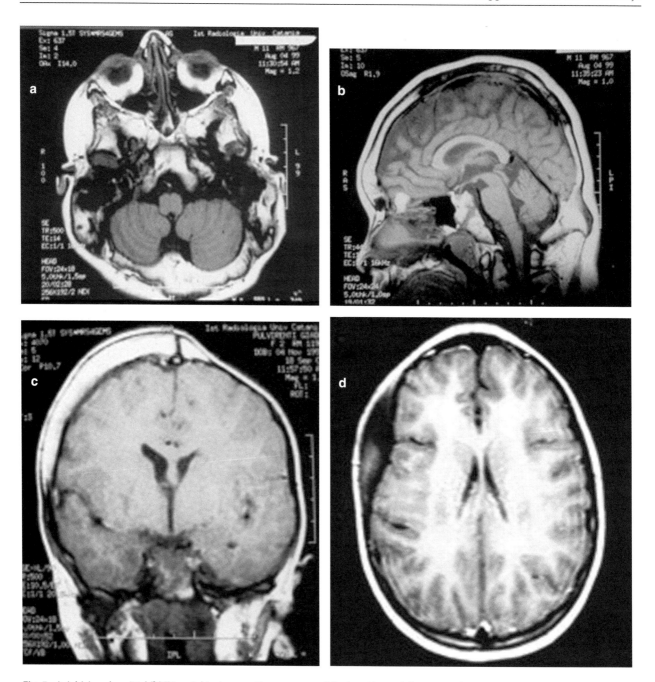

**Fig. 5.** Axial (**a**) and sagittal (**b**) T1-weighted magnetic resonance of the head in a adolescent with Proteus syndrome showing dispropor-tionate overgrowth of the posterior fossa (**a**) and fronto-parietal (**b**) bones; coronal (**c**) T1-weighted magnetic resonance images of the head (same child shown in Figs. 1a, 3a–b, 4 and 6b) showing disproportionate overgrowth of the right inner table of the bones of the parietal cranial vault; (**d**) axial T1-weighted magnetic resonance and coronal computerised tomography images of the head in an adoles-cent with Proteus syndrome: note the mass effect (**d**) of the bony overgrowth (**e**) on the right temporal lobes of the brain.

teus syndrome vs. the proportionate overgrowth (even severe) seen in patients not classified as Pro-teus syndrome (Biesecker 2001).

*Uncommon bony abnormalities* include cervical spine fusion, angular kyphosis with spinal stenosis, clinodactyly, cubitus valgus, radial head subluxation,

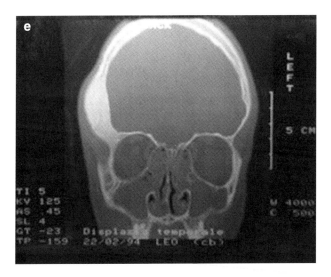

**Fig. 5.** (Continued)

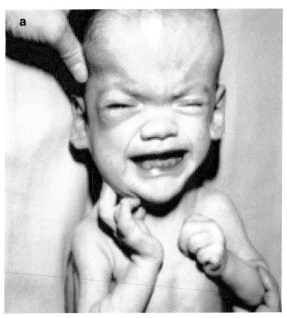

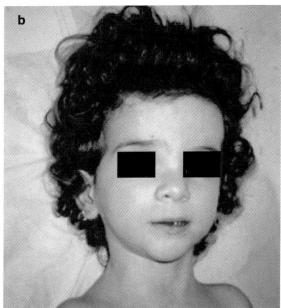

**Fig. 6.** Facial phenotype in Proteus syndrome: (**a**) severe facial dysmorphism in a 6-month child showing dolichocephalism, long face, down slanting of the palpebral fissures with congenital ptosis, low nasal bridge and wide nostrils accompanied by a severe degree of craniofacial distortion due to skull overgrowth; (**b**) moderate facial dysmorphism with high forehead, hypertelorism, low nasal bridge, large nose and philtrum, long face (the other associated features of this girl are shown in Figs. 1a, 3a–b, 4 and 5c) (Clinical and photographic follow-up of the case shown in Fig. 6b have been published by Schepis et al. 2008) [Figs. 6a and b are by courtesy of professors G. Sorge and T. Mattina (Catania), respectively].

elbow ankylosis, pectus excavatum, hip dysplasia, coax valga – plana – vara, genu recurvatum, absent patella, tibial bowing, fibular bowing, gaps between the first and second toes, highly arched palate, and mandibular prognatism (reviewed by Cohen et al. 2002 and Taybi and Lachman 1996).

According to Cohen (1993) and Kreiborg et al. (1991) four types of abnormal *craniofacial growth* (Figs. 5–6) can act singly or in various combinations: a) hyperostoses; b) unilateral condylar hyperplasia; c) abnormal cranial remodelling (secondary to hemimegalencephaly); and d) craniosynostosis (Cohen et al. 2002). Notably, hyperostoses are bony overgrowths rather than true tumours and may occur in calvarial, facial, nasal, alveolar, and mandibular bones (Cohen et al. 2002, Taybi and Lachman 1996).

*Other organs.* Although limb overgrowth is most common in Proteus syndrome, perhaps any organ may be involved. Splenomegaly and enlargement of the thymus have been rarely recorded.

*Orbit and eyes* are frequently involved and show several abnormalities (the true frequency of which is unknown) of whom some are secondary to exostoses, such as strabismus, "enlarged eye" or nystagmus, but other lesions, such as epibulbar tumours, posterior segment hamartomas, retinal coloboma, heterochromic irides, and others, may also be found (Bouzas et al. 1993).

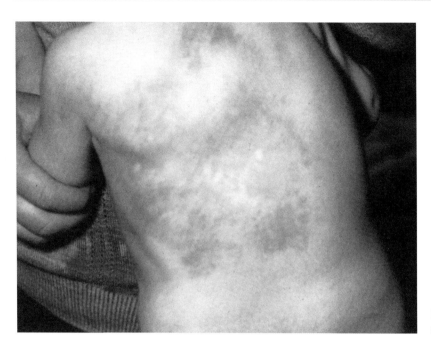

**Fig. 7.** Large nevus extending on the left side of the back.

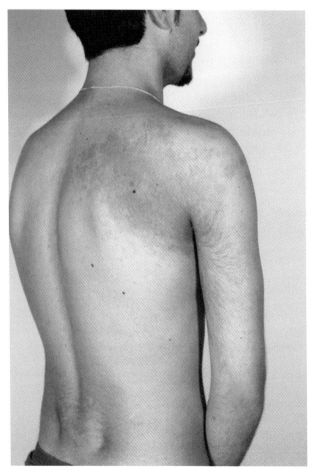

About 12–13% of patients with Proteus syndrome have cystic *lung* changes potentially lethal. Other pulmonary problems may be secondary to skeletal abnormalities (e.g., scoliosis) or tumours.

A variety of *renal abnormalities* have been recorded including nephrogenic diabetes insipidus, kidney cysts, vascular malformations of the bladder and kidney, ureterectasis, heminephronomegaly, duplicated renal systems and hydronephrosis.

*Miscellaneous abnormalities* include rectal polyposis, muscular atrophy, mixed bronchial hamartomas and vocal cord nodules.

## Nervous system abnormalities

Although the intelligence is usually normal in Proteus syndrome, there have been several instances of mental retardation. According to Cohen et al. (2002) *mental deficiency* has been evident in 20% of cases and *seizures* have been documented in approximately 13%. Ohtahara syndrome has been also documented (Bastos et al. 2008).

**Fig. 8.** Bilateral patchy areas of dermal hypoplasia in the lumbar region of an adolescent with Proteus syndrome (same patient shown in Fig. 5d and e): this phenomenon is regarded as an *Elattoproteus* phenotype (see text).

**Table 2.** Tumours in Proteus syndrome

*Uncommon tumours*
Meningioma
Multiple meningiomas
Optic nerve tumour
Pinealoma
Monomorphic adenoma (parotid gland)
Intraductal papilloma & epithelial hyperplasia (breast)
Unilateral breast hyperplasia
Goiter (thyroid)
Cyst or cystadenoma (ovary)
Leiomyoma
Giant cyst (kidney)
Sacrococcygeal teratoma
Mesothelioma
Papillary adenocarcinoma
Papillary adenoma (appendix testis)
Cystadenoma (bilateral epididymis)
Endometrial carcinoma

*Multiple tumours in the same patient*
Meningioma and optic nerve tumour
Multiple meningiomas
Multiple meningiomas and leiomyoma of the bladder
Monomorphic adenoma (parotid) and intraductal papilloma (breast)
Meningioma, multiple leiomyomas of the uterus and ovarian cysts
Bilateral ovarian serous cystadenomas
Endometrial carcinoma and unilateral breast hyperplasia

Adapted from Cohen et al. (2002) and Turner et al. (2004).

A number of cases have had *brain abnormalities* including micro and macrocephaly, hemimegalencephaly, thickened leptomeninges, dural ectasia, polymicrogyria, heterotopic grey matter nodules in the subcortical and periventricular white matter, heterotopic neurons in the cortex and white matter, double cortex, dilated ventricles, hydrocephalus, subependimal periventricular calcified nodules, porencephalic cysts, subarachnoid cysts, arachnoid cysts of the posterior fossa, cystic brain lesions, Dandy-Walker complex anomalies, cortical atrophy, absence of (or thickened) corpus callosum, abnormal signal lesions (hypodense at CT or hyperintense at MRI) in the periventricular white matter, hypoplastic white matter, cavum Vergae cavities, dural sinus thrombosis, meningiomas, astrocytomas, spinal cord stenosis, spinal cord lipomas and syringohydromyelia (Anik et al. 2007; and reviewed in Cremin et al. 1987, Dietrich et al. 1998, Taybi and Lachman 1996, Turner et al. 2004).

According to our own and other authors (Biesecker 2001, Cohen et al. 2002, Mayatepek et al. 1989, Turner et al. 2004) experience mental handicap correlates with a more severe phenotype (see Fig. 6b): the worst (in terms of mosaic lesions) and wider the body involvement the poorer is the cognitive outcome.

Neurological complications can ensue because of primary brain abnormalities (e.g., malformations) or are due to compression secondary to bony

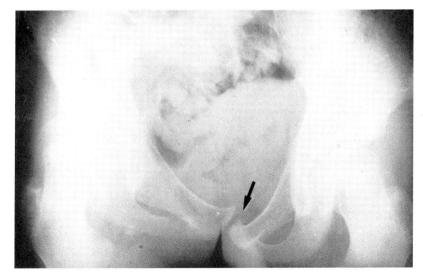

**Fig. 9.** X-ray films show pubic fracture (black arrow).

overgrowth or (benign) tumour localisations in the CNS.

## Facial dysmorphism

A distinctive *facial phenotype* (Fig. 6) including dolichocephalism, long face, minor down slanting of the palpebral fissures and/or minor congenital ptosis, low nasal bridge, wide or anteverted nostrils, and an open mouth at rest accompanied by several degree of craniofacial distortion due to skull vergrowth has been associated with severe mental deficiency, seizures and/or brain malformations (see also above) (Cohen et al. 2002, Rizzo et al. 1990).

## Natural history

Tissue overgrowth is progressive in nature, but usually appears to plateau after puberty and during adolescence (Cohen 1993, Gordon 1995). Most epidermal nevi and vascular malformations are reported to appear in the first month of life and have little tendency for expansion or development of additional lesions. Subcutaneous lipomas and cerebriform connective tissue nevi are commonly noted in the first year of life, progressively increase in size with additional lesions at new locations (Tweede et al. 2005). Genital development of males with Proteus syndrome may be normal, hypotrophic or hypertrophic. Evolution and prognosis is related to the severity of the single clinical features of the patients. Seizures and severe mental delay are usually associated with a poor prognosis (Cohen 1993) as well as tumours. Because the potential for malignant transformation remains unknown, patients with Proteus syndrome should be carefully monitored.

## Causes of death

Early death is most often caused by (or attributed to) pulmonary embolism and/or asphyxia (usually due to vascular abnormalities – see above under skin manifestations), pneumonia (and congestive hart failure), laryngospasm, postoperative causes (mainly spinal surgery), surgical convalescence and immobil-

ity, cerebellar abscesses, sepsis with cerebral abscess, respiratory emphysematous pulmonary disease, complications during epileptic seizures or by sudden and unexplained causes (Cohen 2001, Horie et al. 1995, Kontras 1974, Newman et al. 1994, Slavotinek et al. 2001; reviewed in Cohen et al. 2002 and Turner et al. 2004). Some of these cases occurred in children under 10 years of age (due to pulmonary embolism, pneumonia, epileptic seizures, cerebellar abscess) or teenagers (pulmonary embolism, postoperative death, respiratory empyshematous disease and laryngospasm) (reviewed by Cohen et al. 2002).

## "Elattoproteus syndrome"

Happle et al. (1999) suggested the designation *Elattoproteus syndrome* for a disorder that he considered to be an inverse form of Proteus syndrome (OMIM™ 2005). He described a 7-year-old boy with partial lipohypoplasia and patchy dermal hypoplasia involving large areas of his body. These areas of deficient growth were similar to those described in many cases of Proteus syndrome. Paradoxically, however, he had only a few rather mild lesions of disproportionate overgrowth. The presence of hyperostosis of the external auditory meatus was taken as a highly characteristic sign of Proteus syndrome (Cohen 1993, Smeets et al. 1994). Happle (1999) proposed to explain this unusual phenotype by the contemporary occurrence (twin spotting) of allelic mutations giving rise to either over- and deficient growth of somatic tissues (the latter called "*elatton*" which means *minus*). Patients affected by Proteus syndrome may show classic overgrowth or a mixture of Pleioproteus (from the Greek "*pleion*" which means *plus*) and Elattoproteus lesions or even an isolated elattoproteus phenotype (Fig. 8).

## Pathogenesis/molecular genetics

Proteus syndrome is by definition sporadic (Table 1). In some cases, the disorder has suggested somatic mosaicism – lethal in the non-mosaic state – as the origin of the disease (Cohen 1993, Cohen et al. 2002, Happle 1993, Say and Carpenter 1988): the hypothesis was raised after two instances of mo- nozygotic twins discordant for Proteus syndrome (Holmes 1997, Schwartz et al. 1991). Differences have also been found in the normal vs. the affected areas of another Proteus patient (Schwartz 1991) as occurs in other mosaic/localised autosomal domi- nant conditions (Ruggieri 2001, Ruggieri and Huson 2001). This mechanism has been also suggested for Schimmelpenning-Feuerstein-Mims syndrome (one of the epidermal nevus syndromes) (OMIM # 165630) and the McCune-Albright syndrome (OMIM # 174800) and proved in the case of the lat- ter condition. Rescue of a lethal gene by chimerism with normal embryos (Bennet 1978) is an experi- mental model of this mode of inheritance.

A possible vertical transmission either from fa- ther to son (Goodship et al. 1991) or from mother to son (Krüger et al. 1993) has been reported. How- ever both cases are not convincing as neither the parents nor their children have Proteus syndrome after critical re-evaluation (see also Cohen et al. 2002). In the case of Goodship et al. (1991) the 7- month-old son had left hemimegalencephaly with ipsilateral ventricular enlargement and gross cortical abnormalities, a lymphangioma over the right lum- bar region (surgically removed), a mass over the right lateral rib cage (clinically thought to be a lipoma), an epidermal nevus on the left side of the face and neck, seizures and developmental delay while his fa- ther had only mild facial asymmetry secondary to numerous operative procedures undergone during infancy for a right facial lymphangioma. In the fam- ily of Krüger et al. (1993) a mentally normal 2.5- year-old son with mild hypertrophy of the left side of the upper lip and cheek (with impaired mimic ex- pression in this region), hypertrophy of the left arm, partial gigantism of the left middle finger, and a large subcutaneous swelling (diagnosed by ultra- sound as a lipoma) in the upper left abdomen had a mother with mild facial asymmetry with hypertro- phy of the right lower cheek (and impaired mimic expression in that region).

Another discussed possibility has been "*paradomi- nant inheritance*" as proposed by Happle (1993, 2006): according to this hypothesis heterozygosity for a paradominant mutation would confer pheno-

typic normality and the allele may be transmitted unperceived for generations. The gene carrier would exhibit the disease phenotype when a somatic muta- tion occurred during embryogenesis, giving rise to a cell line that would be either hemizygous, from al- lelic loss, or homozygous, from a point mutation. The occurrence of Proteus syndrome either as an isolated phenotype (Aylsworth et al. 1987) or along with other mosaic skin disorders (Toro-Sola 1987) in consanguineous families (Aylsworth et al. 1987, Toro-Sola 1987) could be explained by such hypoth- esis (Danarti and Happle 2003).

The molecular pathology of Proteus syndrome remains elusive to date. There have been few investi- gations into the molecular basis of this disorder. Zhou et al. (2000) and Eng et al. (2001) examined the PTEN gene (phosphatase and tensin homologue gene) in patients with Proteus syndrome and Proteus- like syndromes and identified heterozygosity for a single base transversion resulting in arg 335-to-ter substitution in the PTEN gene product in two of nine patients with Proteus syndromes and in three of five patients with Proteus-like syndromes (the au- thors postulated that a second hit [arg 335-to-ter] could have occurred early in embryonic development and may even represent germ-line mosaicism). These findings were in line with other reports Smith et al. (2002) but were not confirmed by other au- thors (Barker et al. 2001, Biesecker et al. 2001, Cohen et al. 2003) who believe that, to date, no re- ported patient with a PTEN mutation has Proteus syndrome (Cohen et al. 2003). Similar conclusions were drawn by Thiffault et al. (2004) who screened affected and unaffected tissue from patients with Proteus syndrome finding no mutations neither in the PTEN gene nor in the GPC3. According to our experience in two of the 25 patients fulfilling the di- agnostic criteria for Proteus syndrome followed at our Institutions we detected PTEN gene mutations by means of DHPLC analysis and DNA sequencing (unreported data). Even though the cause(s) of Pro- teus syndrome, presently remain unknown there may exist a subgroup of Proteus patients which might harbour mutations of gene(s) involved in tissue overgrowth (see chapter on PTEN hamartomas-tu- mour syndromes – PHTS). This has been recently demonstrated in a widespread epidermal nevus lesion of a 3-year-old boy with Proteus syndrome who was found to harbour a novel germline p.Y68D mutation of the PTEN gene inherited from his mother who had cowden disease (Loffeld et al. 2006).

Other considered candidate genes have been the insulin-like growth factors (IGF) binding proteins (BP) whose local unbalance might cause disproportionate growth of tissues or the high mobility group protein gene HMGIC in the multiple aberration region (MAR) at 12q15 which has been associated to lipomas growth.

## Diagnosis

### Diagnostic criteria

The First National Conference on Proteus Syndrome for Parents and Families was held at NIH in Bethesda in 1998, and participants developed recommendations for diagnostic criteria (summarised in Table 1), differential diagnosis, and guidelines for the evaluation of patients (Table 3) (Biesecker 2006, Biesecker et al. 1999, Cohen 2005, Cohen et al. 2002). Turner et al. (2004) by reassessing the Proteus syndrome literature re-emphasised several of the criteria originally proposed by Biesecker et al. (1998) further delineating particular criteria which had generated confusion, adding more detail to the list of criteria and simplifying their overall organisation (Turner et al. 2004).

The revised diagnostic criteria (Table 1) include general and specific criteria, manifestations, and category of the signs required to make a diagnosis. As clinical manifestations can be numerous and with variable degree of severity category of signs in order of importance is necessary to make the diagnosis (see categories A, B and C). The relative frequency (indicated as common or uncommon) was avoided in the updated criteria (Table 1). General criteria (all mandatory) for the diagnosis of Proteus syndrome are: a) mosaic distribution of lesions; b) sporadic occurrence; and c) progressive course. At the present time, the single category sign in A appears to be sufficient for diagnosis. Either two category signs from B or three from C also appear to be sufficient for

diagnosis. Conversely, the use of combined partial criteria from B and C is no longer recommended (Cohen et al. 2002, Turner et al. 2004).

## Application and utility of diagnostic criteria (overgrowth vs. connective tissue naevi vs. epidermal naevi)

Among the 250 cases reassessed by Turner et al. (2004) in the Proteus syndrome literature by applying existing diagnostic criteria the areas that generated most confusion included disproportionate overgrowth, cerebriform connective tissue naevi and less commonly epidermal naevi. While the latter two criteria are discussed extensively in other sections, overgrowth is further examined here below.

*Overgrowth* is defined as a body part that has grown excessively and is larger than normal. Overgrowth can be asymmetric or symmetric, progressive or non-progressive, and distorting or non-distorting (Turner et al. 2004). The distinction of proportionate vs. disproportionate overgrowth is generally obvious by the time an individual is two to three years of age (Fig. 3) but can be difficult to assess in infancy. According to Turner et al. (2004) if the overgrowth is subtle, mild or needs measurement to be appreciated, the disproportionate overgrowth criterion (for Proteus syndrome) is negative. Notably, typical non Proteus patients have: 1) asymmetric growth that is apparent at birth (vs. Proteus cases whose body parts size is normal at birth – the latter finding often ignored or forgotten by parents or physicians when recalling birth data); 2) degree of asymmetry not substantially changing over time (vs. Proteus patients who develop severe, rapid, and relentlessly, postnatal overgrowth); 3) rate of growth comparable to the normal tissue (Biesecker 2006, Cohen 2005).

## Differential diagnosis

According to Turner et al. (2004) reported cases of Proteus syndrome that meet the existing criteria have usually a higher incidence of premature death and other complications (scoliosis, megaspondily, CNS abnormalities, tumours, otolaryngology complications, pulmonary cystic malformations, dental and ophthalmic complications) compared to those in the non-Proteus group. In making a differential diagnosis the cerebriform connective tissue nevi are considered pathognomonic while specific tumours occurring before the second decade including ovarian cystadenoma and parotid monomorphic adenoma (see Table 2) and lung cysts are highly specific (OMIM™ 2005, Turner et al. 2004).

The differential diagnosis includes syndromes associated with hemihypertrophy, local or generalized hypertrophies, vascular syndromes or syndromes with hyperpigmentation and/or lipomatoses such as the syndromes of Klippel-Trenaunay, Parkes Weber, Maffucci, Neurofibromatosis type 1, McCune-Albright, the epidermal nevus syndromes, Bannayan-Riley-Ruvalcaba, encephalocraniocutaneous lipomatosis, symmetric lipomatosis, and possibly other less frequent disorders (Goodship et al. 1991, McCall et al. 1992, Rizzo et al. 1993, Martinez-Granero et al. 1998, Biesecker et al. 1999) which may overlap some features with Proteus syndrome. The reader is refereed to the single chapters in this book for differential diagnostic criteria.

Recently, a new phenotype with segmental overgrowth, provisionally called SOLAMEN syndrome (Segmental Overgrowth, Lipomatosis, Arteriovenous Malformation, and Epidermal Nevus), has been delineated (Caux et al. 2007). A loss of the PTEN wild-type allele restricted to the atypical lesions was demonstrated in one affected patient (Caux et al. 2007). This new phenotype is in some aspects reminiscent of the diagnosis of Proteus syndrome.

A further newly delineated phenotype previously considered as part of the spectrum of Proteus syndrome has been named CLOVE syndrome and is characterised by congenital lipomatous overgrowth, vascular malformations and epidermal nevus with enlarged body structures without progressive bony overgrowth (Sapp et al. 2007).

## Management and follow-up

The management of patients with Proteus syndromes needs to be individualized and should always include studies of the soft tissues, the skeleton and the plastic deformities. Guidelines for evaluation of patients are listed in Table 3. Among the numerous complications associated with Proteus syndrome, there are several that are now recognised to be common and therefore define some cohorts of individuals who are at risk of frequent and, in some cases, severe complications (Turner et al. 2004).

Ultrasound studies of the masses visible or palpable at examination and, more in general, of the abdomen and pelvis is the mainstay of initial patient evaluation and should be accompanied by standard ultrasound recording and heart ultrasound examination even in the absence of symptoms. That could be followed by a full abdominal MR study to rule out intra-abdominal masses, which, if present may be aggressive.

High-resolution chest CT may be useful to evaluate pulmonary cystic malformations. This is particularly true for patients who develop unexplained or persistent symptoms suggestive of pulmonary involvement.

X-rays studies of the entire skeleton should be performed in all cases diagnosed. Local or generalized hyperplasia or exostosis, asymmetry of the structures of each hemibody, fractures and other anomalies are best seen with X-ray imaging (Fig. 5) (Velazquez-Fragua and Pascual-Castroviejo 2003, Taybi and Lachman 1996).

The combined use of computerised tomography (CT) and magnetic resonance (MR) studies disclose and characterise skull and spine lesions and abnormalities of the central nervous system (CNS) (Dietrich et al. 1998, Martinez-Granero et al. 1998, DeLone et al. 1999). This is particularly important for inner skull table overgrowth which could progress silently passing unnoticed until a nervous system complication ensues (Fig. 5a, b, d). In addition, because of the number of CNS complications (>40% according to Turner et al. 2004) and cognitive impairment (>30%) linked to Proteus syndrome baseline brain MRIs and early educational intervention should be considered when the diagnosis is made.

As ophthalmologic complications were frequent in a recent literature meta-analysis (>40%) periodic ophthalmologic evaluation are indicated (Table 3).

**Table 3.** Guidelines for patient evaluation

Serial clinical photography
Initial ultrasound examination of head, heart, abdomen and pelvis; periodic ultrasound scanning of abdomen and gonads
Initial skeletal survey with targeted follow-up radiographs
Dermatology consultation; biopsy when indicated
MRI of chest and abdomen even in absence of symptoms
MRI of head and spinal cord even in absence of symptoms (baseline for CNS abnormalities and serially
until adolescence for monitoring of cranial vault bony overgrowth)
MRI of all clinically affected areas
Orthopaedic consultation; operation when indicated
Ongoing clinical genetic/paediatric management
Other consultations as indicated (specifically, ophthalmologist, pneumologist, otolaryngologist
and dentist)
Referral to family support group[a]

[a]Proteus Syndrome Foundation, 6235 Whetstone Drive, Colorado Springs, CO 80918 http://www.kumc.edu/gec/support/proteus.htm
Adapted from Biesecker (2001), Biesecker et al. (1998), Cohen et al. (2002) and Turner et al. (2004).

Breathing difficulties and malocclusion (Table 3) suggest the need for periodic evaluations by an otolaryngologist, pneumologist and a dentist. Although the urologic and renal complications are less frequent, physicians should be aware of them and promptly evaluate symptoms (Turner et al. 2004). Reproductive complications occur and can include malignancies (Gordon et al. 1995). Therefore, periodic testicular and ovarian ultrasounds in males and females should be considered.

Patients with Proteus syndrome and/or their parents should make their health carers aware of the risk of developing lethal disease complications. Symptoms warranting investigation (looking for pulmonary embolism a major contributor to the early mortality of Proteus syndrome) include calf pain, calf or leg swelling, shortness of breath, chest or abdominal pain and any neurological sign and/or symptoms. Even though at this time there are insufficient data to recommend prophylactic anticoagulation therapy (Biesecker et al. 1998, Turner et al. 2004) have successfully treated venous thrombosis and pul-

monary embolism by standard anticoagulation therapy. Patients undergoing surgical procedures should be evaluated for coagulophatic potential.

## Treatment

Patients with visceral manifestations of either Proteus syndrome or overgrowth not meeting Proteus criteria should be treated in a similar manner (Lublin et al. 2002, Ozturk et al. 2000). Lesions involving the ovaries and testes, because of the high incidence of neoplasms, should be managed aggressively (e.g., orchiectomy, orchidopexy, oophorectomy, ovarian cystectomy). Gastrointestinal manifestations (most commonly caused by lipomas and vascular malformations) and renal involvement (overgrowth caused by enlarging cysts or neoplasms) may be managed conservatively with frequent follow-up to minimise abdominal explorations. Determining when to operate on visceral organs can be a challenging decision. The most frequent internal organs operations in a recent series reporting on 80 personal observations (of Proteus and non Proteus cases) and reviewing the existing literature (Lublin et al. 2002) were inguinal hernia repair, partial colectomy, retroperitoneal mass resection, splenectomy, partial bladder resection, nephrectomy, tonsillectomy, parotid mass excision, mastectomy, and heart and lung transplantation.

All patients undergoing surgery should have a thorough preservative assessment of their airway and pulmonary reserve because of the relatively high frequency of tonsillar hypertrophy and pulmonary cystic involvement (reviewed in Lublin et al. 2002).

Recently, rapamycin (sirolimus) has been used to interfere with progressive overgrowth of hamartomas severely affecting the chest, mediastinum, abdomen and pelvis in a 9 month-old boy with Proteus syndrome (Marsh et al. 2008).

## References

Anik Y, Anik I, Gonullu E, Inan N, Demirci A (2007) Proteus syndrome with syringohydromyelia and arachnoid cyst. Childs Nerv Syst 23: 1199–1202.

Aylsworth AS, Lin AE, Friedman PA (1987) New observations with genetic implications in two syndromes (1) father to son transmission of the Nager acrofacial dysostosis syndrome; and (2) parental consanguinity in the Proteus syndrome. Am J Med Genet 41(Suppl): A43.

Azouz EM, Costa T, Fitch N (1987) Radiological findings in the Proteus syndrome. Pediatr Radiol 17: 481–485.

Barker K, Martinez A, Wang R, Bevan S, Murday V, Shipley J, Houlston R, Harper J (2001) PTEN mutations are uncommon in Proteus syndrome. J Med Genet 38: 480–481.

Barona-Mazuera MR, Hidalago-Galvan LR, Orozco-Covarrubias ML, Duran-McKinser C, Tamayo-Sanchez L, Ruiz-Maldonado R (1997) Proteus syndrome: new findings in seven patients. Pediatr Dermatol 14: 1–5.

Bastos H, da Silva PF, de Albuquerque MA, Mattos A, Riesgo RS, Ohlweiler L, Winckler MI, Bragatti JA, Duarte RD, Zandoná DI (2008) Proteus syndrome associated with hemimegalencephaly and Ohtahara syndrome: Report of two cases. Seizure 17: 378–382.

Becktor KB, Becktor JP, Karnes PS, Keller EE (2002) Craniofacial and dental manifestations of Proteus syndrome: a case report. Cleft Palate Craniofac J 39: 233–245.

Biesecker L (2006) The challenges of Proteus syndrome: diagnosis and management. Eur J Hum Genet 14: 1151–1157

Biesecker LG, Peters KF, Darling TN, Choyke P, Hill S, Schimke N, Cunningham M, Meltzer P, Cohen MM Jr (1998) Clinical differentiation between Proteus syndrome and hemihyperplasia: description of a distinct form of hemihyperplasia. Am J Med Genet 79: 311–318.

Biesecker LG, Happle R, Mulliken JB, Weksberg R, Graham JM Jr, Vilkoen DL, Cohen MM Jr (1999) Proteus syndrome: diagnostic criteria, differential diagnosis, and patient evaluation. Am J Med Genet 84: 389–395.

Biesecker LG (2001) The multifaceted challenges of Proteus syndrome. JAMA 285: 2240–2243.

Biesecker LG, Rosenberg MJ, Vacha S, Turner JT, Cohen MM (2001) PTEN mutations and Proteus syndrome. Lancet 358: 2079.

Bouzas EA, Krasnewich D, Kontroumanidis M, Papadimitrou A, Marini JC, Kaiser-Kupfer MI (1993) Ophthalmologic examination in the diagnosis of Proteus syndrome. Ophthalmology 100: 334–338.

Caux F, Plauchu H, Chibon F, Faivre L, Fain O, Vabres P, Bonnet F, Selma ZB, Laroche L, Gerard M, Longy M (2007) Segmental overgrowth, lipomatosis, arteriovenous malformation and epidermal nevus (SOLAMEN) syndrome is related to mosaic PTEN nullizygosity. Eur J Hum Genet Mar 28 [Epub ahead of print].

Child FJ, Werring DJ, Vivier AW (1998) Proteus syndrome: diagnosis in adulthood. Br J Dermatol 139: 132–136.

Clark RD, Donnai D, Rogers J, Cooper J, Baraitser M (1987) Proteus syndrome: an expanded phenotype. Am J Med Genet 27: 99–117.

Clark RD (1994) Proteus syndrome. In: Huson SM, Hughes RAC (eds.) The Neurofibromatoses. A Pathogenic and Clinical Overview. London: Chapman & Hall Medical, pp. 402–413.

Cohen MM Jr, Hayden PW (1979) A newly recognized hamartomatous syndrome. In: O'Donnell JJ, Hall BD (eds.) Penetrance and variability in malformativi syndromes. Birth Defects 15(B): 291–296.

Cohen MM Jr (1986) The elephant man did not have neurofibromatosis. Proc Greenwood Genet Ctr 6: 187–192.

Cohen MM Jr (1988a) Invited historical comment: further diagnostic thought about the Elephant Man. Am J Med Genet 29: 777–782.

Cohen MM Jr (1988b) Understanding Proteus syndrome, unmasking the Elephant Man, and stemming elephant fever. Neurofibromatosis 1: 260–280.

Cohen MM Jr (1993) Proteus syndrome: clinical evidence for somatic mosaicism and selective review. Am J Med Genet 47: 645–652.

Cohen MM Jr (1995) Putting a foot in one's mouth or putting a foot down nonspecificity vs. specificity of the connective tissue nevus in Proteus syndrome. Proc. Greenwood Cent 14: 11–13.

Cohen MM Jr (1999) Thanos syndrome does not exist. Am J Med Genet 86: 101.

Cohen MM Jr (2001) Causes of premature death in Proteus syndrome. Am J Med Genet 101: 1–3.

Cohen MM Jr, Neri G, Weksberg R (2002) Proteus syndrome. In: Cohen MM Jr, Neri G, Weksberg R (eds.) Overgrowth Syndromes. New York: Oxford University Press, pp. 75–110.

Cohen MM Jr, Turner JT, Biesecker LG (2003) Proteus syndrome: misdiagnosis with PTEN mutations. Am J Med Genet 122A: 323–324.

Cohen MM Jr (2005) Proteus syndrome: an update. Am J Med Genet C Semin Med Genet 137: 38–52.

Costa T, Fitch N, Azouz EM (1985) The Proteus syndrome: report of two cases of pelvic lipomatosis. Pediatrics 76: 984–989.

Cremin BJ, Viljoen DL, Wynchank S, Beighton P (1987) The Proteus syndrome: the magnetic resonance and radiological features. Pediatr Radiol 17: 486–488.

Danarti R, Happle R (2003) Paradominant inheritance of twin spotting: phacomatosis pigmentovascularis as a further possible example. Eur J Dermatol 13: 612.

Dean JCS, Cole GF, Appleton Burn JRE, Roberts SA, Donnai D (1990) Cranial hemihypertrophy and neurodevelopmental prognosis. J Med Genet 27: 160–164.

De Lone DR, Brown WD, Gentry LR (1999) Proteus syndrome: craniofacial and cerebral MRI. Neuroradiology 41: 840–843.

Dietrich RB, Glidden DE, Roth GM, Martin RA, Demo DS (1998) The Proteus syndrome: CNS manifestations. AJNR Am J Neuroradiol 19: 987–990.

Eberhard DA (1994) Two-year old boy with Proteus syndrome and fatal pulmonary thromboembolism. Pediatr Pathol 14: 771–779.

Eng C, Thiele H, Zhou XP, Gorlin RJ, Hennekam RC, Winter RM (2001) PTEN mutations and proteus syndrome. Lancet 358: 2079–2080.

Goodship J, Redfearn A, Milligan D, Gardner-Medwin D, Burn J (1991) Transmission of Proteus syndrome from father to son? J Med Genet 28: 781–785.

Gordon PL, Wilroy RS, Lasater OE, Cohen MM Jr (1995) Neoplasms in Proteus syndrome. Am J Med Genet 57: 74–78.

Gorlin RJ, Cohen MM Jr, Hennekam RCM (2001) Proteus syndrome (and encephalocraniocutaneous lipomatosis). In: Gorlin RJ, Cohen MM Jr, Hennekam RCM (eds.) Syndromes of the Head and Neck, 4th ed. New York: Oxford University Press, pp. 480–483.

Graetz I (1928) Ueber einen Fall von sogenannter "totaler halbseitiger Korphypertophie" Z Kinderheilk 45: 381–403.

Happle R (1987) Lethal genes surviving by mosaicism: a possible explanation for sporadic birth defects involving the skin. J Am Acad Dermatol 18: 899–906.

Happle R (1991) How many epidermal nevus syndromes exist? A clinical-genetic explanation. J Am Acad Dermatol 25: 550–556.

Happle R (1993) Mosaicism in human skin. Understanding the patterns and mechanisms. Arch Dermatol 129: 1460–1470.

Happle R (1995a) Epidermal nevus syndromes. Semin Dermatol 14: 111–121.

Happle R (1995b) Lipomatosis and partial lipohypoplasia in Proteus syndrome: a clinical clue for twin spotting? Am J Med Genet 56: 332–333.

Happle R, Steijlen PM, Theile U, Karitzky D, Tinschert S, Albrecht-Nebe H, Kuster W (1997) Patchy dermal hypoplasia as a characteristic feature of Proteus syndrome. Arch Dermatol 133: 77–80.

Happle R (1999) Elattoproteus syndrome: delineation of an inverse form of Proteus syndrome. Am J Med Genet 84: 25–28.

Happle R (2004) The manifold faces of proteus syndrome. Arch Dermatol 140: 1001–1002.

Happle R (2006) Principles of genetics, mosaicism and molecular biology. In: Harper J, Oranje A, Prose N (eds.) Textbook of Pediatric Dermatology. 2nd ed. Oxford: Blackwell Science, pp. 1221–1246.

Ho N, Roig C, Diadori P (1999) Epidermal nevi and localised cranial defects. Am J Med Genet 83: 187–190.

Hoeger PH, Martinez A, Maerker J, Harper JI (2004) Vascular anomalies in Proteus syndrome. Clin Exp Dermatol 29: 222–230.

Hoey SE, Eastwood D, Monsell F, Kangesu L, Harper JI, Sebire NJ (2008) Histopathological features of Proteus syndrome. Clin Exp Dermatol 33: 234–238.

Holmes LB (1997) Personal communication

Horie Y, Fujita H, Mano S, Kuwajima M, Ogawa K (1995) Regional Proteus syndrome: report of an autopsy case. Pathol Int 45: 530–535.

Howard M, Ford P (1980) The True History of the Elephant Man. London: Allison & Busby

Kontras SB (1974) Case report no. 19. Synd Ident 2: 1–3.

Kreiborg S, Cohen MM Jr, Skovby F (1991) Craniofacial characteristics of Proteus syndrome: two modes of abnormal growth. Proc Finn Dent Soc 87(1): 183–188.

Krüger G, Pelz L, Wiedermann HR (1993) Transmission of Proteus syndrome from mother to son? Am J Med Genet 45: 117–118.

Loffeld A, McLellan NJ, Cole T, Payne SJ, Fricker D, Moss C (2006) Epidermal naevus in Proteus syndrome showing loss of heterozygosity for an inherited PTEN mutation. Br J Dermatol 154: 1194–1198.

Lublin M, Schwartzentruber DJ, Lukish J, Chester C, Biesecker LG, Newman KD (2002) Principles of the surgical management of patients with Proteus syndrome and patients with overgrowth not meeting the Proteus criteria. J Pediatr Surg 37: 1013–1020.

Marsh DJ, Trahair TN, Martin JL, Chee WY, Walker J, Kirk EP, Baxter RC, Marshall GM (2008) Rapamycin treatment for a child with germline PTEN mutation. Nat Clin Pract Oncol Apr 22 [Epub ahead of print].

Martinez-Granero MA, Roche Herrero MC, De Ceano-Vivas la Calle M, Martinez-Bermejo A, Pascual-Castroviejo I, Contreras-Rubio F (1998) Síndrome de Proteus y lipomatosis encefalocraneocutanea: una misma hamartomatosis? A propósito de un caso severo. An Esp Pediatr 49: 503–506.

Mayatapek E, Kurczynski TW, Ruppert ES, Hennessy JR, Brinker RA, French BN (1989) Brief clinical report: expanding the phenotype of Proteus syndrome. A severely affected patient with new findings. Am J Med Genet 32: 402–406.

McCall S, Ramzy MI, Cure JK, Pai GS (1992) Encephalocraniocutaneous lipomatosis and the Proteus syndrome: distinct entities with overlapping manifestations. Am J Med Genet 43: 662–668.

McMullin GP, Super M, Clarke MA (1993) Cranial hemihypertrophy with ipsilateral naevoid streaks, intellectual handicap and epilepsy: a report of two cases. Clin Genet 44: 249–253.

Nazzaro V, Cambiaghi S, Montagnani A, Brusasco A, Cerri A, Caputo R (1991) Proteus syndrome: ultrastructural study of linear verrucous and depigmented nevi. J Am Acad Dermatol 25: 377–383.

Newman B, Urbach AH, Orenstein D, Dickman PS (1994) Proteus syndrome: emphasis on the pulmonary manifestations. Pediatr Radiol 24: 189–193.

Okumura K, Sasaki Y, Ohyama M, Nishi T (1986) Bannayan syndrome – generalised lipomatosis associated with megalencephaly and macrodactyly. Acta Pathol Jpn 36: 269–277.

Online Mendelian Inheritance in Man (OMIM)™ (2005) McKusick Catalogue of Mendelian Disorders in Human. Baltimore, Johns Hopkins University Press: http://www.ncbi.nlm.nih.gov/omim

Ozturk H, Karnak I, Turgay Sakarya M, Cetinkursum S (2000) Proteus syndrome: Clinical and surgical aspects. Ann Genet 43: 137–142.

Raman R, Kumar V, Arianayagan S, Peh SC (1989) A unilateral mesenchymal disorder of the head. J Cranio-Max-Fac Surg 17: 143–145.

Reardon W, Harding B, Winter RM, Baraitser M (1996) Brief clinical report: hemihypertrophy, hemimegalencephaly, and polydactyly. Am J Med Genet 66: 141–144.

Rizzo R, Pavone L, Sorge G, Parano E, Baraitser M (1990) Proteus syndrome: report of a case with severe brain impairment and fatal course. J Med Genet 27: 399–402.

Rizzo R, Pavone L, Micali G, Nigro F, Cohen MM Jr (1993) Encephalocraniocutaneous lipomatosis, Proteus syndrome, and somatic mosaicism. Am J Med Genet 47: 653–655.

Ruggieri M (2001) Mosaic (segmental) neurofibromatosis type 1 (NF1) and type 2 (NF2): no longer neurofibromatosis type 5 (NF5). Am J Med Genet 101: 178–180.

Ruggieri M, Huson SM (2001) The clinical and diagnostic implications of mosaicism in the neurofibromatoses. Neurology 56: 1434–1443.

Sampaio C, Martinez A, Barker K, Monsell F, Houlston R, Harper J (2006) Proteus syndrome. In: Harper J, Oranje A, Prose M (eds.) Textbook of Pediatric Dermatology. 2nd ed. Oxford: Blackwell Science, pp. 1143–1150.

Sapp JC, Turner JT, van de Kamp JM, van Dijk FS, Lowry RB, Biesecker LG (2007) Newly delineated syndrome of congenital lipomatous overgrowth, vascular malformations, and epidermal nevi (CLOVE syndrome) in seven patients. Am J Med Genet A 143: 2944–2958.

Say B, Carpenter NJ (1988) Report of a case resembling the Proteus syndrome with a chromosome abnormality. Am J Med Genet 31: 987–989.

Schepis C, Greco D, Siragusa M, Romano C (2008) Cerebriform plantar hyperplasia: the major cutaneous feature of Proteus syndrome. Int J Dermatol 47: 374–376.

Schwartz CE, Brown AM, Der Kaloustian VM, McGill JJ, Saul RA (1991) DNA fingerprinting: the utilization of minisatellite probes to detect a somatic mutation in the proteus syndrome. EXS 58: 95–105.

Seward GR (1994) Did the elephant man have neurofibromatosis type 1? In: Huson SM, Hughes RAC (eds.) The Neurofibromatoses. A Pathogenic and Clinical Overview, Chapman & Hall Medical, London, pp. 382–401.

Sigaudy S, Fredouille C, Gambarelly D, Porlier A, Cassin D, Piquet C, Philip N (1998) Prenatal ultrasonographic findings in Proteus syndrome. Prenat Diagn 18: 1091–1094.

Skovby F, Graham JM Jr, Sonne-Holm S, Cohen MM Jr (1993) Compromise of the spinal canal in Proteus syndrome. Am J Med Genet 47: 656–659.

Slavotinek AM, Vacha SJ, Peters KF, Biesecker LG (2001) Sudden death caused by pulmonary thromboembolism in Proteus syndrome. Clin Genet 58: 386–389.

Smeets E, Fryns JP, Cohen MM Jr (1994) Regional Proteus syndrome and somatic mosaicism. Am J Med Genet 51: 29–31.

Smith JM, Kirk EPE, Theodosopoulos G, Marshall GM, Walker J, Rogers M, Field N, Brereton JJ, Marsh DJ (2002) Germline mutation of the tumour suppressor PTEN in Proteus syndrome. J Med Genet 39: 937–940.

Sugarman JL (2004) The epidermal nevus syndromes. Semin Cut Med Surg 23: 145–157.

Sugarman JL, Frieden IJ (2004) Epidermal nevus syndromes. In: Roach ES, Miller VS (eds.) Neurocutaneous disorders. New York: Cambridge University Press, pp. 88–104.

Taybi H, Lachman RS (1996) Proteus syndrome. In: Taybi H, Lachman RS (eds.) Radiology of Syndromes, Metabolic Disorders, and Skeletal Dysplasia. 4th ed. St. Louis: Mosby, pp. 403–405.

Temtany SA, Rogers JG (1976) Macrodactyly, hemihypertrophy, and connective tissue nevi: report of a new syndrome and review of the literature. J Pediatr 89: 924–927.

Thanos C, Stewart RE, Zonana J (1977) Craniosynostosis, bony exostoses, epibulbar dermoids, epidermal nevus, and slow development. Synd Ident 5: 19–21.

Thiffault I, Schwartz CE, Der Kaloustian V, Foulkes WD (2004) Mutation analysis of the tumour suppressor

PTEN and the glypican 3 (GPC3) gene in patients diagnosed with Proteus syndrome. Am J Med Genet 130A: 123–127.

Tibbles JAR, Cohen MM (1986) The Proteus syndrome: the Elephant Man diagnosed. Br Med J 293: 683–685.

Toro-Sola MA (1987) Proteus syndrome and Klippel-Tranaunay-Weber with Sturge-Weber sequence in a consanguineous Puerto Rican family. Am J Med Genet 41(Suppl): A108.

Treves F (1885a) A case of congenital deformity. Trans Pathol Soc Lond 36: 494–498.

Treves F (1885b) Congenital deformity, in Reports of Societies Pathological of London, 17 March 1885. Br Med J 1: 595–596.

Treves F (1923) The Elephant Man and other Reminiscences. London: Cassell.

Turner JT, Cohen MM Jr, Biesecker LG (2004) Reassessment of the Proteus syndrome literature: application of diagnostic criteria to published cases. Am J Med Genet 130A: 111–122.

Tweede JV, Turner JT, Biesecker LG, Darling TN (2005) Evolution of skin lesions in Proteus syndrome. J Am Acad Dermatol 52: 834–838.

Unsigned comment (1884) Congenital deformity, in Reports of Societies: Pathological Society of Londin, 6 December 1884. Br Med J 11: 1140.

Unsigned comment (1886) The Elephant Man. A commentary on a letter in The Times from Mr Carr Gomm. Br Med J ii: 1188–1189.

Unsigned comment (1890) Death of the Elephant Man. Br Med J i: 916–917.

Velázquez Fragua R, Pascual-Castroviejo I (2003) Dos casos de síndrome de Proteus. An Pediatr 58: 496–501.

Vujevich JJ, Mancini AJ (2004) The epidermal nevus syndromes: multisystem disorders. J Am Acad Dermatol 50: 957–961.

Wiedemann HR, Burgio GR, Aldenhoff P, Kunze J, Kaufmann HJ, Schirg E (1983) The Proteus syndrome. Partial gigantism of the hands and/or feet, nevi, hemihypertrophy, subcutaneous tumors, macrocephaly or other skull anomalies and possible accelerated growth and visceral affections. Eur J Pediatr 140: 5–12.

Wieland E (1907) Zur Pathologie der dystrophischen Form des angeborenen partiellen Riesenwuchses. Jahrbuch fur Kinderheilkunde 65: 519–584.

Zhou XP, Marsh DJ, Hampel H, Mulliken JB, Gimm O, Eng C (2000) Germline and germline mosaic PTEN mutations associated with a Proteus-like syndrome of hemihypertrophy, lower limb asymmetry, arteriovenous malformations and lipomatosis. Hum Molec Genet 9: 765–768.

# Chapter 32

# EPIDERMAL NEVUS SYNDROMES

Jeffrey L. Sugarman

Departments of Dermatology and Community and Family Medicine, University of California, San Francisco, USA

## Introduction

The term epidermal nevus syndrome (ENS) was proposed by Solomon et al. (1968) to describe the association of epidermal hamartomas and extra-cutaneous abnormalities. Although many continue to use the term "epidermal nevus syndrome", it is now understood that this is not one disease, but rather a heterogeneous group each with distinct genetic profiles but defined by a common cutaneous phenotype: the presence of epidermal and adnexal hamartomas (epidermal nevi (EN)) that are associated with extra-cutaneous anomalies. The majority of the extra-cutaneous manifestations involve the brain, eye, and skeletal systems.

Advances in molecular biology have revealed that the manifestations of ENS are due to genomic mosaicism. The varied clinical manifestations of ENS may be due in large part to the functional effects of specific genetic defects and the timing of the mutation in fetal development. Unfortunately, since only a small minority of the genetic abnormalities causing EN have been discovered, complete biologic classification is impossible at the present time, and thus our descriptions and understanding continue to be primarily clinical. Once the genetic bases of different types of EN are more clearly delineated, the patterns of associated malformations are likely to be clarified more completely (Sugarman and Frieden 2004).

As our understanding of diseases involving epidermal nevi has widened, there have been efforts to classify them into subsets based on both their cutaneous features and their extra-cutaneous associations (Happle 1995). This section of the textbook describes the major ENS including nevus sebaceus syndrome (Schimmelpenning-Feuerstein-Mims Solomon syndrome, discussed in Chapter 33), inflammatory linear verrucous epidermal nevus (ILVEN, discussed in

Chapter 34), nevus comedonicus syndrome (discussed in Chapter 35), Becker syndrome (pigmented hairy epidermal nevus syndrome, discussed in Chapter 36), and CHILD syndrome (discussed in Chapter 37). Other syndromes which are generally considered as ENS including Proteus syndrome, and phakomatosis pigmentokeratotica are discussed in other places in this textbook (Chapters 31 and 22, respectively). Another prominent subset of ENS, keratinocytic ENS, and less common subsets of ENS are considered in this introductory chapter.

## Overview of clinical manifestations

The cutaneous features of EN depend in part on the predominant cell type involved, the degree of cellular differentiation, the body site of involvement, and the age of the patient. EN follow linear patterns known as "the lines of Blaschko" (Fig. 1). Blaschko's lines refer to the S-shaped or V-shaped whorled, streaked, and linear patterns that are recognized in many different cutaneous disorders. Blaschko meticulously recorded these lines (Blaschko 1901) that do not follow any known nervous, vascular or lymphatic structures in the skin (Jackson 1976). Rather, they are felt by some to represent the dorso-ventral migratory pathways of the neuroectoderm during embryogenesis (Moss et al. 1995).

In the first comprehensive review of ENS, Solomon (1975) emphasized that although some hamartomas have more sebaceous differentiation [i.e. nevus sebaceus (NS)], and others more epidermal differentiation (i.e., keratinocytic epidermal nevi), many show differentiation toward several cutaneous appendages. This concept had been previously proposed by Mehregan and Pinkus (1965) who described the clinical and histological characteristics of

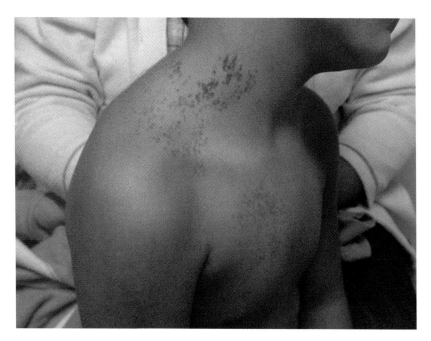

**Fig. 1.** Keratinocytic epidermal nevus following the lines of Blaschko.

NS from infancy to adulthood, building on Jadassohn's (1895) original work. Jadassohn initially used the term "organ-naevus" (organoid nevus) as a label in order to differentiate hamartomas composed of keratinocytes and epidermal appendages from nevocellular (melanocytic) nevi.

The association of EN with CNS abnormalities has been recognized for many years. Schimmelpenning (1957) and subsequently Feuerstein and Mims (1962) were among the first to describe the association. Solomon (1975) provided the first comprehensive review of the associated neurologic (and other organ system) abnormalities. Since then, many reports and reviews have provided more detail and insight into the spectrum of the neurologic, ocular and skeletal (and other) abnormalities associated with ENS (see Chapters 31, 33–37). Estimates of the true incidence of extra-cutaneous involvement in all patients with EN are probably as low as 5–15%, but have been hampered by ascertainment bias, the paucity of accompanying histological data on the EN, and inconsistency in obtaining imaging studies documenting the CNS abnormalities. In addition, definitions of clinical findings vary considerably in different reports. Finally, different ENS are likely to have distinct patterns of neurologic (as well as ocular and skeletal) involvement.

Data on the incidence of extra-cutaneous features in some of the other subsets is sparse secondary to their relative rarity and the more recent characterization of some of these syndromes (Sugarman 2004, 2007).

## Keratinocytic epidermal nevus

Keratinocytic (verrucous) EN are a common form of EN (Rogers 1992) chacterized by papillated or verrucous epidermal hyperplasia without a significant sebaceous component. They are usually present at the time of birth but many have their onset during early infancy, sometimes extending over adjacent areas of skin for the first few months to years of life. Initially they may be flat, but over time they often become more elevated, verrucous and darker in color (Fig. 1). Acral lesions often have a more warty appearance (Solomon 1975).When the nail matrix is affected, the nail may be dystrophic. In the body folds, lesions are softer and less verrucous. The distribution and extent of EN varies widely: they can be solitary, multiple, large or small, and are commonly found on the trunk or extremities. Lesions may be either unilateral (so-called "nevus unius lateris"), or bilateral, usually stopping abruptly at the dorsal and ventral midline.

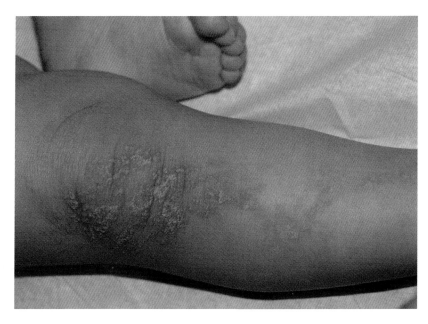

**Fig. 2.** Epidermolytic keratinocytic epidermal nevus.

When they are symmetric and bilateral they have been referred to as systematized EN or ichthyosis histrix. They are less common on the head and neck (Solomon 1975, Atherton et al. 1989).

"Keratinocytic epidermal nevus syndrome" has been left out of Happle's characterization of defined subsets of ENS (Happle 1991). The keratinocytic EN itself likely represents a heterogeneous group that awaits more specific classification. Therefore, this "subset" may not represent one true syndrome because it likely encompasses several unique syndromes awaiting characterization as specific molecular defects are identified and as specific clinical features are better characterized. For example, while the epidermolytic type of keratinocytic EN may have similar clinical features compared to other keratinocytic EN, it has a distinctive surface scale that may offer a subtle but distinct clinical clue distinguishing it from other keratinocytic EN (Fig. 2). In addition, it is clearly histologically distinct from other keratinocytic EN displaying acanthokeratolysis with large clumps of keratohyaline. Furthermore, it is also genetically distinct, harboring mutations in keratin 1 and 10 (as discussed below).

Clearly, keratinocytic EN are associated with extra-cutaneous manifestations but the extra-cutaneous features of keratinocytic EN have been diffi-cult to separate from those of other ENS such as NS (as discussed in Chapter 33). For example, Gurecki et al. (1996) reviewed 23 cases of biopsy proven EN with accompanying neurologic abnormalities. Cases of keratinocytic nevi and NS were approximately equal in numbers. All cases of neonatal seizures (55% of the patients) had major hemispheric malformations; 53% had mental retardation or developmental delays. Of these, most were considered moderately or severely impaired. The most common CNS structural abnormalities were hemiatrophy (26%), vascular anomalies (26%), cranial bone deformities (26%) hemimegalencephaly (22%), gyral abnormalities (22%), and posterior fossa abnormalities (9%). Two patients had CNS tumors, which included gliomatosis cerebri and leptomeningeal hemangioma. Imaging revealed no abnormalities in only 13% (Gurecki et al. 1996). Unfortunately, it was impossible to separate the neurologic manifestations associated with the patients with NS from those with keratinocytic EN.

## Porokeratotic eccrine nevus

PEN was originally described as "comedo nevus of the palm" by Marsden et al. (1979) and subsequently termed porokeratotic eccrine ostial and dermal duct nevus (Abell and Read 1980). Happle prefers the term porokeratotic eccrine nevus as it is simpler and contains the relevant information regarding the pathology. Since the original description, there have been at least 25 reported cases of PEN. PEN consists of verrucous, keratotic papules with keratin filled invaginations representing eccrine ducts located on the palms and soles. The majority of cases present at birth or soon after. There have been 3 reports of widespread cutaneous involvement (Sassmannshausen et al. 2000, Dogra et al. 2002).

## Endocrine abnormalities associated with ENS

The fascinating association of epidermal nevi with endocrine abnormalities may provide insight into the genetic basis of nevus sebaceous as well as providing new information on the regulation of calcium and phosphate metabolism. Sugarman and Reed (1969) were the first to report the association of ENS with hypophosphatemic rickets. Since then, there have been nearly two dozen cases of hypophosphatemic vitamin D-resistant rickets associated with NS syndrome (Olivares et al. 1999). Olivares found that CNS abnormalities were present in 36% of his 14 cases and 86% of these children had mental retardation. Rickets, muscle weakness and bone pain developed at an early age in many of the patients.

The rickets is thought to result from abnormal phosphate excretion secondary to defective renal tubular reabsorption of phosphate. Some authors have proposed the theory that this condition is analogous to the rare association of hypophosphatemic vitamin D-resistant rickets associated with mesenchyme-derived neoplasms (tumor-induced osteomalacia), in which the tumor produces a putative phosphaturic factor that leads to osteomalacia (Sugarman 2004).

There have been two reports of at least partial reversal of the hypophosphatemia with excision of a portion of an epidermal nevus (Aschinberg et al. 1977, Ivker et al. 1997). In one compelling case report, a 12 year old patient with a large facial EN and vitamin D-resistant hypophosphatemic rickets im-

proved following excision of several fibroangiomatous epidermal nevi. Serum phosphate concentrations and tubular reabsorption of phosphorus both increased significantly. These authors then homogenized the epidermal nevi that had been initially removed, and infused them into the femoral vein of a dog. Two hours after the infusion, the tubular reabsorption of phosphorus decreased dramatically. Control infusions had no effect on phosphorus reabsorption. Based on these findings, they speculated that the epidermal nevus produces a phosphaturic factor that leads to osteomalacia. However, it is not clear why removal of only a very small part of the epidermal nevus could correct the hypophosphatemia in their patient (Aschinberg et al. 1977). In addition, several verrucous epidermal nevi were subsequently removed without any further improvement. In the second case, serum phosphate levels increased after excision of a portion of an epidermal nevus but the supplemental phosphate dosage was also increased several times. Unfortunately, it is not clear from their report how much supplemental phosphate the patient was taking before and after the excisions leaving doubt about whether the increase in serum phosphate could be solely attributed to the removal on the epidermal nevi. Other investigators have found no association between removal of all or part of an epidermal nevus and remission of the hypophosphatemia. While there is strong evidence that a humoral factor mediates phosphate wasting in tumor induced osteomalacia (Drezner 2000), the evidence for a factor secreted by the cells of an epidermal nevus is scant.

A phosphate-regulating gene (PHEX) has been cloned, which is thought to be responsible for renal phosphate wasting in X-linked hypophosphatemia and has led to new insights regarding the pathogenesis of tumor induced osteomalacia. Its normal function is thought to inactivate the putative phosphaturic factor phosphatonin leading to phosphate wasting and osteomalacia (Drezner 2000). It could be speculated that the genetic mosaic that exists in those cases of ENS involving hypophosphatemia involves a mutation in the PHEX or a related gene in cutaneous or extracutaneous tissues leading to unopposed phosphatonin and phosphate wasting.

Recently, the phosphaturic factor responsible for tumor induced osteomalacia (TIO) has been identified. These tumors secrete large amounts of fibroblast growth factor-23 (FGF-23) (Jonsson et al. 2003). Similarly, patients with autosomal dominant hypophosphatemic rickets have increased levels of circulating FGF-23 due to the production of a mutant FGF-23 that makes it resistant to cleavage and degradation. It appears likely that the hypophosphatemic rickets seen associated with NS is due to either overproduction of FGF-23 (wild type or mutant) or involves another molecule regulating the phosphate homeostasis and skeletal mineralization axis. Heike described a patient with ENS with hypophosphatemic rickets and asymmetric skeletal abnormalities who had elevated levels of FGF-23 in his circulation (Heike et al. 2005). Hoffman et al. reported a case of an adolescent with nevus sebaceous syndrome and hypophosphatemic rickets in which FGF-23 levels were elevated. Treatment with the somatostatin agonist, octreotide, in addition to excision of the nevus led to normalization of FGF-23 levels and improvement in the hypophosphatemia (Hoffman et al. 2005).

There has also been a case of phakomatosis pigmentokeratotica associated with hypophosphatemic vitamin D-resistant rickets (Saraswat et al. 2003). Yu et al. (2000) reported a case of ENS associated with the syndrome of inappropriate anti-diuretic hormone (SIADH). Their case involved an infant with seizures, hyponatremia and SIADH. There have been several reported cases of central precocious puberty associated with ENS (Tay et al. 1996).

## EN and neoplasms

Several cutaneous malignancies including basal cell carcinoma (BCC), squamous cell carcinoma, and adnexal carcinomas have been described in association with EN. Malignant transformation of EN may occur whether or not they are associated with other organ system abnormalities (Mehregan and Pinkus 1965, Solomon et al. 1968). In the past, NS was thought to have a 10–15% risk of malignant transformation, most commonly to BCC. More recently, the magnitude of malignant potential of NS has been questioned. Cribier et al. (2000) retrospectively analyzed 596 cases of NS, 79% of which were located on the scalp. They found benign tumors in 14% of these, the most common of which included syringocystadenoma papilliferum (5%), trichoblastoma (5%), trichilemmoma (3%), and sebaceoma (2%), but found BCC in only 0.8% of cases. Interestingly, many of the cases of trichoblastoma (a benign neoplasm) had originally been classified as BCC but were re-diagnosed using new criteria. Similarly, a retrospective analysis of 155 cases of NS by Jaqueti et al. (2000) found neoplasms in 21% with trichoblastoma being most common (7.5%), followed by syringocystadenoma papilliferum (6%), and sebomatricoma (5%). Smaller numbers of apocrine hidrocystoma and apocrine poroma were also found. There were no cases of malignant neoplasm found. The decreasing incidence of tumors developing in NS could be the result of more frequent early excision for cosmetic reasons, but the data from Jaqueti suggest otherwise; 61% of their cases were from adults. It seems likely that most of the tumors arising in NS that have in the past been interpreted as BCC are in fact examples of primitive follicular induction or trichoblastomas, and not authentic BCC (Sugarman 2004).

## Extra-cutaneous histopathology

While there is much analysis in the literature of the histopathological features of *cutaneous* lesions in ENS, pathologic descriptions of *CNS* findings in such patients are rare. Prayson et al. (1993) examined the clinicopathologic features of 3 patients with ENS who underwent surgical resections for chronic epilepsy. Microscopic examination of resected cortical tissue demonstrated severe diffuse cortical dysplasia characterized by a disorganized cortical architectural pattern, a haphazard orientation of cortical neurons, and increased molecular layer neurons. There was also prominent cortical astrocytosis. Gyral fusion was seen in 1 patient. Pial glioneuronal hamartomas were observed in 1 patient. Neuronal heterotopia was observed in all 3 patients. Similarly, Pavone et al. (1991) noted a disturbed laminar pattern of the cerebral cortex on microscopic analysis of a patient with neurological involvement. In addition, they noted atypical giant neurons, heterotopic neurons in both the white matter and the subarachnoid space, areas of marked astrocyte proliferation infiltrating into adjacent structures and small angioma-like conglomerations of blood vessels. From an architectural standpoint, this may be analogous to the hamartomatous structures observed microscopically in EN (Sugarman 2004).

The cortical dysplasia seen in individuals with ENS likely represents derangement in neuronal migration, much of which occurs in the first two trimesters of gestation. It is well recognized that cortical dysplasia is associated with epilepsy and may be at least partly responsible for the increased incidence of seizures in ENS. In addition, cortical dysplasia has also been associated with certain low-grade neoplasms including ganglioneuromas, implicating a common underlying etiology for the abnormal neuronal migration in patients with ENS and the development of these tumors (Prayson et al. 1999). It appears that at least in a subset of patients with neurological involvement, primary vascular anomalies may lead to secondary CNS pathology. For example, infarcts, atrophy, porencephaly, and calcifications are best explained in some cases by prior ischemia or hemorrhage (Pavone et al. 1991).

## Genetic basis and pathogenesis

Many lines of evidence suggest that the pathogenesis and clinical expression of ENS is based on genomic mosaicism. Mosaicism is the mixture of more than one genotypically distinct cell lineage within one organism. Epidermal cells are thought to originate in the neural crest and move to the periphery of the growing embryo by directional proliferation (Moss et al. 1995). A somatic mutation occurring during the migration of embryonic ectoderm will only be clinically apparent if the mutation leads to a recognizable difference from the surrounding normal cells, which often follow Blaschko's lines. Thus, Blaschko's lines are believed to be a cutaneous ex-

pression of mosaicism. In this conceptual framework, mutations which occur earlier in development would lead to more extensive cutaneous involvement and a greater likelihood of other organ system involvement. In addition, the biologic severity of a particular mutation is also likely to determine the extent and severity of clinical involvement.

Careful analysis of the cutaneous patterns of certain skin diseases may provide new insights into basic questions of craniofacial development. Haggstrom analyzed photographs of over 100 of infantile hemangiomas affecting the face. The patterns observed allowed the authors to speculate on the possibility of a different developmental map of the facial segments. It also added to the concept that the distribution of infantile hemangiomas is not random. There are 5 distinct embryonic primordia in the developing face that appear between days 21 and 31 of the developing human fetus. Segments 2 and 3 correspond with the previously recognized maxillary and mandibular prominences. Segments 1 and 4 may differ from standard human embryology texts. The frontotemporal segment (Seg. 1) encompasses the lateral forehead, anterior temporal scalp, and lateral frontal scalp. The segment (Seg. 4) encompasses the medial frontal scalp, nasal bridge, nasal tip, ala, and philtrum, and is substantially narrower on the forehead than the previously described frontonasal prominence (Haggstrom et al. 2006). Careful consideration of the patterns observed in epidermal nevi may similarly provide clues to craniofacial development. The inferior border of the maxillary segment (Seg. 2) at the border with the mandibular segment (Seg. 3) is a common location for nevus sebaceus (Fig. 3a). This is recapitulated in the more "full blown" cases in Fig. 3b–d but always carefully respecting the affected facial segment(s). Figure 3a and b show a nevus sebaceus following Blaschko's lines but affecting only Segment 2. However, Fig. 3c and d show a nevus sebaceus also following Blaschko's lines but affecting Segments 2 and 4 (the fronto-nasal segment). One could propose, based on purely clinical grounds, that the mosaic clone of cells causing the nevus sebaceus originated in a neural crest precursor to segments 2 and 4. Furthermore, segments 2 and 4 arose from a common neural crest precursor after

Segments 1 and 3 had "split off" and committed to their geographic fates. Ultimately, this concept also has implications for the patterns of extra-cutaneous manifestations that may accompany epidermal nevi.

The concept of lethal genes surviving by mosaicism has been proposed by Happle (1987) to explain the sporadic inheritance, asymmetric clinical distribution in multiple organs, the lack of diffuse involvement of entire organs, and the equal sex ratio of affected individuals that characterize the features of ENS. Happle postulated that these syndromes are due to the action of a gene product that if present in the germ line would be lethal, but is clinically manifested only when present in a subpopulation of cells, thereby surviving by mosaicism.

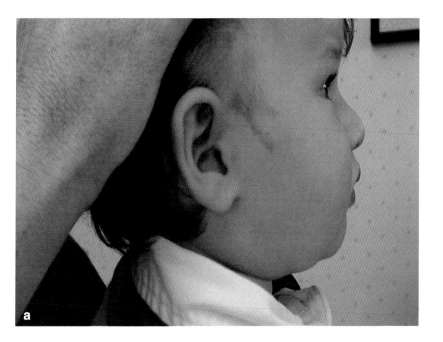

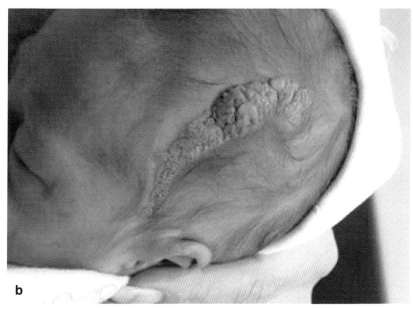

Fig. 3. (a) Form fruste of nevus sebaceous involving facial segment 2; (b) Nevus sebaceus involving facial segment 2; (c) Nevus sebaceus involving facial segments 2 and 4 (courtesy of Maureen Rogers); (d) Nevus sebaceus involving facial segments 2 and 4 (courtesy of Maureen Rogers).

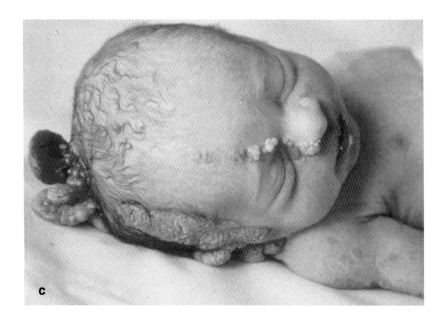

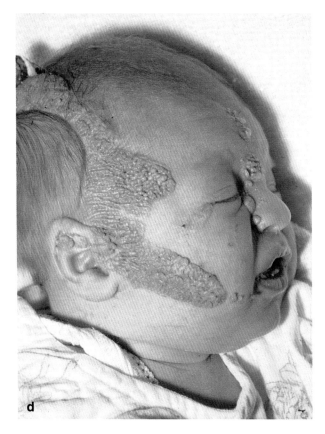

**Fig. 3.** (Continued)

Several specific examples have provided evidence that genetic mosaicism can cause the cutaneous phenotype of EN. There was a case of chromosomal mosaicism in a woman with a widespread verrucous epidermal nevus and multiple trichilemmal cysts in whom it was discovered that 5% of her lymphocytes contained a translocation between 1p36 and 9q34 (Iglesias Zamora and Vazquez-Doval 1997). Stosiek et al. (1994) performed cytogenetic analysis on keratinocytes from two patients with EN and found a translocation at the same breaking point in chromosome 1. Paller et al. (1994) found point mutations in 50% of the keratin 10 alleles of epidermal cells from patients with EN (of the epidermolytic type) while finding no mutations in adjacent clinically normal skin. They also found the same mutations in 50% of the keratin 10 alleles in all the cell types examined from their offspring. Similarly, Moss et al. (1995) has provided evidence of a keratin 10 mutation in affected cells of an individual with linear EN while showing that cells from unaffected adjacent epidermis had no mutation. This is not surprising, as keratins 1 and 10 are obligate partners providing function to the epidermis in a cell type-specific manner.

Mosaicism in ENS may also involve a nonlethal gene defect as demonstrated by the following two examples of epidermolytic hyperkeratosis (EHK) and Aperts syndrome. In the mosaic form of EHK, there is an EN of the epidermolytic type. Keratin 1 gene mosaicism has been identified in an epidermal nevus (of the epidermolytic type) in a woman whose son has EHK and the identical genomic mutation (Happle 1987). This demonstrates that if the keratin 1 gene defect is also present in the germ cells, this nonlethal mutation may be transmitted to the next generation as EHK (also referred to as generalized bullous congenital ichythyosiform erythroderma). Munro and Wilkie (1998) have suggested that nevus comedonicus represents a mosaic condition for a mutation in fibroblast growth factor receptor2 (FGFR2), which if present in the germ line, would result in Apert's syndrome (see Chapter 35 for discussion). Activating FGFR3 mutations have been found in a significant percentage of Keratinocytic EN, almost exclusively at coden 248 (R248c) (Hafner et al. 2006a, b).

Despite the characterization of distinct epidermal nevus syndromes, classification of the majority of the molecular defects seen in ENS has not yet occurred. Investigation of the role of other FGF mutations in ENS may provide insight into the pathogenesis of the cutaneous and extra-cutaneous features of these syndromes. It is well documented that FGFs play a vital role in embryonic development. They function as important signaling molecules between epithelial and mesenchymal boundaries (Ornitz and Itoh 2001). Mutations in FGFs have been associated with developmental defects in cutaneous, neuronal, skeletal, and ocular systems. Future analysis of mutations from different EN will undoubtedly clarify the role of genetic aberrations in the pathogenesis of the ENS.

## References

Abell E, Read SI (1980) Porokeratotic eccrine ostial and dermal duct naevus. Br J Dermatol 103: 435–441.

Aschinberg LC, Solomon LM, Zeis PM, Justice P, Rosenthal IM (1977) Vitamin D-resistant rickets associated with epidermal nevus syndrome: demonstration of a phosphaturic substance in the dermal lesions. J Pediatr 91: 56–60.

Atherton DJ, Kahana M et al. (1989) Naevoid psoriasis. Br J Dermatol 120: 837–841.

Blaschko A (1901) Die Nervenverteilung in der Haut in ihrer Beziehung zu den Erkrankungen der Haut. Wien Leipzig: Braumuller. (Supplement to the proceeding German Dermatological Society 7th Congress in Breslau.)

Cribier B, Scrivener Y, Grosshans E (2000) Tumors arising in nevus sebaceus: a study of 596 cases. J Am Acad Dermatol 42: 263–268.

Dogra S, Jain R, Mohanty SH, Handa S (2002) Porokeratotic eccrine ostial and dermal duct nevus: unilateral systematized involvement. Pediatr Dermatol 19: 568–569.

Drezner MK (2000) PHEX gene and hypophosphatemia. Kidney Int 57: 9–18.

Feuerstein RC, Mims LC (1962) Linear nevus sebaceus with convulsions and mental retardation. Am J Dis Child 104: 675–679.

Gurecki PJ, Holden KR, Sahn EE, Dyer SS, Cure JK (1996) Developmental neural abnormalities and seizures in epidermal nevus syndrome. Dev Med Child Neurol 38: 716–723.

Hafner C, Vogt T, Hartmann A (2006a) FGFR3 mutations in benign skin tumors. Cell Cycle 5: 2723–2728.

Hafner C, van Oers JM, Vogt T, Landthaler M, Stoehr R, Blaszyk H, Hofstaedter F, Zwarthoff EC, Hartmann A (2006b) Mosaicism of activating FGFR3 mutations in human skin causes epidermal nevi. J Clin Invest 116: 2201–2207.

Haggstrom AN, Lammer EJ, Schneider RA, Marcucio R, Frieden IJ (2006) Patterns of infantile hemangiomas: new clues to hemangioma pathogenesis and embryonic facial development. Pediatrics 117: 698–703.

Happle R (1987) Lethal genes surviving by mosaicism: a possible explanation for sporadic birth defects involving the skin. J Am Acad Dermatol 16: 899–906.

Happle R (1991) How many epidermal nevus syndromes exist? A clinicogenetic classification. J Am Acad Dermatol 25: 550–556.

Happle R (1995) Epidermal nevus syndromes. Semin Dermatol 14: 111–121.

Heike CL, Cunningham ML, Steiner RD, Wenkert D, Hornung RL, Gruss JS, Gannon FH, McAlister WH, Mumm S, Whyte MP (2005) Skeletal changes in epidermal nevus syndrome: does focal bone disease harbor clues concerning pathogenesis? Am J Med Genet A 139: 67–77.

Hoffman WH, Jueppner HW, Deyoung BR, O'dorisio MS, Given KS (2005) Elevated fibroblast growth factor-23 in hypophosphatemic linear nevus sebaceous syndrome. Am J Med Genet A 134: 233–236.

Iglesias Zamora ME, Vazquez-Doval FJ (1997) Epidermal naevi associated with trichilemmal cysts and chromosomal mosaicism. Br J Dermatol 137: 821–824.

Ivker R, Resnick SD, Skiolmore RA (1997) Hypophosphatemic vitamin D-resistant rickets, precocious puberty, and the epidermal nevus syndrome. Arch Dermatol 133: 1557–1561.

Jackson R (1976) The lines of Blaschko: a review and reconsideration: observations of the cause of certain unusual linear conditions of the skin. Br J Dermatol 95: 349–360.

Jadassohn J (1895) Bermerkungen zur Histologie der systematisierten nevi und uber "Talgdrusen-Naevi". Arch Derm Syph 33: 355–394.

Jaqueti G, Requena L, Sanchez Yus E (2000) Trichoblastoma is the most common neoplasm developed in nevus sebaceus of Jadassohn: a clinicopathologic study of a series of 155 cases. Am J Dermatopathol 22: 108–118.

Jonsson KB, Zahradnik R, Larsson T, White KE, Sugimoto T, Imanishi Y, Yamamoto T, Hampson G, Koshiyama H, Ljunggren O, Oba K, Yang IM, Miyauchi A, Econs MJ, Lavigne J, Juppner H (2003) Fibroblast growth factor 23 in oncogenic osteomalacia and X-linked hypophosphatemia. N Engl J Med 348: 1656–1663.

Marsden RA, Fleming K, Dawber RP (1979) Comedo naevus of the palm – a sweat duct naevus? Br J Dermatol 101: 717–722.

Mehregan AH, Pinkus H (1965) Life History of Organoid Nevi. Special Reference to Nevus Sebaceus of Jadassohn. Arch Dermatol 91: 574–588.

Moss C, Jones DO, Beight A, Bowden PE (1995) Birthmark due to cutaneous mosaicism for keratin 10 mutation. Lancet 345: 596.

Munro CS, Wilkie AO (1998) Epidermal mosaicism producing localised acne: somatic mutation in FGFR2. Lancet 352: 704–705.

Olivares JL, Ramos FJ, Carapeto FJ, Bueno M (1999) Epidermal naevus syndrome and hypophosphataemic rickets: description of a patient with central nervous system anomalies and review of the literature. Eur J Pediatr 158: 103–107.

Ornitz DM, Itoh N (2001) Fibroblast growth factors. Genome Biol 2: Reviews 3005.

Paller AS, Syder AJ, Chan YM, Yu QC, Hutton E, Tadini G, Fuchs E (1994) Genetic and clinical mosaicism in a type of epidermal nevus. N Engl J Med 331: 1408–1415.

Pavone L, Curatolo P, Rizzo R, Micali G, Incorpora G, Garg BP, Dunn DW, Dobyns WB (1991) Epidermal nevus syndrome: a neurologic variant with hemimegalencephaly, gyral malformation, mental retardation, seizures, and facial hemihypertrophy. Neurology 41: 266–271.

Prayson RA, Estes ML, Morris HH (1993) Coexistence of neoplasia and cortical dysplasia in patients presenting with seizures. Epilepsia 34: 609–615.

Prayson RA, Kotagal P, Wyllie E, Bingaman W (1999) Linear epidermal nevus and nevus sebaceus syndromes: a clinicopathologic study of 3 patients. Arch Pathol Lab Med 123: 301–305.

Rogers M (1992) Epidermal nevi and the epidermal nevus syndromes: a review of 233 cases. Pediatr Dermatol 9: 342–344.

Saraswat A, Dogra S, Bhansali A, Kumar B (2003) Phakomatosis pigmentokeratotica associated with hypophosphataemic vitamin D-resistant rickets: improvement in phosphate homeostasis after partial laser ablation. Br J Dermatol 148: 1074–1076.

Sassmannshausen J, Bogomilsky J, Chaffins M (2000) Porokeratotic eccrine ostial and dermal duct nevus: a case report and review of the literature. J Am Acad Dermatol 43: 364–367.

Schimmelpenning GW (1957) Clinical contribution to symptomatology of phacomatosis. Fortschr Geb Rontgenstr Nuklearmed 87: 716–720.

Solomon LM, Fretzin DF, Dewald RL (1968) The epidermal nevus syndrome. Arch Dermatol 97: 273–285.

Solomon LM (1975) Epidermal nevus syndrome. Mod Probl Paediatr 17: 27–30.

Stosiek N, Ulmer R, von den Driesch P, Claussen U, Hornstein OP, Rott HD (1994) Chromosomal mosaicism in two patients with epidermal verrucous nevus. Demonstration of chromosomal breakpoint. J Am Acad Dermatol 30: 622–625.

Sugarman JL (2004) Epidermal nevus syndromes. Semin Cutan Med Surg 23: 145–157.

Sugarman JL (2007) Epidermal nevus syndromes. Semin Cutan Med Surg 26: 221-230.

Sugarman GI, Reed WB (1969) Two unusual neurocutaneous disorders with facial cutaneous signs. Arch Neurol 21: 242–247.

Sugarman JL, Frieden IJ (2004) Epidermal nevus syndromes. In: Roach EM, Allen VS (eds.) Neurocutaneous disorders. New York: Cambridge University Press, pp. 88–104.

Tay YK, Weston WL, Ganong CA, Klingensmith GJ (1996) Epidermal nevus syndrome: association with central precocious puberty and woolly hair nevus. J Am Acad Dermatol 35: 839–842.

Yu TW, Tsau YK, Young C, Chiu HC, Shen YZ (2000) Epidermal nevus syndrome with hypermelanosis and chronic hyponatremia. Pediatr Neurol 22: 151–154.

# Chapter 33

# SCHIMMELPENNING-FEUERSTEIN-MIMS SYNDROME (NEVUS SEBACEOUS SYNDROME)

Ignacio Pascual-Castroviejo and Martino Ruggieri

Paediatric Neurology Service, University Hospital La Paz, University of Madrid, Madrid, Spain (IPC); Institute of Neurological Science, National Research Council, Catania and Department of Paediatrics, University of Catania, Catania, Italy (MR)

## Introduction

Nevus sebaceous (NS) is a relatively common type of cutaneous lesion characterised by epidermal acanthosis and hyperplasia of the sebaceous glands that, when coupled with extracutaneous manifestations (mostly of the central nervous, ocular or skeletal systems), gives the name to a complex malformation syndrome (NS syndrome) first described by Jadassohn in 1895 and later recognised as a neurocutaneous disorder by Schimmelpenning (Happle 2004, Schimmelpenning 1957, 1983).

NS is an epidermal hamartoma located in the skin regions where the sebaceous glands are more abundant: scalp, forehead and ocular and palpebral regions followed to a lesser degree by any other part of the body (Solomon and Esterly 1975). Typically, the clinical and histopathological features of NS change with age: in *infancy and childhood* (before puberty) the nevi are relatively flat (due to the quiescence of sebaceous glands) showing mild to moderate papillated epidermal hyperplasia and fairly small subjacent abnormal follicular-sebaceous glands; at *puberty* (under hormonal influence), NS often thickens and develop papillomatous hyperplasia of the overlying epidermis with large numbers of mature sebaceous glands; benign and malignant neoplastic changes characterise a *third stage* in a minority of cases (Sugarman 2004).

Both the site and extension of NS appear to influence the risk of the associated extracutaneous disease likely reflecting the dorso-ventral migratory pathways of the neuroectoderm during embryogenesis (Menascu and Donner 2008, Sarnat and Flores-Sarnat 2004, Sugarman 2004) (see also chapter 1).

## Historical perspective and terminology

**Josef Jadassohn** was born in Liegnitz, Germany on 10th September 1863 and studied medicine in Gottingen, Heidelberg, and Leipzig before obtaining his doctorate in 1887 at Breslau. He was subsequently assistant to professor Albert LS. Neisser in the dermatological department of the Allerheilimgen-Hospital in Breslau until 1892. In 1896 he was appointed extraordinarius and director of the university skin clinic in Bern where he was elevated to ordinaries in 1903. In 1917 he assumed the chair of dermatology in Breslau, holding this tenure until he was emerited in 1931. He died in Schlesien on 24th March 1936 (Who named it? 2006). Jadassohn a fine clinician, meticulous scientist (he was one of the first to employ immunology techniques in the study of skin disorders) and notable teacher first described the NS syndrome with complete features in a patient, and some clinical signs in his father, three sisters and one paternal aunt (Jadassohn 1895).

Other reports of patients with NS syndrome may date back to 1927 as reported by Warnke et al. (2003) who discovered, in the Wax Moulage Museum of Skin Diseases and Disorders in the Department of Dermatology at the University of Kiel, Germany, a wax moulage (labelled as "Naevus Sebaceous" and dated 1st December 1927) which was an original impression of a living patient showing several sebaceous nevi of the left head and neck following the lines of Blaschko. Robinson (1932) first applied the term "*naevus sebaceous of Jadassohn*".

**Gustav Wilhelm Schimmelpenning** was born on 18th December 1928 in Oldenburg in northern Germany growing up partly in Norway because of the Norwegian origins of his mother and studying medicine in Kiel, Toronto and Munster before specialising in neuropsychiatry in Munster where he was appointed assistant at the department of neurology and psychiatry under professor Mauz (Happle 2004). He then headed the Allgeneimes Krankenhaus Ochsenzoll in Hamburg (from 1968) and the chair of psychiatry of Kiel (from 1971) retiring from his academic life in 1994 (Happle 2004). Schimmelpenning, in 1957, while training in neurology and psychiatry, comprehensively described a case of a 17-year-old girl with a sebaceous nevus involving her left head and neck and associated ipsilateral ocular lesions including coloboma of the upper lids, fibrous bone dysplasia with increased density of the frontal and parietal cranial bones and the anterior cranial fossa, dilated ventricles (at pneumencephalography), epileptic seizures first appeared at age 12 years and mental retardation (Schimmelpenning 1957). He concluded that this combination of anomalies represented a new "phacomatosis" (Happle 2004, Schimmelpenning 1957). Twenty-five years later he published a follow-up study of the same patient (Schimmelpenning 1983).

The history of Schimmelpenning syndrome exemplifies a rule that has prevailed over the last five decades: namely, that the scientific community will not recognise a new entity until it has been rediscovered in other places (Grosshans and Tomb 1992, Happle 2004). **Richard C. Feuerstein** and **Leroy C. Mims**, two American physicians from California reported, without knowing of Schimmelpenning's publication, two cases of "linear sebaceous nevus with convulsions and mental retardation" (Feuerstein and Mims 1962). Some authors considered this to be the first report on that neurocutaneous phenotype (Happle 2004) and called it "*Feuerstein-Mims syndrome*" (Besser 1976, Brihaye et al. 1988). Paradoxically, this eponym designation even reappeared in the German medical literature (Wauschkuhn and Rohde 1971). Mehregan and Pinkus (1965) applied the term "*organoid nevi*" as a generalized term that included other epidermal nevi syndromes and is not limited to linear NS, although this was the principal lesion. Clancy et al. (1985) questioned whether there is a real difference in the subclassification of organoid nevi into the epidermal nevus syndrome, nevus unis lateris, linear verrucous epidermal nevus, and linear sebaceous nevus. All of these lesions can be associated with neurological abnormalities. Further confusion was generated by the introduction of the new term "*epidermal nevus syndrome*" by the American dermatologist Laurence Solomon (Solomon et al. 1968) who erroneously lumped together quite different phenotypes under this umbrella name (Happle 1999, 2004) (see also chapter 32).

Other eponyms in the literature have been Schimmelpenning syndrome; Feuerstein-Mims syndrome; Schimmelpenning-Feuerstein-Mims syndrome; epidermal nevus syndrome of Solomon, Fretzin and Dewald; Solomon syndrome; linear nevus sebaceous syndrome; organoid nevus phakomatosis; organoid nevus syndrome; Jadassohn disease; Jadassohn sebaceous nevus syndrome; and Jadassohn nevus phacomatosis (reviewed in Happle 2004). As a consequence of this confusing nomenclature, Schimmelpenning syndrome has two different entries in the OMIM catalogue (OMIM # 163200 and OMIM # 165630) (OMIM 2006).

The term "*Schimmelpenning/nevus sebaceous syndrome*" seems historically justified and practically sufficient to distinguish this entity from other epidermal nevus syndromes (Happle 2004, Sugarman 2004) (see chapter 32). The rather long-winded term "Schimmelpenning-Feuerstein-Mims-Solomon syndrome" gives credit to all those who rediscovered the syndrome but also contributed, in one way or the other, to its further delineation (Happle 2004, Who named it? 2006).

## Incidence and prevalence

The prevalence of NS ranges from 1 to 3 per 1000 live births (Solomon and Esterly 1975). Males and females are similarly affected. The largest series published to date is that of Rogers (1992) with 233 cases.

## Clinical manifestations

### Skin anomalies

Histological rather than clinical characteristics of the lesions appear to be actually more decisive to distinguish the type of epidermal nevus: the typical epidermal nevus of the NS type has (besides the papillated epidermal hyperplasia) a predominance of (subjacent) abnormal follicular-sebaceous glands (Sugarman 2004). The clinical and histological appearance of the lesions also change with age (Mehregan 1984, Sugarman 2004, Sugarman and Frieden 2004): from birth to puberty the nevi are relatively flat (due to the quiescence of sebaceous glands) showing mild to moderate epidermal hyperplasia and rather small follicular-sebaceous glands; at puberty (under hormonal influence), the naevi most often thickens and develop papillomatous hyperplasia of the overlying epidermis with increasing numbers of more mature sebaceous glands; benign and malignant neoplastic changes characterise a third stage in a minority of cases (Sugarman 2004). The naevi are typically congenital and also are rarely familial. However, familial NS presentations unassociated with extracutaneous disease has been reported (Meschia et al. 1992).

The cutaneous distribution of NS usually follows the linear patterns known as "lines of Blaschko" (Blaschko 1901). These lines do not follow the segmental trajectory of the peripheral sensory nerves, but instead reflect the streams or trends of growth of embryonic tissues (Montgomery 1901). This view is commonly held although still remains unproven (Moss et al. 1993, Moss 1999).

NS was the first described type of epidermal nevus and likely the most common variety, representing approximately one-half of all epidermal naevi (Rogers 1992, Sugarman 2004). Nearly two thirds of NS are localized to the scalp and the remaining one-third to the face. In some patients the NS may more extensively involve the neck and rarely the chest. NS most frequently is present at birth and shows a salmon to yellow colour. There is a lack of hair in the area of the nevus and the hair of the surrounding zones shows a colourless appearance. The lesion is typically flat during the initial stages of infancy (Fig. 1) but, at puberty often thickens (see above) (Fig. 2) (Mehregan and Pinkus 1965). During this stage the lesion may assume a verrucous nature that can be seen even in the first years of life (Figs. 3–5).

The third stage characterized by the presence of benign or malignant neoplasms, may occur in as many as 10–15% of patients with NS (Mehregan 1984, Morioka 1985).

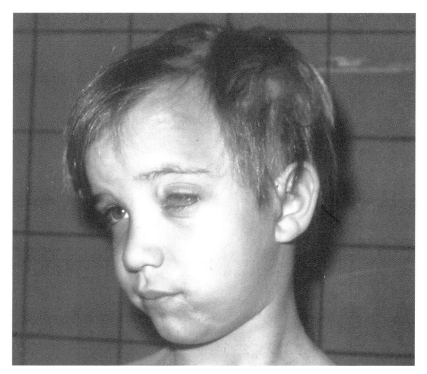

**Fig. 1.** An 8-year-old child shows a sebaceous nevus on the left hemifacies, scalp and orbit involving the eye.

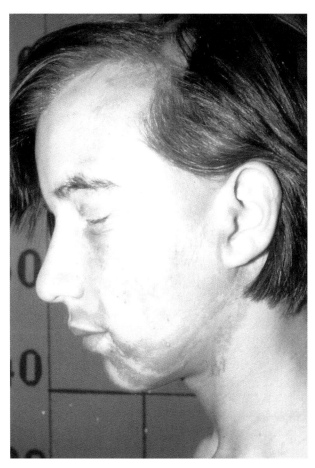

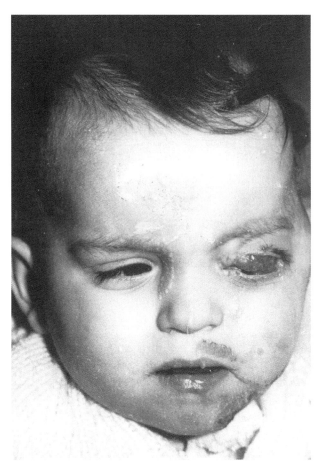

**Fig. 2.** Same patient as in Fig. 1 at 17 years of age showing cutaneous lesions on the left face. Note the moderate verrucous appearance of the sebaceous nevi that follow Blaschko's lines.

**Fig. 3.** A 6-month-old child with sebaceous nevi on both sides of the face, although with predominant extension on the left side. Note the coloboma of the internal zone of the eyelid and the lipoma of the orbit.

The other most common form of epidermal nevus is the keratinocytic or verrucous nevus (Rogers 1992, Sugarman 2004). The *keratinocytic type* most commonly appear at birth or during early infancy as linear whorled to pink or slightly hyperpigmented plaques. This form of nevus may appear anywhere in the body, as a unilateral (nevus unis lateris) or bilateral lesion. *Nevus verrucous* may be solitary, multiple, small or large, and is most frequently found on the trunk or extremities. In their unilateral presentation, lesions usually stop abruptly on the ventral and dorsal midline (Fig. 6). In unilateral presentation, overgrowth of all subjacent structures with asymmetry of the affected organs is commonly seen. This overgrowth is more active during the stage of darkening colour of the cutaneous lesion and may stop

after a few years during which the nevus start to fade (Fig. 7). Verrucous epidermal naevi are commonly present at birth or at early ages as different type of cutaneous lesions that often extend over adjacent areas of skin or organs included in the anatomical region such as eyes, eyelids and the orbital tissues (Fig. 8). Although verrucous naevi most commonly are unilateral, these can also be bilateral. Other types of epidermal nevus are not commonly associated with neurological disease.

## Central nervous system (CNS) anomalies

The most common NS associated neurological abnormalities are seizures, mental retardation, and/or cognitive developmental delay (Sugarman 2004).

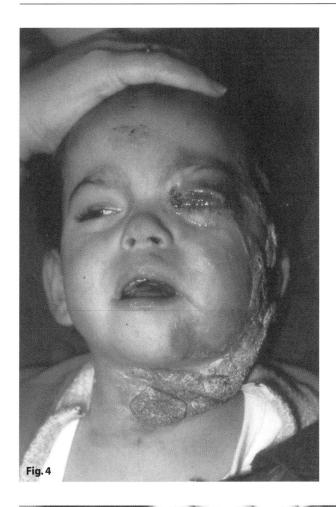

Fig. 4

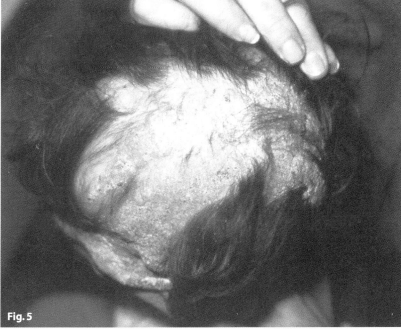

Fig. 5

**Figs. 4 and 5.** Same patient as in Fig. 3 at 1 year of age shows severe verrucous lesions of some parts of the sebaceous nevi on the left face, neck and scalp.

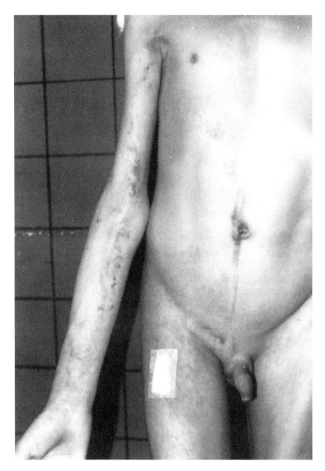

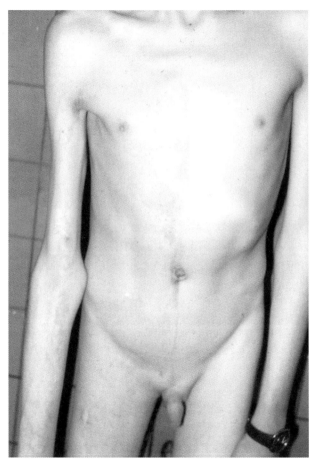

**Fig. 6.** A 6-year-old child shows a nevus unis lateris with verrucous appearance on the right extremities and the right skin of the trunk with cessation of the nevus in the midline.

**Fig. 7.** Same patient as in Fig. 6 at 9 years of age shows the same type of lesions although lighter and with marked decrease of the verrucous component.

## Epilepsy

Seizures and developmental delay are the two main neurological abnormalities of patients who have associated hemimegalencephaly with NS. The seizure disorders in these patients are often of early onset and almost always occur during the first 8 months of life. In some infants, the seizures begin within the first week of life. They are often resistant to medical therapy causing severe neurological sequelae. The severity of the neurological disease is related to the presence of many types of seizures, such as focal, generalized, and infantile spasms that are followed by Lennox-Gastaut syndrome (Alonso et al. 1988,

Herbs and Cohen 1971, Kurokawa et al. 1981, Lopez Martín and Pascual-Castroviejo 1976). Major hemispheric malformations predispose patients to neonatal seizures, infantile spasms and the Lennox-Gastaut variant. In a review of the British literature (Gurecki et al. 1996) more than 50% of patients with epidermal naevi of the NS and keratinocytic types had seizures. Previous reports of seizures in NS syndrome varied from 38 to 96% (Baker et al. 1987, Barth et al. 1977, Clancy et al. 1985, Rogers 1992, Rogers et al. 1989, Solomon and Esterly 1975). Onset of seizures usually occurs earlier than in other neurocutaneous syndromes (Clancy et al. 1985).

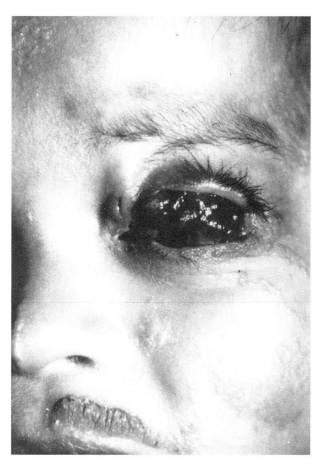

**Fig. 8.** A 6-month-old child with left facial sebaceous nevi (some with verrucous growth) and associated orbital, eyelid and ocular tumor.

## Cognitive deficit

Cognitive impairment and other neurological features, such as monoparesis, hemiparesis or quadriparesis, cranial nerve palsy, deafness, cortical blindness, segmental dysesthaesia, hyperactivity, or different levels of mental retardation are related with the early presentation and severity of the seizures and the nature, location and extension of the cerebral lesion, that is mostly of malformative origin, but that can be of tumoral or vascular origin as well. Thirteen of the 22 patients with epidermal nevus in a review of the English literature (Prensky et al. 1987) were considered to be retarded. Most were severely or deeply retarded but at least 3 had an IQ of 50 or above.

Mental impairment occurred in 10 of the 19 patients with skin-biopsy proven epidermal nevus, and nine of these had moderate or severe cognitive impairment (Sugarman 2004). Other reviews have reported variable proportions of cognitive delay between 64 and 90% (Baker et al. 1987, Clancy et al. 1985, Eichler et al. 1989, Solomon and Esterly 1975). Gurecki et al. (1996) found some degree of global impairment in 21 of the 23 patients with sebaceous and keratinocytic naevi: 16 had moderate to severe neurologic involvement. We agree with these findings, but the similarities of our results may be due to patients studied in neurology departments where these are referred, because of neurological problems rather than cutaneous disease.

## Brain malformations

The incidence of CNS abnormalities is most common in those patients with cutaneous lesions on the head or face (Edelsetin et al. 2005, Holden and Dekaban 1992, Rogers 1992). The association between abnormal neuronal migration and gliomatosis cerebri (Choi and Kudo 1981), or unilateral megalencephaly and NS syndrome, appears to be well established (Boltshauser and Navratil 1978, Cavenagh et al. 1993, Pavone et al. 1991, Vles et al. 1985, Vigevano et al. 1984). Unilateral megalencephaly or hemimegalencephaly in NS syndrome most often is associated with severe neurological features such as seizure disorders, mental retardation and contralateral motor disease (Flores-Sarnat 2001, Flores-Sarnat et al. 2003). The ipsilateral lateral ventricle can appears enlarged or collapsed. Additional imaging features include cortical agyria, pachygyria, polymicrogyria, corticosubcortical heterotopias and gliosis in the subjacent white matter (Fitz et al. 1978), loss of demarcation between cortical grey matter and subcortical white matter (Fig. 9) (Pascual-Castroviejo et al. 2003, Zhang et al. 2003), and grey matter bands with periventricular heterotopia (Williams and Casaer 1994). Lack of horizontal layering may be indicative of underlying histological abnormalities of loss of demarcation between white and grey matter (reviewed in Edelstein et al. 2005).

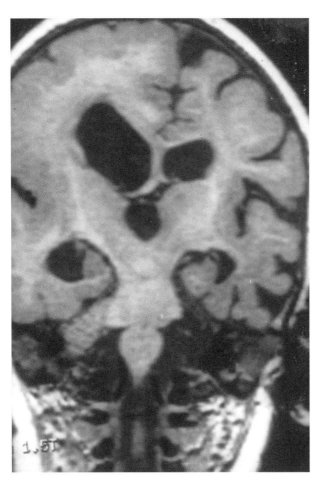

**Fig. 9.** A coronal T1-weighted MRI image shows right hemimega-lencephaly hemispheric and ventricular asymmetry, cortical pachy-gyria and poor delineation between cortical grey matter and sub-cortical white matter.

MR imaging is the preferred structural imaging technique and plays an important role in delineating the CNS structural abnormalities. Other functional neuroimaging techniques, such as magneto encephalography and single-photon emission CT (SPECT), may help to identify epileptogenic foci and cortical regions related to the epileptic foci (Zhag et al. 2003). In addition to unilateral hemimegalencephaly, other less frequent CNS abnormalities, such as tumours, agenesis of the corpus callosum, Dandy-Walker syndrome, Arnold-Chiari malformation, myelomeningocele, or lymphatic or vascular malformations have been reported (Andriola 1976, Baker et al. 1987, Chatkupt et al. 1993, Dobyns and Garg

1991, Dodge and Dobyns 1995, Gurecki et al. 1996, Hennekam et al. 1999, Pavone et al. 1991). Mall et al. (2000) described three patients with NS syndrome and lipoma in the CNS of whom two presented with intraspinal and one pontocerebellar location.

A subgroup of patients with skin lesions localized in the head and neck may represent a more sharply defined entity within the phenotypic spectrum of NS syndrome. This relationship has important diagnostic implications for the clinician. In a review of the literature in English, no consistent relationship between laterality of the nevus and laterality of CNS abnormalities was found, supporting the mosaicism pathogenic theory (Gurecki et al. 1996). However, a relationship between scalp, forehead, eyes, and face NS and subjacent abnormalities, is evident. Cerebral arteriography showed, in one of our cases, vascular anomalies in the subjacent area of the brain to the NS consisting of absence of the anterior cerebral artery (both anterior cerebral arteries were originated from the contralateral internal carotid artery) that caused blood supply deficit due to a poor collateral vascularisation (Figs. 10 and 11).

## Non CNS extracutaneous manifestations

NS may be associated with clinical and imaging manifestations localized anywhere in the body. Extracutaneous manifestations are mostly associated with cutaneous manifestations in adjacent areas. In patients with skin lesions, the anterior portion of the skull, forehead, face, ocular and palpebral regions are, besides the CNS, the structures most frequently involved.

The percentage of individuals with NS who have extracutaneous non CNS findings is not precisely known, and many estimates in the literature are overstated due to ascertainment bias and to lumping of several epidermal naevus syndromes (reviewed in Sugarman 2004).

### Eye abnormalities

Ocular and palpebral abnormalities were observed in 29 of the 74 cases reviewed by Gurecki et al. (1996). Strabismus, lipodermoids and coloboma are the

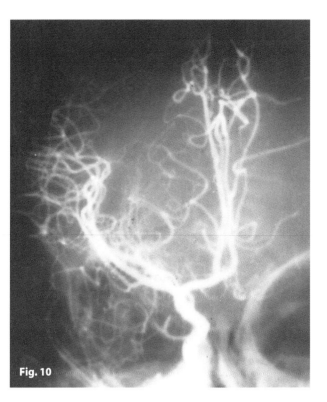
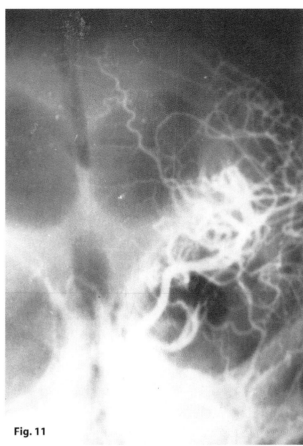

**Figs. 10 and 11.** Coronal views of conventional carotid arteriography of both sides in the same patient shown in Figs. 3–5. Both anterior cerebral arteries originate in the right carotid artery. Very poor vascularization of the left frontal lobe (both lateral and third ventricle were visible two days after pneumoencephalography).

most frequent lesions, followed by corneal opacities, exo/esotropia, retinal changes including scarring, degeneration, and detachment, ptosis, macrophthalmia, and conjunctival growths. In the review of 131 cases with "epidermal NS" by Rogers et al. (1989), 9% had ocular anomalies. Review of smaller series of NS described percentages of ocular anomalies over 30%. Solomon and Esterly (1975) observed ocular abnormalities in 33% of their 60 patients. Gurecki et al. (1996) found ocular and orbital involvement in 9 of 23 (39%) patients, with bilateral involvement in four cases. Ocular involvement in our series were always associated with NS affecting the orbit or the surrounding areas.

Loss of vision in the involved eye may be common. Response to palpebral and ocular surgical treatment is not usually followed by success because all palpebral, orbital and eye structures may be involved, and although most sebaceous naevi of the orbital region and the eye are benign, these are infiltrating lesions and complete removal is very difficult. Most of them regress shortly after surgical treatment but they can lead to loss of vision or even of the eye. Optic nerve hypoplasia has been associated with NS in some cases (Katz et al. 1987).

## Skeletal anomalies

These were found in 50% of 74 patients with NS reviewed by Grebe et al. (1993). Most of these anomalies could be attributed to tissue overgrowth and

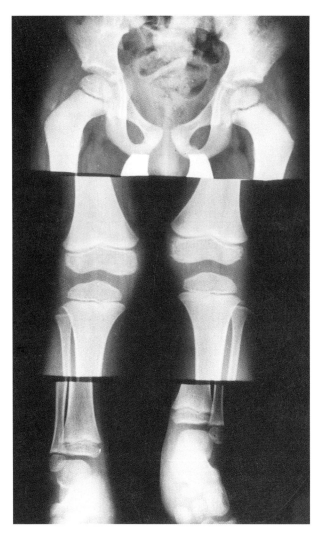

**Fig. 12.** X-ray study of the lower limbs with measurements of limbs of the same patient as in Figs. 6 and 7 shows asymmetry with overgrowth of all bones on the right side.

were ipsilateral to the cutaneous NS maintaining the asymmetry with respect to the unaffected side during life, without further growth after age six or eight, at least in the patients of our series. Skeletal manifestations of NS syndrome were reported in the classic paper of Salomon and Esterly (1975) who distinguished primary anomalies that affected the complete formation and the bone size (hyper-or hypoplasia) and secondary anomalies that included kyphoscoliosis, skull/craniofacial asymmetry, possibly related to localized or generalized hemihypertrophy.

Other described anomalies, such as pes equinovarus, genu valgus, short stature, ankylosis, or microcephaly, do not appear to be directly related to the nevus. Although skeletal asymmetry can be found in any hypertrophic area, extremities are involved most frequently. X-ray study with measurement of the limbs reveals the asymmetry, even in cases that clinically do not show overt difference in size (Fig. 12).

## Other organs abnormalities

Less common is to find NS associated with anomalies that involve other organs. Grebe et al. (1993) described two patients, a newborn who had multiple verrucous epidermal nevi on several areas of the body, and several other anomalies, including bony duplications of the lower limbs and hypoplastic left heart syndrome, and another patient with associated genitourinary, cardiac, skeletal defects and severe CNS involvement. In a review of 74 patients these authors (Grebe et al. 1993) recorded different types of cardiac malformations in 12% of their patients. Genitourinary abnormalities, such as hydronephrosis, double collecting system, horseshoe kidney, cystic kidney, hypospadias, cryptorchidism, testicular and paratesticular tumors, nephroblastomatosis, ureteropelvic junction obstruction, and vitamin D-resistant rickets, were noted in 10% of cases (Grebe et al. 1993).

During recent years, several patients were described with associated hypophosphatemic rickets with endocrine abnormalities, such as precocious puberty (Ivker et al. 1997, Moss et al. 1991, Tay et al. 1996) and the syndrome of inappropriate anti-diuretic hormone (Yu et al. 2000). Olivares et al. (1999) observed that at least 14 cases of hypophosphatemic vitamin-D resistant rickets had been described in association with NS, and 86% of these patients had in addition mental delay.

## Pathology

The histological features of the lesions change with age and may appear different in the various zones of the nevus. Therefore, several skin biopsies may be necessary to ascertain all components of the skin lesion in a given case. During the first stage of the natural history, early in life, the epidermis is acanthotic, but pigment is still only slightly increased; small and poorly formed hair follicles are often represented only by cords of basaloid cells; sebaceous glands are increased, but may not be prominent; apocrine glands may not be developed yet. During the second stage, sebaceous glands proliferate and often the apocrine glands dilate, but the hair follicles remain primordial. In the third stage, the hair follicles remain primordial strands, but large clumps of sebaceous glands occur in the dermis, and apocrine glands can be located aberrantly through the thickness of the skin (Mehregam 1984, Prensky 1987).

## Pathogenesis and molecular genetics

The association of Blaschko's lines with genetic mosaicism has led to the hypothesis that this pattern of lines represents genetically abnormal skin contrasting with genetically normal skin (Happle et al. 1996). Only for linear epidermolytic hyperkeratosis has it been possible to show mutant cells confined to the abnormal streaks. The hypothesis proposed by Moss (1999) to explain this paradox is that disorders following Blaschko's lines are due to mutations in genes expressed in epidermal cells (keratinocytes and melanocytes) rather than in dermal fibroblasts. Notably, most disorders following Blaschko's lines are epidermal. The Blaschko's lines represent the routes of embryonic cell migration. Epidermal cells originate in the neural crest and move to the periphery of the growing embryo by directional proliferation (keratinocytes) or migration (melanocytes) (Moss 1999). Postnatally, the final location of either cellular type in the basal layer is two dimensionally fixed: keratinocytes proliferate only outwards towards the skin surface whilst melanocytes do not proliferate at all. Mutations occurring earlier in development theoretically would cause more extensive cutaneous and subcutaneous lesions, and the severity of a specific mutation may

determine the extent and severity of clinical and radiological features.

Most cases of NS syndrome are sporadic, and only a few familial presentation have been published. Confusion has been generated by lumping different types of epidermal naevi under the umbrella term of "epidermal nevus syndrome". As a consequence the NS (Schimmelpenning-Feuerstein-Mims) syndrome still has two different entries in the OMIM catalogue (OMIM # 163200 and OMIM # 165630) (OMIM 2006).

Several particular genes have been identified in selected sebaceous naevi by investigating epidermal cells (see also chapter 32). Point mutations in 50% of the keratin 10 alleles of epidermal cells from patients with NS vs. no mutations in the unaffected adjacent epidermis were found by Paller et al. (1994). Translocation in chromosome 1 was found by cytogenetic analysis on keratinocytes from two patients with NS by Stosiek et al. (1994). Moss et al. (1995) found in a patient with NS mosaicism for keratin 10 mutations in affected cells vs. lack of mutations in cells derived from unaffected adjacent epidermis. Zamora and Vazquez-Doval (1997) reported a woman with a large verrucous epidermal nevus and multiple trichilemmal cysts who showed chromosomal mosaicism and a translocation between 1p36 and 9q34 in 5% of her lymphocytes.

A possible recent explanation for this hitherto unravelled mutational epidermal framework reflecting genetic mosaicism could be that of Taibjee et al. (2004) who hypothesized that pigmentary mosaic phenotypes could arise through disparate karyotype abnormalities specifically disrupting either expression or function of pigmentary genes. In their study (Taibjee et al. 2004) they cross-compared karyotype abnormalities in pigmentary mosaic disorders following the lines of Blaschko with 76 pigmentary and candidate pigmentary gene loci, either in humans or animals, showing extensive (88%) overlaps between cytogenetic abnormalities and one or more pigmentary genes as well as significant (74%) overlaps between pigmentary genes and one or more karyotype abnormalities supporting the hypothesis of a pathogenic role for the individual chromosomal abnormalities in causing the pigmentary lesions (besides chance occurrence).

## Differential diagnosis

The differential diagnosis during the first two or three years of life may include focal dermal hypoplasia (Goltz's syndrome) and incontinentia pigmenti (IP) of Bloch and Sulzberger, but features of lesions in these two diseases have many differences with those of EN and both of these syndromes are inherited as an X-linked dominant trait and the women are almost exclusively affected. Differential diagnosis with Conradi-Humermann's syndrome, which can be X-linked or autosomal dominantly inherited, and that shows hyperkeratotic papules in a swirling pattern associated with chondrodysplasia congenita punctata, other skeletal defects and cataracts, may be necessary in some young patients.

Recently, a newly defined constellation of congenital anomalies including nevus sebaceous has been reported and named SCALP syndrome [nevus sebaceous, central nervous system anomalies, aplasia cutis congenita, limbal dermoid, and pigmented (melanocytic) nevus] (Demerdjieva et al. 2007, Lam et al. 2008). Another new type of epidermal nevus (nevus marginatus) (Hafner et al. 2008) should be distinguished from the typical nevus sebaceous: it consists of a linear nevus showing a flattish central area characterised by sebaceous hyperplasia and elevated margins showing features of a common nonorganoid Keratinocytic EN.

## Management and prognosis

The management of patients with NS syndrome needs to be individualized and with possible collaboration of several specialists, such as dermatologists, paediatric neurologists, dermatopathologists, plastic surgeons, ophthalmologists, paediatricians, and occasionally others, such as paediatric endocrinologists.

Dermatologists commonly classify the type of NS and investigate the mosaicism. Performing histological investigation or identifying the changes of the cutaneous and subcutaneous tissues. If there is no neurologic involvement, circumscribed skin lesions can be removed by a plastic surgeon because of a tendency to bleed from minor trauma, and the

possibility of tumour formation during adult life, as well as for cosmetic reasons (especially for the protection of psychological development) (Dodge et al. 1992). Several surgical techniques have been used, such as simple excision for small EN or cryosurgery (Pierini and García-Díaz 1986). Oral or topical medication have been also administered, especially corticosteroids, that have been also used intralesionally. Other topical agents have been used to treat NS, although results are not optimistic in every case and lesions commonly recur when treatments are discontinued. Topical calcipotriol, a synthetic analogue of vitamin D that exerts an immunosuppressive effect on lymphoid cells, inhibits proliferation and promotes differentiation of keratinocytes, has been used for treatment of inflammatory linear verrucous epidermal nevus (Micali et al. 1995, Zvulunov et al. 1997).

Neurologic symptoms, especially the most severe, most commonly appear during the first months of life. These include seizures that are refractory to antiepileptic drug therapy. Seizures frequently originate in organic focus caused by vascular, tumoral or structural changes (i.e., hemimegalencephaly) lesions (Winstom et al. 2008). Patients with focalised lesions or with megalencephaly may improve after surgical treatment. These patients usually show severe mental retardation. Most patients with ENS without CNS lesion, however, present no significant loss of motor and/or mental function later during childhood or in adult life. Mental retardation has been reported between 64 and 90% of subjects with ENS (Solomon and Sterly 1975, Clancy et al. 1985, Baker et al. 1987, Prensky et al. 1987, Eichler et al. 1989, Gurecki et al. 1996).

Ophthalmologic involvement with tumors of the eye and/or other orbital components most times need early surgical excision of ocular lesions that in any way impair vision. Recurrence of lesions, however, often occurs.

Asymmetry of the limbs frequently needs orthopaedic treatment.

Bone abnormalities, muscle weakness, caused by vitamin D-resistant rickets, may improve with L-.25-dihydroxy vitamin D3 and phosphorus (Oranje et al. 1994).

# References

Alonso Luengo O, Ortiz Ocaña JM, Gomez de los Terreros I, Nieto Barrera M (1988) Nevus sebáceo de Jadassohn con espasmos infantiles asociados. An Esp Pediatr 28: 266–268.

Andriola M (1976) Nevus unis lateris and brain tumor. Am J Dis Child 130: 1259–1261.

Baker RS, Ross PA, Baumann RJ (1987) Neurologic complications of the epidermal nevus syndrome. Arch Neurol 44: 227–232.

Barkham MC, White N, Brundler MA, Richard B, Moss C (2007) Should naevus sebaceus be excised prophylactically? A clinical audit. J Plast Reconstr Aesthet Surg 60: 1269–1270.

Barth PG, Vark J, Kalsbeek GL, Blom A (1977) Organoid nevus syndrome (linear nevus sebaceous of Jadassohn): clinical and radiological study of a case. Neuropädiatrie 8: 418–428.

Besser FS (1976) Linear sebaceous naevi with convulsions and mental retardation (Feuerstein-Mims' syndrome), vitamin-D-resistant rickets. Proc R Soc Med 69: 518–520.

Blaschko A (1901) Die Nervenverteilung in ther Haut in ihrer Beziehung zu den Erkrankungen der Haut. In: Beilage zu den Verhandlungen der Deutschen Dermatologischen Gesellschaft VII Congress, Breslau. Table 16. Wien Leipzig: Braumuller.

Boltshauser E, Navratil F (1978) Organoid nevus syndrome in a neonate with hemimacrocephaly. Neuropädiatrie 9: 195–196.

Brihaye J, Brihaye-van Geertruyden M, Retif J, Mercier AM (1988) Late occurrence of additional ocular and intracranial pathologies in the linear naevus sebaceous (Feuerstein-Mims) syndrome. Acta Neurochir (Wien) 92: 132–137.

Cavenagh EC, Hart BL, Rose D (1993) Association of linear sebaceous nevus syndrome and unilateral megalencephaly. Am J Neuroradiol 14: 405–408.

Chatkupt S, Ruzicka PO, Lastra CR (1993) Myelomeningocele, spinal arteriovenous malformations and epidermal nevi syndrome: a possible rare association? Dev Med Child Neurol 35: 737–741.

Choi B, Kudo M (1981) Abnormal neuronal migration and gliomatosis cerebri in epidermal nevus syndrome. Acta Neuropathol (Berlin) 53: 319–325.

Clancy RR, Kurtz MB, Baker D, Sladky JT, Honig PJ, Younkin DP (1985) Neurologic manifestations of the organoid nevus syndrome. Arch Neurol 42: 236–240.

Demerdjieva Z, Kavaklieva S, Tsankov N (2007) Epidermal nevus syndrome and didymosis aplasticosebacea. Pediatr Dermatol 24: 514–516.

Dobyns WB, Garg BP (1991) Vascular abnormalities in epidermal nevus syndrome. Neurology 41: 276–278.

Dodge NN, Dobyns WB (1995) Agenesis of the corpus callosum and Dandy-Walker malformation associated with hemimegalencephaly in the sebaceous nevus syndrome. Am J Med Genet 56: 147–150.

Edelstein S, Naidich TP, Newton TH (2005) The rare phakomatoses. In: Tortori-Donati P (ed.) Pediatric Neuroradiology. Brain. Berlin: Springer-Verlag, pp. 819–854.

Eichler C, Flowers FP, Ross J (1989) Epidermal nevus syndrome: case report and review of clinical manifestations. Pediatr Dermatol 6: 316–320.

Fenerstein RC, Mims LC (1962) Linear nevus sebaceous with convulsions and mental retardation. Am J Dis Child 104: 675–679.

Fizt CR, Harwood-Nash DC, Boldt DW (1978) The radiographic features of unilateral megalencephaly. Neuroradiology 15: 145–148.

Flores-Sarnat L (2002) Hemimegalencephaly. 1. Genetic, clinical, and imaging aspects. J Child Neurol 17: 373–384.

Flores-Sarnat L, Sarnat HB, Dávila-Gutierrez G, Alvarez A (2003) Hemimegalencephaly: Part 2. Neuropathology suggests a disorder of cellular lineage. J Child Neurol 18: 776–785.

Grebe TA, Rimsza ME, Richter SF, Hansen RC, Hoyme HE (1993) Further delineation of the epidermal nevus syndrome: two cases with new findings and literature review. Am J Med Genet 47: 24–30.

Grosshans E, Tomb R (1992) 1492–1992: 500 years ago Christopher Columbus rediscovered America. From the rediscovery of skin diseases already described. Ann Dermatol Venereol 119: 7–9.

Gurecki PJ, Holden KR, Sahn EE, Dyer DS, Cure JK (1996) Developmental neural abnormalities and seizures in epidermal nevus syndrome. Dev Med Child Neurol 38: 716–723.

Hafner C, Landthaler M, Happle R, Vogt T (2008) Nevus marginatus: a distinct type of epidermal nevus or merely a variant of nevus sebaceus? Dermatologo 216: 236–238.

Happle R (1991) How many epidermal nevus syndromes exist? A clinicogenetic classification. J Am Acad Dermatol 25: 550–556.

Happle R (2004) Gustav Schimmelpenning and the syndrome bearing his name. Dermatology 209: 84–87.

Happle R, Hoffmann R, Restano L, Caputo R, Tadini G (1996) Phacomatosis pigmentokeratotica: a melanocytic-epidermal twin nevus syndrome. Am J Med Genet 65: 363–365.

Hennekam RC, Kwa VI, van Amerongen A (1999) Arteriovenous and lymphatic malformations, linear verrucous epidermal nevus and mild overgrowth: another hamarto-neoplastic syndrome? Clin Dysmorph 8: 111–115.

Herbs BA, Cohen ME (1971) Linear nevus sebaceous. A neurocutaneous syndrome associated with infantile spasms. Arch Neurol 24: 317–322.

Holden KR, Dekaban AD (1972) Neurological involvement in nevus unis lateris and nevus linearis sebaceous. Neurology 22: 879–887.

Ivker R, Resnick SD, Skidmore RA (1997) Hypophosphatemic vitamin D-resistant rickets, precocious puberty, and the epidermal nevus syndrome. Arch Dermatol 133: 1557–1561.

Jadassohn J (1895) Bemerkunzen zur Histologie der Systematisierten Naevi und Umber "Taldrusen-Naevi". Arch Dermatol Syph 33: 355–394.

Katz B, Wiley C, Lee V (1987) Optic nerve hypoplasia and the syndrome of nevus sebaceous of Jadassohn. Ophthalmology 94: 1570–1576.

Kurokawa T, Sasaki K, Hanai T, Goya N, Komaki S (1981) Linear nevus sebaceous syndrome. Report of a case with Lennox-Gastaut syndrome following infantile spasms. Arch Neurol 38: 375–377.

Lam J, Dohil MA, Eichenfield LF, Cunningham BB (2008) SCALP syndrome: sebaceous nevus syndrome, CNS malformations, aplasia cutis congenita, limbal dermoid, and pigmented nevus (giant congenital melanocytic nevus) with neurocutaneous melanosis: a distinct syndromic entity. J Am Acad Dermatol 58: 884–888.

Lopez Martín V, Pascual-Castroviejo I (1976) EEG en el nevus sebaceous of Jadassohn. Presentación de cuatro casos y revisión de la literatura. An Esp Pediatr 9: 519–525.

Mall V, Heinen F, Uhl M, Willens E, Korinthemberg R (2000) CNS lipoma in patients with epidermal nevus syndrome. Neuropediatrics 31: 175–179.

Marioka S (1985) The natural history of nevus sebaceous. J Cutan Pathol 12: 200–213.

Mehregan AH (1984) Sebaceous tumors of the skin. J Cutan Pathol 12: 196–199.

Mehregan AH, Pinkus H (1965) Life history of organoid nevi. Special reference to nevus sebaceous of Jadassohn. Arch Dermatol 91: 574–588.

Menascu S, Donner EJ (2008) Linear nevus sebaceous syndrome: case reports and review of the literature. Pediatr Neurol 38: 207–201.

Meschia JF, Junkins E, Hofman KJ (1992) Familial systematized epidermal nevus syndrome. Am J Med Genet 44: 664–667.

Micalli C, Nasca MR, Musameci ML (1995) Effect of topical calcipotriol on inflammatory linear verrucous epidermal nevus. Pediatr Dermatol 12: 386–387.

Montgomery DW (1901) The cause of the streaks in naevus linearis. J Cutan Genitourin Dis 19: 455–464.

Morioka S (1985) The natural history of nevus sebaceous. J Cutan Pathol 12: 200–213.

Moss C (1999) Cytogenetic and molecular evidence for cutaneous mosaicism: the ectodermal origin of Blaschko lines. Am J Med Genet 85: 330–333.

Moss C, Parkin JM, Comaish JS (1991) Precocious puberty in a boy with widespread linear epidermal naevus. Brit J Dermatol 125: 178–182.

Moss C, Larkins S, Blight A, Farndon P, Davison EV (1993) Epidermal mosaicism and Blaschko's lines. J Med Genet 30: 752–755.

Moss C, Jones DO, Blight A, Bowden PE (1995) Birthmark due to cutaneous mosaicism for keratin 10 mutation (letter) Lancet 345: 596.

Olivares JL, Ramos EJ, Carapeto FJ, Bueno M (1999) Epidermal naevus syndrome and hypophosphataemic rickets: description of a patient with central nervous system anomalies and review of the literature. Eur J Pediatr 158: 103–107.

Oranje AP, Przyrembel H, Meradji M, Loonen MCB, de Klerk JBC (1994) Solomon's epidermal nevus syndrome (Type: linear nevus sebaceous) and hypophosphatemic vitamin D-resistant rickets. Arch Dermatol 130: 1167–1171.

Paller AS, Syder AJ, Chan Y-M, Yu Q-C, Hutton E, Tadini G, Fuchs E (1994) Genetic and clinical mosaicism in a type of epidermal nevus. N Engl J Med 331: 1408–1415.

Pascual-Castroviejo I, Pascual-Pascual SI, Viaño J, Martínez V, Palencia R (2003) Malformaciones del desarrollo cortical y su repercusión clínica en una serie de 144 casos. Rev Neurol 37: 327–344.

Pavone L, Curatolo P, Rizzo R, Micali G, Incorpora G, Garg BP, Dobyns WB (1991) Epidermal nevus síndrome: A neurologic variant hemimegalencephaly, gyral malformation, mental retardation, seizures, and facial hemihypertrophy. Neurology 41: 266–271.

Pierini AM, García-Díaz R (1986) Therapy for LIBEN (letter). Pediatr Dermatol 3: 349.

Prensky AN (1987) Linear sebaceous nevus. In: Gomez MR (ed.) Neurocutaneous Diseases. A Practical Approach. Stoneham: Butterworths, pp. 335–344.

Rogers M (1992) Epidermal nevi and the epidermal nevus syndromes: a review of 233 cases. Pediatr Dermatol 9: 342–344.

Rogers M, McCrossin I, Commens C (1989) Epidermal nevi and the epidermal nevus syndrome: A review of 131 cases. J Am Acad Dermatol 20: 476–488.

Sarnat HB, Flores-Sarnat L (2004) Integrative classification of morphology and molecular genetics in central nervous system malformations. Am J Med Genet A 126: 386–392.

Schimmelpenning GW (1957) Clinical contribution to symptomatology of phacomatosis. Fortschr Geb Rontgenstr Nuklearmed 87: 716–720.

Schimmelpenning GW (1983) Long-term observation of a case of organoid naevus phakomatosis (Schimmelpenning-Feuerstein-Mims syndrome). Rofo 139: 63–67.

Solomon LM, Fretzin DF, Dewald RL (1968) The epidermal nevus syndrome. Arch Dermatol 97: 273–285.

Solomon LM, Sterly NB (1975) Epidermal and other congenital organoid nevi. Curr Probl Pediatr 6: 1–55.

Stosiek N, Ulmer R, von den Driesch P, Clausen U, Hornstein OP, Rott HD (1994) Chromosomal mosaicism in two patients with epidermal verrucous nevus. Demonstration of chromosomal breakpoint. J Am Acad Dermatol 30: 622–625.

Sugarman JL (2004) Epidermal nevus syndromes. Semin Cutan Med Surg 23: 145–157

Sugarman JL, Frieden IJ (2004) Epidermal nevus syndromes. In: Roach ES, Miller VS (eds.) Neurocutaneous Disorders. Cambridge: Cambridge University Press, pp. 88–104.

Taibjee SM, Bennett DC, Moss C (2004) Abnormal pigmentation in hypomelanosis of Ito and pigmentary mosaicism: the role of pigmentary genes. B J Dermatol 151: 269–282.

Tay YK, Weston WL, Ganong CA, Klingensmith GJ (1998) Epidermal nevus syndrome: association with central precocious puberty and woolly hair nevus. J Am Acad Dermatol 35: 839–842.

Vigevano F, Aicardí J, Lini M, Pasquinelli A (1984) La síndrome del nevo sebáceo lineare: Presentazione di una casistica multicentrica. Boll Lega It Epilepsia 45/46: 59–63.

Vles JC, Degraeuwe P, De Cock P, Casaer P (1985) Neuroradiological findings in Jadassohn nevus phakomatosis: a report of four cases. Eur J Pediatr 144: 290–294.

Warnke PH, Hauschild A, Schimmelpenning GW, Terheyden H, Sherry E, Springer IN (2003) The sebaceous nevus as part of the Schimmelpenning-Feuerstein-Mims syndrome – an obvious phacomatosis first documented in 1927. J Cutan Pathol 30: 470–472.

Wauschkuhn J, Rohde B (1971) Systematized sebaceous, pigmented and epithelial nevi with neurologic symptoms. Neuroectodermal Feuerstein-Mims syndrome. Hautarzt 22: 10–13.

Who Named it? (2006) A biographical dictionary of medical eponyms. http://www.whonamed.it.com

Williams G, Casaer P (1994) More association of linear sebaceous nevus syndrome and unilateral megalencephaly. Am J Neuroradiol 15: 196–197.

Winston KR, Kang J, Laoprasert P, Kleinschmidt-DeMasters BK (2008) Hemispherectomy in a premature neonate with linear sebaceous nevus syndrome. Pediatr Neurosurg 44: 159–164.

Yu TW, Tsau YK, Young C, Chiu HC, Shen YZ (2000) Epidermal nevus syndrome with hypermalanosis and chronic hyponatremia. Pediatr Neurol 22: 151–154.

Zamora ME, Vazquez-Doval FJ (1997) Epidermal naevi associated with trichilemmal cysts and chromosomal mosaicism. Brit J Dermatol 137: 821–824.

Zhang W, Simos PG, Ishibashi H, Wheless JW, Castillo EM, Breier JI, Baumgartner JE, Fitzgerald ME, Papanicolaou AC (2003) Neuroimaging features of epidermal nevus syndrome. Am J Neuradiol 24: 1468–1470.

Zvulunov A, Grunwald MH, Halvi S (1997) Topical calcipotriol for treatment of inflammatory linear verrucous epidermal nevus. Arch Dermatol 133: 567–568.

# INFLAMMATORY LINEAR VERRUCOUS EPIDERMAL NEVUS (ILVEN)

Martino Ruggieri and Jeffrey L. Sugarman

Institute of Neurological Science, National Research Council, Catania and Department of Paediatrics, University of Catania, Catania, Italy (MR); Department of Dermatology and Community and Family Medicine, University of California, San Francisco, USA (JLS)

## Introduction

The term ILVEN (*inflammatory linear verrucous epidermal nevus*) describes a distinct variety of keratinocytic epidermal nevus which presents as linear, pruritic, erythematous, and hyperkeratotic papules that often coalesce into plaques, with a raised scaly surface, occurring unilaterally in narrow linear patterns following the lines of Blaschko (Lee and Rogers 2001, Rogers 2006, Sugarman 2004, Vujevich and Mancini 2004). The nevus can be present at birth, but most frequently arises in infancy (Lee and Rogers 2001). It appears clinically as inflammatory (Rogers 2006) but histologically demonstrates ortho-hyperkeratosis alternating with parakeratotic hyperkeratosis. Affected patients are generally otherwise normal but there have been multiple reports of ILVEN associated with ipsilateral skeletal abnormalities (often representing incorrectly diagnosed cases of CHILD syndrome) (Lee and Rogers 2001, Rogers 2006) and isolated case reports in association with systemic and/or nervous system malformations and neurological dysfunction.

## Historical perspective and terminology

The term ILVEN was first introduced by Altman and Mehregan (1971) because of the inflammatory appearance of a linear verrucous nevus, which was psoriasiform on histopathology (Rogers 2006). Originally described by Unna in 1896 (Schwartz and Jozwiack 2007) ILVEN had been previously reported as *dermatitic epidermal naevus* (Kaidbey and Kurban 1971) until its delineation as a distinct entity in 25 patients (Altman and Mehregan 1971).

Recently, Hofer (2006) and Happle (2006) have discussed the nosologic problem of whether ILVEN and linear psoriasis (LP) are separate entities or the former would represent a mosaic form of psoriasis vulgaris. In this respect they have proposed (Happle 2006, Hofer 2006) two different classification systems for lumping (Hofer 2006) or splitting (Happle 2006) the two conditions (see below).

## Prevalence and incidence

ILVEN represents approximately 6% of all cases of epidermal nevus and epidermal syndromes (Rogers et al 1989). Neither side is predominant. Initially, a female preponderance with a female: male ratio of 4:1 was reported (Altman and Mehregan 1971) but further studies indicated that the sexes might be equally affected (Lee and Rogers 2001, Morag and Metzker 1985, Rogers et al. 1989, Schwartz and Jozwiack 2007). Children are most commonly affected, often prior to the age 2; however, adult onset of the condition has been reported (Goldman and Don 1994, Kawaguchi et al. 1999, Kosann 2003).

## Clinical manifestations

### Skin involvement

ILVEN presents as erythematous, extremely pruritic papules that often coalesce into plaques, with a raised scaly surface, occurring in narrow or, more often, wide linear patterns following the lines of Blaschko (Fig. 1). The lower limb, with or without extension to the buttock or inguinogenital area, is

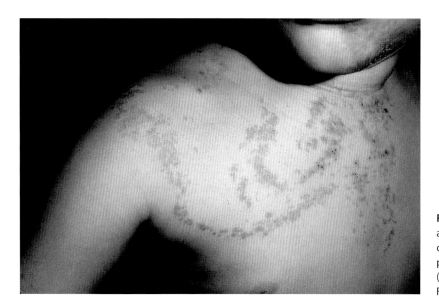

**Fig. 1.** A child with erythematous, hyperkeratotic papules (coalesced into plaques in certain areas) in a wide linear and whorled pattern along the Blaschko's lines (ILVEN) (courtesy of J. L. Sugarman UCSF, San Francisco, USA).

the commonest site of involvement but lesions may involve the arm, the shoulder (Fig. 1), the genital area and rarely other sites (Morag and Metzker 1985, Rogers et al 1989). It is almost always unilateral but widespread bilateral lesions have been reported (Cheesbrough and Kilby 1978, Landwehr and Starink 1983).

In most cases the onset is in the first 5 years of life, often under 1 year and occasionally at birth (Altman and Mehregan 1971, Morag and Metzker 1985, Rogers et al. 1989). Rarely the onset is in later childhood or even adult life (Altman and Mehregan 1971, Cheesbrough and Kilby 1978, Kosann 2003, Rogers 2006). In the original series of Altman and Mehregan (1971) 50% of patients were noted to have lesions by age 6 months with over 75% of cases developing lesions by age 5 years; the oldest onset of ILVEN reported is at age 49 years (Altman and Mehregan 1971). Once established, the lesions are persistent, usually accompanied by severe pruritus, with no tendency to remission or improvement with time and are resistant to standard treatment (Rogers 2006). All these features may help to distinguish ILVEN clinically from psoriasis (Sugarman 2004).

In the series of Lee and Rogers (2001) some of the eight patients with associated anomalies had cutaneous abnormalities including haemangioma, macular hyperpigmentation and psoriasis.

## Extracutaneous involvement

### Systemic involvement

Patients with ILVEN are generally otherwise normal but there have been multiple reports of ILVEN associated with ipsilateral skeletal abnormalities (Barr and Plank 1980, Golitz and Weston 1979, Grosshans and Laplanche 1981) although others have called into question the association of ILVEN with extracutaneous manifestations. In a 13 year follow-up study (Lee and Rogers 2001), only 2 out of 23 ILVEN cases had foot and skeletal deformities: in both cases these were mild, bilateral and thought to be coincidental. It has therefore been suggested (Lee and Rogers 2001, Rogers 2006, Sugarman 2004) that the original reports associating ILVEN with severe skeletal defects (in particular hypoplasia or aplasia of limb bones) were in fact incorrectly diagnosed cases of CHILD syndrome.

ILVEN has been reported to be associated with other diseases including autoimmune thyroiditis (Dereure et al. 1994), asymmetric (psoriatic-like) arthritis of large and small joints and dactylitis (Al-Enezi et al. 2001), Fanconi anemia (Unal et al. 2004), and lichen amyloidosis (Zhuang et al. 1996).

In sporadic cases, ILVEN has been seen in association with congenital anomalies including bilateral branchial cleft sinuses (Tom et al. 1985) (in this specific case the ILVEN was explained as a cutaneous reaction to residual branchial remnants), ipsilateral undescended testicle (Oskay and Kutluay 2003) (in this case however the ILVEN diagnosis was later contested and re-diagnosed as an epidermal nevus of the epidermolytic type by Happle) (Happle 2004), melanodontia (Miteva et al. 2001). One infant had congenital dislocation of the ipsilateral hip and Fallot tetralogy of the heart (Schwartz and Jozwiack 2006). Nevus depigmentosus and ILVEN may occur together, as may ILVEN and melanodontia (Schwartz and Jozwiack 2006).

### Nervous system involvement

In the series of Lee and Rogers (2001) of the eight ILVEN patients with associated extracutaneous abnormalities, two had neurological dysfunction including epilepsy and developmental delay and were thought to be likely coincidental. Surve et al. (1999) reported on a boy with an ILVEN distributed over the lower trunk and left lower limb who presented at age 10 years with seizures and later developed right sided hemiplegia and aphasia: at imaging he showed an infarct in the right thalamus and in the left pons and bilateral vertebral artery occlusion with good collateral circulation.

It our experience, histologically proven cases of ILVEN (localised to the right chest, flank, buttocks and proximal end of lower limbs) negative to NSDHL gene testing (see chapter 37), manifested with psychomotor delay associated with central nervous system (CNS) abnormalities. These CNS abnormalities included posterior fossa malformations (specifically, megacisterna magna and Chiari 1 malformation) (Figs. 2 and 3) and absent corpus callosum. These individuals had minor muskuloskeletal abnormalities consisting of mild to moderate (thoracic and lumbosacral) kyphoscoliosis and mild dysmorphic signs including hypertelorism, low set ears and coarse face (unreported data). It is possible that these associated findings could be coincidental due to their prevalence in the population but it may be more likely that all these phenomena might be (non specific but) secondary to genetic mosaicism (see below).

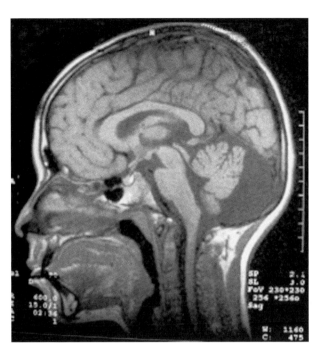

**Fig. 2.** Sagittal T1-weighted MR showing a megacisterna magna in a child with ILVEN.

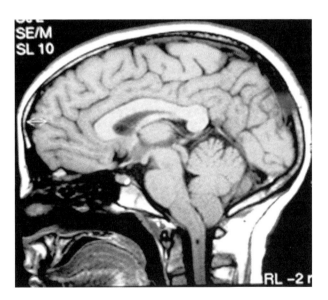

**Fig. 3.** Sagittal T1-weighted MR shows a Chiari malformation in a patient with ILVEN.

## Pathology

The most distinctive histopathology findings are sharply demarcated alternating areas of hypergranulosis with overlying orthokeratotic hyperkeratosis and hypogranulosis with overlying parakeratotic hyperkeratosis (Rogers 2006). Psoriasiform epidermal hyperplasia with close-set elongation of the red ridges and spongiosis, exocytosis and even microabscess formation may be seen. An upper dermal perivascular lymphohistiocytic inflammatory infiltration is a regular feature; this infiltrate may extend to the overlying irregularly hyperplastic epidermis (Kosann 2003). Absent *involucrin* expression has been reported and also may be helpful in differentiating ILVEN from psoriasis (Ginarte et al. 2000). Sometimes the histopathology is less specific, mimicking a chronic eczema or lichen simplex chronicus.

## Pathogenesis and molecular genetics

The electrophoresis pattern of protein extracted from scales in an ILVEN differs from that of normal stratum corneum and of a psoriatic scale (Adrian and Baden 1980) and is not identical in each case of ILVEN (Bernhart et al. 1984). A distinctive pattern of clonal dysregulation of growth has been suggested in these nevi. The report of a patient with ILVEN and autoimmune thyroiditis, raised the question of autoimmune involvement in the inflammatory component of ILVEN (Dereure et al. 1994).

Familial cases have been reported (Alsaleh et al. 1994, Goldman and Don 1994, Hamm and Happle 1986, Moulin et al. 1975). Moulin et al. (1975) reported ILVEN in a 39-year-old woman and her 13-year-old nephew. Hamm and Happle (1986) observed ILVEN in a 47-year-old mother and her 17-year-old daughter. Alsaleh et al. (1994) reported a family with 4 members (two siblings, mother and maternal grandfather) affected in 3 generations: the mother had localised ILVEN, whereas both the siblings and the maternal grandfather had the systemic form of the condition (there is no systemic form). Goldman and Don (1994) reported on a 40-year-old mother and her 10-year-old daughter. The exact role of transmission is not yet clear. Hamm and Happle (1986) have suggested, among the different possible explanations, X-linked inheritance with extreme lyonisation.

Happle (2002) hypothesised that transposable elements or retrotransposons (i.e., particles of retroviral origin that are interspersed in large numbers in the genome of plants and animals), which are partly activating and partly silencing a neighbouring gene by demethylation or methylation at an early development stage, could be responsible for the development of ILVEN. That could also explain (Happle 2002) the usual sporadic occurrence of the disorder and the occasional familial aggregation (Alsaleh et al. 1994, Goldman and Don 1994, Hamm and Happle 1986, Moulin et al. 1975).

Recently, Hofer (2006) subdivided the reported cases of ILVEN and LP into four different groups: (1) ILVEN with or without concomitant psoriasis, only in part reacting to antipsoriatic treatment; (2) ILVEN without concomitant psoriasis; (3) LP with concomitant psoriasis vulgaris, with both groups 2 and 3 reacting successfully to antipsoriatic treatment; and (4) LP without concomitant psoriasis vulgaris and with a family history of psoriasis (very rarely reported). On this basis, he proposed to lump ILVEN and LP hypothesising that inflammatory linear verrucous eruptions besides nevoid psoriasis/LP may represent segmental type 1/type 2 mosaic forms of psoriasis, which, if a (verrucous) epidermal nevus exists, shows a high affinity of occurrence in close context to such nevus (Hofer 2006). Happle (2006) however, advocated to split the two disorders observing that ILVEN is usually far more itchy and tends to be unresponsive to the classical, time-honoured methods of antipsoriatic treatment. In contrast to Hofer's view (Hofer 2006) he proposed to distinguish the following three categories (Happle 2006): (1) cases that undoubtedly represent LP; (2) cases that undoubtedly represent ILVEN; and (3) cases that can so far not be categorised with certainty (in these latter doubtful cases, immunohistochemical techniques may perhaps be helpful). In addition, he coined the terms of *linear psoriasis (LP) of the isolated type* (in which disseminated lesions of psoriasis vulgaris are constantly absent), and *linear psoriasis (LP) of the superimposed type* (in which a pronounced linear involvement is, either intermittently or constantly, associated with psoriasis vulgaris) so as to further distinguish the LP phenotypes which would be explained either from loss of heterozygosity or from any other mutation occurring at one of the many gene loci involved in psoriasis.

## Differential diagnosis

The differential diagnosis includes nevoid psoriasis (also known as linear psoriasis), lichen striatus, linear lichen planus, the erythematous scaly lesions which may occur in Goltz syndrome and a non-inflammatory epidermal nevus on which psoriasis has become superimposed as a Koebner phenomenon or irritation and maceration in flexures, such as the napkin area has occurred.

Non-inflammatory epidermal naevi are usually asymptomatic, are more commonly associated with other abnormalities and do not show a predilection for the buttock and leg area (Lee and Rogers 2001).

The differentiation of ILVEN from naevoid/linear psoriasis is a difficult and evolving area (Sotiriadis et al. 2006): Hofer (2006) and Happle (2006) have recently attempted to construct a classification system which may aid in diagnosis advancing our understanding of the relationship between these entities (see above "pathogenesis and molecular genetics). The CHILD syndrome includes non-pruritic, erythematous, verrucous areas, segmentally distributed or occasionally in Blaschko's lines. Limb defects are on the ipsilateral side of the most prominent cutaneous lesions. Cases of ILVEN reported in association with severe limb defects are more likely cases of CHILD syndrome.

Lichen striatus is usually less pruritic and less scaly than ILVEN, differs from it histologically and, unlike ILVEN, is self-limiting.

## Management

Treatment of ILVEN has been unsatisfactory. Once established, the lesions persist and do not improve with time. Some relief from pruritus and lessening in thickness and degree of inflammation may be achieved with the use of potent topical or intralesional corticosteroids; however, this is usually short-lived on cessation of therapy. Similarly prompt recurrence is likely to follow electrodessication, cryotherapy, $CO_2$ laser therapy and superficial dermabrasion (Michel et al. 2001). However, long-lasting resolution has been reported following cryotherapy and disappearance of all symptoms (erythema, excoriation, granulation, and pruritus) with residual pale pigmentation has been reported with carbon dioxide laser therapy (Ulkur et al. 2004). Topical calcitriol and/or calcipotriol, has been reported to be effective in one case report, although this agent would have to be used with caution in children (Bohm et al. 2003). For small, circumscribed or narrow lesions surgical excision may be the treatment of choice (Lee et al. 2001).

## References

Al-Enezi S, Huber AM, Krafchik BR, Laxer RM (2001) Inflammatory linear verrucous epidermal nevus and arthritis: a new association. J Pediatr 138: 602–604.

Alsaleh OA, Nanda A, Hassab-el-Naby HM, Sakr MF (1994) Familial inflammatory linear verrucous epidermal nevus (ILVEN). Int J Dermatol 33: 52–54.

Altman J, Mehregan AH (1971) Inflammatory linear verrucous epidermal nevus. Arch Dermatol 104: 385–389.

Barr RJ, Plank CJ (1980) Verruciform xanthoma of the skin. J Cutan Pathol 7: 422–428.

Bohm M, Luger TA, Traupe H (2003) Successful treatment of inflammatory linear verrucous epidermal naevus with topical natural vitamin D3 (calcitriol). Br J Dermatol 148: 824–825.

Cheesbrough MJ, Kilby PE (1978) The inflammatory linear verrucous epidermal naevus – a case report. Clin Exp Dermatol 3: 293–298.

Dereure O, Paiilet C, Bonnel F, Guilhou JJ (1994) Inflammatory linear verrucous epidermal naevus with auto-immune thyroiditis: coexistence of tow auto-immune epithelial inflammation). Acta Derm Venereol 74: 208–209.

Ginarte M, Fernandez-Redondo V, Toribio J (2000) Unilatreal psoriasis: a case individualized by means of involucrin. Cutis 65: 167–170.

Goldman K, Don PC (1994) Adult onset of inflammatory linear verrucous epidermal nevus in a mother and her daughter. Dermatology 189: 170–172.

Golitz LE, Weston WL (1979) Inflammatory linear verrucous epidermal nevus. Association with epidermal nevus syndrome. Arch Dermatol, pp. 1208–1209.

Grosshans E, Laplanche G (1981) Verruciform xanthoma or xanthomatous transformation of inflammatory epidermal nevus? J Cutan Pathol 8: 382–384.

Hamm H, Happle R (1986) Inflammatory linear verrucous epidermal nevus (ILVEN) in a mother and her daughter. Am J Med Genet 24: 685–690.

Happle R (2002) Transposable elements and the lines of Blaschko: a new perspective. Dermatology 204: 4–7.

Happle R (2004) A further case of non-ILVEN. Clin Exp Dermatol 29: 98–99.

Happle R (2006) Linear psoriasis and ILVEN: is lumping or splitting appropriate? Dermatology 212: 101–102.

Hofer T (2006) Does inflammatory lenear verrucous epidermal nevus represent a segmental type 1/type 2 mosaic of psoriasis? Dermatology 212: 103–107.

Kaidbey KH, Kurban AK (1971) Dermatitic epidermal nevus. Arch Dermatol 104: 166–171.

Kawaguchi H, Takeuchi M, Nakajima H (1999) Adult onset of inflammatory linear verrucous epidermal nevus. J Dermatol 26: 599–602.

Kosann MK (2003) Inflammatory linear verrucous epidermal nevus. Dermatol Online J 9: 15.

Landwehr AJ, Starink TM (1983) Inflammatory linear verrucous epidermal nevus. Dermatologica 166: 107–109.

Lee BJ, Mancini AJ, Renucci J, Paller AS, Bauer BS (2001) Full-thickness surgical excision for the treatment of inflammatory linear verrucous epidermal nevus. Ann Plast Surg 47: 285–292.

Lee SH, Rogers M (2001) Inflammatory linear verrucous epidermal naevi: a review of 23 cases. Australas J Dermatol 42: 252–256.

Michel JL, Has C, Has V (2001) Resurfacing $CO_2$ laser treatment of linear verrucous epidermal nevus. Eur J Dermatol 11: 436–439.

Miteva LG, Dourmishev AL, Schwartz RA (2001) Inflammatory linear verrucous epidermal nevus. Cutis 68: 327–330.

Morag C, Metzker A (1985) Inflammatory linear verrucous epidermal nevus: report of seven cases and review of the literature. Pediatr Dermatol 3: 15–18.

Moulin G, Biot A, Valignat P, Bouchet B, Meurnier F (1975) Nevus èpidermique verruquex inflammatoire familial. Bull Soc Fr Dermatol Syphilol 82: 130–131.

Oskay T, Kutluay L (2003) Inflammatory linear verrucous epidermal naevus associated with undescended testicle. Clin Exp Dermatol 28: 557–558.

Rogers M (2006) Epidermal naevi. In: Harper J, Oranje A, Prose N (eds.) Textbook of Pediatric Dermatology. 2nd ed. Oxford: Blackwell Science, pp. 955–972.

Rogers M, McCrossin I, Commens C (1989) Epidermal nevi and the epidermal nevus syndrome. A review of 131 cases. J Am Acad Dermatol 20: 476–488.

Schwartz RA, Jozwiak S (2007) Epidermal nevus syndrome. E-medicine: instant access to the minds of medicine: http://www.emedicine.com/DERM/topic732.htm

Sotiriadis D, Patsatsi A, Lazaridou E, Kastanis A, Devliotou-Panatgiotidou D (2006) Is inflammatory linear verrucous epidermal nevus a form of linear naevoid psoriasis? J Eur Acad Dermatol Venereol 20: 484–484.

Sugarman JL (2004) Epidermal nevus syndromes. Semin Cut Med Surg 23: 145–157.

Surve TY, Muranjan MN, Deshmukh CT, Warke CS, Bharucha BA (1999) Inflammatory linear verrucous epidermal nevus syndrome with bilateral vertebral artery occlusion. Indian Pediatr 36: 820–823.

Tom DW, Alper JC, Bogaars H (1985) Inflammatory linear epidermal nevus caused by branchial cleft sinuses in a woman with numerous congenital anomalies. Pediatr Dermatol 2: 318–321.

Ulkur E, Celikoz B, Yuksel F, Karagoz H (2004) Carbon dioxide laser therapy for an inflammatory linear verrucous epidermal nevus: a case report. Aesth Plast Surg 28: 428–430.

Unal S, Ozbek N, Kara A, Alikasifoglu M, Gumruk F (2004) Five Fanconi anemia patients with unusual organ pathologies. Am J Hematol 77: 50–54.

Vissers WH, Muys L, Erp PE, de Jong EM, van de Kerkhof PC (2004) Immunohistochemical differentiation between inflammatory linear verrucous epidermal nevus (ILVEN) and psoriasis. Eur J Dermatol 14: 216–220.

Vujevich JJ, Mancini AJ (2004) The epidermal nevus syndromes: multisystem disorders.

Zhuang L, Zhu W (1996) Inflammatory linear verrucose epidermal nevus coexisting with lichen amyloidosis. J Dermatol 23: 415–418.

# Chapter 35

# NEVUS COMEDONICUS SYNDROME

Jeffrey L. Sugarman

Departments of Dermatology and Community and Family Medicine, University of California, San Francisco, USA

## Introduction

Nevus comedonicus (NC) is a hamartoma of pilosebaceous units. It often appears as wide keratin filled invaginations of the epidermis. Many have noted its resemblance to open or closed comedones, which has given rise to the moniker NC. NC is considered in the family of epidermal nevi because it contains hamartomatous epidermal and adnexal elements. NC occurs less frequently than other epidermal nevi, accounting for less than 2% of epidermal nevi in one study (Rogers 1992). NC is usually found on the face and trunk but has been reported in other locations (Lefkowitz et al. 1999). Although, NC usually presents as an isolated clinical finding, it has been reported in association with extra-cutaneous anomalies (the nevus comedonicus syndrome). There have been recent advances in the understanding of the genetic basis of NC, which has served to clarify the relationship between NC and the associated extra-cutaneous manifestations. There are many reports of treatment approaches to NC but no controlled clinical trials have been performed to this point. This chapter discusses various facets of NC, including historical background and epidemiology, cutaneous and extra-cutaneous features, histopathology, genetic basis, pathogenesis, and management.

## Historical perspective and terminology

Kofmann, in 1895, first described nevus comedonicus (Kofmann 1895). There were two additional European reports the following year (Selhorst 1896, Thibierge 1896). White objected to the label "comedone" arguing that there are not true comedones in NC and preferred the label "nevus follicularis keratosus" (White 1914). Other historical terms for NC are comedone nevus, acne nevus, nevus acneiformis unilateralis, and nevus zoniforme. Rogers reviewed 233 cases of epidermal nevi and classified them according to their predominant component. Four out of 233 or 1.7% were follicular nevi felt to represent NC (Rogers 1992).

## Overview of clinical manifestations

NC appears clinically as collections of dilated follicular openings often containing keratin plugs. NC usually follows linear patterns known as "the lines of Blaschko", which as discussed elsewhere in this section, refer to the S-shaped or V-shaped whorled, streaked, and linear patterns that are recognized in many different cutaneous disorders. The involved hamartomatous follicular openings many be pinhead sized to large and dilated. NC is present at birth but becomes visible in infancy (Fig. 1). It is less common for NC to manifest during adolescence. It may manifest as a small isolated "nevus" (Fig. 2), or as extensive lesions (Fig. 3). NC often occurs on the face and trunk. There have been reports of NC occurring in other locations. Ghaninezhad reported a case of NC on the scalp (Ghaninezhad et al. 2006). Harper has reported a case of NC of the wrist and palm and reviewed five other similar cases (Harper and Spielvogel 1985). Some cases of NC on the palm or wrist may in fact be of eccrine origin and more appropriately labeled porokeratotic eccrine nevus (see below). NC is most often unilateral although bilateral cases have been reported (Wakahara et al. 2003). NC may be complicated by hypertrophy of follicular units with extensive plugging (Fig. 4a, b), super-

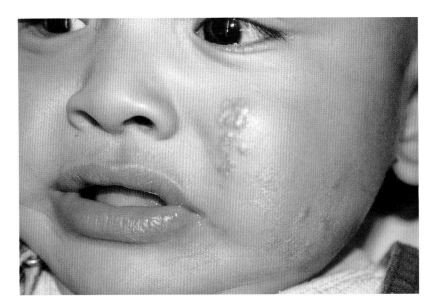

**Fig. 1.** Isolated nevus comedonicus on the face of an infant.

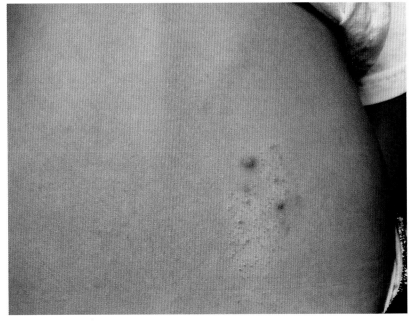

**Fig. 2.** A small isolated nevus comedonicus on the back that became apparent during early adolescence starting with open and closed comedones and eventual inflammatory lesions.

infection with bacteria, and scarring (Cestari et al. 1991). NC may also be complicated by chronic inflammation, presumably by similar mechanisms as those leading to inflammation in acne vulgaris. If one looks carefully at the clinical features of NC, it becomes clear that this group is likely more heterogeneous than previously thought (compare Figs. 1–5). As mentioned earlier, the phenotype of NC ranges from widened follicular invaginations to large closed comedones filled with follicular debris.

These latter cases are much more likely to be complicated by inflammation and scarring. Vasiloudes reviewed five cases of inflammatory NC in children and described the associated prominent and persistent inflammatory changes. These were resistant to treatment and required surgical removal in two children (Vasiloudes et al. 1998). Köse et al. (2008) reported co-occurrence of three different epidermal naevi including sebaceous nevus, nevus comedonicus and Becker's nevus.

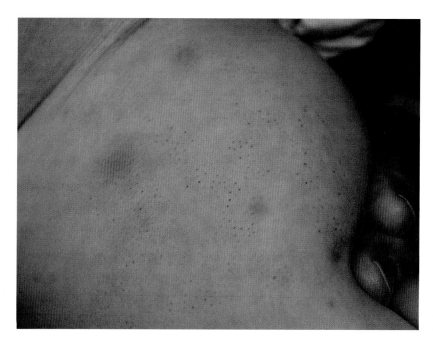

**Fig. 3.** Nevus comedonicus involving a large area containing numerous dilated follicular openings.

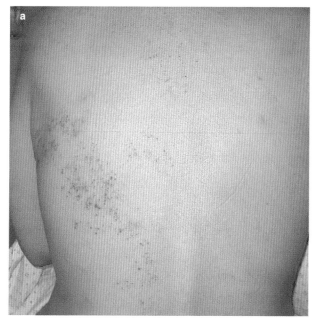

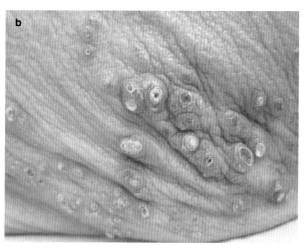

**Fig. 4.** (**a**) Large nevus comedonicus containing numerous dilated follicular openings, as well as others with keratin plugs (courtesy of T. Miller). (**b**) Close-up view of keratotic plugs in a nevus comedonicus (courtesy of T. Miller).

## Extra-cutaneous manifestations

While most cases of NC are confined to the skin, NC can occur in association with extra-cutaneous manifestations. This association is referred to as ne-

vus comidonicus syndrome (NCS). The extra-cutaneous anomalies are often ipsilateral to the NC. In a review of 35 patients with epidermal nevus syndrome, 8% of these were NCS (Vidaurri-de la Cruz et al. 2004). Electroencephalographic (EEG)

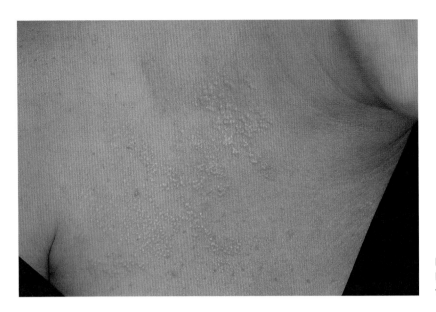

**Fig. 5.** Collections of closed comedone-like lesions present since childhood and resistant to topical therapy.

abnormalities, Alagille syndrome (arteriopathic dysplasia), occult spinal dysraphism, accessory breast tissue, ipsilateral cataract, corneal changes, and skeletal anomalies have been associated with nevus comedonicus (Ahn et al. 2008, Engber 1978, Filosa et al. 1997, Happle 1995, Patrizi et al. 1998, Woods et al. 1994). These extra-cutaneous associations have lead Happle and others to purport that NCS is a distinct entity. The skeletal defects include supernumerary or missing digits, syndactyly, scoliosis, hemivertebrae, and absence of the fifth ray of a hand (Patrizi et al. 1998). Seo described a case of NC involving both skeletal and neurologic abnormalities which included mental retardation and EEG changes (Seo et al. 2001).

## Histopathology

Histologically, rudimentary hair follicles are dilated to form epidermal invaginations which are filled with keratin in concentric lamellae. The follicular walls are comprised of several layers of keratinocytes. Scattered hair shafts and small sebaceous lobules may be seen in early lesions, while in older lesions, hyperkeratosis and ossification may be seen (Lefkowitz et al. 1999). Epidermolytic hyperkeratosis has also been reported in associated with NC (Schecter et al. 2004). Some reported cases of NC occurring in acral locations may in fact represent porokeratotic eccrine

nevus (also known as porokeratotic eccrine ostial and dermal duct nevus) (Abell and Read 1980). Histologically, both the eccrine nevus and NC display widened and plugged epidermal invaginations. The keratotic plugs resemble those seen in NC but arise from eccrine ducts rather than pilosebaceous units. Overlap lesions involving both eccrine and pilosebaceous units have also been described (Resnik et al. 1993, Kroumpouzos et al. 1999). Although these lesions share overlapping clinical and histopathological features, they are surely genetically distinct entities.

Benign adnexal and malignant tumors are rare in NC but have been reported. Lee reported NC associated with hidradenoma papilliferum and syringocystadenoma papilliferum (Lee et al. 2002). Trichilemmal cysts have been reported to arise in NC (Leppard 1977). Other follicular tumors including trichofolliculoma and pilar sheath acanthoma have been documented within a NC (Dudley et al. 1986). A case of multiple basal cell carcinomas and a rudimentary toe was reported by Alpsoy et al. (2005).

## Pathogenesis and molecular genetics

Many lines of evidence suggest that the pathogenesis and clinical expression of epidermal nevi (including NC) is based on genomic mosaicism. Mosaicism is the mixture of more than one genotypically distinct cell lineage within one organism. Epidermal cells are thought to originate in the neural crest and move to the periphery of the growing embryo by directional proliferation (Moss et al. 1995). A somatic mutation occurring during the migration of embryonic ectoderm will only be clinically apparent if the mutation leads to a recognizable difference from the surrounding normal cells, which often follow Blaschko's lines. Thus, Blaschko's lines are believed to be a cutaneous expression of mosaicism. In this conceptual framework, mutations which occur earlier in development would lead to more extensive cutaneous involvement and a greater likelihood of other organ system involvement. In addition, the biologic severity of a particular mutation is also likely to determine the extent and severity of clinical involvement (Sugarman and Frieden 2004).

The concept of lethal genes surviving by mosaicism has been proposed by Happle (1987) to explain the sporadic inheritance, asymmetric clinical distribution in multiple organs, the lack of diffuse involvement of entire organs, and the equal sex ratio of affected individuals that characterize the features of epidermal nevus syndromes (including NCS). Happle postulated that these syndromes are due to the action of a gene product that if present in the germ line would be lethal, but is clinically manifested only when present in a subpopulation of cells, thereby surviving by mosaicism. However, as we shall see, mosaicism in some of the epidermal nevus syndromes may involve a non-lethal gene defect.

Munro and Wilkie (1998) reported on a 14 year old boy with a NC who had a mutation in the fibroblast growth factor receptor 2 (FGFR2) identical to that found in Apert's syndrome. The mutation was found in DNA analysis from the NC, but not from uninvolved skin or peripheral blood lymphocytes. This suggests that NC represents a mosaic condition for a mutation in FGFR2, which if present in the germ line, would result in Apert's syndrome. It also provides a framework for understanding the association of nevus comedonicus with skeletal anomalies. Apert's syndrome is characterized by skeletal anomalies such as craniosynostosis, syndactyly, fusion of cervical vertebrae and severe acne. Individuals with

NC and skeletal anomalies (i.e. NCS) are likely mosaic for FGFR2 in both skin and extra-cutaneous tissues. The mutational event leading to NCS likely occurs earlier in development than in individuals without extra-cutaneous involvement resulting in a more severe manifestation of the disease. In addition, because the product of a single gene may be involved in the formation of different structures at distinct times during embryogenesis, a single genetic defect may cause anomalies of multiple structures in different organs during development (Sugarman 2004).

The follicular structure is created and maintained by complex signaling pathways involving interaction between the epithelium and mesodermal structures. Fibroblast Growth Factors (FGFs) are therefore well suited as candidate genes for involvement in disorders that disrupt this process. It is well documented that FGFs play a vital role in embryonic development. They function as important signaling molecules between epithelial and mesenchymal boundaries (Ornitz and Itoh 2001). Mutations in FGFs have been associated with developmental defects in neuronal, skeletal, and ocular, and cardiovascular systems. There are 2 isoforms of FGFR2 and the expression of the two isoforms is regulated in a tissue-specific manner, with FGFR2b expression restricted to epithelial lineages and FGFR2c expression restricted to mesenchymal lineages. The mesenchymally expressed ligands, FGF7 and FGF10, can activate only epithelially expressed FGFR2b. Epithially expressed FGF2, FGF4, FGF6, FGF8, and FGF9 are specific for mesenchymally expressed FGFR2c. The most common mutation seen in Aperts syndrome (S252W mutation in FGFR2) renders mutant FGFRs abnormally susceptible to non specific activation by multiple FGFs allowing autocrine signaling in tissues that express these ligands (Ibrahimi et al. 2005). Presumably, this allows aberrant development and expression of pilosebaceous units leading to the phenotype of NC. In addition to mutations in FGFR2, there may be other mutations involved in the pathogenesis of NC as the heterogeneous phenotype seen in NC may very well be due to heterogeneity in genotype.

## Management

Generally, children with small isolated NC and a normal physical exam do not require further work-up. Diagnostic and screening laboratory investigations should be performed if extra-cutaneous abnormalities are suspected after history and physical exam.

The management of the patient with NCS needs to be individualized, and should always include a thorough history including prenatal history, developmental history, family history and physical exam. Careful and complete cutaneous examination should include the mucosa and areas covered by hair. A careful neurological exam is important, as is examination of the eyes, especially the conjunctiva, sclerae, and extra-ocular eye movements. Skeletal exam should include evaluation for kyphoscoliosis and evaluation of gait. Limb length and size should be measured to ascertain any asymmetry. Shoe wear patterns can serve as a clue to uneven weight distribution. Referral to appropriate subspecialists should be considered.

Referral to a medical geneticist rarely may be warranted for further evaluation including gene testing regarding the possibility of transmission of a more generalized form of this disease (Apert's syndrome) to future offspring.

Prophylactic excision of NC for cosmetic reasons may sometimes be warranted. However, simple excision may not always be practical because of the location or size of the NC. In addition, the disfigurement from the surgery itself may limit its utility. Consequently, there have been attempts at medical treatment and non-surgical ablation of NC. Unfortunately, because epidermal nevi (including NC) involve not only the epidermis but also appendageal structures in the underlying dermis, removal of the epidermis alone may result in recurrence (Solomon and Esterly 1975, Paller 1987). Despite this, many alternative treatments have been reported. Unfortunately, the efficacy of these therapies is uncertain due to the lack of controlled trials (e.g. Fig. 5). Many of the following therapeutic interventions are based on individual case reports where long-term follow-up is lacking. Stripping of the keratin plugs using a pore strip cosmetic pack has been reported to produce excellent results (Inoue et al. 2000). This technique will need to be repeated periodically as the follicular units will become plugged again over time. The combination of topical tazarotene and calcipotriene has been reported to improve the appearance of an extensive NC (Deliduka and Kwong 2004). As our understanding of the pathogenesis of NC expands, future management may be directed toward specific molecular defects.

## References

Abell E, Read SI (1980) Porokeratotic eccrine ostial and dermal duct naevus. Br J Dermatol 103: 435–441.

Ahn SY, Oh Y, Bak H, Ahn SK (2008) Co-occurrence of nevus comedonicus with accessory breast tissue. Int J Dermatol 47: 530–531.

Alpsoy E, Durusoy C, Ozbilim G, Karpuzoglu G, Yilmaz E (2005) Nevus comedonicus syndrome: a case associated with multiple basal cell carcinomas and a rudimentary toe. Int J Dermatol 44: 499–501.

Cestari TF, Rubim M, Valentini BC (1991) Nevus comedonicus: case report and brief review of the literature. Pediatr Dermatol 8: 300–305.

Deliduka SB, Kwong PC (2004) Treatment of nevus comedonicus with topical tazarotene and calcipotriene. J Drugs Dermatol 3: 674–676.

Dudley K, Barr WG, Armin A, Massa MC (1986) Nevus comedonicus in association with widespread, well-differentiated follicular tumors. J Am Acad Dermatol 15: 1123–1127.

Engber PB (1978) The nevus comedonicus syndrome: a case report with emphasis on associated internal manifestations. Int J Dermatol 17: 745–749.

Filosa G, Bugatti L, Ciattaglia G, Salaffi F, Carotti M (1997) Naevus comedonicus as dermatologic hallmark of occult spinal dysraphism. Acta Derm Venereol 77: 243.

Ghaninezhad H, Ehsani AH, Mansoori P, Taheri A (2006) Naevus comedonicus of the scalp. J Eur Acad Dermatol Venereol 20: 184–185.

Happle R (1987) Lethal genes surviving by mosaicism: a possible explanation for sporadic birth defects involving the skin. J Am Acad Dermatol 16: 899–906.

Happle R (1995) Epidermal nevus syndromes. Semin Dermatol 14: 111–121.

Harper KE, Spielvogel RL (1985) Nevus comedonicus of the palm and wrist. Case report with review of five previously reported cases. J Am Acad Dermatol 12: 185–188.

Ibrahimi OA, Chiu ES, McCarthy JG, Mohammadi M (2005) Understanding the molecular basis of Apert syndrome. Plast Reconstr Surg 115: 264–270.

Inoue Y, Miyamoto Y, Ono T (2000) Two cases of nevus comedonicus: successful treatment of keratin plugs with a pore strip. J Am Acad Dermatol 43: 927–929.

Kofmann S (1895) Ein Fall von seltener Lokalisation und Verbreitung von Comedonen. Arch Dermatol Syphilis (Wein) 32: 177–178.

Köse O, Caliṣkan E, Kurumlu Z (2008) Three different epidermal naevi with no organ involvement: sebaceous naevus, naevus comedonicus and Becker's naevus. Acta Derm Venereol 88: 67–69.

Kroumpouzos G, Stefanato CM, Wilkel CS, Bogaars H, Bhawan J (1999) Systematized porokeratotic eccrine and hair follicle naevus: report of a case and review of the literature. Br J Dermatol 141: 1092–1096.

Lee HJ, Chun EY, Kim YC, Lee MG (2002) Nevus comedonicus with hidradenoma papilliferum and syringocystadenoma papilliferum in the female genital area. Int J Dermatol 41: 933–936.

Lefkowitz A, Schwartz RA, Lambert WC (1999) Nevus comedonicus. Dermatology 199: 204–207.

Leppard BJ (1977) Trichilemmal cysts arising in an extensive comedo naevus. Br J Dermatol 96: 545–548.

Moss C, Jones DO, Blight A, Bowden PE (1995) Birthmark due to cutaneous mosaicism for keratin 10 mutation. Lancet 345: 596.

Munro CS, Wilkie AO (1998) Epidermal mosaicism producing localised acne: somatic mutation in FGFR2. Lancet 352: 704–705.

Ornitz DM, Itoh N (2001) Fibroblast growth factors. Genome Biol 2: S300–S305.

Paller AS (1987) Epidermal nevus syndrome. Neurol Clin 5: 451–457.

Patrizi A, Neri I, Fiorentini C, Marzaduri S (1998) Nevus comedonicus syndrome: a new pediatric case. Pediatr Dermatol 15: 304–306.

Resnik KS, Kantor GR, Howe NR, Ditre CM (1993) Dilated pore nevus. A histologic variant of nevus comedonicus. Am J Dermatopathol 15: 169–171.

Rogers M (1992) Epidermal nevi and the epidermal nevus syndromes: a review of 233 cases. Pediatr Dermatol 9: 342–344.

Schecter AK, Lester B, Pan TD, Robinson-Bostom L (2004) Linear nevus comedonicus with epidermolytic hyperkeratosis. J Cutan Pathol 31: 502–505.

Selhorst S (1896) Naevus acneiformis unilateralis. British J Dermatol Syphilis 8: 419–421.

Seo YJ, Piao YJ, Suhr KB, Lee JH, Park JK (2001) A case of nevus comedonicus syndrome associated with neurologic and skeletal abnormalities. Int J Dermatol 40: 648–650.

Solomon LM, Esterly NB (1975) Epidermal and other congenital organoid nevi. Curr Probl Pediatr 6: 1–56.

Sugarman JL (2004) Epidermal nevus syndromes. Semin Cutan Med Surg 23: 145–157.

Sugarman JL, Frieden IJ (2004) Epidermal nevus syndromes. Neurocutaneous disorders. R. E. M. VS. New York: Cambridge University Press, pp. 88–104.

Thibierge G (1896) Naevus acneique uniteralen bandes et en plaques (naevus a comedons). Annual Dermatology Syphiligr (Paris) 7: 1298–1303.

Vasiloudes PE, Morelli JG, Weston WL (1998) Inflammatory nevus comedonicus in children. J Am Acad Dermatol 38: 834–836.

Vidaurri-de la Cruz H, Tamayo-Sanchez L, Duran-McKinster C, de la Luz Orozco-Covarrubias M, Ruiz-Maldonado R (2004) Epidermal nevus syndromes: clinical findings in 35 patients. Pediatr Dermatol 21: 432–439.

Wakahara M, Kiyohara T, Kumakiri M, Kuwahara H, Fujita T (2003) Bilateral nevus comedonicus: efficacy of topical tacalcitol ointment. Acta Derm Venereol 83: 51.

White C (1914) Nevus follicularis Keratosus. J Cutan Dis 32: 187–190.

Woods KA, Larcher VF, Harper JI (1994) Extensive naevus comedonicus in a child with Alagille syndrome. Clin Exp Dermatol 19: 163–164.

# Chapter 36

# BECKER'S NEVUS SYNDROME (PIGMENTARY HAIRY EPIDERMAL NEVUS)

Martino Ruggieri and Simone Gangarossa

Institute of Neurological Science, National Research Council, Catania and Department of Paediatrics, University of Catania, Catania, Italy (MR); Paediatric Unit, AUSL 2, Ragusa, Italy (SG)

## Introduction

Becker nevus syndrome is a phenotype characterised by the simultaneous occurrence of: (1) a circumscribed patch of (light or dark brown) hyperpigmentation with a sharply outlined but irregular border (resolving into small spots reminiscent of an archipelago) and hypertrichosis (with increased smooth muscle bundles) with slight acanthosis (the so-called *Becker's nevus*); (2) associated unilateral hypoplasia of one or more of the following: breast, underlying musculature (mostly the shoulder girdle), underlying adipose tissue (lipoatrophy) and limb (usually the arm); and (3) underlying skeletal anomalies including vertebral defects and scoliosis, fused or accessory cervical ribs, pectus excavatum or carenatum, and internal tibial torsion (Danarti et al. 2004, Happle et al. 1997, Sugarman 2004). All of these anomalies tend to show a regional correspondence to the nevus and are mostly ipsilateral (Danarti et al. 2004).

## Historical perspective and terminology

The cutaneous anomaly known as Becker nevus was first delineated by **Samuel William Becker**, an American physician born in Indianapolis, USA, in June 1924 (Who named it? 2006) who in 1948 described two young men with acquired melanosis and hypertrichosis in a unilateral distribution (Becker 1949). In the past, several authors had reported cases of Becker nevus associated with other (developmental) anomalies such as unilateral hypoplasia of breast or scoliosis (Glinik et al. 1983, Mascarò et al. 1970, Moore and Schosser 1985). However, this association did not receive much attention until 1995 when the term "*pigmentary hairy epidermal nevus syndrome*" was proposed by Happle (1995). Later, Happle and Koopman (1997) by reviewing the spectrum of associated anomalies proposed the new designation of "*Becker nevus syndrome*" recently revisited by Danarti et al. (2004).

## Incidence and prevalence

Approximately 60 cases have been reported in the literature so far with a female:male ratio of 1.5:1.0 (Alfaro et al. 2007, Danarti et al. 2004, Happle and Koopman 1997, Sugarman 2004). This has been partially explained by the fact that the associated ipsilateral breast hypoplasia frequently occurs and is far more conspicuous in female than in male patients (Danarti et al. 2004).

## Clinical manifestations

### Skin manifestations

#### Becker nevus

This cutaneous anomaly, which is also known under the term "*pigmentary hairy epidermal nevus*" (Copeman and Jones 1965) constitutes the hallmark of the syndrome, although it mostly occurs as an isolated skin abnormality (Happle and Koopman 1997). It can be categorised as a particular type of androgen-dependent organoid epidermal nevus (Sugarman 2004), which often involves the thorax or the scapular re-

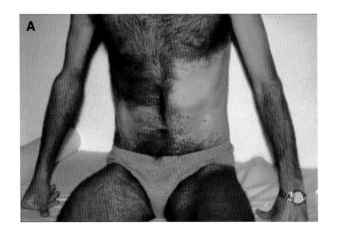

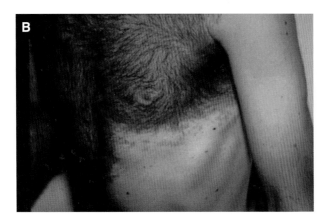

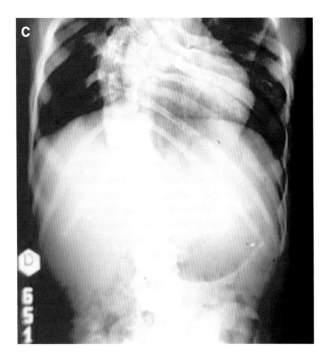

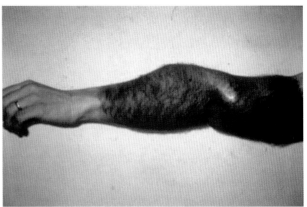

**Fig. 2.** Pigmentary hairy nevus of the left arm.

gion (Happle and Koopman 1997) but may affect any area of the body usually in a mosaic (checkerboard) (Fig. 1) pattern (Danarti et al. 2004).

Clinically, the nevus is characterised by the presence of light or dark brown maculae with a sharply outlined but irregular and bizarre borders that resolve into small spots reminiscent of an archipelago (Fig. 1a, b). In male patients, the lesion shows increased hairiness after puberty (Fig. 2) (Danarti et al. 2004, Happle and Koopman 1997). A systematised involvement that may be either unilateral or bilateral has likewise been described (Fig. 3) (Panizzon et al. 1984). Involvement of the head may result in asymmetric hair growth within the nevus, asymmetric growth of beard or pronounced acne-lesions within the nevus (Danarti et al. 2004). Cases with localised scleroderma have been also reported (Fegeler and Schreiner 1954, Rufli 1972, Smolle 1983).

Because an increased number of androgen receptors (Downs et al. 1998, Formingon et al. 1992) and androgen receptor messenger RNA (Nirdé et al. 1999), as compared with unaffected skin, has been reported (Danarti et al. 2004) the "full blown" picture of Becker nevus is in general observed exclusively in adolescent or adult men (Happle and Koopman 1997). The intralesional presence of acne (reviewed in Danarti et al. 2004) and the occurrence

**Fig. 1.** Becker nevus syndrome: (**A**) Pigmentary hairy nevus of the thorax arranged in a checkerboard pattern; (**B**) close up view of the nevus showing areolar hypoplasia; (**C**) X-ray films of the spine in an anteroposterior view showing right curved scoliosis.

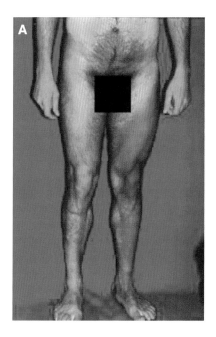 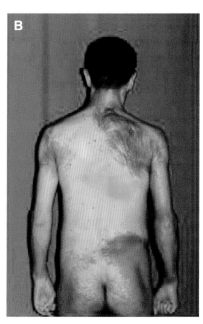

**Fig. 3.** (**A**) Capillary nevus of the left thigh and the lower abdomen associated to pigmentary hairy nevus of the right scapula (**B**); note (**B**) the capillary malformation over the right lumbar region and right buttock.

of Becker nevus in a patient with an accessory scrotum (Szylit et al. 1986) further reflects the pathogenic role of androgens in this disorder (Danarti et al. 2004). In women and pre-pubertal boys the lesion is much less conspicuous because the pigmentation is less intense and hairiness is absent or only mild (Happle and Koopman 1997).

Histopathological examination shows slight epidermal acanthosis and regular elongation of reteridges, variable hyperkeratosis, and acanthosis. The basal cell layer is hyperpigmented and melanophages are present in the papillary dermis (Danarti et al. 2004). The arrector pili muscles are increased in number and size, often resulting in histopathological appearance indistinguishable from smooth muscle hamartomas. Neither epidermis nor dermis contain any increase or aggregation of melanocytes (Copeman and Jones 1965, Haneke 1979).

## Other cutaneous anomalies

These include so far: patchy hypoplasia of ipsilateral extramammary fatty tissue, hypoplasia of the contralateral labius minus, an accessory scrotum, sparse hair of the ipsilateral axilla, patchy cutaneous hypoplasia of the ipsilateral temporal region, and supernumerary nipples (reviewed in Danarti et al. 2004).

## Unilateral hypoplasia of breast

In affected women this is the most frequently reported anomaly to be associated with Becker's nevus (Danarti et al. 2004, Happle and Koopman 1997) but has also been reported in men usually in the form of hypoplastic areola (reviewed in Danarti et al. 2004). In female patients it may involve the entire breast including the fatty tissue (Fig. 4) or only the nipple and areola (Danarti et al. 2004).

## Maxillofacial abnormalities

Ipsilateral segmental odontomaxillary dysplasia, ipsilateral absence of the right maxillary lateral incisor and canine teeth, facial asymmetry and polyostotic fibrous dysplasia of the right maxillae and mandible have been reported in isolated cases (reviewed by Danarti et al. 2004, Happle and Koopman 1997). Because of the closer regional relationship of the cutaneous and extracutaneous lesions the authors assumed a common origin (Danarti et al. 2004).

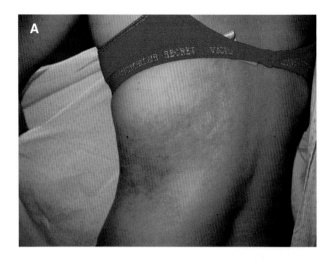

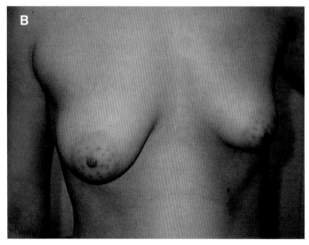

**Fig. 4.** Pigmentary hairy nevus of the left side of the body in a women with Becker's nevus syndrome associated to ipsilateral hypoplasia of the breast (courtesy of J. L. Sugarman, UCSF, San Franciso, USA).

## Musculoskeletal anomalies

They include scoliosis (Fig. 1c), vertebral defects (including hemivertebrae, cleft vertebrae and spina bifida occulta), fused or accessory cervical ribs, pectus excavatum or carenatum, asymmetry of scapulae, short limb or other forms of limb asymmetry, bilateral internal tibial torsion, ipsilateral hypoplasia of the shoulder girdle (including absence of the pectoralis major muscle), hypoplasia of the sternocleidomastoideus muscle and umbilical hernia (reviewed in Danarti et al. 2004, Happle and Koopman 1997).

## Miscellaneous findings

Bilateral congenital cataract has been reported in one woman so far (Domjan and Torok 1999).

## Natural history

The associated extracutaneous lesions are congenital and thus non progressive. The natural history of the Becker's nevus within the syndromic constellation is the same as in the isolated naevi: in pre-pubertal boys the pigmentation may be less intense and the hairiness absent or mild as occurs in women whilst in men there is an increase of hairiness after puberty.

## Pathogenesis and molecular genetics

Both Becker's nevus and mammary hypoplasia can be explained as hormone-dependent developmental abnormalities caused by disturbances of receptor activity (Danarti et al. 2004, Downs et al. 1998, Formingon et al. 1992, Nirdé et al. 1999). The development of breast, areola and nipple are essentially oestrogen-dependent in both sexes: hypoplasia of these structures could be caused by an excess of androgen receptors in the region of the nevus counteracting the effect of estrogens (Crone and James 1997, Danarti et al. 2004). The associated musculoskeletal anomalies, however, are difficult to explain solely by this pathogenic mechanism (Danarti et al. 2004) and could be better explained by regional (mosaic) correspondence between the area of the nevus and the associated anomaly (Happle and Koopman 1997). For example, the frequently occurring hypoplasia of breast as well as the skeletal defects were almost always ipsilateral and the associated Becker's nevus involved the thorax.

*Paradominant patterns of inheritance.* Happle and Koopman (1997) suggested that Becker nevus syndrome might represent a paradominant phenomenon (the disorder would become apparent when a post-zygotic mutation occurred in the developing embryo) on the basis of: (1) the sporadic occurrence of isolated Becker's nevus in most but not all cases (there are few families with several affected members) (reviewed in Danarti et al. 2004); (2) Mendelian inheritance patterns which do not explain why the disease always occurs in mosaic patterns; (3) mosaicism for chromosomal abnormalities which has been documented in fibroblasts derived from a Becker's nevus in one sporadic case (Lambert et al. 1994); and (4) the familial occurrence of Becker's nevus syndrome in a father and his eldest son both affected by Becker's nevus and scoliosis, whereas another son and a daughter had isolated Becker's nevus (Maessen-Visch et al. 1997). Interestingly, Wagner et al. (1989) have observed a case of Becker's nevus arranged in close proximity to unilateral nevoid telangiectasia. In one of our Becker's nevus syndrome patients the Becker's nevus, arranged in a checkerboard pattern in the chest and shoulder (Fig. 1), was associated to a capillary malformation of one thigh and ipsilateral buttock (Fig. 3) (unpublished data). These associations could be taken as possible examples of twin spotting, implying allelic loss by somatic recombination (Happle 1993).

The concept of paradominant inheritance implies that both Becker's nevus and Becker's nevus syndrome originate from regional loss of heterozygosity occurring at an early stage of embryogenesis and resulting in a mosaic population of homozygous cells. Heterozygous individuals would be, as a rule, phenotypically normal, and the responsible mutation would, therefore, be transmitted unperceived through many generations. This would explain why Becker's nevus syndrome virtually always occurs sporadically but may show, by way of exception, a familial aggregation (Danarti et al. 2004, Happle and Koopman 1997).

## Differential diagnosis

The most characteristic manifestations of Becker's nevus syndrome are Becker's nevus, ipsilateral hypoplasia of breast and ipsilateral skeletal defects with sporadic contralateral anomalies. Although scoliosis certainly belongs to the spectrum of this phenotype it seems important to realise that in a given case of co-occurrence of Becker's nevus and very mild scoliosis is not sufficient to firmly establish a diagnosis of Becker's nevus syndrome (Happle and Koopman 1997).

Becker's nevus syndrome cab be easily from other epidermal nevus syndromes such as Schimmelpenning-Feuerstein-Mims syndrome, CHILD syndrome or Proteus syndrome (Happle 1995, Happle and Koopman 1997).

The Becker's nevus syndrome must not be confused with "Becker syndrome" a familial phenotype characterised by discrete or confluent brown macules on the neck and forearms (Becker and Reuter 1939, Bleehen et al. 1992).

## Management and follow-up

There are no special issues relating to management besides the treatment of Becker's nevus in those who seek for this. Ultrasound scans can be obtained to search for underlying abnormalities ipsilateral or contralateral to the lesion.

## Genetic counselling

All but one case (Maessen-Visch et al. 1997) of Becker nevus syndrome reported so far have been sporadic (Danarti et al. 2004, Happle and Koopman 1997). Lambert et al. (2004) described mosaicism involving a small extra chromosome predominantly present in fibroblasts derived from the area of Becker's nevus. Some cases (Wagner et al. 1989) including one of ours were suggestive of twin spotting as a pathogenic mechanism (Happle and Koopman 1997). Happle and Koopman (1997) and Danarti et al. (2004), by reviewing the existing literature, have suggested paradominant inheritance (see above). Thus, an affected individual with Becker's nevus syndrome could be given a small but proven risk of passing the isolated nevus or the full blown syndrome to the offspring in one generation.

## References

Alfaro A, Torrelo A, Hernández A, Zambrano A, Happle R (2007) Becker nevus syndrome. Actas Dermosifiliogr 98: 624–626.

Becker SW, Reuter MJ (1939) A familial pigmentary anomaly. Arch Dermatol 40: 987–998.

Becker SW (1949) Concurrent melanosis and hypertrichosis in distribution of nevus unius unilateralis. Arch Dermatol Syph 60: 155–160.

Bleehen SS, Ebling FJC, Champion CH (1992) Disorders of skin colours. In: Champion RH, Burton JL, Ebling FJG (eds.) Rook/Wilkinson/Ebling Textbook of Dermatology. 5th ed. Oxford: Blackwell Scientific Publications, pp. 1561–1622.

Copeman PWJ, Jones EW (1965) Pigmented hairy epidermal nevus (Becker). Arch Dermatol 92: 249–251.

Crone AM, James MP (1997) Giant Becker's nevus with ipsilateral areolar hypoplasia and limb asymmetry. Clin Exp Dermatol 22: 240–241.

Danarti R, Koning A, Salhi A, Bittar M, Happle R (2004) Becker's nevus revisited. J Am Acad Dermatol 51: 965–969.

Domjan K, Torok L (1999) Becker-naevus syndroma. Borgyogy Venereol 75: 3–5 [in Hungarian].

Downs AM, Mehta R, Lear JT, Peachey RD (1998) Acne in Becker's naevus: an androgen-mediated link? Clin Exp Dermatol 23: 191–192.

Fegeler F, Schreiner H (1954) Familiares Vorkommen von systematisierten Pigmentnaevi mit circumscripter Sklerodermie im gleichen Hautsegment. Hautarzt 5: 253–255.

Formigòn M, Alsina MM, Mascarò JM, Rivera F (1992) Becker's nevus and ipsilateral breast hypoplasia: androgen-receptor study in two patients. Arch Dermatol 128: 992–993.

Glinik SE, Alper JA, Bogaars H, Brown JA (1983) Becker's melanosis: associated abnormalities. J Am Acad Dermatol 9: 509–514.

Haneke E (1979) The dermal component in melanosis naeviformis Becker. J Cutan Pathol 6: 53–58.

Happle R (1993) Mosaicism in human skin. Understanding the patterns and mechanisms. Arch Dermatol 129: 1460–1470.

Happle R (1995) Epidermal nevus syndromes. Semin Dermatol 14: 111–121.

Happle R, Koopman RJJ (1997) Becker nevus syndrome. Am J Med Genet 68: 357–361.

Lambert JR, Willems P, Abs R, Van Roy B (1994) Becker's nevus associated with chromosomal mosaicism and congenital adrenal hyperplasia. J Am Acad Dermatol 30: 655–657.

Maessen-Visch MB, Hulsmans RFHJ, Hulsmans FJH, Neumann HAM (1997) Melanosis naeviformis of Becker and scoliosis: a coincidence? Acta Derm Venereol 77: 135–136.

Mascarò JM, Galy de Mascarò G, Pinol Aguadé J (1970) Historia natural del nevus de Becker. Med Cutan Ibero Latinoamer 4: 437–445.

Moore JA, Schosser RH (1985) Becker's hypomelanosis and hypoplasia of the breast and pectoral major muscle. Pediatr Dermatol 3: 34–37.

Nirdé P, Dereure O, Belon C, Lumbroso S, Guilhou JJ, Sultan C (1999) The association of Becker nevus with hypersensitivity to androgens. Arch Dermatol 135: 212–214.

Rufli T (1972) Melanosis Becker mit lokalisierter Sklerodermie. Dermatologica 145: 222–229.

Smolle J (1983) Becker'sche Melanosis und oberflachliche zirkumskripte Sklerodermie. Akt Dermatol 39: 187–188.

Sugarman JL (2004) Epidermal nevus syndromes. Semin Cut Med Surg 23: 145–157.

Szylit JA, Grossman ME, Luyando V, Olarte MR, Nagler H (1986) Becker's nevus and an accessory scrotum: a unique occurrence. J Am Acad Dermatol 14: 905–907.

Vujevich JJ, Mancini AJ (2004) The epidermal nevus syndromes: multisystem disorders. I Am Acad Dermatol 50: 957–961.

Wagner RF Jr, Grande DJ, Bhawan J, Hellerstein MK, Longrope C (1989) Unilateral dermatomal superficial telangiectasia overlapping Becker's melanosis. Int J Dermatol 28: 595–596.

Who named it? (2006) http://www.whonamedit.com

# Chapter 37

# CHILD SYNDROME

Ramón Ruiz-Maldonado, Luz Orozco-Covarrubias, Carola Duran-McKinster, and Marimar Saez-De-Ocariz

Department of Dermatology, National Institute of Paediatrics, Mexico City, Mexico

## Introduction

*CHILD syndrome* (OMIM # 308050) is an acronym designation for **C**ongenital **H**emidysplasia with **I**chthyosiform nevus and **L**imb **D**efects. This X-linked dominant, male-lethal trait is characterized by: (1) congenital unilateral inflammatory erythematous patches often covered in dry yellowish scales which usually undergo spontaneous partial regression during childhood; (2) psoriasiform epidermal hyperplasia with marked hyperkeratosis and parakeratosis, with sparse perivascular lymphocytic infiltrates at skin histology; and (3) ipsilateral hypoplasia of the limbs (but also of the skeleton) and/or other organs (e.g., lungs, thyroid, muscles, cranial nerves, brain, brainstem, cerebellum and spinal cord, etc.). Other associate extra-cutaneous manifestations include cardiovascular and neurological deficits (related to the underlying central visceral and/or nervous system abnormalities) (Happle et al. 1980, Tang and McCreadle 1974, Taybi and Lachman 1996). CHILD syndrome is caused by mutations in the gene encoding NSDHL (3β-hydrosteroid dehydrogenase-like protein) at Xq28 (Konig et al. 2000, 2002). Emopamil-binding protein (EBP) gene defects (responsible for the Conradi-Hunermann-Happle syndrome/X-linked dominant chondrodysplasia punctata – EBP/CDPX2 gene on Xp11) (OMIM # 302960) (see chapter 38) have been also described (OMIM$^{TM}$ 2006). Both enzymes are involved in cholesterol biosynthesis.

## Historical perspective and eponyms

The acronym designation was first introduced by Happle et al. (1980) who reviewed 18 cases that were earlier reported under various designations and added two further cases.

The earliest reported case is that of *Otto Sachs* published in 1903 (Sachs 1903a) and only recently diagnosed in retrospect by Bittar and Happle (2004). In 1901, Otto Sachs, while working as a resident on Albert Neisser's team at the Breslau Department of Dermatology, presented at a session of the Breslau Dermatological Association, a case of "nevus papillomatous of the right axilla and the fingers of the right hand (with demonstration of moulages, photographs, and microscopical slides)" (Sachs 1902). When Sachs moved to Vienna to become a resident and, later, senior physician at the Imperial-Royal Hospital he presented again this case (1903a) and later he comprehensively published it under the title of "Contributions to the histology of soft nevi (a case of pointed condyloma on the fifth finger of the right hand, xanthoma-like nevus verrucosus of the right axillary region and several linear nevi scattered over the body)" (Bittar and Happle 2004, Sachs 1903b). In his report of 1903a, Sachs gave a classical (documented) description of the clinical and histopathological features of CHILD nevus and associated limb hypoplasia (Bittar and Happle 2004).

Another case diagnosed in retrospect (Happle et al. 1996) was that of Zellweger and Uehlinger in 1948 that paradoxically described this male-lethal phenotype in a boy. Earlier reports describing this entity had been published under the name "unilateral ichthyosiform erythroderma" (Rossman et al. 1963), "congenital unilateral ichthyosiform erythroderma" (Cullen et al. 1969) and "ichthyosis-limb reduction syndrome" (Taybi 1996, Spitz 2005, Sugarman 2004).

## Incidence and prevalence

Over 30 cases of child syndrome have been reported (Spitz 2005, Sugarman 2004). The sex ratio calculated on the 29 cases reported until 1987 (Hebert et al. 1987) was 28 females: 1 male. As an exception to the rule that CHILD syndrome is observed only in females, two cases have been reported in boys (Happle et al. 1996, Zelleweger and Uehlinger 1948).

## Clinical manifestations

### Skin abnormalities

The skin lesions are present since birth or manifest soon after birth and may progress during the first year of life and then partially (spontaneously) regress in childhood: they may persist in skin folds (ptychotropism) (Spitz 2005) or periods of aggravation and improvement may occur alternately (Happle et al. 1908). Most patients present with a sharply demarcated, unilateral, inflamed and hyperkeratotic, thickened plaque with scaling covering a large portion of one side of the body (Figs. 1 and 2). The existence of normal thin skin strips in the affected body side and strips of diseased skin (following the lines of Blaschko) in the "unaffected" body side have been reported (Emami et al. 1992). In the affected side flexural folds are preferentially involved (e.g., the vulva, axillae and the gluteus folds). Exceptionally, a heterozygous carrier of a NSDHL mutation may exhibit a bilateral "quasi symmetric" CHILD nevus (Konig et al. 2002).

### Skin appendages

Unilateral impaired hair growth and linear areas of alopecia on the affected side may also be present (Spitz 2005). Nail dystrophy (often leading to destruction of nails and replacement by keratotic claw-

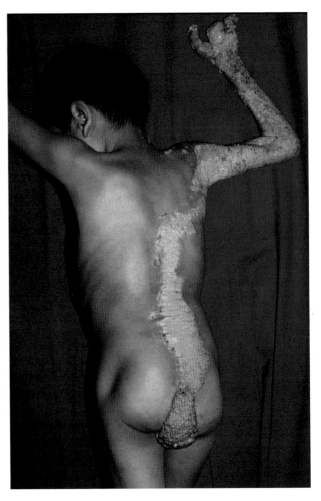

**Fig. 1.** CHILD syndrome: Extensive, unilateral, verrucose epidermal nevus, vegetating new growth in the intergluteal fold, and patch of alopecia in the scalp.

like material) or onychorrhexis are other associated features which may also be present.

### Ipsilateral bone anomalies

#### Hypoplasia/aplasia of limbs

Ipsilateral body hypoplasia most frequently affects skeletal structures and varies from hypoplasia of some metacarpals or phalanges to shortening or complete absence of an extremity causing asymmetry (Taybi 1996). Sometimes, the hands or feet are

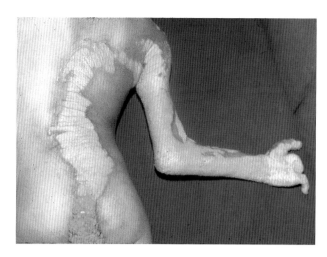

**Fig. 2.** CHILD syndrome: missing finger in the epidermal nevus involved arm.

grossly deformed and/or hypoplasia of long bones mat result in contractures.

## Skeletal hypoplasia of the head and trunk

Unilateral hypoplasia of bones may involve any other part of the skeleton (Happle et al. 1980, Spitz 2005) including the calvarium, mandible, scapula, clavicle, pelvis, ribs, and vertebrae (including hemivertebrae or fused vertebrae) (Taybi 1996). Scoliosis may be due to the asymmetry of limbs as well as to one or more genuine vertebral defect(s). Radiologically there is either unilateral hypoplasia or aplasia of a limb or unilateral hypoplasia of any skeletal segment.

## Punctate calcifications of cartilage

In some cases punctate epiphyseal calcifications have been observed when x-rays have been obtained soon after birth (Happle et al. 1980, Taybi 1996). In addition to that, stippled calcifications of the pelvis, sella turcica, ribs, vertebrae, larynx or thyroid cartilage have been recorded. Stippling usually disappeared at age two years (Happle et al. 1980).

## Ipsilateral central nervous system anomalies

Associated ipsilateral hypoplasia has been reported in the brain, cranial nerves, pons, medulla, cerebel-

lum, and spinal cord (Baden and Rex 1970, Cullen et al. 1963, Shear et al. 1971, Tang and McCreadie 1974, Zellweger and Uehlinger 1948). EEG anomalies have been recorded on the affected side in some of these cases. One case showed associated mild cognitive deficits (Happle et al. 1980) and another decreased sensation to touch and heat on the affected side (Pereiro Mignens et al. 1960).

## Ipsilateral anomalies of internal organs

Ipsilateral anomalies (mostly consistent of hypoplasia) have been found in any part of the body including the heart; lungs (Lewis and Messner 1970); kidneys (hydroureter, hydronephrosis or absence of the ipsilateral kidney) (Happle et al. 1980, Rossman et al. 1963, Tang and McCreadie 1974); muscles; adrenal gland; ovary; and fallopian tube. Associated cardiovascular defects include single ventricle, atrial and ventricular septum defects, single coronary ostium, and Shone complex: these have the cause of early death in many CHILD cases (Baden and Rex 1970, Falek et al. 1969, Happle et al. 1980, Lipsitz et al. 1979, Tang and McCreadie 1974). In one instance unaffected relatives and siblings died of complications of cardiovascular defects (Falek et al. 1969).

## Contralateral and miscellaneous anomalies

The unilateral distribution of defects is not absolute (Happle et al. 1980). There can be minor associated skin and visceral abnormalities on the contralateral side such as cleft lip, umbilical hernia, minimal (bilateral) hearing loss, laryngeal hypoplasia, and short trachea (Taybi 1996).

## Pathology

The cutaneous nevus in CHILD syndrome shows a psoriasiform epidermal hyperplasia, sometimes with aspect of verruciform xanthoma. In the patient seen at our Department of Dermatology, a biopsy of the cauliflower-like verrucous nevus located in the intergluteal fold showed a striking digit-like and lace-like

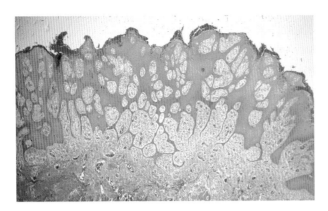

**Fig. 3.** CHILD syndrome. Histopathology of the vegetating inter-gluteal new growth: impressive acanthosis with sebaceous-cells digitiform epidermal invasion.

sebaceous-cell hyperplasia, substituting most of the epidermis: these were compatible with nevus sebaceous (Fig. 3).

## Pathogenesis and molecular genetics

### Familial occurrence

Almost all cases so far reported have been observed in girls (Happle 1990, Peter and Meinecke 1993), and transmission from mother to daughter has been described (Happle et al. 1990) as well as transmission in multiple generations (Bittar et al. 2006). Remarkably, however, the first published case that could retrospectively be classified as CHILD syndrome was a boy (Zellweger and Uehlinger 1948) and Happle et al. (1996) described a further case of a 2-year-old boy of Egyptian origin born to healthy unrelated parents. In this latter case (Happle et al. 1996), at birth, a severely deformed right leg and an inflammatory ichthyosiform skin lesion involving the right side of the body were noted. Despite dermal abrasion of parts of the lesion involving the trunk, the CHILD nevus had completely recurred in the treated area 8 months later. Some functional improvement was achieved by orthopedic surgical correction of the dislocated right knee joint and right foot. Happle et al. (1996) explained the occurrence of CHILD syndrome in males as likewise caused either by post zygotic mutations or by half-chromatid mutation.

## Pathogenesis

The molecular basis of CHILD syndrome has recently been elucidated. The predominant unilateral and mosaic distribution of lesions may be explained by the Lyon effect of random X chromosome inactivation (Happle et al. 1980). CHILD syndrome is caused by a mutation in the NSDHL gene encoding a 3β-hydrosteroid dehydrogenase-like protein at Xq28 (Konig et al. 2000, 2002). In some cases mutations have been found in the EBP gene which is responsible for the Conradi-Hunermann-Happle syndrome on Xp11. Either proteins function in cholesterol biosynthetic pathway (the EBP protein functions downstream of NSDHL in a later step of cholesterol biosynthesis) (Konig et al. 2000). Previous studies of peroxisomal morphology and function in CHILD syndrome have shown that fibroblasts from affected skin accumulated cytoplasm lipids, lamellated membranes and vacuolar structures. Peroxisomes contain enzymes catalyzing a number of indispensable functions mainly related to cholesterol metabolism. Notably, however, the majority of peroxisomal functions are preserved in CHILD syndrome (Emami et al. 1992). CHILD syndrome may be considered among the developmental disorders associated with mutations affecting cholesterol synthesis (Happle et al. 1996). A defective response to Hedgehog signaling is now thought to play a role in disorders of cholesterol biosynthesis that share some of the skeletal and cardiovascular defects seen in CHILD syndrome (Sugarman 2004).

## Natural history

The ichthyosiform erythroderma is usually present at birth, but may also develop during the first weeks of life. In most cases, the extent of the dermatosis remains unchanged and may persist especially in skin folds (ptychotropism) (Spitz 2005). Sometimes, spontaneous improvement is observed or periods of aggravation and improvement may occur alternately (Happle et al. 1908). Involvement of new skin areas has been observed until the age of nine years. The outcome, depending on which organs are affected, can range from normal life span to incompatible with life (Spitz 2005).

## Differential diagnosis

Although CHILD syndrome is genetically well characterized with mutations in the gene of the cholesterol synthesis pathway NSDHL located at Xq28, from a clinical perspective a number of epidermal nevi should be included in the differential diagnosis of patients who present with unilateral inflammatory epidermal verrucous nevi associated to ipsilateral skeletal and/or visceral abnormalities. In a recent publication, among 443 epidermal nevi we found that 408 where isolated lesions and 35 where a component of complex syndromes. No relationship was found between the extension and/or location of nevi and the degree of systemic involvement (Vidaurri de La Cruz et al. 2004).

The clinical distinction between CHILD and *Proteus syndromes* is made on the basis of the strict lateralization of the epidermal nevus (which is clinically different in either syndrome) and the predomi-

nant associated skeletal/visceral hypoplasia/absence in CHILD syndrome and the cerebriform connective tissue nevus of the palms and soles in Proteus syndrome (Fig. 4). Sometimes the differential diagnosis with the Elattoproteus syndrome could be difficult because of the hypotrophic/hypoplastic tissue which characterizes this variant of the Proteus syndrome.

*Sebaceous nevus syndrome* is more frequently found on the head. In infants it presents as a usually small, orange-yellow patch devoid of hair that becomes thicker in puberty. Rarely there may be large, vegetating lesions. Our case with CHILD syndrome had a vegetating lesion clinically similar to a nevus sebaceous (Fig. 5). Of note, 66 of our patients with epidermal nevus syndromes had associated brain abnormalities consisting in brain dysgenesis, ventriculomegaly, microcephaly, developmental delay and scizures (Barona-Mazuera et al. 1997).

The *nevus comedonicus syndrome* is characterized by a plaque or linear lesion covered by comedons or "black heads". Our three patients with this condition had musculoskeletal disorders. There should be no problem to distinguish this condition from CHILD syndrome.

*Phakomatosis pigmentokeratotica* is defined as the association of an organoid nevus with sebaceous differentiation following Blaschko's lines with a speckled lentiginous nevus in a checkerboard pat-

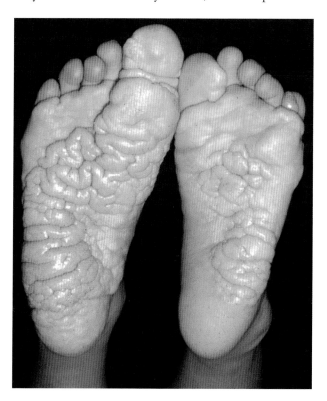

**Fig. 4.** Proteus syndrome: typical folded soles.

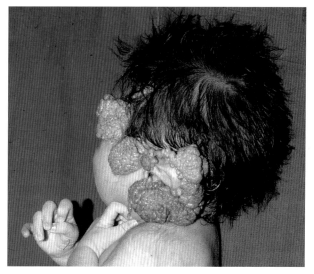

**Fig. 5.** Nevus sebaceous: vegetating lesion similar to those found in skin folds of CHILD syndrome.

tern. Neurological deficits and/or musculoskeletal alterations may be associated.

If punctate epiphyseal calcifications are present, the CHILD syndrome may be confused with *X-linked Conradi-Hunermann-Happle chondrodysplasia punctata* caused by mutations in the EBP gene, since asymmetric shortening of limbs, as well as congenital ichthyosiform erythroderma and limitation to the female sex are features of both conditions. In contrast to the CHILD syndrome, however, the ichthyosiform erythroderma of X-linked dominant chondrodysplasia punctata affects both sides of the body, the hyperkeratoses are always distributed in a linear or patchy pattern along the Blaschko's lines, and widespread atrophic skin lesions, arranged in the same pattern are children observed in older child (Happle 1979, Spitz 2005). Screening for mutations in the NSDHL and EBP genes should rule any further clinical/imaging dilemmas (see also chapter 38 for further discussion).

## Management and follow-up

In the suspect (or at the time of diagnosis) of a CHILD syndrome a skeletal survey should be planned in search of ipsilateral (but also contralateral) bone anomalies. Ultrasound examination of the heart and internal organs could help in revealing underlying organs/systems malformations but a full body magnetic resonance imaging (MRI) study should be obtained to detect minimal (ipsilateral and contralateral) anomalies. A full ophthalmologic examination is advisable even though no eye abnormalities have been recorded so far in CHILD syndrome. Laboratory investigations must be dictated by clinical or imaging findings. DNA must be extracted for mutational analysis of the NSDHL and EBP genes.

Clinical, laboratory and imaging follow-up controls are usually dictated by previous or new findings.

## Treatment

In practically all keratinization disturbances small, localized lesions are treated surgically or with destructive methods: lasers, cryotherapy, electrodessication. Larger or multiple lesions require systemic retinoids, namely *acitretin* from 0.5 to 2 mg/kg/day.

For vegetating, condyloma-like lesions like the ones in our patient with CHILD syndrome, topical 5-fluorouracil, imiquimod, or podophillin may be temporarily effective.

Musculoskeletal and neurological alterations require specialized treatment and rehabilitation.

## Genetic counseling

For the practical purpose of genetic counseling it should be borne in mind that: (a) CHILD syndrome is an X-linked dominant condition and thus is transmitted from mother to daughter with a 50% rate of occurrence in each pregnancy; (b) a male affected with CHILD syndrome bears a risk to transmit the trait to his daughters (provided the assumed underlying postzygotic mutation has occurred early and involves the gonads, too); (c) a transmission of this phenotype from mother to son should be not possible (in apparent contrast with this idea, cases of alleged transmission of other X-linked dominant conditions from mother to son have been demonstrated) (Happle et al. 1996, Hecht et al. 1982, Kurczynski et al. 1982).

## References

Baden HP, Rex JH (1970) Linear ichthyosis associated with skeletal abnormalities: new entity. Arch Dermatol 102: 126–128.

Barona-Mazuera del Rosario M, Hidalgo-Galvan LR, de la Luz Orozco-Covarrubias, Duran-McKinster C, Tamayo-Sanchez L, Ruiz-Maldonado R (1997) Proteus syndrome: new findings in seven patients. Ped Dermatol 14: 1–5.

Bittar M, Happle R (2004) CHILD sìndrome avant la lettre. J Am Acad Dermatol 50: 34–37.

Bittar M, Happle R, Grzeschik KH, Leveleki L, Hertl M, Bornholdt D, König A (2006) CHILD syndrome in 3 generations: the importance of mild or minimal skin lesions. Arch Dermatol 142: 348–351.

Cullen S, Harris DE, Carter CH, Reed WB (1969) Congenital ichthyosiform erythroderma. Arch Dermatol 99: 724–729.

Emami S, Rizzo WB, Hanley KP, Taylor JM, Goldyne ME, Williams ML (1992) Peroxisomal abnormality in fibroblasts from evolved skin of CHILD syndrome: Case study and review of peroxisomal disorders in relation to skin disease. Arch Dermatol 128: 1213–1222.

Falek A, Heath CW, Ebbin AJ, McLean WR (1969) Unilateral limb and skin deformities with congenital heart disease in two siblings: a lethal syndrome. J Pediatr 73: 910–913.

Happle R (1979) X-linked dominant chondrodysplasia punctata. Review of literature and report of a case. Hum Genet 53: 65–73.

Happle R (1990) Psychotropism as a cutaneous feature of the CHILD syndrome. J Am Acad Dermatol 23: 763–766.

Happle R (1991) CHILD syndrome is not ILVEN. J Med Genet 28: 214.

Happle R, Koch H, Lenz W (1980) The CHILD syndrome: Congenital hemidysplasia with ichthyosiform erythroderma and limb defects. Eur J Pediatr 134: 27–33.

Happle R, Kerlic D, Steijlen PM (1990) CHILD-Syndrom bei Mutter und Tochten. Hautarzt 41: 105–108.

Happle R, Mittag, Kuster W (1995) The CHILD nevus: a distinct skin disorder. Dermatology 191: 210–216.

Happle R, Effendy I, Magahed M, Orlow SJ, Kuster W (1996) CHILD syndrome in a boy. Am J Med Genet 62: 192–194.

Hebert AA, Esterly NB, Holbrook KA, Hall JC (1987) The CHILD syndrome: Histologic and ultrastructural studies. Arch Dermatol 123: 503–509.

Hecht F, Hecht BK, Austin WJ (1982) Incontinentia pigmenti in Arizona Indians including transmission from mother to son inconsistent with the half chromatid migration model. Clin Genet 21: 293–296.

Herman GE (2003) Disorders of cholesterol biosynthesis: prototypic metabolic malformation syndromes. Hum Molec Genet 12(R1): R75–R88.

König A, Happle R, Borholdt D, Engel H, Grzeschik KH (2000) Mutations in the NSDHL gene, encoding a 3-beta-hydroxysteroid dehydrogenase, cause CHILD syndrome. Am J Med Genet 90: 339–346.

König A, Happle R, Fink-Puches R, Soyer HP, Borholdt D, Engel H, Grzeschik KH (2002) A novel missense mutation of NSDHL in an unusual case of CHILD syndrome showing bilateral, almost symmetric involvement. J Am Acad Dermatol 46: 594–596.

Kurczynski TW, Berns JS, Johnson WE (1982) Studies of a family with incontinentia pigmenti variably expressed in both sexes. J Med Genet 19: 447–451.

Lewis RG, Messner DG (1970) Prosthetic fitting of congenital unilateral ichthyosiform erythroderma. A case report. Interclin Inform Bull 9: 1–6.

Lipsitz PJ, Suser F, Weinberg S, Valderama E (1979) Congenital unilateral ichthyosis in a newborn. Amer J Dis Child 133: 76–78.

OMIM™ (2006) Online Mendelian Inheritance in Man. Baltimore: Johns Hopkins University. http://www.ncbi.nlm.nih.gov/omim

Pereiro Miguerns M, Pena Guitian J, Vieites Faya F (1960) Lesiones psoriasiform de distribucion linear acompanadas de malformaciones congenitas. Actas Dermosifiliogr (Madrid) 51: 213–219.

Peter C, Meinecke P (1993) CHILD-Syndrom: Fallbericht einer meltenen Genodermatose. Hautarzt 44: 590–593.

Prayson RA, Kotagal P, Wyllie E, Bingaman W (1999) Linear epidermal nevus and nevus sebaceous syndrome. A clinicopathologic study of 3 patients. Arch Pathol Lab Med 123: 301–305.

Rossman RE, Shapiro EM, Freeman RG (1963) Unilateral ichthyosiform erythrodermia. Arch Dermatol 88: 567–571.

Sachs O (1902) Ein 8-jähriges Mädchen mit einem Naevus papillomatous der rechten Achselhöhle und der Finger der rechten Hand (mit Demonstration von Moulagen, Photographien und mikroskopischen Präparaten). Arch Dermatol Syphilis (Vienna) 60: 147.

Sachs O (1903a) Demonstration der Mikroskopischen Praparate eines Naevus verrucosus der Achselhöhle eines 8-jährigen Mädchens mit dem Befunde xanthomahnlicher Zellen in Anordnung von Naevuszellen. Arch Dermatol Syphilis 66: 212.

Sachs O (1903b) Beitrage zur Histologie der weichen Naevi. (Ein Fall von sptiztem kondylom am kleinen Finger der rechten Hand, xanthomartigen Naevus verrucosus der rechten Achsellhöhle und mehreren über den Körper verstreuten Naevi lineares). Arch Dermatol Syphilis (Vienna) 66: 101–126.

Shear CS, Nyhan WL, Kirman BH, Stern J (1971) Self-mutilative behavior as a feature of the de Lange syndrome. J Pediatr 78: 506–509.

Spitz JL (2005) Genodermatoses. A Clinical Guide to Genetic Skin Disorders. Philadelphia: Lippincott Williams & Wilkins.

Sugarman JL (2004) Epidermal nevus syndromes. Semin Cut Med Surg 23: 145–157.

Tang TT, McCreadie SR (1974) Congenital hemidysplasia with ichthyosis. Birth Defects Orig Art Ser 10: 257–261.

Taybi H (1996) Child syndrome. In: Taybi H, Lachman RS (eds.) Radiology of Syndromes, Metabolic Disorders and Skeletal Dysplasia. 4th ed. St. Louis: Mosby, pp. 84–85.

Vidaurri-de la Cruz H, Tamayo-Sanchez L, Duran McKinster C, Orozco-Covarrubias L, Ruiz-Maldonado R (2004) Epidermal nevus syndromes: clinical findings in 35 patients. Pediatr Dermatol 21: 432–439.

Vujevich JJ, Mancini AJ (2004) The epidermal nevus syndromes: multisystem disorders. J Am Acad Dermatol 50: 957–961.

Zellweger H, Uehlinger E (1948) Ein Fall von halbseitiger Knochencondromotase (Ollier) mit Naevus ichthyosiform. Helvet Paediatr Acta 2: 153–163.

# Chapter 38

# CHONDRODYSPLASIA PUNCTATA (CDP)
# CONRADI-HUNERMANN-HAPPLE TYPE (CDPX2)

Martino Ruggieri and Ignacio Pascual-Castroviejo

Institute of Neurological Science, National Research Council, Catania and Department of Paediatrics, University of Catania, Catania, Italy (MR);
Paediatric Neurology Service, University Hospital La Paz, University of Madrid, Madrid, Spain (IPC)

## Introduction

*Punctate epiphyses* are small calcifications in cartilaginous epiphysis or in certain other cartilaginous structures, such as the larynx and vertebrae (Spranger et al. 2002). These lesions appear initially during infancy or prenatally in some patients and usually disappear by 3–5 years of age

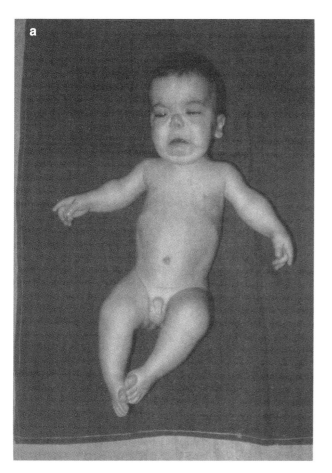
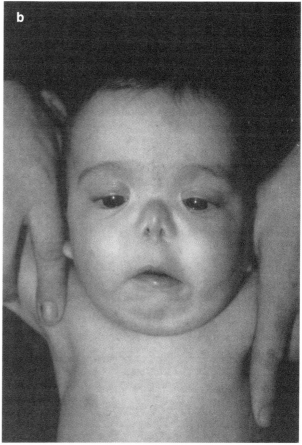

Fig. 1. (a) General apearance of a 8-month-old patient with RCDP. He shows symmetrical shortening of the proximal parts of the upper and lower limbs, joint contractures, narrow thorax and typical dysmorphic facial characteristics. (b) Facial features of the patient who shows exophthalmos and bilateral cataracts, prominent forehead, hypoplasia of the midface, short nose with anteverted nares and long philtrum. (c) Lateral spinal radiograph of the same patient shows dorso-lumbar kyphosis and antero-posterior shortening of $L_{12}$ (arrowhead).

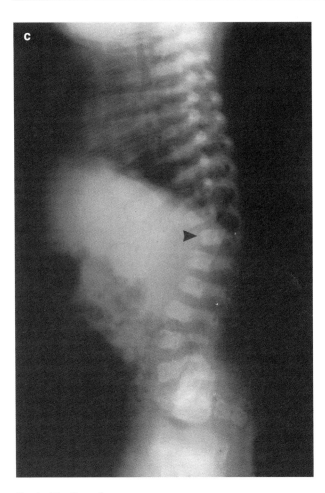

**Fig. 1.** (Continued)

**Table 2.** Other genetic disorders associated with puncta

| Name |
| --- |
| Acrodysotosis |
| Binder syndrome |
| CHILD syndrome |
| De Barsy syndrome |
| De Lange syndrome |
| Fibrochondrogenesis |
| Galactosialidosis |
| GM1-gangliosidosis |
| Ichthyosis X-linked |
| Keutel syndrome |
| Mucolipidosis 2 |
| Osebold-Remondini syndrome |
| Pacman dysplasia |
| Smith-Lemli-Opitz syndrome |
| Trisomy 18 and 21 |
| Turner syndrome |

(Basbug et al. 2005, Brookhyser et al. 1999, Duff et al. 1990, Gray et al. 1990, Mayden et al. 1996). A certain group of chondrodysplasias in which the puncta are a consistent and important part of the manifestations of the disease have been considered as Chondrodysplasia punctata (CDP) in the international nomenclature and classification of the osteochondrodysplasias (Lachman 1998) (Table 1).

**Table 1.** Skeletal dysplasia with neonatal calcific stippling or fragmented ossification of the skeleton

| Name | Abnormal structure/pathway | Inheritance | OMIM |
| --- | --- | --- | --- |
| **Chondrodysplasia punctata (CDP) syndromes and related disorders** | | | |
| Greenberg dysplasia | cholesterol biosynthesis | AR | 215140 |
| Dappled diaphysis dysplasia | ? | AR | |
| CDP syndrome | | | 215105 |
| CDPX1, X-linked recessive | arylsulfatase E | XLR | 302950 |
| CDPX2, Conradi-Hunermann-Happle type | cholesterol biosynthesis | XLD | 302960 |
| CDP, brachitelephalangic type BCDP) | arylsulfatase E | XLR | 302940 |
| CDP, tibial-metacarpal type | ? | AD? | 118651 |
| CDP, (Vitamin-K dependent) | | AD | 118650 |
| CDP, rhizomelic type (RCDP1) | peroxisome | AR | 215100 |
| CDP, rhizomelic type (RCDP2) | peroxisome | AR | 222765 |
| CDP, rhizomelic type (RCDP3) | peroxisome | AR | 600121 |
| Zellweger syndrome | peroxisome | AR | |

Adapted from Lachman (1998) and Spranger et al. (2002).

Molecular studies have shown considerable heterogeneity of disorders with punctate calcifications (Braverman et al. 1997, Daniele et al. 1998, Heymans et al. 1985, Kumada et al. 2001, Motley et al. 2002, Ofman et al. 1998, Wanders 2004, Purdue et al. 1997, Spranger 1971, White et al. 2003, Spranger et al. 2002). They have also been demonstrated that fragmented ossification of the bones can be expression if the same pathological mechanisms that cause punctate calcifications.

Tables 1 and 2 summarise the conditions with fragmented prenatal ossification of the bones and conditions associated with punctate calcifications. In this chapter we will deal only with the *CDP Conradi-Hunermann-Happle type* as one of the main features is a disorder of cornification in the skin (i.e., ichthyosiform erythroderma in Blaschko's lines in infancy which resolves with follicular atrophoderma and/or hyperpigmentation) and hair (coarse, patchy alopecia) associated to eye and central nervous system abnormalities (e.g., mental retardation).

In the CDP Conradi-Hunermann-Happle type the puncta may be asymmetric. In the Zellweger syndrome the puncta are often in the patella, which is less commonly seen in other disorders. In rhizomelic CDP stippling is sparse in the spine and the puncta are mostly in the ends of the long bones (Fig. 1). In the brachitelephalangic type the puncta are mainly in the distal phalanges. The pattern of puncta in some cases does not fit well with any of the conditions listed in Table 1. In most of the other genetic syndromes and in the acquired disorders associated with punctate epiphysis the puncta most commonly affect the tarsus (Hall 2002, Lachman 1996, Spranger et al. 2002).

# CONRADI–HUNERMANN–HAPPLE SYNDROME

## Introduction

The *Conradi-Hünermann-Happle syndrome* (CHH) or *CDPX2* (X-linked dominant chondrodysplasia punctata 2) (OMIM # 302960) is a rare X-linked dominant disorder characterised by distinctive skeletal (punctate calcification of the bones with asymmetric, rhizomelic shortening of the limbs), cutaneous (neonatal ichthyosiform erythroderma distributed along the lines of Blaschko followed after age 3–6 months by follicular atrophoderma) and ocular (microcornea, microphthalmia) anomalies distributed in a mosaic pattern (Williams et al. 2006). Neurological abnormalities include hypotonia, developmental delay, seizures and mental retardation. The cause of DCPX2 was unknown until Derry et al. (1999) found a missense mutation (G107R) in the mouse gene encoding delta-8, delta-7 sterol isomerase emopamil-binding protein/EBP in a CDPX2 model mouse and mutations of the human EBP gene in humans (Braverman et al. 1999, Silve et al. 1996) located on chromosome Xp11.22-23.

## Historical perspective and terminology

Chondrodysplasia punctata (CDP) was first described by Conradi (1914). Hünermann (1931) reported the same osseous lesions as an abortive form of chondrodystrophy. Happle (1979) defined the mosaic distribution pattern of lesions. Kalter et al. (1989) suggested the designation Conradi–Hunermann syndrome be reserved for the X-linked dominant form of the disorder. Sheffield (2001) traced the legitimacy of a tripartite eponym for this disorder: *Conradi-Hunermann-Happle* (OMIM 2006).

## Incidence and prevalence

Is a rare disorder which equally affects males and females in all racial groups (Savarirayan et al. 2004,

Spranger et al. 2002, Stoll et al. 1989). The phenotype of CDPX2 is variable among affected females even within the same family due to X-inactivation.

## Clinical features

### Skin manifestations

CHH presents at birth with ichthyosiform erythroderma distributed along the lines of Blaschko (Happle 1979, Happle et al. 1977, Hoang et al. 2004). The erythema and scaling usually resolves spontaneously during the first 3–6 months of life, leaving atrophic patches ("follicular atrophoderma"), often with post-inflammatory pigmentary changes, also in a Blaschkoid distribution (Williams et al. 2006). Other cutaneous features include coarse and lustreless hair, patches of scarring alopecia and flattening or splitting of the nails (Williams et al. 2006).

### Skeletal dysplasia

Neonate or young infants may exhibit the typical radiographic signs consisting of asymmetric punctate calcifications as well as variable asymmetric proximal limb shortening (Fig. 2a, b). As with the skin manifestations these skeletal changes are asymmetric, reflecting the mosaic pattern of disease expression: this feature contrast with most other CDP syndromes in which the findings are symmetrical, with the exception of CHILD syndrome, in which they are unilateral and ipsilateral to the skin manifestations (see below). The stippling may be widespread and involve the cartilage of the vertebrae and trachea typically resolving during the first months of life. Patients with CDPX2 have short stature, neck shortening and asymmetric, rhizomelic shortness of the limbs, scoliosis and craniofacial anomalies (frontal bossing, high arched palate, nasal hypoplasia

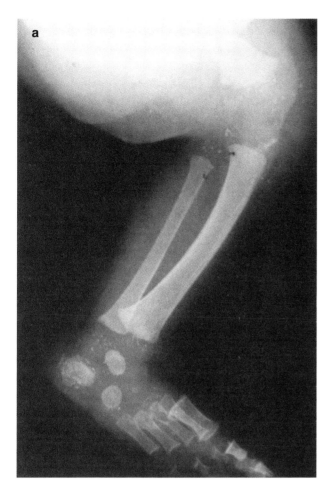

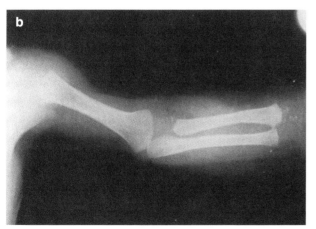

**Fig. 2.** CDPX2. Two radiographs of an infant girl that show chondrodysplasia punctata: (**a**) In lower limbs (knees and feet); (**b**) in one upper limb (shoulder, elbow and wrist).

with flat nasal bridge) as a result of their skeletal dysplasia (Happle 1981, Milunsky et al. 2003, Silengo et al. 1980).

## Ocular involvement

Asymmetric or sectorial cataracts are present in approximately 30% of patients. Microcornea and microphthalmia may also be present.

## Central nervous system manifestations

Neurological abnormalities include hypotonia, developmental delay, seizures and mental retardation (the latter more rarely as intelligence is usually normal in CHH patients). Brain malformations have been also reported including cortical dysplasia, hemimegalencephaly and posterior fossa malformations (Powers et al. 1999, Sigirci et al. 2005, Sztriba et al. 2000, Williams et al. 2001). Some patients may have sensorineural deafness. Typically, the spinal dysplasia may produce cord compression (Fig. 3) and secondary neurological deficits (Figs. 4, 5) (Bams-Mengerink et al. 2006, Khanna et al. 2001).

## Systemic manifestations

Other, less common manifestations include hydronephrosis, and other renal defects, congenital heart disease, joint contractures, postaxial polydactyly, and conductive deafness (Happle 1981, Milunsky et al. 2003, Silengo et al. 1980).

## Pathology

Ichthyosis and keratotic follicular plugs containing dystrophic calcifications in newborns are distinctive histopathological features of CDPX2 (Hoang et al. 2004). Focal pigmentation of the basal layer and needle-like calcium inclusions in vacuoles may be seen on electron microscopy.

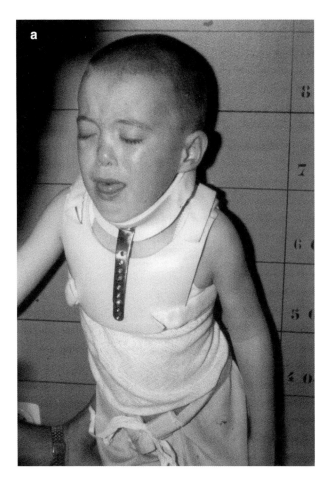
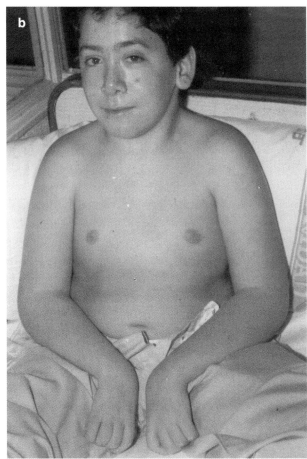

**Fig. 3.** Photographs of a girl (**a**) and a boy (**b**) with typical facial characteristics that are very similar in both patients – who are not relatives – and who also have severe cervical spinal stenosis.

## Molecular genetics

CDPX2 syndrome is caused by the emopamil-binding protein (EBP) gene, located on chromosome Xp11.22-23. The prevalence of CDPX2-associated EBP mutations in exon 2, and the existence of two potential mutational hotspots were first reported by Metzemberg et al. (1999). The cause of DCPX2 was unknown until Derry et al. (1999) found a missense mutation (G107R) in the mouse gene encoding delta-8, delta-7 sterol isomerase emopamil-binding protein/EBP in a CDPX2 model mouse and mutations of the human EBP gene in humans (Braverman et al. 1999, Silve et al. 1996). EBP mutations, other chromosomal alterations, such as deletions, frame-shifts, nonsense or missense mutations, and intronic mutations causing abnormal splicing can be also found (Ikegawa et al. 2000). CDPX2 is presumed to be lethal in males (De Raeve et al. 1989, Happle 2003, Sutphen et al. 1995, Wettke-Schafer and Kantner 1983). Hypomorphic alleles within the EBP gene cause a phenotype quite different from CDPX2, possibly a novel clinical genetic entity (Happle 2003, Ikegawa 2004).

The EBP gene encodes the *3β-hydroxysteroid-Δ8, Δ7-isomerase enzyme* that catalyses an intermediate step in the conversion of lanosterol to cholesterol. As a result of this defect, affected patients have elevated tissue and blood levels of the

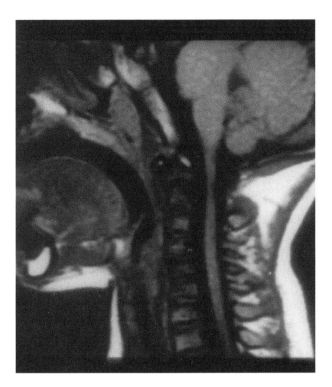

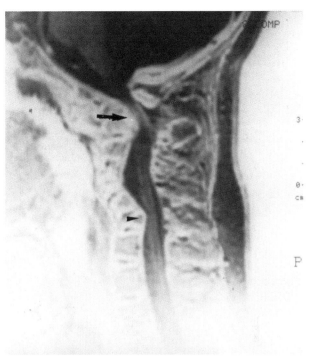

**Fig. 4.** MR sagittal view of the posterior fossa and the upper cervical region of the same girl as in Fig. 3a shows stenosis of the upper part of the spinal canal and thinning of the spinal cord.

**Fig. 5.** MR In $T_2$-weighted sagittal view of the upper cervical region of the same boy shown in Fig. 3b demonstrating severe stenosis of the spinal canal at different levels with compression of the spinal cord at $C_1$ (arrow) and narrowing of the anterior arachnoid space at $C_6$ (arrowhead).

cholesterol intermediates 8(9)-cholesterol, and 8-dehydrocholesterol.

## Pathogenesis

Cholesterol is an essential constituent of cell membranes, and it is also an intermediate in steroid hormone biosynthesis. Dietary cholesterol may be sufficient for most of these functions, supplying the sterol to tissues in the form of circulating LDL cholesterol (Williams et al. 2006). However, tissues such as suprabasal epidermis, which lack LDL receptors are likely to be vulnerable to mutations that impair sterol biosynthesis (Ponec et al. 1983, Williams et al. 1987), and this may partly account for the organs primarily affected in CHH and CHILD syndromes (Williams et al. 2006). In a similar way cataract formation has been associated with hyocholesterolemia while skeletal defects are more difficult to explain.

Alternatively, some or all the manifestations of CHH and CHILD syndromes may reflect the role of sterols in regulating gene transcription both through their participation in the formation of active hedgehog proteins and through the activation of nuclear hormone receptor, LXR, by its oxygenated sterol precursors or metabolites. Target genes of the hedgehog signalling pathway regulate some aspects of morphogenesis such as Wnt gene family and bone morphogenic proteins (Cohen et al. 2003). In addition, activation of LXR by oxygenated metabolites of cholesterol regulates cellular lipogenesis and epidermal differentiation and skin permeability barrier maturation.

A third pathologic mechanism is the atrophic residua left after resolution of the scaling disorder in CHH which is likely explained by reduced viability of the keratinocyte populations in which the mutant X chromosome is active (Williams et al. 2006). In the same way, skewed patterns of X-inactivation may account for much of the observed intra- and interfamilial variability.

## Similarities and overlaps with CHILD syndrome

CHH is closely related to another X-linked dominant disorder known as *CHILD syndrome* (congenital hemidysplasia with ichthyosiform erythroderma and limb defects), which is caused by mutations in the NSDHL gene, encoding for an enzymatic protein crucial in a step of the cholesterol synthesis just proximal to the $\Delta 8$, $\Delta 7$ sterol isomerase step associated to CHH (Wilson et al. 2006). CHILD syndrome (discussed more fully in chapter 37) is also characterised by cutaneous and skeletal abnormalities: however a striking unilateral distribution of skin lesions with a sharp midline demarcation is seen in CHILD syndrome with the skin changes usually persisting throughout life, in contrast to the transient ichthyosiform erythroderma of CHH. Partial (or even total) resolution of the dermatosis can occur in CHILD syndrome as well (Happle 1990). Alopecia and nail abnormalities are commonly seen in CHILD syndrome. Epiphyseal stippling may be noted during infancy in both CHH and CHILD syndromes. Limb reduction defects (at times resulting in the absence of a limb) occur on the same side as the skin abnormalities in CHILD syndrome, and the associated skeletal abnormalities are usually more severe in CHILD syndrome (Williams et al. 2006). Cardiac, renal and nervous system malformations can also be seen in both syndromes, although they are always distributed ipsilaterally in CHILD syndrome. Happle (1995) has also suggested that the CHILD syndrome should be considered a "naevus" rather than an "ichthyosis", because the skin lesions resemble an inflammatory linear epidermal nevus clinically. Thus, given the clinical similarities between the two disorders, as well as their causation by mutations affecting sequential steps in the same enzymatic pathway, and also in view of reports of patients with typical features of CHILD syndrome harbouring mutations in the EBP gene rather than in the NSDLH gene (Grange et al. 2000) some authors (Williams et al. 2006) have proposed that there should be no distinction between the two syndromes and both conditions may be considered "*disorders of cornification*" (DOC) (Williams et al. 2006).

## Diagnosis

The diagnosis is usually made following sterol analysis revealing elevations of 8(9)-cholesterol and 8-dehydrocholesterol (Kelley et al. 1999, Kolb-Mäurer et al. 2008). Ikegawa et al. (2000) reported that mutations resulting in a truncated EBP protein gene result in typical CDPX2, an incompatible form with survival of males, while missense mutations result in atypical phenotypes. The occurrence of CDPX2 in boys with a normal gonosome constitution XY is uncommon but compatible with a concept of X-linked dominant transmission with lethality for male embryos (Happle 1985). By contrast, XXY males (Sutphen et al. 1995) can be explained either by a postzygotic mutation or by a gametic half-chromatid mutation (Happle 1995).

## Differential diagnosis

CDPX-linked recessive type (brachytelencephalangic) or CDPX1 Sheffield type of CDP (OMIM # 392940 or 302950) is also known as CDPX1. The main clinical manifestations of CDPX1, namely the mild or Sheffield type, symmetrical and brachytelencephalangic CDP, are facial anomalies (Fig. 3) similar to those found in Binder maxillo-facial dysostosis and hypoplasia of the distal phalanges of the fingers. Growth and mental development are normal or mildly affected and the prognosis is good (Sheffield et al. 1976). It may be difficult to recognize in adulthood the characteristic punctate epiphyseal changes that are resolved in the first 2 years of life. Franco et al. (1995) demonstrated that mutations in the arylsulfatase E gene, mapped to Xp22.3, cause a subset of CDPX1, although genetic heterogeneity was suggested. Cervical spinal stenosis with chronic myelopathy (Figs. 4 and 5) that started during the first years of life has been reported (Pascual-Castroviejo et al. 2004). Surgical decompression may be necessary in these cases, preferably if it is performed at an early age.

# References

Bams-Mengerink AM, Majoie CBLM, Duran M, Wanders RJA, Van Hove J, Scheurer CD, Barth PG, Poll-The BT (2006) MRI of the brain and cervical spinal cord in rhizomelic chondrodysplasia punctata. Neurology 66: 798–803.

Basbug M, Serin IS, Ozcelik B, Gunes T, Akcakus M, Tayyar M (2005) Prenatal ultrasonographic diagnosis of rhizomelic chondrodysplasia punctata by detection of rhizomelic shortening and bilateral cataracts. Fetal Diagn Ther 20: 171–174.

Braverman N, Steel G, Obie C, Moser A, Moser H, Gould SJ, Valle D (1997) Human PEX7 encodes the peroxisomal PTS2 receptor and is responsible for rhizomelic chondrodysplasia punctata. Nat Genet 15: 369–376.

Braverman N, Lin P, Moebius FF, Obie C, Moser A, Glossmann H, Wilcox WR, Rimoin DL, Smith M, Kratz L, Kelley RI, Valle D (1999) Mutations in the gene encoding 3 beta-hydroxysteroid-delta8, delta 7-isomerase cause X-linked dominant Conradi–Hünermann syndrome. Nat Genet 22: 291–294.

Brookhyser KM, Lipson MH, Moser AB, Moser HW, Lachman RS, Rimoin DL (1999) Prenatal diagnosis of rhizomelic chondrodysplasia punctata due to isolated alkyldihydroacetonephosphate acyltransferase synthase deficiency. Prenat Diagn 19: 383–385.

Cohen MM Jr (2003) Craniofacial anomalies: Clinical and molecular perspectives. Ann Acad Med Singapore 32: 244–251.

Conradi E (1914) Vorzeitiges Auftreten von Knocken und eigenartigen Verkalgunskernen bei chondrodystrophia featalis hypoplastica: histologische und Roentgenuntersuchungen. J Kinderheilk 80: 86–97.

Daniele A, Parenti G, d'Addio M, Andria G, Ballabio A, Meroni G (1998) Biochemical characterization of arylsulfatase E and functional analysis of mutations found in patients with X-linked chondrodysplasia punctata. Am J Hum Genet 62: 562–572.

De Raeve L, Song M, De Dobbeleer G, Spehl M, Van Regemorter N (1989) Lethal course of X-linked dominant chondrodysplasia punctata in a male newborn. Dermatologica 178: 167–170.

Derry JM, Gormally E, Means GD, Zhao W, Meindl A, Kelley RI, Boyd Y, Herman GE (1999) Mutations in a delta 8-delta 7 sterol isomerase in the tattered mouse and

X-linked dominant chondrodysplasia punctata. Nat Genet 22: 286–290.

Duff P, Harlass FE, Milligan DA (1990) Prenatal diagnosis of chondrodysplasia punctata by sonography. Obstet Gynecol 76: 497–500.

Franco B, Meroni G, Parenti G, Levilliers J, Bernard L, Gebbia M, Cox L, Maroteaux P, Sheffield L, Rappold GA, et al. (1995) A cluster of sulfatase genes on Xp22.3: mutations in chondrodysplasia punctata (CDPX) and implications for warfarin embryopathy. Cell 81: 15–25.

Grange DK, Kratz LE, Braverman NE, Kelley RI (2000) CHILD syndrome caused by deficiency of 3beta-hydroxysterol delta8, delta7 isomerase. Am J Med Genet 90: 336–338.

Gray RGF, Green A, Schutgens RBH, Wanders RJA, Farndon PA, Kennedy CR (1990) Antenatal diagnosis of rhizomelic chondrodysplasia punctata in the second trimester. J Inherit Metab Dis 13: 380–382.

Hall CM (2002) International nosology and classification of constitutional disorders of bone (2001). Am J Med Genet 113: 65–77.

Happle R (1979) X-linked dominant chondrodysplasia punctata. Hum Genet 53: 65–73.

Happle R (1981) Cataracts as a marker of genetic heterogeneity in chondrodysplasia punctata. Clin Genet 19: 64–66.

Happle R (1985) Lyonization and the lines of Blaschko. Hum Genet 70: 200–206.

Happle R (1990) Psychotropism as a cutaneous feature of the CHILD syndrome. J Am Acad Dermatol 23: 763–766.

Happle R (1995) X-linked dominant chondrodysplasia punctata/ichthyosis/cataract syndrome in males. Am J Med Genet 57: 493.

Happle R (2003) Hypomorphic alleles within the EBP gene cause a phenotype quite different from Conradi–Hünermann–Happle syndrome. Am J Med Genet 122A: 279.

Happle R, Matthias HH, Macher E (1977) Sex-linked chondrodysplasia punctata? Clin Genet 11: 73–76.

Happle R, Mittag H, Kuster W (1995) The CHILD nevus: a distinct skin disorder. Dermatology 191: 210–216.

Hertzberg BS, Kliewer MA, Decker M, Miller CR, Bowie JD (1999) Antenatal ultrasonographic diagnosis of rhizomelic chondrodysplasia punctata. J Ultrasound Med 18: 715–718.

Heymans HAS, Oorthuys JWE, Nelck G, Wanders RJA, Schutgens RBH (1985) Rhizomelic chondrodysplasia punctata: another peroxisomal disorder. N Engl J Med 313: 187–188.

Hoang MP, Carder KR, Pandya AG, Bennett MJ (2004) Ichthyosis and keratotic follicular plugs containing dystrophic calcification in newborns: distinctive histopathologic features of X-linked dominant chondrodysplasia punctata (Conradi–Hünermann–Happle syndrome). Am J Dermatopathol 26: 53–58.

Hünermann C (1931) Chondrodystrophia calcificans congenital als abortive Form der Chondrodystrophia. Z Kinderheilk 51: 1–19.

Ikegawa S (2004) Hypomorphic alleles within the EBP gene cause a phenotype quite different from Conradi–Hünermann–Happle syndrome. Am J Med Genet 130: 106.

Ikegawa S, Ohashi H, Ogata T, Honda A, Tsukahara M, Kubo T, Kimizuka M, Shimode M, Hasegawa T, Nishimura G, Nakamura Y (2000) Novel and recurrent EBP mutations in X-linked dominant chondrodysplasia punctata. Am J Med Genet 94: 300–305.

Kalter DC, Atherton DJ, Clayton PT (1989) X-linked dominant Conradi-Hunermann syndrome presenting as congenital erythroderma. J Am Acad Dermatol 21: 248–256.

Kelley RI, Wilcox WG, Smith M, Kratz LE, Moser A, Rimoin DS (1999) Abnormal sterol metabolism in patients with Conradi–Hünerman–Happle syndrome and sporadic lethal chondrodysplasia punctata. Am J Med Genet 83: 213–219.

Khanna AJ, Braverman NE, Valle D, Sponseller PD (2001) Cervical stenosis secondary to rhizomelic chondrodysplasia punctata. Am J Med Genet 99: 63–66.

Kolb-Mäurer A, Grzeschik KH, Haas D, Bröcker EB, Hamm H (2008) Conradi-Hünermann-Happle syndrome (X-linked dominant chondrodysplasia punctata) confirmed by plasma sterol and mutation analysis. Acta Derm Venereol 88: 47–51.

Kumada S, Hayashi M, Kenmochi J, Kurosawa S, Shimozawa N, Kratz LE, Kelley RI, Taki K, Okaniwa M (2001) Lethal form of chondrodysplasia punctata with normal plasmalogen and cholesterol biosynthesis. Am J Med Genet 98: 250–255.

Lachman RS (1996) Chondrodysplasia punctata, Conradi–Hünermann type (CP-CH); X-linked dominant (Happle) type. In: Taybi H, Lachman RS (eds.) Radiology of Syndromes, Metabolic Disorders and Skeletal Dysplasias. 4th ed. St. Louis: Mosby, pp. 777–780, 785.

Lachman RS (1998) International nomenclature and classification of the osteochondrodysplasias (1997). Pediatr Radiol 28: 737–744.

Mayden Argo K, Toriello HV, Jelsema RD, Znidema LJ (1996) Prenatal findings in chondrodysplasia punctata, tibia-metacarpal type. Ultrasound Obstet Gynecol 8: 350–354.

Metzemberg AB, Kelley R, Smith D, Kupacz K, Sutphen R, Sheffield L (1999) Mutations in chondrodysplasia punctata, X-linked dominant type (CDPX2). Am J Hum Genet 65: A480.

Milunsky JM, Maher TA, Metzenberg AB (2003) Molecular, biochemical, and phenotypic analysis of a hemizygous male with a severe atypical phenotype for X-linked dominant Conradi–Hünermann–Happle syndrome and mutation in EBP. Am J Med Genet 116A: 249–254.

Motley AM, Brites P, Gerez L, Hogenhout E, Haasjes J, Benne R, Tabak HF, Wanders RJ, Waterham HR (2002) Mutational spectrum in the PEX7 gene and functional analysis of mutant alleles in 78 patients with rhizomelic chondrodysplasia punctata type 1. Am J Hum Genet 70: 612–624.

Ofman R, Hettema EH, Hogenhout E, Caruso U, Muijser AO, Wanders RJ (1998) Acyl-CoA: dihydroxyacetonephosphate acyltransferase: Cloning of the human cDNA and resolution of the molecular basis in rhizomelic chondrodysplasia punctata type 2. Hum Mol Genet 7: 847–853.

Pascual-Castroviejo I, Pascual-Pascual SI, Garcia-Peñas JJ, Hernández-Moneo JL (2004) Compresión de la médula cervical en la condrodisplasia punctata: Presentación de dos casos. Rev Neurol 39: 826–829.

Ponec M, Havekes L, Kempenaar J, Vermeer BJ (1983) Cultured human skin fibroblasts and keratinocytes differences in the regulation of cholesterol synthesis. J Invest Dermatol 81: 125–130.

Powers JM, Kenjarski TP, Moser AB, Moser HW (1999) Cerebellar atrophy in chronic rhizomelic chondrodysplasia punctata: a potential role for phytanic acid and calcium in the death of its Purkinje cells. Acta Neuropathol 98: 129–134.

Purdue PE, Zhang JW, Skoneczny M, Lazarow PB (1997) Rhizhomelic chondrodysplasia punctata is caused by deficiency of human PEX7, a homologue of the yeast PTS2 receptor. Nat Genet 15: 381–384.

Savarirayan R, Boyle RJ, Masel J, Rogers JG, Sheffield LJ (2004) Longterm follow-up in chondrodysplasia punctata, tibia-metacarpal type, demonstrating natural history. Am J Med Genet 124A: 148–157.

Sheffield LJ (2001) Comment on Traupe's tribute to Rudolf Happle. Am J Med Genet 101: 283.

Sheffield LJ, Danks DM, Mayne V, Hutchinson LA (1976) Chondrodysplasia punctata-23 cases of a mild and relatively common variety. J Pediatr 89: 916–923.

Sigirci A, Alkam A, Kutlu R, Gülcan H (2005) Multivoxel magnetic resonance spectroscopy in a rhizomelic chondrodysplasia punctata case. J Child Neurol 20: 698–701.

Silengo MC, Luzzatti L, Silverman FN (1980) Clinical and genetic aspects of Conradi–Hünermann disease. Pediatrics 97: 911–917.

Silve S, Dupuy PH, Labit-Lebouteiller C, Kaghad M, Chalon P, Rahier A, Taton M, Lupker J, Shire D,

Loison G (1996) Emopamil-binding protein, a mammalian protein that binds a series of structurally diverse neuroprotective agents, exhibits delta 8 -delta 7 sterol isomerase activity in yeast. J Biol Chem 271: 2234–2240.

Spranger JW, Opitz JM, Bidder U (1971) Heterogeneity of chondrodysplasia punctata. Humangenetik 11: 190–212.

Spranger JW, Brill PW, Poznaski AK (2002) Chondrodysplasia punctata syndromes and other conditions with fragmented prenatal ossification. In: Spranger JW, Brill PW, Poznaski AK (eds.) Bone dysplasia. An atlas of genetic disorders of skeletal development. 2nd edn. München: Urban & Fisher, pp. 57–79.

Stoll C, Dott B, Roth M, Alembik Y (1989) Birth prevalence rates of skeletal dysplasias. Clin Genet 35: 88–92.

Sutphen R, Amar MJ, Kousseff BG, Toomey KE (1995) XXY male with X-linked dominant chondrodysplasia punctata (Happle syndrome). Am J Med Genet 57: 489–492.

Sztriba L, Al-Gazali LI, Wanders RJA, Ofman R, Nork M, Lestringant GG (2000) Abnormal myelin formation in rhizomelic chondrodysplasia punctata type 2 (DHAPAT deficiency). Dev Med Child Neurol 42: 492–495.

Wanders RJ (2004) Metabolic and molecular basis of peroxisomal disorders: a review. Am J Med Genet A 126: 355–375.

Wettke-Schafer R, Kantner G (1983) X-linked dominant inherited diseases with lethality in hemizygous males. Human Genet 64: 1–23.

White AL, Modaff P, Holland-Morris F, Pauli RM (2003) Natural history of rhizomelic chondrodysplasia punctata. Am J Med Genet 118A: 332–342.

Williams DW III, Elster AD, Cox TD (1991) Cranial MR imaging in rhizomelic chondrodysplasia punctata. Am J Neuroradiol 12: 363–365.

Williams ML, Mommaas-Kienhuis AM, Rutherford SL, Grayson S, Vermeer BJ, Elias PM (1987) Free sterol metabolism and low density lipoprotein receptor expression as differentiation markers of cultured human keratinocytes. J Cell Physiol 132: 428–440.

Williams ML, Bruckner AL, Nopper AJ (2006) Generalized disorders of cornification (the Ichthyoses). In: Harper J, Oranje A, Prose N (eds.) Textbook of Pediatric Dermatology. 2nd edn. Oxford: Blackwell Science, pp. 1304–1358.

Zizka J, Charvat J, Baxova A, Balicek P, Kozlowski K (1998) Brachytelephangic chondrodysplasia punctata with distinctive phenotype and normal karyotype. Am J Med Genet 76: 213–216.

# Chapter 39

# SJÖGREN–LARSSON SYNDROME

Martino Ruggieri and Ignacio Pascual-Castroviejo

Institute of Neurological Science, National Research Council, Catania and Department of Paediatrics, University of Catania, Catania, Italy (MR); Paediatric Neurology Service, Hospital La Paz, University of Madrid, Madrid, Spain (IPC)

## Introduction

Sjögren–Larsson syndrome (SLS) is a metabolic disorder with neurocutaneous features inherited as an autosomal recessive trait (OMIM # 270200) characterized by a clinical triad of congenital ichthyosis, gradually developing spastic di- or tetraplegia and mental retardation (Gordon 2007; Rizzo 2006, 2007).

SLS patients have impaired oxidation of long-chain aliphatic alcohols to corresponding fatty acids caused by deficient activity of the microsomal enzyme, fatty aldehyde dehydrogenase (FALDH) (OMIM # 609523) (Rizzo 2007, Rizzo et al. 1988, Rizzo and Craft 1991) whose gene (ALDH3A2) has been mapped to chromosome 17p11.2 (Pigg et al. 1994, Rizzo and Carney 2005).

Recently, beneficial effects of the leukotriene $B_4$ ($LTB_4$) have been described (Rizzo 2006, 2007; Zalewska 2006; Willemse et al. 2000).

## Historical perspective and eponyms

SLS was first described by Sjögren in 1956 and by Sjögren and Larsson (1957) in 28 Swedish patients nearly completely ascertained from highly consanguineous families in a remote area of Sweden (Chaves-Carballo 1987). Although earlier descriptions (Pardo-Castelló and Faz 1932, Pisani and Cacchione 1935, Laubenthal 1938, Bredmose 1940, Soderhjelm 1957) of the syndrome have been found, the Swedish cohort (Sjögren and Larsson 1957) remains the largest and most completely studied group (Chaves-Carballo 1987). As suggested by Sjögren (1956) and Sjögren and Larsson (1957) in Sweden

likely the mutation was introduced in around the 13th century (Zalewska 2006).

**Karl Gustaf Torsten Sjögren** was a Swedish physician, psychiatrist and inheritance researcher, born on January 30, 1896 in Södertälje and died on July 27, 1974. After graduating from the Gymnasium in Stockholm in 1914, Sjögren studied medicine at the University of Uppsala. He graduated from that university in 1918, and in 1925 became a licentiate of medicine in Stockholm. He was conferred doctor of medicine at the University of Lund in 1931. During the years 1922–1927 he held positions in neurology, psychiatry and medicine in Stockholm. He was assistant in the State Institute of Race Biology in Uppsala 1926–1927. From 1929 he had an appointment at the university clinic in Lund, where he trained in psychiatry, and in 1931 became head physician in 1931. From 1932 to 1935 he was head physician and hospital director at the Lillehagen hospital in Gothenburg, and during years 1935–1945 was physician-in-chief at the psychiatric department of the Sahlgrenska sjukhuset in Gothenburg. Sjögren was instrumental in establishing the psychiatric unit at this hospital. He was called to the chair of psychiatry at the Karolinska Institute in 1945, and from 1946 was a member of the scientific council of Medicinalstyrelsen. In 1951 he was elected member of Vetenskapsakademin – the Academy of Science. He is remembered as one of the pioneers of modern Swedish psychiatry (Who named it? 2006).

**Tage Konrad Leopold Larsson** was a Swedish physician, born 1905 (Who named it? 2006).

In 1988 (Rizzo et al. 1988) SLS was shown to be an inborn error of lipid metabolism caused by deficient activity of fatty alcohol oxidoreductase. Later studies identified a defect in FALDH, a component of the fatty alcohol: NAD oxidoreductase enzyme complex (Rizzo and Craft 1991). The FALDH gene was cloned in 1994 (Pigg et al. 1994) and patients with SLS were found to have mutations in this gene (reviewed by Rizzo 2007, Rizzo and Carney 2005). Enzymatic and genetic testing provided a reliable mean for diagnosing SLS and determining carrier status (Rizzo 2006).

Eponyms for SLS include icthyosis, spastic neurologic disorder and oligophrenia; fatty alcohol: NAD-oxidoreductase deficiency; fatty alcohol dehydrogenase deficiency; and FALDH deficiency.

## Incidence and prevalence

The prevalence of SLS is estimated at 0.4 per 100,000 for the Swedish population (8.3 for the area of Vasterbotten) and the incidence for the period 1901 to 1977 was 0.6 per 100,000 births (10.3 for the area of Vasterbotten) (Iselius and Jagell 1989, Jagell et al. 1981a). It occurs more rarely worldwide (Rizzo 2006, Williams et al. 2006, Zalewska 2006). There is no apparent racial or sexual predilection (Rizzo 2006, Zelewska 2006).

## Clinical manifestations

The main clinical features are cutaneous, manifested as ichthyosis, and neurological with spastic di- or tetraplegia and mental retardation (Jagell and Heijbel 1982, Jagell et al. 1981b, Sjögren and Larsson 1957, van Domburg et al. 1999, Willemsen et al. 2001a).

Dermatological and neurological manifestations appear during the first months of life and increase progressively. In some infants the syndrome is incomplete, and atypical cases in older children are reported. Most patients are born pre-term and a spastic diplegia caused by the prematurity can be suspected during the first months of life when the patient is the first affected case in the family. Willemsen et al. (1999) observed in a series of 15 patients, that all SLS children were born before or at the 38th week of gestation, and mean gestational age was 35.3 weeks (S.D. 2.4 weeks): pre-term birth was found in 73% of the children. Pregnancies were uncomplicated in most children and birth weight

was normal for gestational age in all patients. A possible explanation for pre-term birth in SLS could be the defective inactivation of leukotriene $B_4$ ($LTB_4$) (see also pathogenesis).

## Skin manifestations

The cutaneous features in SLS show a characteristic appearance with prominent generalized hyperkeratosis and remarkable brownish yellow color.

Typically, *newborns* exhibit a combination of hyperkeratosis and scale with variable erythema. This may resemble an exaggerated pattern of neonatal desquamation, and only rarely (15% of cases) is there a colloidon membrane. The first cutaneous symptom, however, is the congenital erythema (con-

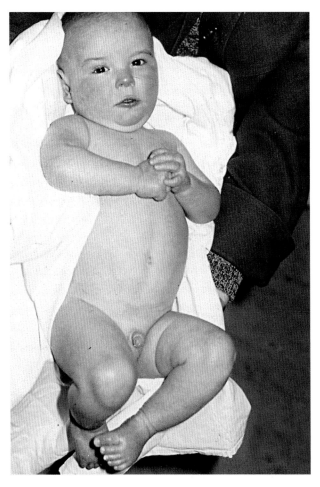

**Fig. 1.** A 4-month-old boy with SJS shows congenital erythema mainly located in the face, hands and feet.

genital nonbullous ichthyosiform eythroderma) (Chaves-Carballo 1987) (Fig. 1), which is usually no longer evident after one year of age. Thereafter the skin gradually becomes thickened and scaly (during the first year of life).

After the neonatal period, *infants* may exhibit a fine, dandruff-like or more prominent, lamellar-like scale, similar to a mild lamellar ichthyosis phenotype.

The cornification disorder is usually fully developed by *1 year of age*. There may be extensive yellow-

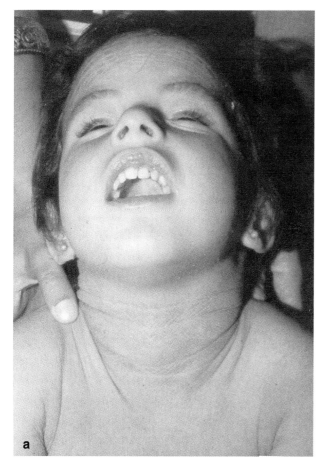

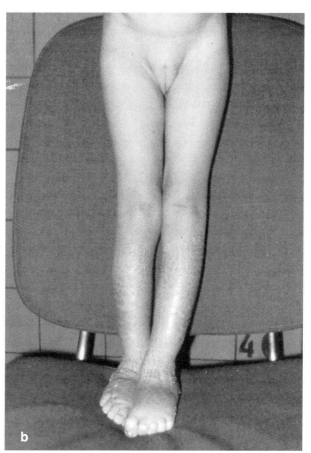

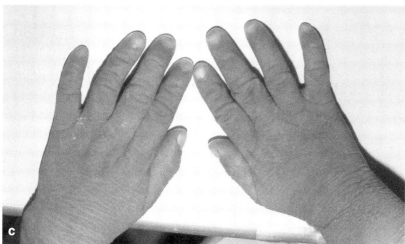

Fig. 2. (a) Photograph of the characteristic abnormalities of the skin of the neck and frontal region of a 6-year-old girl. The skin of the neck shows wrinkled hyperkeratosis. The skin of the frontal region shows the typical ichthyosis. (b) Spastic diplegia and ichthyosis in both legs and feet. (c) The hands of a 2-year-old girl with SJS show severe yellowish brown wrinkled hyperkeratosis.

ish hyperkeratosis or lichenification, especially of the major flexures. The hyperkeratosis is usually generalized (Fig. 2), but the abdomen, back, neck, flexures and dorsal surfaces of the hands and feet are often most prominently affected. The central face is spared. A distinctive cutaneous sign is periumbilical hyperkeratosis with yellow discoloration and radiating furrows. All patients with SLS suffer from severe pruritus. The presence of pruritus is strongly suggestive of SLS as usually, pruritus, is not a common finding in other ichthyosis. The pruritus is caused by the accumulation of leukotriene B4 and its omega-hydroxy degradation products (Rizzo 2006, 2007) (see also below pathogenesis). Excoriations due to pruritus are often present in patients with SLS (Rizzo 2006).

Mild hyperkeratosis with desquamation of the palms and soles is usually present (60% of cases), but the hair, nails and sweat glands are generally not affected. Over time the hyperkeratosis and lichenification may increase, and dark brown or gray pigmentation may develop in most of the hyperkeratotic areas, especially on the neck and axillary rim. Skin margins are exaggerated, especially over the major flexures. Scales on the trunk and extremities may become larger and more lamellar (Williams et al. 2006). Severity of the ichthyosis may not be apparent if the patient bathes before examination (as bathing rehydrates the skin). Likewise the ichthyosis may not be evident after the application of moisturizing lotions (Rizzo 2006, Zalewska 2006).

Persistent, aberrant Mongolian spots have been also reported (Inamadar and Palit 2007, Willemsen and Rotteveel 2008).

## Nervous system involvement

Because the dermatological manifestations of SLS in early infancy are non-specific, the diagnosis may not be suspected until the neurological signs are manifest. The neurological manifestations usually become apparent in the first or second year and are characterized by spastic diplegia or paraplegia and mental retardation (Figs. 2b and 3).

The first signs are characterized by development of an abnormal gait, with pyramidal signs, in

the first 2 years of life (usually between 4 and 30 months of age). In infants with SLS hypertonia is the most common neurological finding on physical examination. Variable hypotonia occasionally precedes hypertonia (Rizzo 2006). The legs are more severely affected then the arms in all SLS patients with gradual worsening. Some patients can walk a short distance, but almost all require a wheelchair in everyday life. As expected, deep tendon reflexes are

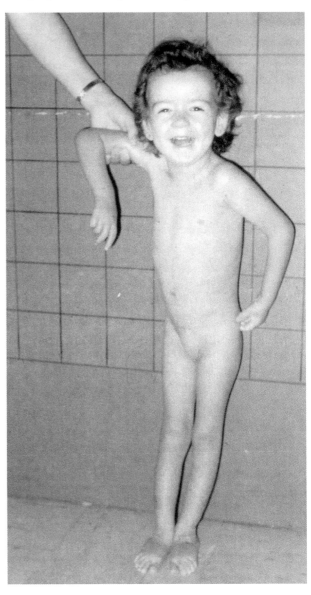

**Fig. 3.** A 4-year-old girl with SLS shows spastic diplegia, ichthyosis in both legs and feet, skin of axilary region with wrinkled hyperkeratosis and friendly attitude.

exaggerated, clonus is easily elicited, and plantar responses (Babinski) are extensor. In a recent study Verhoog et al. (2008) recorded limitations in gross motor performance (except for lying and rolling) in a cohort of 17 SLS patients (aged 1 to 35 years). In most of these patients spasticity was present (bilaterally) in hamstrings, hip adductors, and gastronomic muscles. All patients above 4 years had contractures in lower extremities (Verhoog et al. 2008).

Language is retarded and none of the severely affected children can speak with more than short sentences consisting of stammered, single, often incomprehensible syllables, showing pseudobulbar dysarthria. Most patients are able to answer just simple questions but only seldom speak on their own accord (Chaves-Carballo 1987).

Cognitive defects are seen in almost all patients. The mental retardation can be qualified as mild to moderate because the patients' mood is good however IQ scores are below 50 in the majority of cases, between 50 and 60 in about one third and only rarely are scores above 70. Mental performance is characterized by a marked slowness. SLS is not neurodegenerative. Developmental skills, once gained, are usually maintained over time. Phenotypic variability among siblings has been however recorded (Lossos et al. 2006). After puberty the neurological alterations usually remain stable. However, if contractures ensue patients may soon loose the ability to ambulate.

Epileptic seizures can occur in 30–40% of cases.

## Eye abnormalities

The ocular abnormalities in SLS have been studied by Willemsen et al. (2000a). Photophobia, macular dystrophy and decreased visual acuity are the most prominent features. The presence of distinctive crystals in the macular area of the retina is a cardinal (pathognomonic) sign of SLS: essentially all patients develop juvenile macular dystrophy of the retina, manifesting as "glistening white dots" which often impair the central vision (Aslam and Sheth 2007). Glistening dots usually become apparent after 1–2 years of age and increase in number thereafter. Ophthalmologic and fundus photography show that the crystals are located in the innermost layers of the retina (Fuijkschot et al. 2008, Willemsen et al. 2005). Additional ocular findings include corneal dystrophy, amblyopia, macular degeneration, keratitis, blepharitis and cataracts (Jagell et al. 1980, Willemsen et al. 2000a).

Photophobia causes squinting in bright sunlight. Patients with decreased vision acuity may require corrective lenses (Aslam and Sheth 2007, Rizzo 2006).

## Other features

Short stature is common owing to a combination of growth delay and leg contractures (Gordon 2007, Rizzo 2006). Other secondary features described in some patients, besides small stature, include kyphosis and dental enamel hypoplasia (Forsberg et al. 1983).

## Neurophysiologic investigation

The EEG findings are abnormal but non specific, usually showing generalized epileptiform activity. EEG showed a slow background activity, without other abnormalities in a study of 19 children, adolescents and adult patients (Willemsen et al. 2001a). No peripheral and spinal sensory conduction disorders or motor conduction velocity abnormalities are commonly observed: in some patients however values outside the reference ranges can be recorded (Gordon 2007, Rizzo 2006).

## Imaging studies

CT studies reveal diffuse or patchy cerebral white matter hypodensities, most marked in the frontal areas. No enhancement is present after contrast administration (van der Knaap and Valk 2005).

MRI and $^1$MR spectroscopy ($^1$H-MRS) studies have shown to be almost pathognomonic of SLS (Mano et al. 1999; Miyanomae et al. 1995; van Somburg et al. 1999; Willemsen et al. 2000, 2001a, 2004; Pirgon et al. 2006). MRI shows widespread periventricular low signal on $T_1$-weighted images and high signal areas on $T_2$-weighting, most prominent around the trigones, mild ventricular enlargement, diffuse brain atrophy and a mildly hypoplastic corpus cal-

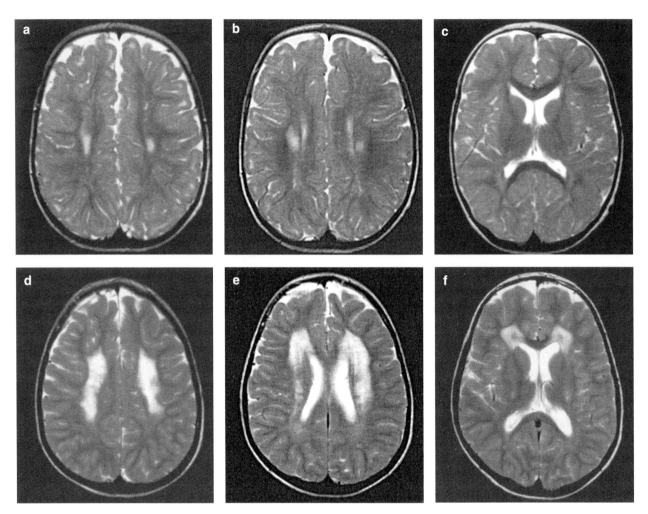

**Fig. 4.** Axial T2-weighted images of the brain in a 2-year-old boy (**a–c**) and a 8 year-old boy (**d–f**) with SLS. At younger ages there is evidence of: (**a–c**) high signal in the directly subcortical white matter in all areas; and (**b, c**) focal signal abnormalities in the periventricular white matter (note that the myelination is incomplete in **a–c**). At older ages the myelination is still incomplete (**d–f**) and there are prominent signal abnormalities (with a sharp delimitation) in the periventricular and deep white matter, most pronounced in the frontoparietal regions (**d–f**). The corpus callosum is largely spared (**f**) (reprinted with permission from van der Knaap and Valk 2005; the original figures were courtesy of Prof. M.A.A.P. Willemsen, Department of Paediatric Neurology, University Medical Centre, Nijmegen, The Netherlands).

losum along with an arrest of myelination or dysmyelination secondary to accumulation of free lipids in the periventricular white matter. Broadly speaking, MRI studies show three types of white matter abnormalities (van der Knaap and Valk 2005, Willemsen et al. 2004) (Fig. 4): (1) mild delay of the process of myelination which appear not to reach completion in SLS patients; (2) in some patients, symmetrical periventricular rims of markedly increased signal intensity, most often in the frontal and parietal lobes; and (3) in other patients, symmetrical periventricular rims of slightly to mildly increased signal intensity predominantly in the poste-

rior areas. All these changes become apparent during the process of myelination and seem to be stable. Their severity among individuals varies.

Cerebral $^1$H-MRS of these lesions reveals high lipid peak in the "lipid region" (between 0.8 and 1.6 ppm) and low B-acetyl aspartate peaks. Metabolic maps derived from $^1$H-MRS data revealed a spatial distribution of the peaks' maximum height around the anterior and posterior regions (Willemsen et al. 2004). A clear relationship between the degree of the MRI abnormality and the neurological features could not be demonstrated (Willemsen et al. 2001a, 2004).

## Molecular genetics and pathogenesis

SLS is an autosomal recessive inherited disorder caused by deficient activity of microsomal fatty aldehyde (FALDH). This enzyme catalyses the oxidation of different long and medium-chain fatty aldehyde, whether or not derived from fatty alcohols, to the corresponding carboxylic acids (Rizzo 2007, Rizzo and Carney 2005, Willensen et al. 2000). It has been suggested that FALDH deficiency may lead to an accumulation of fatty alcohols or aldehyde-modified macromolecules with structural consequences for cell-membrane integrity, and elevated concentrations of biologically highly active lipids (Rizzo and Craft 1991).

The first clue to the cause of SLS was the discovery by Rizzo et al. (1988) of impaired ability of SLS cultured fibroblasts to oxidize alcohols to fatty acids. Subsequently, they determined that this was attributable to deficiency of the FALDH component of the fatty-alcohol-nicotinamide-adenine dinucleotide reductase (FO) enzyme complex which consists of two separate proteins that sequentially catalyze the oxidation of fatty alcohol to fatty aldehyde and then to fatty acid (Rizzo et al. 1989, 1991). Rizzo's group (Pigg et al. 1994) subsequently mapped FALDH gene to chromosome 17p11.2. The gene consists of 10 exons and nine introns, and spans ~31 kb. The cDNA for FALDH encodes a protein of 485 amino acids. Genomic organization and tissue-dependent expression have subsequently been elucidated (Chang and Yoshida 1997, Rogers et al. 1997). Mutation analysis has identified many different mutations in the FALDH gene in SLS patients (De Laurenzi et al. 1996, Rizzo et al. 1999, Sillén et al. 1997, Tsukamoto et al. 1997). The disease does not affect genetic carriers for SLS (Rizzo 2006, Rizzo and Carney 2005).

The pathogenesis of the cornification disorder has been recently clarified (reviewed in Rizzo 2006, 2007; Williams et al. 2006). Overall, tissue dysfunction is thought to be due to lipid storage in membranes (Rizzo 2006). In cultured skin keratinocytes, elevated fatty alcohol is diverted into the synthesis of wax ester lipids. Accumulation of fatty alcohol and wax esters in the intercellular membrane lamella in the stratum corneum may cause disruption of the epidermal water barrier, which critically depends on the lipid composition and which causes the skin to dry out, resulting in ichthyosis (Gordon 2007; Rizzo 2006, 2007; Williams et al. 2006).

Fatty alcohol may likewise alter the normal integrity of myelin membranes in the brain, leading to white matter disease and spasticity (van der Knaap and Vlak 2005, Rizzo 2006). In addition, fatty aldehydes which are reactive molecules, can form covalent Schiff-base derivatives with phospatidylethanolamine, which may influence membrane properties and alter the function of membrane-bound proteins or membrane enzymes (Rizzo 2006).

Other additional pathogenic compounds, which can contribute to the skin and neurological diseases in SLS, are the polyunsaturated fatty acids whose levels in the plasma are low in SLS patients (Rizzo 2006).

Recently, defective metabolism of leukotriene B4 (LTB4) has been reported in SLS patients (Willemsen et al. 2001b) and has been postulated to play a role in the pathogenesis (Williams et al. 2006).

## Pathology

The histological findings in the skin of SLS patients are non specific and include acanthosis, papillomatosis, hyperkeratosis, and thickening of the granular layer. Electron microscopy can reveal abnormal lamellar inclusions in the cytoplasm of the spinous and granular layers with increased numbers of mitochondria in the basal cell layer: these changes however are not diagnostic (Williams et al. 2006).

Only a few reports on postmortem findings in SLS are available with disparate results (Barr and Galindo 1965, Sylvester 1969, Mc Lennan et al. 1974, Silva et al. 1980, Yamaguchi and Handa 1998). The main findings in all patients were (reviewed in Chaves-Carballo 1987, Willemsen et al. 2004): (a) asymmetrical atrophy of the caudate and status marmoratus of the right corpus striatum (Barr and Galindo 1965); (b) neuronal loss in the caudate, lentiform nuclei and hypothalamus as well as patchy or diffuse disseminated loss of myelin in the frontal lobes along with marked gliosis of central gray matter and cortical-subcortical boundaries; (c) loss of myelin in myelinated tracts of the spinal cord being (to a lesser degree); (d) inconsistent loss of gray matter, including basal ganglia with a tendency toward accumulation of astrocytes, lipoid substances and lipofuscin-like pigments (Yamaguchi and Handa 1998).

Maia (1974) found destruction of axons and vacuolization and fragmentation of myelin sheaths with partial tumefaction of axons (sausage appearance) in peripheral nerves (i.e., sural nerves). Sylvester (1969), McLennon et al. (1974) and Silva et al. 1980) described variability in severity of lesions but not in type and distribution of lesions (Chaves-Carballo 1987).

Pathological examination of eye (McLennan et al. 1974) revealed reduction in the number of ganglion cells in the posterior segment, particularly in the section passing through the perimaculari area with reduced number of axons in the retina and optic nerve, no visible myelin in the optic nerve and no evidence of pigmentary lesion in the macula.

## Diagnosis

Although the phenotype in most SLS children is unmistakable, diagnosis is challenging in some atypical cases and in infants under 1 year of age when the full spectrum of signs and symptoms is not present (Williams et al. 2006). The clinical suspect of the diagnosis should be confirmed by genetic or biochemical testing (Rizzo 2006, 2007). Demonstrating accumulation of FALDH substrates such as plasma free fatty alcohols, or elevated urinary LTB4 and 20-OH-LTB4 one can obtain a presumptive diagnosis. However the most direct and definite measure is to assay FALDH activity in cultured cells (that can be easily done in a variety of cell types) and/or to identify a mutation in the FALDH gene (ALDH3A2). Although SLS homozygotes have FALDH activities less than 10% of normal, asymptomatic heterozygotes have activity levels ~50% of normal.

A histochemical assay of alcohol dehydrogenase activity in the epidermis of routine skin biopsies has been also described (Judge et al. 1990, Lake et al. 1991).

Outside the founder's mutation in Swedish patients, numerous FALDH mutations have been found and therefore extensive mutational analysis is often required to identifying the underlying defect in SLS.

Prenatal diagnosis is possible by assaying FALDH activity in cells obtained by amniocentesis of chorionic villus samples and by identifying known mutations (Gordon 2007; Rizzo 2006, 2007; Rizzo et al. 1994; van der Brink et al. 2005).

A form of ichthyosis of intermediate severity closely resembling the non-scaly hyperkeratosis of the SLS has been reported in a family (originating from the county of Nordland, Norway) in which the two affected sisters and the affected brother lacked di- or quadriplegia and mental retardation (*Sjögren–Larsson-like ichthyosis without CNS or eye involvement*; OMIM # 270220) (Gedde-Dahl et al. 1984).

## Management

Recently, Willemsen et al. (2000a, 2001b) described beneficial effects of the leukotriene $B_4$ ($LTB_4$) synthesis inhibitor zileuton in the treatment of SLS. Zileuton was administered in 600 mg doses three times daily, over 5 weeks in a 9-year-old patient (Willemsen et al. 2000a). Favorable effects were found on pruritus score, general well-being, and background activity of EEG studies. Neuropsychological tests results, cerebral MRI and MRI spectroscopy did not change significantly in five SLS patients after 3 months with zileuton (Willemsen et al. 2001b).

Topical calcipotriol (Fernandez-Vozmediano et al. 2003) and more in general topical moisturizing creams and keratolytic agents are the mainstay of the therapy (Rizzo 2006, Zalewska 2006). Daily water bath help keeping the skin hydrated. Systemic retinoids markedly benefit ichthyosis: however their use in children with SLS may be limited because of their potential adverse effects. Experience in treating the spasticity in SLS with Baclofen is not encouraging and data on Botulinum toxin injections are controversial (Gordon 2007; Rizzo 2006, 2007).

## References

Aslam SA, Sheth HG (2007) Ocular features of Sjögren–Larsson syndrome. Clin Experiment Ophthalmol 35: 98–99.

Baar HS, Galindo J (1965) Pathology of the Sjögren–Larsson syndrome. J Maine Med Assoc 56: 223–226.

Bredmose GV (1940) Et tilfaelde af mongoloid idioti og ichtyosis med neurohistologiske forandringer. Nord Med 5: 440–442.

Chang C, Yoshida A (1997) Human fatty aldehyde dehydrogenase gene (ALDH10): organization and tissue-dependent expression. Genomics 40: 80–85.

Chaves-Carballo E (1987) Sjögren–Larsson syndrome. In: Gomez MR (ed.) Neurocutaneous diseases. A practical approach. Boston: Butterworths, pp. 119–224.

De Laurenzi V, Rogers GR, Hamrock DJ, Marekov LN, Steinert PM, Compton JG, Markova N, Rizzo WB (1996) Sjögren–Larsson syndrome is caused by a common mutation in the fatty aldehyde dehydrogenase gene. Nat Genet 12: 52–57.

De Laurenzi V, Rogers GR, Tarcsa E, Carney G, Marekov L, Bale SJ, Compton JG, Markova, Steinert PM, Rizzo WB (1997) Sjögren–Larsson syndrome is caused by a common mutation in northern European and Swedish patients. J Invest Dermatol 109: 79–83.

Fernandez-Vozmediano JM, Armario-Hita JC, Gonzalez-Cabrerizo A (2003) Sjögren–Larsson syndrome: treatment with topical calcipotriol. Pediatr Dermatol 20: 179–180.

Forsberg H, Jagell S, Reuterving CO (1983) Oral conditions in Sjögren–Larsson syndrome. Swed Dent J 7: 141–151.

Fuijkschot J, Cruysberg JR, Willemsen MA, Keunen JE, Theelen T (2008) Subclinical changes in the juvenile crystalline macular dystrophy in Sjögren-Larsson syndrome detected by optical coherence tomography. Ophthalmology 115: 870–875.

Gedde-Dahl T Jr, Rajka G, Larsen TE, Jellum E (1984) Autosomal recessive ichthyosis in Norway. II. Sjögren–Larsson-like ichthyosis without CNS or eye involvement. Clin Genet 25: 242–244.

Gordon (2007) Sjögren–Larsson syndrome. Dev Med Child Neurol 49: 152–154.

Inamadar AC, Palit A (2007) Persistent, aberrant Mongolian spots in Sjögren–Larsson syndrome. Pediatr Dermatol 24(1): 98–99.

Iselius L, Jagell S (1989) Sjögren–Larsson syndrome in Sweden: distribution of the gene. Clin Genet 35(4): 272–275.

Jagell S, Polland W, Sandgren O (1980) Specific changes in the fundus typical for the Sjögren–Larsson syndrome. An ophthalmological study of 35 patients. Acta Ophthalmol (Copenh) 58: 321–330.

Jagell S, Gustavson KH, Holmgren G (1981a) Sjögren–Larsson syndrome in Sweden: a clinical, genetical and epidemiological study. Clin Genet 19: 233–256.

Jagell S, Hallmans G, Gustavson KH (1981b) Zinc and copper concentration in serum of patients with congenital ichthyosis, spastic di- or tetraplegia and mental retardation (Sjögren–Larsson syndrome). Ups J Med Sci 86: 291–295.

Jagell S, Heijbel J (1982) Sjögren–Larsson syndrome: physical and neurological features. A survey of 35 patients. Helv Paediatr Acta 37: 519–530.

Judge MR, Lake BD, Smith VV, Besley GT, Harper JI (1990) Depletion of alcohol (hexanol) dehydrogenase activity in the epidermis and jejunal mucosa in Sjögren–Larsson syndrome. J Invest Dermatol 95: 632–634.

Lake BD, Smith VV, Judge MR, Harper JI, Besley GT (1991) Hexanol dehydrogenase activity shown by enzyme histochemistry on skin biopsies allows differentiation of Sjögren–Larsson syndrome from other ichthyoses. J Inherit Metab Dis 14: 338–340.

Laubenthal F (1938) Uber einige Sonderformen des "angehorenen Schwachsinns". Z Ges Neurol Psychiatr 163: 233–238.

Lossos A, Khoury M, Rizzo WB, Gomori JM, Banin E, Zlotogorski A, Jaber S, Abramsky O, Argov Z, Rosenmann H (2006) Phenotypic variability among adult siblings with Sjögren–Larsson syndrome. Arch Neurol 63: 278–280.

Maia M (1974) Sjögren–Larsson syndrome in two sibs with peripheral nerve involvement and bisalbuminaemia. J Neurol Neurosurg Psychiatr 37: 1306–1315.

Mano R, Ono J, Kaminaga T, Imai K, Sakurai K, Harada K, Nagai T, Rizzo WB, Okada S (1999) Proton MR Spectroscopy of Sjögren–Larsson syndrome. Am J Neuroradiol 20: 1671–1673.

McLennan JE, Gilles FH, Robb RM (1974) Neuropathological correlation in Sjögren–Larsson syndrome. Oligophrenia, ichthyosis, spasticity. Brain 97: 693–703.

Miyanomae Y, Ochi M, Yoshioka H, Takaya K, Kizaki Z, Inoue E, Furuya S, Naruse S (1995) Cerebral MRI and spectroscopy in Sjögren–Larsson syndrome: case report. Neuroradiology 37: 225–228.

Pardo-Castellò V, Faz H (1932) Ichthyosis-Little's disease. Arcj Dermatol Syph (Chicago) 26: 915.

Pigg M, Jagell S, Sillen A, Weissenbach J, Gustavson KH, Wadelius C (1994) Sjögren–Larsson syndrome gene is close to D17S805 as determined by linkage analysis and allelic association. Nat Genet 8: 381–384.

Pirgon O, Aydin K, Atabek ME (2006) Proton magnetic resonance spectroscopy findings and clinical effects of montelukast sodium in a case with Sjögren–Larsson syndrome. J Child Neurol 21: 1092–1095.

Pisani D, Cacchione A (1935) Frenastenia e dermatosi. Riv Sper Freniat 58: 722–736.

Rizzo WB (1999) Sjögren–Larsson syndrome: explaining the skin-brain connection. Neurology 52: 1307–1308.

Rizzo WB (2006) Sjögren–Larsson syndrome. E-medicine from webMD. http://www.emedicine.com/ped/topic2111.httm

Rizzo WB (2007) Sjögren–Larsson syndrome: molecular genetics and biochemical pathogenesis of fatty aldehyde dehydrogenase deficiency. Mol Genet Metab 90: 1–9.

Rizzo WB, Craft DA (1991) Sjögren–Larsson syndrome. Deficit activity of the fatty aldehyde dehydrogenase component of fatty alcohol: NAD+ oxidoreductase in cultured fibroblasts. J Clin Invest 88: 1643–1648.

Rizzo WB, Carney G (2005) Sjögren–Larsson syndrome: diversity of mutations and polymorphisms in the fatty aldehyde dehydrogenase gene (ALDH3A2). Hum Mutat 26: 1–10.

Rizzo WB, Damman AL, Craft DA (1988) Sjögren–Larsson syndrome. Impaired fatty alcohol oxidation in cultured fibroblasts due to deficient fatty alcohol: nicotinamide adenine dinucleotide oxidoreductase activity. J Clin Invest 81: 738–744.

Rizzo WB, Carney G, Lin Z (1999) The molecular basis of Sjögren–Larsson syndrome: mutation analysis of the fatty aldehyde dehydrogenase gene. Am J Hum Genet 65: 1547–1560.

Rogers GR, Markova NG, De Laurenzi V, Rizzo WB, Compton JG (1997) Genomic organization and expression of the human fatty aldehyde hydrogenase gene (FALDH). Genomics 39: 127–135.

Sillén A, Jagell S, Wadelius C (1997) A missense mutation in the FALDH gene identified in Sjögren–Larsson syndrome patients origination from the northern part of Sweden. Hum Genet 100: 201–203.

Silva CA, Saraiva A, Goncales V, de Sousa G, Martins R, Cruz C (1980) Pathologial findings in one of two siblings with Sjögren–Larsson syndrome. Eur Neurol 19: 166–170.

Sjögren T (1956) Oligophrenia combined with congenital ichthyosiform erythrodermia, spastic syndrome and macular-retinal degeneration. A clinical and genetic study. Acta Genet Stat Med 6: 80–91.

Sjögren T, Larsson T (1957) Oligophrenia in combination with congenital ichthyosis and spastic disorders. Acta Psychiatr Neurol Scand 32 (Suppl 113): 1–113.

Sylvester PE (1969) Pathological findings in Sjögren–Larsson syndrome. J Ment Defic Res 13: 267–275.

Tsukamoto N, Chang C, Yoshida A (1997) Mutations associated with Sjögren–Larsson syndrome. Ann Hum Genet 61: 235–242.

van der Brink DM, van Miert JM, Wanders RJ (2005) A novel assay for the prenatal diagnosis of Sjögren–Larsson syndrome. J Inherit Metab Dis 28: 965–969.

Van der Knaap M, Valk J (2005) Magnetic resonance of myelinisation and myelin disorders, 3rd ed. Berlin: Springer Verlag, pp. 383–386.

Van Domburg PH, Willemsen MA, Rotteveel JJ, de Jong JG, Thijssen HO, Heerschap A, Cruysberg JR, Wanders RJ, Gabreels FJ, Steijlen PM (1999) Sjögren–Larson syndrome. Clinical and MRI/MRS findings in FALDH-deficit patients. Neurology 52: 1345–1352.

Verhoog J, Fuijkschot J, Willemsen M, Ketelaar M, Rotteveel J, Gorter JW (2008) Sjögren-Larsson syndrome: motor performance and everyday functioning in 17 patients. Dev Med Child Neurol 50: 38–43.

Willemsen MA, Rottveel JJ, van Domburg PH, Gabreëls FJM, Mayatepek E, Sengers RCA (1999) Preterm birth in Sjögren–Larsson syndrome. Neuropediatrics 30: 325–327.

Willemsen MA, Rotteweel JJ, Steijlen PM, Heerschap A, Mayatepe E (2000a) 5-Lipoxygenase inhibition: a new treatment strategy for Sjögren–Larsson syndrome. Neuropediatrics 31: 1–3.

Willemsen MA, Cruysberg JR, Rotteveel JJ, Aandekerk AL, van Domburg PH, Deutman AF (2000b) Juvenile macular dystrophy associated with deficient activity of fatty aldehyde dehydrogenase in Sjögren–Larsson syndrome. Am J Ophthalmol 130: 782–789.

Willemsen MA, Ijlst L, Steijlen PM, Rotteveel JJ, deJong JGN, van Domburg PH, Mayatepek E, Gabreels FJ, Wanders RJ (2001a) Clinical, biochemical and molecular genetic characteristics of 19 patients with the Sjögren–Larsson syndrome. Brain 124: 1426–1437.

Willemsen MA, Lutt MAJ, Steijlen PM, Cruysberg JRM, van der Graaf M, Nijhuis-van der Sanden MWG, Pasman JW, Mayatepek E, Rotteveel JJ (2001b) Clinical and biochemical effects of Zileuton in patients with the Sjögren–Larsson syndrome. Eur J Pediatr 160: 711–717.

Willemsen MA, Van Der Graaf M, Van Der Knaap MS, Heerschap A, Van Domburg PH, Gabreels FJ, Rotteveel JJ (2004) MR imaging and proton MR spectroscopic studies in Sjögren–Larsson syndrome: characterization of the leukoencephalopathy. Am J Neuroradiol 25: 649–657.

Willemsen MA, Telen T, Fuijckschot J, Rotteveel JJ, Cruysberg JRM (2005) The crystalline retinopathy in Sjögren–Larsson syndrome: new insights by a novel imaging technique. Eur J Paediatr Neurol 9: 272 (Abstract).

Willemsen MA, Rotteveel JJ (2008) Mongolian spots in Sjögren-Larsson syndrome. Pediatr Dermatol 25: 285.

Williams ML, Bruckner AL, Nopper AJ (2006) Generalized disorders of cornification (the Ichthyoses). In: Harper J, Oranje A, Prose N (eds.) Textbook of Pediatric Dermatology, 2nd ed. Oxford: Blackwell Science, pp. 1304–1358.

Yamaguchi K, Handa T (1998) Sjögren–Larsson syndrome: postmortem brain abnormalities. Pediatr Neurol 18: 338–341.

Zalewska A (2006) Sjögren–Larsson syndrome. E-medicine from webMD. http://www.emedicine.com/derm/topic706.httm

# Chapter 40

# KID SYNDROME (KERATITIS-ICHTHYOSIS-DEAFNESS)

Luz Orozco-Covarrubias, Marimar Saez-De-Ocariz, Carola Durán-McKinster, and Ramón Ruiz-Maldonado

Department of Dermatology, National Institute of Paediatrics, Mexico City, Mexico

## Introduction

Keratitis-ichthyosis-deafness (KID) *syndrome* is a genetically determined disorder of keratinization, a congenital ichthyosiform dermatosis with additional extracutaneous features (keratitis and deafness). Because of the association of ichthyosis or ichthyosiform dermatosis with central and/or peripheral nervous system involvement, KID syndrome has been (and is) traditionally defined as a neuroichthyosis or neurocutaneous disorder.

Disorders of keratinization have in common an abnormal differentiation of the epidermis with aberrant formation of the cornificial layer. There has been a long debate between several authors over whether KID syndrome represents an ichthyosis or an erythrokeratoderma, however the acronym prevailed (Caceres-Rios et al. 1996, Traupe 1989a, b).

The familial occurrence of KID syndrome recorded in the literature has suggested: (1) an autosomal dominant mode of inheritance (OMIM # 148210) with vertical transmission in a father and his daughter (Grob et al. 1987) and in a mother and her daughter (Nazarro et al. 1990) and additional families reported by Langer et al. (1990) and Messmer et al. (2005); (2) an autosomal recessive transmission with additional features including hepatic disease (progressive cirrhosis necessitating liver transplantation), growth failure and mental retardation (*Desmons syndrome*) (OMIM # 242150) (Caceres-Rios et al. 1996, Cremers et al. 1977, Desmons et al. 1971, Wilson et al. 1991). In the autosomal dominant form, hepatic disease, growth problems and cognitive deficit are not features, and heterozygous mutations have been identified in the connexin-26 gene (GJB2) located on chromosome 13q11-q12 (Richard et al.

2002, van Geel et al. 2002, van Steensel et al. 2002).

## Historical perspective and eponyms

The association of keratitis, ichthyosis and deafness was described in 1915 by Frederick S. Burns in a 16-year old boy with congenital keratoderma, ocular and mucosal involvement, and deafness (Burns 1915). Between 1915 and 1981 several cases were reported in the literature under different names.

The term KID syndrome, coined by Skinner et al. in 1981, is firmly entrenched in the medical literature. However there have been multiple arguments about the features of the disease calling for a change in terminology. Some of these arguments are: (a) the ichthyosis is an ichthyosis-like hyperkeratosis (Traupe 1989b), an erythrokeratoderma at birth, or hystrix-like ichthyosis (Nousari et al. 2000); (b) the associated deafness is highly variable (van Steensel et al. 2002); and (c) the keratitis can be absent at the time of ophthalmologic examination.

The features of ectodermal dysplasia in KID syndrome are another argument that suggests an overlap between disorders of cornification and ectodermal dysplasias (Caceres-Rios et al. 1996).

## Prevalence and incidence

Kid syndrome is a very rare disorder with world wide distribution: there are about 100 cases reported in the literature. Caceres-Rios et al. (1996) considered in the late 90s that about 15 cases did not correspond to KID syndrome. The male to female proportion is equal.

## Clinical manifestations

The variability of expression in patients with KID syndrome results in a broad clinical spectrum.

### Skin and annexes

Cutaneous manifestations are usually present at birth (Fig. 1) as a transient generalized scaly erythema, or during the first weeks of life as a dry, rough skin. Scaling is diffuse, minimal and transient. The permanent skin changes of the syndrome gradually develop during infancy, usually in the first months of life (Harms et al. 1984, Langer et al. 1990, Ney et al. 1990). The skin becomes thick and has a leathery appearance (Ney et al. 1990). The typical symmetrical, erythrokeratodermic, well demarcated (Fig. 2), non scaling plaques develop later. A verrucous surface has been also described (Grob et al. 1987). Erythrokeratodermic plaques affect predominantly the elbows and knees. Facial involvement with verrucous hyperkeratotic coalescent plaques (Fig. 3) located on the ears, cheeks, forehead, nose, and perioral skin gives patients with Kid syndrome a peculiar facies. Diffuse involvement of the scalp, extremities and trunk may be present. The trunk, if involved, has only slight scaling. Follicular keratoses (spiny hyperkeratosis) over extensor surfaces of the limbs, scalp and nose

have been described (Langer et al. 1990). Some degree of palmo-plantar hyperkeratosis is present in all patients with KID syndrome (Fig. 4). The typical reticulated pattern occurs in almost half of the cases (Caceres-Rios et al. 1996).

Development of hyperplastic nodules on the affected areas increases the incidence of malignancies in adult life, particularly of squamous cell carcinomas, that may be in situ or invasive. Squamous cell carcinomas may develop even in childhood and in mucous areas (tongue), besides skin (Baden et al. 1977, Grob et al. 1987, Hazen et al. 1989, Lancaster et al. 1969, Madariaga et al. 1986, van Steensel et al. 2002).

Scarring alopecia of the scalp, brows, lashes and even the body hair (Fig. 1), affects almost all patients (Caceres-Rios et al. 1996). Follicular hyperkeratosis may also be the cause of alopecia.

Progressive nail dystrophy (Fig. 5) may occur, nails show leukonychia and shedding. Dental abnormalities such as delayed eruption and small teeth are possible features (Caceres-Rios et al. 1996, Grob et al. 1987, Muramoto et al. 1987, Pincus et al. 1975).

### Nervous system manifestations

Congenital sensorineural not progressive deafness is present in all patients. Hearing impairment is gener-

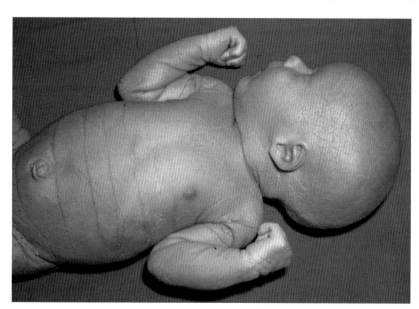

**Fig. 1.** Generalized fine scales, erythema and alopecia. Note the leathery appearance in a 21 days-old boy with KID syndrome.

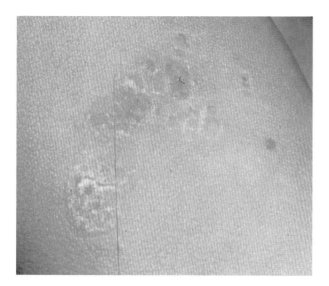

**Fig. 2.** KID syndrome: a well demarcated plaque of erythrokeratoderma.

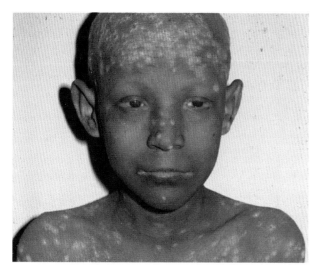

**Fig. 3.** Verrucous hyperkeratotic coalescent plaques in a 10 year-old boy with KID syndrome.

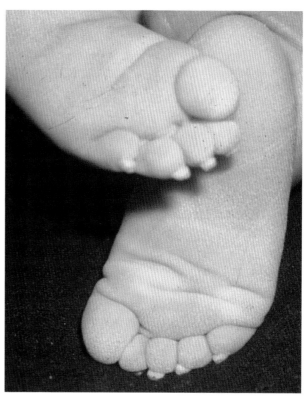

**Fig. 4.** Plantar hyperkeratosis in a 2 year-old girl with KID syndrome.

ally bilateral and severe, but it can be moderate and unilateral. In most patients sensorineural deafness is evident from the first months of life, but may be undetected until the child experiences learning delay (Harms et al. 1984, Langer et al. 1990, Ney et al. 1990, Pincus et al. 1975, Szymko et al. 2002). Todt et al. (2006) reported on the clinical pattern, audiovestibular and neuroimaging findings in 4 patients with identical HID (hystrix-like ichthyosis, deafness)/KID-associated mutation D50N of Connexin 26 (see below). The audiological test results demonstrated profound sensorineural hearing loss in all of the patients. Neurotological testing revealed inconsistent abnormalities in dynamic posturography (sensory organization test), but the vestibular ocular reflex upon caloric irrigation was normal in all patients. Vestibular-evoked myogenic potential testing for otolith function (saccule) showed a regular response in 1 patient and pathologic responses in 3 patients, while subjective haptic vertical (utricular function) testing was normal in all of the patients. CT showed an extended (in length), but very thin (in diameter) bony lining between the basal portion of the internal auditory canal and the vestibule in the 3 scanned patients. They concluded (Todt et al. 2006) that semicircular canals were functionally intact and utricular function was normal in subjects with the autosomal dominant D50N mutation of Connexin 26, in contrast to saccular function which was generally compromised and hearing loss which was profound.

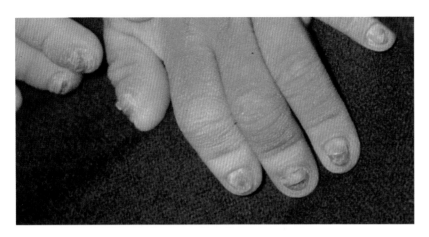

**Fig. 5.** Nail dystrophy in KID syndrome.

Most patients with KID syndrome are intellectually normal. Mental retardation reported in some patients (Caceres-Rios et al. 1996) is questionable: the degree of deafness, blindness and disfigurement may be determinant of severe limitations in these patients. Mental retardation is a constant feature of the autosomal recessive form of KID syndrome (Desmons syndrome) (OMIM # 242150).

Other, less frequently reported, neurological abnormalities are peripheral neuropathy (Beare et al. 1972, Grob et al. 1987), microcephaly (Ney et al. 1990), cerebellar hypoplasia (Jureka et al. 1985) and Dandy-Walker malformation (Boudghene-Stambouli et al. 1994, Lenane et al. 2006).

## Ocular lesions

Vascularizing keratitis starting with photophobia and ending in blindness, is present in up to 95% of patients. Photophobia and blepharitis, present at birth or starting later, may progress to corneal vascularization. By the second decade of life epithelial scarring and neovascularization lead to blindness (Baden and Alper 1977, Caceres-Rios et al. 1996, Harms et al. 1984).

Other eye abnormalities include loss of eyebrows and lashes, thickened and keratinized eyelids, trichiasis, recurrent corneal epithelial defects, superficial and deep corneal stromal vascularization with scarring, keracinjunctivitis sicca and limbal insufficiency (Messmer et al. 2005).

## Other abnormalities

Non specific immune defects in KID syndrome are: increased susceptibility to viral, bacterial, fungal and parasite infections (Caceres-Rios et al. 1996), increased IgE and IgG levels, chemotaxis deficiencies and lymphocyte proliferative response (Caceres-Rios et al. 1996, Harms et al. 1984, Helm et al. 1990, Pincus et al. 1975, Stalder and Litoux 1988). Their significance is not yet clear. Candida infections are particularly common and may be fatal in infants (Gilliam and Williams 2002). Alopecia, nail dystrophy and body malodor may be associated to chronic skin fungal and bacterial infections.

Other occasional abnormalities are: oral leukoplakia, short heel cords, hypohidrosis, short stature, breast hypoplasia, cryptorchidism, malignant histiocytoma, multiple hair follicle tumors, multiple eccrine poromas, arthropathy, inguinal hernia, pes cavus, Hirschprung disease and nephritic syndrome (Caceres-Rios et al. 1996).

## Pathology

There are not uniform findings: skin biopsy specimens show epidermal orthohyperkeratosis, acanthosis and papillomatosis with focal parakeratosis, follicular plugging and keratin horns (De Berker et al. 1993). Vacuolization of the granular layer has been described (Harms et al. 1984). In the upper dermis there is moderate inflammatory infiltrate of mononuclear cells. Hair follicles are atrophic or plugged

(Ney et al. 1990). No significant abnormalities have been found in ultrastructural studies (Harms et al. 1984, Langer et al. 1990). Pseudoepitheliomatous hyperplasia and malignancies may develop in proliferating keratosis (McGregor et al. 1990).

In the inner ear, the organ of Corti is immature or atrophic (Schnyder 1977).

Ocular abnormalities such as corneal dyskeratosis with peripheral hypertrophy and atrophy or absent in the center, and absence of the Bowman membrane have been demonstrated (De Berker et al. 1993).

The histopathology abnormalities support the involvement of ectodermal derived tissues in KID syndrome.

## Pathogenesis and molecular genetics

Most cases of KID syndrome are sporadic. According to the reported familial cases of KID syndrome in the literature two forms have been identified (Wilson et al. 1991): (1) *an autosomal dominant form* (OMIM # 148210) with well demonstrated vertical transmission in a father and his daughter (Grob et al. 1987) in mothers and her daughters (Kelley et al. 2008, Nazarro et al. 1990) and additional families reported by Senter et al. (1978), Langer et al. (1990), Kone-Paut et al. (1998) and Messmer et al. (2005); (2) an *autosomal recessive form*, which has additional features including hepatic disease (progressive cirrhosis necessitating liver transplantation), growth failure and mental retardation (*Desmons syndrome*) (OMIM # 242150) (Cacer-Rios et al. 1996, Cremers et al. 1977, Desmons et al. 1971, Wilson et al. 1991). A low incidence of affected sibs in reported cases and 2 sibships of 9 with only 1 affected member (Beare et al. 1972, Cram et al. 1979) support the existence of a dominant form. In the autosomal dominant form, hepatic disease, growth problems and cognitive deficit are not features, and heterozygous mutations have been identified in the connexin-26 gene (GJB2) (Richard et al. 2002, van Geel et al. 2002, van Steensel et al. 2002).

Mutations in gap junction proteins (*connexins*) have been reported in several epidermal diseases sometimes accompanied by deafness including GJB2, GJB6 (OMIM # 604418), GJB3 (OMIM # 603324), GJB5 (OMIM # 604493), GJB4 (OMIM # 605425) and GJA4 (OMIM # 121012): in KID syndrome heterozygous missense mutations in the connexin gene GJB2 (OMIM # 121011), located on chromosome 13q11-q12, encoding the gap junction protein 26 (Cx26) have been demonstrated (Richard et al. 2002, van Steensel et al. 2002). The most common mutation until now is in codon 50 (D50N) substituting the aspartic acid with an aspargine. The spectrum of mutations seems to produce a wide phenotypic variability (van Geel et al. 2002).

Similar mutations in the GJB2 gene cause another congenital sensorineural syndrome with keratopachydermia and constrictions of fingers and toes (*Vohwinkel syndrome* or *keratoderma hereditarium mutilans*/KHM) (OMIM # 124500).

No specific tissue abnormalities to elucidate the underlying etiology in KID syndrome have been found. However, Richard et al. (2002) found that mutant CX26 is incapable of forming gap junction plaques at the cell membranes or impairs the function of gap junction channels. In the skin, cornea and inner ear, these mechanisms likely alter the exchange of signals and small molecules between cells, thus leading to disturbed epithelial homeostasis and differentiation. In addition, decreased host defense and increased carcinogenic potential in KID illustrated that gap junction communication plays not only a crucial role in epithelial homeostasis and differentiation but also in immune response and epidermal carcinogensis (OMIM™ 2006).

Nonspecific immunologic abnormalities such as increased IgE and IgG, deficiencies of chemotaxis and lymphocyte response have been reported (Caceres-Rios et al. 1996, Harms et al. 1984, Helm et al. 1990, Pincus et al. 1975) suggesting an associated immunologic impairment.

Because of findings of glycogen storage in different tissues (Jureka et al. 1985, Muramoto et al. 1987), KID syndrome has been also considered as a primary genetic defect of carbohydrate metabolism.

## Animal models

Cohen-Salmon et al. (2002) used targeted ablation of Cx26 in the mouse inner ear epithelial network to selectively disrupt Cx26 expression. The inner ears of homozygous mutant mice developed normally, and these mice had a hearing impairment, but not vestibular dysfunction. On postnatal day 14, soon after the onset of hearing, cell death appeared and eventually extended to the cochlear epithelial network and sensory hair cells. Cell death initially affected only the supporting cells of inner hair cells (IHC), suggesting that apoptosis could be triggered by the IHC response to sound stimulation. The authors concluded (Cohen-Salmon et al. 2002) that Cx26-containing epithelial gap junctions are essential for cochlear function and cell survival and that prevention of cell death in the sensory epithelium is essential in restoring auditory function in patients with hereditary sensorineural deafness.

## Diagnosis

The diagnosis of KID syndrome is clinical, based on the cutaneous alterations and supported by the evidence of sensorineural deafness and keratitis. Caceres-Rios et al. (1996) suggested major and minor diagnostic criteria for this syndrome (Table 1).

Erythrokeratoderma with variable expression is always present. Mild to severe congenital hearing loss is always present too. The ocular affection may first develop later in childhood even in adolescence. Keratitis should not be a sign of early diagnosis. Because of its frequency and appearance alopecia and reticulated palmo-plantar hyperkeratosis should be

**Table 1.** Diagnostic criteria for KID syndrome

| |
| --- |
| **Major criteria** |
| Erythrokeratoderma (100%) |
| Neurisensorial deafness (100%) |
| Vascularizing keratitis |
| Reticulated palmo-plantar hyperkeratosis |
| Alopecia |
| **Minor criteria** |
| Susceptibility to infections |
| Dental dysplasia |
| Hypohidrosis |
| Growth delay |

Adapted and modified from Caceres-Rios et al. (1996).

considered as mayor criteria. Minor criteria may or may not be present.

## Differential diagnosis

The differential diagnosis of KID syndrome includes congenital erythrokeratodermias and other ichthyosiform conditions with hearing loss. Hystrix-like ichthyosis and deafness – HID syndrome – (Schnyder 1977), in which mild keratitis also occurs, the cutaneous alteration is a true ichthyosis.

Erythrokeratodermias such as erythrokeratodermia variabilis (EKV) and progressive symmetric erythrokeratoderma (PSEK) are not associated with keratitis and hearing loss.

Refsum disease and Rud syndrome (Ruiz-Maldonado 1987) are ichthyosiform conditions with deafness. Other syndrome characterized by similar skin changes and deafness associated with neutral lipid storage have no keratitis (Williams et al. 1985).

## Treatment and prognosis

There is no specific treatment for patients with KID syndrome. Mild cleansers, emollients and keratolytics may be beneficial. Symptomatic therapy of keratoconjunctivities may be indicated.

The control of skin infections with intermittent antibiotic therapy and/or systemic antifungal agents plays an important roll in controlling odor and avoiding complications.

Oral retinoids have been used in several patients with variable results. Hyperkeratosis responds partially to etretinate 2 mg/kg/day, but palmo-plantar keratoderma is recalcitrant. The ocular side effects of retinoids (isotretinoin) may aggravate keratitis and neovascularization (Hazen et al. 1986). Close ophthalmologic follow-up should be done.

Early audiologic assessment should be performed; speech therapy, hearing aids and coclear implants may improve communication. Recently (Choung et al. 2008), cochlear implantation has proven effective in a child with KID syndrome.

Progressive vascularizing keratitis has been successfully treated with topical cyclosporine (Derse et al.

2002). Corneal transplant has failed to improve vision because of revascularization (Nazarro et al. 1990).

Surgical treatment of hyperplastic lesions may be needed. Bening multiple hair follicle tumors (Kim et al. 2002) do not require treatment. Squamous cell carcinoma of the skin and/or tongue reported in about 10% of patients (Hazen et al. 1989) is the most severe malignant complication of the disease, requiring Mohs microsurgery.

A fatal course of KID syndrome in the first year of life, due to severe infections of the skin lesions and septicemia, was reported in at least 5 patients (Gilliam and Williams 2002, Janecke et al. 2005).

## References

Baden EP, Alper JC (1977) Ichthyosiform dermatosis, keratitis and deafness. Arch Dermatol 113: 1701–1704.

Beare JM, Nevin NC, Froggatt P, Kernohan DC, Allen IV (1972) Atypical erythrokeratoderma with deafness, physical retardation and peripheral neuropathy. Br J Dermatol 87: 308–314.

Boudghene-Stambouli O, Merad-Boudia A, Abdelali S (1994) KID syndrome, pachydermatoglyphy and Dandy-Walker syndrome. Ann Dermatol Venereol 121: 99–102.

Burns FS (1915) A case of generalized congenital keratoderma with unusual involvement of eyes, ears and nasal and buccal mucous membranes. J Cutan Dis 33: 255–260.

Caceres-Rios H, Tamayo-Sánchez L, Durán Mckinster C, Orozco ML, Ruiz-Maldonado R (1996) Keratitis, ichthyosis and deafness (KID syndrome): Review of the literature and proposal of a new terminology. Pediatr Dermatol 13: 105–113.

Choung YH, Shin YR, Kim HJ, Kim YC, Ahn JH, Choi SJ, Jeong SY, Park K (2008) Cochlear implantation and connexin expression in the child with keratitis-ichthyosis-deafness syndrome. Int J Pediatr Otorhinolaryngol 72: 911–915.

Cohen-Salmon M, Ott T, Michel V, Hardelin J-P, Perfettini I, Eybalin M, Wu T, Marcus DC, Wangemann P, Willecke K, Petit C (2002) Targeted ablation of connexin26 in the inner ear epithelial gap junction network causes hearing impairment and cell death. Curr Biol 12: 1106–1111.

Cram DL, Resneck JS, Jackson WB (1979) A congenital ichthyosiform syndrome with deafness and keratitis. Arch Dermatol 115: 467–471.

Cremers CW (1977) Retrospective study of the cause of deafness in 60 students at the Institute for the Deaf and 33 of their deaf relatives. Acta Otorhinolaryngol Belg 31: 591–592.

De Berker D, Branford WA, Soucek S, Michaels L (1993) Fatal keratitis, ichthyosis and deafness syndrome (KIDS). Aural, ocular and cutaneous histopathology. Am J Dermatopathol 15: 64–69.

Derse M, Wannke E, Payer H, Rohrbach JM, Zierhut M (2002) Successful topical cyclosporin A in the therapy of progressive vascularising keratitis in keratitis-ichthyosis-deafness (KID) syndrome (Senter syndrome). Klin Monals Augenheild 219: 383–386.

Desmons F, Bar J, Chevillard Y (1971) Erythrodermie ichthyosiforme congenitale seche, surdi-mutite, hepatomegaly, de transmission recessive autosomique: etude d'ue famille. Bull Soc Derm Syph 78: 585–588.

Gilliam A, Williams ML (2002) Fatal septicaemia in an infant with keratitis, ichthyosis and deafness syndrome. Pediatr Dermatol 19: 232–236.

Grob JJ, Breton A, Bonafe JL, Sauvan-Ferdni M, Bonerandi JJ (1987) Keratitis, ichthyosis and deafness (KID) syndrome: vertical transmission and death from multiple squamous cell carcinomas. Arch Dermatol 123: 777–782.

Harms M, Gilarde S, Levy PM, Saurat JH (1984) KID syndrome (keratitis, ichthyosis and deafness) and chronic mucocutaneous candidiasis: case report and review of the literature. Pediatr Dermatol 2: 1–7.

Hazen PG, Carney JM, Langston RHS, Meisler DM (1986) Corneal effects of isotretinoin: possible exacerbation of corneal neovascularization in a patient with keratitis, ichthyosis and deafness (KID) syndrome. J Am Acad Dermatol 14: 141–142.

Hazen PG, Carney P, Lynch WS (1989) Keratitis, ichthyosis and deafness syndrome with development of multiple cutaneous neoplasms. Cameo 28: 190–191.

Helm K, Lane AT, Orosz J, Metlay L (1990) Systemic cytomegalovirus in a patient with keratitis, ichthyosis and deafness (KID) syndrome. Pediatr Dermatol 7: 54–56.

Janecke AR, Hennies HC, Gunther B, Gansl G, Smolle J, Messmer EM, Utermann G, Rittinger O (2005) GJB2 mutations in keratitis-ichthyosis-deafness syndrome including its fatal form. Am J Med Genet 133A: 128–131.

Jureka W, Aberer E, Mainitz M, Jurgensen O (1985) Keratitis, ichthyosis and deafness syndrome with glycogen storage. Arch Dermatol 121: 799–801.

Kelly B, Lozano A, Altenberg G, Makishima T (2008) Connexin 26 mutation in keratitis-ichthyosis-deafness (KID) syndrome in mother and daughter with combined conductive and sensorineural hearing loss. Int J Dermatol 47: 443–447.

Kim HH, Kim JS, Piao YJ et al. (2002) Keratitis, ichthyosis and deafness syndrome with development of multiple hair follicle tumours. Br J Dermatol 143: 139–143.

Kone-Paut I, Hesse S, palix C, Rey R, Remediani K, Garnier JM, Berbis P (1998) Keratitis, ichthyosis and deafness (KID)-syndrome: report of three cases and a review of the literature. Br J Dermatol 122: 689–697.

Lancaster L, Fournet LF (1969) Carcinoma of the tongue in a child. J Oral Maxillofac Surg 27: 269–270.

Langer K, Konrad K, Wolff K (1990) Keratitis, ichthyosis and deafness (KID) syndrome: report of three cases and a review of the literature. Br J Dermatol 122: 689–697.

Lenane P, Cammisuli S, Chitayat D, Krafchik B (2006) What syndrome is this? KID syndrome (keratitis, ichthyosis, deafness). Pediatr Dermatol 23: 81–83.

Madariaga J, Fromowitz F, Phillip SM, Hoover HC (1986) Squamous cell carcinoma in congenital ichthyosis with deafness and keratitis. Cancer 57: 2026–2029.

McGregor J, Markey A, Allen M (1990) Keratitis, ichthyosis and deafness (KID)-syndrome: an histopathological and immunohistochemical study. 28th Annual Meeting of the American Society of Dermatopathology, November 28–30, 1990; 307 (Abstract).

Messmer EM, Kenyon KR, Rittinger O, Janecke AR, Kampik A (2005) Ocular manifestations of keratitis-ichthyosis-deafness (KID) syndrome. Ophthalmology 112: e1.

Muramoto T, Shirai T, Sakamato K (1987) KID syndrome: congenital ichthyosiform dermatosis with keratitis and deafness. J Dermatol 14: 158–162.

Nazarro V, Blanchet-Bardon C, Lorette G, Civatte J (1990) Familial occurrence of KID (keratitis, ichthyosis, deafness) syndrome; case reports of a mother and daughter. J Am Acad Dermatol 23: 385–388.

Ney E, Tamayo L, Laterza A, Ruiz-Maldonado R (1990) Sindrome KID (queratitis-ictiosis y sordera). Comunicación de 5 casos. Dermatol Rev Mex 34: 22–26.

Nousari HC, Kimyai-Asadi A, Pinto JL (2000) KID syndrome associated with features of ichthyosis hystrix. Pediatr Dermatol 17: 115–117.

OMIM™ (2006) Online Mendelian Inheritance in Man. Baltimore: Johns Hopkins University Press. http://www.ncbi.nlm.nih.gov/omim

Pincus SH, Thomas IT, Clark RP, Ochs HD (1975) Defective neutrophil chemotaxis with variant ichthyosis, hyperimmunoglobulinemia E and recurrent infections. J Pediatr 87: 907–908.

Richard G, Rovan F, Willoughby CE, Brown N, Chung P, Ryynanen M, Jabs EW, Bale J, DiGiovanna JJ, Uitto J, Russell L (2002) Missense mutations in GJB2 encoding connexin 26 cause the ectodermal dysplasia keratitis-ichthyosis-deafness syndrome. Am J Hum Genet 70: 1341–1348.

Ruiz-Maldonado R (1987) Neuroichthyosis. In: Gomez MR (ed.) Neurocutaneous Diseases. A Practical Approach. Boston: Butterworth Publishers, pp. 214–218.

Schnyder UW (1977) Ichthyosis hystrix typus Rheydt (ichthyosis hystrix gravior mit praktischer Taubheit). Z Hautkr 52: 763–766.

Senter TP, Jones KL, Sakati N, Nyhan WL (1978) Atypical ichthyosiform erythroderma and congenital neurosensory deafness – a distinct syndrome. J Pediatr 92: 68–72.

Skinner BA, Greist MC, Norins AL (1981) The keratitis, ichthyosis, and deafness (KID) syndrome. Arch Dermatol 117: 285–289.

Stalder JF, Litoux P (1988) A case for diagnosis: KID syndrome (Keratitis, ichthyosis and deafness). Ann Dermatol Venereol 15: 357–358.

Szymko YM, Russel LJ, Bale SJ, Griffith AJ (2002) Auditory manifestations of keratitis ichthyosis-deafness (KID) syndrome. Laryngoscope 112: 272–280.

Todt I, Hennies HC, Küster W, Smolle J, Rademacher G, Mutze S, Basta D, Eisenschenk A, Ernst A (2006) Neurotological and Neuroanatomical Changes in the Connexin-26-Related HID/KID Syndrome. Audiol Neurotol 11: 242–248.

Traupe H (1989a) The ichthyosis. A guide to clinical diagnosis, genetic counseling and therapy. Berlin: Springer, pp. 191–197.

Traupe H (1989b) Not an ichthyosis at all: the keratitis, ichthyosis-like hyperkeratosis, and deafness (KID) syndrome. In: Traupe H (ed.) The Ichthyosis A guide to clinical diagnosis, genetic counseling and therapy. Berlin: Springer, pp. 198–200.

van Geel M, van Steensel MA, Kuster W, Hennies HC, Happle R, Steijlen PM, Konig A (2002) HID and KID syndromes are associated with the same connexin 26 mutation. Br J Dermatol 146: 938–942.

van Steensel M, van Geel M, Nahuys M, Smitt JHS, Steijlen PM (2002) A novel connexin 26 mutation in a patient diagnosed with keratitis-ichthyosis-deafness syndrome. J Invest Dermatol 118: 724–727.

Williams ML, Koch TK, O'Donnell JJ, Frost PH, Epstein LB, Grizzard WS, Epstein CJ (1985) Ichthyosis and neutral lipid storage disease. Am J Med Genet 20: 711–726.

Wilson GN, Squires RH, Weinberg AG (1991) Keratitis, hepatitis, ichthyosis, and deafness: report and review of KID syndrome. Am J Med Genet 40: 255–259.

# Chapter 41

# PAPILLON–LEFÈVRE SYNDROME (PLS)

**Christer Ullbro**

Department of Pedodontics, Institute of Postgraduate Dental Education, Jonkoping, Sweden

## Introduction

In 1924 two French pediatricians, MM Papillon and P Lefèvre, published an article with the title "Deux cas de keratodermie palmaire et plantaire symetrique familiale (Maladie de Meleda) chez le frere et la soeur. Coexistance dans les deux cas d'alterations dentaires graves" (Papillon and Lefèvre 1924). They reported the first two known cases, a brother and a sister, with transgradient palmoplantar hyperkeratosis, an aggressive periodontal inflammation, and premature loss of primary and permanent teeth. The two children, being products of a first cousin mating, showed the classical clinical characteristics that later have been known as the cardinal symptoms of Papillon–Lefèvre syndrome (PLS). Today, several hundred cases have been reported in the literature and the awareness of the clinical variance of the disease has been acknowledged. The genetics behind the syndrome has been identified although the biological mechanism causing the skin and the periodontal lesions is still undisclosed.

## Historical perspective and terminology

Papillon and Lefèvre envisioned PLS being a variant of mal de Meleda. Both conditions belong to a heterogeneous group of skin disorders called palmoplantar keratodermas or keratoses (PPKs). The PPKs are characterized by hyperkeratotic lesions primarily affecting the palms of the hands and the soles of the feet. Hyperkeratosis refers to hypertrophy of the horny layer of the epidermis causing gross thickening of the skin.

The biological mechanism of PPK appears to be genetically as well as clinically heterogenous (Stevens et al. 1996). Historically PPK classifica-

tions have been based on pattern of inheritance, clinical expression, histology and co occurrence with associated clinical features (Itin 1992, Paller 1999). Stevens et al. (1996) classified PLS as a type IV palmoplantar keratosis, using the clinical site of the lesions, the associated lesions, the histopathological findings as well as the suggested molecular mechanisms in their classification. Application of modern molecular biology techniques has led to an increased understanding of the genetic basis of these disorders, and classification based upon molecular pathology has been achieved (Ratnavel and Griffiths 1997). More recently, the specific gene defects responsible for many of the hereditary PPKs have been identified (Kimayi-Asadi et al. 2002).

PLS differs from other PPKs by the presence of early-onset and aggressive periodontitis. Haneke (1979) used the following criteria to classify a case as PLS: (i) presence of palmoplantar hyperkeratosis, (ii) loss of primary and permanent teeth, and (iii) autosomal recessive inheritance.

## Clinical manifestations

### Skin abnormalities

The dermatological affection is one of the cardinal signs in PLS. Hyperkeratosis develops in pressure areas, such as palms, soles, knuckles, ankles, elbows and knees. Onychogryphosis as well as retardation of somatic development and follicular hyperkeratosis has also been reported (Haneke 1979). The keratotic plaques are symmetric, usually diffuse but focal callosities with punctate lesions have been reported. The lesions are thick and scaly and may involve the entire surfaces of the palms and soles, sometimes ex-

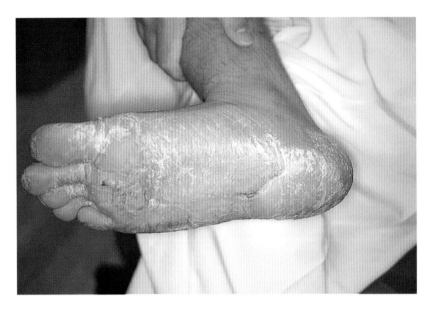

**Fig. 1.** Severe thickening of plantar skin in a 15 year old boy.

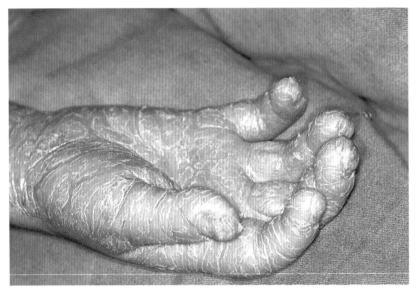

**Fig. 2.** Severe hyperkeratosis with scaling and cracking of palmar skin in a 6 year old boy.

tending to the dorsal surface of the hands and feet (Siragusa et al. 2000). Frequently the feet are more severely involved and the thickening and cracking of the plantar skin may be so severe that walking is difficult (Fig. 1). Occasionally the hyperkeratosis of the hands is limited to accentuation of the palmar creases although severe hyperkeratosis with scaling and cracking of the palmar skin may occur (Fig. 2). Transgression onto the elbows and knees are common. Aggravation of the skin lesions in very young males compared to young females has been reported (Ullbro et al. 2006).

Histological examination with light microscopy shows mild hyperkeratosis, focal hyperparakeratosis, hypergranulosis, mild acanthosis and irregular elongation and widening of the rete ridges in the epidermis. The upper dermis expresses, a slight perivascular chronic inflammatory cell infiltrate composed mostly of mononuclear cells, similar to that seen in chronic dermatitis (Nazarro et al. 1988). Electron microscopy reveals non-specific histological changes in the affected skin, with lipid like vacuoles in the corneocytes and granulocytes, a reduction in tonofilaments, and irregular keratohyalin granules (Lucker et al. 1994). The mitotic activity index of the cutaneous epidermal cells appears unremarkable (Lu et al. 1987).

There is no association with the palmoplantar keratoses and malignancy in patients with PLS, even though cases with malignant melanoma developing in the hyperkeratotic palmar epidermis (Hacham-Zadeh and Goldberg 1982, Nakajima et al. 2008) and one case with ocular surface squamous neoplasia (Murhty et al. 2005) have been reported. Saatci (2006) describes a 7-year-old boy with PLS who in addition to the classic dental and dermatologic findings had bilateral, almost symmetric, hypertrophic-looking corneal leukoma.

## Abnormalities of other systems and organs

The early onset aggressive periodontal disease is another cardinal sign of PLS. The premature and extensive tooth loss has a severe impact on oral health often resulting in functional as well as cosmetic handicaps. In the primary dentition, treatment options are restricted due to the very young patient's inability to cooperate to meticulous oral hygiene measurements and to conservative periodontal treatment. In the permanent dentition the extent and the severity of the periodontal disease are more variable and conservative periodontal treatment has in many cases been proven successful (Preus 1988, Wiebe et al. 2001). Ability to obtain and maintain good oral hygiene is crucial in order to reach a successful outcome in this treatment. Whenever deemed necessary the conservative periodontal treatment has to be combined with antibiotics in order to cure episodes of periodontal inflammation (Ullbro et al. 2005).

An increased susceptibility to infection, besides the periodontal inflammation, has been reported in approximately 20% of patients with PLS (Bergman and Friedman-Birnbaum 1988, Haneke et al. 1975). Patients with PLS are not known to be unusually susceptible to viral infections (Pham et al. 2004) instead painful fissures and recurrent pyogenic infections of the skin seem to be the most common medical complications (Haneke et al. 1975). However, a number of PLS patients with abscesses or pseudotumors of the liver have been described (Czauderna

et al. 1999, Almuneef et al. 2003) as well as one case with xanthogranulomatous pyelonephritis and hepatitis (Mansur 2006).

There have been reports of PLS patients with other stigmata such as growth retardation (Ressa 1970), non-symptomatic intracranial calcifications (Gorlin et al. 1964), and mental retardation (Haneke 1979, Hart and Shapira 1994). Furthermore, coinheritance of PLS and albinism type 1 have been reported by Hewitt et al. (2004b) and Hattab and Amin (2005).

## Nervous system abnormalities

Asymptomatic ectopic intracranial calcification of the falx cerebri, tentorium and dura mater have been reported either in sporadic PLS cases (Brownstein and Skolnik 1972, Gorlin et al. 1964, Landow et al. 1983, Posteraro 1992) and in a family with PLS (Verma et al. 1979). Notably, however, Lundgren and Renvert (2004) found intracranial calcification in only 2 out of 15 examined patients with PLS. The aetiology or possible consequences of these calcifications are obscure.

## Natural history

The palmoplantar keratoses usually develop during the first year of life. It starts with redness and thickening of the palms of the hands and soles of the feet. It is a common finding that the gravity of hyperkeratosis varies significantly between affected individuals even between those in the same family (Krebs 1978, Gorlin et al. 1964). Factors such as seasonal variations, the concurrent level of periodontal inflammation, as well as the individuals' age have been alleged to influence the severity of the skin lesions (Gorlin et al. 1964, Hattab et al. 1995). The skin lesions are reported to decrease with age, even though some degree of palmoplantar keratosis appears to remain throughout life (Hart and Shapira 1994). Ullbro et al. (2003) found no correlation between the level of periodontal inflammation and severity of skin affections.

In young patients with PLS, the oral mucosal and gingival tissues appear normal prior to the eruption of the deciduous teeth. After eruption, the gingival tissues become inflamed and the inflammation leads to rapid destruction of the periodontal tissues (Haneke 1979, Lu et al. 1987). As a result of the periodontal destruction in PLS patients most of the deciduous teeth are shed spontaneously and prematurely at an early age. The gingival tissues resume normal appearance following the loss of the decidu-

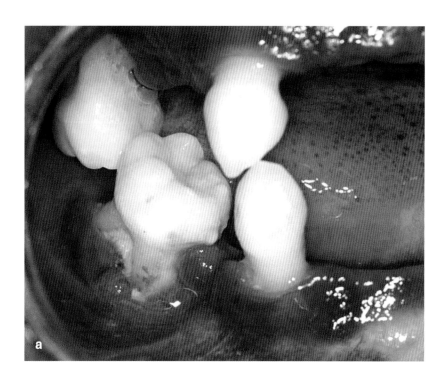

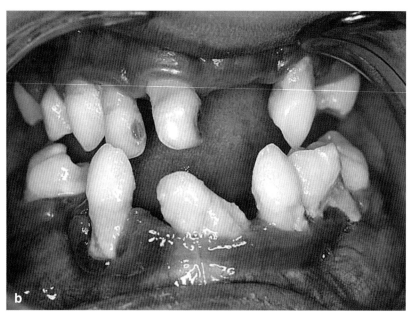

Fig. 3. Severe periodontal inflammation in the primary dentition of a 3-year-old girl (a), a 5-year-old boy (b), and a 8-year-old boy (c) with PLS.

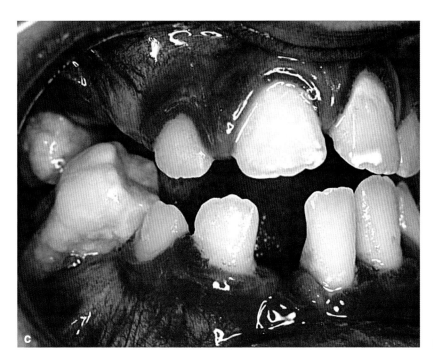

**Fig. 3.** (Continued)

ous teeth. After eruption of permanent teeth, the inflammatory process often repeats itself leading to devastating periodontal destruction (Fig. 3). In the permanent dentition the extent and the severity of the periodontal disease are more variable than in the primary dentition and a number of patients are able to preserve some or most of their teeth into their adult life (Preus 1988, Wiebe et al. 2001). Nevertheless, many patients with PLS will become edentulous by their early teens (Gorlin et al. 1964).

## Molecular genetics and pathogenesis

Autosomal recessive transmission for the PLS disorder was early on suggested by Decker and Jansen (1956). Gorlin et al. (1964) confirmed this hypothesis after noting that parents were not affected, and similar pathology was diagnosed in affected siblings. The observed rate of consanguinity in families with PLS was also noted to be far greater than that for the general population. Between 2 and 4 people per 1000 are heterozygous for the PLS gene and therefore, carriers of the disorder. This results in a population prevalence of 1 case per 1–4 million people

(Gorlin et al. 1964). It is calculated that 1/3 of all cases of PLS are the result of consanguinity (Gorlin et al. 1990).

By using homozygosity linkage mapping Fischer et al. (1997) and Laass et al. (1997) located the gene for PLS to chromosome 11q14. In 1999 two research groups were able to identify the mutation linked to PLS as a lack-of-function mutation of the gene encoding cathepsin C (Hart et al. 1999, Toomes et al. 1999). Today more than 41 different mutations of the cathepsin C gene have been identified in patients with PLS, all of them homozygous (Hart et al. 2000, Noack et al. 2008, Selvaraju et al. 2003), However, compound heterozygous mutations in patients with PLS as well as "symptomless mutations" in the cathepsin C gene in homozygous individuals have also been described (Allende et al. 2003, Hewitt et al. 2004, Noack et al. 2004). Heterozygous carriers of the mutation are clinically unaffected (Nakano et al. 2001) although one heterozygous patient presented with plantar hyperkeratosis without periodontal disease (Cury et al. 2002). Biochemical analysis has demonstrated almost no cathepsin C activity in leukocytes from patients with PLS (Zhang et al. 2002, de Haar et al. 2004).

The cathepsin C gene is normally expressed in those epithelial regions frequently affected by PLS such as the palms, soles, knees, and keratinized oral gingiva (Rao et al. 1997). Nuckols and Slavkin (1999) suggested that cathepsin C may be essential for establishing or maintaining the structural organization of the epidermis of the extremities and the integrity of the tissues surrounding the teeth, and that it might also participate indirectly in the processing of proteins such as keratins. The exact mechanism by which cathepsin C gene mutations cause or are involved in PPK is unclear since its role in the epidermis has not yet been studied in detail.

Cathepsin C is a lysosomal cysteine proteinase functioning as a central coordinator in degradation of proteins and as an activator of various serine proteases in immune and inflammatory cells (Rao et al. 1997). It activates the serine proteases, granzymes A and B in cytotoxic lymphocytes and natural killer cells, which are required for the cytotoxic lymphocytes granule-mediated apoptosis of tumor cells and infected cells (Pham and Ley 1999). It also activates tryptase (Sheth et al. 2003) and chymase (Caughey 2002) in mast cells, and cathepsin G, elastase and proteinase 3 in neutrophils (Adkison et al. 2002). This activation is essential for the phagocytic destruction of bacteria (de Haar et al. 2004). Furthermore, activation of serine proteases is important for local activation and deactivation of cytokines and other inflammatory mediators, and for extracellular matrix degradation (Murphy et al. 1992, Turk et al. 2001, Hewitt et al. 2004). Cathepsin C functions by removing dipeptides from the amino terminus of the protein substrate, as well as having endopeptidase activity (Turk et al. 2001).

The importance of cathepsin C in the defence of the organism has been studied on cell lines from cathepsin C-deficient mice, which fail to activate serine proteinases in immune and inflammatory cells (Wolters et al. 2001). According to these findings cathepsin C is required for the activation of the serine proteases, granzymes A and B in cytotoxic lymphocytes and natural killer cells. This activation is essential for the cytotoxic lymphocytes granule-mediated apoptosis of tumor cells and infected cells (Pham and Ley 1999). Based on the phenotype seen in cathepsin C-deficient mice, patients with PLS would have generalized immunodeficiency as a result of the loss of activation of these serine proteases (Pham et al. 2004). However, PLS patients are not known to be unusually susceptible to viral infections (Pham et al. 2004). In their investigations Pham et al. (2004) report that patients with PLS have well-preserved cytotoxic lymphocyte function. A similar result was shown by Meade et al. (2006) who concluded that loss-of-function mutations in cathepsin C do not affect lymphokine activated killer cell function. However, Meade et al. (2006) found that resting natural killer (NK) cells in humans with PLS have a cytolytic defect and contain inactive granzyme B. This finding indicates that cathepsin C is required for the granzyme B activation in unstimulated human NK cells.

## Diagnosis, follow up and management

The diagnosis of Papillon–Lefèvre syndrome is made through clinical examination of the skin and oral tissue. A pedigree will reveal the mode of inheritance and by using mutation analysis it is possible to identify the mutation through blood or tissue samples.

### Palmoplantar hyperkeratosis – treatment of skin lesions

Mild to moderate palmoplantar hyperkeratosis can be treated with lubricants and topical agents like 20% urea cream, or 12% lactic acid, with or without 6% salicylic acid, in petroleum jelly. PLS patients with severe palmoplantar hyperkeratosis may, in addition to topical treatment, receive systemic medication with synthetic retinoids (acitrecin 0.5 mg/kg/day, Neo-Tigason, Roche, Basel, Switzerland), which have been proven effective (Nazzaro et al. 1988). The retinoids down-regulate the expression of metalloproteinases, cytokines and skin-derived anti-leukoproteinase (Nagpal et al. 1996). However, case reports have indicated that long-term retinoid medication may increase the risk of adverse side effects such as hyperostoses, severe skeletal changes, teratogenicity, and liver toxicity (Sillevis Smitt and de Mari 1984, DiGiovanna et al. 1986, Halkier-Sorensen and Andresen 1989) and the use of the drugs has, consequently, been restricted.

## Treatment of PLS periodontitis

Treatment of PLS periodontitis was early on restricted to extraction of severely affected teeth (Rosenthal 1951). In order to create an edentulous period free of infection prior to eruption of the permanent teeth, Baer and McDonald (1981) extracted all primary teeth at a young age followed by treatment with systemic tetracycline while the permanent teeth were erupting. This treatment approach has successfully been used by others as well (Tinnanoff et al. 1986, Preus and Gjermo 1987). The extraction of all primary teeth is indicated due to the severe inflammation that in most cases affects the primary dentition. The gramnegative periopathogenic bacteria Actinobacillus actinomycetem comitans (*A.a.*) seems to be an important periopathogen in PLS periodontitis and it would therefore be valid to employ antimicrobials that target this microorganism in the treatment of the periodontal disease. However, posttreatment improvement of clinical and radiological conditions, in spite of recurrent findings of *A.a.*, suggests that other microbes might be implicated as well (Kleinfelder et al. 1996).

Other treatment modalities reported in PLS patients are rinsing or subgingival irrigation with chlorhexidine solutions (Rüdiger et al. 1999, Wiebe et al. 2001, Lundgren and Renvert 2004), and frequent professional prophylaxis including scaling and rootplaning (Kressin et al. 1995). Some authors have found that synthetic retinoids improve the periodontal condition (Kressin et al. 1995), while others find them ineffective (Lundgren et al. 1996).

## Differential diagnosis

The scaly erythematous lesions over knees, elbows and interphalangeal joints are sometimes misdiag-

nosed as psoriasis although the histological findings are different (Lucker et al. 1994).

Mutations of the cathepsin C gene have been confirmed in patients with PLS and Haim-Munk syndrome. The latter condition has a phenotypic expression similar to PLS, plus in addition arachnodactyly, atrophic changes of the nails, and deformity of the phalanges of the hand (Haim and Munk 1965). The associated occurrence of severe early-onset periodontitis and PPK is unique to PLS and Haim–Munk syndrome (Hart et al. 2000b) and is a diagnostic distinction between other conditions with palmoplantar keratoses. However, this has been challenged by the reports of families affected by PLS and Haim–Munk syndrome in which some family members manifest the typical skin and periodontal lesions, whereas other siblings manifest the palmoplantar keratosis without any involvement of periodontal tissues either in the primary or the permanent dentition (Bullon et al. 1993). Bullon et al. (1993) reported a family with 6 children where 4 were affected by PLS by having palmoplantar lesions although only two of the 4 children had periodontal inflammation. Haneke (1979), Rateitshak-Pluss and Schroeder (1984), and Nguyen et al. (1986) reported patients with palmoplantar keratoses with periodontal inflammation in the permanent, but not in the primary dentition. On the contrary, Ullbro et al. (2003) did not find any patients without periodontal inflammation in the primary dentition. Whether the reported difference is the result of genetic variance is not known.

Mutations of the cathepsin C gene have also been reported in patients with prepubertal periodontitis, which is characterized by a periodontal condition similar to PLS periodontitis, but without the dermatological effects. It has been suggested that prepubertal aggressive periodontitis could be an allelic variant of PLS (Hart et al. 2000a, Noack et al. 2004) or a genetically heterogeneous disease that, in some families, manifests as partially penetrant PLS (Hewitt et al. 2004b). Conditions with aggressive periodontal disease are not always a consequence of cathepsin C mutations and there is no proof that patients will experience aggressive periodontitis because they have a low activity of cathepsin C (Hewitt et al. 2004a).

## Genetic counseling

PLS is inherited with an autosomal recessive trait and if both parents are carriers of the defective gene there is a 25% risk that their child will be born with the disorder.

## References

Adkison AM, Raptis SZ, Kelley DG, Pham CT (2002) Dipeptidyl peptidase I activates neutrophil-derived serine proteases and regulates the development of acute experimental arthritis. J Clin Invest 109: 363–371.

Allende LM, Moreno A, de Unamuno P (2003) A genetic study of cathepsin C gene in two families with Papillon–Lefèvre syndrome. Mol Genet Metab 79: 146–148.

Almuneef M, Al Khenaizan S, Al Ajaji S, Al-Anazi A (2003) Pyogenic liver abscess and Papillon–Lefèvre syndrome: not a rare association. Pediatrics 111: 85–88.

Baer PN, McDonald RE (1981) Suggested mode of periodontal therapy for patients with Papillon–Lefèvre syndrome. Periodontal Case Rep 3: 10.

Bergman R, Friedman-Birnbaum R (1988) Papillon–Lefèvre syndrome: a study of the long-term clinical course of recurrent pyogenic infections and the effects of etretinate treatment. Br J Dermatol 119: 731–736.

Brownstein MH, Skolnik P (1972) Papillon–Lefèvre syndrome. Arch Dermatol 106: 533–534.

Bullon P, Pascual A, Fernandez-Novoa MC, Borobio MV, Muniain MA, Camacho F (1993) Late onset Papillon–Lefèvre syndrome? A chromosomic, neutrophil function and microbiological study. J Clin Periodontol 20: 662–667.

Caughey GH (2002) New developments in the genetics and activation of mast cell proteases. Mol Immunol. 38: 1353–1357.

Cury VF, Costa JE, Gomez RS, Boson WL, Loures CG, De ML (2002) A novel mutation of the cathepsin C gene in Papillon–Lefèvre syndrome. J Periodontol 73: 307–312.

Czauderna P, Sznurkowska K, Korzon M, Roszkiewicz A, Stoba C (1999) Association of inflammatory pseudotumor in the liver of Papillon–Lefèvre syndrome – case report. Eur J Pediatr Surg 9: 343–346.

Decker G, Jansen LH (1956) Hyperkeratosis palmo-plantaris with periodontosis (Papillon–Lefèvre). Dermatologica 113: 207–219.

de Haar SF, Jansen DC, Shoenmaker T, De Vree H, Everts V, Beertsen W (2004) Loss of function mutations in cathepsin C in two families with Papillon–Lefèvre syndrome are associated with deficiency of serine proteinases in PMNs. Hum Mutat 23: 524.

DiGiovanna JJ, Helfgott RK, Gerbert LH, Peck GL (1986) Extraspinal tendon and ligament calcification associated with long-term therapy with ertretinate. N Engl J Med 315: 1177–1182.

Fischer J, Blanchet-Bardon C, Prud'homme JF, Pavek S, Steijlen PM, Dubertret L, Weissenbach J (1997) Mapping of Papillon–Lefèvre syndrome to the chromosome 11q14 region. Eur J Hum Genet 5: 156–160.

Gorlin RJ, Sedano H, Anderson VE (1964) The syndrome of palmo-plantaris hyperkeratosis and premature periodontal destruction of the teeth. J Pediatr 65: 895–908.

Gorlin RJ, Cohen MM Jr, Levin LS (1990) Syndromes of the head and neck. 3rd ed. New York: Oxford University Press, 853–854.

Hacham-Zadeh S, Goldberg L (1982) Malignant melanoma and Papillon–Lefèvre syndrome. Arch Dermatol 118: 2.

Haim S, Munk J (1965) Keratosis palmo-plantaris congenita, with periodontosis, arachnodactyly and peculiar deformity of the terminal phalanges. Br J Dermatol 77: 42–54.

Halkier-Sorensen L, Andresen J (1989) A retrospective study of bone changes in adults treated with etretinate. J Am Acad Dermatol 20: 83–87.

Haneke E (1979) The Papillon–Lefèvre syndrome: keratosis palmoplantaris with periodontopathy. Report of a case and review of the cases in the literature. Hum Genet 51: 1–35.

Haneke E, Hornstein OP, Lex C (1975) Increased susceptibility to infections in the Papillon–Lefèvre syndrome. Dermatologica 150: 283–286.

Hart PS, Zhang Y, Firatli E, Uygur C, Lotfazar M, Michalec MD, Marks JJ, Lu X, Coates BJ, Seow WK, Marshall R, Williams D, Reed JB, Wright JT, Hart TC (2000a) Identification of cathepsin C mutations in ethnically diverse Papillon–Lefèvre syndrome patients. J Med Genet 37: 927–932.

Hart TC, Shapira L (1994) Papillon–Lefèvre syndrome. Periodontol 6: 88–100.

Hart TC (1996) Genetic risk factors for early-onset periodontitis. J Periodontol 67: 355–366.

Hart TC, Hart PS, Bowden DW, Michalec MD, Callison SA, Walker SJ, Zhang Y, Firatli E (1999) Mutations of the cathepsin C gene are responsible for Papillon–Lefèvre syndrome. J Med Genet 36: 881–887.

Hart TC, Hart PS, Michalec MD, Zhang Y, Firatli E, Van Dyke TE, Stabholz A, Zlotogorski WA, Shapia L, Soskolne WA (2000b) Haim-Munk syndrome and Papillon–Lefèvre syndrome are allelic mutations in cathepsin C. J Med Genet 37: 88–94.

Hathway R (1982) Papillon–Lefèvre syndrome. Br Dent J 153: 370–371.

Hattab FN, Rawashdeh MA, Yassin OM, al-Momani AS, al-Ubosi MM (1995) Papillon–Lefèvre syndrome: a review of the literature and report of 4 cases. J Periodontol 66: 413–420.

Hewitt C, McGormick D, Linden G, Turk D, Stern I, Wallace I, Southern L, Zhang L, Howard R, Bullon P, Wong M, Widmer R, Gaffar KA, Awawdeh L, Briggs J, Yaghmai R, Jabs EW, Hoeger P, Bleck O, Rudiger SG, Petersilka G, Battino M, Brett P, Hattab F, Al-Hamed M, Sloan P, Toomes C, Dixon M, James J, Read AP, Thakker N (2004a) The role of cathepsin C in Papillon–Lefèvre syndrome, prepubertal periodontitis, and aggressive periodontitis. Human Mutat 23: 222–228.

Hewitt C, Wu CL, Hattab FN, Amin W, Ghaffar KA, Toomes C, Sloan P, Pead AP, James JA, Thakker NS (2004b) Coinheritance of two rare genodermatoses (Papillon–Lefèvre syndrome and oculocutaneous albinism type 1) in two families: a genetic study. Br J Dermatol 151: 1261–1265.

Itin PH (1992) Classification of autosomal dominant palmoplantar keratoderma: past-present-future. Dermatology 185: 163–165.

Kimyai-Asadi A, Kotcher LB, Jih MH (2002) The molecular basis of hereditary palmoplantar keratodermas. J Am Acad Dermatol 47: 327–343.

Krebs A (1978) Papillon–Lefèvre syndrome. Dermatologica 156: 59–63.

Kressin S, Herforth A, Preis S, Wahn V, Lenard HG (1995) Papillon–Lefèvre syndrome – successful treatment with a combination of retinoid and concurrent systematic periodontal therapy: case reports. Quintessence Int. 26: 795–803.

Laass MW, Hennies HC, Preis S, Stevens HP, Jung M, Leigh IM, Wienker TF, Reis A (1997) Localisation of a gene for Papillon–Lefèvre syndrome to chromosome 11q14-q21 by homozygosity mapping. Hum Genet 101: 376–382.

Landow RK, Cheung H, Bauer M (1983) Papillon–Lefèvre syndrome. Int J Dermatol 22: 177–179

Lu HK, Lin CT, Kwan HW (1987) Treatment of a patient with Papillon–Lefèvre syndrome. A case report. J Periodontol 58: 789–793.

Lucker GP, Van de Kerkhof PC, Steijlen PM (1994) The hereditary palmoplantar keratoses: an updated review and classification. Br J Dermatol 131: 1–14.

Lundgren T, Crossner CG, Twetman S, Ullbro C (1996) Systemic retinoid medication and periodontal health in patients with Papillon–Lefèvre syndrome. J Clin Periodontol 23: 176–179.

Lundgren T, Renvert S (2004) Periodontal treatment of patients with Papillon–Lefèvre syndrome. A 3-year follow-up. J Clin Periodontol 31: 933–938.

Mansur AT, Goktay F, Demirok N (2006) A case of Papillon–Lefèvre syndrome associated with xanthogranulomatous pyelonephritis and hepatitis. J Dermatol 33: 59–63.

Meade JL, de Wynter EA, Brett P, Sharif SM, Woods CG, Markham AF, Cook GP (2006) A family with Papillon–Lefèvre syndrome reveals a requirement for cathepsin C in granzyme B activation and NK cell cytolytic activity. Blood 107: 3665–3668.

Murphy G, Atkinson S, Ward R, Gavrilovic J, Reynolds JJ (1992) The role of plasminogen activators in the regulation of connective tissue metalloproteinases. Ann NY Acad Sci 667: 1–12.

Murthy R, Honovar SG, Vemuganti GK, Burman S, Naik M, Parathasaradhi A (2005) Ocular squamous neoplasia in Papillon–Lefèvre syndrome. Am J Ophthalmol 139: 207–209.

Nagpal S, Thacher SM, Patel S, Friant S, Malhotra M, Shafer J, Krasinski G, Asano AT, Teng M, Duvic M, Chandraratna RA (1996) Negative regulations of two hyperproliferative keratinocyte differentiation markers by a retinoic acid receptor-specific retinoid: insight into the mechanism of retinoid action in psoriasis. Cell Growth Differ 7: 1783–1791.

Nakajima K, Nakano H, Takiyoshi N, Rokunohe A, Ikenaga S, Aizu T, Kaneko T, Mitsuhashi Y, Sawamura D (2008) Papillon-Lefèvre Syndrome and Malignant Melanoma. A High Incidence of Melanoma Development in Japanese Palmoplantar Keratoderma Patients. Dermatology 217: 58–62.

Nakano A, Nomura K, Nakano H, Ono Y, LaForgia S, Pulkkinen L, Hashimoto I, Uitto J (2001) Papillon–Lefèvre syndrome: mutations and polymorphism in the cathepsin C gene. J Invest Dermatol 116: 339–343.

Nazzaro V, Blanchet-Gardon C, Mimoz C, Revuz J, Puissant A (1988) Papillon–Lefèvre syndrome. Ultrastructure study and successfully treatment with acitretin. Arch Dermatol 124: 533–539.

Nguyen TO, Greer KE, Fisher GB Jr, Cooper PH (1986) Papillon–Lefèvre syndrome. Report of two patients treated successfully with isotretinoin. J Am Acad Dermatol 15: 46–49.

Noack B, Gorgens H, Hoffman T, Fanghanel J, Kocher T, Eickholz P, Schackert HK (2004) Novel mutations in the cathepsin C gene in patients with pre-pubertal aggressive periodontitis and Papillon–Lefèvre syndrome. J Dent Res 83: 368–370.

Noack B, Görgens H, Schacher B, Puklo M, Eickholz P, Hoffmann T, Schackert HK (2008) Functional Cathepsin C mutations cause different Papillon-Lefèvre syndrome phenotypes. J Clin Periodontol 35: 311–316.

Nuckols GH, Slavkin HC (1999) Paths of glorious proteases. Nat Genet 23: 378–380.

Paller AS (1999) The molecular bases for the palmoplantar keratodermas. Ped Dermatol 16: 483–486.

Papillon MM, Lefèvre P (1924) Deux cas de keratodermie palmaire et plantaire symétrique famiale (maladie de

Meleda) chez le frere et la soeur: coexistance dans les deux cas d'alterations dentaires graves. Bull Soc Fr Dermatol Syphiligr 31: 82–87.

Pham CT, Ley TJ (1999) Dipeptidyl peptidase I is required for the processing and activation of granzymes A and B *in vivo*. Proc Natl Acad Sci USA 96: 8627–8632.

Pham CT, Ivanovich JL, Raptis SZ, Zehnbauer B, Ley TJ (2004) Papillon–Lefèvre syndrome: correlating the molecular, cellular, and clinical consequences of cathepsin C/dipeptidylpeptidase I deficiency in humans. J Immunol 173: 7277–7281.

Posteraro AF (1992) Papillon–Lefèvre syndrome. J Am Dent Assoc 76: 16–19.

Preus HR, Gjermo P (1987) Clinical management of prepubertal periodontitis in 2 siblings with Papillon–Lefèvre syndrome. J Clin Periodontol 14: 156–160.

Preus HR (1988) Treatment of rapidly destructive periodontitis in Papillon–Lefèvre syndrome. Laboratory and clinical observations. J Clin Periodontol 15: 639–643.

Rao NV, Rao GV, Hoidal JR (1997) Human dipeptidyl-peptidase 1. Gene characterization, localization and expression. J Biol Chem 272: 10260–10265.

Rateitschak-Pluss EM, Schroeder HE (1984) History of periodontitis in a child with Papillon–Lefèvre syndrome. A case report. J Periodontol 55: 35–46.

Ratnavel RC, Griffiths WA (1997) The inherited palmoplantar keratodermas. Br J Dermatol 137: 485–490.

Ressa P (1970) Keratoderma of the Papillon–Lefèvre type associated with diffuse hyperkeratosis follicularis. Arch Anat Microsc Exp 59: 195–197.

Reynaldo Arosemena M, Abdiel Leon R (1984) Papillon–Lefèvre syndrome. Presentation of a case. Med Cutan Ibero Lat Am 12: 245–249

Rosenthal SL (1951) Periodontosis in a child resulting in exfoliation of the teeth. J Periodontal Res 22: 101–104.

Saatci P, Arli AO, Demir K, Saatci AO, Kavakcu S (2006) Corneal involvement in Papillon–Lefèvre syndrome. J Pediatr Ophtalmol Strabismus 43: 167–169.

Selvaraju V, Markandaya M, Prasad PV, Sathyan P, Sethuraman G, Srivastava SC, Thakker N, Kumar A (2003) Mutation analysis of the cathepsin C gene in Indian families with Papillon–Lefèvre syndrome. BMC Medical Genetics 4: 5.

Sheth PD, Pedersen J, Walls AF, McEuen AR (2003) Inhibition of dipedtidyl pedtidase I in the human mast cell line HMC-1: blocked activation of trypytase, but not of the predominant chymotryptic activity. Biochem Pharmacol 66: 2251–2262.

Sillevis Smitt JH, de Mari F (1984) A serious side-effect of etretinate (Tigason). Clin Exp Dermatol 9: 554–556.

Siragusa M, Romano C, Batticane N, Batolo D, Schepis C (2000) A new family with Papillon–Lefèvre syndrome: effectiveness of etretinate treatment. Cutis 65: 151–155.

Stevens HP, Kelsell DP, Bryant SP, Bishop T, Spurr NK, Weissenbach J, Marger D, Marger RS, Leigh IM (1996) Linkage of an American Pedigree with Palmoplantar Keratoderma and Malignancy (Palmoplantar Ectodermal Dysplasia Type III) to 17q24. Arch Dermatol 132: 640–651.

Tinanoff N, Tanzer JM, Kornman KS, Maderazo EG (1986) Treatment of periodontal component of Papillon–Lefèvre syndrome. J Clin Periodontol 13: 6–10.

Toomes C, James J, Wood AJ, Wu CL, McGormick D, Lench N, Hewitt C, Moynihan L, Roberts E, Woods CG, Markham A, Wong M, Widmer R, Ghaffar KA, Pemberton M, Hussein IR, Temtamy SA, Davies R, Read AP, Sloan P, Dixon MJ, Thakker NS (1999) Loss-of-function mutations in the cathepsin C gene result in periodontal disease and palmoplantar keratosis. Nat Genet 23: 421–424.

Turk D, Janjic V, Stern I, Podobnik M, Lamba D, Dahl SW, Lauritzen C, Pedersen J, Turk V, Turk B (2001) Structure of human dipeptidyl peptidase I (cathepsin C): exclusion domain added to an endopeptidase framework creates the machine for activation of granular serine proteases. EMBO Journal 20: 6570–6582.

Ullbro C, Crossner C-G, Nederfors T, Alfadley A, Thestrup-Pedersen K (2003) Dermatological and oral findings in a cohort of 47 patients with Papillon–Lefèvre syndrome. J Am Acad Dermatol 48: 345–351.

Ullbro C, Brown A, Twetman S (2005) Preventive periodontal regimen in Papillon-Lefèvre Syndrome. Pediatr Dent 27: 226–232.

Ullbro C, El-Samadi S, Boumah C, Al-Yousef N, Wakil S, Twetman S, Alfadley A, Thestrup-Pedersen K, Meyer B (2006) Phenotypic Variation and Allelic Heterogeneity in Young Patients with Papillon–Lefèvre Syndrome. Acta Derm Venereol 86: 3–7.

Verma KC, Chaddha MK, Joshi RK (1979) Papillon–Lefèvre syndrome. Int J Dermatol 18: 146–149.

Wiebe CB, Hakkinen L, Putnins EE, Walsh P, Larjava HS (2001) Successful periodontal maintenance of a case with Papillon–Lefèvre syndrome: 12 year follow-up and review of the literature. J Periodontol 72: 824–830.

Wolters PJ, Pham CT, Muilenburg DJ, Ley TJ, Caughey GH (2001) Dipeptidyl peptidase I is essential for activation of mast cell chymases, but not tryptases, in mice. J Biol Chem 276: 18551–18556.

Woods EC, Wallace WRJ (1941) A case of alveolar atrophy of unknown origin in a child. Am J Oral Surg 27: 676–682.

Zhang Y, Hart PS, Moretti AJ, Bouwsma OJ, Fisher EM, Dudlicek L, Pettenati MJ, Hart TC (2002) Biochemical and mutational analyses of the cathepsin C gene (CTSC) in three North American families with Papillon–Lefèvre syndrome. Hum Mutat 20: 75.

# Chapter 42

# RICHNER–HANHART SYNDROME (TYROSINE TRANSAMINASE DEFICIENCY)

Luz Orozco-Covarrubias, Marimar Saez-De-Ocariz, Carola Durán-McKinster, and Ramón Ruiz-Maldonado

Department of Dermatology, National Institute of Paediatrics, Mexico City, Mexico

## Introduction

There are two types of tyrosinemia: *tyrosinemia type 1* due to *fumarylacetoacetase* deficiency which is a hepatorenal form without skin abnormalities, and *tyrosinemia type II* or *Richner–Hanhart Syndrome* due to hepatic cytosolic *aminotransferase* deficiency, which is the oculocutaneous form of the disease we will discuss in this chapter.

Richner–Hanhart syndrome (R-HS) is an inborn error of tyrosine metabolism (OMIM # 276600) also known as tyrosine transaminase (TAT) deficiency: the TAT gene is located on chromosome 16q22.1-q22.3 (Barton et al. 1986, Goldsmith 1985, Huhn et al. 1998, Natt et al. 1986, Westphal et al. 1988). Skin lesions including painful punctate keratosis of digits, palms, and soles, herpetiform corneal ulcers and associated mental retardation (and in some cases seizures) make of this syndrome a neurocutaneous disorder.

## Historical perspective and eponyms

R-HS syndrome was clinically described in 1938 by Richner, a Swiss ophthalmologist born in September 6th 1908 (Richner 1938, Who named it? 2006). **Hermann Richner's** father belonged to the leadership of a trade company in Zurich. Due to his illness the family Richner in 1910 moved to Davos where the father died two years later. He started his medical studies in Geneva and continued them in Zurich, excepted one semester in Kiel. He graduated 1934 and received his doctor's degree two years later (*Vererbung der Netzhautablösung* 1936). In 1938 Richner described skin lesions of the keratotic type in a brother and sister: only the brother had corneal lesions (Richner 1938). Hanhart, a Swiss internist and geneticist, born in March 14th 1891, first reported in 1947 that the parents of his patient with palmar and plantar keratosis and corneal lesions were second cousins and described associated severe mental and somatic retardation (Hanhart 1947): he classified the inheritance of the syndrome as autosomal recessive. After qualifying in medicine from the University of Zurich in 1916, **Ernst Hanhart** worked as a country practitioner, but in 1921 became an assistant in the Zurich policlinic. Working under professors Otto Nägeli (1871–1938) and Wilhelm Löffler (1887–1972), Hanhart became interested in human genetics and became a specialist in hereditary disorders. Hanhart worked extensively on the effects of consanguinity and investigated Swiss families with inherited disorders in isolated communities. He was appointed professor at the University of Zurich in 1942 and was a founding member of the Swiss Society of Genetics. Hanhart achieved an international reputation, but in 1954 he had to resign after having been crippled in a criminal attack (Prader 1971, Who named it? 2006).

The pedigree reported by Hanhart (1947) was reproduced by Waardenburg et al. (1961) who described children of a first-cousin marriage, one with the full syndrome and one with only corneal changes. More than 30 years after of the original clinical description R-HS was associated with an inborn error of tyrosine metabolism (Burns 1972, Goldsmith et al. 1973).

## Prevalence and incidence

The R-HS is a rare inborn error of tyrosine metabolism. There are about 100 cases reported from several countries, the majority are Italian or of Italian ancestry. Cases of non-Italian ancestry are from Switzerland, Spain, France, Norway, United States, Germany (Turkish origin), United Arab Emirates and Japan, between others (Goldsmith et al. 1979). Both sexes are equally affected.

## Clinical manifestations

Richner–Hanhart syndrome usually presents with eye, skin and central nervous system alterations.

### Eye involvement

Eye manifestations are usually the initial sign of tyrosinemia type II, often before the skin lesions. Photophobia, redness and lacrimation may be present during the first months of life or even during the first decade of life, after the skin lesions. Eye examination reveals bilateral mild corneal herpetiform erosions, dendritic ulcers that may progress to severe ulcerative keratitis, corneal and conjunctival plaques with prominent neovascularization and blindness. Corneal scarring, nystagmus, exodeviation and glaucoma have been reported as long term effects, related with untreated cases (Gipson et al. 1975, Irons and Harvey 1986, Macsai et al. 2001).

### Cutaneous manifestations

Skin lesions may appear during early childhood (Fig. 1) or be delayed until the second decade of life after the eye lesions, or never appear. There are also families with skin but no eye damage. Cutaneous symptoms may begin as painful blisters and painful palmar and plantar erosions with crusts and hyperkeratosis that may lead to refusal to walk. Typically plantar hyperkeratosis is focal, and on the weight-bearing surfaces. In the palms affects fingertips and, thenar and hypothenar eminences (Fig. 2). Erythema

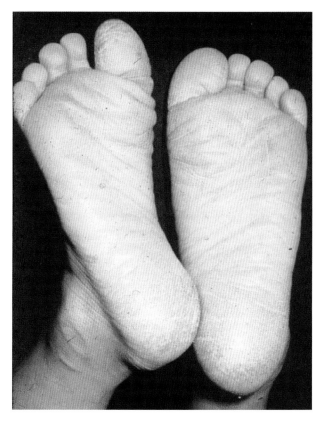

**Fig. 1.** Plantar hyperkeratosis in an 8 year-old with Richner–Hanhart syndrome.

may or may not be present. Cutaneous lesions are painful and tender, non pruritic and sometimes associated with palmo-plantar hyperhidrosis (Hunziker 1980, Rehak et al. 1981). Hyperkeratotic lesions in aberrant areas such as the elbows, knees and tongue have also been reported (Larregue et al. 1979). Hair and nails are unaffected.

### Nervous system involvement

The complete oculo-cutaneous neurological triad of the R-HS is an inconstant feature because of the variability in the neurological symptoms. Mild to moderate mental retardation of unknown origin is the most common feature. In the absence of a restricted diet, mental retardation may be progressive and severe. Language defects may be more prominent than mathematical defects in patients of R-HS

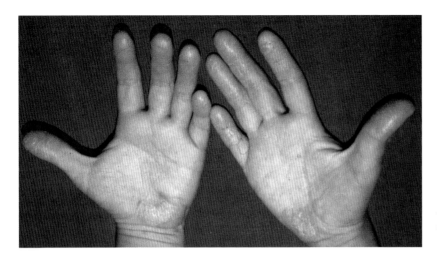

**Fig. 2.** Hyperkeratotic, erosive and erythematous lesions associated with hyperhidrosis on fingertips and hypothenar eminences of palmar surfaces in Richner–Hanhart syndrome.

(Goldsmith and Laberge 2005). Other central nervous system alterations include self-mutilating behavior, fine coordination disturbances, convulsions, nystagmus, tremor and ataxia particularly in adult cases (Burns 1972, Pelet et al. 1979, Kato et al. 1993).

## Other organs

Involvement of other organs has been limited to one case with multiple congenital anomalies (Burns 1972).

## Histopathology

Light microscopy of hyperkeratotic lesions shows non-specific changes such as acanthosis with hypergranulosis and hyperkeratosis with parakeratosis (Goldsmith et al. 1973). Electron microscopy of eosinophilic cytoplasmic inclusions in the malphigian layer of the thickened epidermis have been interpreted as tonofilament condensation (Bonhert and Anton-Lamprecht 1982). Recent ultrastructural observations have shown that the cytoplasm of squamous cells and Merkel cells is vacuolated due to the presence of minute tyrosine crystals and that corneocytes contain lipid droplets. Tyrosine crystals have also been demonstrated in the cornea (al-Hemidan and al-Hazzaa 1995, el-Shoura and Tallab 1997, Shimizu et al. 1990).

## Molecular genetics and pathogenesis

RH-S is inherited as an autosomal recessive trait caused by mutations in the gene of the hepatic tyrosine aminotransferase (TAT) which is located on chromosome 16q22.1-q22.3 (Barton et al. 1986, Natt et al. 1986). Until now several different mutations have been identified (Huhn et al. 1998, Westphal et al. 1988) in the TAT gene. Both sexes are equally affected. Consanguinity has been demonstrated in several families (Goldsmith 1985, Goldsmith and Laberge 2005).

Tyrosine aminotransferase (TAT) is a pyridoxine-dependent enzyme that catalyzes the conversion of tyrosine to para-hydroxyphenylpyruvate (PHPPA).

Deficiency of the hepatic cytosolic TAT enzyme leads to accumulation of tyrosine, resulting in increase of plasma (tyrosinemia) and urine (tyrosyluria) tyrosine levels. The increase of urinary tyrosine metabolites such as p-hydroxyphenylacetic acid, N-acetyltyrosine, and p-tyramine is due to the continued tyrosine transamination by the mitochondrial muscular enzyme, aspartate amino transferase (Irons and Harvey 1986, Larregue et al. 1979). The levels of tyrosine in affected tissues may be increased. The excessive saturation of tyrosine in plasma may lead to accumulation of tyrosine in tissues such as the skin and eyes. Clinical manifestations of RH-S are due either to tyrosine or to metabolites. The mechanism of tissue damage may be due to intracellular crystallization of tyrosine. Tyrosine crystals destabilize lysosomes and provoke erythrocyte membranes lyses, releasing cellular proteolytic enzymes that may be the initial step of the inflammatory cascade. Polymorphonuclear-cell infiltrates have been associated with skin lesions (Gipson et al. 1975; Goldsmith 1975, 1976, 1978a, b).

## Diagnosis

Clinically, the diagnosis of tyrosinemia II must be considered in an infant of Italian ancestry with photophobia, redness and lacrimation, during the first months of life. The diagnosis of tyrosinemia II depends upon the demonstration of increased tyrosine in blood, tyrosinemia (normal $<0.18 \,\mu m$) and tyrosine metabolites in urine.

## Differential diagnosis

Presence of focal palmoplantar keratoses and painful blisters should be considered as a differential diagnosis of different forms of focal hereditary palmoplantar keratodermas and blistering diseases, such as epidermolysis bullosa. The eye lesions are frequently first diagnosed as herpetic ulceration.

## Treatment and prognosis

Treatment of tyrosinemia type II consists in a restricted diet in tyrosine and phenylalanine. Early dietary intervention can prevent ocular and cutaneous signs, improve neurological symptoms and prevent mental retardation (Barr 1991, Goldsmith and Laberge 2005). As in other palmoplantar keratodermas topical keratolytics may help. Oral retinoids have provided satisfactory control (Fraser et al. 1987). Diet is difficult to follow up but if strict dietary treatment is not observed, ocular, cutaneous, and neurological changes progress.

## References

Al-Hemidan AL, al-Hazzaa SA (1995) Richner–Hanhart syndrome (Tyrosinemia type II). Case report and literature review. Ophthal Genet 16: 21–26.

Barr DGD, Kirk JM, Laing SC (1991) Outcome of tyrosinaemia type II. Arch Dis Child 66: 1249–1250.

Barton DE, Yang-Feng TL, Francke V (1986) The human tyrosine aminotransferase gene mapped to the long arm of chromosome 16 (region 16q22-q24) by somatic cell hybrid analysis and in situ hybridization. Hum Genet 72: 221.

Bonhert A, Anton-Lamprecht I (1982) Richner–Hanhart's syndrome: ultrastructural abnormalities of epidermal keratinization indicating a causal relationship to high intracellular tyrosine levels. J Invest Dermatol 79: 68–74.

Burns PR (1972) The tyrosine aminotransferase deficiency: an unusual cause of corneal ulcers. Am J Opthalmol 73: 400.

el-Shoura SM, Tallab TM (1997) Richner–Hanhart's syndrome: new ultrastructural observations on skin lesions of two cases. Ultrastruct Pathol 21: 51–56.

Fraser NG, MacDonald J, Griffiths WAD, McPhie JL (1987) Tyrosinaemia type II (Richner–Hanhart syndrome) report of two cases treated with etretinate. Clin Exp Dermatol 12: 440–443.

Gipson IK, Burns RP, Wolfe-Lande JD (1975) Crystals in corneal epithelial lesions of tyrosine fed rats. Invest Ophthalmol 14: 937.

Goldsmith LA, Kang E, Bienfang DC, Jimbow K, Gerald R, Baden HP (1973) Tyrosinaemia with plantar and palmar keratosis and keratitis. J Pediatr 83: 798–805.

Goldsmith LA (1975) Hemolysis and lysosomal activation by solid state tyrosine. Biochem Biophys Res Commun 64: 558.

Goldsmith LA (1976) Haemolysis induced by tyrosine crystals. Modifiers and inhibitors. Biochem J 158: 17.

Goldsmith LA (1978a) Molecular biology and molecular pathology of a newly described molecular disease-tyrosinemia II (the Richner–Hanhart syndrome). Exp Cell Biol 46: 96.

Goldsmith LA (1978b) Tyrosine-induced skin disease. Br J Dermatol 98: 119.

Goldsmith LA, Thorpe J, Roe CR (1979) Hepatic enzymes of tyrosine metabolism in tyrosinaemia II. J Invest Dermatol 73: 530–532.

Goldsmith LA (1985) Tyrosinemia II. A large North Carolina kindred. Arch Intern Med 145: 1697–1700.

Goldsmith LA, Laberge C (2005) Tyrosinemia and related disorders. In: Scriver CR, Beaudet AL, Sly WS, Valle D (eds.) The metabolic basis of inherited disease. 10th ed. New York: McGraw-Hill, pp. 547–562.

Hanhart E (1947) Neue Sonderformen von keratosis palmoplantaris, u. a. eine regelmässig-dominate Form mit systematisierten Lipomen, ferner zwei einfach rezessive, mit Schwachsinn und mit Hornhautveränderungen des Auges (Ektodermalsyndrom). Dermatologica 94: 286–308.

Huhn R, Stoermer H, Klingele B et al. (1998) Novel and recurrent tyrosine aminotransferase gene mutations in tyrosinemia type II. Hum Genet 102: 305–313.

Hunziker N (1980) Richner–Hanhart syndrome and tyrosinemia type II. Dermatologica 160: 180–189.

Irons M, Harvey LL (1986) Metabolic syndromes with dermatological manifestations. Clin Rev Allergy 4: 101–124.

Kato M, Suzuki N, Koeda T (1993) A case of tyrosinemia type II with convulsion and EEG abnormality. No To Hattatsu 25: 558–562.

Larregue M, de Giacomoni PH, Bressieux JM, Odievre M (1979) Syndrome de Richner–Hannart ou tyrosinose oculo-cutanee. Ann Dermatol Vénéréol 106: 53–62.

Macsai MS, Schwartz TL, Hinkle D, Hummel MB, Mulhern MG, Rootman D (2001) Tyrosinemia type II: nine cases of ocular signs and symptoms. Am J Ophthalmol 132: 522–527

Natt E, Kao PT, Rettenmeier R, Scherer G (1986) Assignment of the human tyrosine aminotransferase gene to chromosome 16. Hum Genet 72: 225.

Pelet B, Anteneri L, Faggioni R, Spahr A, Gautier (1979) Tyrosinemia without liver or renal damage with plantar and palmar keratosis and keratitis (hypertyrosinemia). Helv Paediatr Acta 34: 177.

Prader A (1971) Eulogy. Prof Ernst Hanhart 80th year. Schweizerische medizinische Wochenschrift 101/11: 402.

Rehak A, Selim MM, Yadau G (1981) Richner–Hanhart syndrome (Tyrosinemia II). Br J Dermatol 104: 469–475.

Richner H (1938) Hornhautaffektionen bei keratoderma palmare et plantare hereditarium. Klin Monatsbl Augenheilkd 100: 580–588.

Shimizu N, Ito M, ItoK, Nakamura A, Sato Y, Maruyama T (1990) Richner–Hanhart's syndrome: electron microscopic study of the skin lesions. Arch Dermatol 126: 1342.

*Vererbung der Netzhautablösung.* Würzburg (1936) Offprint from Graefes Archiv für Ophthalmologie 135: 49–66 [Medical thesis Zürich with curriculum vitae]

Waardenburg PJ, Franceschetti A, Klein D (1961) Genetics and ophthalmology. Springfield III: Charles C Thomas Publishers, pp. 515–517

Westphal EM, Natt E, Grimm T, Odievre M, Scherer G (1988) The human tyrosine aminotransferase gene: characterization of restriction fragment length polymorphisms and haplotype analysis in a family with tyrosinemia type II. Hum Genet 79: 260–264.

Who named it? (2006) A dictionary of medical biographies. http://www.whonamedit.com

# Chapter 43

# DARIER'S DISEASE

Marimar Saez-De-Ocariz, Luz Orozco-Covarrubias, Carola Durán-McKinster, and Ramón Ruiz-Maldonado

Department of Dermatology, National Institute of Paediatrics, Mexico City, Mexico

## Introduction

*Darier's disease* is an autosomal dominant acantholytic disorder (OMIM # 124200) characterized by a peculiar keratinization of the epidermis, nails, and mucous membranes, resulting in a persistent eruption of keratotic papules predominantly in seborrheic areas (upper and central trunk, flexures, scalp and forehead), palmar pits and nail dystrophy. Involvement may be severe, with widespread itchy malodorous crusted plaques, painful erosions, blistering, and mucosal lesions. Secondary infection is common. Sun, heat, and sweating exacerbate the disease, which never remits (even though oral retinoids may reduce hyperkeratosis). Neuropsychiatric abnormalities including mild mental retardation, epilepsy, and schizophrenia have been reported in some families (Burge and Wilkinson 1992, Jacobsen et al. 1999): whether this association is due to pleiotropism of the mutated gene or reflects coincidence is not clear (OMIM 2006). Several variants have been described (see below).

Ultrastructural and immunologic studies suggest the disease results from an abnormality in the desmosome-keratin filament complex leading to a breakdown in cell adhesion. The disease is caused by mutations in a gene, located on chromosome 12q23-q24.1, which encodes the sarcoplasmic/endoplasmic reticulum $Ca^{++}$-ATPase isoform 2 protein (SERCA2). SERCA2 is a calcium ($Ca^{++}$) ATPase pump that maintains a low cytoplasmic and high extracellular $Ca^{++}$ level by actively transporting calcium ions from the cytoplasm into the lumen of the endoplasmic reticulum: this process is necessary for normal epidermal differentiation and formation (specifically for cell cycle exit and onset of terminal differentiation) (Ahn et al. 2003; Bale and Toro 2000; Berridge 1997; Craddock et al. 1993; Dhitavat et al. 2004; Foggia et al. 2006; Hovanaian 2004; Ikeda et al. 1998; Jacobsen et al. 1999; Lytton and Madennan 1988; Maclennan et al. 1997; Ringpfeil et al. 2001; Ruiz-Perez et al. 1999; Sakuntabhai et al. 1999a, b, 2000; Sehgal and Srivastava 2005; Sheridan et al. 2002; Takahashi et al. 2001; Wakem et al. 1996). The precise mechanism by which decreased activity of the SERCA2-gated calcium pump leads to the pathological changes in Darier's disease is still under investigation (Kwork and Liao 2006): recent tentative explanations have been stress-induced limitation of SERCA levels as extra demands are made on the pump (Byrne 2006) or deficiency in SERCA-gated ER $Ca^{++}$ replenishment due to somatic mutation accumulation (Muller et al. 2006). Notably, family members with conformed identical ATP2A2 mutations can exhibit differences in the clinical severity of disease, suggesting that other genes or environmental factors affect the expression of Darier's disease (OMIM 2006).

## Historical background and eponyms

Darier's disease is also known as keratosis *follicularis* or Darier-White disease because of its first independent description by Darier and White in 1889 (Darier 1889, White 1889).

**Ferdinand-Jean Darier** was a French dermatologist, born on April 26, 1856 in Budapest and died in 1938. He came from a Huguenot family who had emigrated from Dauphine, France. His parents moved to Budapest before his birth, and returned to Geneva when he was eight years of age. By this time he was fluent in Hungarian, French and German. Although he commenced medical studies in Geneva at the early age of 15, he decided to leave for Paris. He became an externe in 1878, Interne des Hôpitaux de Paris in 1880 and later a naturalized Frenchman and settled in Paris. Following his doctoral thesis in Paris in 1885, he joined Ranvier's laboratory in the Collège de France. Darier was head of a medical department in the Hôpital Saint-Louis from 1909 to 1922. He was one of the most brilliant dermatologists of his day, both in clinics and histology. He was the last surviving member of the celebrated «Big Five» – Ernest Henri Besnier (1831–1909), Louis-Anne-Jean Brocq (1856–1928), Darier, Raymond Jacques Adrien Sabouraud (1864–1938), all dermatologists, and Jean Alfred Fournier (1832–1915), whose prime interest was in venereal disease. This group made the Paris school of dermatology one of the most famous of its time. Following his training in Louis Antoine Ranvier's (1835–1922) laboratory in histology he became Médecin des Hôpitaux and worked at La Roche Foucauld, La Pitié, Broca, and finally St. Louis. Although an outstanding clinical dermatologist, Darier's international reputation was based to a large extent upon his endeavors in the field of histopathology. In addition to the conditions that bear his name, he published seminal papers on atrophic lichen planus and cutaneous sarcoidosis, tuberculosis and leprosy. Darier held the conviction that investigations of cutaneous histopathology were an essential part of the diagnostic process. He made extensive use of material of this type in his articles and lectures, and founded the Museum of Histology at the Hôpital St. Louis. He was an innovator in the use of radiotherapy, chemotherapy and vaccines, and his enthusiasm was evident in his lectures, which attracted large audiences. Besides being an extremely cultivated and charming person as well a collector of art crafts he had a very keen sense of humor. In 1921 Darier retired to his country estate in the village of Longpont-sur-Orge, a small town in the Parisian suburban area. He was mayor of the village from 1925 to 1935 and was much concerned with local issues. At the age of 70, Darier was the chief editor of the greatest French dermatological encyclopedia: *Nouvelle Pratique Dermatologique*, 8 volumes published in 1936. This was the standard text of its time (Graham-Little 1938, Mitchell 1960, Who named it? 2006).

**James Clarke White** was an American physician born on July 7, 1833 in Belfast, Maine and died on January 5, 1916 in Boston. He graduated in medicine from Harvard in 1856 and subsequently worked some time in Massachusetts General Hospital, before going to Europe for further studies. After a year, mostly spent in Vienna as a pupil of Ferdinand Ritter von Hebra (1816–1880), he settled in practice in Boston. In 1858 White was appointed instructor in chemistry at the medical school, in 1864 university lecturer in skin diseases, and in 1866 adjunct professor of chemistry. In 1867 White became a physician to the Massachusetts General Hospital, after having been for some years previous chemist to this institution. In 1870 he resigned his former positions, and became physician to the department of skin disease. White, an outstanding personality in American dermatology, in 1871 assumed the first chair of dermatology in America, at Harvard Medical School. Besides this he concerned himself with comparative anatomy, botany, and chemistry. White was one of the publishers of Boston Medical and Surgical Journal, of which he was editor. He was an extraordinarily prolific writer. White was a member of the American Academy of Arts and Sciences, and of various medical societies (Who named it? 2006).

Other eponyms are hypertrophic Darier disease and vesicobullous segmental Darier disease.

## Incidence and prevalence

Darier's disease has a worldwide distribution. Estimates of prevalence vary from 1 in 100,000 in Denmark (Svendsen and Alberchtsen 1959) to 3.8 in 100,000 inhabitants in Slovenia (Godie et al. 2005) and 1 in 30,000 in England and Scotland (Tavadia et al. 2002) with an estimated incidence varying from 3.1 (Goh et al. 2005) to 4 new cases per million per 10 years (Wilkinson et al. 1977). Males and females are almost equally affected: one recent study however recorded a male to female ratio of 4:1 (Goh et al. 2005). The ratio of affected vs. unaffected family members was 0.355 in one study (Godie et al. 2005). Onset is usually before the 3rd decade (>60% of cases according to Godie et al. 2005), however, patients may manifest as early as age 4 years or as late as age 70 years.

## Clinical manifestations

The onset of Darier's disease occurs generally between the ages of 6 and 20 years with a peak around puberty. The majority of patients first become aware of lesions in the second decade of life, although minor lesions or nail or palmar changes may be detected earlier (Burge et al. 1992). The disease is equally prevalent in males and females, although the clinical expression is milder in females (Munro 1992).

Most patients have the classical seborrheic distribution of papules, but there is considerable variation in the severity even within families, from isolated nail or palmar changes, to universal and grossly disfiguring involvement (Burge and Wilkinson 1992, Munro 1992). Burge and Wilkinson (1992) found in their large study of 163 patients with Darier's disease, that 26% of the patients had mild disease, 65% had moderate disease and 9% had severe disease.

The distinctive lesion of Darier's disease is a firm, rough, mildly greasy keratotic papule, either skin-colored, yellow-brown or brown (Fig. 1). Seborrheic areas of the trunk and face, particularly the scalp margins (Fig. 2), temples, ears and scalp, are most often involved. Coalescent papules form irregular warty fissured plaques or papillomatous masses, which, in the flexures, become vegetating and malodorous. Flexural involvement most notably affects the anogenital region, the groins and the natal cleft. On the scalp, the heavy crusting simulates seborrhea, but has a characteristic spiny feeling on palpation. Loss of hair is exceptional. The external auditory meatus may be blocked by keratotic debris. Limb involvement usually takes the form of scattered papules, but confluent lesions on lower legs and arms may be a problem. On the dorsa of the hands and feet, discrete papules are clinically indistinguishable from acrokeratosis verruciformis of Hopf (Fig. 3). The palms and soles may show minute pits or, in older subjects, punctate or filiform keratosis (Burge 1994, Burge and Wilkinson 1992, Sehgal and Srivastava 2005).

Mucous membrane lesions, such as white umbilicated or cobblestone papules affecting the hard palate may be seen in 15% of the patients with Darier's disease (Burge and Wilkinson 1992). Other mucosal involvement: tongue, buccal mucosa, gums, epiglottis, pharyngeal walls (Macleod and Munro 1991), vulva,

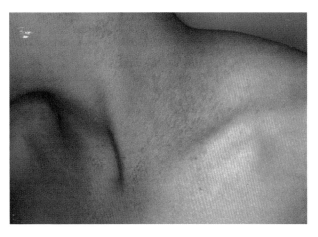

**Fig. 1.** The characteristic greasy keratotic papules of Darier's disease.

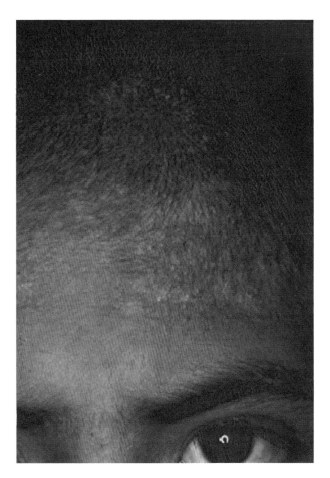

**Fig. 2.** Note the involvement of the scalp and the scalp margins.

esophagus (Al Robaee et al. 2004) or rectum, although uncommon, may be pronounced in some families. The confluence of these papules may mimic leukoplakia.

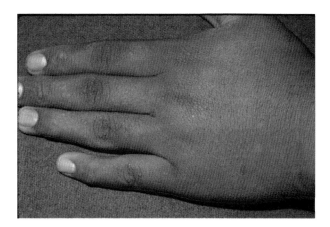

**Fig. 3.** Warty papules on the dorsa of the hands.

Nail involvement includes red or white longitudinal lines of varying width, extending from the base of the nail across the lunula to the free margin of the nail, nail fragility, V-shaped notches at the free edge of the nail, longitudinal ridging of the nail, painful splits, and subungual hyperkeratotic fragments (Burge and Wilkinson 1992, Richert 2000, Sehgal and Srivastava 2005, Zaias and Ackerman 1973).

## Clinical variants

The disease pattern may be classified as:

a) *Seborrheic*: it is the most common disease pattern, being observed in nearly 90% of the patients and is characterized by keratotic papules located on the center of the chest, back, hair margin, supraclavicular fossae and neck, scalp and ears (Fig. 4). There is usually a clear cut-off point at the sacrum, with involvement of the buttocks being clearly unusual (Burge and Wilkinson 1992).

b) *Flexural*: this pattern predominates in up to 6% of patients with Darier's disease (Burge and Wilkinson 1992) and it is characterized by malodorous, fleshy, papillomatous masses in the axillae and groins with extension to the perineum. There may be mild involvement with keratotic papules on the trunk.

c) *Linear or nevoid*: it presents with keratotic lesions disposed in a unilateral, linear, zosteriform or lo-

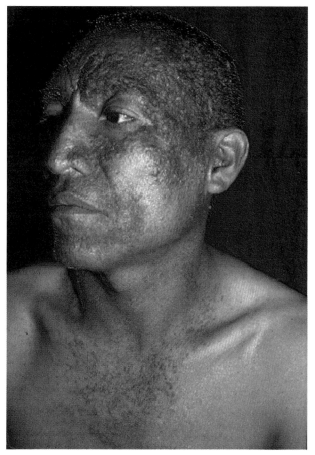

**Fig. 4.** Moderate to severe seborrheic pattern in an adult male.

calized pattern, possessing features of dyskeratotic acantholysis. Debate is often created about whether it is a localized Darier's disease or an acantholytic dyskeratotic epidermal nevus. Since the lesions follow Blaschko lines, are commonly of late onset and display photoaggravation, it is suggested they are nevoid forms of Darier's disease due to genetic mosaicism for this autosomal disorder, representing a type 2 segmental manifestation of the disease (Boente et al. 2004, Happle et al. 1999, Itin et al. 2000, O'Malley et al. 1997).

d) *Acral*: it is characterized by warty to convex, brownish to skin-colored papules on the dorsa of the hands and feet (Happle et al. 1999, Hur et al. 1994, Romano et al. 1999). This clinical pattern may be the sole manifestation of the disease, but it may also precede the development of Darier's disease in up to 13% of the patients (Burge and Wilkinson 1992).

e) *Familial hemorrhagic variant*: it is expressed consistently by all affected members within families and is characterized by hemorrhagic macules on hands and feet (Foresman et al. 1993, Jorg et al. 2000). Macules usually have angular outlines and are occasionally associated with blistering (Burge et al. 1992).

f) *Comedonal*: some patients present with multiple comedones or nodulocystic acne with deep pitted scars. A typical histology of Darier's disease may be found in these lesions (Derrick et al. 1995).

g) *Other patterns*: vesiculobullous (Colver and Gawkrodger 1992, Speight 1998, Telfer et al. 1990), cornifying (Katta et al. 2000), or Darier's disease restricted to sun-exposed areas (Kimoto et al. 2004) have been described in literature.

Some authors have described the occurrence of café-au-lait (Soroush and Gurevitch 1997) and leukodermic macules (Bleiker and Burns 1998, Gupta and Shaw 2003), or Darier's disease localized to the cervix (Adam 1996), breast (Fitzgerald and Lewis-Jones 1997) and vulva (Salopek et al. 1993). Typical histological features of Darier's disease have been demonstrated in all these lesions.

## Histopathological features

The characteristic changes in Darier's disease on light microscopy are: a peculiar form of dyskeratosis resulting in the formation of "corps ronds" and grains (eosinophilic dyskeratotic cells confined to the granular layer and the stratum corneum, respectively); suprabasal acantholysis leading to the formation of suprabasal clefts or lacunae (Fig. 5); and irregular upward projection into the lacunae of papillae lined with a single layer of basal cells (villi). The extent of the cleavage is variable and is occupied by acantholytic cells of diverse morphology (Sehgal and Srivastava 2005, Johnson and Honig 1997).

Electron microscopy studies reveal basal cell vacuolation, a decreased number of desmosomes on the lateral border of the basal cells, separation of

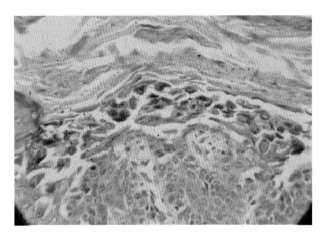

**Fig. 5.** Eosinophilic dyskeratotic cells in the granular layer ("corps ronds"), suprabasal acantholysis with cleft formation.

tonofilaments from their insertion on the cell membrane, and large circular aggregates around the nucleus (Burge and Schomberg 1992, Sehgal and Srivastava 2005, Watt et al. 1984).

The hyperkeratotic papules on the dorsa of the hands and feet reveal church-spurt-like epidermal changes. On serial sectioning, they show mild dyskeratotic changes and often suprabasal clefts, as well (Johnson and Honig 1997).

The histopathologic evidence suggests that Darier's disease is not a disorder of keratinization, but a disruption of the desmosomal junction, resulting in adhesion problems and acantholysis. Darier's disease shows haplo-insufficiency (a deficiency of one copy of the gene) and this suggests that, in complex membrane structures in which ATPases function, they are insufficient, so that a combination of half the normal gene product with another factor, such as UVB or mechanical trauma, may cause the clinical phenotype (Hedblad et al. 1991, Ruiz-Perez et al. 1999).

## Pathogenesis and molecular genetics

Darier's disease is an autosomal dominant disorder (OMIM # 124200) determined by mutations in a gene of variable penetrance located on chromosome 12q23-24.1 (Craddock et al. 1993, Ruiz-Perez et al.

1999). The Darier's disease gene encodes the sarcoplasmic/endoplasmic reticulum calcium ATPase type 2 (SERCA2) (Bale and Toro 2000, Sakuntabhai et al. 1999b). SERCA2 is member of a family of ion pumps that maintains low intracellular (and high extracellular) calcium levels (Foggia and Hovnanian 2004, Maclennan et al. 1997). This calcium ATPase pump has two isoforms which differ only in the C-terminal domains: SERCA2a is expressed in cardiac and smooth muscle, whereas SERCA2b is more widely expressed in the body, including the epidermis (Lytton and Maclennon 1988, Ruiz-Perez et al. 1999). Darier's disease is caused by a variety of missense, nonsense, frameshift and splicing mutations, that result in an abnormally expressed protein (Sakuntabhai et al. 2000, Sehgal and Srivastava 2005, Sheridan et al. 2002).

Keratinocyte differentiation, adhesion and motility are directed by extracellular $Ca^{++}$ concentration increases, which in turn increase intracellular $Ca^{++}$ levels. Normal keratinocytes, in contrast to most non-excitable cells, require $Ca^{++}$ release from both Golgi and endoplasmic reticulum $Ca^{++}$ stores for efficient $Ca^{++}$ signaling. Mutations in ATP2A2 have been suggested to cause acantholysis in Darier's disease through haploinsufficiency, resulting in impaired uptake of cytosolic calcium into the endoplasmic reticulum, and consequent disruption of calcium signaling (Sakuntabhai et al. 1999b), conferring a direct effect on the established calcium-dependent assembly of desmosomes (Dhitavat et al. 2004, Ringpfeil et al. 2001). A compensatory upregulation of the human secretory pathway $Ca^{++}$ ATPase hSPCA1, encoded by the ATP2C1 gene, maintains viability and partially compensate for defective SERCA2 ATPase in Darier's disease keratinocytes (Foggia et al. 2006, Pani and Singh 2008).

The control of cytoplasmic calcium signaling however is complex (Ahn et al. 2003, Berridge 1997, Hovnanian 2004) and the sequence and details of the pathogenic mechanism in Darier's disease needs to be elucidated. Byrne in 2006 has reviewed the mechanistic links between stress, calcium pumps and calcium levels: according to one hypothesis the disease manifests in stress-induced lesions because SERCA levels become limiting as extra demands are made on the pump in time of stress. Muller et al. (2006), using a novel animal model for depleted keratinocyte SERCA-gated $Ca^{++}$ stores, showed that keratinocytes from Darier-like lesions retain their distinctive phenotype after culture, thus hypothesizing that deficiencies in SERCA-gated ER $Ca^{++}$ replenishment might be due to somatic mutation accumulation.

To date comparison of molecular data and phenotypic features, such as severity and type of disease, occurrence of mucosal involvement, or association with neuropsychiatric disorders, has not revealed consistent or obvious genotype-phenotype correlations (Ringpfeil et al. 2001, Sakuntabhai et al. 1999a). For instance, in the study conducted by Jacobsen et al. (1999), mutation analysis in patients with Darier's disease and neuropsychiatric phenotypes revealed a non-random clustering of mutations in the 3' end of the gene and a predominance of the missense type of mutations (70 vs. 38% in Darier's patients). On the other hand, Ruiz-Perez et al. (1999) did not find any specific class of mutation associated with neuropsychiatric features, whereas they found a clear association with the familial hemorrhagic variant where all families tested had a missense mutation.

## Associated features

The wide expression of SERCA2 might suggest that ATP2A2 mutations could cause a multisystemic disease. Fortunately there are no consistent extracutaneous manifestations of Darier's disease.

Transgenic mice haplo-insufficient for SERCA2 display impaired cardiac contractility (Periasamy et al. 1999) and an increased incidence of gastroesophageal and other squamous cancers (Liu et al. 2001). Tavadia et al. (2001) found no evidence for altered cardiac function in 10 patients with two-dimensional color and Doppler echocardiography, nor consistent defects in platelet function in 12 patients using bleeding time and aggregation studies. These facts suggest that SERCA2 function in humans appears to be largely compensated by other genes or epigenetic factors, as there is no evidence of a consistent cardiac problem and an increased incidence of cancer has not been documented, and that the skin is sensitive to defects in SERCA2 function to which other organs and/or systems seem immune (Sehgal and Srivastava 2005).

Isolated reports have recorded the involvement of bones and other systems: chronic renal failure, epilepsy, cataract, corneal opacity, and mental retardation (Al-Homrany et al. 1997, Sehgal and Srivastava 2005).

The assessment of neuropsychiatric features in Darier's disease remains problematic. Despite a number of clinical studies having described the co-occurrence of various neurological and psychiatric symptoms in Darier's disease, including mood disorders, a high prevalence of epilepsy, mental retardation and a slowly progressive encephalopathy, it is hard to confirm that mild defects are due to the disease without careful psychometric testing (Ruiz-Perez et al. 1999).

A higher frequency of bipolar affective disorders, depression (Cordeiro et al. 2000), schizophrenia, psychosis, and suicidal tendencies have all been recorded in Darier's disease patients (Burge et al. 1992, Sehgal and Srivastava 2005). Co-segregation of bipolar affective disorder and Darier's disease has prompted to look for the gene of bipolar disorder in chromosome 12. Even when initial linkage studies have implicated the region 12q23-q24.1 as harboring a susceptibility gene for bipolar affective disorder (Craddock et al. 1994, Ewald et al. 1994, Jones et al. 2002, Sidenberg et al. 1994), new data has shown no evidence for the involvement of ATP2A2 in producing susceptibility to bipolar disorder (Jacobsen et al. 2001).

Most patients with Darier's disease are of normal intellect, but clinical experience suggests that mild degrees of learning difficulty are common. Mental retardation, usually of mild-moderate severity has been reported repeatedly in association with Darier's disease patients or their families (Burge 1994, Jacobsen et al. 1999, Svedsen and Alberchtsen 1959).

Epilepsy has been described at an increased prevalence in a cohort of patients with Darier's disease compared with the general population (42.9/1000 vs. 1–7/1000 in general population), although this association is not clearly related with a specific subtype of epilepsy (Burge et al. 1992).

There is one report in the literature of unilateral Darier's disease associated with contralateral migraine headache, both responsive to isotretinoin, and recurrent concurrently after discontinuation of isotretinoin (Rotunda et al. 2005). The authors suggest the findings of Darier's disease and migraine in this patient may represent a true pathogenic relationship, or reflect an alteration in calcium homeostasis lowering migraine headache threshold. It should be kept in mind that migraine is a potential co-morbid condition with Darier's disease.

The nature of the association of neuropsychiatric disorders with Darier's disease remains elusive. It is now believed that Darier's disease gene has pleiotropic effects in brain and that mutations in SERCA2 are implicated in the pathogenesis of neuropsychiatric disorders (Jacobsen et al. 1999). Neuropsychiatric features may be an intrinsic, but inconsistent consequence of defective ATP2A2 expression along with concomitant genetic and environmental factors (Ruiz-Perez et al. 1999).

## Natural history

The disease usually runs a chronic relapsing course with exacerbations and remissions, and general health is normally unaffected. Only one third of patients note improvement with age (Burge and Wilkinson 1992).

Seasonal variations have a definitive effect on the natural history of the disease. Almost all patients have worse symptoms during the summer, due to the heat and humidity. Other precipitating factors are UVB light exposure (Burge and Schomberg 1992, Burge and Wilkinson 1992, Kimoto et al. 2004, Sehgal and Srivastava 2005), mechanical trauma, oral lithium, phenol and steroids for nevoid disease (Burge and Wilkinson 1992, Sehgal and Srivastava 2005). Despite the absence of consistent immunologic abnormalities, the frequent occurrence of herpes simplex and various bacteriologic infections may exacerbate the condition. Occasionally, spontaneous remissions may occur and the course may be influenced by treatment (Burge and Wilkinson 1992).

## Complications

Cell mediated immunity of Darier's disease patients with bacterial and viral infections is usually normal, except for a few reports in which defects in cell-mediated immunity have been reported (Burge and Wilkinson 1992, Sehgal and Srivastava 2005). An increased susceptibility to herpes simplex infection, Kaposi's varicelliform eruption (Hur et al. 1994) and pox virus infections occasionally complicate the chronic course of the disease. There may also be an increased incidence of chronic pyogenic infection. Salivary gland swelling is an unusual complication in certain families. Histologic examination of the salivary ducts revealed squamous metaplasia with Darier like changes (Burge and Wilkinson 1992).

## Differential diagnosis

In mild forms, acne and seborrheic dermatitis may be confused, unless the warty papules are carefully sought. Flexural Darier's disease may overlap clinically and histologically with benign familial pemphigus but patients with intertriginous Darier's disease have changes typical of Darier's disease elsewhere and the age of onset is usually earlier (Johnson and Honig 1997). The localized form of Darier's disease needs to be differentiated from epidermal nevi.

*Acrokeratosis verruciformis of Hopf* is a rare autosomal dominant genodermatosis. It usually develops during early childhood affecting both sexes equally (OMIM # 101900) (OMIM 2006). Typically, lesions are warty to convex, brownish to skin-colored papules on the dorsa of the hands and feet, forearms and legs (Bukhari 2004). Although histology of acrokeratosis verruciformis lesions shows no evidence of dyskeratosis, a possible relationship with Darier's disease has long been postulated on the basis of clinical similarity. Recently, it was demonstrated that SERCA2 is mutated in AV, providing evidence that AV and Darier's disease are allelic disorders (Dhitavat et al. 2003) even though genetic heterogeneity is likely (Wang et al. 2006).

## Treatment

The treatment of Darier's disease corresponds to its severity. Both itching and body malodor are a usual complaint in patients with Darier's disease (Burg and Wilkinson 1992) and may be particularly distressing problems.

Many patients with mild disease require no treatment other than emollients, simple hygiene and advice to avoid sunburn. Topical tretinoin and isotretinoin, adapalene and tazarotene have been reported as effective. In practice, irritancy limits the value of most topical preparations and extra emollients are needed. Antiseptics may help with infected plaques which may respond to topical steroid-antibiotic combinations (Burge 1999, Burge and Wilkinson 1992, Sehgal and Sivristava 2005, Wicks 2002).

For those with more severe disease, oral retinoids are usually effective. Both acitretin and isotretinoin may be used (Christophersen et al. 1992). Dermabrasion in limited areas may prove useful to smooth the keratotic papules and plaques (Sehgal and Sivristava 2005). Laser therapy has also shown some promising results (Beier and Kauffman 1999). Severe inflammatory exacerbations of Darier's disease occur in some patients, and have responded to cyclosporin. In a recent report, radiotherapy treatment for bronchial carcinoma in a patient with Darier's disease cleared the lesions after initial aggravation, and may also be considered for some patients (MacManus et al. 2001).

It is expected that knowledge on the molecular aspects of Darier's disease will yield more successful therapies in the near future.

## References

Adam AE (1996) Ectopic Darier's disease of the cervix: an extraordinary cause of an abnormal smear. Cytopathology 7: 414–421.

Ahn W, Lee MG, Kim KH, Muallem S (2003) Multiple effects of SERCA2b mutations associated with Darier's disease. J Biol Chem 278: 20795–20801.

Al-Homrany M, Taliab T, Bahamadan KA (1997) Darier-White disease in a French patient with systemic involvement. Afr J Med Sci 26: 195–196.

Al Robaee A, Hamadah IR, Khuroo S, Alfadley A (2004) Extensive Darier's disease with esophageal involvement. Int J Dermatol 43: 835–839.

Bale SJ, Toro JR (2000) Genetic basis of Darier-White disease: bad pumps cause bumps. J Cutan Med Surg 4: 103–106.

Beier C, Kaufmann R (1999) Efficacy of erbium YAG laser ablation in Darier's disease and Hailey–Hailey disease. Arch Dermatol 135: 423–427.

Berridge MJ (1997) Elementary and global aspects of calcium signaling. J Physiol 499: 291–306.

Bleiker To, Burns DA (1998) Darier's disease with hypopigmented macules. Br J Dermatol 138: 913–914.

Boente MC, Frontini MV, Primic NB, Asial RA (2004) Linear Darier disease in two siblings. An example of loss of heterozygosity. Ann Dermatol Venereol 131: 805–809.

Bukhari I (2004) Acrokeratosis verruciformis of Hopf: a localized variant. J Drugs Dermatol 3: 687–688.

Burge S (1994) Darier's disease – the clinical features and pathogenesis. Clin Exp Dermatol 19: 193–205.

Burge S (1999) Management of Darier's disease. Clin Exp Dermatol 24: 53–56.

Burge S, Schomberg K (1992) Adhesion molecules and related proteins in Darier's disease. Br J Dermatol 127: 335–343.

Burge SM, Wilkinson JD (1992) Darier-White disease: a review of the clinical features in 163 patients. J Am Acad Dermatol 27: 40–50.

Byrne CR (2006) The focal nature of Darier's disease lesions: calcium pumps, stress, and mutation? J Invest Dermatol 126: 702–703.

Christophersen J, Geiger JM, Danneskiold-Sansoe P, Kragballe K, Larsen FG, Laurberg G, Serup J, Thomsen K (1992) A double-blind comparison of acitretin and etretinate in the treatment of Darier's disease. Acta Derm Venereol 72: 150–152.

Colver GB, Gawkrodger DJ (1992) Vesiculobullous Darier's disease. Br J Dermatol 126: 416–417.

Cordeiro Q Jr, Werebe DM, Vallada H (2000) Darier's disease: a new paradigm for genetic studies in psychiatric disorders. Sao Paulo Med J 118: 201–203.

Craddock N, Dawson E, Burge S, Parfitt L, Mant B, Roberts Q, Daniels J, Gill M, McGuffin P, Powell J (1993) The gene for Darier's disease maps to chromosome 12q23-q24.1. Hum Mol Genet 2: 1941–1943.

Craddock N, Owen M, Burge S, Kurian B, Thomas P, McGuffin P (1994) Familial cosegregation of major affective disorder and Darier's disease (keratosis foliculalis). Br J Psychiatry 164: 355–358.

Darier J (1889) Psorospermose folliculaire végétante. Ann Dermatol Syphilol 10: 597–612.

Derrick EK, Darley CR, Burge S (1995) Comedonal Darier's disease. Br J Dermatol 132: 453–455.

Dhitavat J, Macfarlane S, Dode L, Leslie N, Sakuntabhai A, MacSween R, Saihan E, Hovnanian A (2003) Acrokeratosis verruciformis of Hopf is caused by mutation in ATP2A2: evidence that it is allelic to Darier's disease. J Invest Dermatol 120: 229–232.

Dhitavat J, Fairclough RJ, Hovnanian A, Burge S (2004) Calcium pumps and keratinocytes: lessons from Darier's disease and Hailey–Hailey disease. Br J Dermatol 150: 821–828.

Ewald H, Mors O, Flint T, Fruse TA (1994) Linkage analysis between maniac depressive illness and the region on chromosome 12q involved in Darier's disease. Psychiatr Genet 4: 195–200.

Fitzgerald DA, Lewis-Jones MS (1997) Darier's disease presenting as isolated hyperkeratosis of the breast. Br J Dermatol 7: 414–421.

Foggia L, Hovnanian A (2004) Calcium pump disorders of the skin. Am J Med Genet C Semin Med Genet 131C: 20–31.

Foggia L, Aronchik I, Aberg Km Brown B, Hovnanian A, Mauro TM (2006) Activity of the hSPCA1 Golgi $Ca^{2+}$ pump is essential for $Ca^{2+}$ response and cell viability in Darier disease. J Cell Sci 119: 671–679.

Foresman PL, Goldsmith LA, Ginn L, Beck AL (1993) Hemorrhagic Darier's disease. Arch Dermatol 129: 511–512.

Godie A, Milikovic J, Kansky A, Vidmat G (2005) Epidemiology of Darier's disease in Slovenia. Acta Dermatoven APA 14: 43–48.

Goh BK, Ang P, Goh CL (2005) Darier's disease in Singapore. Br J Dermatol 152: 284–288.

Graham-Little EG (1938) Obituary. Br J Dermatol 50: 384–389.

Gupta S, Shaw JC (2003) Unilateral Darier's disease with unilateral guttate leukoderma. J Am Acad Dermatol 48: 955–957.

Happle R, Itin PH, Brun AM (1999) Type 2 segmental Darier's disease. Eur J Dermatol 9: 449–451.

Hedblad MA, Nakatani T, Beitner H (1991) Ultrastructural changes in Darier's disease induced by ultraviolet irradiation. Acta Derm Venereol 71: 108–112.

Hovnanian A (2004) Darier's disease: form dyskeratosis to endoplasmic reticulum calcium ATPase deficiency. Biochem Biophys Res Commun 322: 1237–1244.

Hur W, Lee WS, Ahn SK (1994) Acral Darier's disease: report of a case complicated by Kaposi's varicelliform eruption. J Am Acad Dermatol 30: 860–862.

Ikeda S, Shigihara T, Ogawa H, Haake A, Polakowska R, Roublevskaia I, Wakem P, Goldsmith LA, Epstein E Jr (1998) Narrowing of the Darier's disease gene interval on chromosome 12q. J Invest Dermatol 110: 847–848.

Itin PH, Buchner SA, Happle R (2000) Segmental manifestation of Darier's disease. What is the genetic background in type 1 and type 2 mosaic phenotypes? Dermatology 200: 254–257.

Jacobsen N, Lyons I, Hoogendoorn B, Burge S, Kwok PY, O'Donovan MC, Craddock N, Owen MJ (1999) ATP2A2 mutations in Darier's disease and their relationship to neuropsychiatric phenotypes. Hum Mol Genet 8: 1631–1636.

Jacobsen NJ, Franks EK, Elvidge G et al. (2001) Exclusion of the Darier's disease gene, ATP2A2, as a common susceptibility gene for bipolar disorder. Mol Psychiatry 6: 92–97.

Johnson B, Honig P (1997) Congenital Diseases (Genodermatoses). In: Elder D, Elenitsas R, Jaworsky C, Johnson B (eds.) Lever's Histopathology of the Skin. 8th ed. Philadelphia: Lippincott-Raven, pp. 132–134.

Jones I, Jacobsen NJ, Green EK, Elvidge GP, Owen MJ, Craddock N (2002) Evidence for familial cosegregation of major affective disorder and genetic markers flanking the gene for Darier's disease. Mol Psychiatry 7: 424–427.

Jorg B, Erhard H, Rutten A (2000) A hemorrhagic acral form of dyskeratosis follicularis Darier. Hautarzt 51: 857–861.

Katta R, Reed J, Wolf JE (2000) Cornifying Darier's disease. Int J Dermatol 39: 844–845.

Kimoto M, Akiyama M, Matsuo I (2004) Darier's disease restricted to sun-exposed areas. Clin Exp Dermatol 29: 37–39.

Kwork PI, Liao W (2006) Keratosis follicularis (Darier disease). e-Medicine from WebMD. http://www.emedicine.com/DERM/topic209.htm

Liu LH, Boivin GP, Prasad V, Periasamy M, Shull GE (2001) Squamous cell tumors in mice heterozygous for a null allele of ATP2A2 encoding the sarco(endo)plasmic reticulum $Ca^{2+}$-ATPase isoform 2 $Ca^{2+}$ pump. J Biol Chem 276: 26737–26740.

Lytton J, MacLennan DH (1988) Molecular cloning of cDNAs from human kidney coding for two alternatively spliced products of the cardiac $Ca^{2+}$-ATPase gene. J Biol Chem 263: 15024–15031.

Maclennan DH, Rice WJ, Green NM (1997) The mechanism of $Ca^{2+}$ transport by sarco (endo)plasmic reticulum $Ca^{2+}$ ATPases. J Biol Chem 272: 28815–28818.

Macleod RJ, Munro CS (1991) The incidence and distribution of oral lesions in patients with Darier's disease. Br Dent J 171: 133–136.

MacManus MP, Cavalleri G, Ball DL, Beasley M, Rotstein H, McKay MJ (2001) Exacerbation, then clearance of mutation-proved Darier's disease of the skin after radiotherapy for bronchial carcinoma: a case of radiation-induced epidermal differentiation? Radiat Res 156: 724–730.

Mitchell JH (1960) Some French dermatologists I have known. Arch Dermatol 81: 962–968.

Muller EJ, Caldelari R, Kolly C, Williamson L, Baumann D, Richard G, Jensen P, Girling P, Delprincipe F, Wyder M, Balmer V, Suter MM (2006) Consequences of depleted SERCA2-gated calcium stores in the skin. J Invest Dermatol 126: 721–723.

Munro CS (1992) The phenotype of Darier's disease: penetrance and expressivity in adults and children. Br J Dermatol 127: 126–130.

O'Malley MP, Haake A, Goldsmith L, Berg D (1997) Localized Darier's disease. Implications for genetic studies. Arch Dermatol 133: 1134–1138.

OMIM TM (2006) Online Mendelian Inheritance in Man. Baltimore: Johns Hopkins University Press: http://www.ncbi.nlm.nih.gov/omim

Pani B, Singh BB (2008) Darier's disease: a calcium-signaling perspective. Cell Mol Life Sci 65: 205–211.

Periasamy M, Reed TD, Liu LH, Ji Y, Loukianov E, Paul RJ, Nieman ML, Riddle T, Duffy JJ, Doetschman T, Lorenz JN, Shull GE (1999) Impaired cardiac performance in heterozygous mice with a null mutation in the sarco(endo)plasmic reticulum $Ca^{2+}$-ATPase isoform 2 (SERCA2) gene. J Biol Chem 274: 2556–2562.

Richert B (2000) Nail localization of dermatoses. Rev Prat 50: 2231–2235.

Ringpfeil F, Raus A, DiGiovanna J, Korge B, Harth W, Mazzanti C, Uitto J, Bale SJ, Richard G (2001) Darier disease – novel mutations in ATP2A2 and genotype-phenotype correlation. Exp Dermatol 10: 19–27.

Romano C, Massai L, Alessandrini C et al. (1999) A case of acral Darier's disease. Dermatology 199: 365–368.

Rotunda AM, Cotliar J, Haley JC, Craft N (2005) Unilateral Darier's disease associated with migraine headache responsive to isotretinoin. J Am Acad Dermatol 52: 175–176.

Ruiz-Perez V, Carter S, Healy E (1999) ATP2A2 mutations in Darier's disease: variant cutaneous phenotypes are associated with missense mutations, but neuropsychiatric features are independent of mutation class. Hum Mol Genet 8: 1621–1630.

Sakuntabhai A, Burge S, Monk S, Hovnanian A (1999a) Spectrum of novel ATP2A2 mutations in patients with Darier's disease. Hum Mol Genet 8: 1611–1619.

Sakuntabhai A, Ruiz-Perez V, Carter S, Jacobsen N, Burge S, Monk S, Smith M, Munro CS, O'Donovan M, Craddock N, Kucherlapati R, Rees JL, Owen M, Lathrop GM, Monaco AP, Strachan T, Hovnanian A et al. (1999b) Mutations in ATP2A2, encoding a $Ca^{2+}$ pump, cause Darier's disease. Nat Genet 21: 271–277.

Sakuntabhai A, Dhitavat J, Burge S, Hovnanian A (2000) Mosaicism for ATP2A2 mutations causes segmental Darier's disease. J Invest Dermatol 115: 1144–1147.

Salopek TG, Krol A, Jimbow K (1993) Case report of Darier's disease localized to the vulva in a 5 year-old girl. Pediatr Dermatol 10: 146–148.

Sehgal V, Srivastava G (2005) Darier's (Darier-White) disease/keratosis follicularis. Int J Dermatol 44: 184–192.

Sheridan AT, Hollowood K, Sakuntabhai A, Dean D, Hovnanian A, Burge S (2002) Expression of sarco/endo-plasmic reticulum $Ca^{2+}$-ATPase type 2 isoforms (SERCA2) in normal human skin and mucosa, and Darier's disease skin. Br J Dermatol 147: 670–674.

Sidenberg DG, Berg D, Bassett AS, King N, Petronis A, Kamble AB, Kennedy JL et al. (1994) Genetic linkage evaluation of twenty-four loci in an eastern Canadian family segregating Darier's disease (keratosis follicularis). J Am Acad Dermatol 31: 27–30.

Soroush V, Gurevitch AW (1997) Darier's disease associated with multiple café-au-lait- macules. Cutis 59: 193–195.

Speight EL (1998) Vesiculobullous Darier's disease responsive to oral prednisolone. Br J Dermatol 139: 934–935.

Svendsen I, Alberchtsen B (1959) The prevalence of dyskeratosis follicularis in Denmark. An investigation into heredity in 22 families. Acta Derm Venereol 39: 256–259.

Takahashi H, Atrsuta Y, Sato K (2001) Novel mutation of ATP2A2 gene in Japanese patients of Darier's disease. J Dermatol Sci 26: 169–172.

Tavadia S, Tait RC, McDonagh TA, Munro CS (2001) Platelet and cardiac function in Darier's disease. Clin Exp Dermatol 26: 696–699.

Tavadia S, Mortimer E, Munro CS (2002) Genetic epidemiology of Darier's disease: a population study in the west of Scotland. Br J Dermatol 146: 107–109.

Telfer NR, Burge SM, Ryan JJ (1990) Vesiculobullous Darier's disease. Br J Dermatol 122: 831–834.

Wakem P, Ikeda P, Haake A, Polakowska R, Ewing N, Sarret Y, Duvic M, Berg D, Bassett A, Kennedy JL, Tuskis A, Epstein EH Jr, Goldsmith LA (1996) Localization of the Darier's disease gene to a 2-cm portion of 12q23-24.1. J Invest Dermatol 106: 365–367.

Wang PG, Gao M, Lin GS, Yang S, Lin D, Liang YH, Zhang GL, Zhu YG, Cui Y, Zhang KY, Huang W, Zhang XJ (2006) Genetic heterogeneity in acrokeratosis verruciformis of Hopf. Clin Exp Dermatol 31: 558–563.

Watt FM, Mattey DL, Garrod DR (1984) Calcium-induced reorganization of desmosomal components in cultured human keratinocytes. J Cell Biol 99: 2211–2215.

White JC (1889) A case of keratosis (icthyosis) follicularis. Cutan Genitourin Dis 7: 201–209.

Who named it? (2006) A dictionary of medical biographies. http://www.whonamedit.com

Wicks G (2002) Meeting the complex care needs of a patient with Darier's disease. J Wound Care 11: 330–332.

Wilkinson JD, Marsden RA, Dawber RPR (1977) Review of Darier's in the Oxford region. Br J Dermatol Suppl 15: 15–16.

Zaias N, Ackerman AB (1973) The nail changes in Darier-White disease. Arch Dermatol 107: 193–197.

# Chapter 44

# DYSKERATOSIS CONGENITA

Marimar Saez-De-Ocariz, Luz Orozco-Covarrubias, Carola Durán-McKinster, and Ramón Ruiz-Maldonado

Department of Dermatology, National Institute of Paediatrics, Mexico City, Mexico

## Introduction

Dyskeratosis congenita (DKC) is a rare genodermatosis with multisystemic, life-threatening complications characterized by atrophy and pigmentation of the skin, nail dystrophy, leukoplakia of the oral mucosa, bone marrow failure and a predisposition to malignancy. Other clinical manifestations may include continuous lacrimation due to atresia of the lacrimal ducts, lung fibrosis, liver cirrhosis, osteoporosis and various neurological abnormalities including mental retardation and basal ganglia calcification (Chan 2006, Mason et al. 2005, Scoggings et al. 1971, Walne et al. 2005). The clinical picture often resembles that of a premature aging syndrome and tissues affected are those with a high cell turnover.

Most reported cases have been in males, although either the full syndrome and some partial forms with only pigmentary changes have occurred in females (Sirinavin and Trowbridge 1975). X-linked (Zinsser-Cole-Engman syndrome) (OMIM # 305000), autosomal dominant (Dyskeratosis congenita Scoggins type) (Scoggins et al. 1971) (OMIM # 127550) and autosomal recessive (OMIM # 224230) forms are recognized (Bessler et al. 2004, Mason et al. 2005, Walne et al. 2005) and the disease has been linked to mutations in at least four distinct genes, three of which have been identified (Bessler et al. 2004, Dokal and Vulliamy 2003, Elliot et al. 1999, Heiss et al. 1998, Hofer et al. 2005, Knight et al. 1999b, Marrone and Dokal 2004, Marrone and Mason 2003, Marrone et al. 2004, Mochizuki et al. 2004, Tchou and Kohn 1982, Vulliamy et al. 2004). The gene that is mutated in the *X-linked form* (OMIM # 305000) of the disease is DKC1 located on chromosome Xq28: the DKC1-encoded protein, *dyskerin*, is a component of small

nucleolar ribonucleoprotein particles, which are important in ribosomal RNA processing, and of the telomerase complex. The *autosomal dominant form* (OMIM # 127550) is due to mutations in the gene for the RNA component of telomerase (*TERC*) located on chromosome 3q21-q28. The gene or genes involved in the *autosomal recessive form* (OMIM # 224230) remain elusive, although genes whose products are required for telomere maintenance remain strong candidates.

## Historical perspective and eponyms

Dyskeratosis congenita was first described in 1906 by Zinsser, and later by Cole et al. (1930) and Engman (1926). The X-linked form is still named Zinsser-Cole-Engman syndrome while the autosomal dominant form is also named Scoggings syndrome (Scoggins et al. 1971) (OMIM™ 2006).

**Ferdinand Zinsser** was a German dermatologist, born on February 11, 1865, in New York and died in 1952. He was the son of Friedrich Zinsser (born 1837) and Auguste Balser. His father had studied medicine in Giessen and Würzburg and emigrated to America after receiving his doctorate. The family later returned to Germany and settled in Wiesbaden. Ferdinand Zinsser studied at the Universities of Bonn, Munich, and Heidelberg, where he obtained his doctorate in 1891. He worked in the university medical clinic in Leipzig under Hans Curschmann (1875–1950) as well as in the university dermatological clinic in Bern under Edmund Lesser (1852–1918). In 1904 he became Docent in dermatology at the academy of practical medicine in Cologne and in 1908 professor. In 1919 he was appointed ordentlicher Professor of skin and venereal diseases at the newly founded university. He was emerited in 1931.

**Harold Newton Cole** was a Professor of Dermatology at Western Reserve University in the 1920s and 1930s. He was born in 1884 in New Orleans, Louisiana and died in 1968.

**Martin Feeney Engman** was an American dermatologist, born on August 20, 1869 in New Orleans, Louisiana and died in 1953. Engman attended the University of New York, where he obtained his doctorate in 1891, before continuing his studies at Heidelberg, Paris, Berlin, and Hamburg. He settles as a specialist of dermatology in St. Louis, representing dermatology at the Washington University, St. Louis, from 1905.

## Prevalence and incidence

Dyskeratosis congenita is a rare syndrome with approximately 200 cases reported in the literature (Chan 2006). Because the disorder is primarily X-linked recessive, the male to female ratio is approximately 10:1. Cases have been reported equally in all races.

## Clinical manifestations

### Skin and annexes and mucosa

The essential features of the syndrome are:

1) extensive areas of atrophy and netlike pigmentation of the skin;
2) nail dystrophy, with failure of the nails to form a nail plate;
3) white thickened plaques in the oral and occasionally the anal mucosa.

The nail changes are usually the first to appear and are found in 98% of the patients. Initial changes include longitudinal ridging and splitting, followed by pterygia (Fig. 1). Complete nail loss can be seen in some patients. Between the ages of 5 and 13 years the nails become dystrophic and are shed: they may be reduced to horny plugs or be completely destroyed. There may be recurrent episodes of suppura-

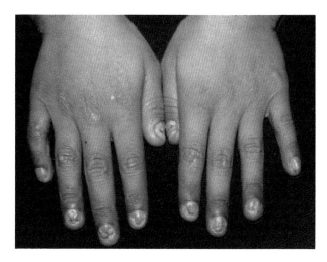

**Fig. 1.** Nail changes in dyskeratosis congenita. There is longitudinal ridging and splitting in some nails, and pterygia formation in others.

tive paronichya (Dokal 2000, Fistoral and Itin 2002, Knight et al. 1998, Sirinavin and Trowbridge 1975).

The dermatological changes are the most consistent features (Knight et al. 1998). Pigmentary changes may appear simultaneously or 2 or 3 years after the nail changes, and reach their full development in 3–5 years. Fine, reticulate, gray-brown pigmentation is most conspicuous on the neck and thighs, but involves most of the trunk (Fig. 2). The skin is atrophic, and telangiectases may give a poikilodermatous appearance. The skin of the face is red and atrophic, with irregular macular pigmentation, while that of the dorsa of the hands and feet is diffusely atrophic, transparent and shining. The palms

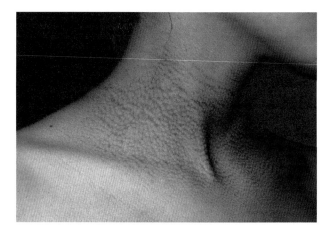

**Fig. 2.** Fine, brown, netlike pigmentation on the neck.

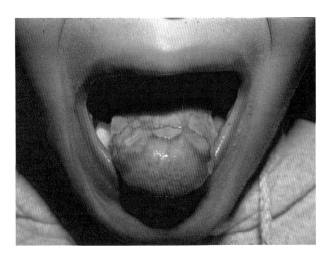

**Fig. 3.** Erosions and leukoplakia on the tongue.

and soles may be hyperkeratotic with disappearance of dermal ridges, and may form trauma induced bullae (Dokal 2000, Fistoral and Itin 2002, Knight et al. 1998, Sirinavin and Trowbridge 1975).

The onset of mucous membrane lesions may coincide with, or follow, the nail and skin changes. Leukoplakia may be present in any mucosal site. Small blisters and erosions of the lingual and buccal mucous membranes are followed by irregular white patches especially on the lateral portions of the tongue in about 85% of the patients (Fig. 3). Involvement of the urethra, glans penis, vagina, rectum and anus may also be seen (Knight et al. 1998). Mucosal surfaces such as the esophagus (Arca et al. 2003, Brown et al. 1993), urethra, and lacrimal duct (Woog et al. 1985) may become constricted and stenotic (Knight et al. 1998), resulting in dysphagia, dysuria and epiphora.

In patients with dyskeratosis congenita, the hair may be normal or sparse and dry. Premature canities and cicatricial alopecia have occasionally been noted (Hofer et al. 2005).

## Teeth

Oro-dental findings include defective and irregularly implanted teeth, early caries, gingival recession, short-blunted roots, gingival bleeding, tooth mobility and severe alveolar bone loss resembling juvenile periodontitis (Yavuzyilmaz et al. 1992).

## Lung

Another recognized complication is interstitial pneumonia (Imokawa et al. 1994, Utz et al. 2005) or progressive pulmonary disease, including infections and fibrosis (Imokawa et al. 1994, Kilic et al. 2003, Knight et al. 1998, Utz et al. 2005).

## Bone

Osteoporosis, similar to that seen in normal aging, is found in some patients and may lead to bone fractures (Hofer et al. 2005, Kelly and Stelling 1982).

## Eye

Ophtalmologic manifestations include blepharitis, conjuctivitis, obliteration of the lacrimal puncta, nasolacrimal duct obstruction, ectropian, loss of eyelashes and retinal vasculopathy with haemorrhages (Nazir et al. 2008, Teixeira et al. 2008).

## Neurological manifestations

General physical and mental growth is sometimes retarded (Knight et al. 1998, Pai et al. 1989). Intracranial calcifications have seldom been reported (Duprey and Steger 1988, Kelly and Stelling 1982, Lieblich et al. 1981, Mills et al. 1979). If present, they tend to be extensive located in the basal ganglia, dentate nuclei and cortex or throughout the cerebral hemispheres (Lieblich et al. 1981). According to Mills et al. (1979), calcifications consist of aggregates of laminated, perivascular concretions surrounded by focal reactive gliosis; they may account for global developmental deficits. Additional nervous system anomalies are Chiari 1 malformation (Cakmak et al. 2008).

## Associated features

### Hematological abnormalities

Bone marrow failure occurs in 50–90% of patients during the second or third decades of life. It presents as aplastic anemia, thrombocytopenia and pancytopenia and is a major cause of mortality (Knight et al. 1998).

Many cases have shown blood dyscrasias, myeloid aplasia, refractory anemia or pancytopenia. Hematological manifestations are usually added to the clinical picture from the age of 10 years. The resulting infection or hemorrhage are important causes of death. Rarely, neutropenia can be an early finding (Yel et al. 1996).

## Malignancies

They tend to develop during the third or fourth decade of life in at least 12% of the patients (Davidson and Connor 1988); most commonly as squamous cell carcinoma in the areas of leukoplakia of the mouth, anus, cervix, vagina, esophagus and atrophic skin. Myelodysplasia and acute myelogenous leukemia, Hodgkin's disease and pancreatic adenocarcinoma have also been observed (Connor and Teague 1981, Knight et al. 1998).

## Immune dysfunction

Immune system abnormalities are not classically considered as a part of the disease complex in dyskeratosis congenita. However, both humoral and cellular immune defects have been reported in these patients (Knudson et al. 2005, Solder et al. 1998, Wiedemann et al. 1984). In patients with TERC mutations, severe B lymphopenia and hypogammaglobulinemia have been noted and are likely a consequence of replicative failure and premature senescence of lymphocytes (Knudson et al. 2005). Evidence of cellular immune dysfunction was indicated by skin tests anergy and absent lymphocyte proliferation in a patient with dyskeratosis congenita that developed *Pneumocystis carinii* pneumonia and disseminated candidiasis (Wiedemann et al. 1984).

## Hoyeraal-Hreidarsson syndrome

Hoyeraal-Hreidarsson syndrome represents the severe infantile variant of dyskeratosis congenita, also characterized by missense DKC1 mutations (Knight et al. 1999a). It is an X-linked recessive, progressive, multisystemic disorder affecting boys, reported up to 2003 in 12 pedigrees (Sznajer et al. 2003). It is characterized by intrauterine growth retardation, microcephaly, cerebellar hypoplasia, ataxia, delayed myelination of cerebral white matter and hypoplastic corpus callosum (Akaboshi et al. 2000), mental retardation, progressive combined immune deficiency and aplastic anemia (Aalfs et al. 1995). Patients may also have early digestive disorders with chronic, bloody diarrhea and feeding problems (Sznajer et al. 2003). It is believed that affected individuals die before characteristic mucocutaneous features develop (Yaghmai et al. 2000). Almost all cases have died before 4 years, though there is one patient alive at his 12th year of age (Ozdemir et al. 2004). To date bone marrow transplantation using a conditioning regimen has allowed prompt engraftment with adequate immune reconstitution in one infant (Cossu et al. 2002).

## Histopathological features

The cutaneous changes are unimpressive and not pathognomonic. The areas of netlike pigmentation show as their only constant feature melanophages in the upper dermis. Other findings such as epidermal atrophy, basal cell vacuolization and lymphocytic infiltrates of the upper dermis are either absent or mild and not diagnostic. The connective tissue is usually normal (Johnson and Honig 1997).

Oral biopsies may show squamous cell carcinoma in situ or invasive squamous cell carcinoma (Johnson and Honig 1997).

## Pathogenesis and molecular genetics

Dyskeratosis congenita is usually determined by an X-linked recessive gene, localized to Xq28 (OMIM # 305000), however both autosomal dominant (OMIM # 127550) (Scoggins et al. 1971, Tchou and Kohn 1982) and autosomal recessive (OMIM # 224230) forms (Elliot et al. 1999) have also occurred.

Dyskeratosis congenita can originate through 3 different genetic mechanisms:

(1) Mutations in the DKC1 gene, which result in X-linked recessive dyskeratosis congenita.
(2) Mutations in the RNA component of telomerase (TERC) which result in autosomal dominant dyskeratosis congenita.
(3) Mutations in other, currently uncharacterized gene(s), which result in autosomal recessive dyskeratosis congenita.

X-linked recessive Dyskeratosis congenita is predominantly caused by missense mutations clustered in exons 3, 4 and 11, in the DKC1 gene, located at Xq28 (Heiss et al. 1999). The DKC1 gene is highly conserved across species barriers and is the ortholog of rat NAP57 and *Saccharomyces cervisiae* CBF5 (Heiss et al. 1999). This gene encodes the protein dyskerin (Knight et al. 1999b), a component of both small nucleolar ribonucleoprotein (snuRNP) particles (which are important in ribosomal RNA processing), and the telomerase complex (Mochizuki et al. 2004).

The autosomal dominant form of the disease is due to mutations in the RNA component of telomerase (TERC) (Dokal and Vulliamy 2003, Marrone et al. 2004, Vulliamy et al. 2004). Telomerase (a ribonucleoprotein complex that is required to synthesize DNA repeats at the ends of each chromosome) (Vulliamy et al. 2004) prevents the progressive shortening of chromosomes that occurs with successive replications. Tissues with high replication rates (bone marrow, skin and digestive tract) are thought to be more vulnerable to telomerase dysfunction. Mutations in TERC are predicted to either disrupt secondary structure or alter the template region (Bessler et al. 2004, Marrone and Mason 2003).

The gene(s) involved in the recessive forms of the disease remain elusive, though genes whose products are required for telomere maintenance are strong candidates (Marrone and Mason 2003).

Regarding molecular findings, dyskeratosis congenita was initially described as a disorder of defective ribosomal biogenesis. Subsequently, dyskerin and TERC were shown to closely associate with each other in the telomerase complex. Dyskeratosis congenita has since then, been considered as a telomerase deficiency disorder characterized by shorter telomeres. Telomerase deficiency in humans (through DKC1 and TERC mutations) results in multiple abnormalities including premature aging, bone marrow failure and altered immunity (Hofer et al. 2005, Marrone and Dokal 2004).

The premature aging features due to shorter telomeres are also found in a variety of otherwise unrelated progeroid symptoms and are characterized by an alopecia-osteoporosis-fingernail atrophy group of symptoms. Fingernail atrophy, osteoporosis, alopecia and gray hair resemble the natural changes that occur in normal aging (Hofer et al. 2005).

Dysfunction also leads to chromosome instability and this theoretically plays a role in tumorigenesis. Identification of the gene(s) involved in autosomal recessive dyskeratosis congenita will help to further define the pathophysiology of dyskeratosis congenita, as well as expand the understanding of telomere function, aging and cancer (Hofer et al. 2005, Marron and Dokal 2004).

## Differential diagnosis

Because of the relatively late onset of the characteristic features of dyskeratosis congenita, its diagnosis is often delayed for some years (Morrison 1974).

Dyskeratosis congenita has often been confused with Rothmund-Thompson syndrome, characterized by erythema of the face, buttocks and limbs in infancy, progressively succeeded by poikiloderma. Nail changes are unusual and leukoplakia does not occur.

In anhidrotic ectodermal dysplasia the dental changes, distinctive facies, sparse or absent hair and normal nails provide points of differentiation.

Fanconi's anemia is universally autosomal recessive. It is associated with pigmentary abnormalities, pancytopenia and an increased incidence of neoplasia (leukemia). However, patients with FA have a more generalized hypermelanosis, often in association with bony defects involving the thumb (Auerbach 1995).

Naegeli-Franceschetti-Jadassohn syndrome differs by lack of leukoplakia and bone marrow involvement as well as autosomal dominant inheritance.

Patients with chronic graft-versus-host disease may develop poikiloderma-like skin changes and lacy white patches on the oral mucosa. However GVHD is usually diagnosed by the history of a bone marrow, hematopoietic stem cell or solid organ transplant (Treister et al. 2004).

## Treatment

Close surveillance of all mucosal surfaces is indicated, in order to monitor the development of squamous cell carcinoma within areas of leukoplakia. Sun and tobacco avoidance are advisable.

Bone marrow failure requires supportive transfusions with blood products. Erythropoietin and granulocyte colony stimulating factor have been used successfully to improve hematological parameters in the short term (Erduran et al. 2003, Yel et al. 1994). Aplastic anemia associated with dyskeratosis congenita can be successfully treated by allogeneic bone marrow transplantation; however this approach does not reverse other systemic manifestations of the syndrome (Langston et al. 1996, Phillips et al. 1992).

Oral retinoids have been reported to cause regression of lesions in leukoplakia and so may reduce the incidence of malignancy. In our hands painted bleomycin has also met success for the treatment of oral leukoplakia.

## Prognosis

The prognosis is usually poor, for either blood dyscrasia or carcinoma may prove fatal. However in patients with nail dystrophy and pigmentation only, the expectation of life is normal.

Average survival in X-linked and autosomal recessive dyskeratosis congenita is 33 years. The autosomal dominant form is milder, median survival being greater than 50 years with no reported deaths due directly to the dyskeratosis congenita (Drachtman and Alter 1995).

## References

Aalfs CM, van den Berg H, Barth PG, Hennekam RC (1995) The Hoyeraal-Hreidarsson syndrome: the fourth case of a separate entity with prenatal growth retardation, progressive pancytopenia and cerebellar hypoplasia. Eur J Pediatr 154: 304–308.

Akaboshi S, Yoshimura M, Hara T, Kageyama H, Nishikwa K, Kawakami T, Ieshima A, Takeshita K (2000) A case of Hoyeraal-Hreidarsson syndrome: delayed myelination and hypoplasia of corpus callosum are other important signs. Neuropediatrics 31: 141–144.

Arca E, Tuzun A, Tastan HB, Akar A, Kose O (2003) Dyskeratosis congenita with esophageal and anal stricture. Int J Dermatol 42: 555–557.

Auerbach AD (1995) Fanconi anemia. Dermatol Clin 13: 41–49.

Bessler M, Wilson DB, Mason PJ (2004) Dyskeratosis congenita and telomerase. Curr Opin Pediatr 16: 23–28.

Brown KE, Kelly TE, Myers BM (1993) Gastrointestinal involvement in a woman with dyskeratosis congenita. Dig Dis Sci 38: 181–184.

Cakmak SK, Gönül M, Kiliç A, Gül U, Koçak O, Demiriz M (2008) A case of dyskeratosis congenita with Chiari 1 malformation, absence of inferior vena cava, webbed neck, and low posterior hair neck. Int J Dermatol 47: 377–379.

Chan EF (2006) Dyskeratosis congenita. E-medicine from WebMD. http://emedicine.com/derm/topic111.htm

Cole HN, Rauschkolb JC, Toomey J (1930) Dyskeratosis congenita with pigmentation, dystrophia unguis and leukokeratosis oris. Arch Dermatol Syphilol 21: 71–95.

Connor JM, Teague RH (1981) Dyskeratosis congenita: report of a large kindred. Br J Dermatol 105: 321–325.

Cossu F, Vulliamy TJ, Marrone A, Badiali M, Cao A, Dokal I (2002) A novel DKC1 mutation, severe combined immunodeficiency (T+B-NK-SCID) and bone marrow transplantation in an infant with Hoyeraal-Hreidarsson syndrome. Br J Haematol 119: 765–768.

Davidson HR, Connor JM (1988) Dyskeratosis congenita. J Med Genet 25: 843–846.

Dokal I (2000) Dyskeratosis congenita in all its forms. Br J Haematol 110: 768–779.

Dokal I, Vulliamy T (2003) Dyskeratosis congenita: its link to telomerase and aplastic anemia. Blood Rev 17: 217–225.

Drachtman RA, Alter BP (1995) Dyskeratosis congenita. Dermatol Clin 13: 33–39.

Duprey PA, Steger JW (1988) An unusual case of dyskeratosis congenita with intracranial calcifications. J Am Acad Dermatol 19: 760–762.

Elliot AM, Graham GE, Bernstein M, Mazer B, Terbi AS (1999) Dyskeratosis congenita: an autosomal recessive variant. Am J Med Genet 83: 178–182.

Engmann MF (1926) A unique case of reticular pigmentation of the skin with atrophy. Arch Dermatol Syphilol 13: 685–687.

Erduran E, Hacisalihoglu S, Ozoran Y (2003) Treatment of dyskeratosis congenita with granulocyte-macrophage-colony-stimulating factor and erythropoietin. J Pediatr Hematol Oncol 25: 333–335.

Fistoral SK, Itin PH (2002) Nail changes in genodermatoses. Eur J Dermatol 12: 119–128.

Heiss NS, Knight SW, Vulliamy TJ, Klauck SM, Wieman S, Masson PJ, Poustka A, Dokal I (1998) X-linked dyskeratosis congenita is caused by mutations in a highly conserved gene with putative nucleolar functions. Nat Genet 19: 32–38.

Heiss NS, Girod A, Salowsky R, Wiemman S, Pepperkok R, Poutska A (1999) Dyskerin localizes to the nucleolus and its mislocalization is unlikely to play a role in the pathogenesis of dyskeratosis congenita. Hum Mol Genet 8: 2515–2524.

Hofer AC, Tran RT, Aziz OZ (2005) Shared phenotypes among segmental progeroid syndromes suggest underlying pathways of aging. J Gerontol A Biol Sci Med Sci 60: 10–20.

Imokawa S, Sato A, Toyoshima M, Yoshitomi A, Tamura R, Suda T, Suganuma H, Yagi T, Iwata M, Hayakawa H, Chida K (1994) Dyskeratosis congenita showing usual interstitial pneumonia. Intern Med 33: 226–230.

Johnson B Jr, Honig P (1997) Congenital Diseases (Genodermatoses). In: Elder D, Elenitsas R, Jaworsky C, Johnson B (eds.) Lever's Histopathology of the Skin. 8th ed. Philadelphia: Lippincott-Raven, p. 122.

Kelly TE, Stelling CB (1982) Dyskeratosis congenita: radiologic features. Pediatr Radiol 12: 31–36.

Kilic S, Kose H, Ozturk H (2003) Pulmonary involvement in a patient with dyskeratosis congenita. Pediatr Int 45: 740–742.

Knight S, Vulliamy TJ, Copplestone A, Gluckmann E, Mason P, Dokal I (1998) Dyskeratosis Congenita (DC) Registry: identification of new features of DC. Br J Haematol 103: 990–996.

Knight SW, Heiss NS, Vulliamy TJ, Aalfs CM, McMahon C, Richmond P, Jones A, Hennekam RC, Poustka A, Mason PJ, Dokal I (1999a) Unexplained aplastic anaemia, immunodeficiency, and cerebellar hypoplasia (Hoyeraal-Heidarsson syndrome) due to mutations in the dyskeratosis congenita gene, DKC1. Br J Haematol 107: 335–339.

Knight W, Heiss NS, Vulliamy TJ, Greschner S, Stavrides G, Pai GS, Lestringant G, Varma N, Mason PJ,

Dokal I, Poustka A (1999b) X-linked dyskeratosis congenita is predominantly caused by missense mutations in the DKC1 gene. Am J Hum Genet 65: 50–58.

Knudson M, Kulkarni S, Ballas ZK, Bessler M, Goldman F (2005) Association of immune abnormalities with telomere shortening in autosomal-dominant dyskeratosis congenita. Blood 105: 682–688.

Langston AA, Sanders JE, Deeg HJ, Crawford SW, Anasetti C, Sullivan KM, Flowers ME, Storb R (1996) Allogeneic marrow transplantation for aplastic anemia associated with dyskeratosis congenita. Br J Haematol 92: 758–765.

Lieblich LM, Auerbach R, Auerbach AD (1981) Dyskeratosis congenita and intracranial calcifications. Arch Dermatol 117: 523.

Marrone A, Mason PJ (2003) Dyskeratosis congenita. Cell Mol Life Sci 60: 507–517.

Marrone A, Dokal I (2004) Dyskeratosis congenita: molecular insights into telomerase function, ageing and cancer. Expert Rev Mol Med 6: 1–23.

Marrone A, Stevens D, Vulliamy T, Dokal I, Mason PJ (2004) Heterozygous telomerase RNA mutations found in dyskeratosis congenita and aplastic anemia reduce telomerase activity via happloinsufficiency. Blood 104: 3936–3942.

Mason PJ, Wilson DB, Bessler M (2005) Dyskeratosis congenita – a disease of dysfunctional telomere maintenance. Curr Mol Med 5: 159–170.

Mills SE, Cooper PH, Beacham BE, Greer KE (1979) Intracranial calcifications and dyskeratosis congenita. Arch Dermatol 115: 1437–1439.

Mochizuki Y, He J, Kulkarni S, Bessler M, Mason PJ (2004) Mouse dyskerin mutations affect accumulation of telomerase RNA and small nucleolar RNA, telomerase activity, and ribosomal RNA processing. Proc Natl Acad Sci USA 101: 10756–10761.

Morrison JG (1974) Dyskeratosis congenita: two extremes. S Afr Med J 48: 223–225.

Nazir S, Sayani N, Phillips PH (2008) Retinal hemorrhages in a patient with dyskeratosis congenita. J AAPOS May 1 [Epub ahead of print].

OMIM$^{TM}$ (2006) Online Mendelian Inheritance in Man. Baltimore: Johns Hopkins University Press. http://www.ncbi.nlm.nih.gov/omim

Ozdemir MA, Karakukcu M, Kose M, Kumandas S, Gumus H (2004) The longest surviving child with Hoyeraal-Hreidarsson syndrome. Haematologica 89: ECR38.

Pai GS, Morgan S, Whetsell C (1989) Etiologic heterogeneity in dyskeratosis congenita. Am J Med Genet 32: 63–66.

Phillips RJ, Judge M, Webb D, Harper JI (1992) Dyskeratosis congenita: delay in diagnosis and successful treatment of pancytopenia by bone marrow transplantation. Br J Dermatol 127: 278–280.

Scoggins RB, Prescott KJ, Asher GH, Blayclock WK, Bright RW (1971) Dyskeratosis congenita with Fanconi-type anemia: investigations of immunologic and other defects. Clin Res 19: 409 (Abstract).

Sirinavin C, Trowbridge AA (1975) Dyskeratosis congenita: clinical features and genetic aspects. Report of a family and review of the literature. J Med Genet 12: 339–354.

Solder B, Weiss M, Jager A, Belohradsky BH (1998) Dyskeratosis congenita: multisystemic disorder with special consideration of immunologic aspects. A review of the literature. Clin Pediatr 37: 521–530.

Sznajer Y, Baumann C, David A, Journel H, Lacombe D, Perel Y, Blouin P, Segura JF, Cezard JP, Peuchmaur M, Vulliamy T, Dokal I, Verloes A (2003) Further delineation of the congenital form of X-linked dyskeratosis congenita (Hoyeraal-Hreidarsson syndrome). Eur J Pediatr 162: 863–867.

Tchou PK, Kohn T (1982) Dyskeratosis congenita: an autosomal dominant disorder. J Am Acad Dermatol 6: 1034–1039.

Teixeira LF, Shields CL, Marr B, Horgan N, Shields JA (2008) Bilateral retinal vasculopathy in a patient with dyskeratosis congenita. Arch Ophthalmol 126: 134–135.

Treister N, Lehmann LE, Cherrick I, Guinan EC, Woo SB (2004) Dyskeratosis congenita vs. chronic graft versus host disease: report of a case and review of the literature. Oral Surg Oral Med Oral Pathol Oral Radiol Endod 98: 566–571.

Utz JP, Ryu JH, Myers JL, Michels VV (2005) Usual interstitial pneumonia complicating dyskeratosis congenita. Mayo Clin Proc 80: 817–821.

Vulliamy T, Marrone A, Szydlo R, Walne A, Mason PJ, Dokal I (2004) Disease anticipation is associated with progressive telomere shortening in families with dyskeratosis congenita due to mutations in TERC. Nat Genet 36: 437–438.

Walne AJ, Marrone A, Dokal I (2005) Dyskeratosis congenita: a disorder of defective telomere maintenance? Int J Hematol 82: 184–189.

Wiedemann HP, McGuire J, Dwyer JM, Sabetta J, Gee JB, Smith GJ, Loke J (1984) Progressive immune failure in dyskeratosis congenita. Report of an adult in whom Pneumocystis carinii and fatal disseminated candidiasis developed. Arch Intern Med 144: 397–399.

Woog JJ, Dortzbach RK, Wexler SA, Shahidi NT (1985) The role of aminocaproic acid in lacrimal surgery in dyskeratosis congenita. Am J Ophtalmol 100: 728–732.

Yaghmai R, Kimyai-Asadi A, Rostamiani K, Heiss NS, Poustka A, Eyaid W, Bodurtha J, Nousari HC, Hamosh A, Metzenberg A (2000) Overlap of dyskeratosis congenita with the Hoyeraal-Hreidarsson syndrome. J Pediatr 136: 390–393.

Yavuzyilmaz E, Yamalik N, Yetgin S, Kansu O (1992) Oral-dental findings in dyskeratosis congenita. J Oral Pathol Med 21: 280–284.

Yel L, Pritchard SL, Junker AK (1994) Positive response to granulocyte-colony-stimulating factor in dyskeratosis congenita before matched unrelated bone marrow transplantation. Am J Pediatr Hematol Oncol 16: 186–187.

Yel L, Tezcan I, Sanal O, Ersoy F, Berkel AI (1996) Dyskeratosis congenita: unusual onset with isolated neutropenia at an early age. Acta Paediatr Jpn 38: 288–290.

Zinsser F (1906) Atrophia cutis reticularis cum pigmentione, dystrophia unguium et leukokeratosis oris. Ikonogr Dermatol (Hyoto) 5: 219–223.

# Chapter 45

# NEVOID BASAL CELL CARCINOMA (GORLIN) SYNDROME

**Robert J. Gorlin**[†]

[†]The late professor R. J. Gorlin, Department of Oral Pathology, University of Minnesota, Minneapolis, USA

## Introduction

Nevoid basal cell carcinoma syndrome (NBCCS) is characterized by large numbers of basal cell cancers and epidermal cysts of the skin, odontogenic keratocysts of the jaws, palmoplantar pits, calcified dural folds, various neoplasms or hamartomas which include medulloblastoma, ovarian fibroma, lymphomesenteric cysts, fetal rhabdomyoma, etc., and various stigmata of maldevelopment (rib and vertebral anomalies, cortical defects of bone, cleft lip and/or palate, etc.).

## Historical perspective and eponyms

Satinoff and Wells (1969), examining a cache of related mummies housed in Torino, Italy, found impressive evidence that NBCCS existed during dynastic Egyptian times. The material derived from a single family, whose mummies dated from approximately 1000 BC, exhibited bifid ribs, short 4th metacarpals, and numerous jaw cysts. While wandering through a medical museum housing material that dated from the middle of the 19th century and housed in the basement of the Academic Health Center in Amsterdam, Netherlands, Dr. Raoul Hennekam and I, in 1995, noted that several family members had huge numbers of bifid ribs.

The syndrome has been variously known as basal cell nevus syndrome, Gorlin-Goltz syndrome*, Gorlin syndrome, and nevoid basal cell carcinoma syndrome. None of these terms is entirely satisfactory because only one facet of the syndrome has been selected in naming it. For example, basal cell

*There may be confusion with Goltz-Gorlin syndrome which is *focal dermal hypoplasia*, an unrelated disorder.

carcinomas are relatively uncommon in African-Americans with the syndrome. The term *nevus* does not reflect the truly cancerous nature of the skin lesions although only a small number of basal cell carcinomas become aggressive. Eponyms imply priority of description (and are often wrong, frequently chauvinistic, and say absolutely nothing about the disorder). Furthermore, they serve to plague residents who are required to memorize them.

The earliest reports of the syndrome are apparently those of Jarisch (1894) and White (1894). The disorder was then essentially forgotten until the 1950s. The reader is referred to the reports of Binkley and Johnson (1951), Howell and Caro (1959), and Gorlin and Goltz (1960) for early development of the syndrome. Approximately every five years (1987, 1995, 1999, 2004), Gorlin updated the expansion of the syndrome. For comprehensive, systematic surveys, the reader is referred to Evans et al. (1993), Shanley et al. (1994), Kimonis et al. (1997, 2004), LoMuzio et al. (1999a), Bakaeen et al. (2004), Manfredi et al. (2004) and Gorlin (2004). For historic reviews, one should consult Howell (1980) and Gorlin (1987, 2004). Gorlin (2004) discussed how he happened to discover the syndrome and gave personal reminiscences regarding individual patients.

## Incidence and prevalence

Maddox (1962) and Maddox et al. (1964) indicated that about 0.4% of all cases of basal cell carcinomas represent the syndrome. This figure is clearly too high in light of findings cited below. Rahbari and Mehregan (1982) found that 2% of those younger than 45 years of age with basal cell carcinomas have NBCCS. Evans et al. (1991a, b) calculated that the minimal prevalence was 1 per 57,000. An almost identical value was found by Pratt and Jackson (1987). Chevenix-Trench et al. (1993) indicated that in Australia, they found a minimal prevalence of 1 per 164,000. The frequency among Korean patients has been cited as 1 per 14,000,000 (Ahn et al. 2004).

## Clinical manifestations

### Skin abnormalities

Basal cell carcinomas appear as early as two years of age. They are especially common on the nape in those having received radiation for medulloblastoma (vide infra). Most patients experience a proliferation of lesions between puberty and 35 years (Shanley et al. 1994) (Table 1). Rayner et al. (1977) found that only about 10% of those over 30 years with NBCCS do not have a basal cell tumor. Surely a relationship to increased sun exposure exists (Goldstein et al. 1993) because only 40% of African–Americans with the syndrome manifest basal cell carcinomas. The percent among Italians and Koreans is considerably less than in England (Ahn et al. 2004). Blacks usually have but a few skin lesions in contrast to the myriad basal cell carcinomas evident in Caucasians (90%) (Daramola et al. 1980, Goldstein et al. 1994, Korczak et al. 1997). It should be emphasized that melanotic skin pigmentation does not protect against ionizing radiation (vide infra).

The basal cell carcinomas, which vary from a few to literally thousands, especially following radiation, range in size from 1 to 10 mm in diameter and vary in color from pearly to flesh-colored to pale brown to reddish brown and may be mistaken for skin tags, nevi, or molluscum contagiosum (Fig. 1) (Golitz et al. 1980). They may be isolated or grouped. The areas most commonly involved are the face, back, and chest. A basal cell carcinoma is less often found below the waist or on the extremities. Those on the eyelid are especially difficult to deal with (Honovar et al. 2001). New lesions appear from time to time, but most remain static in growth. A 2005 edition of Guinness Book of World Records indicated that a man with nevoid basal cell carcinoma

**Table 1.** Diagnostic findings in adults with nevoid basal cell carcinoma syndrome

*50% or greater frequency*
Enlarged occipitofrontal circumference (macrocephaly, frontal-parietal bossing)
Multiple basal cell carcinomas
Odontogenic keratocysts of jaws
Epidermal cysts of skin
High-arched palate
Palmar and/or plantar pits
Rib anomalies (splayed, fused, partially missing, bifid, etc.)
Spina bifida occulta of cervical or thoracic vertebrae
Calcified falx cerebri
Calcified diaphrgma sellae (bridged sella, fused clinoids)
Hyperpneumatization of paranasal sinuses

*49–15% frequency*
Brain ventricle asymmetry
Calcification of tentorium cerebelli and petroclinoid ligament
Calcified ovarian fibromas
Short fourth metacarpals
Kyphoscoliosis or other vertebral anomalies
Lumbarization of sacrum
Narrow sloping shoulders
Prognathism
Pectus excavatum or carinatum
Pseudocystic lytic lesion of bones (hamartomas)
Strabismus (exotropia)
Syndactyly
Synophrys

*14% or less but not random*
Medullablastoma
True ocular hypertelorism
Meningioma
Lymphomesenteric cysts
Cardiac fibromas
Fetal rhabdomyoma
Ovarian fibrosarcoma
Marfanoid build
Anosmia
Agenesis of corpus callosum
Cyst of septum pellucidum
Cleft lip and/or palate
Low-pitched female voice
Polydactyly, postaxial—hands or feet
Sprengel deformity of scapula
Vertebral body fusion

(Continued)

**Table 1.** (Continued)

Congenital cataract, glaucoma, coloboma of iris, retina, optic
   nerve medullated retinal nerve fibers
Subcutaneous calcification of skin (possibly underestimated
frequency)
Minor kidney malformations
Hypogonadism in males
Mental retardation

Modified from Gorllin R. J. (1995).

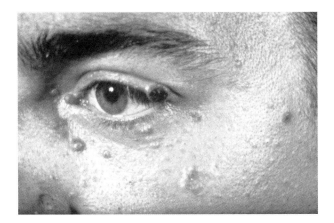

**Fig. 1.** Patient with nevoid basal cell carcinoma syndrome. Note
numerous lesions around eye. Those cancers, which occur on the
thin eyelid skin, are especially difficult to control.

seen at Mayo Clinic in Rochester, Minnesota, held
the record for the most surgical operations-970 over
40 years. It is only after puberty that the basal cell
cancers may become aggressive and invade locally. It
must be emphasized that only a small fraction of the
lesions become invasive. Increase in size, bleeding,
ulceration, and crusting indicate invasion of the underlying skin. Radiation therapy causes proliferation
of basal cell carcinomas followed by invasion several
years later (Gorlin 1987). Death has resulted in
rare instances from invasion of the brain or lung.
Even less often have metastases been documented
(Murphy 1975, Goldberg et al. 1977, Winkler and
Guyuron, 1987, Berardi et al. 1991, Tawfik et al.
1999, Adem and Nassar, 2004, Gorlin, personal observations, 2005). Several examples of unilateral or
even quadrant involvement with basal cell carcinomas likely represent postzygotic somatic mutation
(Shelley et al. 1969, Horio and Komura, 1978,

Camissa et al. 1985, Gutierrez and Mora 1986,
Wirth and Tilgen 1983, Jiminez Acosta et al. 1992,
Zarour et al 1993). Involvement of the external
ear canal has made for especially difficult therapy
(Winkler and Guyuron 1987, Lobo et al. 1997).

Multiple basaloid follicular hamartomata have
been noted in patients with the syndrome, predomi-
natly on the upper back and chest, neck, and face.
The relationship to nevoid basal cell carcinomas has
been hotly debated, but Grachtchouk et al. (2003)
believe that lower levels of activation of the *Patched*
gene results in multiple basaloid follicular hamartomata (see Differential diagnosis). Small keratin-
filled cysts (milia), found intermixed with basal cell
carcinomas in 30–50% of affected individuals, are
analogous to odontogenic keratocysts (vide infra).

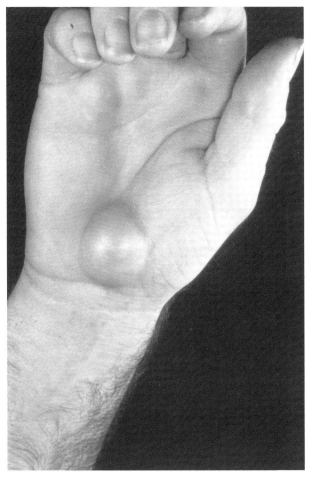

**Fig. 2.** Epidermoid inclusion cyst of extremity.

Larger (1–2 cm) often multiple epidermal cysts resembling odontogenic keratocysts, arise on the limbs (Fig. 2) and trunk in about 50% of Caucasians with NBCCS (Leppard 1983, Barr et al. 1986, Shanley et al. 1994, Baselga et al. 1996). In African–Americans, about 35% exhibit these cysts (Goldstein et al. 1994), but more studies are needed to test any racial difference. Multiple cysts (milia) are located on the palpebral conjunctiva in about 40%. This figure has been ascertained by the author by questioning members of support groups. They cause little discomfiture and are often ignored.

Acrochordons (Chiritescu and Maloney 2001) and sebaceous nevi, Xin et al. 1999, Rogers and Wilson 2000) have also been reported.

The nevoid basal cell carcinoma cannot be differentiated histopathologically from the usual sporadic basal cell carcinoma. The tumor is composed of nests and islands or sheets of large, deeply-stained nuclei with distinct cell membranes (Fig. 3). At the periphery of each lesion, the epithelial cells are well-polarized, suggestive of cutaneous basal cells. About 30% of patients have two or more types of basal cell carcinoma patterns (solid, superficial, morphea-like, cystic, adenoid, fibroepithelial).

Calcified foci may be noted not only within the basal cell tumor (Fig. 3) but also in normal skin (Murphy 1969). Perhaps this reflects the "turning on" of the *bone morphogenetic protein* gene.

Palmar and, somewhat less often, plantar pits (about 1–2 mm in diameter) (Fig. 4) are asymmetri-

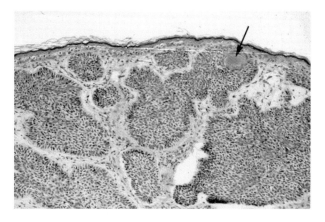

**Fig. 3.** Photomicrograph of nevoid basal cell carcinoma lesion. Arrow points to small bit of calcium deposited within the tumour.

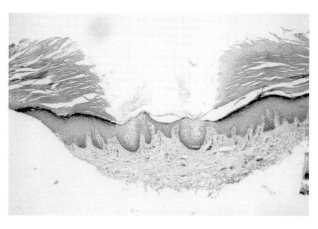

**Fig. 4.** Photomicrograph of palmar pit. Note that cells at base of pit exhibit dyshesion.

cally present in 65–80% (Nicolai 1979, Evans et al. 1993, Shanley et al. 1994, Ahn et al. 2004) and occur with equal frequency in African-Americans and Caucasians. They are best visualized if the patient wets the hands in warm water before examination. Individuals whose occupations involve manual labor may have more obvious pits because of ingrained dirt or grease. The pits may be present in children, but a careful age-related study is lacking. Rarely, basal cell carcinomas arise in these pits (Holubar et al. 1970, Howell and Mehregan 1970, Taylor and Wilkins 1970, Gorlin 1987).

Louise Wilson, (personal communication, 2005) asked Raoul Hennekam if a random swatch of hair is part of the syndrome. Initially skeptical, we asked support groups whether members noted this. We were surprised to find that several exhibited these hair swatches: on the lateral neck, wrist, above the knee, etc. (personal observation, 2005).

## Craniofacial features

Relative macrocephaly (occipital frontal circumference greater than the 95th centile for height) is found in 50% (Bale et al. 1997, Kimonis et al. 1997). Head circumference due to frontal and biparietal bossing is greater than 60 cm in adults (Soeckermann et al. 1991). Only rarely is hydrocephalus reported. Frontal bossing, which has been noted in 25%, may cause the eyes to appear sunken. The eyebrows are highly arched in about 40% (Dahl et al. 1976a, Shanley et al. 1994). Broad nasal bridge is noted in 60%. Mild mandibular prognathism, reported as "pouting lower lip", is seen in about 35% of both Caucasians (Gorlin 1987) and African-Americans (Goldstein et al. 1994). The coronoid processes may be elongated (Leonardi et al. 2002). Milia (small keratin-filled cysts) appear scattered among the basal cell carcinomas in at least 50–60%, especially around the eyes, eyelids, nose, malar region, and upper lip. Cleft lip and/or palate has been found in 3–9% (Taicher and Shteyer 1978, Gorlin et al. 1987, Ruprecht et al. 1987, deLeón et al. 1990, Soekermann et al. 1991, Evans et al. 1993, Shanley et al. 1994, Lambrecht and Kreusch 1997, Ahn et al. 2004).

## Mean height

Height in both males and females is significantly greater than normal (M=183 cm, F=174 cm), compared to their unaffected first degree relatives. About 15% are extremely tall (Springate 1986). The shoulders are frequently narrowed and sloped (Pratt and Jackson 1987, Chevenix-Trench et al. 1993). See *Skeletal Radiographic Findings*.

## Odontogenic keratocysts

Multiple cysts of both the upper and lower jaws (Fig. 5) start to appear at about 8 years of age and increase in number from puberty onward (Myong et al. 2001). The cysts may be the initial presentation (Dowling et al. 2000, Veenestrat-Knol et al. 2005). They average 6 in number and have ranged from 1 to 30 cysts. Mandibular cysts are three times as common as maxillary examples. In a population-based study, Evans et al. (1993) noted odontogenic keratocysts in 90% of those over 40 years and in 30% in those over 20 years with an overall frequency of over 65%. They peak during the second and third decades but continue to appear throughout life (Gorlin 1987, Chevenix-Trench et al. 1993). There is no racial predilection (Goldstein et al. 1994). In children, the cysts can cause displacement of permanent tooth germs (Shear 1985). The cysts may reach enormous size, causing marked tooth displacement and jaw expansion (Fig. 5) but only rarely cause fractures (Southwick and Schwartz 1979). About one-third do not produce significant symptoms. Approximately 50% present with swelling, 25% with mild pain, and 15% with unusual taste following rupture (Chevenix-Trench et al. 1993, Palacios et al. 2004). Rarely, they perforate the cortex and extend into soft tissues. In the maxilla, the sinuses may be

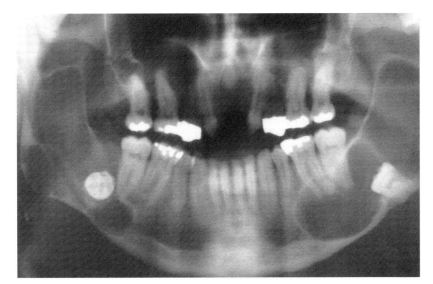

**Fig. 5.** Bilateral odontogenic keratocysts. Notice displacement of teeth and extension of cysts into coronoid processes.

invaded. In the mandible, the cysts may extend throughout the molar-ramus area up to the coronoid process. The condyle is never involved. The cysts may cross the midline (Gorlin 1987). Computerized tomography has been employed in estimating the size of jaw cysts (MacSweeney et al. 1985, Palacios et al. 2004). In a random series of odontogenic keratocysts, about 10% are syndrome-associated (Kakarantza-Angelopoulou and Nicolatou 1990).

There is marked tendency (over 60%) for these cysts to recur following surgery (Donatsky and Hjorting-Hansen 1980). Recurrence appears to result from several causes: incomplete removal, retention of epithelial islands and/or satellite microcysts which occur with great frequency in the connective tissue capsule, and from proliferation of the basal layer of the epithelium (Woolgar et al. 1987, Dominguez and Keszler 1988, Myong et al. 2001).

Odontogenic keratocysts, present as multilocular or invaginated cysts (along with micro-daughter cysts or epithelial rests in 25–50% of the cases), with parakeratinized or, rarely, orthokeratinized (4%), stratified squamous epithelium consisting of 5–8 rows of cells having irregularly oriented, well-defined flat basal epithelial cell layer, palisaded nuclei, but not rete ridges (Fig. 6). The contents may be a clear serum-like substance or a cheesy material which consists of keratinous debris. The epithelial lining may become detached and float in the cyst cavity. Some of the larger keratocysts expand in size to include dental

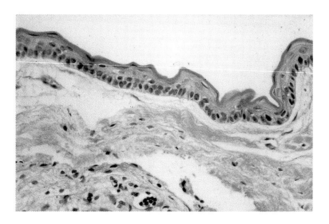

**Fig. 6.** Photomicrograph of odontogenic keratocyst. Notice that the cyst wall consists of but few cells in thickness. Lining is either keratinised or parakeratinised.

follicles. Budding of epithelium into the connective tissue and suprabasilar splitting are noted in at least 50%. Rarely are inflammatory cells found in the underlying connective tissue. The cyst capsule is thin and difficult to enucleate. Some cysts exhibit foci of calcification in the wall (Cotton et al. 1982). Woolgar et al. (1987) and Dominguez et al. (1996) found significant differences between syndrome keratocysts and isolated keratocysts. Syndrome-related keratocysts were found to have a markedly increased number of satellite cysts, solid islands of epithelial proliferation, odontogenic rests within the capsule, and mitotic figures in the epithelial lining of the main cavity. Immunologic differences between syndrome and solitary keratocysts have also been found (Li et al. 1995). Woolgar et al. (1987) noted that syndrome keratocysts tend to occur at a much earlier age than nonsyndromal keratocysts. Most authors believe that odontogenic keratocysts arise from the dental lamina (Shanley et al. 1994).

LoMuzio et al. (1999b) found that all isolated cysts are p53 and cyclin D1 negative while most cysts in the syndrome are immunopositive for p53 and overexpress cyclin D1 oncoproteins. Shear (2002) noted p53 positivity was more often found in syndrome-associated cysts but it was non-diagnostic. Ling et al. (2001) found p53 even less diagnostic than Shear (2002). Scintigraphic studies have been carried out (Ly 2002).

There have been very few reports of ameloblastoma arising in odontogenic keratocysts (Clendenning et al. 1964, Maddox et al. 1964, Cernéa et al. 1969, Happle 1973, Jensen 1978, Jeanmougin et al. 1979, Schultz et al. 1987, R. Gopalakrishnan, unpublished, 2005). The case of Jensen (1978), we suspect, really represents proliferated odontogenic rests.

Squamous cell carcinoma has arisen from a cyst wall in a few examples (Ramsden and Barrett, 1978, Moos and Rennie 1987, Hasegawa et al. 1989).

## Eyes

Various ophthalmologic problems occur with a frequency of perhaps 10–25% which is far greater than that in the normal population. These include strabismus (15%), anterior segment dysgenesis, cataract(5%) and Peter's anomaly, microphthalmia with orbital cyst, hamartoma, coloboma of iris, choroid and optic nerve, ectopic pupil, and nystagmus (Schlieter 1973, Gorlin 1987, Evans et al. 1991b, Manners et al. 1996, Roggi et al. 2005). As mentioned earlier, multiple transient cysts of the palpebral conjunctivae are noted in about 40% (Levine et al. 1987). Medullated retinal nerve fibers have been described by a few authors (DeJong et al. 1985, Tafi et al. 1986, De Potter et al. 2000). Epiretinal membranes were reported (Yoshida et al. 2004).

## Cardiac fibroma

Cardiac fibromas may be present at any age, from birth to 60 years. They are discrete, well-circumscribed, firm, not encapsulated, grey-white, 3–4 cm in diameter, and, in some cases, exhibit central calcification. The tumor is most often located in the left anterior ventricular wall. In those cases in which the tumor projects into the ventricle, the hemodynamics is impeded. Arythymias result, due to involvement of the interventricular septum (Hogge et al. 1994). However, in most cases, there are no symptoms and most examples have been discovered purely by chance. As of this writing, approximately 25 examples have been noted.

In a population-based study, Evans et al. (1993) estimated that cardiac fibromas were seen in about 3% of individuals with the syndrome. Conversely about 5% of those with cardiac fibromas have NBCCS. Microscopically, the tumors are composed of fibroblasts embedded in a dense matrix of collagen and elastic fibers. The tumor is poorly cellular and unencapsulated. The reader is referred to the cases of Edlund and Holmdahl (1957), Cawson and Kerr (1964), Lincoln et al. (1968), Osano et al. (1969), Hess and Bink-Boelkins (1976), Bunting and Remensnyder (1977), Littler (1979), Jamieson et al. (1981), Reiter et al. (1982), Williams et al. (1982), Harris and Large (1984), Jones et al. (1986), Gorlin (1987), Lacro and Jones (1987), Back et al. (1988), Cotton et al. (1991), Herman et al. (1991), Coffin (1992), Evans et al. (1993), Burket et al. (1994), Aszterbaum et al. (1998), Doede et al. (2004).

## Ovarian fibromas and fibrosarcomas

In general, ovarian fibromas are rare, accounting for only 4% of all ovarian tumors. Less than 10% have been noted in women less than 30 years, and their occurrence in prepubertal females is truly rare. Initially it was difficult to know the absolute frequency of ovarian fibromas in nevoid basal cell carcinoma syndrome as they do not present unless they become large and calcified and twist on their pedicles (Bosch-Banyeras et al. 1989). However, there have been ultrasound studies performed which have rather well established their frequency in the syndrome. A population-based study suggested a 25% incidence (Evans et al. 1993). Shanley et al. (1994) and Kimonis et al. (1997, 2004) found ovarian fibro-

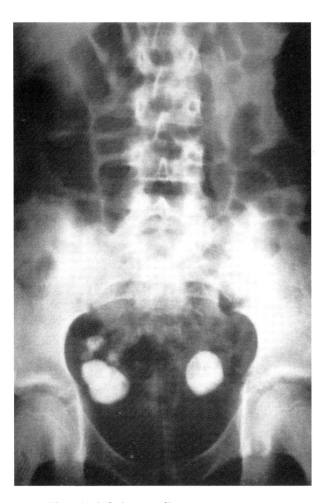

**Fig. 7.** Bilateral calcified ovarian fibromas.

mas with ultrasound in 15–17%. The fibromas associated with the syndrome are more often bilateral (75%), multinodular and calcified (Fig. 7), often overlapping medially (Johnson et al. 1986, Seracchioli et al. 2001). Several such cases have been erroneously diagnosed as calcified uterine leiomyomas. They may present before menarche (Raggio et al. 1983, Johnson et al. 1986). In contrast, ovarian fibromas not associated with this syndrome are typically unilateral, and only 10% are calcified. The reader is referred to a paper by Gorlin (1987) for cases reported prior to 1986. Rarely, the ovarian fibroma in the syndrome may be virilizing or renin-secreting (Ismail and Walker 1990, Yoshizumi et al. 1990, Fox et al. 1994). We suspect that the patients described by Reiter et al. (1982) had ovarian fibromas. Virilization was found in both mother and daughter.

Ovarian fibrosarcoma has also been described (Jackson and Gardere 1971, Rittersma 1972, Ryan and Burkes 1973, Lindeberg et al. 1982, Kraemer et al. 1984, Gorlin 1987, Seracchioli et al. 2003) as well as other tumors. However, I have not been able to obtain this material for personal microscopic review.

## Fetal rhabdomyoma

Schweisguth et al. (1968) first reported fetal rhabdomyoma of the newborn. Originally interpreted as an intercostal rhabdomyosarcoma, immunological reexamination in 1986 showed its true nature. Dahl et al. (1976b) reported examples on the thigh and chest wall in a newborn child. Gorlin (1987) reviewed examples of fetal rhabdomyoma on the thigh and chest wall in newborn children with NBCCS. He further noted that he had occasion to see an adult male with the syndrome who had a fetal rhabdomyoma of intercostal muscles. Klijanienko et al. (1988) described a presternal example in a one-year-old. Subsequently, additional fetal rhabdomyomas appeared at the angle of the mandible at six years and in the cervical area at 26 years. DiSanto et al. (1992) reported a six-year-old female child with fetal rhabdomyoma of the posterior mediastinum and retroperitoneum. Hardisson et al. (1996) noted a retroperitoneal neural variant in a 15-year-old male.

Fetal rhabdomyoma of the tongue in association with cleft lip-palate was found by Watson et al. (2004).

Among the various types of rhabdomyoma: adult, fetal and genital, fetal is the least common of the three types. They tend to arise in the head and neck region of young male infants, particularly in the retroauricular region. Local recurrence is not a feature. As the reader will note, among the examples described associated with the syndrome, there is no predilection for site or age. Differentiation into strap-like rhabdomyoblasts may only be evident toward the periphery of the lesions.

## Mesenteric cysts

Single or multiple chylous or lymphatic mesenteric cysts have been documented in several examples of NBCCS. Most examples have been without symptoms, only have been found at laparatomy and, hence, are underestimated in frequency (Clendenning and Bloch 1964, Cernéa et al. 1969, Rossi et al. 1979, Southwick and Schwartz 1979, MacSweeney et al. 1985, Gorlin 1987).

The thin-walled cysts measure 2–14 cm in diameter. The contents are chylous but may contain hemorrhagic turbid fluid. Microscopically, the wall of the cyst is composed of fibrous connective tissue and smooth muscle. A layer of lymphocytic cells is often located beneath the endothelial lining. The cysts may be calcified and show up on an axial CT scan of the abdomen.

## Miscellaneous tumors

There seems to be an increase in several other neoplasms or hamartomas: leiomyomas of the bowel of the bowel and mesentery (Kahn and Gordon 1967, Taylor et al. 1968, Helseth and Mylius 1986); leiomyosarcoma (Garcia-Prats et al. 1994, Seracchioli et al. 2003); liposarcoma (O'Malley et al. 1997); lymphangioma (Rossi et al. 1979); adrenal cystic lymphangioma (Mortelé et al. 1999); melanoma (Summerly and Hale 1965; Kedem et al. 1970, (Bansal et al. 1975), craniopharyngioma (Mortimer et al. 1984); mesenchymoma (Schlieter 1973, Wolthers and Stellfeld 1987, Koch et al. 2002); rhabdomyosarcoma (Beddis et al. 1983); Hodgkin lymphoma (Neblett et al. 1971, Potaznik and Steinherz 1984, Zvulunov et al. 1995; non-Hodgkin lymphoma (Schulz-Butulis et al. 2000); adenoid cystic carcinoma (Yilmaz et al. 2003); schwannoma (O'Malley et al. 1997); cyst of lung (Totten 1980); paratesticular pseudotumor (Watson and Harper 1992); seminoma (Zaun 1981); and a host of other neoplasms cited by Gundlach and Kiehn (1979), Stieler et al. (1987), Zvulunov et al. (1995), Schulz-Butulis et al. (2000), Gorlin (2001), and Yilmaz et al. (2003). No doubt, some of these tumors have only chance association.

## Kidney anomalies

Approximately 5% have minor kidney anomalies. These have included horseshoe kidney, L-shaped kidney, unilateral renal agenesis, renal cysts, and duplication of renal pelvis and ureters. Because most of these findings have been diagnosed on laparoscopy or at autopsy, their frequency is probably higher (Santis et al. 1983, Coffin 1992, Gorlin 1995, Veenestra-Knol et al. 2005).

## Hypogonadism

Approximately 5–10% of males exhibit such signs of hypogonadotrophic hypogonadism as anosmia, cryptorchidism, female pubic escutcheon, gynecomastia, and/or scanty facial or body hair (Cernéa et al. 1969, Wallace et al. 1973, Rayner et al. 1977, Gorlin 1987). Shanley et al. (1994), in their survey, noted that 10% exhibited anosmia.

We are aware of two female patients with NBCCS who had classic Turner syndrome. We suspect that this was chance association (Andreev and Zlaatkov 1971, Kittler and Binder 2000).

## Neurological findings

### Medulloblastoma, other brain tumors, and seizures

The association of nevoid basal cell carcinoma syndrome (NBCCS) with medulloblastoma has been known since 1963 when this relationship was pointed out by Herzberg and Wiskemann (1963). The tumor characteristically presents during the first two years of life (Gorlin 1987, Korczak et al. 1997) as opposed to seven to eight years in the general population, reflecting Knudson's hypothesis. There have been various studies concerning the incidence of medulloblastoma in NBCCS (Lacombe et al. 1990). Evans et al. (1993) determined that 1–2% of 173 consecutive cases of medulloblastoma had the syndrome. Stavrou et al. (2000) found that about 4% of a large series of medulloblastoma had NBCCS. Conversely, a population study of NBCCS patients determined that 3–5% had medulloblastoma. There was a 3M:1F sex predilection. Because medulloblastoma presents so early in patients with NBCCS as opposed to those in the general population, children who exhibit with the tumor, especially those that are less than 5 years of age, should be carefully examined for signs of the syndrome (Kimonis et al. 1997).

As far as we can tell, all examples of medulloblastoma in the syndrome have been of the desmoplastic variety (Fig. 8) (Schofield et al. 1995, Amlashi et al. 2003). There is some evidence that medulloblastoma associated with NBCCS behaves more benignly than those found as isolated examples (Schofield et al. 1995, Amlashi et al. 2003, Su et al. 2003). Stavrou et al. (2000) noted that both of his medulloblastoma patients with NBCCS had calcification of the meninges.

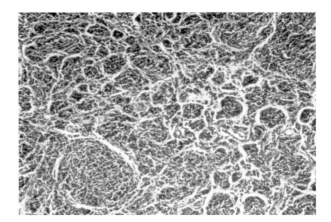

**Fig. 8.** Medulloblastoma of the desmoplastic type characteristic of those having nevoid basal cell carcinoma syndrome.

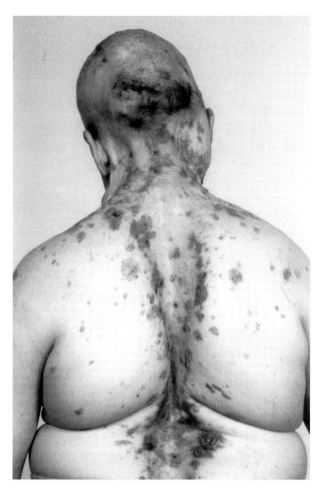

**Fig. 9.** Patient who as a child had medulloblastoma and was subsequently radiated from base of skull along spine. Within months to years following radiation, huge numbers of basal cell carcinomas appeared in areas of radiation.

Radiation therapy of medulloblastoma to the base of the skull and along the spine often results in huge numbers of invasive basal cell carcinomas appearing in the radiation field (Fig. 9) (i.e., from nape to base of spine) (Frentz 1987, O'Malley et al. 1997, Walter et al. 1997, Evans et al. 1998). Clinically, a "rash" appears from six months to three years following radiation therapy. This rash represents activated basal cell cancers which often become markedly invasive within another ten years. It should be pointed out that numerous small radiolucencies of bone ("flame lucencies") which are really hamartomas, may be confused with intracalvarial spread of medulloblastoma (Gorlin et al. 1995).

Brain tumors other than medulloblastoma are infrequent. The next most common is meningioma (Gorlin 1987, Albrecht et al. 1994); but other tumors have included astrocytoma (Cawson and Kerr 1964, Hermans et al. 1965, Evans et al. 1993); craniopharyngioma (Tamoney 1969); and oligodendroglioma. (Kirsch and Selle 1969). These tumors may well be secondary to radiation therapy, especially meningioma (O'Malley et al. 1997). A malignant-appearing meningioma was reported by Albrecht et al. (1994).

Cysts of the brain have been described: colloid cyst of the third ventricle, arachnoid cyst, cyst of choroid plexus, intraparenchymal cyst, cysts of the septum pellucidum (Kahn and Gordon 1967, Neblett et al. 1971, Murphy and Tenser 1982, Naguib et al. 1982, Lindeberg et al. 1982, Cramer and Niederdellmann 1983, Lambrecht et al. 1985, Pearlman and Herzog 1990, Nishimo et al. 1991, Albrecht et al. 1994, Goldstein et al. 1994, Snider 1994, Takanashi et al. 2000, Kantarci et al. 2003). Vermian dysgenesis has been reported in a mother and daughter (Snider 1994, Kantarci et al. 2003, Ozturk et al. 2003).

Seizures have occasionally been reported unassociated with brain tumors and possibly due to focal neuronal heterotopia (Hogan et al. 1996). The corpus callosum has been thinned (Kantarci et al. 2003, Ozturk et al. 2003). Empty sella syndrome may be seen (Takanashi et al. 2000).

## Pathogenesis and molecular genetics

The syndrome has autosomal dominant inheritance with complete penetrance and variable expressivity. There are many large pedigrees involving several generations. About 60% of the patients do not have an affected parent. A paternal age effect has been demonstrated in cases of such new mutations (Jones et al. 1975). The nevoid basal cell carcinoma syndrome nicely fits Knudson two-hit hypothesis. In the case of *isolated basal cell carcinoma*, both hits must affect the same cell; hence the low frequency of basal cell carcinomas (Bonifas et al. 1994, Cowan et al. 1997). Rayner et al. (1977) noted the increase of susceptibility of the skin of patients with the syndrome to the oncogenic effect of tissue-damaging physical agents; they also noted that radiotherapy is contraindicated as a form of treatment of the basal cell carcinomas. Sunlight appears to play some role in the syndrome as the lesions are more often found on the head, neck, and other sun-exposed areas. Furthermore, African–Americans with the syndrome manifest skin tumors less frequently and at a later age (Cotton et al. 1982).

The first hit or mutation is present in each cell in the inherited form; the second, in most cases, represents radiation damage. Nevoid basal cell carcinomas are basically the same in origin as ordinary basal cell cancers, but they differ in their earlier onset of appearance and are less related to sun exposure than ordinary basal cell cancers. In sporadic cases, both copies of *PTCH1* may be inactivated somatically during postnatal life, frequently during ultraviolet-mutgenesis.

The mutated gene, *Patched1*, has been mapped to chromosome band 9q22.3 (Farndon et al. 1992; Reis

et al. 1992; Wicking et al. 1997a, b; Boutet et al. 2003). The gene has 23 exons and 12 transmembrane-spanning domains coding for 2 large hydrophilic extra-cellular loops where *Sonic Hedgehog* ligand-binding occurs. Mutations can occur throughout the *PTCH1* gene (Reifenberger 2004).

In the event that a mutation occurs in *Patched*, the second loop is not formed, and *Sonic Hedgehog* cannot be attached (Fig. 10). A few examples of deletion of this area of chromosome 9 have been seen in patients with the syndrome (Shimkets et al. 1996, Haniffa et al. 2004, Midro et al. 2004, Boonen et al. 2005). I have personally seen two such individuals who were severely mentally retarded (Biljsma and Gorlin 1999).

The widespread developmental anomalies as well as other neoplasms and loss of heterozygosity at this site suggest mutation of a tumor-suppressing gene (Bale et al. 1994, Levenat et al. 1996). The gene, *Patched1*, which modifies the Hedgehog-signalling pathway, is mutated not only in the syndrome but in ordinary isolated basal cell carcinomas (Gailani et al. 1992, 1996; Hahn et al. 1996; Undén et al. 1996, 1997; Bale 1997; Gailani and Bale 1997; Lench et al. 1997; Aszterbaum et al. 1998; Villavicencio et al. 2000; Lam et al. 2002; Fujii et al. 2003). *Patched*, in the absence of its ligand, *Sonic Hedgehog*, acts as cell-cycle regulator, normally inhibiting expression of downstream genes (*Smoothened*, among others) which control cellular patterning and growth (Bale et al. 1994, 1998, Johnson et al. 1996, Sidransky 1996, Taipale et al. 2000, Bale and Yu 2001). In the case of a C-terminal truncation caused by a mutation in *Patched*, *Smoothened* is no longer repressed. As noted above, in accordance with the Knudson two-hit hypothesis, there is an inherited point (germline) mutation with subsequent loss of its homologue by mitotic non-disjunction, deletion, or mitotic recombination, i.e., random somatic events. In the syndrome, various tumors and hamartomas (basal cell carcinomas, odontogenic keratocysts, medulloblastomas, ovarian fibromas) exhibit loss of heterozygosity (Schofield et al. 1995, Lench et al. 1996, Vortmeyer et al. 1999, Barreto et al. 2000, Matsumara et al. 2000, Minami et al. 2001, Koch et al. 2002, Shear 2002, Agaram et al. 2004). However, other lesions

**HEDGEHOG ABSENT**     **HEDGEHOG PRESENT**

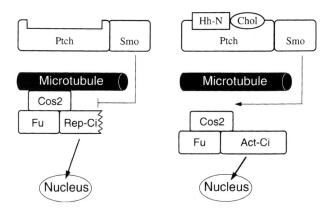

**Fig. 10.** Molecular basis for nevoid basal cell carcinoma syndrome. Normally, the *Patched gene* acts as a receptor for *Sonic Hedgehog*. Under normal conditions, the *Patched gene* suppresses the adjacent gene, *Smoothened*. This prevents detachment of costal 2 from the microtubules. However, with attachment of *Sonic Hedgehog* and its cholesterol moiety, the inhibition of *Smoothened* ceases, and the costal 2-fused complex is released and causes several genes, among them *Patched*, to be produced by the nucleus which causes inhibited basal cell multiplication.

do not exhibit loss of heterozygosity (e.g., palmar pits) (Matsumura et al. 2000). Loss of heterozygosity of the *Patched* locus has been observed in almost 90% of hereditary basal cell carcinomas. Various physical anomalies (bifid rib, macrocephaly) apparently need only one hit. The reader is referred to superb detailed reviews of the molecular aspects of this syndrome by Cohen (1999, 2003).

Oski et al. (2004) in a study of PTCH1 gene mutations and expression of SHH, PTCH, SMD, and GLI-1 in odontogenic keratocysts, found the PTCH mutation not only in the syndrome cysts but in isolated keratocysts as well. Patients with NBCCS inherit one defective copy of PTCH1, and frequently the second copy is mutated during basal cell carcinogenesis.

Analysis of over 60 different gene mutations in the syndrome indicates deletions, insertions, splice-site alterations, and nonsense and missense mutations with no hot spots identified for mutations. About 70% of germline *Patched* mutations are rearrangements (Wicking et al. 1994, 1997a, b; Hasenpusch-Theil et al. 1998; Zedan et al. 2001; High and Zedan 2005; Tanioka et al. 2005). Over 80% appear to result in truncation of the Patched 1 protein (Boutet ct al. 2003). As noted earlier, the gene is large, consisting of 23 exons which span 34 KB. It encodes a transmembrane glycoprotein composed of 1447 amino acids with 12 hydrophobic transmembrane domains. Using single strand confirmation polymorphism analysis or heteroduplex analysis, only about 50% of mutations can be detected. However, Lamb et al. (2002), using denaturating high-performance liquid chromatography, found that 90% of patients had mutations. There are no genotype-phenotype correlations (Wicking 1997b, Reifenberger 2004). Prenatal diagnosis has been accomplished (Bialer et al. 1994, Petrikovsky et al. 1996).

The *Hedgehog* signalling pathway is much more involved with regard to (1) *Hedgehog's* complex with cholesterol and a palmitate moiety (the cholesterol is attached at the C-terminal, and the palmitate at the end-terminal) and (2) downstream signalling. An intracellular complex of *costal 2, fused, suppressor of fused*, and a short form of *cubitus interruptus* (GLI

protein in vertebrates) (Ruiz I Altaba et al. 1987, Bale and Yu 2001) is tethered to microtubules. Release of this complex from the microtubules is effected by the *Hedgehog*-cholesterol-palmitate ligand which, in turn, allows transcription of *Patched (PTC), Wingless (WNT)*, and *decapentaplegic (BMP)* genes (Cohen 1999, 2003).

Various disorders related to defects in the extended pathway include Smith–Lemli–Opitz syndrome, Greig cephalopolysyndactyly, Pallister–Hall syndrome, and polyaxial polydactyly, type A. Mutations in both *Sonic Hedgehog* and *Patched* genes have been shown to cause holoprosencephaly (Ming et al. 2002, Debeer and Devriendt 2005).

In the presence of *Sonic Hedgehog*, the pathway acts in at least two ways to regulate target genes. One is to activate GLI1-2 transcription factors, and the other is to inhibit formation of GLI repressors, mostly from GLI3 to repress target genes (Ruiz y Altaba 1987, Taipale et al. 2000). Finally, it is noteworthy that about 30% of basal cell carcinomas in patients with NBCCS have mutations in *p53 gene* (Ling et al. 2001).

## Differential diagnosis

Basaloid follicular hamartomas have been reported with alopecia and myasthenia gravis on several occasions (Ridley and Smith 1981, Mehregan and Baker 1985, Starink et al. 1986, Weltfriend et al. 1987, Miyakawa et al. 1988, Gartmann et al. 1989, Brownstein 1992, Mascaro et al. 1995, Requena et al. 1999). However, the reader should review the discussion of this entity earlier. Bazex syndrome consists of basal cell carcinomas (especially of the face), follicular atrophoderma (especially of hands, feet, and elbows), hypotrichosis, and generalized hypohidrosis or anhidrosis of the face and head (Plosila et al. 1981, Metha and Potdur 1985, Vabres and de-Prost 1993, Goeteyn et al. 1994, Rapelenoro et al. 1994, Lacombe and Taïeb 1995, Kidd et al. 1996, Inoue et al. 1998). Bazex syndrome has dominant inheritance. Vabres et al. (1995) mapped the gene of Bazex syndrome to Xq24-q27.

Oley et al. (1992) reported a possible X-linked dominant syndrome of basal cell carcinomas, sparse hair and milia, but Vabres and DeProst (1993) argued that this represents Bazex syndrome. Rombo syndrome, named after a family, resembles Bazex syndrome, but there is neither follicular atrophoderma nor sweating abnormalities. It, too, has autosomal dominant inheritance (Michaëlson et al. 1981, Ashinoff et al. 1993). Rasmussen syndrome consists of trichoepitheliomas, milia, and cylindromas (Rasmussen 1971).

## Management

Diagnostic radiographic study is mandated.

## Radiographic findings

### Skull

Lamellar calcification of the falx cerebri (Fig. 11) is found in 55–95% (Ratcliffe et al. 1995a). A calcified falx is especially significant in the younger patient (under 20 years). Calcification of the tentorium cerebelli has been noted in 20–40%, the petroclinoid ligament in 20%, and the diaphragma sellae in 60–80%. Radiographically, the sella turcica appears bridged, i.e., as if there were fusion of the anterior and posterior clinoid processes (Dunnick et al. 1978; Lovin et al. 1991; Kimonis 1997, 2004; Stavrou et al. 2000).

Focal thinning of the skull, which we have interpreted as corresponding to flame-shaped lucen-

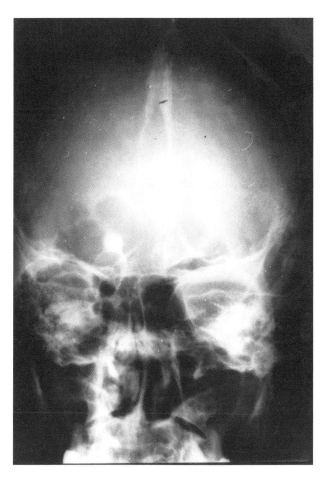

**Fig. 11.** Note layered calcification of falx cerebri.

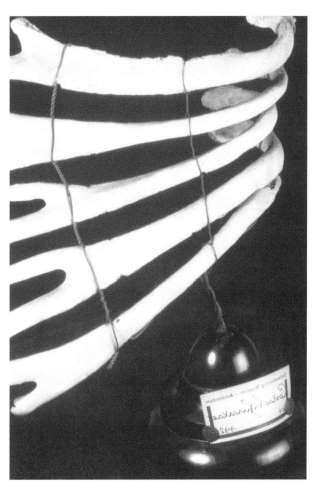

**Fig. 12.** Multiple bifid ribs.

cies, has been noted in the calvaria (Hawkins et al. 1979).

## Skeletal radiographic findings

Fused, splayed, hypoplastic or bifid ribs (Fig. 12) have been documented in 45–60% (Ratcliffe et al. 1995b). Kyphoscoliosis with or without pectus has been noted in 25–40% (Kimonis et al. 1997, 2004). Spina bifida occulta of the cervical or thoracic vertebrae was reported in 60% (Ratcliffe et al. 1995a). However, Kimonis et al. (1997, 2004) found spina bifida occulta in only about 20% of their series. Sprengel deformity and/or unusual narrow sloping shoulders have been noted in 10–40% (Cernéa et al. 1969; Rayner et al. 1977; Pratt and Jackson 1987; Kimonis et al. 1997, 2004; Reifenberger 2004). Other anomalies seen in about 40% include cervical or upper thoracic vertebral fusion, hemivertebra, and lumbarization of the sacrum. Various other bony anomalies have been reported in about 5%. Sclerotic bone lesions were described by Yee et al. (1993) and Hawkins et al. (1979).

Rarely one finds pre-or postaxial polydactyly of hands or feet, hallux valgus, and syndactyly of fingers 2–3 or 3–4 (Cernéa et al. 1969, Doede et al. 2004). Other examples have been cited by Gorlin (1987). Specifically, Shanley et al. (1994) found syndactyly in 3% and polydactyly in 4%. Although the 4th metacarpal has been alleged to be short, this is a poor sign because about 10% of the normal population has a positive sign (Gorlin 1987, Chevenix-Trench et al. 1993). Small pseudocystic bone lesions (flame-shaped lucencies) have been identified in phalanges, metapodial bones, carpal and tarsal bones, long bones, pelvis, and calvaria in 30% (Novak and Bloss 1976; Dunnick et al. 1978; Hermann and Som 1981; DelaPlaza 1983; Blinder et al. 1984; Dereume et al. 1985; Kimonis et al. 1997, 2004; Ly 2002). Calvarial and other osseous involvement may give the impression that medulloblastoma has spread to bone (Miller and Cooper 1972, Hawkins et al. 1979, Blinder et al. 1984). Histologically, the flame-like lesions are hamartomas, consisting of fibrous connective tissue, nerves and blood vessels. Subcutaneous calcification of fingers and scalp has been rare.

Prenatal diagnosis by sonography and other means has been accomplished (Bale et al. 1993, Hogge et al. 1994, Petrikovsky et al. 1996).

## Skin management

Patients with nevoid basal cell carcinoma syndrome involves visits to a dermatologist every two to three months, especially during adolescence. Earlier visits are indicated for the young child at risk. Surgical (Mohs) excision and split-thickness grafting can be used for larger skin cancers (Mohs et al. 1980, Rowe et al. 1989, Stockfleth et al. 2002). Carbon dioxide laser resurfacing may be useful following multiple Mohs surgeries (Doctoroff et al. 2003). However, incompletely treated carcinomas growing under the laser-induced scarring can be a problem (A. Oseroff, personal communication, 2005). $CO_2$ laser has also been used for nodular lesions. Intralesional application of interferon-2b has been used to remove papular lesions of small size (Kopera et al. 1996).

Management of superficial multicentric basal cell carcinomas without folllicular involvement can be accomplished by total body application of a topical 0.1% tretinoin cream and 5-fluourouracil twice daily (Peck et al. 1988, Altucci and Gronemeyer 2001, DiGiovanna 2001). This regimen is essentially free of side effects, may uncover clinically imperceptible lesions, and may slow or prevent new tumors. For lesions around the eyes, only 5-fluorouracil is applied. The patient should be examined every three months, and lesions manifesting growth or those which have become invasive should be excised or curretted. This approach has been extensively discussed by Strange and Lang (1992) and DiGiovanna (2001).*

---

*Oral etretinate should not be taken by females of child-bearing potential and, if used, a negative pregnancy test should be obtained prior to starting therapy. Adequate contraception should be used during and for at least two months after stopping etretinate therapy. Pseudotumor cerebri (benign intracranial hypertension may result from etretinate and isotretinoin and hepatotoxicity has occurred in 1–2% of those taking oral etretinate. The FDA has not specifically approved either etretinate or isotretinoin for use in treatment of NBCCS, so, if these medications are prescribed, the risks versus benefits of each must be discussed with the patients.

The efficacy of 5% imiquimod (Aldera) cream has been demonstrated. Imiquimod is a cytokine inducer, as is interferon-alpha. The cream is applied 5–7 days per week for 12 weeks (Kagy and Amonette 2000, Stockfleth et al. 2002, Micali et al. 2003). There is usually mild erythema and erosion and bleeding at week 3. Although no huge controlled studies have been published, the present evidence would indicate that this mode of treatment is markedly helpful. Successful imiquimod treatment requires an inflammatory response. Some patients with the syndrome report minimal inflammation, and they tend to have little benefit.

Photodynamic therapy (PDT) is also an extremely effective form of treatment of diffuse basal cell cancers and basaloid follicular hamartomas (Cairnduff et al. 1994, Thissen et al. 2000, Oseroff et al. 2005). Topical PDT involves application of photosensitizing topical 20% delta-aminolevulinic acid for 24 hours under occlusion. There is accumulation of the sensitizer within the malignant cells which are then treated with red light, usually produced by a laser, which subsequently kills these cells. Minimal morbidity is expressed. Scabs formed over the basal cell carcinomas usually fall off by 2 weeks following PDT with minimal scarring (Itkin and Gilchrest 2004, Oseroff et al. 2005). After 4–7 hours there is an average of 95% tumor response in adults. This appears to be the treatment of choice for children (Oseroff et al. 2005). It works best for superficial and thin nodular disease (<2 mm thick). Systemic photophorin II, a light sensitizer composed of porphyrin linked by ether bonds, has been given systemically in numerous clinical trials. A side effect is prolonged cutaneous photosensitivity to bright sunlight. Patients should be instructed to avoid sunlight for 6–8 weeks after injection. There is also damage to normal skin (Wilson et al. 1992).

## Odontogenic keratocyst management

Odontogenic keratocysts can be particular vexing because, as with the basal cell carcinomas, one never reaches a "safe time" in life after which they do not appear. Although jaw fracture is very rare, the cysts can be extremely destructive and push various anatomic structures out of the way. A panoramic radiograph of the jaws is mandated annually from the age of 8 years onward. If keratocysts are found, they should be completely removed by an oral/maxillofacial surgeon or otolaryngologist who has extensive experience with their removal because recurrence is frequent (Posnick et al. 1994).

Small odontogenic keratocysts should be completely removed surgically. Mucoperiosteal flaps are raised, the cystic cavity unroofed with a dental handpiece and bur and the cysts enucleated.

Adjunctive therapies for odontogenic keratocysts such as cryotherapy or Carnoy's solution are indicated (Blanchard 1997, Blanas et al. 2000, Schmidt and Pogrel 2001). The latter is especially safe and generally effective in reducing recurrence. The solution is applied for two minutes following enucleation. It is important to emphasize that recurrence is lower with smaller cysts, so early attention is needed. Large cysts require marsupialization or decompression following secondary enucleation. There must be strict adherence to follow-up protocol (every year for the first five years, then every other year). Although almost self-evident, dental implants are contraindicated. Elaborate bridgework should be avoided because of cyst recurrence.

## Other management

For infants at risk, medulloblastoma should be excluded by annual magnetic resonance imaging until 8 years of age. Although rare, cardiac fibroma should be excluded by a chest radiograph periodically. In children at risk, the presumptive diagnosis of NBCCS can often by achieved by radiographic means (calcification of falx, rib anomalies, calcification of ovarian fibromas, etc.). Definitive presymptomatic diagnosis can be often achieved by molecular genetic studies. These are done by a number of laboratories: Dr. Sherri Bale at Gene Diagnosis (sherrib@genedx.com) or that of Dr. Allen Bale at Yale University School of Medicine (bale@biomed.med.yale.edu).

The patient may also desire help from a support group. We are fortunate in having superb ones in the

United States (BCCNS Life Support Network, Kristi Schmitt Burr, info@bccns.org); England (Gorlin Syndrome Group, Margaret Costello, gorlin. group@ btconnect.com) and the Netherlands (Willem Breurken, gorlin@planet.nl.

There is a toll-free telephone connection in the United States at 866-834-1895.

## Genetic counseling

The nevoid basal cell carcinoma syndrome has autosomal dominant inheritance with complete penetrance and remarkably variable expressivity (Reifenberger 2004). There is no sexual predilection. About one-half of the cases represent new mutations. The mutated gene, *Patched*, has been mapped to chromosome band 9q22.3 (Farndon et al. 1992, 1994; Chidambaram et al. 1996; Wicking et al. 1997a). The accuracy with which the mutation can be detected has ranged in commercial labs from 65 to 85%. In some cases, the diagnosis is so obvious as to preclude molecular confirmation of the diagnosis (Table 2). A web page of *PTCH* mutation database is available at: http://www. cybergene.se/cgi-bin/w3-msql/ptchbase/index.html

**Table 2.** Diagnostic criteria for NBCCS

Diagnosis based on two major or one major and two minor criteria

*Major criteria*

1. More than 2 BCCs or one under age of 20 years
2. Odontoggenic keratocyst
3. Three or more palmar pits
4. Bilamellar calcification of falx cerebri
5. Bifid, fused or splayed ribs
6. First degree relative with NBCCS

*Minor criteria*

1. Macrocephaly adjusted for height
2. Frontal bossing, cleft lip/palate, hypertelorism
3. Sprengel deformity, pectus, syndactyly of digits
4. Bridging of sella turcica, hemivertebrae, flame-shaped radiolucencies
5. Ovarian fibroma
6. Medulloblastoma

Based on V.E. Kimonis et al. (1997)

## Acknowledgements

The text of this chapter was critically reviewed by Dr. Erv Epstein (San Francisco) and Dr. Allan Oseroff (Buffalo, NY). The author is indebted to them for their many suggestions.

## References

Adem K, Nassar A (2004) Fine needle aspiration of lytic bone lesions in a 63-year–old woman — pathologic diagnosis: Metastatic basal cell carcinoma to the bone in Gorlin syndrome. Arch Pathol Lab Med 128: 819–820.

Agaram NP, Collins BM, Barnes L (2004) Molecular analysis to demonstrate that odontogenic keratocysts are neoplastic. Arch Pathol Lab Med 128: 313–317.

Ahn SG, Lim YS, Kim DK, Kim SG, Lee SH, Yoon JH (2004) Nevoid basal cell carcinoma syndrome: a retrospective analysis of 33 affected Korean individuals. Int J Oral Maxillofac Surg 33: 458–562.

Albrecht S, Goodman JC, Rajagopalan S, Levy M, Cech PA, Cooley LD (1994) Malignant meningioma in Gorlin's syndrome. Cytogenetic and p53 gene analysis. J Neurosurg 81: 466–471.

Altucci L, Gronemeyer H (2001) The promise of retinoids to fight against cancer. Nat Rev Cancer 1: 181–193.

Amlashi SFA, Riffaud L, Brassier G, Morandi X (2003) Nevoid basal cell carcinoma syndrome: relation with desmoplastic medulloblastoma in infancy. Cancer 98: 618–624.

Andreev VC, Zlatkov NB (1971) Basal cell nevus syndrome and Turner's syndrome in a patient. Int J Dermatol 10: 13–16.

Ashinoff R, Jacobson M, Belsito DV (1993) Rombo syndrome: a second case report and review. J Am Acad Dermatol 28: 1101–1104.

Aszterbaum M, Rothman A, Johnson RL, Fisher M, Xie J, Bonifas JM, Zhang X, Scott MP, Epstein EH (1998) Identification of mutations in the human *PATCHED* gene in sporadic basal cell carcinomas and in patients with the basal cell nevus syndrome. J Invest Derm 110: 885–888.

Bakaeen G, Rajab LD, Sawairi FA, Hamdan MAM, Dallal WD (2004) Nevoid basal cell carcinoma syndrome: a review of the literature and report of a case. Int J Paediatr Dent 14: 279–287.

Back LM, Brown AS, Barot LR (1988) Congenital cardiac tumors in association with orofacial clefts. Ann Plast Surg 20: 558–561.

Bale AE (1997) The nevoid basal cell carcinoma syndrome: genetics and mechanism of carcinogenesis. Cancer Invest 15: 180–186.

Bale AE, Bialer M, Gailani M (1993) Prenatal presymptomatic and preimplantation diagnosis of Gorlin syndrome [Abst #1381]. Am J Hum Genet 53.

Bale AE, Gailani MR, Leffell DJ (1994) Nevoid basal cell carcinoma syndrome. J Invest Dermatol 103: Suppl 126S–130S.

Bale AE, Yu KP (2001) The hedgehog pathway and basal cell carcinomas. Hum Molec Genet 10: 757–762.

Bale SJ, Amos CI, Parry DM, Bale AE (1991) Relationship between head circumference and heights in normal adults and in the nevoid basal cell carcinoma syndrome and neurofibromatosis, type 1. Am J Med Genet 40: 206–210.

Bale SJ, Falk RT, Rogers GR (1998) Patching together the genetics of Gorlin syndrome. J Cutan Med Surg 3: 31–34.

Bansal MP, Sengupta SR, Krishnan EC (1975) Basal cell naevus syndrome. Indian J Cancer 12: 214–218.

Barr RJ, Headley JL, Jensen JL, Howell JB (1986) Cutaneous keratocysts of nevoid basal cell carcinoma syndrome. J Am Acad Dermatol 14: 572–576.

Barreto DL, Gomez RS, Bale AE, Boson WL, DeMarco L (2000) PTCH gene mutations in odontogenic keratocysts. J Dent Res 79: 1418–1422.

Baselga E, Dzwierzynski WW, Neuberg M, Troy JL, Esterly NL (1996) Cutaneous keratocysts in naevoid basal cell carcinoma syndrome. Br J Derm 135: 810–812.

Beddis IR, Mott MG, Bullimore J (1983) Nasopharyngeal rhabdomyosarcoma and Gorlin's naevoid basal cell carcinoma syndrome. Med Pediatr Oncol 11: 178–179.

Berardi RS, Korbe J, Melton J, Chen H (1991) Pulmonary metastasis in nevoid basal cell carcinoma syndrome. Int Surg 76: 64–66.

Bialer MG, Gailani MR, McLaughlin JA, Petrikovsky B, Bale AE (1994) Prenatal diagnosis of Gorlin syndrome. Lancet 344: 477.

Bijlsma EK, Gorlin RJ: Two patients with nevoid basal cell carcinoma syndrome and an interstitial deletion on chromosome 91. XX David W. Smith Workshop on Malformations and Morphogenesis. Schlangenbad, Germany, 3–9 August, 1999.

Binkley GW, Johnson HH (1951) Epithelioma adenoides cysticum: Basal cell nevi, agenesis of the corpus callosum, and dental cysts. Arch Dermatol Syph 63: 73–84.

Blanas N, Freund B, Schwartz M, Furst IM (2000) Systematic review of the treatment and prognosis of the odontogenic keratocyst. Oral Surg Oral Med Oral Pathol Oral Radiol Endod 90: 553–558.

Blanchard SB (1997) Odontogenic keratocysts: review of the literature and report of a case. J Periodontol 68: 306–311.

Blinder G, Barke Y, Petz M, Bar-Ziv J (1984) Widespread osteolytic lesions of the long bones in basal cell nevus syndrome. Skel Radiol 12: 195–198.

Bonifas JM, Bare JW, Kerschmann RL, Master SP, Epstein EH (1994) Parental origin of chromosome 9q22.3q31 lost in basal cell carcinomas from basal cell nevus syndrome patients. Hum Molec Genet 3: 447–448.

Boonen SE, Stahl D, Kreiborg S, Rosenberg T, Kalscheuer V, Larsen LA, Tommerup N, Brøndum-Nielsen K, Tümer Z (2005) Delineation of an interstitial 9q22 deletion in basal cell nevus syndrome. Am J Med Genet 132A: 324–328.

Bosch-Banyeras JM, Lucaya X, Bernet M, Iriondo L, Capdevila A, Bau A, Zuagnabar A, Bosch J (1989) Calcified ovarian fibromas in prepubertal girls. Eur J Pediatr 148: 749–750.

Boutet N, Bignon Y, Drouin-Garraud V, Sarda P, Longy M, Lacombe D, Gorry P (2003) Spectrum of PTCH1 mutations in French patients with Gorlin syndrome. J Invest Dermatol 121: 478–481.

Brownstein MH (1992) Basaloid follicular hamartoma: solitary and multiple types. J Am Acad Dermatol 27: 237–240.

Bunting PD, Remensnyder JP (1977) Basal cell nevus syndrome. Plast Reconstr Surg 60: 895–901.

Burke AP, de Christenson MR, Templeton PA, Virmani R (1994) Cardiac fibroma: clinocopathologic correlates and surgical treatment. J Thorac Cardiovasc Surg 108: 862–870.

Cairnduff F, Stringer MR, Hudson EJ, Ash DV, Brown SB (1994) Superficial photodynamic therapy with topical 5 aminolaevulinic acid for superficial primary and secondary skin cancer. Br J Cancer 69: 605–608.

Camisa C, Rossana C, Little L (1985) Naevoid basal-cell carcinoma syndrome with unilateral neoplasms and pits. Br J Dermatol 113: 365–367.

Cawson RA, Kerr GA (1964) The syndrome of jaw cysts, basal cell tumours and skeletal anomalies. Proc R Soc Med 57: 799–801.

Cernéa P, Kuffer R, Baumont M, Brocheriou C, Guilbert F (1969) Naevomatose baso-cellulaire. Rev Stomatol (Paris) 70: 181–226.

Chen Y, Hsieh C, Eng H, Huang C (2004) Ovarian fibroma in a 7-month-old infant: a case report and review of the literature. Pediatr Surg Int 20: 894–897.

Chevenix-Trench G, Wicking C, Berkman J, Sharp H, Hockey A, Haan E, Oley C, Ravine D, Turner A, Goldgar D, Searle J, Wainwright B (1993) Further localization of the gene for nevoid basal cell carcinoma syndrome in 15 Australasian families: linkage and loss of heterozygosity. Am J Hum Genet 53: 760–767.

Chidambaram A, Goldstein AM, Gailani MR, Gerrard B, Bale SJ, DiGiovanna JJ (1996) Mutations in the human homologue of the *Drosophila patched* gene in Caucasian and African-American nevoid basal cell carcinoma syndrome patients. Cancer Res 56: 4599–4601.

Chiritescu E, Maloney ME (2001) Acrochordons as a presenting sign of nevoid basal cell carcinoma syndrome. J Am Acad Dermatol 44: 789–794.

Clendenning WE, Block MB, Radde JC (1964) Basal cell nevus syndrome. Arch Dermatol 90: 38–53.

Coffin C (1992) Congenital cardiac fibroma associated with Gorlin syndrome. Pediatr Pathol 1: 255–262 (same patient as in Herman et al).

Cohen MM Jr (1999) Nevoid basal cell carcinoma syndrome: molecular biology and new hypotheses. Int J Oral Maxillofac Surg 28: 216–233.

Cohen MM Jr (2003) The Hedgehog signalling network. Am J Med Genet 123A: 5–28.

Cotton JL, Kavey RW, Palmier CE, Tunnessen WW (1991) Cardiac tumors and the nevoid basal cell carcinoma syndrome. Pediatrics 87: 725–727.

Cotton S, Super S, Sunder R, Chaudhry A (1982) Nevoid basal cell carcinoma syndrome. J Oral Med 37: 69–73.

Cowan R, Hoban P, Kelsey A, Birch JM, Gattamenini R, Evans DGR (1997) The gene for the naevoid basal cell carcinoma syndrome acts as a tumour-suppressor gene in medulloblastoma. Br J Cancer 76: 141–145.

Cramer H, Niederdellmann H (1983) Cerebral gigantism associated with jaw cyst-basal cell naevoid syndrome in two females. Arch Psychiatr Nervenkr 233: 111–124.

Dahl E, Kreiborg S, Jensen BL (1976a) Craniofacial morphology in the nevoid basal cell carcinoma syndrome. Int J Oral Surg 5: 300–310.

Dahl I, Angervall I, Sävesödervergh J (1976b) Foetal rhabdomyoma. J Acta Pathol Microbiol Scand [Sect. A] 84: 107–112.

Daramola JO, Komolafe OF, Ajagbe HA, Lawoyen DO (1980) Syndrome of multiple jaw cysts, skeletal anomalies, and basal cell nevi: Report of a case. J Natl Med Assoc 72: 259–262.

Debeer P, Devriendt K (2005) Early recognition of basal cell naevus syndrome. Eur J Pediatr 164: 123–125.

DeJong PT, Bistervels B, Cosgrove J, De Grep G, Leys A, Goffin M (1985) A sign of multiple basal cell nevi (Gorlin's) syndrome. Arch Ophthalmol 103: 1833–1836.

DelaPlaza R (1983) Two cases of nevoid basal cell carcinoma syndrome. Plast Reconstr Surg 71: 114–119.

deLeón GA, Zaeri N, Donner RM, Karmazin N (1990) Cerebral rhinocele, hydrocephalus, and cleft lip and palate in infants with cardiac fibroma. J Neurol Sci 99: 27–36.

De Potter P, Stanescu D, Caspers-Velu L, Hofmans A (2000) Combined hamartoma of the retina and retinal pigment epithelium in Gorlin syndrome. Arch Ophthalmol 118: 1004–1005.

Dereume JL, de Sélys R, Bataille S (1985) Syndrome basocellulaire. Dermatologica 170: 293–296.

DiGiovanna JJ (2001) Retinoid chemoprevention in patients at high risk for skin cancer. Med Pediatr Oncol 36: 564–567.

DiSanto S, Abt AB, Boal DK, Krummel TM (1992) Fetal rhabdomyoma and nevoid basal cell carcinoma syndrome. Pediatr Pathol 12: 441–447.

Doctoroff A, Oberlender SA, Purcell SM (2003) Full-face carbon dioxide laser resurfacing in the management of a patient with the nevoid basal cell carcinoma syndrome. Derm Surg 29: 1236–1240.

Doede T, Seidel J, Riede FT, Vogt L, Mohr FW, Schier F (2004) Occult, life threatening cardial tumor and syndactylism in Gorlin-Goltz syndrome. J Pediatr Surg 39: E17–E19.

Dominguez FR, Keszler A (1988) Comparative study of keratocysts associated and non-associated with nevoid basal cell carcinoma syndrome. J Oral Pathol 17: 39–42.

Dominguez M, Brunner M, Hafen E, Basler K (1996) Sending and receiving the Hedgehog signal: control by the Drosophila Gli protein Cubitus interruptus. Science 272: 1621–1625.

Donatsky O, Hjorting-Hansen E (1980) Recurrence of the odontogenic keratocyst in 13 patients with the nevoid basal cell carcinoma syndrome in a 6 year follow-up. Int J Oral Surg 9: 173–179.

Dowling PA, Fleming P, Saunders ID, Gorlin RJ, Napier S (2000) Odontogenic keratocysts in a 5-year-old. Initial manifestations of nevoid basal cell carcinoma syndrome. Pediatr Dent 22: 53–55.

Dunnick NR, Head GL, Peck GL, Yoder FW (1978) Nevoid basal carcinoma syndrome: radiographic manifestations including cystlike lesions of the phalanges. Radiology 127: 331–334.

Edlund S, Holmdahl K (1957) Primary tumour of the heart. Acta Paediatr Scand 46: 59–63.

Evans DGR, Birch HM, Orton CI (1991a) Brain tumours and the occurrence of severe invasive basal cell carcinoma in first degree relatives with Gorlin syndrome. Br J Neurosurg 5: 643–646.

Evans DGR, Farndon PA, Burnell LD, Gattamenini R, Birch JM (1991b) The incidence of Gorlin syndrome in 173 consecutive cases of medulloblastoma. Br J Cancer 64: 959–961.

Evans DGR, Ladusans EJ, Rimmer S, Burnell LD, Thakker N, Farndon PA (1993) Complications of the naevoid basal cell carcinoma syndrome: results of a population based study. J Med Genet 30: 460–464.

Farndon PA, Del Mastro RG, Evans DGR, Kilpatrick MW (1992) Location of gene for Gorlin syndrome. Lancet 339: 581–582.

Farndon PA, Morris D, Hardy C, McConville C, Weissenbach J, Kilpatrick MW, Reis A (1994) Analysis of 133 meioses places the genes for nevoid basal cell carcinoma (Gorlin) syndrome and Fanconi anemia group C in a 2.6-cM interval and contributes to the fine map of 9q22.3. Genomics 23: 486–489.

Fox R, Eckford S, Hirschkowitz L (1994) Refractory gestational hypertension due to a renin-secreting ovarian fibrothecoma associated with Gorlin's syndrome. Br J Obstet Gynaecol 101: 1015–1017.

Frentz G, Munch-Petersen B, Wulf HC, Niebuhr E, Bang F (1987) The nevoid basal cell carcinoma syndrome: sensitivity to ultraviolet and X-ray irradiation. J Am Acad Dermatol 17: 637–643.

Fujii K, Kohno Y, Sugita K, Nakamura M, Moroi Y, Urabe K, Fureie M, Yamada M (2003) Mutations in the human homolog of Drosophila patched in Japanese nevoid basal cell carcinoma syndrome patients. Hum Mutat 21: 451–452.

Gailani MR, Bale AE (1997) Developmental genes and cancer: role of patched in basal cell carcinoma of skin. J Nat Cancer Inst 89: 1103–1109.

Gailani MR, Bale SJ, Leffell DJ, DiGiovanna JJ, Peck GL, Poliak S, Drum MA, Mulvihill J, Bale AE (1992) Developmental defects in Gorlin syndrome related to a putative tumor suppressor gene on chromosome 9. Cell 69: 111–117.

Gailani MR, Stähle-Bäckdahl M, Leffell DJ, Glynn M, Zaphiropoulos PG, Pressman C, Undén AB, Dean M, Brash D, Bale AE (1996) The role of the human homologue of Drosophila patched in sporadic basal cell carcinoma. Nat Genet 14: 78–81.

Garcia-Prats MD, Lopez-Carreira M, Mayordomo JI, Ballestin C, Rivera F, Diaz-Puente MT, Munoz M, Cortes-Funes H, Martinez-Telle F (1994) Leiomyosarcoma of the soft tissues in a patient with nevoid basal-cell carcinoma syndrome. Tumori 80: 401–404.

Gartmann H, Groth W, Quinkler C (1989) Multiple basaloid follikuläre Hamartome bei zwei Mitgliedern einer Familie mit Gorlin-Goltz-Syndrom. Z Hautkrankh 64: 915–918.

Goeteyn M, Geerts ML, Kint A, DeWeert J (1994) The Bazex-Dupré-Christol syndrome. Arch Dermatol 130: 337–342.

Goldberg HM, Pratt-Thomas HR, Harvin HS (1977) Metastasizing basal cell carcinoma. Plast Reconstr Surg 59: 750–753 (Case 1).

Goldstein AM, Bale SJ, Peck GL, DiGiovanna JJ (1993) Sun exposure and basal cell carcinomas in the nevoid basal cell carcinoma syndrome. J Am Acad Dermatol 29: 34–41.

Goldstein AM, Pastakia B, DiGiovanna JJ, Poliak S, Santucci S, Kase R, Bale AE, Bale SJ (1994) Clinical findings in two African–American families with the nevoid basal cell carcinoma syndrome (NBCC). Am J Med Genet 50: 272–281.

Golitz LE, Norris DA, Leukens CA, Charles DN (1980) Multiple basal cell carcinomas of the palms after radiation therapy. Arch Dermatol 116: 1159–1163.

Gorlin RJ, Goltz R (1960) Multiple nevoid basal cell epitheliomata, jaw cysts, bifid rib-a syndrome. N Engl J Med 262: 908–911.

Gorlin RJ (1987) Nevoid basal-cell carcinoma syndrome. Medicine 66: 98–113.

Gorlin RJ (1995) Nevoid basal cell carcinoma syndrome. Dermatol Clin 13: 113–125.

Gorlin RJ (1999) Nevoid basal cell carcinoma (Gorlin) syndrome: unanswered issues. J Lab Clin Med 134: 551–552.

Gorlin RJ (2004) Nevoid basal cell carcinoma (Gorlin) syndrome. Genet Med 6: 530–534.

Grachtchouk V, Grachtchouk M, Lowe J, Johnson T, Wei L, Wang A, de Sauvage F, Dlugosz A (2003) The magnitude of hedgehog signaling activity defines skin tumor phenotype. EMBO 22: 2741–2751.

Gundlach KKH, Kiehn M (1979) Multiple basal cell carcinomas and keratocysts–the Gorlin and Goltz syndrome. J Maxillofac Surg 7: 299–307.

Gutierrez MM, Mora RG (1986) Nevoid basal cell carcinoma syndrome: a review and case report of a patient with unilateral basal cell nevus syndrome. J Am Acad Dermatol 15: 1023–1030.

Hahn H, Wicking C, Zaphiropoulos P, Gailani MR, Shanley S, Chidambiram A, Vorechovsky I et al. (1996) Mutations of the human homolog of Drosophila patched in the nevoid basal cell carcinoma syndrome. Cell 85: 841–851.

Haniffa MA, Leech SN, Lynch SA, Simpson NB (2004) NBCCS secondary to an interstitial chromosome 9q deletion. Clin Exp Dermatol 29: 542–544.

Happle R (1973) Naevobasaliom und Ameloblastom. Hautarzt 24: 290–294.

Hardisson D, Jimenez-Heffernan JA, Nistal M, Picazo ML, Tovar JA, Contreras F (1996) Neural variant of fetal rhabdomyoma and naevoid basal cell carcinoma syndrome. Histopathology 29: 247–252.

Harris SA, Large DM (1984) Gorlin's syndrome with a cardiac lesion and jaw cysts with some unusual histologic features: a case report and review of the literature. Int J Oral Surg 13: 59–64.

Hasegawa K, Amagasa T, Shioda S, Kayano T (1989) Basal cell nevus syndrome with squamous cell carcinoma of the maxilla. J Oral Maxillofac Surg 47: 629–633.

Hasenpusch-Theil K, Bataille V, Laehdetie J, Obermayr F, Sampson JR, Frischauf A (1998) Gorlin syndrome: identification of 4 novel germ-line mutations of the human *patched (PTCH)* gene. Hum Mutat 11: 480.

Hawkins JC III, Hoffman HJ, Becker LE (1979) Multiple nevoid basal cell carcinoma syndrome (Gorlin's syndrome): possible confusion with metastatic medulloblastoma. J Neurosurg 50: 100–102.

Helseth A, Mylius EA (1986) Gorlins syndrome. Tidsk Norsk Laegeforen 106: 2851.

Herman TE, Siegel MJ, McAlister WH (1991) Cardiac tumor in Gorlin syndrome. Nevoid basal cell carcinoma syndrome. Pediatr Radiol 21: 234–235 (Same case as Coffin).

Hermann G, Som P (1981) Multiple basal cell nevus syndrome. Case report 135. Skel Radiol 6: 62–64.

Hermans EH, Grosfeld JCM, Spaas JAJ (1965) The fifth phacomatosis. Dermatologica 130: 446–476.

Herzberg JJ, Wiskemann A (1963) Die fünfte Phakomatose. Basalzellnaevus mit familiärer Belastung und Medulloblastom. Dermatologica 126: 106–123.

Hess J, Bink-Boelkens MTE (1976) Fibroma cordis bij een zvigeling met het basocellulaire naevussyndroom. Ned Tijdschr Geneesk 120: 1796–1799.

High A, Zedan W (2005) Basal cell nevus syndrome. Curr Opin Oncol 17: 160–166.

Hogan RE, Tress B, Gonzales MF, King JO, Cook MJ (1996) Epilepsy in the nevoid basal cell carcinoma syndrome (Gorlin syndrome): report of a case due to focal neuronal heterotopia. Neurology 46: 574–576.

Hogge WA, Blank C, Roochvarg LB, Hogge JS, Wulfsberg EA, Raffel LJ (1994) Gorlin syndrome (naevoid basal cell carcinoma syndrome): prenatal detection in a fetus with macrocephaly and ventriculomegaly. Prenat Diagn 14: 725–727.

Holubar K, Matros H, Smalik AV (1970) Multiple basal epitheliomas in basal cell nevus syndrome. Arch Dermatol 101: 679–682.

Honovar SG, Shields JA, Shields CL, Eagle RC Jr, Demirci H, Mahmood EZ (2001) Basal cell carcinoma of the eyelid associated with Gorlin–Goltz syndrome. Ophthalmology 108: 1115–1123.

Horio T, Komura J (1978) Linear unilateral basal cell nevus with comedo-like lesions. Arch Dermatol 114: 95–97.

Howell JB (1980) The roots of nevoid basal cell carcinoma syndrome. Clin Exp Dermatol 5: 339–348.

Howell JB, Caro MR (1959) Basal cell nevus: its relationship to multiple cutaneous cancers and associated anomalies of development. Arch Dermatol 79: 67–80.

Howell JB, Mehregan A (1970) Pursuit of the pits in the nevoid basal cell carcinoma syndrome. Arch Dermatol 102: 586–597.

Inoue Y, Ono T, Kayashima K, Johno M (1998) Hereditary perioral pigmented follicular atrophoderma associated with milia and epidermal cysts. Br J Dermatol 139: 713–718.

Ismail SM, Walker SM (1990) Bilateral virilizing sclerosing stromal tumors of the ovary in a pregnant woman with Goorlin's syndrome: implications for pathogenesis of ovarian stromal neoplasms. Histopathology 17: 159–163.

A, Gilchrest BA (2004) δ-aminolevulinic acid and blue light photodynamic therapy for treatment of multiple basal cell carcinomas in two patients with nevoid basal cell carcinoma syndrome. Derm Surg 30: 1054–1061.

Jackson R, Gardere S (1971) Nevoid basal cell carcinoma syndrome. Canad Med Assoc J 105: 850–859.

Jamieson SW, Gaudiani VA, Reitz BA, Oyer PE, Stinson EB, Shumway NE (1981) Operative treatment of an unresectable tumor of the left ventricle. J Thorac Cardiovasc Surg 81: 795–799.

Jarisch W (1894) Zur Lehre von den Hautgeschwülsten. Arch Dermatol (Berlin) 28: 162–222.

Jeanmougin M, Zeller J, Wechsler J, Revuz J, Touraine R (1979) Naevomatose basocellulaire et améloblastome. Ann Dermatol Venereol (Paris) 106: 691–693.

Jensen MJ (1978) Gorlin's syndrome with ameloblastoma. Oral Surg 45: 325–326.

Jiménez Acosta FJ, Redondo E, Baez O, Hernandez B (1992) Linear unilateral basaloid follicular hamartoma. J Am Acad Dermatol 27: 316–319.

Johnson AD, Hebert AA, Esterly NB (1986) Nevoid basal cell carcinoma syndrome: bilateral ovarian fibromas in a 3 1/2 year old girl. J Am Acad Dermatol 14: 371–374.

Johnson RL, Rothman A, Xie J, Goodrich LV, Bare JW, Quinn JM, Myers RM, Cox DR, Epstein EH, Scott MP (1996) Human homolog of *patched*, a candidate gene for the basal cell nevus syndrome. Science 272: 1668–1671 [same case as Jamieson et al].

Jones KL, Smith DW, Harvey MAS, Hall BD, Quan L (1975) Older paternal age in fresh gene mutation data. Additional disorders. J Pediatr 86: 84–88.

Jones KL, Wolf PL, Jensen P, Dittrich H, Benirschke K, Bloor C (1986) The Gorlin syndrome: a genetically determined disorder associated with cardiac tumors. Am Heart J 111: 1013–1015.

Kagy MK, Amonette R (2000) The use of imiquimod 5% cream for the treatment of superficial basal cell carcinomas in a basal cell nevus syndrome patient. Derm Surg 26: 577–578.

Kahn LB, Gordon W (1967) Basal cell naevus syndrome. S Afr Med J 41: 832–835.

Kakarantza-Angelopoulou E, Nicolatou O (1990) Odontogenic keratocysts. Clinicopathologic study of 87 cases. J Oral Maxillofac Surg 48: 593–600.

Kantarci M, Ertas U, Alper F, Sutbeyaz Y, Karasen RM, Onbas O (2003) Gorlin's syndrome with a thin corpus callosum and a third ventricular cyst. Neuroradiol 45: 390–392.

Kedem A, Even-Paz Z, Freund M (1970) Basal cell nevus syndrome associated with malignant melanoma of the iris. Dermatologica 140: 99–106.

Kidd A, Carson L, Gregory DW, deSilva D, Holmes J, Dean JCS, Haites N (1996) A Scottish family with Bazex-Dupré-Christol syndrome: follicular atrophoderma, congenital hypotrichosis, and basal cell carcinoma. J Med Genet 33: 493–497.

Kimonis VE, Goldstein AM, Pastaku B, Yang ML, Kase R, DiGiovanna JJ, Bale AE, Bale SJ (1997) Clinical manifestations in 105 persons with nevoid basal cell carcinoma syndrome. Am J Med Genet 69: 299–308.

Kimonis VE, Mehta SG, DiGiovanna JJ, Bale SJ, Pastakia B (2004) Radiological features in 82 patients with nevoid basal cell carcinoma (NBCC or Gorlin). Genet Med 6: 495–502.

Kirsch T, Selle G (1969) Kieferzysten und Hautveränderungen-ein wenig bekanntes Syndrome. Dtsch Zahnärtzl Z 24: 938–942.

Kittler H, Binder M (2000) A patient with nevoid basal cell carcinoma syndrome and Turner syndrome. Br J Dermatol 143: 1105–1106.

Klijanienko J, Caillaud JM, Micheau C, Flamant F, Schwaab G, Avril MF, Ponzio-Prion A (1988) Naevomatose basocellulaire associée a un rhabdomyome foetal multifocale. Presse Méd 17: 2247–2250.

Koch CA, Chrousos GP, Chandra R, Evangelista RS, Gilbert JC, Hobuhara K, Zhuang Z, Vortmeyer AO (2002) Two-hit model for tumorigenesis of nevoid basal cell carcinoma (Gorlin) syndrome in associated hepatic mesenchymal tumor. Am J Med Genet 109: 74–76.

Kopera D, Cerroni L, Fink-Puches R, Kerl H (1996) Different treatment modalities for the management of a patient with the nevoid basal cell carcinoma syndrome. J Am Acad Dermatol 23: 937–939.

Korczak JF, Brahim JS, Giovanna JJ, Kase RG, Wexler LH, Goldstein AM (1997) Nevoid basal cell carcinoma syndrome with medulloblastoma in an African–American boy: a rare case illustrating gene-environment interaction. Am J Med Genet 69: 309–314.

Kraemer BB, Silver EG, Sneige N (1984) Fibrosarcoma of the ovary: a new component in the nevoid basal cell carcinoma syndrome. Am J Surg Pathol 8: 231–236.

Lacombe D, Taïeb A (1995) Overlap between Bazex syndrome and congenital hypotrichosis and milia. Am J Med Genet 56: 423–424.

Lacombe D, Chateil JF, Fontan D, Battin J (1990) Medulloblastoma in the nevoid basal cell carcinoma syndrome. Genetic Couns 1: 237–277.

Lacro RV, Jones KL (1987) The Gorlin syndrome: a genetically determined disorder associated with cardiac tumor. J Thorac Cardiovasc Surg 94: 919.

Lam C, Leung C, Lee K, Xie J, Lo F, Au T, Tong S, Poone M, Chan L, Luk N (2002) Novel mutations in the PATCHED gene in basal cell nevus syndrome. Mol Genet Metab 76: 57–61.

Lambrecht JT, Kreusch T (1997) Examine your orofacial cleft patients for Gorlin–Goltz syndrome. Cleft Palate Craniofac J 34: 342–350.

Lambrecht JT, Sojka-Raytscheff A, Brix F (1985) Computertomographische Befunde des Hirnschädels bei Patienten mit Gorlin-Goltz-Syndrom. Dtsch Zahnärtzl Z 40: 529–530.

Lench NJ (1996) Investigation of chromosome 9q22.3-q31 DNA marker loss in odontogenic keratocysts. Eur J Cancer 32B: 202–206.

Lench NJ, Telford EAR, High AS, Markham AF, Wicking C, Wainwright BJ (1997) Characterization of human patched germ line mutations in naevoid basal cell carcinoma syndrome. Hum Genet 100: 497–502.

Leonardi R, Caltabiano M, LoMuzio I, Gorlin RJ, Bucci P, Pannone G, Canfora M, Sorge G (2002) Bilateral hyperplasia of the mandibular coronoid processes in patients with nevoid basal cell carcinoma syndrome. Am J Med Genet 110: 400–403.

Leppard BJ (1983) Skin cysts in the basal cell naevus syndrome. Clin Exp Dermatol 8: 603–612.

Levanat S, Gorlin RJ, Fallet S, Johnson DR, Fantasia JE, Bale AE (1996) A two-hit model for developmental defects in Gorlin syndrome. Nat Genet 12: 85–87.

Levin JD, Talarico CL, Wegert SL, Gaynor LF, Sutley S (1991) Gorlin's syndrome with associated odontogenic cysts. Pediatr Radiol 21: 584–587.

Levine DJ, Robertson DB, Varma VA (1987) Familial subconjunctival epithelial cysts associated with the nevoid basal cell carcinoma syndrome. Arch Dermatol 123: 23–24.

Li TJ, Browne RM, Matthews JB (1995) Epithelial cell proliferation in odontogenic keratocysts: a comparative immunocytochemical study of Ki67 in simple, recurrent and basal cell naevus syndrome (BCNS)-associated lesions. J Oral Pathol Med 24: 221–226.

Lincoln JCR, Tynan MJ, Waterston DJ (1968) Successful excision of an endocardial fibroma of the left ventricle in a 10-month-old infant. J Thorac Cardiovasc Surg 56: 63–70 [Same case as Littler].

Lindeberg H, Halaburt H, Larsen PØ (1982) The naevoid basal cell carcinoma syndrome. J Maxillofac Surg 10: 246–249.

Ling G, Ahmadian A, Posson A, Undén AB, Afink G, Williams C, Uhlen M, Toftgård R, Lundberg J, Ponten F (2001) *PATCHED* and p53 gene alterations in sporadic and hereditary basal cell cancer. Oncogene 20: 7770–7778.

Littler BO (1979) Gorlin's syndrome and the heart. Br J Oral Surg 17: 135–146 [Same case as Lincoln et al].

Lobo CJ, Timms MS, Puranik VC (1997) Basal cell carcinoma of the external auditory canal and Gorlin–Goltz syndrome. A case report. J Laryngol Otol 111: 850–851.

LoMuzio L, Nocini PF, Savoia A, Consolo U, Procaccini M, Zelanti L, Pannone G, Bucci P, Dolci M, Bambin F, Solda P, Favia G (1999a) Nevoid basal cell carcinoma syndrome. Clinical findings in 37 Italian affected individuals. Clin Genet 55: 34–40.

LoMuzio L, Staibano S, Pannone G, Bucci P, Nocini PF, Bucci E, DeRosa G (1999b) Expression of cell cycle and apoptosis-related proteins in sporadic odontogenic keratocysts and odontogenic keratocysts associated with the nevoid basal cell carcinoma syndrome. J Dent Res 78: 1345–1353.

Ly JQ (2002) Scintigraphic findings in Gorlin's syndrome. Clin Nucl Med 27: 913–914.

MacSweeney JE, Manhore AR, Forbes A, Lees WR (1985) Gorlin's syndrome. J Roy Soc Med 78: 253–255.

Maddox WD (1962) Multiple basal tumors, jaw cysts, and skeletal defects: A clinical syndrome. MS Thesis, University of Minnesota.

Maddox WD, Winkelmann RK, Harrison EG, Devine KD, Gibilisco JA (1964) Multiple nevoid basal cell epitheliomas, jaw cysts and skeletal defects. JAMA 188: 106–111.

Manfredi M, Vescovi P, Bonanini M, Porter S (2004) Nevoid basal cell carcinoma syndrome: a review of the literature. Int J Oral Maxillofac Surg 33: 117–124.

Manners RM, Morris RJ, Francis PJ, Hatchwell E (1996) Microphthalmos in association with Gorlin's syndrome. Br J Ophthalmol 80: 378.

Mascaro JM Jr, Ferrando J, Bombi JA, Lambruschini N, Mascaro JM (1995) Congenital generalized follicular hamartoma associated with alopecia and cystic fibrosis in three siblings. Arch Dermatol 131: 454–458.

Matsumura Y, Nishigori C, Murakami K, Miyachi Y (2000) Allelic loss at the *PTCH* gene locus in jaw cysts but not in palmar pits in patients with basal cell nevus syndrome Arch Dermatol Res 292: 475–476.

Mehregan AH, Baker S (1985) Basaloid follicular hamartoma: three cases with localized and systematized unilateral lesions. J Cutan Pathol 12: 55–65.

Metha VR, Potdur R (1985) Bazex syndrome: follicular atrophoderma and basal cell epitheliomas. Int J Dermatol 24: 444–446.

Micali G, Lacarrubba F, Nasca MR, DePasquale R (2003) The use of imiquimod 5% cream for the treatment of basal cell carcinoma as observed in Gorlin's syndrome. Clin Exp Dermatol 28(Suppl 1): 19–23.

Michaëlsson G, Olson E, Westermark P (1981) The Rombo syndrome: a familial disorder with vermiculate atrophoderma, milia, hypotrichosis, trichoepitheliomas, basal cell carcinomas and peripheral vasodilation with cyanosis. Acta Dermatovenereol (Stockholm) 61: 497–503.

Midro AT, Panasiuk B, Tümer Z, Stankiewicz P, Silahtaroglu A, Lupski JR et al. (2004) Interstitial deletion 9q22.32-9q33.2 associated with additional familial translocation t(9;17)(q34.11;p11.2) in a patient with Gorlin–Goltz syndrome and features of nail-patella syndrome. Am J Med Genet 124A: 179–191.

Miller RF, Cooper RR (1972) Nevoid basal cell carcinoma syndrome. Histogenesis of skeletal lesions. Clin Orthop Rel Res 89: 246–272.

Minami M, Urano Y, Ishigami T, Tsuda H, Husaka J, Arase S (2001) Germline mutations with nevoid basal cell carcinoma syndrome. J Dermatol Surg 27: 21–26.

Ming JE, Kupas ME, Roessler E, Brunner HG, Golabi M, Stratton RF, Sujansky E, Bale SJ, Muencke M (2002) Mutations in *patched-1*, the receptor for *Sonic Hedgehog*, are associated with holoprosencehaly. Human Genet 110: 297–301.

Miyakawa S, Araki Y, Sugawara M (1988) Generalized trichoepitheliomas with alopecia and myasthenia gravis. J Am Acad Dermatol 19: 361–362.

Mohs FE, Jones DL, Koranda FC (1980) Microscopically controlled surgery for carcinomas in patients with nevoid basal cell carcinoma syndrome. Arch Dermatol 116: 777–779.

Moos KF, Rennie JS (1987) Squamous cell carcinoma arising in a mandibular cyst in a patient with Gorlin's syndrome. Br J Oral Maxillofac Surg 25: 280–284.

Mortelé KJ, Hoier MR, Mergo PJ, Ros PR (1999) Bilateral adrenal cystic lymphangiomas in nevoid basal cell carcinoma (Gorlin–Goltz) syndrome: US, CT and MR findings. J Comput Assist Tomogr 23: 562–564.

Mortimer PS, Geaney DP, Liddell K, Dawber RPR (1984) Basal cell naevus syndrome and intracranial meningioma. J Neurol Neurosurg Psychiatr 47: 210–212.

Murphy KJ (1969) Subcutaneous calcification in the naevoid basal-cell carcinoma syndrome: Response to parathyroid hormone and relationship to pseudo-hypoparathyroidism. Clin Radiol 20: 287–293.

Murphy KJ (1975) Metastatic basal cell carcinoma with squamous appearance in nevoid basal cell carcinoma syndrome. Br J Plast Surg 28: 331–334.

Murphy MJ, Tenser RB (1982) Nevoid basal cell carcinoma syndrome and epilepsy. Ann Neurol 11: 372–376.

Myong H, Hong SP, Hong SD, Lee JI, Lim CY, Chuong PH, Lee JH, Choi JY, Seo BM, Kim MJ (2001) Odontogenic keratocyst: review of 256 cases for recurrence and clinicopathology parameters. Oral Surg Oral Med Oral Pathol Oral Radiol Endod 91: 328–333.

Naguib MG, Sung JH, Erickson DL, Gold LHA, Seljeskog EL (1982) Central nervous system involvement in nevoid basal cell carcinoma syndrome. Neurosurg 11: 52–56.

Neblett CR, Waltz TA, Anderson DW (1971) Neurological involvement in the nevoid basal cell carcinoma syndrome. J Neurosurg 35: 577–584.

Nicolai JP (1979) The basal cell naevus syndrome and palmar cysts. Hand 11: 99–101.

Nishimo H, Gomez MR, Kelly PJ (1991) Is colloid cyst of the third ventricle a manifestation of nevoid basal cell carcinoma syndrome? Brain Dev 13: 368–370.

Novak KD, Bloss N (1976) Röntgenologische Aspekte des Basalzell-Naevus Syndromes (Gorlin-Goltz Syndrom). Roefo 124: 11–16.

Oley CA, Sharpe H, Chevenix-Trench 804.

Olivieri C, Maraschio P, Caselli D, Martini C, Beluffi G, Masarati E, Danesino C (2003) Interstitial deletion of chromosome 9, int del(9)(q22.31-q31.2 including the genes causing multiple basal cell nevus syndrome and Robinow/brachydactyly 1. Eur J Pediatr 162: 100–103.

O'Malley S, Weitman D, Olding M, Sekhar L (1997) Multiple neoplasms following craniospinal irradiation for medulloblastoma in a patient with nevoid basal cell carcinoma syndrome. J Neurosurg 86: 286–288.

Osano M, Yashiro K, Oikawa T, Takeuchi Y, Matsuo N, Inoue T, Yamamoto H (1969) Intramural fibroma of the heart. Pediatrics 43: 605–608.

Oseroff AR, Shieh S, Frawley NP, Cheney R, Blumenson LE, Pivnick EK, Bellnier DA (2005) Treatment of diffuse basal cell carcinomas and basaloid follicular hamartomas in nevoid basal cell carcinoma syndrome by wide-area 5-aminolevulinic acid photodynamic therapy. Arch Dermatol 141: 60–70.

Oski K, Kumamoto H, Ichinohasama R, Sato T, Takahashi N, Ooye K (2004) PTC gene mutations and expression of SHH, PTC, SMO, and GLI-1 in odontogenic keratocysts. Int J Oral Maxillofac Surg 33: 584–592.

Ozturk A, Oguz KK, Tümer C, Balci S (2003) Neuroradiological findings in a mother and daughter with Gorlin syndrome. Clin Dysmorphol 12: 145–146.

Palacios E, Serou M, Restrepo S, Rojas R (2004) Odontogenic keratocysts in nevoid basal cell carcinoma (Gorlin's) syndrome: CT and MRI evaluation. ENT-Ear Nose Throat J 83: 40–42.

Pearlman RL, Herzog JL (1990) Arachnoid cyst in a patient with basal cell nevus syndrome. J Am Acad Dermatol 23: 519–520.

Peck GL, DiGiovanna JJ, Sarnoff DS, Gross EG, Butkus D, Olsen TG, Yoder FW (1988) Treatment and prevention of basal cell carcinoma with oral isotretinoin. J Am Acad Dermatol 19: 176–185.

Petrikovsky BM, Bialer MG, McLaughlin JA, Bale AE (1996) Sonographic and DNA-based prenatal detection of Gorlin syndrome. J Ultrasound Med 15: 493–495.

Plosila M, Kiistala R, Niemi KM (1981) The Bazex syndrome: follicular atrophoderma with multiple basal cell carcinomas, hypotrichosis and hypohidrosis. Clin Exp Dermatol 6: 31–41.

Posnick JC, Clokie CML, Goldstein JA (1994) Maxillofacial considerations for diagnosis and treatment in Gorlin's syndrome: access osteotomies for cyst removal and orthognathic surgery. Ann Plast Surg 32: 512–518.

Potaznik D, Steinherz P (1984) Multiple nevoid basal cell carcinoma syndrome and Hodgkin's disease. Cancer 53: 2713–2715.

Pratt MD, Jackson R (1987) Nevoid basal cell carcinoma syndrome. J Am Acad Dermatol 16: 964–970.

Raggio M, Kaplan AL, Harberg JF (1983) Recurrent ovarian fibromas with basal cell nevus syndrome (Gorlin syndrome). Obstet Gynecol 61(Suppl): 95–96.

Rahbari H, Mehregan AH (1982) Basal-cell nevus epithelioma [cancer in children and teenagers]. Cancer 49: 350–353.

Ramsden RT, Barrett A (1978) Gorlin's syndrome. J Laryngol Otol 89: 615–621.

Rapelenoro R, Taieb A, Lacombe D (1994) Congenital hypotrichosis and milia: report of a large family suggesting X-linked dominant inheritance. Am J Med Genet 52: 487–490.

Rasmussen JE (1971) A syndrome of trichoepitheliomas, milia and cylindromas. Arch Dermatol 111: 610–614.

Ratcliffe JF, Shanley S, Ferguson J, Chevenix-Trench G (1995a) The diagnostic implication of falcine calcification on plain skull radiographs of patients with basal cell naevus syndrome and the incidence of falcine calcification in their relatives and two control groups. Br J Radiol 68: 361–368.

Ratcliffe JF, Shanley S, Chevenix-Trench G (1995b) The prevalence of cervical and thoracic congenital skeletal abnormalities in basal cell naevus syndrome: a review of cervical and chest radiographs in 80 patients with BCNS. Br J Radiol 68: 596–599.

Rayner CRW, Towers JF, Wilson JSP (1977) What is Gorlin's syndrome? The diagnosis and management of basal cell naevus syndrome based on a study of thirty-seven patients. Br J Plast Surg 30: 62–67.

Reifenberger J (2004) Hereditäre Tumorsyndrome. Hautarzt 55: 942–951.

Reis A, Küster W, Linss G, Gebel E, Hamn H, Fuhrmann W, Wolff G, Groth W, Gustafson G et al.(1992) Localisation of gene for the naevoid basal-cell carcinoma syndrome. Lancet 339: 617.

Reiter C, Hiss J, Müller-Hartburg W (1982) Herzfibrom bei familiärem Gorlin-Syndrom mit Virilisierung. Wien Klin Wochenschr 94: 430–434.

Requena L, Farina MC, Robledo M, Sangueza O, Sanchez Yus E, Villanueva A, Marquina A, Tamarit A (1999) Multiple hereditary infundibulocystic basal cell carcinomas: a genodermatosis different from nevoid basal cell carcinoma syndrome. Arch Dermatol 135: 1227–1235.

Ridley CM, Smith N (1981) Generalized hair follicle hamartomata with alopecia and myasthenia gravis. Clin Exper Dermatol 6: 283–289.

Rittersma J (1972) Het basocellulaire nevus syndrom. Thesis. Groningen.

Roggi NK, Salt A, Collin JRO, Michalski A, Farnson PA (2005) Gorlin syndrome: the *PTCH* gene links ocular developmental defects and tumor formation. Br J Ophthalmol 89: 998–992.

Rossi R, Libertino JA, Dowd JB, Braasch JW (1979) Neurocutaneous syndromes and retroperitoneal tumors. Urology 13: 292–294.

Rowe DE, Carroll RJ, Day CLJ (1989) Mohs surgery is the treatment of choice for recurrent (previously-treated) basal cell carcinoma. J Dermatol Surg Oncol 15: 424–431.

Ruiz i Altaba A, Sanchez P, Dahmane N (1987) Gli and hedgehog in cancer: tumours, embryos, and stem cells. Nat Rev Cancer 2: 361–372.

Ruprecht A, Austermann KH, Umstadt H (1987) Cleft lip and palate, seldom seen features of the Gorlin-Goltz syndrome. Dermatomaxillofac Radiol 16: 99–103.

Ryan DE, Burkes EJ Jr (1973) The multiple basal cell nevus syndrome in a Negro family. Oral Surg 36: 831–840.

Santis HR, Nathanson NR, Bauer SB (1983) Nevoid basal cell carcinoma syndrome associated with renal cysts and hypertension. Oral Surg 55: 127–132.

Satinoff MI, Wells C (1969) Multiple basal cell naevus syndrome in ancient Egypt. Med Hist 13: 294–297.

Schlieter F (1973) Die 5. Phakomatose – Verlaufsbeobachtungen bei einem Kind mit Orbitalzyste und Hirnmissbildung. Klin Mbl Augenheilk 163: 184–192.

Schmidt BL, Pogrel MA (2001) The use of enucleation and liquid nitrogen cryotherapy in the management of odontogenic keratocysts. J Oral Maxillofac Surg 59: 720–725.

Schofield D, West DC, Anthony DC, Marshal R, Sklar J (1995) Correlation of loss of heterozygosity at chromosome 9q with histological subtype in medulloblastomas. Am J Pathol 146: 472–480.

Schultz SM, Twickler DM, Wheeler DE, Hogan TD (1987) Ameloblastoma with basal cell nevus (Gorlin) syndrome: CT findings. J Comput Assist Tomogr 11: 901–904.

Schulz-Butulis BA, Gilson R, Garley M, Keeling JH (2000) Nevoid basal cell carcinoma syndrome and non-Hodgkin's lymphoma. Cutis 66: 35–38.

Schweisguth O, Gerard-Marchant R, Lemerle J (1968) Naevomatose basocellulaire; association à un rhabdomyosarcome congénital. Arch Fr Pédiatr 25: 1083–1093.

Seracchioli R, Bagnoli A, Colombo FM, Missiroli S, Venturoli S (2001) Conservative treatment of recurrent ovarian fibromas in a young patient affected by Gorlin syndrome. Hum Reprod 16: 1261–1263.

Seracchioli R, Coloboma FM, Bagnoli A, Trengia V, Venturoli S (2003) Primary ovarian leiomyosarcoma as a new component in the nevoid basal cell carcinoma syndrome: a case report. Am J Obstet Gynecol 188: 1093–1095.

Shanley S, Ratcliffe J, Hockey A, Haan E, Oley C, Ravine D, Martin N, Wicking C, Chevenix-Trench G (1994) Nevoid basal cell carcinoma syndrome: review of 118 affected individuals. Am J Med Genet 50: 282–290.

Shear M (1985) The odontogenic keratocyst: recent advances. Dtsch Zahnärztl Z 40: 510–513.

Shear M (2002) The aggressive nature of the odontogenic keratocyst: is it a benign cystic neoplasm? Part 2. Proliferation and genetic studies. Oral Oncol 38: 323–331.

Shelley WB, Rawnsley HM, Beerman H (1969) Quadrant distribution of basal cell nevi. Arch Dermatol 100: 741–743.

Shimkets R, Gailani MR, Sue VM, Yang-Feng T, Pressman CL, Levanat S, Goldstein A, Demin M, Bale AE (1996) Molecular analysis of chromosome 9q deletions in two Gorlin syndrome patients. Am J Hum Genet 59: 417–422.

Sidransky D (1996) Is human *patched* the gatekeeper of common skin cancers? Nat Genet 14: 7–8.

Snider RL (1994) Unusual presentation of a third ventricular cyst in a patient with basal cell nevus syndrome. Pediatr Dermatol 11: 323–326.

Soekermann D, Fryns JP, Caesar P, Van den Berghe (1991) Increased head circumference and facial cleft as presenting signs of the nevoid basal-cell carcinoma syndrome. Genet Couns 2: 157–162.

Southwick GJ, Schwartz RA (1979) The basal cell nevus syndrome. Disasters occurring among a series of 36 patients. Cancer 44: 2294–2305.

Springate JE (1986) The nevoid basal cell carcinoma syndrome. J Pediatr Surg 21: 908–910.

Starink TM, Lanc EB, Meijer CJLM (1986) Generalized trichoepitheliomas with alopecia and myasthenia gravis: clinicopathologic and immunohistochemical study and comparison with classic and desmoplastic trichoepithelioma. J Am Acad Dermatol 15: 1104–1112.

Stavrou T, Dubovsky EC, Reaman GH, Goldstein AM, Vezina G (2000) Intracranial calcifications in childhood medulloblastoma: relation to nevoid basal cell carcinoma syndrome. AJNR Am J Neuroradiol 21: 790–794.

Stieler W, Plewig G, Küster W (1987) Basalzellnävus-Syndrom mit Plattenepithelkarzinom des Larynx. Z Hautkrankh 63: 113–120.

Stockfleth E, Ulrich C, Hauschild A, Lischner S, Meyer T, Christopher E (2002) Successful treatment of basal cell carcinomas in nevoid basal cell carcinoma syndrome with topical 5% imiquimod. Eur J Dermatol 12: 569–572.

Stoelinga PJ (2001) Long-term follow-up on keratocysts treated according to a defined protocol. Int J Oral Maxillofac Surg 30: 14–25.

Strange PR, Lang PG Jr (1992) Long-term management of basal cell nevus syndrome with topical tretinoin and 5-fluorouracil. J Am Acad Dermatol 27: 842–845.

Su CW, Link L, Hou JW, Jung SN, Zen EC (2003) Spontaneous recovery from a medulloblastoma by a female with Gorlin-Goltz syndrome. Pediatr Neurol 28: 231–234.

Summerly RM, Hale AJ (1965) Basal cell naevus syndrome. St. Johns Hosp Derm Soc 51: 77–79.

Tafi A, Ghisolfi A, Bandi A, Mazzacane D, Bertholdi G (1986) The Gorlin-Goltz 5th phakomatosis: ophthalmological aspects of a case. J Fr Ophtalmol 9: 135–138.

Taicher S, Shteyer A (1978) The basal cell nevus syndrome associated with cleft lip and cleft palate. J Oral Surg 36: 799–802.

Taipale J, Cooper MK, Maiti T, Beachy PA (2002) *Patched* acts catalytically to suppress the activity of (italics) Smoothened. Nature 418: 892–897.

Takanashi J, Fujii K, Takano H, Sugita K, Kohno Y (2000) Empty sella syndrome in nevoid basal cell carcinoma syndrome. Brain Dev 22: 272–279.

Tamoney HJ Jr (1969) Basal cell nevoid syndrome. Am Surg 35: 279–283.

Tanioka M, Takahashi K, Kawabata T, Kosugi S, Murakami K, Miyachi Y, Nishigori C, Iizuka T (2005) Germline mutations of the *PTCH* gene in Japanese patients with nevoid basal cell carcinoma syndrome. Arch Dermatol Res 296: 303–308.

Tawfik O, Casparian JM, Garrigues N, Smith S, Kestenbaum T, Chamberlin F, Khan QS (1999) Neuroendocrine differentiation of a metastatic basal cell carcinoma in a patient with basal cell nevus syndrome. J Cutan Pathol 26: 306–310.

Taylor WB, Anderson DE, Howell JB, Thurston CS (1968) The nevoid basal cell carcinoma syndrome. Arch Dermatol 98: 612–614.

Taylor WB, Wilkins JW (1970) Nevoid basal cell carcinomas of the palm. Arch Dermatol 102: 654–655.

Thissen MR, Schroeter CA, Neumann HA (2000) Photodynamic therapy with delta-aminolaevulinic acid for nodular basal cell carcinomas using a prior debulking technique. Br J Dermatol 142: 338–339.

Totten JR (1980) The multiple nevoid basal cell carcinoma: report of its occurrence in four generations of a family. Cancer 46: 1456–1462.

Undén AB, Holmberg E, Lundh-Rozell B, Ståhle-Bäckdahl M, Zaphiropoulos P, Toftgård R, Vořchovsky I (1996) Mutations in the human homologue of *Drosophila patched (PTCH)* in basal cell carcinoma and the Gorlin syndrome: different *in vivo* mechanisms of *PTCH* interaction. Cancer Res 56: 4562–4565.

Undén AB, Ståhle-Bäckdahl M, Holmberg E, Larsson C, Toftgård R (1997) Fine mapping of the locus for nevoid basal cell carcinoma syndrome on chromosome 9q. Acta Dermatol Venereol (Stockh) 77: 4–9.

Vabres P, deProst Y (1993) Bazex-Dupré-Christol syndrome: a possible diagnosis for basal cell carcinomas, coarse sparse hair, and milia. Am J Med Genet 45: 786.

Vabres P, Lacombe D, Rabinowitz LG, Aubert G, Anderson CE, Taieb A, Bonife JL, Hors-Cayla MC (1995) The gene for Bazex-Dupré-Christol syndrome maps to chromosome Xq. J Invest Dermatol 105: 87–91.

Veenestra-Knol HE, Scheewe JH, van der Vlist G, Van Doorn ME, Ausems MG (2005) Early recognition of basal cell naevus syndrome. Eur J Pediatr 164: 126–130.

Villavicencio EH, Waterhouse DO, Iannacone PM (2000) The *Sonic Hedgehog-Patched*-Gli pathway to human development and disease. Am J Hum Genet 67: 1047–1054.

Vortmeyer AO, Stavrou T, Selby D, Li G, Weil RJ, Park W, Moon Y, Chandra R, Goldstein AM, Zhuang Z

(1999) Deletion analysis of the adenomatous polyposis coli and *PTCH* gene loci in patients with sporadic and nevoid basal cell carcinoma syndrome-associated medulloblastoma. Cancer 85: 2662–2667.

Wallace DC, Murphy KJ, Kelly L, Ward WH (1973) The basal cell naevus syndrome. Report of a family with anosmia and a case of hypogonadotrophic hypopituitarism. J Med Genet 10: 30–33.

Walsh N, Ackerman AB, Brownstein MH (1993) Basaloid follicular hamartoma: solitary and multiple types. J Am Acad Dermatol 29: 125–129.

Walter AW, Pivnick EK, Bale AE, Kun LE (1997) Complications of the nevoid basal cell carcinoma syndrome. J Pediatr Hematol Oncol 19: 258–262.

Watson J, Depasquale K, Ghaderi M, Zwillenberg S (2004) Nevoid basal cell carcinoma syndrome and fetal rhabdomyoma. ENT-Ear Nose Throat J 83: 716–718.

Watson RA, Harper BN (1992) Paratesticular fibrous pseudotumor in a patient with Gorlin's syndrome: nevoid basal cell carcinoma syndrome. J Urol 148: 1254–1255.

Weltfriend S, David M, Ginzberg A (1987) Generalized hair follicle hamartoma: The third case in association with myasthenia gravis. Am J Dermatopathol 9: 428–432.

White JC (1894) Multiple benign cystic epitheliomas. J Cutan Genitourin Dis 12: 477–484.

Wicking C, Shanley S, Smyth I, Gillies S, Negus K, Graham S, Suthers G, Haites N, Ewards M, Wainwright JB, Chevenix-Trench G (1997a) Most germline mutations in the nevoid basal cell carcinoma syndrome lead to premature termination of the *PATCHED* protein, and no genotype-phenotype correlations are evident. Am J Hum Genet 60: 21–26.

Wicking C, Gillies S, Smyth I, Shanley S, Fowles L, Ratcliffe J, Wainwright B, Chevenix-Trench G (1997b) De novo mutations of the *Patched* gene in nevoid basal cell carcinoma syndrome help to define the clinical phenotype. Am J Med Genet 73: 304–307.

Wicking C, Berkman J, Wainwright B, Chevenix-Trench G (1994) Fine genetic mapping of the gene for nevoid basal cell carcinoma syndrome. Genomics 22: 505–511.

Williams DB, Danielson GK, McGoon DC, Feldt RH, Edwards WD (1982) Cardiac fibroma: long term survival after excision. J Thorac Cardiovasc Surg 84: 230–236.

Wilson BD, Mang TS, Stoll H, Jones C, Cooper M, Dougherty TJ (1992) Photodynamic therapy for the treatment of basal cell carcinoma. Arch Dermatol 128: 1597–1601.

Winkler PA, Guyuron B (1987) Multiple metastases from basal cell naevus syndrome. Br J Plast Surg 40: 528–531.

Wirth H, Tilgen W (1983) Linearer unilateraler Basalzellnävus. Hautarzt 34: 620–664.

Wolthers OD, Stellfeld M (1987) Benign mesenchymoma of the trachea of a patient with the nevoid basal cell carcinoma syndrome. J Laryngol Otol 101: 522–526.

Woolgar JA, Rippin JW, Taylor M et al. (1987) The odontogenic keratocyst and its occurrence in the nevoid basal cell carcinoma syndrome. Oral Surg Oral Med Oral Pathol 64: 727–730.

Xin H, Matt D, Qin JZ, Boni R (1999) The sebaceous nevus. A nevus with deletions of the *PTCH* gene. Cancer Res 59: 1834–1836.

Yee KC, Tan CY, Bhatt KB, Davies AM (1993) Sclerotic bone lesions in Gorlin's syndrome. Br J Radiol 66: 77–80.

Yilmaz B, Goldberg LH, Schechter NR, Kemp BL, Ruiz H (2003) Basal cell nevus syndrome concurrent with adenoid cystic carcinoma of salivary gland. J Am Acad Dermatol 48(Suppl 5): S64–S66.

Yoshida S, Yoshikawa H, Yoshida A, Nakamura T, Noda Y, Gondoh H, Fukagawa S, Moroi Y, Urabe K, Furue M, Ishibashi T (2004) Bilateral epiretinal membranes in nevoid basal cell carcinoma syndrome. Acta Ophthalmol Scand 82: 488–490.

Yoshizumi J, Vaughan RS, Jasani B (1990) Pregnancy associated with Gorlin's syndrome. Anaesthesia 45: 1046–1048.

Zarour H, Grab JJ, Choux R, Collet-Villette AM, Bonerandi J (1993) Hamartome baso-cellulaire et annexiel unilatérale linéare. Ann Dermatol Venereol 119: 901–903.

Zaun H (1981) Basalzellnävussyndrom mit ungewöhnlicher Begleitsymptomatik. Hautarzt 32: 455–458.

Zedan W, Robinson PA, High AS (2001) A novel polymorphism in the PTC gene allows easy identification in basal cell nevus syndrome lesions. Diagn Molec Pathol 10: 41–45.

Zvulunov A, Strother D, Zirbel G, Rabinowitz L, Esterly NB (1995) Nevoid basal cell carcinoma syndrome. Report of a case with associated Hodgkin's disease. J Pediatr Hematol Oncol 17: 66–70.

# Chapter 46

# MULTIPLE ENDOCRINE NEOPLASIA TYPE 2B

Electron Kebebew, Jessica E. Gosnell, and Emily Reiff

Department of Surgery and UCSF Comprehensive Cancer Center, University of California, San Francisco , USA

## Introduction

Multiple endocrine neoplasia type 2 (MEN 2) is a distinct hereditary syndrome that has an autosomal pattern of inheritance (OMIM 2005). There have been 500–1000 MEN 2 kindreds reported in the literature. The MEN 2 syndrome consists of three variants: MEN 2A, MEN 2B and familial medullary thyroid cancer (Table 1). Patients with MEN 2B develop medullary thyroid cancer (100%), pheochromocytoma, mucocutaneous neuromas and have characteristic physical features. MEN 2B accounts for 5–10% of MEN 2 cases. In patients with MEN 2B, neuromas may involve the skin, musculoskeletal system, gastrointestinal tract and eyes (Schimke et al. 1968, Williams and Pollock 1966a).

Patients with MEN 2B often develop aggressive medullary thyroid cancer within the first decade of life. Although MEN 2B is uncommon, early genetic screening and diagnosis offers the only chance at curative treatment. Because the penetrance of MEN 2B is 100%, clinical awareness of this syndrome and its physical manifestation is essential. Genetic screening identifies 95–99% of gene carriers at risk of developing MEN 2. This has resulted in prophylactic treatment of gene carriers who have no clinical evidence of disease and has improved patient outcome (Kebebew et al. 2000).

In this chapter, we review the clinical manifestation, pathogenesis, and management of MEN 2B. We also review the common physical and neurocutaneous findings that can be used to identify affected or at-risk patients before they develop medullary thyroid cancer and pheochromocytoma.

## Historical perspective and Terminology

The MEN 2 syndrome was originally described by Sipple (1961), who reported an association of pheochromocytoma with medullary thyroid carcinoma. **John H. Sipple** was born in 1930 in Lakewood, Ohio and graduated from Cornell University Medical College in 1955. He trained in internal medicine at the State University of New York Medical Center (SUNY) in Syracuse. He then did a fellowship in pulmonary medicine at the Johns Hopkins Hospital in Baltimore, Maryland. In 1962 he returned to Syracuse to practice Pulmonary and Internal Medicine, and was appointed clinical professor of medicine at SUNY Medical Center in 1977. Dr. Sipple became a governor of the Upstate New York region of the American College of Physicians and president of the Internist Associates of Central New York (Who named it? 2007).

The triad of medullary thyroid carcinoma, pheochromocytoma, and parathyroid hyperplasia or adenoma, in association with elevated calcitonin and catecholamine levels (MEN 2A) was originally known as Sipple's syndrome (Boord 2004). Another eponym for MEN 2 is Wagenmann-Froboese syndrome (OMIM 2005). Wageman (1922) and Froboese (1923) described in part a clinical syndrome of multiple mucosal neuromas, pheochromocytoma, medullary carcinoma of the thyroid, and asthenic body build with muscle wasting of the extremities (marfanoid habitus). Williams and Pollock (1966) further characterized this MEN 2B phenotype with a description of true mucosal neuromas, intestinal ganglioneuromatosis, pheochromocytoma, and medullary thyroid carcinoma (Boord 2004, Gorlin et al. 2001) in two unrelated patients (OMIM 2005). The father of one of the

**Table 1.** The MEN 2 syndrome and its variants and affected sites

| MEN 2 syndrome variants | Affected sites |
|---|---|
| MEN 2A | Families with medullary thyroid cancer, parathyroid disease, or both; rarely some families may have cutaneous lichen amyloidosis |
| MEN 2A (1) | Families with medullary thyroid cancer and pheochromocytoma, parathyroid disease, or both |
| MEN 2A (2) | Families with medullary thyroid cancer and pheochromocytoma in at least one member; objective evidence against the presence of parathyroid disease in affected and at-risk members |
| MEN 2A (3) | Families with medullary thyroid cancer and parathyroid disease in at least one member; objective evidence against the presence of pheochromocytoma in affected and at-risk members |
| MEN 2B | Families with medullary thyroid cancer, pheochromocytoma, mucosal neuromas, musculoskeletal abnormalities usually without parathyroid disease |
| Familial medullary thyroid cancer (FMTC) | Only medullary thyroid cancer; families with at least four members with medullary thyroid cancer and no objective evidence of pheochromocytoma or parathyroid disease on screening of affected and at-risk members |
| Other | Families with fewer than four members with medullary thyroid cancer but none with pheochromocytoma or parathyroid disease on biochemical screening or families with clinical screening results that could not be confirmed |

patients had very thick lips and eyelids, and tongue lesions as did his daughters. He also had medullary thyroid cancer and died at 38 years old after an abdominal operation, having had symptoms suggestive of a pheochromocytoma (OMIM 2007, Williams and Pollock 1966). Other eponyms for MEN 2B are MEN type 3, Mucosal neuromata with endocrine tumours, Mucosal Neuroma syndrome, Wagenmann-

Froboese syndrome, or Ganglioneuromatosis of the alimentary tract (OMIM 2007).

## Incidence and prevalence

The precise incidence and prevalence of MEN 2 is unknown. Based on the National Cancer Institute's Surveillance, Epidemiology and End Result program, the age-adjusted annual incidence of medullary thyroid cancer in the United States ranges from 0.1 to 1.6 cases per million (NCI 2005). Because MEN 2B accounts for 5–10% of all MEN 2 cases and MEN 2 accounts for 25% of all medullary thyroid cancer cases, the estimated annual age-adjusted incidence is 4 cases per 100 million. The prevalence of thyroid cancer in the United States is 0.1%; therefore, the estimated prevalence of MEN 2B is 0.0025%.

## Clinical manifestations of MEN 2B

### Neurocutaneous and physical manifestations

Although medullary thyroid cancer and pheochromocytoma account for most of the morbidity and mortality associated with MEN 2B, the neurocutaneous manifestations and non-endocrine physical findings are important in identifying at-risk individuals early in life. Moreover, some of these physical

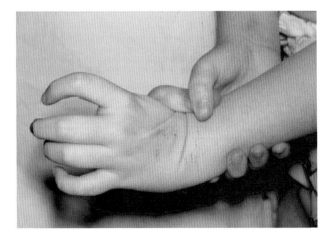

**Fig. 1.** A 11 year-old boy with MEN 2B demonstrates laxity in his first metacarpal joint with complete hyperextension causing no pain.

features contribute greatly to the poor quality of life that these patients endure (O'Riordain et al. 1995).

Patients with MEN 2B are often described as having a marfinoid body habitus with a tall and thin frame, disproportionately long limbs, joint laxity and severe muscular wasting (Fig. 1) (O'Riordain et al. 1995). Weakness especially of the proximal muscles of the extremities seen in 15% simulates a myopathic state. In infancy, there is often a history of profound difficulty in feeding with failure to thrive. The distinct facies is elongated and characterized by a wide-eyed expression, broad-base nose, and large nodular lips with submucosal nodules on the vermilion border (Gorlin et al. 2001). Some patients with MEN 2B will also have thickened lips and eye-

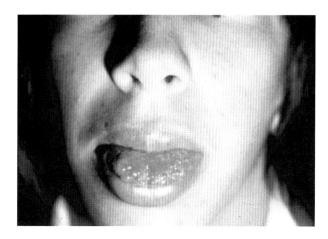

**Fig. 3.** Mucosal neuroma in the anterior tongue in a patient with MEN 2B.

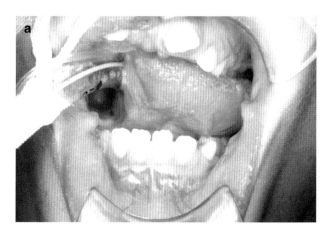

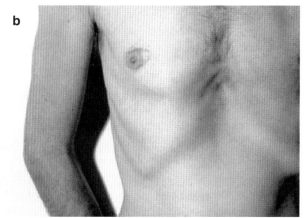

**Fig. 2.** (**a**) Abnormal dentition in a young girl with MEN 2B about to undergo total thyroidectomy and lymph node dissection for her medullary thyroid cancer, and (**b**) Pectus excavatum in a patient with MEN 2B.

lids, the latter resulting in eversion of the upper eyelids. Surgical resection of the lips reveals enormous enlargement of the diameter of the peripheral nerves. The lower face appears long. Circumoral and midfacial lentiginosis have been occasionally seen. Slit-lamp examination often reveals corneal nerve thickening with medullated nerve fibers (O'Riordain et al. 1995).

Patients with MEN 2B often have skeletal abnormalities such as pectus excavatum, talipes equinovarus, pes cavus, slipped femoral epiphysis, aseptic necrosis of lumbar spine, dorsal scoliosis, kyphoscoliosis, lordosis and abnormal dentition (Fig. 2). Almost 100% of patients with MEN 2B have mucosal neuromas (Pujol et al. 1997). Mucosal neuromas are benign tumors of the nerve sheath that may be located anywhere on the mucosal surfaces in the body, but are most common and visible in the anterior portion of the tongue, lips, palate and gums (Fig. 3). They are present at birth or develop early in childhood and are commonly non-pigmented or palewhite, painless papules that measure a few millimeters to one centimeter in size. The presence of these tumors is considered a pathognomonic feature in MEN 2B and any patient found to have one should be screened for MEN 2B by genetic testing (Kebebew and Duh 1998). On light and electron microscopy, the mucosal nodules are plexiform neuromas – that is, uncapsulated masses of convoluted myelinated and unmyelinated nerves surrounded by a tickened perineurium which elaborate calcitonin (Gorlin et al. 2001). In contrast to neurofibromas histochemical investigation demonstrates absence of both specific and non-specific cholinesterase activity and epithelial membrane antigen negativity.

Cutaneous neuromas are uncommon and when present, are usually located on the face and trunk, appearing as small, well-demarcated papules covered by normal dermis (Truchot et al. 2001). Histologic examination shows an increased number and size of well-circumscribed clusters of small dermal nerves without surrounding inflammation.

Ganglioneuromas throughout the gastrointestinal tract are present in up to 50% of patients with MEN 2B and contribute to dysmotility, abdominal pain, constipation and megacolon. In infancy, gastrointestinal complaints such as constipation or diarrhea may, in fact, be the heralding symptoms of MEN 2B and should be considered in the differential diagnosis.

## Medullary thyroid cancer

Medullary thyroid cancer develops within the first decade of life in essentially all patients with MEN 2B and is the leading cause of death. In patients with MEN 2B, medullary thyroid cancer is commonly multicentric, bilateral and lymph node metastasis are commonly present (Kebebew et al. 2000). Medullary thyroid cancer originates from the parafollicular or C-cells (calcitonin secreting) of the thyroid gland. C-cells are concentrated in the posterior and upper one-third of each thyroid lobe. In patients with advanced medullary thyroid cancer, hoarseness and stridor may indicate local invasion, or systemic symptoms from vasoactive hormone secretion may induce flushing and diarrhea, usually in patients with liver metastases (Kebebew et al. 2000).

## Pheochromocytoma

Pheochromocytomas, which occur in 20–50% of patients with MEN 2B, are tumors of the adrenal medulla that are derived from the neural crest. They secrete excess catecholamines and usually cause paroxysmal hypertension, headache, palpitations and sweating. They are more likely to be bilateral and extra-adrenal in MEN 2B patients than in patients with sporadic pheochromocytoma. Pheochromocytomas in patients with MEN 2B are usually benign.

In the past, pheochromocytomas accounted for most of the morbidity and mortality in patients with MEN 2B, but this has decreased because of the improved diagnostic accuracy of biochemical testing for elevated catecholamines and metabolites, precise localizing studies, and better perioperative care (Kebebew and Duh 1998).

## Natural history

Most patients with MEN 2B come to clinical attention within the first two decades of life. The neurocutaneous manifestation especially oral mucosal neuromas usually develop during the first decade of life. Medullary thyroid cancer and pheochromocytoma usuall present after puberty. Most patients with MEN 2B present with aggressive medullary thyroid cancer, so that most will have persistent or recurrent disease even after complete surgical treatment and are at risk for developing systemic disease. About half of the patients with MEN 2B will develop pheochromocytoma that are commonly bilateral. Most patients with MEN 2B eventually die from metastatic medullary thyroid cancer in the 4th or 5th decade of life.

## Pathogenesis and molecular genetics

The RET (REarranged during Transfection) proto-oncogene is responsible for MEN 2 (Lodish and Stratakis 2008). The RET proto-oncogene encodes a transmembrane, tyrosine-kinase receptor-protein that regulates cell growth, migration, and differentiation in neural crest-derived cells located in the thyroid, adrenal medulla, parathyroid glands, enteric and sympathetic nervous system (Pachnis et al. 1993). Activating germline point mutations in the RET proto-oncogene are thought to result in constitutively stimulated tyrosine kinase activity. Point mutations in the extracellular and intracellular domains have been identified in the MEN 2 syndrome, but all of the mutations documented in MEN 2B patients have been in the intracellular, tyrosine-kinase binding domain (Brandi et al. 2001). Ligands that bind the RET receptor are members of the glial cell-derived neurotrophic factor (GDNF) family (GDNF, persephin, neurturin, artemin) (Baloh et al. 2000). Activation of the RET receptor results in transphosophorylation of numerous tyrosine residues that activate signaling pathways important in cell growth, migration and differentiation. Most cases of MEN 2B occur as a result of germline mutations most commonly in exon 16 (codon 918), and less commonly in exon 14 (codon 883) (Brandi et al. 2001, Machens et al. 2003).

Genotype–phenotype associations have been observed in the MEN 2 syndrome. In MEN 2A, 85% of the RET mutations are present in exon 11 (codon 634) and in MEN 2B, 95% of mutations involve codon 918 (Brandi et al. 2001, Eng et al. 1996, Machens et al. 2003). Because MEN 2B has an autosomal dominant pattern of inheritance, 50% of offspring will be affected with MEN 2B. Of these affected patients, virtually all will develop medullary thyroid cancer and approximately 50% will develop or may already have pheochromocytomas. Almost all patients with MEN 2B have a constellation of distinct phenotypic features. Half of the MEN 2B cases are discovered as hereditary cases; the others present as the index case in which there is a *de novo* RET germline mutation and no other affected family members (Norum et al. 1990).

## Diagnosis, follow-up and management

The presence of mucosal neuromas are enough to diagnose most patients with MEN 2B and occur within the first decade of life. Mucosal neuromas are extremely rare, perhaps unheard of, outside of the MEN 2B syndrome. Other phenotypic features such as a tall, lanky, marfanoid body habitus, and a narrow face are also commonly present but not specific to MEN 2B. If diagnosed clinically all patients will have medullary thyroid cancer with or without pheochromocytoma in association with the phenotypic features of MEN 2B.

Today, with the implementation of genetic screening for RET germline mutations, some patients may have none of the obvious phenotypic features, no medullary thyroid cancer, and pheochromocytoma if diagnosed at infancy or at a very young age.

## Medullary thyroid cancer

Fine needle aspiration biopsy and cytologic examination of neck masses are accurate for diagnosing medullary thyroid cancer, especially when used with immunohistochemical staining for the presence of amyloid, calcitonin, and carcinoembryonic antigen.

Surgical treatment consisting of total thyroidectomy and removal of cervical lymph nodes and is the only effective treatment for medullary thyroid cancer. Unlike follicular cells of the thyroid gland, the C-cells do not trap iodine so radioiodine ablation is not effective. Chemotherapy and external-beam radiation therapy are generally ineffective. Basal and stimulated serum calcitonin measurement is indispensable as a tumor marker to detect persistent or recurrent medullary thyroid cancer after surgical resection. The mortality due to medullary thyroid cancer in patients with MEN 2B patients is 20–33% at 10 years follow up (Brauckhoff et al. 2004, O'Riordain et al. 1995).

## Pheochromocytoma

The diagnosis of pheochromocytoma is established by measuring 24-hour urinary levels of catecholamine and metabolites. All patients diagnosed with medullary thyroid cancer should have biochemical testing to exclude a diagnosis of pheochromocytoma before thyroidectomy because an undiagnosed pheochromocytoma may result in hypertensive crisis and death during the operation (Sutton et al. 1981). Imaging studies including CT scans, MRI and MIBG scans are used to localize the tumor and rule out bilateral or extra-adrenal disease, which are frequently found in patients with MEN 2B (Kebebew and Duh 1998). Laparoscopic adrenalectomy, preceded by meticulous preoperative preparation with alpha and beta-blockade is the optimal treatment approach and reduces perioperative morbidity and mortality (Lairmore et al. 1993).

## Differential diagnosis

Because of the distinct physical features of patient with MEN 2B they can easily be distinguished from the other types of MEN 2 syndrome. In young patients who may not have the characteristic features of MEN 2B, testing for germline RET mutation in codons 833 and 918 are specific for MEN 2B.

## Genetic counseling

Because MEN 2B is an autosomal dominant hereditary syndrome with an early and 100% penetrance, affected individuals and at risk family should have early genetic counseling. Fortunately, the responsible gene for the MEN 2 syndrome is known and performing direct DNA sequencing for RET mutations is accurate.

Genetic counseling should focus in patient education, comprehensive family history collection and review of medical records. Genetic screening is more accurate than basal or stimulated calcitonin measurement for screening patients at risk for MEN 2. In a family with a known RET germline mutation, MEN 2 can be safely ruled out if no RET mutation is identified in that individual. At least two separate blood samples should show the same RET germline mutation before a patient is determined to be a gene carrier. RET germline mutations in codons 918 and 883 have the earliest age for presenting with medullary thyroid cancer, as early as 9 months of age (Machens et al. 2003). Because MEN 2B cases have germline RET mutations in codons 918 and 883, family members should be screened at birth or before the age of 1 year. All patients found to be gene carriers should have prophylactic thyroidectomy with central neck node dissection as soon as the diagnosis is made and screening for pheochromocytoma (Gertner and Kebebew 2004).

## Summary

Although MEN 2B is an uncommon hereditary syndrome, most patients develop aggressive medullary thyroid cancer and pheochromocytomas. The physical and neurocutaneous features of MEN 2B patients are specific, and should increase the index of suspicion because half of the MEN 2B cases present as the index case and can be recognized early in childhood if one is aware of these features. Early genetic screening and diagnosis affords patients with MEN 2B the only chance at curative treatment for medullary thyroid cancer and pheochromocytoma, and permits other family members to be screened. Family members of a patient with a known RET mutation who are found to be negative for the RET proto-oncogene mutation can be assured that they are not at risk for developing MEN 2 and require no further follow-up.

## References

Baloh RH, Enomoto H, Johnson EM Jr, Milbrandt J (2000) The GDNF family ligands and receptors – implications for neural development. Curr Opin Neurobiol 10: 103–110.

Boord JBBL (2004) Multiple endocrine neoplasia type 2. In: Roach ESMV (ed.) Neurocutaneous disorders. New York: Cambridge University Press, pp. 105–111.

Brandi ML, Gagel RF, Angeli A, Bilezikian JP, Beck-Peccoz P, Bordi C, Conte-Devolx B, Falchetti A, Gheri RG, Libroia A, Lips CJ, Lombardi G, Mannelli M, Pacini F, Ponder BA, Raue F, Skogseid B, Tamburrano G, Thakker RV, Thompson NW, Tomassetti P, Tonelli F, Wells SA Jr, Marx SJ (2001) Guidelines for diagnosis and therapy of MEN type 1 and type 2. J Clin Endocrinol Metab 86: 5658–5671.

Brauckhoff M, Gimm O, Weiss CL, Ukkat J, Sekulla C, Brauckhoff K, Thanh PN, Dralle H (2004) Multiple endocrine neoplasia 2B syndrome due to codon 918 mutation: clinical manifestation and course in early and late onset disease. World J Surg 28: 1305–1311.

Eng C, Clayton D, Schuffenecker I, Lenoir G, Cote G, Gagel RF, van Amstel HK, Lips CJ, Nishisho I, Takai SI, Marsh DJ, Robinson BG, Frank-Raue K, Raue F, Xue F, Noll WW, Romei C, Pacini F, Fink M, Niederle B, Zedenius J, Nordenskjold M, Komminoth P, Hendy GN, Mulligan LM et al. (1996) The relationship between specific RET proto-oncogene mutations and disease phenotype in multiple endocrine neoplasia type 2. International RET mutation consortium analysis. JAMA 276: 1575–1579.

Froboese C (1923) Das aus markhaltigen nervenfascern bestehende gangliezellenlose echte neurom in rankenformzugleich ein beitrag zu den nervosen Geschwulsten der zunge und des augenlides. Virchows Arch Pathol Anat 240: 312–327.

Gertner ME, Kebebew E (2004) Multiple endocrine neoplasia type 2. Curr Treat Options Oncol 5: 315–325.

Gorlin R, Cohen MM Jr, Hennekam RCM (2001) Multiple endocrine neoplasia type 2B (multiple mucosal neuroma syndrome, MEN type 3). In: Gorlin RJ CMJ, Hennekam RCM (eds.) Syndromes of the Head and Neck. Oxford/New York: Oxford University Press, pp. 462–468.

Kebebew E, Duh QY (1998) Benign and malignant pheochromocytoma: diagnosis, treatment, and follow-Up. Surg Oncol Clin N Am 7: 765–789.

Kebebew E, Ituarte PH, Siperstein AE, Duh QY, Clark OH (2000) Medullary thyroid carcinoma: clinical characteristics, treatment, prognostic factors, and a comparison of staging systems. Cancer 88: 1139–1148.

Lairmore TC, Ball DW, Baylin SB, Wells SA Jr (1993) Management of pheochromocytomas in patients with multiple endocrine neoplasia type 2 syndromes. Ann Surg 217: 595–601; discussion 601–593.

Lodish MB, Stratakis CA (2008) RET oncogene in MEN2, MEN2B, MTC and other forms of thyroid cancer. Expert Rev Anticancer Ther 8: 625–632.

Machens A, Niccoli-Sire P, Hoegel J, Frank-Raue K, van Vroonhoven TJ, Roeher HD, Wahl RA, Lamesch P, Raue F, Conte-Devolx B, Dralle H (2003) Early malignant progression of hereditary medullary thyroid cancer. N Engl J Med 349: 1517–1525.

NCI (2005) Surveillance, epidemiology and end results. Vol. 2005.

Norum RA, Lafreniere RG, O'Neal LW, Nikolai TF, Delaney JP, Sisson JC, Sobol H, Lenoir GM, Ponder BA, Willard HF et al. (1990) Linkage of the multiple endocrine neoplasia type 2B gene (MEN2B) to chromosome 10 markers linked to MEN2A. Genomics 8: 313–317.

OMIM (2007) Online Mendelian inheritance in man. A Catalog of autosomal recessive, autosomal dominant and X-linked diseases in man. Baltimore, Johns Hopkins University.

O'Riordain DS, O'Brien T, Crotty TB, Gharib H, Grant CS van Heerden JA (1995) Multiple endocrine neoplasia type 2B: more than an endocrine disorder. Surgery 118: 936–942.

Pachnis V, Mankoo B, Costantini F (1993) Expression of the c-ret proto-oncogene during mouse embryogenesis. Development 119: 1005–1017.

Pujol RM, Matias-Guiu X, Miralles J, Colomer A, de Moragas JM (1997) Multiple idiopathic mucosal neuromas: a minor form of multiple endocrine neoplasia type 2B or a new entity? J Am Acad Dermatol 37: 349–352.

Schimke RN, Hartmann WH, Prout TE, Rimoin DL (1968) Syndrome of bilateral pheochromocytoma, medullary thyroid carcinoma and multiple neuromas. A possible regulatory defect in the differentiation of chromaffin tissue. N Engl J Med 279: 1–7.

Sutton MG, Sheps SG, Lie JT (1981) Prevalence of clinically unsuspected pheochromocytoma. Review of a 50-year autopsy series. Mayo Clin Proc 56: 354–360.

Truchot F, Grezard P, Wolf F, Balme B, Perrot H (2001) Multiple idiopathic mucocutaneous neuromas: a new entity? Br J Dermatol 145: 826–829.

Wagenmann A (1922) Multiple neurome des auges und der Zunge. Ber Dtsch Ophthal 43: 282–285.

Who named it? (2007) A biographic dictionary for medical eponyms. http://www.whonamedit.com

Williams ED, Pollock DJ (1966) Multiple mucosal neuromata with endocrine tumours: a syndrome allied to Von Recklinghausen's disease. J Pathol Bacteriol 91: 71–80.

# Chapter 47

# TURCOT SYNDROME

**Laura Papi**

Department of Clinical Physiopathology, Medical Genetics Unit, University of Florence, Florence, Italy

## Introduction

Turcot syndrome is an inherited cancer syndrome characterized by the occurrence of primary tumors of the central nervous system and multiple colorectal adenomas and/or colorectal adenocarcinoma. In Turcot patients the most frequent brain tumors are astrocytomas, glioblastomas and medulloblastomas; ependymoma, spongioblastoma, gliosarcoma and oligodendroglioma have also been reported (Hamada et al. 1998).

## Historical background and terminology

In 1949, Crail described the first case of adenomatous polyposis coli associated with medulloblastoma of the brain stem and papillary carcinoma of the thyroid gland. However, the syndrome derived its eponym in 1959 from two cases reported by Turcot et al. which described colonic polyposis associated with cerebral tumors in two sibs born from a consanguineous marriage. One sibling developed a medulloblastoma involving the spinal cord and adenocarcinomas of the sigmoid colon and rectum; his sister had a cerebral glioblastoma multiforme and a pituitary adenoma. Since then, several cases resembling those of Turcot and Crail have been reported in the literature. They encompass a broad spectrum of colorectal findings, from a single adenoma to typical adenomatous polyposis, as well as various histopathologic types of central nervous system (CNS) tumors.

The mode of inheritance of Turcot syndrome had been controversial; some authors reported autosomal dominant inheritance and others supported an autosomal recessive pattern.

In recent times, the etiology of Turcot syndrome has been clarified by the development of molecular genetic analysis: it is now known that it can be caused by mutations in either adenomatous polyposis coli (*APC*) or in one of the genes responsible of Lynch syndrome or "Hereditary non-polyposis colorectal cancer" (HNPCC); indeed some cases may be due to autosomal recessive inheritance of two mutations in the same HNPCC gene.

Recently, the syndrome has been divided in two subgroups based on the clinical and pathologic aspects, as well as on the genetic abnormalities (Paraf et al. 1997). *Turcot syndrome type 1* comprise patients presenting with few polyps of the colon and developing colorectal cancer and glial tumors. These patients have mutations in the DNA mismatch repair (MMR) genes, such as *hMSH2*, *hMLH1*, *hMSH6* and *hPMS2* (Lucci-Cordisco et al. 2003). Patients with germline mutations in MMR genes do not appear to have an increased risk of medulloblastoma, and sporadic medulloblastomas do not show microsatellite instability, the hallmark of MMR mutations (Hamilton et al. 1995). On the other hand, *Turcot syndrome type 2* is characterized by hundreds to thousands of polyps in the colon and has a greatly increased risk of medulloblastoma (Hamilton et al. 1995, Paraf et al. 1997). These patients tend to have mutations in the *APC* gene on chromosome 5q21 (Hamilton et al. 1995). Although the distinction between these two forms of TS is attractive, it might be an oversimplification. Indeed, there are reports of medulloblastoma, colon cancer and glioblastoma occurring in the same patient (McLaughlin et al. 1998) and the family originally described by Turcot et al. (1968) included a glial tumor as well as a medulloblastoma in two sibs born from a consanguineous marriage.

# TURCOT SYNDROME TYPE 1

## Incidence and prevalence

The incidence of Turcot syndrome type 1 is unknown. The incidence of Lynch syndrome/HNPCC is 1: 800–2000.

## Clinical manifestations

Turcot syndrome type 1 consist of patients diagnosed with Lynch syndrome or hereditary nonpolyposis colorectal cancer (HNPCC) [OMIM 114500] and brain tumors.

HNPCC is the most frequent autosomal dominant predisposition to the development of colorectal cancer. It is characterized by young-age onset of mostly right-sided colon cancer as well as tumors in a variety of extracolonic sites. Apart from a lifetime risk of colorectal cancer of about 80%, individuals with HNPCC have an increased risk to develop tumors of the endometrium, stomach, small intestine, pancreas, hepatobiliary system, urinary tract, ovary, brain, and skin (Aarnio et al. 1995, 1999; Davis and Cohen 1995; Vasen et al. 1996a, b; Rodriguez-Bigas et al. 1997; Lin et al. 1998; Watson et al. 1998; Vasen 2005). However, it is well known that a few subset of HNPCC families can have unique tumor spectrums, for example an increased predisposition to sebaceous cancers (which is often referred to as *Muir-Torre syndrome*) or to central nervous neoplasms, mainly gliomas (*Turcot syndrome*).

## Natural history

HNPCC is associated with an increased risk of colorectal cancer and other cancers (Table 1) (Aarnio et al. 1995, 1999; Davis and Cohen 1995; Vasen et al. 1996b; Rodriguez-Bigas et al. 1997; Lin et al. 1998; Watson et al. 1998; Vasen 2005). Colon cancers have more often a proximal location and it is usual the occurrence of multiple tumors (synchronous or meta-

**Table 1.** Cumulative life-time risk for specific types of cancer in HNPCC

| Cancer | General population Risk (%) | HNPCC Risk (%) | Mean age of onset (range) (years) |
|---|---|---|---|
| Colon | 5–6 | 80 | 44 (15–90) |
| Endometrium | 2–3 | 20–60 | 46 (24–78) |
| Stomach | 1 | 11–19 | 56 (23–82) |
| Ovary | 1–2 | 9–12 | 42 (19–65) |
| Hepatobiliary tract | 0.6 | 2–7 | Not determined |
| Urinary tract (ureter and renal pelvis) | 1 | 4–5 | 57 (40–73) |
| Small bowel | 0.01 | 1–4 | 49 (23–69) |
| Central nervous system | 0.6 | 1–4 | 43 (2–79) |

chronous). Moreover, HNPCC-associated colon cancers have the following pathological characteristics: poor differentiation, high frequency of the mucinous histotype and of tumor-infiltrating lymphocytes.

In HNPCC, both colon and endometrial cancers have a relatively good prognosis compared to the sporadic counterpart (Watson et al. 1998, Maxwell et al. 2001).

## Molecular genetics

HNPCC is caused by germline mutations in human homologues of the bacterial mismatch repair (MMR) genes MutL and MutS: *MSH2*, *MLH1*, *MSH6*, and *PMS2* (Table 2) (Fishel et al. 1993, Bronner et al. 1994, Nicolaides et al. 1994, Miyaki et al. 1997). The vast majority of HNPCC-causing mutations have been reported in *MSH2* and *MLH1* (Peltomaki and Vasen 1997). Accordingly, mutations in these genes give rise to the "classical" HNPCC phenotype (Wijnen et al. 1997, Giardiello et al. 2001), whereas *MSH6* mutations have been described in families with more atypical HNPCC (Kolodner et al. 1999, Wijnen et al. 1999). Only a few *PMS2* germline mutations have been described so far (Hamilton et al.

**Table 2.** Mismatch repair system genes in bacteria and human

| E. coli | H. sapiens | Chromosome | Role in HNPCC predisposition |
|---------|-----------|------------|------------------------------|
| MutS | MSH2 | 2p21 | Typical HNPCC, Muir-Torre syndrome, Turcot syndrome |
| | MSH6 | 2p21 | Atypical and typical HNPCC |
| | MSH3 | 5q11.2–q13.2 | No predisposing mutation known |
| | MSH4 | 1p31 | No predisposing mutation known |
| | MSH5 | 6p22.3–p21.3 | No predisposing mutation known |
| MutL | MLH1 | 3p21 | Typical HNPCC, Turcot syndrome |
| | PMS2 | 7p22 | Turcot syndrome |
| | PMS1 | 2q31–33 | No predisposing mutation known |
| | MLH3 | 14q24.3 | Atypical HNPCC? |

1995, Liu et al. 1996). Specific germ-line MMR mutations do not appear to be associated with the development of brain tumors; in Turcot syndrome patients, inactivating mutations have been found in *MLH1*, *MSH2* and *PMS2* (Hamilton et al. 1995).

The mismatch repair system is one of the best characterized mechanisms involved in maintaining the genome integrity, by repairing damaged DNA. The primary function of the MMR system is to eliminate base-base mismatches and insertion/deletion loops which arise during DNA duplication (Peltomaki 2001). Insertion/deletion loops classically results in the shortening or lengthening of repetitive sequences in microsatellites. This is termed "*microsatellite instability*" (MSI) and is seen in tumor cells, which harbor biallelic MMR mutations.

In humans, MMR proteins function as heterodimers (Peltomaki 2005). The predominant mismatch-binding factor in humans is MutSα that include two proteins, MSH2 and MSH6; another mismatch-binding factor, called MutSβ, consisting of MSH2 and MSH3, is present at a lesser amounts in humans. MutSα is primarily responsible for the repair of base–base mismatches and 1-bp insertion/

deletion loops, while MutSβ mainly repairs insertion/deletion loops with 2–8 nucleotides. The MutS complexes initiate DNA repair by mismatch recognition but their interaction with the downstream repair proteins is dependent upon MutL activity. The major species providing MutL activity in humans is the heterodimer MutLα, consisting of MLH1 and PMS2 (Fig. 1).

Nearly all HNPCC-associated tumors exhibit MSI (Fig. 2) (Aaltonen et al. 1994). Inactivation of both alleles of *hMSH2* or *hMLH1* is necessary to generate the MSI phenotype, and this occurs through several routes. Loss of heterozygosity (LOH) is often coupled with point mutations of *hMSH2* or *hMLH1*, consistent with the two-hit model of tumor suppressor gene inactivation. Epigenetic mechanisms may also play a role because *hMLH1* can be silenced through hypermethylation of CpG islands in its promoter (Esteller et al. 2001). DNA mismatch repair gene defects in HNPCC syndrome are presumed to lead to tumor development as a result of the accumulation of widespread mutations within short repetitive sequences. Because most stretches of microsatellite DNA lie in noncoding sequences, many such alterations are unlikely to be functionally significant. However, genes with simple repetitive sequences (such as polyA tracts or CA-repeat) in coding exons are particularly susceptible targets. The type II TGF-β receptor gene was the first such target to be identified, and frameshift mutations occurred in a short GT-repeat sequence or a stretch of 10 adenines as a consequence of either an insertion or deletion of the repeated nucleotides (Markowitz et al. 1995). This finding provided independent validation of the importance of the TGF-β signaling pathway in colorectal tumorigenesis because TGF-β is a potent inhibitor of colonic epithelial cell growth (Kurokowa et al. 1987, Markowitz et al. 1996). Additional mutational targets include the apoptosis regulator BAX (Rampino et al. 1997), the insulin-like growth factor II receptor (Souza et al. 1996), the cell cycle–regulated transcription factor E2F-4 (Yoshitaka et al. 1996), TCF-4,33 caspase 5 (Schwartz et al. 1999), the intestinal homeobox factor CDX2 (Wicking et al. 1998), and even the mismatch repair genes hMSH3 and hMSH6 themselves (Malkhosyan et al. 1996). The latter provides a unique positive feedback loop in which tumors with MSI can enhance their own phenotype. Although the relative importance of these alterations in tumorigenesis is unknown, they are likely to play a pathogenic role because no mutations of short repeat sequences are identified in genes (e.g. histone) that are not intimately linked to the tumorigenic process (Ouyang et al. 1997).

## Diagnosis

Because sporadic colorectal cancer is common, some "colon cancer" families may occur by chance clustering. Therefore, strict clinical selection criteria have been created in order to diagnose HNPCC (Table 3). The "*Amsterdam criteria*" (Vasen et al. 1991) were originally designed for research purposes and are generally thought too stringent as they will exclude small

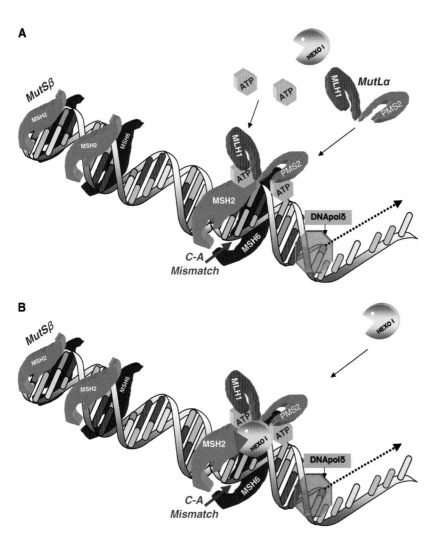

**Fig. 1.** A model for human mismatch repair. (**A**) MutS dimer clamps to DNA and functions as a mismatch sensor. When a mismatch is recognized, ADP is exchanged for ATP and the stable MutS clamp recruits other MutS in the region to help fix the problem. The MutS-ATP complex recruit a MutL dimer. (**B**) MutS-MutL complex binds and activates endonuclease activity in order to finishing the repair job. (**C**) MutS-MutL complex targets hEXOI to the mismatch. hEXOI digests the DNA strand containing the mismatch. (**D**) DNA polymerase synthesise a new DNA filament. (**E**) The repair job is finished. (modified from: Gruber 2006).

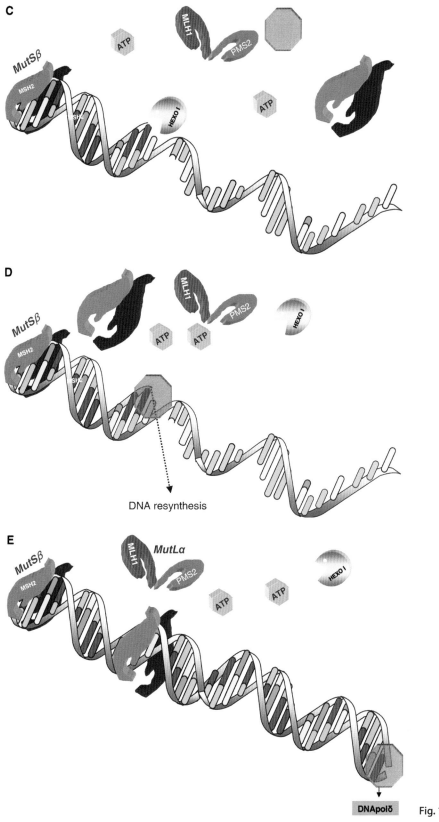

DNA resynthesis

**Fig. 1.** (Continued)

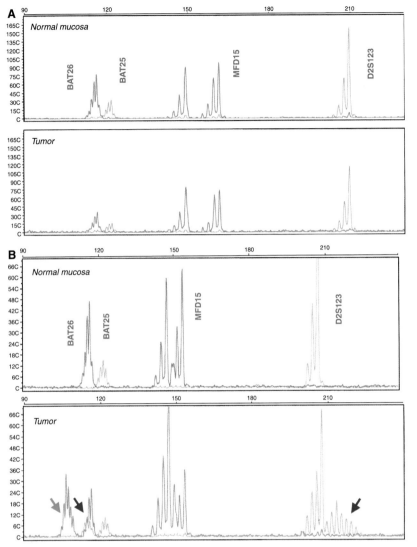

**Fig. 2.** Analysis with four microsatellites (BAT26, BAT25, MFD15 and D2S123) of two colon cancers compared with the normal mucosa. (**A**) MSS-colon carcinoma. (**B**) MSI-H colon carcinoma; microsatellites BAT26, BAT25 and D2S123 show instability (arrows).

families or families with HNPCC associated cancers. Therefore, the "*Amsterdam II Criteria*" were created in 1999 (Vasen et al. 1999) to take into account other HNPCC associated cancers (endometrial, small bowel, ureter and renal pelvis). The accuracy of the diagnosis based on clinical criteria depend on the accuracy of the reported family history; therefore it is unreliable unless the diagnosis are confirmed by pathologic reports.

The diagnosis of HNPCC can also be made on the basis of *molecular genetic testing* to detect a germline mutation in one of the several MMR genes. Molecular genetic testing is often preceded by microsatellite instability and immunohistochemical testing of the tumor tissue. Microsatellites are stretches of DNA with repetitive nucleotide sequences (e.g. CTCTCT or TTTTTT) that are particularly prone to acquiring errors when MMR function is impaired. HNPCC-associated tumors, arising in cells with defective MMR gene function, show an inconsistent number of microsatellite repeats when compared to normal tissue (Fig. 2), a finding named "microsatellite instability". To assess MSI, a panel of microsatellites is used: a tumor is classified "*MSI-high*" when at least 30% of the tested markers show instability, "*MSI-low*" when fewer than 30% of the

**Table 3.** Diagnostic criteria for HNPCC

Amsterdam criteria I (the classical criteria):

There should be at least three relatives with histologically verified CRC; all the following criteria should be present:

1) one should be a first degree relative of the other two
2) at least two successive generations should be affected
3) at least one CRC should be diagnosed before age 50
4) FAP should be excluded in the CRC case
5) tumors should be verified by pathological examination

Amsterdam criteria II:

There should be at least three relatives with an HNPCC-associated cancer (CRC, cancer of the endometrium, small bowel, ureter or renal pelvis); all the following criteria should be present:

1) one should be a first degree relative of the other two
2) at least two successive generations should be affected
3) at least one cancer should be diagnosed before age 50
4) FAP should be excluded in the CRC case (if present)
5) tumors should be verified by pathological examination

tested markers show instability, and "*MSI-stable*" if no instability is present. Approximately 90% of HNPCC-associated colon cancers are "*MSI-high*" (Thibodeau et al. 1993, Aaltonen et al. 1994, Liu et al. 1996, Cunningham et al. 2001).

Immunohistochemistry (IHC) of the tumor tissue detects the presence or absence of the protein product encoded by MMR genes; it is clinically available for the detection of MLH1, MSH2 and MSH6 proteins. IHC can be performed on tumors showing MSI to help identifying the specific MMR gene most likely to have a germline mutation (Fig. 3) (de Leeuw et al. 2000, Cunningham et al. 2001).

Molecular genetic testing is available on clinical basis for *MLH1*, *MSH2* and *MSH6*. The identification of a HNPCC-causing MMR gene mutation in a family allows to perform predictive testing in at-risk individuals. In general, predictive testing for HNPCC is not performed for at-risk individuals

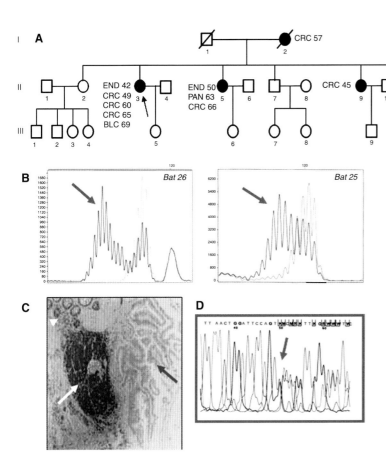

Fig. 3. (**A**) Pedigree of a Lynch family. Clinical diagnosis can be made on the basis of Amsterdam criteria. (**B**) Microsatellite instability (arrows) in two microsatellites in the colon cancer confirmed the diagnosis. Black lines: tumor. Blu and green lines: normal mucosa. (**C**) Immunohistochemical analysis of the colon carcinoma with an anti-MSH2 antibody. Tumor-infiltrating lymphocytes (white arrow) and normal mucosa (white arrowhead) have a positive stain; the tumor has a negative stain (red arrow). (**D**) DNA sequencing revealed a frameshift mutation in exon 10 of the *MSH2* gene (1549delGCinsT). *CRC*: colorectal cancer, *END*: endometrial cancer; *BLC*: bladder cancer; *PAN*: pancreatic cancer.

under the age of 18 years; however, since there have been rare reported cases of HNPCC individuals diagnosed with cancer at very young ages (Huang et al. 2001), and it is recommended that screening begin ten years before the earliest age of onset in the family, in some families, individuals may need to begin screening before the age of 18 years. Predictive testing enables at-risk relatives to be informed about their cancer risks and to benefit from intensive surveillance programs that have been proven to reduce their overall mortality by 65% (Jarvinen et al. 2000).

## Management and follow-up

Management of HNPCC comprises the surveillance for colon cancer and the other HNPCC-related cancers.

*Colon cancer surveillance* can be performed with regular colonoscopy with removal of adenomatous polyps; this approach reduces the colon cancer incidence in affected individuals (Jarvinen et al. 2000). Recommendations for individuals at risk of an HNPCC-related colon cancer are to undergo colonoscopy every one to two years beginning at age 25 or 10 years before the earliest age of diagnosis in the family, whichever is earlier (National Comprehensive Cancer Network, 2003).

*Endometrial and ovarian cancer surveillance* is less well established: annual transvaginal ultrasound examination, endometrial biopsy and CA-125 blood test beginning 25–30 years of age can be considered (National Comprehensive Cancer Network 2003) but its efficacy is still unclear.

*Stomach and duodenum cancer surveillance* is performed by upper endoscopy; however, it has been suggested no benefit from this screening strategy because of the lack of identifiable precursor lesions (Renkonen-Sinisalo et al. 2002).

*Urinary tract cancer surveillance* can be achieved by annual cytology approach, although no data indicate that this screening leads to earlier diagnosis or improved outcome.

At this time, no specific *surveillance* recommendations do exist for *hepatobiliary tract* and *brain tumors*.

## Differential diagnosis

The differential diagnosis includes syndromes associated with increased risk to develop colon cancer such as:

1. *AFAP*, the milder presentation of FAP, is usually associated with less than 100 polyps and with a later age of onset. However, in AFAP polyps of gastric fundus and duodenum also occur, while the extracolonic manifestations of classical FAP may be absent. Moreover, polyps and colon cancers associated with AFAP do not display MSI.
2. *Turcot syndrome due to APC gene mutations:* usually associated with medulloblastomas.
3. *MYH-associated polyposis* may be associated with few adenomatous polyps. However, colon cancers associated with *MYH* gene mutations do not display MSI; moreover, it has an autosomal recessive pattern of inheritance.
4. *Hamartomatous polyp syndromes* (Juvenile polyposis syndrome, Peutz-Jeghers syndrome and PTEN hamartomatous syndromes) are associated with an increased risk of colonic polyps and cancer, but they can usually be distinguished by their extracolonic manifestations as well as the hamartomatous rather than adenomatous pathology.

## Treatment

When colon cancer is detected in a person with HNPCC, full colectomy with ileorectal anastomosis is recommended rather than a segmental/partial colonic resection because of the risk of metacronous cancers (Aarnio et al. 1995, Church and Simmang 2003). However, the diagnosis of HNPCC is often considered only after the treatment of an initial colon cancer, consequently many HNPCC individuals have had their cancer treated with a limited colonic resection. Although it may be difficult, evaluating the tumor biopsy specimen by MSI and IHC, may help to decide the best surgical approach.

The treatment of other HNPCC-associated cancer do not differ from the sporadic ones.

# TURCOT SYNDROME DUE TO BIALLELIC MUTATION IN MMR GENES

Over the past few years, there have been a few reports of families that have presented with a constellation of very early onset of gastrointestinal cancers, together with features of neurofibromatosis type 1 and/or hematologic malignancies. In these patients biallelic mutations of a MMR gene can be found. Homozygous or compound heterozygous for mutations in *MLH1*, *MSH2*, *MSH6* and *PMS2* have been described (Table 4).

A distinctive clinical syndrome caused by biallelic mutations in MMR genes is now emerging. It is characterized by cafè-au-lait spots, an unusual

**Table 4.** Clinical features of families with biallelic mutations in MMR genes

| Gene | Mutation | Gastointestinal tumors (age of onset) | NF1 features | Hematologic malignancies (age of onset) | CNS tumors (age of onset) | Reference |
|------|----------|----------------------------------------|--------------|------------------------------------------|----------------------------|-----------|
| *MLH1* | R226X/ R226X | *Parents*: CRC(26; 33); family history of HNPCC | *Sister 1*: CLS *Sister 2*: CLS | *Brother*: ALL (2) *Sister 1*: NHL (3) *Sister 2*: atypical CML (1) | | Ricciardone et al. (1999) |
| | G67W/G67W | Family history of HNPCC | *Sister 1*: CLS, pseudoarthrosis of the tibia *Sister 2*: CLS, dermal neurofibromas | | *Sister 2*: medulloblastoma (7) | Wang et al. (1999) |
| | delEx16/ delEx16 | Family history of HNPCC | *Proband*: CLS, axillary freckling | | *Proband*: glioma (4) | Vilkki et al. (2001) |
| | R687W/R687W | *Proband*: duodenal adenocarcinoma (11) *Sister 1*: colon polyps and CRC (9) | *Proband*: CLS *Sister 1*: CLS *Sister 2*: CLS, plexiform neurofibroma | | | Gallinger et al. (2004) |
| | P648S/ P648S | Family history of HNPCC | *Proband*: CLS, skin tumor (neurofibroma?) | | | Raevaara et al. (2004) |
| *MSH2* | 1662-1 G>A/ 1662-1 G>A | No family history of HNPCC | *Proband*: CLS | *Proband*: ALL (2) | | Whiteside et al. (2002) |
| | delEx1-6/ Ex3 del 1bp (codon 153) | | | *Sister*: NHL (1) | *Proband*: Glioblastoma (3) | Bougeard et al. (2003) |
| *MSH6* | 3386-3388delGTG/ 3386-3388delGTG | *Proband*: CRC (12) | *Proband*: CLS | | *Proband*: Oligodendroglioma (10) | Menko et al. (2004) |
| | 3634insT/ 3634insT | *Proband*: CRC (8) *Proband*: CRC (19), endometrial (24) | *Sister*: CLS, axillary freckling *Proband*: CLS | *Proband*: lymphoma (5) | *Sister*: Glioblastoma multiforme (8) | Hegde et al. (2005) Plaschke et al. (2006) |

(Continued)

**Table 4.** (Continued)

| Gene | Mutation | Gastointestinal tumors (age of onset) | NF1 features | Hematologic malignancies (age of onset) | CNS tumors (age of onset) | Reference |
|---|---|---|---|---|---|---|
| PMS2 | 1221delG/ 2361delCTTC | *Proband*: CRC (18) | | | *Proband*: Oligodendroglioma (14) *Sister*: neuroblastoma (13) | De Rosa et al. (2000) |
| | 1169ins20/ 1169ins20 | *Proband*: CRC (16) *Sister*: Colon adenomas (20) | *Sister*: CLS *Brother*: CLS | *Brother*: ALL (4) | *Proband*: PNET (21), endometrial (23), brain tumor (24) *Sister*: astrocytoma (7) | Trimbath et al. (2001) |
| | R134X/ 2184delTC | *Proband*: Colon adenomas (13) *Sister*: CRC (11), colon adenomas (14) | *Sister*: CLS | *Proband*: NHL (17) | *Proband*: Glioblastoma (4 and 21) | De Vos et al. (2004) |
| | R802X/ R802X* | *Proband*: Colon adenomas | *Proband*: CLS *Sister*: CLS *Brother*: CLS | | *Proband*: PNET (14) *Sister*: cerebral NHL (10) *Brother*: PNET (8) | De Vos et al. (2004) |
| | R802X/R802X* | *Proband*: CRC (18) | *Proband*: CLS | *Proband*: T-cell leukaemia (2), T-cell lymphoma (14) | | De Vos et al. (2006) |
| | 543delT/ 543delT* | No family history of HNPCC | *Proband*: CLS *Sib*: CLS | | *Proband*: PNET (8) *Sib*: PNET (4) | De Vos et al. (2006) |
| | R802X/R802X* | | *Proband*: CLS *Sib 1*: CLS *Sib 2*: CLS | *Sib 1*: ALL (15) | *Proband*: glioma (15) *Sib 2*: astrocytoma (6), glioblastoma (7) | De Vos et al. (2006) |
| | R802X/R802X* | | *Proband*: not reported *Sib 1*: not reported *Sib 2*: not reported | *Sib 1*: NHL (3) *Sib 2*: ALL (6) | *Proband*: glioblastoma (2) | De Vos et al. (2006) |
| | R802X/R802X* | | *Proband*: CLS | *Proband*: ALL | | De Vos et al. (2006) |
| | Q643X/S46I | *Proband*: duodenal carcinoma (17), colon adenomas (17) Family history of HNPCC | *Proband*: CLS | | *Proband*: glioblastoma (18) | Agostini et al. (2005) |
| | E705K/wt | *Proband*: CRC (13) | | *Proband*: NHL (15) | *Proband*: Astrocytoma (7) | Miyaki et al. (1997) |

*ALL* Acute lymphatic leukaemia; *AML* acute myeloid leukemia; *CML* cronic myeloid leukemia; *NHL* non-Hodgkin's lymphoma; *PNET* primitive neuroectodermal tumor; *CRC* colorectal cancer.

*Consanguineous families of Pakistani origin.

tumor spectrum, colonic polyps or cancer, and a high risk of second primary malignancies. The tumor spectrum is marked by hematologic malignancies, including T-cell lymphoblastic leukemia and non-Hodgkin lymphoma, and CNS tumors such as glioma, medulloblastoma, neuroblastoma and, in case of *PMS2* biallelic mutations, supratentorial primitive neuroectodermal tumors. Other tumors reported in MMR-deficient children include colorectal cancer and multiple colonic polyps in adolescence or early adult life.

Since heterozygous mutations in MMR genes typically cause HNPCC, in the case of MLH1, MSH2 and MSH6 the recessive phenotype occurs in the contest of a family history consistent with HNPCC (Table 3). In contrast, in nine of the ten families that are now known with homozygous or compound heterozygous PMS2 mutations, no history of HNPCC in heterozygotes has been reported. Despite this fact, heterozygous PMS2 mutations have recently been described in adult patients with familial or sporadic colorectal cancer (Nakagawa et al. 2004, Worthley et al. 2005). These apparently conflicting observations are most probably due to the lower penetrance of heterozygous PMS2 mutations than MLH1 and MSH2 ones (Truninger et al. 2005).

A further key distinction between dominant HNPCC and biallelic MMR mutations concern miscrosatellite instability. This is observed in the tumor tissue of patients with dominant HNPCC. However, a very high level of microsatellite instability in normal tissues of individuals carrying biallelic MMR genes mutations has been observed at high frequency (Wang et al. 1999, De Rosa et al. 2000, Vilkki et al. 2001).

In the case of *Turcot Syndrome due to biallelic mutation in MMR genes* a differential diagnosis with Neurofibromatosis type 1 should be considered.

# TURCOT SYNDROME TYPE 2

Turcot syndrome type 2 consist of patients diagnosed with familial adenomatous polyposis (FAP) [OMIM 114500] and medulloblastoma.

*APC-associated polyposis conditions* include the overlapping, often indistinguishable phenotypes of classic familial adenomatous polyposis (FAP), Gardner and Turcot syndromes as well as the phenotype of attenuated FAP (AFAP).

## Incidence and prevalence

The birth frequency of FAP is estimated at roughly 1 in 13,000 to 1 in 18,000 live births (Bisgaard et al. 1994), and is responsible for less than 1% of all CRC cases. The reported prevalence of *APC*-associated polyposis conditions is 2.29–3.2 per 100,000 population (Burn et al. 1991, Jarvinen 1992).

## Clinical manifestations

The hallmark of FAP is the development of hundreds of adenomatous polyps in the colon and rectum, usually in adolescence, with an inevitable progression to colorectal cancer by the age of 35–40 years. Almost 70–80% of tumors occur in the left colon (Bjork et al. 1999). FAP-associated features include upper gastrointestinal tract polyps, congenital hypertrophy of the retinal pigment epithelium, desmoid tumors, and other extracolonic malignancies.

FAP patients are at increased risk for polyps and cancer of the upper gastrointestinal tract. Gastric and duodenal adenomas are present in about 90% of FAP patients by the age of 70 years (Bülow et al. 2004). About two thirds of duodenal adenomas occur in the papilla or periampullary region (Bertoni et al. 1996) and confer an increased risk of small bowel cancer which is the third cause of death in FAP patients (8.2%), following metastatic colorectal cancer (58.2%) and desmoid tumors (10.9%) (Arvanitis et al. 1990).

Benign congenital hypertrophy of the retinal pigment epithelium (CHRPE), a specific FAP lesion, occurs in 70–80% of patients. CHRPE refers to the presence of pigmented fundus lesions (Ruhswurm et al. 1998), usually present at birth, largely preceding the development of intestinal polyposis, asymptomatic and with no malignant potential.

Desmoid tumors are rare, locally invasive fibromatoses that are the second cause of death in FAP

**Table 5.** Extracolonic cancer risk in FAP

| Malignancy | Relative risk | Absolute lifetime risk (%) |
|---|---|---|
| Desmoid | 852 | 15 |
| Hepatoblastoma | 847 | 1.6 |
| Duodenum | 330.8 | 3–5 |
| Ampullary | 123.7 | 1.7 |
| Thyroid | 7.6 | 2 |
| Brain | 7 | 2 |
| Pancreas | 4.5 | 1.7 |

Giardiello et al. (1995), Jagelman et al. (1988), Sturt et al. (2004), Lynch et al. (1996), Bülow et al. (2004), Galiatsatos and Foukes (2006).

patients (Arvanitis et al. 1990). The prevalence of desmoid disease in FAP is 15% (Sturt et al. 2004), with a relative risk of ~850 times that of the general population (Lynch and Fitzgibbons 1996). The majority of tumors occurs within the abdomen (50%), usually involving small bowel mesentery, or in the abdominal wall (48%) (Clark et al. 1999). Desmoids have been linked to trauma, particularly abdominal surgery such as prophylactic colectomy (Soravia et al. 2000). Females have twice the odds of developing desmoids compared to males (Sturt et al. 2004, Bertario et al. 2001).

Extracolonic malignancies associated with FAP are thyroid cancer, hepatoblastoma and CNS tumors (Table 5).

Thyroid cancer has an estimated incidence of 1–2% (Bülow et al. 1997) and, most commonly, its histological type is papillary, with a cribriform pattern (Bülow et al. 1997).

Hepatoblastomas usually affects children under the age of 2.5 yr, with a male: female ratio of 2.3:1 (Hartley et al. 1990). The incidence of hepatoblastoma among children of FAP patients is 1 in 235, compared to 1 in 100,000 in the general population (Hughes and Michels 1992).

In FAP families there is an increased risk of primary central nervous system (CNS) tumors, most commonly medulloblastoma, although anaplastic astrocytomas, ependymomas and pinealoblastomas have also been described (Hamilton et al. 1995). The relative risk for developing a medulloblastoma in patients with *Turcot syndrome* and an APC gene

mutation is 92 times that in the general population (Raffel 2004).

*Gardner syndrome* is a historically coined variant of FAP characterized by the association of gastrointestinal polyposis with osteomas, as well as multiple skin and soft tissue tumors (Gardner and Richards 1953). Although most FAP patients can be found to have at least subtle findings of Gardner syndrome on thorough investigation, the term is usually used to refer to patients and families where the extraintestinal features are particularly prominent. Osteomas typically occur in the mandible, but can also present in the skull and long bones (Bilkay et al. 2000). Epidermal cysts are the most common skin manifestation of Gardner syndrome (Bilkay et al. 2000); other cutaneous features include lipomas, fibromas, and leiomyomas. Dental abnormalities, such as supernumerary and impacted teeth, are seen in 22–30% of FAP patients on panoramic radiographs, and constitute another feature of Gardner syndrome (Bertario et al. 2003).

*Attenuated FAP* (AFAP) is characterized by fewer colonic polyps (average of 30), with a more proximal colonic localization, than classic FAP. The average age of colon cancer diagnosis in individuals with AFAP is age 50–55 years, therefore 10–15 years later than in those with classic FAP (Spirio et al. 1993). Upper gastrointestinal polyps and cancers may be seen in individuals with AFAP (Burt 2003) but the extraintestinal manifestations of FAP are rare.

## Natural history

Colorectal adenomatous polyps begin to appear at an average age of 16 years (range 7–36 years) (Petersen et al. 1991); by age 35 years, 95% of individuals have polyps. When colonic expression is fully developed, hundreds to thousands of colonic adenomatous polyps are typically observed. Without colectomy, colon cancer is inevitable. The average age of colon cancer diagnosis in untreated individuals is 39 years (range 34–43 years), but seven percent of untreated individuals with FAP develop colon cancer by age 21 years (Bussey 1975).

## Molecular genetics

FAP is a highly penetrant autosomal-dominant disorder, caused by a germline mutation in the adenomatous polyposis coli (*APC*) gene, located on chromosome 5q21. *APC* is a tumor suppressor gene, cloned in 1991 (Kinzler et al. 1991, Groden et al. 1991); it has an 8538bp open reading frame, and consists of 15 transcribed exons (Van Es et al. 2001, Fearnhead et al. 2001).

Inactivation of APC represent the first step in colorectal carcinogenesis in FAP patients. APC functions as a key regulator in a complex developmental pathway; APC is a component of a protein

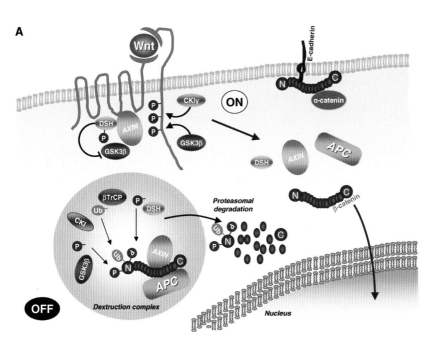

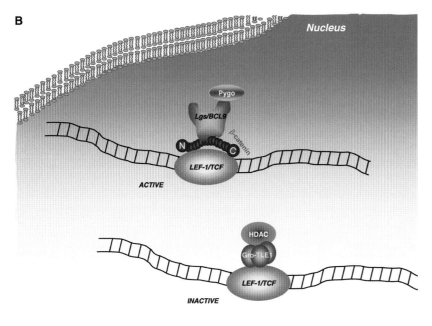

**Fig. 4.** Wnt signaling (see text); modified from Willert and Jones (2006).

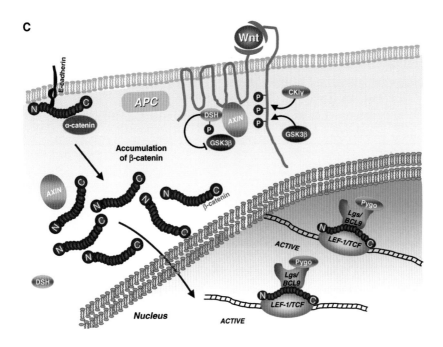

**C**

**Fig. 4.** (Continued)

complex, modulated by the Wnt signaling pathway (Fig. 4), which regulates the phosphorylation and degradation of β-catenin (Goss and Groden 2000, Näthke 2004). In the cytoplasm, APC associates with at least seven proteins, including β-catenin. The control of free β-catenin levels in the cytoplasm by APC defines the role of APC as a tumor suppressor. Normally, free levels of β-catenin are low, as binding of β-catenin by APC sequesters β-catenin and targets the protein for degradation (Fig. 4A). APC only binds β-catenin when β-catenin is hyperphosphorylated. β-catenin is phosphorylated by GSK-3β, a serine/threonine kinase. Free β-catenin associates with members of the Tcf family of transcription factors. When β-catenin associates with Tcf, the complex moves to the nucleus and upregulates the expression of genes that increase the rate of cell division, either by stimulating cell proliferation or by inhibiting apoptosis (Fig. 4B). When APC is inactivated by mutation, levels of cytoplasmic β-catenin rise (Fig. 4C).

Moreover, APC also control the cell cycle, by inhibiting the progression of cells from the $G_0/G_1$ to the S phase (Goss and Groden 2000) and stabilizes microtubules, promoting chromosomal stability (Näthke 2004).

Over 700 different germline APC mutations have been reported, and the most common mutation involves the introduction of a premature stop codon, either by a nonsense mutation (30%), frameshift mutation (68%), or large deletion (2%), leading to truncation of the protein product in the C-terminal region (Béroud and Soussi 1996). The two most frequently mutated codons are at positions 1061 and 1309 (Béroud and Soussi 1996). An updated database of APC gene mutations is available online (URL: http://www.cancer-genetics.org).

A correlation between certain mutations and the phenotypes have been observed (Fig. 5). Mutations at codon 1309 have been associated with a more severe clinical phenotype (patients tend to develop bowel symptoms earlier, have more colorectal polyps and CRCs develop at earlier ages (Friedl et al. 2001, Nugent et al. 1994, Bertario et al. 2003). Mutations occurring in the 5′ end or in the distal part of exon 15 generally result in a milder (attenuated) form of FAP, named AFAP. AFAP is characterized as having fewer polyps (<100), later expression (third or fourth decade) and more proximal location (right colon) (Burt et al. 2004).

As regards extracolonic manifestations, mutations from codons 976–1067 are associated with a

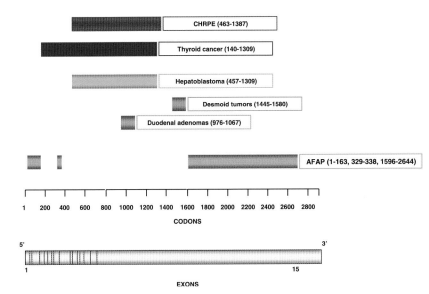

**Fig. 5.** *APC* cDNA and extracolonic genotype-phenotype correlation; modified from Galiatsatos and Foulkes (2006).

three- to four-fold increased risk for developing duodenal adenomas, while those spanning between codons 543 and 1309 are associated with CHRPE (Bertario et al. 2003). Mutations beyond codon 1309 are linked to a six-fold increased risk of desmoid tumors (Bertario et al. 2003), while patients with papillary thyroid cancer often have mutations between codons 140 and 1309 (Cetta et al. 2000). So far, no *APC* germline mutations predisposing to CNS tumors have been described.

## Diagnosis

The diagnosis of APC-associated polyposis conditions relies primarily on clinical findings.

**FAP** is diagnosed clinically in an individual with:

- more than 100 colorectal adenomatous polyps or
- less than 100 colorectal adenomatous polyps and a first degree relative with FAP.

Attenuated FAP is considered in an individual with:

- many colorectal adenomatous polyps

or

- family history of colon cancer in individuals younger than 60 years of age with multiple colorectal adenomatous polyps.

## Management and follow-up

At initial diagnosis of FAP, to establish the extent of the disease, studies should always include:

1. personal medical history and family history with particular attention to FAP features;
2. physical examination with particular attention to extracolonic manifestation of APC-associated polyposis;
3. ophthalmologic evaluation;
4. colonscopy;
5. upper gastrointestinal tract evaluation (endoscopy and small bowel X-ray);
6. molecular genetic testing of *APC* gene to confirm diagnosis if clinical criteria are not satisfied. However, if such a test do not identify a disease causing mutation, the FAP diagnosis is still possible because the mutation detection rate is less than 100% with the available tests.

Recommended *surveillance protocols* for affected individuals and their at-risk relatives are summarized in Table 6.

Strict neurological evaluation has been recommended for FAP families with a member affected by a CNS tumor (*Turcot syndrome*), due to evidence of familial clustering (Hamilton et al. 1995). No guidelines exist, however, and there are no studies so far to determine whether such an intervention could improve survival.

**Table 6.** Surveillance protocols for FAP patients and their first-degree relatives

---

*Proband with clinical diagnosis of FAP*

---

*Total colectomy with IPAA:* Periodic flexible sigmoidoscopy for pouch polyps/cancers every 2 years
*Subtotal colectomy with IRA:* Flexible sigmoidoscopy every 6–12 months.
Upper endoscopy every 1–3 years (depending on polyp burden)
Annual thyroid exam by palpation (consider U/S)
Consider periodic abdominal U/S for pancreatic cancer + desmoid tumor screening

---

*Unaffected first-degree relative of FAP proband*

---

*No mutation identified in the family, or mutation identified but relative refuses genetic testing:*

- Flexible sigmoidoscopy annually starting at age 10–12, biennially from 26 to 35, every third year from 36 to 50.
- Consider eye exam for CHRPE.
- If no polyps by age 50, follow general population colon cancer screening guidelines

*APC mutation carriers:*

- Sigmoidoscopy annually/biannually from age 10 to 12; colonoscopy once polyps are detected
- Upper endoscopy every 1–3 years (depending on polyp burden) beginning by age 25 years
- Annual thyroid exam by palpation (consider U/S)
- Consider periodic abdominal U/S for pancreatic cancer + desmoid tumor screening
- Annual surveillance for hepatoblastoma from birth to age 5 years by physical examination and/or abdominal U/S and serum alpha-fetoprotein

---

*Unaffected first-degree relative of AFAP proband:*

---

- Colonoscopy every 2–3 years beginning at 18–20 years of age.
- Once polyps are detected same recommendations of classical FAP

---

*CHRPE* Congenital hypertrophy of the retinal pigment epithelium; *IPAA* ileal pouch-anal anastomosis; *IRA* ileorectal anastomosis; *U/S* ultrasound.

## Differential diagnosis

The differential diagnosis includes hereditary syndromes associated with increased risk to develop colon cancer. Conditions to consider in differential diagnosis include the following:

1. *MYH-associated polyposis* whose phenotype is similar to FAP and AFAP but displays an autosomal recessive inheritance. If an *APC* mutation is not found in an individual with FAP or AFAP, molecular genetic testing of *MYH* should be considered (Sieber et al. 2003).
2. *HNPCC*: there is a predominance of colon cancer located in the proximal colon and, usually, only few colonic adenomas are present.
3. *Turcot syndrome due to MMR gene mutations*: usually associated with glioblastomas.
4. *Hamartomatous polyp syndromes* (Juvenile polyposis syndrome, Peutz-Jeghers syndrome and *PTEN* hamartomatous syndromes) are associated with an increased risk of colonic polyps and cancer, but they can usually be distinguished by their extracolonic manifestations as well as the hamartomatous rather than adenomatous pathology.

## Treatment

Individuals affected by classical FAP should undergo colectomy after adenomas appear; colectomy is usually recommended when more than 20–30 polyps have occurred. Frequently, in classical FAP, a total colectomy with mucosal proctectomy with ileo-anal pull through is performed. Subtotal colectomy with ileorectal anastomosis is often used in individual affected by AFAP or in instances in which the rectum is spared of polyps.

Endoscopic or surgical removal of duodenal adenomas should be considered if polyps exhibit villous change or severe dysplasia, exceed one centimeter in diameter or cause symptoms.

Treatment of desmoid tumors is very problematic. Surgical removal is associated with high rates of recurrence; treatments with non-steroidal anti-inflammatory drugs, anti-estrogens, cytotoxic chemotherapy and radiation have been attempt (reviewed in Knudsen and Bulow 2001)

The treatment of other FAP-associated cancer do not differ from the sporadic ones.

# References

Aaltonen LA, Peltomaki P, Mecklin JP, Jarvinen H, Jass JR, Lynch HT, Green JS, Lynch HT, Watson, P, Tallqvist G, Juhola M, Sistonen P, Hamilton SR, Kenneth WK, Vogelstein B, de la Chapelle A (1994) Replication errors in benign and malignant tumors for hereditary nonpolyposis colorectal cancer patients. Cancer Res 54: 1645–1648.

Aarnio M, Mecklin JP, Aaltonen LA, Nystrom-Lahti M, Jarvinen HJ (1995) Life-time risk of different cancers in hereditary non-polyposis colorectal cancer (HN-PCC) syndrome. Int J Cancer 64: 430–433.

Aarnio M, Sankila R, Pukkala E, Salovaara R, Aaltonen LA, de la Chapelle A, Peltomaki P, Mecklin JP, Jarvinen HJ (1999) Cancer risk in mutation carriers of DNA-mismatch-repair genes. Int J Cancer 81: 214–218.

Agostini M, Tibiletti MG, Lucci-Cordisco E, Chiaravalli A, Morreau H, Furlan D, Boccuto L, Pucciarelli S, Capella C, Boiocchi M, Viel A (2005) Two PMS2 mutations in a Turcot syndrome family with small bowel cancers. Am J Gastroenterol 100: 1886–1891.

Arvanitis ML, Jagelman DG, Fazio VW, Lavery IC, McGannon E (1990) Mortality in patients with familial adenomatous polyposis. Dis Colon Rectum 33: 639–642.

Béroud C, Soussi T (1996) APC gene: database of germline and somatic mutations in human tumors and cell lines. Nucleic Acids Res 24: 121–124.

Bertario L, Russo A, Sala P, Eboli M, Giarola M, D'amico F, Gismondi V, Varesco L, Pierotti MA, Radice P (2001) Genotype and phenotype factors as determinants of desmoid tumors in patients with familial adenomatous polyposis. Int J Cancer 95: 102–107.

Bertario L, Russo A, Sala P, Varesco L, Giarola M, Mondini P, Pierotti M, Spinelli P, Radice P (2003) Multiple approach to the exploration of genotype-phenotype correlations in familial adenomatous polyposis. J Clin Oncol 21: 1698–1707.

Bertoni G, Sassatelli R, Nigrisoli E, Pennazio M, Tansini P, Arrigoni A, Ponz de Leon M, Rossini FP, Bedogni G (1996) High prevalence of adenomas and microadenomas of the duodenal papilla and periampullary region in patients with familial adenomatous polyposis. Eur J Gastroenterol Hepatol 8: 1201–1206.

Bilkay U, Erdem O, Ozek C, Helvaci E, Kilic K, Ertan Y, Gurler T (2000) Benign osteoma with Gardner syndrome: review of the literature and report of a case. J Craniofac Surg 15: 506–509.

Bisgaard ML, Fenger K, Bulow S, Niebuhr E, Mohr J (1994) Familial adenomatous polyposis (FAP): frequency, penetrance, and mutation rate. Hum Mutat 3: 121–125.

Bjork J, Akerbrant H, Iselius L, Alm T, Hultcrantz R (1999) Epidemiology of familial adenomatous polyposis in Sweden: changes over time and differences in phenotype between males and females. Scand J Gastroenterol 34: 1230–1235.

Bougeard G, Charbonnier F, Moerman A, Martin C, Ruchoux MM, Drouot N, Frebourg T (2003) Early onset brain tumor and lymphoma in MSH2-deficient children. Am J Hum Genet 72: 213–216.

Bronner CE, Baker SM, Morrison PT, Warren G, Smith LG, Lescoe MK, Kane M, Earabino C, Lipford J, Lindblom A (1994) Mutation in the DNA mismatch repair gene homologue hMLH1 is associated with hereditary nonpolyposis colon cancer. Nature 368: 258–261.

Bülow C, Bülow S, Leeds Castle Polyposis Group (1997) Is screening for thyroid carcinoma indicated in familial adenomatous polyposis? Int J Colorectal Dis 12: 240–242.

Bülow S, Björk J, Christensen IJ, Fausa O, Jarvinen H, Moesgaard F, Vasen HF; DAF Study Group (2004) Duodenal adenomatosis in familial adenomatous polyposis. The DAF Study Group. Gut 53: 381–386.

Burn J, Chapman P, Delhanty J, Wood C, Lalloo F, Cachon-Gonzalez MB, Tsioupra K, Church W, Rhodes M, Gunn A (1991) The UK Northern region genetic register for familial adenomatous polyposis coli: use of age of onset, congenital hypertrophy of the retinal pigment epithelium, and DNA markers in risk calculations. J Med Genet 28: 289–296.

Burt RW (2003) Gastric fundic gland polyps. Gastroenterology 125: 1462–1469.

Burt RW, Leppert MF, Slattery ML, Samowitz WS, Spirio LN, Kerber RA, Kuwada SK, Neklason DW, Disario JA, Lyon E, Hughes JP, Chey WY, White RL (2004) Genetic testing and phenotype in a large kindred with attenuated familial adenomatous polyposis. Gastroenterology 127: 444–451.

Bussey HJR (1975) Familial polyposis coli. Family studies, histopathology, differential diagnosis and results of treatment. Baltimore: The Johns Hopkins University Press.

Cetta F, Montalto G, Gori M, Curia MC, Cama A, Olschwang S (2000) Germline mutations of the APC gene in patients with familial adenomatous polyposis-associated thyroid carcinoma: results from a European Cooperative Study. J Clin Endocrinol Metab 85: 286–292.

Chung DC (2000) The Genetic Basis of Colorectal Cancer: Insights Into Critical Pathways of Tumorigenesis. Gastroenterology 119: 854–865.

Church J, Simmang C (2003) Practice parameters for the treatment of patients with dominantly inherited colorectal cancer (familial adenomatous polyposis and hereditary nonpolyposis colorectal cancer). Dis Colon Rectum 46: 1001–1012.

Clark SK, Neale KF, Landgrebe JC, Phillips RK (1999) Desmoid tumours complicating familial adenomatous polyposis. Br J Surg 86: 1185–1189.

Crail HW (1949) Multiple primary malignancies arising in the rectum, brain and thyroid. US Nav Med Bull 49: 123–128.

Cunningham JM, Kim CY, Christensen ER, Tester DJ, Parc Y, Burgart LJ, Halling KC, McDonnell SK, Schaid DJ, Walsh Vockley C, Kubly V, Nelson H, Michels VV, Thibodeau SN (2001) The frequency of hereditary defective mismatch repair in a prospective series of unselected colorectal carcinomas. Am J Hum Genet 69: 780–790.

Davis DA, Cohen PR (1995) Genitourinary tumors in men with Muir-Torre syndrome. J Amer Acad Dermatol 33: 909–912.

de Leeuw WJ, Dierssen J, Vasen HF, Wijnen JT, Kenter GG, Meijers-Heijboer H, Brocker-Vriends A, Stormorken A, Moller P, Menko F, Cornelisse CJ, Morreau H (2000) Prediction of a mismatch repair gene defect by microsatellite instability and immunohistochemical analysis in endometrial tumours from HNPCC patients. J Pathol 192: 328–335.

De Rosa M, Fasano C, Panariello L, Scarano MI, Belli G, Iannelli A, Ciciliano F, Izzo P (2000) Evidence for a recessive inheritance of Turcot's syndrome caused by compound heterozygous mutations within the PMS2 gene. Oncogene 19: 1719–1723.

De Vos M, Hayward BE, Picton S, Sheridan E, Bonthron DT (2004) Novel PMS2 pseudogenes can conceal recessive mutations causing a distinctive childhood cancer syndrome. Am J Hum Genet 74: 954–964.

De Vos M, Hayward BE, Charlton R, Taylor GR, Glaser AW, Picton S, Cole TR, Maher ER, McKeown CM, Mann JR, Yates JR, Baralle D, Rankin J, Bonthron DT, Sheridan E (2006) PMS2 mutations in childhood cancer. J Natl Cancer Inst. 98: 358–361.

Esteller M, Fraga MF, Guo M, Garcia-Foncillas J, Hedenfalk I, Godwin AK, Trojan J, Vaurs-Barriere C, Bignon YJ, Ramus S, Benitez J, Caldes T, Akiyama Y, Yuasa Y, Launonen V, Canal MJ, Rodriguez R, Capella G, Peinado MA, Borg A, Aaltonen LA, Ponder BA, Baylin SB, Herman JG (2001) DNA methylation patterns in hereditary human cancers mimic sporadic tumorigenesis. Hum Mol Genet 10: 3001–3007.

Fearnhead NS, Britton MP, Bodmer WF (2001) The ABC of APC. Hum Mol Genet 10: 721–733.

Fishel R, Lescoe MK, Rao MR, Copeland NG, Jenkins NA, Garber J, Kane M, Kolodner R (1993) The human mutator gene homolog MSH2 and its association with hereditary nonpolyposis colon cancer. Cell 75: 1027–1038.

Friedl W, Caspari R, Sengteller M, Uhlhaas S, Lamberti C, Jungck M, Kadmon M, Wolf M, Fahnenstich J, Gebert J, Moslein G, Mangold E, Propping P (2001) Can APC mutation analysis contribute to therapeutic decisions in familial adenomatous polyposis? Experience from 680 FAP families. Gut 48: 515–521.

Galiatsatos P, Foulkes WD (2006) Familial Adenomatous Polyposis. Am J Gastroenterol 101: 385–398.

Gallinger S, Aronson M, Shayan K, Ratcliffe EM, Gerstle JT, Parkin PC, Rothenmund H, Croitoru M, Baumann E, Durie PR, Weksberg R, Pollett A, Riddell RH, Ngan BY, Cutz E, Lagarde AE, Chan HS (2004) Gastrointestinal cancers and neurofibromatosis type 1 features in children with a germline homozygous MLH1 mutation. Gastroenterology 126: 576–585.

Gardner EJ, Richards RC (1953) Multiple cutaneous and subcutaneous lesions occurring simultaneously with hereditary polyposis and osteomatosis. Am J Hum Genet 5: 139–147.

Giardiello F, Brensinger JD, Petersen GM (2001) AGA Technical review on hereditary colorectal cancer and genetic testing. Gastroenterology 121: 198–213.

Giardiello FM, Offerhaus JGA (1995) Phenotype and cancer risk of various polyposis syndromes. Eur J Cancer 31A: 1085–1087.

Goss KH, Groden J (2000) Biology of the adenomatous polyposis coli tumor suppressor. J Clin Oncol 18: 1967–1979.

Groden J, Thliveris A, Samowitz W, Carlson M, Gelbert L, Albertsen H, Joslyn G, Stevens J, Spirio L, Robertson M et al. (1991) Identification and characterization of the familial adenomatous polyposis coli gene. Cell 66: 589–600.

Gruber SB (2006) New Developments in Lynch Syndrome (Hereditary Nonpolyposis Colorectal Cancer) and Mismatch Repair Gene Testing. Gastroenterology 130: 577–587.

Hamada H, Kurimoto M, Endo S, Ogiichi T, Akai T, Takaku A (1998) Turcot's syndrome presenting with medulloblastoma and familiar adenomatous polyposis: a case report and review of the literature. Acta Neurochir 140: 631–632.

Hamilton SR, Liu B, Parsons RE, Papadopoulos N, Jen J, Powell SM, Krush AJ, Berk T, Cohen Z, Tetu B, Burger PC, Wood PA, Taqi F, Booker SV, Petersen GM, Offerhaus GJA, Tersmette AC, Giardiello FM, Vogelstein B, Kinzler KW (1995) The molecular basis of Turcot's syndrome. N Engl J Med 332: 839–847.

Hartley AL, Birch JM, Kelsey AM, Jones PH, Harris M, Blair V (1990) Epidemiological and familial aspects of hepatoblastoma. Med Pediatr Oncol 18: 103–109.

Hegde MR, Chong B, Blazo ME, Chin LH, Ward PA, Chintagumpala MM, Kim JY, Plon SE, Richards CS (2005) A homozygous mutation in MSH6 causes Turcot syndrome. Clin Cancer Res 11: 4689–4693.

Huang SC, Lavine JE, Boland PS, Newbury RO, Kolodner R, Pham TT, Arnold CN, Boland CR, Carethers JM (2001) Germline characterization of early-aged onset of hereditary non-polyposis colorectal cancer. J Pediatr 138: 629–635.

Hughes LJ, Michels VV (1992) Risk of hepatoblastoma in familial adenomatous polyposis. Am J Med Genet 43: 1023–1025.

Jagelman DG, DeCosse JJ, Bussey HJR (1988) Upper gastrointestinal cancer in familial adenomatous polyposis. Lancet 1: 1149–1151.

Jarvinen HJ (1992) Epidemiology of familial adenomatous polyposis in Finland: impact of family screening on the colorectal cancer rate and survival. Gut 33: 357–360.

Jarvinen HJ, Aarnio M, Mustonen H, Aktan-Collan K, Aaltonen LA, Peltomaki P, De La Chapelle A, Mecklin JP (2000) Controlled 15-year trial on screening for colorectal cancer in families with hereditary nonpolyposis colorectal cancer. Gastroenterology 118: 829–834.

Kinzler KW, Nilbert MC, Su LK, Vogelstein B, Bryan TM, Levy DB, Smith KJ, Preisinger AC, Hedge P, McKechnie D et al. (1991) Identification of FAP locus genes from chromosome 5q21. Science 253: 661–665.

Knudsen AL, Bulow S (2001) Desmoid tumour in familial adenomatous polyposis. A review of literature. Fam Cancer 1: 111–119.

Kolodner RD, Tytell JD, Schmeits JL, Kane MF, Gupta RD, Weger J, Wahlberg S, Fox EA, Peel D, Ziogas A, Garber JE, Syngal S, Anton-Culver H, Li FP (1999) Germ-line MSH6 mutations in colorectal cancer families. Cancer Res 59: 5068–5074.

Kurokowa M, Lynch K, Podolsky DK (1987) Effects of growth factors on an intestinal epithelial cell line: transforming growth factor beta inhibits proliferation and stimulates differentiation. Biochem Biophys Res Comm 142: 775–782.

Liu B, Parsons R, Papadopoulos N, Nicolaides NC, Lynch HT, Watson P, Jass JR, Dunlop M, Wyllie A, Peltomaki P, de la Chapelle A, Hamilton SR, Vogelstein B, Kinzler KW (1996) Analysis of mismatch repair genes in hereditary non-polyposis colorectal cancer patients. Nat Med 2: 169–174.

Lucci-Cordisco E, Zito I, Gensini F, Genuardi M (2003) Hereditary nonpolyposis colorectal cancer and related conditions. Am J Med Genet A 122: 325–334.

Lynch HT, Fitzgibbons R Jr (1996) Surgery, desmoid tumors, and familial adenomatous polyposis: case report and literature review. Am J Gastroenterol 91: 2598–2601.

Malkhosyan S, Rampino N, Yamamoto H, Perucho M (1996) Frameshift mutator mutations. Nature 382: 499–500.

Markowitz S, Roberts A (1996) Tumor suppressor activity of the TGF-β pathway in human cancers. Cytokine Growth Factor Rev 7: 93–102.

Markowitz S, Wang J, Myeroff L, Parsons R, Sun L, Lutterbaugh J, Fan R, Zborowska E, Kinzler K, Vogelstein B, Brattain M, Willson J (1995) Inactivation of the type II TGF-beta receptor in colon cancer cells with microsatellite instability. Science 268: 1336–1338.

Maxwell GL, Risinger JI, Alvarez AA, Barrett JC, Berchuck A (2001) Favorable survival associated with microsatellite instability in endometrioid endometrial cancers. Obstet Gynecol 97: 417–422.

McLaughlin MR, Gollin SM, Lese CM, Albright AL (1998) Medulloblastoma and glioblastoma multiforme in a patient with Turcot syndrome: a case report. Surg Neurol 49: 295–301.

Menko FH, Kaspers GL, Meijer GA, Claes K, van Hagen JM, Gille JJ (2004) A homozygous MSH6 mutation in a child with café-au-lait spots, oligodendroglioma and rectal cancer. Fam Cancer 3: 123–127.

Miyaki M, Konishi M, Tanaka K, Kikuchi-Yanoshita R, Muraoka M, Yasuno M, Igari T, Koike M, Chiba M, Mori T (1997) Germline mutation of MSH6 as the cause of hereditary nonpolyposis colorectal cancer. Nat Genet 17: 271–272.

Nakagawa H, Lockman JC, Frankel WL, Hampel H, Steenblock K, Burgart LJ, Thibodeau SN, de la Chapelle A (2004) Mismatch repair gene PMS2: disease-causing germline mutations are frequent in patients whose tumors stain negative for PMS2 protein, but paralogous genes obscure mutation detection and interpretation. Cancer Res 64: 4721–4727.

Näthke I (2004) APC at a glance. J Cell Sci 117: 4873–4875.

National Comprehensive Cancer Network (2003) Colorectal cancer screening: clinical practice guidelines in oncology. J Nat Comp Cancer Net 1: 72–93.

Nicolaides NC, Papadopoulos N, Liu B, Wei YF, Carter KC, Ruben SM, Rosen CA, Haseltine WA, Fleischmann RD, Fraser CM (1994) Mutations of two PMS homologues in hereditary nonpolyposis colon cancer. Nature 371: 75–80.

Nugent KP, Phillips RK, Hodgson SV, Cottrell S, Smith-Ravin J, Pack K, Bodmer WF (1994) Phenotypic expression in familial adenomatous polyposis: partial prediction by mutation analysis. Gut 35: 1622–1623.

Ouyang H, Shiwaku H, Hagiwara H, Miura K, Abe T, Kato Y, Ohtani H, Shiiba K, Souza R, Meltzer S, Horii A (1997)

The insulin-like growth factor II receptor gene is mutated in genetically unstable cancers of the endometrium, stomach, and colorectum. Cancer Res 57: 1851–1854.

Paraf F, Jothy S, Van Meir EG (1997) Brain tumor-polyposis syndrome: two genetic diseases? J Clin Oncol 15: 2744–2758.

Peltomaki P (2001) Deficient DNA mismatch repair: a common etiologic factor for colon cancer. Hum Mol Genet 10: 735–740.

Peltomaki P (2005) Lynch syndrome genes. Familial Cancer 4: 227–232.

Peltomaki P, Vasen HF (1997) Mutations predisposing to hereditary nonpolyposis colorectal cancer: database and results of a collaborative study. The International Collaborative Group on Hereditary Nonpolyposis Colorectal Cancer. Gastroenterology 113: 1146–1158.

Petersen GM, Slack J, Nakamura Y (1991) Screening guidelines and premorbid diagnosis of familial adenomatous polyposis using linkage. Gastroenterology 100: 1658–1664.

Raevaara TE, Gerdes AM, Lonnqvist KE, Tybjaerg-Hansen A, Abdel-Rahman WM, Kariola R, Peltomaki P, Nystrom-Lahti M (2004) HNPCC mutation MLH1 P648S makes the functional protein unstable, and homozygosity predisposes to mild neurofibromatosis type 1. Genes Chromosomes Cancer 40: 261–265.

Raffel C (2004) Medulloblastoma: molecular genetics and animal models. Neoplasia 6: 310–322.

Rampino N, Yamamoto H, Ionov Y, Li Y, Sawai H, Reed JC, Perucho M (1997) Somatic frameshift mutations in the BAX gene in colon cancers of the microsatellite mutator phenotype. Science 275: 967–969.

Renkonen-Sinisalo L, Sipponen P, Aarnio M, Julkunen R, Aaltonen LA, Sarna S, Jarvinen HJ, Mecklin JP (2002) No support for endoscopic surveillance for gastric cancer in hereditary non-polyposis colorectal cancer. Scand J Gastroenterol 37: 574–577.

Ricciardone MD, Ozcelik T, Cevher B, Ozdag H, Tuncer M, Gurgey A, Uzunalimoglu O, Cetinkaya H, Tanyeli A, Erken E, Ozturk M (1999) Human MLH1 deficiency predisposes to hematological malignancy and neurofibromatosis type 1. Cancer Res 59: 290–293.

Rodriguez-Bigas MA, Boland CR, Hamilton SR, Henson DE, Jass JR, Khan PM, Lynch H, Perucho M, Smyrk T, Sobin L, Srivastava S (1997) A National Cancer Institute workshop on Hereditary Nonpolyposis Colorectal Cancer Syndrome: meeting highlights and bethes daguidelines J Natl Cancer Inst 89: 1758–1762.

Ruhswurm I, Zehetmayer M, Dejaco C, Wolf B, Karner-Hanusch J (1998) Ophthalmic and genetic screening in pedigrees with familial adenomatous polyposis. Am J Ophthalmol 125: 680–686.

Schwartz S, Yamamoto H, Navarro M, Maestro M, Reventos J, Perucho M (1999) Frameshift mutations at mononucleotide repeats in caspase-5 and other target genes in endometrial and gastrointestinal cancer of the microsatellite mutator phenotype. Cancer Res 59: 2995–2302.

Sieber OM, Lipton L, Crabtree M, Heinimann K, Fidalgo P, Phillips RK, Bisgaard ML, Orntoft TF, Aaltonen LA, Hodgson SV, Thomas HJ, Tomlinson IP (2003) Multiple colorectal adenomas, classic adenomatous polyposis, and germline mutations in MYH. N Engl J Med 348: 791–799.

Soravia C, Berk T, McLeod RS, Cohen Z (2000) Desmoid disease in patients with familial adenomatous polyposis. Dis Colon Rectum 43: 363–369.

Souza R, Appel R, Yin J, Wang S, Smolinski KN, Abraham JM, Zou T, Shi Y, Lei J, Cottrell J, Cymes K, Biden K, Simms L, Leggett B, Lynch PM, Frazier M, Powell SM, Harpaz N, Sugimura H, Young J, Meltzer SJ (1996) Microsatellite instability in the insulin-like growth factor II receptor gene in gastrointestinal tumours. Nat Genet 14: 255–257.

Spirio L, Olschwang S, Groden J, Robertson M, Samowitz W, Joslyn G, Gelbert L, Thliveris A, Carlson M, Otterud B (1993) Alleles of the APC gene: an attenuated form of familial polyposis. Cell 75: 951–957.

Sturt NJH, Gallagher MC, Bassett P, Philp CR, Neale KF, Tomlinson IP, Silver AR, Phillips RK (2004) Evidence for genetic predisposition to desmoid tumours in familial adenomatous polyposis independent of the germline APC mutation. Gut 53: 1832–1836.

Thibodeau SN, Bren G, Schaid D (1993) Microsatellite instability in cancer of the proximal colon. Science 260: 816–819.

Trimbath JD, Petersen GM, Erdman SH, Ferre M, Luce MC, Giardiello FM (2001) Café-au-lait spots and early onset colorectal neoplasia: a variant of HNPCC? Fam Cancer 1: 103–108.

Truninger K, Menigatti M, Luz J, Russell A, Haider R, Gebbers JO, Bannwart F, Yurtsever H, Neuweiler J, Riehle HM, Cattaruzza MS, Heinimann K, Schar P, Jiricny J, Marra G (2005) Immunohistochemical analysis reveals high frequency of PMS2 defects in colorectal cancer. Gastroenterology 128: 1160–1171.

Turcot J, Despres J-P, St Pierre F (1959) Malignant tumors of the central nervous system associated with familial polyposis of the colon: report of two cases. Dis Colon Rectum 2: 465–468.

Umar A, Boland CR, Terdiman JP, Syngal S, de la Chapelle A, Ruschoff J, Fishel R, Lindor NM, Burgart LJ, Hamelin R, Hamilton SR, Hiatt RA, Jass J, Lindblom A, Lynch HT, Peltomaki P, Ramsey SD, Rodriguez-Bigas MA, Vasen HF, Hawk ET, Barrett JC, Freedman AN, Srivastava S (2004) Revised Bethesda Guidelines for hereditary nonpolyposis colorectal cancer (Lynch syndrome) and microsatellite instability. J Natl Cancer Inst 96: 261–268.

Van Es JH, Giles RH, Clevers HC (2001) The many faces of the tumor suppressor gene APC. Exp Cell Res 264: 126–134.

Vasen HF (2000) Clinical diagnosis and management of hereditary colorectal cancer syndromes. J Clin Oncol 18: 81S–92S.

Vasen HF (2005) Clinical description of the Lynch syndrome [hereditary nonpolyposis colorectal cancer (HNPCC)]. Familial Cancer 4: 219–225.

Vasen HF, Mecklin JP, Khan PM, Lynch HT (1991) The International Collaboration Group on Hereditary Non-Polyposis Colorectal Cancer (ICG-HNPCC). Dis Colon Rectum 34: 424–425.

Vasen HF, Sanders EA, Taal BG, Nagengast FM, Griffioen G, Menko FH, Kleibeuker JH, Houwing-Duistermaat JJ, Meera Khan P (1996a) The risk of brain tumours in hereditary non-polyposis colorectal cancer (HNPCC). Int J Cancer 65: 422–425.

Vasen HF, Wijnen JT, Menko FH, Kleibeuker JH, Taal BG, Griffioen G, Nagengast FM, Meijers-Heijboer EH, Bertario L, Varesco L, Bisgaard ML, Mohr J, Fodde R, Khan PM (1996b) Cancer risk in families with hereditary nonpolyposis colorectal cancer diagnosed by mutation analysis. Gastroenterology 110: 1020–1027.

Vasen HF, Watson P, Mecklin JP, Lynch HT (1999) New Clinical Criteria for Hereditary Nonpolyposis Colorectal Cancer (HNPCC, Lynch Syndrome) Proposed by the International Collaborative Group on HNPCC. Gastroenterology 116: 1453–1456.

Vilkki S, Tsao JL, Loukola A, Poyhonen M, Vierimaa O, Herva R, Aaltonen LA, Shibata D (2001) Extensive somatic microsatellite mutations in normal human tissue. Cancer Res 61: 4541–4544.

Wang Q, Lasset C, Desseigne F, Frappaz D, Bergeron C, Navarro C, Ruano E, Puisieux A (1999) Neurofibromatosis and early onset of cancers in hMLH1-deficient children. Cancer Res 59: 294–297.

Watson P, Lin KM, Rodriguez-Bigas MA, Smyrk T, Lemon S, Shashidharan M, Franklin B, Karr B, Thorson A, Lynch HT (1998) Colorectal carcinoma survival among hereditary nonpolyposis colorectal carcinoma family members. Cancer 83: 259–266.

Whiteside D, McLeod R, Graham G, Steckley JL, Booth K, Somerville MJ, Andrew (2002) A homozygous germline mutation in the human MSH2 gene predisposes to hematological malignancy and multiple café-au-lait spots. Cancer Res 62: 359–362.

Wicking C, Simms LA, Evans T, Walsh M, Chawengsaksophak K, Beck F, Chenevix-Trench G, Young J, Jass J, Leggett B, Wainwright B (1998) CDX2, a human homologue of Drosophila caudal, is mutated in both alleles in a replication error positive colorectal cancer. Oncogene 17: 657–659.

Wijnen J, Khan PM, Vasen H, van der Klift H, Mulder A, van Leeuwen-Cornelisse I, Bakker B, Losekoot M, Moller P, Fodde R (1997) Hereditary nonpolyposis colorectal cancer families not complying with the Amsterdam criteria show extremely low frequency of mismatch-repair-gene mutations. Am J Hum Genet 61: 329–335.

Wijnen J, de Leeuw W, Vasen H, van der Klift H, Moller P, Stormorken A, Meijers-Heijboer H, Lindhout D, Menko F, Vossen S, Moslein G, Tops C, Brocker-Vriends A, Wu Y, Hofstra R, Sijmons R, Cornelisse C, Morreau H, Fodde R (1999) Familial endometrial cancer in female carriers of MSH6 germline mutations. Nat Genet 23: 142–144.

Willert K, Jones KA (2006) Wnt signaling: is the party in the nucleus? Genes Dev. 20: 1394–1404.

Worthley DL, Walsh MD, Barker M, Ruszkiewicz A, Bennett G, Phillips K, Suthers G (2005) Familial mutations in PMS2 can cause autosomal dominant hereditary nonpolyposis colorectal cancer. Gastroenterology 128: 1431–1436.

Yoshitaka T, Matsubara N, Ikeda M, Tanino M, Hanafusa H, Tanaka N, Shimizu K (1996) Mutations of E2F-4 trinucleotide repeats in colorectal cancer with microsatellite instability. Biochem Biophys Res Commun 227: 553–557.

# Chapter 48

# DEGOS' DISEASE (MALIGNANT ATROPHIC PAPULOSIS)

**Carmelo Schepis, Maddalena Siragusa, Carmelo Amato, and Martino Ruggieri**

Unit of Dermatology, IRCCS OASI Maria Santissima, Troina, Italy (CS) (MS); Unit of Neuroradiology, IRCCS OASI Maria Santissima, Troina, Italy (CA); Institute of Neurological Science, National Research Council, Catania, and Department of Paediatrics, University of Catania, Catania, Italy (MR)

## Introduction

Malignant atrophic papulosis (MAP) also known as Degos' disease (Degos et al. 1942; Kohlmeier 1940, 1941) is a rare, often fatal, multisystem disorder characterised by multiple infarcts in the skin and internal organs. The pathognomonic lesions are secondary to narrowing and occlusion of the lumen by intimal proliferation and thrombosis of small-caliber blood vessels which leads to ischaemia and infarction in the involved organ systems (Amato et al. 2005, Pande and Cheskin 2006, Scheinfeld 2006, Torrelo et al. 2002). MAP may involve the gastrointestinal and genitourinary tracts, central and peripheral nervous system, skin, heart, lungs, pancreas, adrenal glands and kidneys. Systemic manifestations usually develop from weeks to years after the onset of skin lesions, or, in rare instances, they may precede the skin lesions (Scheinfeld 2006).

A *benign (skin) variant* of the disease (associated with prolonged survival and low morbidity) occurs in which the disease process is limited to the skin whilst in the more aggressive *systemic variant* the reported mean survival is approximately 2 years (Notash et al. 2008, Pande and Cheskin 2006). The main causes of morbidity and mortality are related to bowel infarction, bowel perforation, pleuropericardial disease, and central nervous system (CNS) infarction and haemorrhage.

The aetiology is unknown and three possible pathogenic mechanisms have been suggested so far: (1) disturbance in immunity; (2) vital infection: and (3) abnormality in the clotting system of blood (reviewed in Pande and Cheskin 2006 and Scheinfeld 2006). In familial cases (OMIM # 602248) an autosomal dominant model of inheritance has been suggested (Beljaards et al. 1988, Katz et al. 1997, Kisch and Bruynzeel 1984, Moulin et al. 1984, Pande and Cheskin 2006).

## Historical perspective and eponyms

In the years 1940–1941 the German radiologist W. Kohlmeier reported a case of what he believed to be a Buerger's disease with characteristic skin lesions (Kohlmeier 1940, 1940–41). Some months later, Degos independently described a similar case (Degos et al. 1942). Both patients died within one year of diagnosis following sudden intestinal perforation. Degos recognised the serious nature of this syndrome and named it "malignant atrophic papulosis" (Reji et al. 2003, Who named it? 2006).

**Robert Degos** was a French dermatologist born in 1904 and died in 1987 who became an interne of the Hospitaux de Paris in 1926. In 1934 he became chef de clinique under professor Henri Gougerot (1881–1955) in the dermatological department at the Hopital St.-Louis, where he was medicine de l'Hopital from 1946. In 1951 he seceded Gougerot as professor of skin and syphilitic diseases (Who named it? 2006).

The disease is also known as Kohlmeier-Degos-Delort-Tricot disease; Kohlmeier–Degos syndrome; Kohlmeier-Degos disease; papulosis atrophicans maligna; papuleuse maligne atrophiante; lethal cutaneous and gastrointestinal arterioral thrombosis; fatal cutaneointestinal syndrome; tromboangioiitis cutaneointestinalis disseminata; and dermatite papulosquameuse atrophiante.

## Incidence and prevalence

This is a rare disease with fewer than 150 cases reported. Most of the cases are sporadic although member of the same family reportedly have been affected (OMIM # 602248) (Beljaards et al. 1988, Katz et al. 1997, Kisch and Bruynzeel 1984, Moulin et al. 1964, Pande and Cheskin 2006). Both sexes are affected with a 3:1 prevalence in males (Katz et al. 1997). The onset is usually in middle age but infantile cases (with onset from 3 weeks to 17 months of age) have been recorded (Barabino et al. 1990, Henkind and Clark 1968, Horner et al. 1976, Moraga et al. 1980, Moulin et al. 1984, Schneider et al. 1986, reviewed in Torrelo et al. 2002).

## Clinical manifestations

### Skin manifestations

Most patients have cutaneous involvement, and these are the manifestations that prompt the patient to seek clinical evaluation. The disease involve the skin alone in 37% of cases. The typical cutaneous lesions (Fig. 1) are 0.3–10 cm papules with an atrophic (umbilicated) and porcelain-white centre, surrounded by an erythematous telangiectatic border. Such lesions are usually asymptomatic (rarely itch or cause a burning sensation when the rash develops) and appear in crops involving primarily the trunk and limbs sparing the palms, soles, face and scalp (Pande and Cheskin 2006, Torrelo et al. 2002).

The recognition of the skin lesions is crucial to an accurate diagnosis. The early lesions are pinkish papules that appear in bouts, are about 2–5 mm in size, and occur on the trunk and extremities. Within

a few days, these papules become umbilicated with depressed centres. At presentation, most of the papules have reached the atrophic stage and appears as porcelain-white lesions covered with a fine scale and surrounded by a 1- to 2-mm erythematous border (Fig. 2). Individual lesions usually remain stable, without a tendency to spread or coalesce with neighbouring lesions.

### Extracutaneous involvement

MAP may involve the gastrointestinal and genitourinary tracts, central and peripheral nervous system, skin, heart, lungs, pancreas, adrenal glands and kidneys (Shahshahani et al. 2008). Systemic manifestations usually develop from weeks to years after the onset of skin lesions, or, in rare instances, they may precede the skin lesions (Scheinfeld 2006).

### Ocular manifestations

Lesions comparable to those in the skin occasionally may be seen on the conjunctiva and are avascular in origin: these include atrophic lesions of eyelids and conjunctiva, telangiectasia of the conjunctival vessels and episcleral plaques. Severe loss of myelinated nerve fibres in the optic nerve(s) has been demonstrated at magnetic resonance imaging (MRI) and at neuropathology along with obstruction of the cen-

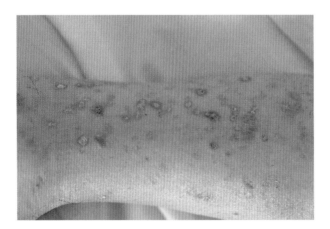

**Fig. 1.** Pinkish papules covered with a fine scale and an erythematous rim over the upper limbs.

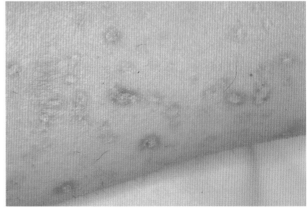

**Fig. 2.** Some lesions appear on the athrophic stage of the disease.

tral retinal arteries (Matsuura et al. 2006). A variety of ocular findings occur however in MAP including congenital posterior subcapsular cataracts, congenital glaucoma (due to angle dysgenesis), visual field defects, ptosis, 3rd cranial nerve palsies, blepharoptosis, and optic atrophy. Additional findings consist in optic neuritis, retinochoroidal colobomas, papilledema, and scleral plaques. Sibillat et al. (1986) reported that ophthalmologic symptoms were present in 35 of 105 extant reports of MAP: the disease manifested in the eye tissues, usually in the conjunctiva. The sclera, the episclera, the retina, the choroid, and/or neuro-ophthalmologic apparatus demonstrated damage consonant with MAP (Scheinfeld 2006, Sibillat et al. 1986)

## Gastrointestinal manifestations

These manifestations most often appear several weeks, months, or even years after a cutaneous eruption, although there are isolated reports of gastrointestinal symptoms preceding the skin lesions. Gastrointestinal manifestations are usually non specific and may include abdominal pain, abdominal distension, nausea, vomiting, diarrhoea, or constipation. Patients with extensive involvement of the gastrointestinal tract also may experience weakness, fatigue, weight loss or symptoms of malabsorption. In late stages of MAP, gastrointestinal haemorrhage, bowel infarction, and perforation may be observed. The liver may be involved and associated with a vasculitis. Affected patients may have enterocutaneous fistulae. Peristomal and/or buccal lesions have been reported.

## Nervous system involvement

Neurological involvement also is common. As with the gastrointestinal symptoms, neurological manifestations are usually non specific. Involvement of both central and peripheral nervous system can occur and can cause paresthesias of the face and extremities, headache, dizziness, seizures, hemiplegia, aphasia, paraplegia, gaze palsy or non specific neurological symptoms such as memory loss (Shahshahani et al. 2008). These manifestations are related to haemorrhagic and/or ischaemic strokes in the brain and/or spinal cord.

## Other organ involvement

MAP infrequently causes symptomatic involvement of other organs (e.g., lungs, heart, etc.), which may require appropriate tests such as radiograms and/or ultrasonography. Chest pain and dyspnoea may occur with involvement of lungs and heart. Other typical pulmonary manifestations include pleuritis and bilateral pleural effusion. Constrictive pericarditis has been reported induced by pericardial vasculitis causing left ventricular wall motion abnormalities. The kidney may be involved and associated with a vasculitis.

## Imaging

Chest radiographs may depict extensive calcification of the pericardium, pleural and/or pericardium involvement, and constrictive pericarditis.

Endoscopy of the gastrointestinal tract (i.e., oesophagus, stomach, duodenum, colon, rectum) can show infracted lesions or ulcers even in asymptomatic patients. Lesions similar to those seen in the skin are most often observed in the small bowel but can also be seen anywhere in the upper and lower gastrointestinal tract.

Laparoscopy of the intestine can show similar type lesions that manifest with white plaques surrounded by red borders on the serosal surface of the bowel and the peritoneum.

MR imaging of the central nervous system (Fig. 3) shows multiple cerebral infarctions accompanied by small haemorrhagic areas and abnormal signal enhancement on fat suppressed T1 weighted images after contrast administration or a saw tooth pattern over the vertebral segments of the spinal cord with patchy and moth-eaten patterns caused by thromboses and endothelial proliferation in subarachnoid vessels (Matsuura et al. 2006). Other patterns include meningovascular abnormalities (Amato et al. 2005), intracerebral bleeding, subdurale haemorrhage and cord infarcts (Scheinfeld 2006). Cerebral

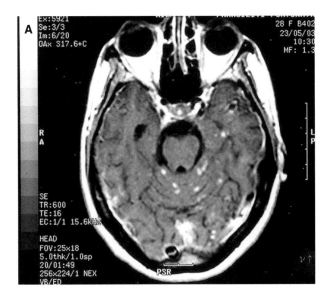

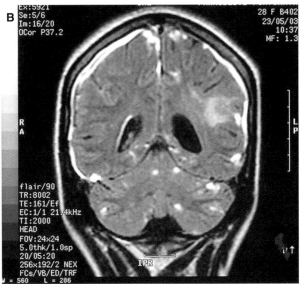

**Fig. 3.** (**A**) Contrast-enhanced T1 axial image shows multiple vasculitic lesions located in the peripheral gray and subarachnoid spaces. (**B**) Contrast-enhanced FLAIR coronal image shows cerebral and cerebellar lesions, right ependimal enhancement and diffuse dural thickening.

angiograms may reveal narrowing and occlusion of small intracranial arteries depicting stenosis, ectasis, and aneurysms of the peripheral branch arteries.

With angiograms, stenosis can be observed in the celiac artery and the small arteries in the kidney.

## Pathology

Early papules in MAP are skin coloured and can demonstrate a superficial and deep perivascular, peri-adnexal, and perineural chronic inflammatory cell infiltrate associated with intestinal mucin deposition. The epidermis of the papules can show a mild vacuolar interface reaction, and, at this early phase, the histological appearance of MAP can mimic tumid lupus erythematous. Histologically, fully developed papules demonstrate wedge-shaped degeneration of collagen. An interface dermatitis can be present but is often limited to the central portion of the tissue examined. Additionally, squamatization of the dermoepidermal junction, melanin incontinence, and epidermal atrophy can manifest. In many cases, an area of capillary dermal sclerosis manifests that mirrors the early stages of lichen sclerosus and atrophicus. Hyperkeratosis, epidermal atrophy, dermoepidermal separation, oedema, and papillary dermal necrosis occur. Fibrinoid necrosis and thrombosis occur in the papillary dermis and in the capillary and venules.

A superficial and deep perivascular lymphocytic infiltrate can gather at the fringe of ischaemic areas (Figs. 4, 5). Marked endothelial swelling and occasional platelet-fibrin thrombi are often noted.

One of the distinctive characteristics of MAP which distinguishes it from other vasculitides is the

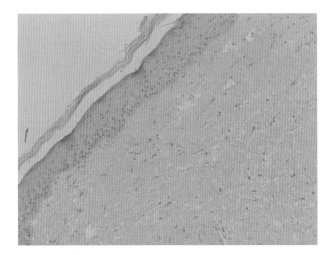

**Fig. 4.** Skin biopsy showing athrophic epidermis, low cellularity and focal necrosis in the mid dermis.

**Fig. 5.** The deep dermis shows a perivascular infiltrate surrounding an arteriolar hyalinosis with endothelial hyperplasia.

paucity or complete absence of inflammatory cells at the periphery of affected vessels.

## Molecular genetics and pathogenesis

The aetiology of MAP is unknown and three possible pathogenic mechanisms have been suggested so far: (1) disturbance in immunity; (2) vital infection: and (3) abnormality in the clotting system of blood (Pande and Cheskin 2006, Scheinfeld 2006). Broadly speaking MAP is a vasculopathy or an endovasculitis different from other vasculitides in that inflammation is not a prominent component of the disease. However, because of the broad overlap in clinical and histological findings High et al. (2004) contended that MAP could not be a specific entity but, rather, a common end point to a variety of vascular insults (including a variant of lupus) (Ball et al. 2003). Scheinfeld (2005, 2006) adduced strong evidence that MAP is a distinct condition because, unlike lupus, (1) it does not involve the face; (2) it does not respond to therapies such as corticosteroids that at least abate lupus; (3) it does mot manifest with photosensitivity; (4) viral inclusions are present in some cells in affected patients; and (5) systemic MAP is universally fatal, usually within 1–2 years, whereas lupus (even if severe) takes years to be fatal.

In familial cases (OMIM # 602248) an autosomal dominant model of inheritance has been suggested (Beljaards et al. 1988, Katz et al. 1997, Kisch and Bruynzeel 1984, Moulin et al. 1964, Pande and Cheskin 2006).

## Management

The skin lesions are not painful, usually do not itch, and generally do not require treatment. Patients who have gastrointestinal or neurological symptoms should undergo an appropriate work-up to detect systemic disease, which is determinant in prognosis. Many medications have been tried for treatment of MAP without success. Antiplatelet drugs (e.g., aspirin, dipyridamole) may reduce the number of new lesions in some patients with only skin involvement. Some believe intravenous immunoglobulins may have a role in treatment.

Surgically treatment usually is required for patients who develop complications such as gastrointestinal bleeding, intestinal perforation, bowel infarction, or intracranial bleeding.

## References

Amato C, Ferri R, Elia M, Cosentino F, Schepis C, Siragusa M, Moschini M (2005) Nervous system involvement in Degos disease. AJNR 26: 646–649.

Ball E, Newburger A, Ackerman AB (2003) Degos' disease, a distinctive pattern of disease, chiefly of lupus erythematous, and not a specific disease per se. Am J Dermatopathol 25: 308–320.

Barabino A, Pesce F, Gatti R, Colotto P, Nobili F, Colacino R, Giampalmo A (1990) An atypical pediatric case of malignant atrophic papulosis (Kohlmeier-Degos disease). Eur J Pediatr 149: 457–458.

Beljaards R, Starink TM, Meuwissen SW (1988) Twee families met maligne atrofische papulosis (zietke van Degos). Ned Tijdschr Geneeskd 132: 269–271.

Degos R, Delort J, Tricot R (1942) Dermatitis papulosuqameuse atrophique. Bull Soc Franc Dermatol Syphil 49: 148–150.

Degos R (1979) Malignant atrophic papulosis. Br J Dermatol 100: 21–35.

Henkind PE, Clark WE (1968) Ocular pathology in malignant atrophic papulosis (Degos' disease). Am J Ophthalmol 65: 164–169.

High WA, Aranda J, Patel SB, Cockerell CJ, Costner MI (2004) Degos' disease is a clinical and histological end point rather than a specific disease? J Am Acad Dermatol 50: 895–899.

Horner FA, Myers GJ, Stumpf DA, Oseroff BJ, Choi BH (1976) Malignant atrophic papulosis (Kohlmeier-Degos disease) in childhood. Neurology 26: 317–321.

Katz SK, Mudd LJ, Roenigk HH Jr (1997) Malignant atrophic papulosis (Degos' disease) involving three generations of a family. J Am Acad Dermatol 37: 480–484.

Kisch LS, Bruynzeel DP (1984) Six cases of malignant atrophic papulosis (Degos' disease) occurring in one family. Br J Dermatol 111: 469–471.

Kohlmeier W (1940) In: Frankfurter Zeischrift fur Pathologie. 54: 413.

Kohlmeier W (1940–41) Multiple hautnekrosen bei Thrombangiitis obliterans. Arch Drmatol Syph 181: 783–792.

Matsuura F, Makino K, Fukushima T, Matsubara N, Shibuya M, Higuchi T, Hashidate H, Yamada M, Shibuya H, Yamazaki M (2006) Optic nerve and spinal cord manifestations of malignant atrophic papulosis (Degos disease). J Neurol Neurosurg Psychiatry 77: 260–262.

Moraga Llop FA, Gonzalez Fernandez J, Gallart Català A, Cabre Piera J, Bosch Castane J, Huguet Redecilla P, Bosch Banyeras JM (1980) Papulosis atrofiante maligna de Degos. An Esp Pediatr 13: 437–440.

Moulin G, Barrut D, Franc MP, Person A (1984) Papulose atrophiante de Degos familiale (mere-fille). Ann Dermatol Venereol 111: 149–155.

Notash AY, Mazoochy H, Mirshams M, Nikoo A (2008) Lethal systemic Degos disease with prominent cardiopulmonary involvement. Saudi Med J 29: 133–137.

Pande H, Cheskin L (2006) Malignant atrophic papulosis. e-Medicine from WebMD. http://www.emedicine.com/med/topic2943.htm

Reji TK, Nithyanandam S, Rawoof BA, Rajendran SC (2003) Malignant atrophic papulosis. Report of a case with multiple ophthalmic findings. Ind J Ophthalmol 51: 260–263.

Scheinfeld N (2005) Degos' disease is probably a distinct entity: a review of clinical and laboratory evidence. J Am Acad Dermatol 52: 375–376.

Scheinfeld NS (2006) Degos disease. E-Medicine from WebMD. http://www.emedicine.com/DERM/topic931.htm

Schneider A, Tschumi A, Egloff B, Ott F, Fanconi A (1986) Maligne atrophiserende Pupulose (Degos syndrom) bei einem Saugling. Helv Pediatr Acta 41: 447–454.

Shahshahani MM, Hashemi P, Nemati R, Nikoo A, Mazoochy H, Rashidi A (2008) A case of Degos disease with pleuropericardial fibrosis, jejunal perforation, hemiparesis, and widespread cutaneous lesions. Int J Dermatol 47: 493–495.

Sibillat M, Avril MF, Charpenter P, Offret H, Bloch-Michel E (1986) Malignant atrophic papulosis (Degos' disease): clinical review. A propos of a case. J Fr Ophthalmol 9: 299–304.

Torrelo A, Sevilla J, Mediero IG, Candelas D, Zambrano A (2002) Malignant atrophic papulosis in an infant. Br J Dermatol 146: 916–918.

Who named it? (2006) A medical dictionary of biographic eponyms. http://www.whonamedit.com

# Chapter 49

# ATAXIA-TELANGIECTASIA

Luciana Chessa, Agata Polizzi, and Martino Ruggieri

Department of Experimental Medicine, University "La Sapienza" Rome, Rome, Italy (LC, AP); Institute of Neurological Science, National Research Council, Catania and Department of Paediatrics, University of Catania, Catania, Italy (MR)

## Introduction

Ataxia Telangiectasia (AT; OMIM #208900) is a multisystemic autosomal recessive disorder characterized by progressive cerebellar ataxia, oculocutaneous telangiectasias, immunodeficiency, recurrent sinopulmonary infections, growth retardation, endocrine abnormalities, hypogonadism and cancer proneness, with laboratory evidence of increased alpha-fetoprotein levels, chromosomal instability and hypersensitivity to ionising radiations (Boder 1985, Taylor et al. 1975, Gatti et al. 1991). This radiohypersensitivity was first noted after exposure of an AT patient to conventional doses of radiation therapy, which proved fatal (Gotoff et al. 1967).

The neurological features of AT characteristically include early onset cerebellar ataxia with degeneration and loss of Purkinje cells, oculomotor apraxia (slow or absent voluntary eye movements), strabismus, nystagmus, choreoathetosis, dystonia, dysarthria and tremors.

At the cutaneous level, café-au-lait spots, hypo- and hyper-pigmented areas, as well as early greying hairs are often noticed. These progeric changes of hair and skin, which usually ensue after the first years of life, along with the typical ocular and body telangiectasias, led many authors to include AT in the group of the classical phakomatoses (Louis-Bar 1941) or neurocutaneous disorders (Gomez 1987, Roach and van Miller 2004). Certainly, from a pathogenic point of view AT is a more complex and somewhat different condition from classical neurocutaneous diseases. However, clinically it features (and is first diagnosed because of) nervous system and skin involvement. Thus, we have maintained its handling in this book.

The clinical diagnosis of AT can be difficult before the appearance of the telangiectasias. Most individuals affected with AT have an abnormal gait in the first few years of life, require the use of a wheelchair during late childhood or adolescence, and survive only into the late teens or twenties. However, individual prognosis may be variable, as some affected individuals have reportedly survived into the sixth decade (Crawford et al. 2000, Saxon et al. 1979a, b).

The discovery of the *ATM* (Ataxia Telangiectasia Mutated) gene that, when mutated, causes the disease has opened the way to a more accurate diagnosis. The typical AT phenotype is caused by biallelic *ATM* mutations that truncate or severely destabilize the gene product. The *ATM* gene is localized at 11q22.3 and encodes for a protein which plays a pivotal role in cell cycle checkpoint regulation and DNA double strand breaks repair (Frappart and McKinnon 2006, Delia et al. 2003, Savitsky et al. 1995, Shiloh 2003, Subba 2007). The ATM protein is present in the nucleus as an inactive dimer and is activated in response to DNA double strand breaks, initiating the cascade phosphorylation of multiple intermediates involved in DNA repair, cell cycle control, regulation of gene expression and stress responses (Bakkenist and Kastan 2003, Shiloh 2003, Zhang et al. 2007).

Occasionally milder cases of the disease, showing later age of onset and/or moderate severity of clinical features, longer life-span and intermediate cellular radiosensitivity (the so-called '*AT variants*') have been reported. In addition, other syndromes showing some AT signs combined with other clinical features (*Nijmegen Breakage syndrome/NBS*, $AT_{Fresno}$, *Ataxia without Telangiectasia, Ataxias with immunodeficiency*) were reported. With the aid of molecular testing, the expanding phenotype of AT (Chun and Gatti 2004) can now be distinguished from other autosomal recessive cerebellar ataxias including Friedreich ataxia, Mre11 deficiency (*AT-like disease*), the Oculomotor apraxias type 1 (AO1) and 2 (AO2) and the Nijmegen breakage syndrome (NBS). On the other hand, some atypical patients with minimal signs and symptoms, such as very mild or very late-onset ataxia, or late-onset spinal muscular atrophy, can now be included in the diagnosis of AT because they either lack ATM protein or ATM kinase activity, and have mutations in the ATM gene (Chun and Gatti 2004).

## Historical perspective and eponyms

The first description of patients with AT was published by Syllaba and Henner in 1926. They reported three adolescent Czech siblings with progressive choreoathetosis and striking ocular telangiectasia as having a variant of Ramsay Hunt's familial double athetosis. There was no post-mortem examination. In 1941, after 15 years gap, a second clinical description was published by Louis-Bar (Louis-Bar 1941), regarding a 9-year-old Belgian boy with progressive cerebellar ataxia and extensive cutaneous telangiectasia distributed in nevoid patches; nor family history neither pathologic studies were reported. The Author identified the syndrome as a previously undescribed entity belonging among the phakomatoses, either a variant of the Sturge-Weber syndrome or a separate new entity (Boder 1987).

**Denise Bar** received her medical qualification from the Free University of Brussels in 1939. Shortly after she married F. Louis, a civil engineer, and began using the hyphenated surname Louis-Bar. In 1940 she became a resident at the Bunge Institute of Neurology, Antwerp, working under the neuropathologist Ludo van Bogaert (1897–1989). In 1943 she was appointed as instructor in pharmacology at the University of Liège, and in 1945 she became a neuropsychiatrist at the department of internal medicine. In 1957 Louis-Bar and her husband

moved to Brussels, where she spent the remainder of her career devoting herself to persons with mental handicap (Beighton and Beighton 1997, Evrard et al. 1990, Who named it? 2006).

Until Martin's paper in 1964 (Martin 1964) which called attention to the report of Syllaba and Henner, Louis-Bar's report was believed to be the first clinical description, and AT was sometimes referred to as the Louis-Bar syndrome (Boder 1987, van Miller 2004). Both of these early case reports were lost in the literature, and the syndrome remained unknown until 1957 when two independent clinicopathological reports – with no knowledge of the two earlier reports (Jabado et al. 2000) – appeared in two widely separated areas of the world. The first clinicopathological study, based on 8 cases from 6 families, was presented by Boder and Sedgwick (1957, 1958), who named for the first time the syndrome ataxia-telangiectasia (later renamed also Boder-Sedgwik syndrome or cephalo-oculocutaneous telangiectasia). This report included the first autopsy of an AT patient, describing the absence of thymus and ovaries. **Elena Boder**, an American physician, obtained her MD in 1932. Besides her contributions to AT she is particularly remembered for her work on dyslexia. **Robert Sedwick** is an American paediatric neurologist (Who named it? 2006). The second paper, by Biemond (1957), was based on four familial cases and two autopsies, without references to the thymus and the ovaries. This report underlined the occurrence of extra pyramidal manifestations in the absence of histopathological findings in the basal ganglia. Both of these initial clinicopathological studies emphasized the "heredofamilial nature of the syndrome" and called attention to severe recurrent sinopulmonary infections as the third major component of the syndrome and as the main cause of death (Boder 1987, Boder and Sedgwik 1977, Bridges and Harden 1982, Gatti 1985, Sedgwik and Boder 1972). Wells and Shy published in the same year a report without autopsy on two sisters with "progressive choreoathetosis with cutaneous telangiectasia" (Wells and Shy 1957). Like Syllaba and Henner, Wells and Shy classified the syndrome as a basal ganglia disorder rather than a cerebellar syndrome. This points out that the choreoathetotic component of AT, now known to occur in about 85% of cases, may be severe enough in older children to overshadow the cerebellar ataxia. In 1958, in a paper based on two non familial cases, Centerwall and Miller provided a further autopsy (Centerwall and Miller 1958). Boder's and Sedgwik' second and third papers on the syndrome differentiated AT clinically and pathologically from Friedreich's ataxia and identified AT as the only predominantly cerebellar degeneration of infancy and childhood (Boder and Sedgwik 1958, Sedgwik and Boder 1963).

With the rapid proliferation of reports in the world literature after 1958 it was possible to develop tabular analysis of known cases that definitively confirmed the syndrome (Boder 1987). The identification of sinopulmonary infections and lymphoid malignancies as further cardinal features of the disease stimulated early immunologic studies, even though AT was not established as an immunodeficiency disease until 1963 (Boder 1987). That despite the absence of thymus was first noted in 1957 (Boder and Sedgwik 1957) and selective deficiency of serum IgA was first reported by Thyeffry et al. (1961).

Formal recognition of a near 25% segregation ratio confirming simple autosomal recessive inheritance was achieved in 1965 (Tadjoedin and Fraser 1965).

In 1967 Swift and co-workers, through systematic epidemiological-genetic studies, definitively established the increased predisposition to cancer among the parents and relatives of AT patients. Hecht et al. (1966), having found increased chromosomal breakage in 20–30% of cultured lymphocytes from AT patients, suggested that chromosomal breakage may predispose AT patients to cancers.

The rapid proliferation of research reports focusing on early immunologic, genetic, cytogenetic, radiobiological, endocrine, oncologic and pathological aspects of AT led to a better definition of the syndrome between the 70 and 80s and established the basis for the major breakthrough in understanding AT, that came in 1995 after the identification of a single gene, called *ATM* (Ataxia Telangiectasia Mutated) which when defective is the underlying cause of the disease (Savitsky et al. 1995, Rasio et al.

1995). Indeed as such a broad spectrum of organs affected in AT, the discovery of ATM was hailed as the medical equivalent of the Rosetta stone, the 18th century discovery that allowed archaeologists to decipher Egyptian hieroglyphics (Nowak 1995).

## Incidence and prevalence

The incidence of AT in the population has been variously estimated at between 1 in 40,000 (in the United States) and 1 in 400,000 live births. The disease is found in all races (Jabado et al. 2000, Swift et al. 1991) and its frequency varies considerably from country to country depending upon the degree of inbreeding and the ability to distinguish it from other neurological disorders (Chun and Gatti 2004). The carrier frequency is estimated at 0.5–2.0% in the general population.

An epidemiological study was conducted on 72 Italian AT families from the Italian Registry for Ataxia Telangiectasia applying the Dahlberg's formula. On the basis of the consanguinity rates a theoretical disease frequency of 1 patient in 7090 conceptions and a heterozygotes frequency from 1.69 to 3.43% were obtained (Chessa et al. 1994).

## Clinical manifestations

### Classical AT phenotype

#### Neurological features

AT is primarily an early onset, progressive, neurodegenerative disorder: thus, neurological signs (and/or symptoms) are usually the presenting problem of patients with AT. *Cerebellar ataxia* is the clinical hallmark of the disease (the *conditio sine qua non* among the many neurological features) and usually considered the earliest manifestation of the disorder and chief complaint that parents raise with doctors.

**Earliest clinical signs.** At first, some newborns with AT are not obviously abnormal at birth and then they walk at a normal age: in these children the diagnosis could be elusive. However, a frequent story is that the early instability of walking fails to improve with age, so that falls and bumps persist despite development. When parents are thoroughly enquired about even subtle signs that had alerted them on "abnormal development" in their children, they almost always recall that either gross motor milestones were reached "slightly after time" or the child was "clumsy", having mild generalised "hypotonia" or sitting unbalance. Children differ – and parent's histories often fail to agree with one another – but the story of stable motor function or small improvements for a time until ages 3–7 years is common. Often these signs prompt referral to a specialists: however at this very young age it is not uncommon for the classical AT phenotype to be confused or misinterpreted with mild cerebral palsy, acute infections or non specific "benign" motor delay (Chum and Gatti 2004, Perlman et al. 2003, Miller 2004). Upon examination AT children under 1 year of age will show head-tilting (apparent after age 6 months), mild truncal ataxia (swaying of the head and trunk on standing and even on sitting) (Leuzzi et al. 1993, Sedgwik and Boder 1972), mild to moderate truncal hypotonia with hypotonic posture, slow voluntary movements with slow handling of objects and unexplained unsteadiness and sitting (and/or aided standing) unbalance. These signs could be very mild or sometimes missed, needing serial close up examinations to be confirmed.

**Gait and posture.** Overt cerebellar ataxia usually becomes apparent between 16 and 18 months of age, after the child learns to walk. The instability of gait has certain unusual characteristics. Most children walk on what seems to be an inappropriately narrow base, and early in the disorder they generally have a regular stride length but err in excessive adduction of the leg during the passing phase or on foot strike, causing a stagger to the outside of the base. Despite this error, children frequently compensate for their missteps well and they prefer to walk quickly or run, the advantages of momentum apparently reducing errant steps or aiding balance in the same manner that riding a bicycle quickly is more stable than riding one slowly (Crawford 1998, Crawford et al. 2000). With the passage of time, each step becomes less predictable and stride length errors are added to the gait cycle. In many, the foot position assumes a dystonic posture (Fig. 1) with excessive varus and sometimes equine, leading to a toe–toe gait. By the age of 2 years the diagnosis could be straightforward as a staggering gait caused by predominantly truncal ataxia is first noted and insidiously becomes associated with other manifestations of cerebellar dysfunction, including dysarthria, muscular hypotonia, slow voluntary movements, hypotonic facies and posture, and drooling. If an MRI scan of the brain (and spine) is obtained before 2 years of age, cerebellar atrophy or other typical AT lesions of the nervous system are usually not apparent. In fact, the imaging of the cere-

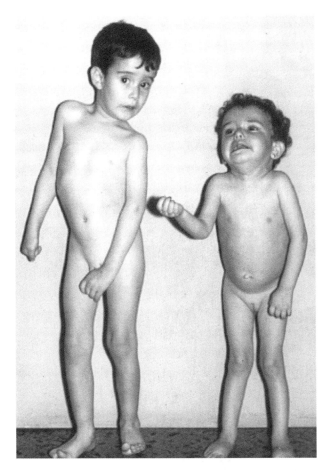

**Fig. 1.** Dystonic posture in two children (siblings) with AT: note the excessive valgus position of legs and feet.

bellum may appear normal for several years after the onset of ataxia (see below under neuroimaging).

Also the instability of sitting often shows highly distinctive features. Children may sway from one direction to another, often tipping to the edge of stability and holding that edge for a prolonged time before correcting or overcorrecting. With time and progression many teenagers will develop smaller abrupt corrections of the trunk that may be either adventitious postural-induced jerks or excessive uncoordinated postural corrections. Head instability has many of the same features, often with prolonged deviation of position to one or the other side, in extreme extension or flexion before correcting or overcorrecting. Though this movement may appear to be related to diminished postural tone, it is notable that attempts to correct this head instability passively will usually meet active resistance.

**Adventitious movements and progression of ataxia.** The ataxia is slowly but inexorably progressive, and children typically may require a wheelchair by age of 12, usually because of excessive unbalance and unsteadiness with frequent falling coupled with slow reflexes that causes serious bodily injuries (Perlman et al. 2003). Differences in personal pref-

erence affect the defined "age of wheelchair dependence" as much or more that does motor capacity. By the toddler age the disorder will be clearly progressive; in addition, by this age, cerebellar (and other systems) atrophy will be also apparent on MRI studies.

Limb ataxia, intention tremor, and segmental myoclonus become apparent as the child matures. Children also have speech and writing problems that impair their social life and school work: most children will enjoy colouring in pre-school years – sometimes doing so very well – but will cease to write for communication by the age of 10 years because of difficulties in legibility and speed.

*Extra pyramidal features* are also frequently observed in patients with AT. Choreoathetosis occurs in about 90% of patients and, when severe, can initially mask the presence of ataxia (Jabado et al. 2000): it may be difficult to distinguish it from dysmetria and intention tremor. At times the choreoathetosis may resemble segmental myoclonus of the extremities and trunk (Miller 2004). From toddler age on, most will have small, "fidgety" choreiform movements of the hands and feet when asked to still. This movement is rarely noted by the parent or the child. With time, difficulties with finger-nose-finger

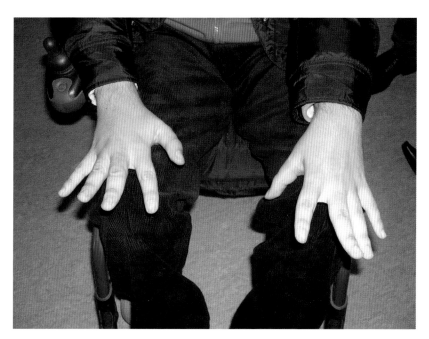

**Fig. 2.** Dystonic posture of the fingers in a 8-year-old child with AT.

can be undermined by end-point dysmetria, intentional or ballistic ataxia, postural instability, or a combination of all of these. Dystonia (typically a progressive dystonia of the fingers) (Fig. 2) is also found, mostly in toddlers and adolescents (Jabado et al. 2000) whereas torsion dystonia of the neck and limbs can occur earlier. Axial muscles are also affected and the patients gradually develop a stooped posture due to dystonia (Bodensteiner et al. 1980).

In the teenage years, the range of abnormal movements increases even further. It is not uncommon to see disabling intention and essential tremor, "overflow" cerebellar phenomena, apparent multifocal and chaotic myoclonus, tics, and advanced chorea. In many patients, motivation appears to have a perverse effect, so that with increasing intent performance diminishes, often with intervening jerks that are not apparent in other circumstances.

**Bulbar function and facial expressiveness.** Abnormalities of articulation are prominent in virtually all AT patients (Crawford 1998). Most children with AT never develop normal speech articulation and prosody. Like the development of gait, worsening of the dysarthria is often noted only after 5 or more years or relative stability. The speech is often slow with emphasis placed inappropriately on words or syllables, in a manner very suggestive of cerebellar dysfunction. There are equal contributions of lingual, labial, and palatal dysfunction to the dysarthria.

Though often unrecognised, progressive difficulty with chewing and swallowing are nearly universal in children with AT, contributing to the development of *"ab ingestis"* sinopulmonary infections. The time required for meals increases and silent aspiration becomes dramatically more prominent in the second decade. Weight for height often drops later in the second decade.

The face is normally expressive in most young children with AT (see Fig. 1). However, virtually all of them will develop hypomimea (Fig. 3) that at first affect the small and subtle facial expression. In school-aged AT children a mask-like appearance may contribute to the impression of mental subnormality, instead of broad and pleasant smiles or

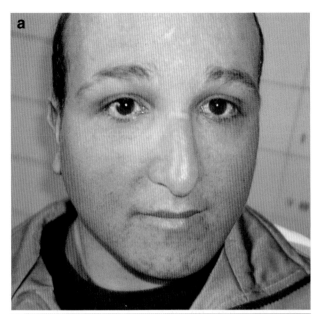

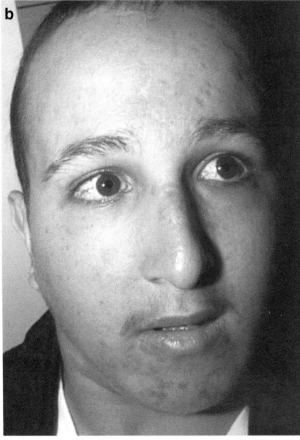

**Fig. 3.** Facial appearance at different ages: note the progression of hypomimea (and of ocular teleangiectasias) from age 22 years (**a**) to age 33 years (**b**).

prominent furrowed-brow-frowns; later in the second decade, these larger expressions become less vigorous.

**Oculomotor signs.** Oculomotor signs are peculiar in AT, as they combine features of cerebellar and extra pyramidal disorders. They are present in virtually all AT patients and precede the appearance of telangiectasias, providing an important diagnostic criterion; most of them are localised to the flocculus (Crawford 1998). The apraxia steadily progresses and may eventually simulate ophthalmoplegia. When the head is fixed, voluntary eye movements are initiated slowly and are frequently interrupted but, in contrast to ophthalmoplegia, can be completed successfully if sufficient time is given. When the head is suddenly turned toward a target, the eyes first deviate tonically in the opposite direction and then slowly follow the direction of the head (Jabado et al. 2000). Eye movements are smooth and full in range on involuntary movements, as when the head is moved passively from side to side. Abnormalities of conjugate gaze are seen only on voluntary movement. Optokinetic nystagmus is absent. Strabismus is seen in many young children with AT but is often transient and corrective surgery is not required. Deficits in eye movement systems that stabilise images on the retina (pursuit, gaze holding, convergence, vestibular and optokinetic slow phases, and cancellation of vestibular slow phases) and that maintain fixation and shift gaze (reflexive and voluntary saccades, impaired fixation, and reduction in vestibular and optokinetic quick phases) are found in AT patients (Lewis et al. 1999, Miller 2004). The progression of these signs also makes it difficult for the patient to read small print. When preparing study cards for school in AT children, it is best to place only a few words in the centre of each card in large print, thereby minimizing the need to initially scan the card for content (Jabado et al. 2000).

In a recent study, Khan et al. (2008) found that saccadic dysfunction without head thrusts and convergence abnormalities are common in AT-like syndrome; older AT-like syndrome have nystagmus with abnormalities in smooth pursuit and vestibular ocular reflex. In AT-like syndrome cases were not recorded conjunctival telangiectasia, head thrusting and manifest strabismus at distance.

**Neuropathy and myelopathy.** Most younger patients with AT have normal muscle strength and deep tendon reflexes. By the age of 10 through adolescence, the neurological features of the disease resemble those of a spinocerebellar degeneration with peripheral neuropathy (manifested by the loss of ankle-deep tendon reflexes) as well as variable loss of vibratory and position sense. Despite the prominent sway that can be seen in standing or sitting, there is usually little enhancement of the instability with eye's closure in Romberg's manoeuvre. Electrophysiological and neuropathologic studies reveal dorsal column demyelination with astrocytes proliferation and severe anterior horn degeneration. Studies of peripheral nerves reveal a primary axonal peripheral polyneuropathy (Stankovich et al. 1998). The neuropathy of AT rarely participates in the overall neurological dysfunction to any meaningful degree, because motor impairments due to central causes are usually limiting at a much earlier age.

The initial varus and equinc foot deformity associated with AT has a dystonic origin. Though similar to the pes cavus foot seen in other neuropathies (Friedreich's ataxia, Charcot-Marie-Tooth, etc.) the foot deformity in AT is often exaggerated with walking; not associated with an inflexible high arch, forefoot atrophy, or hammer toe; and is often found in younger patients despite the retention of ankle tendon reflexes.

A significant portion of older patients develop progressive neurogenic amyotrophy which is thought to be due to the degeneration of anterior horn cells and dorsal root ganglion cells, with signs of spinal muscular atrophy affecting mostly hands and feet. Because flexor muscles are normally stronger than extensor muscles, contractures result in all muscles atrophy; they can be prevented by aggressive exercise. Peripheral and spinal cord involvement, even though characteristics in AT patients, produce signs and symptoms not so prominent as the cerebellar ataxia is.

**Cognitive development.** Cognitive function is usually preserved even into adulthood, but progressive dysarthria may lead to the underestimation of mental capacity, this being one of the reasons for the high figures for mental retardation in the AT literature (Gatti et al. 1991, Miller 2004). Most patients have IQ scores within the average or above. Moderate or severe mental retardation, with IQ scores below 50, is unknown (Gatti et al. 1991). There is however little or no indication in the early decades of life that cognitive function decreases significantly, but rather it seems to "level off". As the development of new skills and the acquisition of new information fail to keep pace with chronological age IQ scores tend to drop, but there is no evidence of mental deterioration. Verbal IQ scores in adult AT are lower than those of control subjects (Mostofsky et al. 2000). Some older patients in their twenties and thirties have an unexpectedly severe loss of short-term memory, suggestive of premature aging (Gatti et al. 1991).

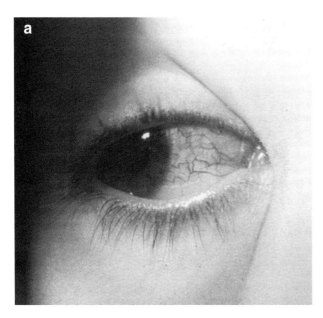

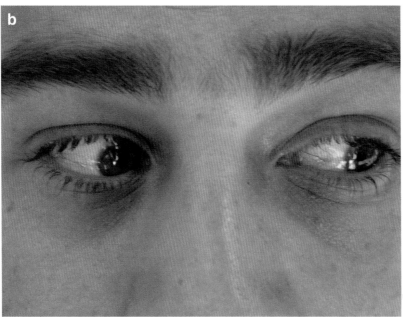

**Fig. 4.** Typical ocular telangiectasias in two AT subjects.

Several of our patients with AT have been able to function intellectually well enough to complete high school and even primary schools despite significant handicaps and extra help support in classes.

## Skin manifestations

*Telangiectasias* are the second hallmark of the disease and are eventually noted in the majority of the AT patients. Rarely they can develop in adulthood or not at all and occasionally they disappear later in life. They consist of dilated vessels, which usually appear between ages 2 and 8 (with a mean of 72 months) (Harding 1988) but can be noted as early as in the first months of life. The most commonly affected area is the conjunctiva, where they first appear in the angle of the eye and then spread toward the border of the cornea (Fig. 4a). With time, they cover the entire conjunctiva bilaterally (Fig. 4b). At close up inspection they are frequently found on the external earlobe, the bridge of the nose, the eyelid, the flexure folds of the neck, the anticubital and popliteal spaces, and, less frequently, on the extremities and on the palate – or even over the entire body (Jabado et al. 2000, Miller 2004). Telangiectasias may reflect progeric changes. It is rare for the telangiectatic vessels in AT to haemorrhage (Gatti et al. 1991).

*Other cutaneous abnormalities*, which may also reflect progeric changes and are sometimes overlooked, include scattered grey hairs and hypertrichosis (the latter occurring particularly over the forearms). Hair changes usually begins with the appearance of occasional grey hairs, even in young-aged/school-aged children, and increases in many to become diffusely grey in the early twenties. We were able to record multiple ($<6$) café-au-lait spots with irregular margins (Fig. 5), hypomelanotic macules and various types of naevi in all of our AT patients (including the subjects in the Italian Registry for AT – see below). Other progeric changes are poichilodermia, loss of subcutaneous fat with sclerosis/sclerodermoid changes of the skin (especially on the face, hand and feet which become atrophic and taut), seborrhoic dermatitis, vitiligo-like hypopigmented areas (which may appear early and be relatively non progressive in a few, whereas many will have more subtle and progressive mottling of hypo-pigmented areas with the passage of time), acanthosis nigricans, senile keratosis and eczema (Cohen et al. 1984, Jabado et al. 2000, Miller 2004). All these manifestations are progressive with age.

Basal cell carcinoma in young adults are common and may be due to abnormal radiosensitivity. Cutaneous granulomas, commonly associated with immune deficiency states (e.g., severe combined immune deficiency or X-linked hypogammaglobulinemia), may uncommonly appear as the initial cutaneous manifestation of AT (Drolet et al. 1997). These granulomas may persist despite treatment with intravenously administered immunoglobulins, topical antibiotic therapy, and topical corticosteroid therapy (Paller 1991).

## Immunodeficiency

Immunodeficiency with variable degrees of severity is present in approximately 60% of children with AT and involves both humoral and cellular responses (Chun and Gatti 2004; Gatti 1982, 1991; Jabado et al. 2000). Conversely, 30% of AT patients have no discernible immunodeficiency (Woods et al. 1992). Thus, the absence of immunologic abnormalities does not preclude a diagnosis of AT.

One of the most striking and consistent pathological features of AT is that the thymus is small or absent, and lacks corticomedullary architecture and Hassal's corpuscles; it is embryonic in appearance (Peterson et al. 1964). A progressive T-cell lymphopenia is commonly noted with an increase in the proportion of γδ T-cell receptor-expressing cells (Fiorilli et al. 1985b). Discordant increases in the NK cell proportions have been also reported (Peter 1983, Porras et al. 1993). Giovanetti et al. (2002) studying 9 AT patients demonstrated that the T-cell receptor (TCR) variable beta (BV)-chain repertoire as well as the B-cell repertoire were restricted by diffuse expansions of some variable genes, indicating that *ATM* mutation limits the generation of a wide repertoire of normally functioning T and B cells.

Disorders of *antibody responses* are associated with low B-lymphocyte counts and abnormalities of immunoglobulins levels. About 80% of AT patients

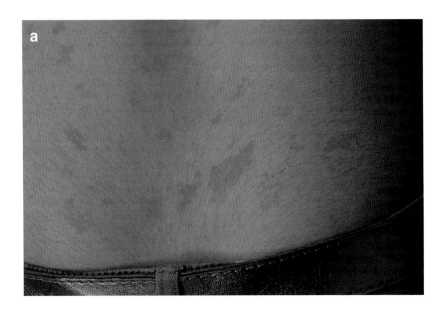

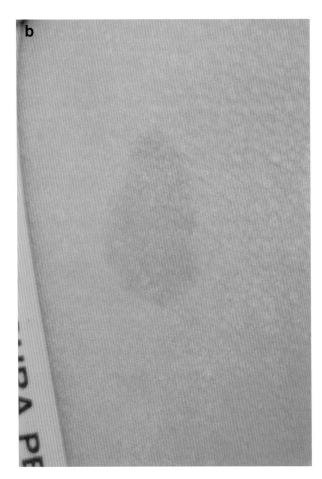

**Fig. 5.** Skin changes in AT individuals may take the form of multiple, middle to large café-au-lait spots (**a**) with irregular shape and margins (**b**).

have low molecular weight monomeric IgM in their serum. Most patients also have a reduced serum concentration of the IgG2 and IgG4 subclasses, while 70% of patients have an extreme deficiency or absence of IgE as well as of serum and secretory IgA. Antibodies against IgA have also been observed in some patients; this may further account for the low or absent serum IgA levels and should serve to caution against the administration of immunoglobulins preparation containing IgA.

Clinical manifestations are characterised by recurrent infections mostly reminiscent of humoral immune deficiencies. Mainly sinopulmonary infections are reported, but otitis and urinary infections are also frequent. The pulmonary infections begin as multiple discrete episodes and become chronic and persistent in one-third of the patients, leading to pulmonary fibrosis and insufficiency (Bott et al. 2007). The unremitting course is similar to that observed in patients with cystic fibrosis. Infections remain the first cause of death in AT patients despite early and aggressive treatment (see later). The bacteria associated with infections are frequently extra cellular high-grade pathogens, such as *Staphylococcus*, *Streptococcus*, and *Haemophylus* species. Opportunistic infections are not characteristics of AT, unlike other primary immune deficiencies. The severity of neurological manifestations is not directly associated with the severity of infections. Despite this, children with AT have major coordination problems and this may affect their ability to cough effectively. Swallowing problems with saliva stagnation and chronic aspiration often lead to pneumonia, and this situation is cumulative and progressive.

Autoimmune manifestations are also reported in patients with AT, mainly of the haematopoietic type with peripheral thrombopenia and haemolytic anaemia. It is also possible that autoimmunity may play a role in the degenerative phase of AT. We have seen these autoimmune disorders in carrier relatives of our AT patients.

## Malignancies and cancer risk

Malignancy is a frequent occurrence in patients with AT and is the second most common cause of death in

these patients. One in three AT individuals will develop a malignancy at some time during their lives. Occasionally an AT patient may present first with cancer, before a diagnosis of AT is suspected. It has been speculated that the frequency of tumours in AT patients could be very high if they will not die young for the infections. In fact, the risk for malignancy in individuals with AT is 38%. Leukaemia and lymphoma account for about 85% of malignancies, with a 70-fold and 250-fold increased incidence of either tumour, respectively. Younger children tend to have acute lymphocytic leukaemia of T-cell origin and older children are likely to have an aggressive T-cell leukaemia. Lymphomas are usually of B-cell type. In older patients chronic T-cell prolymphocytic leukaemia (T-PLL) accounts for 10% of the T-cell malignancies. As individuals with AT begin to live longer, other cancers and tumours, including ovarian cancer, breast cancer, gastric cancer, melanoma, leiomyoma and sarcomas have been observed. After the age of 20, solid tumours are more frequent (mainly epithelial tumours) including dysgerminoma, brain tumours (e.g., astrocytomas, medulloblastoma and glioma), gastric carcinoma, liver carcinoma, retinoblastoma, and pancreatic carcinoma. Their frequencies are only slightly different from those in the general population. Solid gynaecologic tumours (ovarian and uterine) are more common in AT female patients.

The cancer risk of carriers of an *ATM* mutation was established approximately four times that of the general population, primarily because of breast cancer; a prevalent role of missense mutations was noticed (Swift et al. 1991, Easton 1994, Athma et al. 1996, FitzGerald et al. 1987, Stankovic et al. 1998, Geoffrey-Perez et al. 2001, Olsen et al. 2001, Teraoka et al. 2001, Chenevix-Trench et al. 2002, Sommer et al. 2002, Bernstein et al. 2003, Bretsky et al. 2003, Thorstenson et al. 2003). However, the relative risk for cancer in AT heterozygotes is still controversial (Angele and Hall 2000, Miller 2004). Recent studies of molecular epidemiology on 32 French AT families showed no significant difference in the relative risk of breast cancer (BC) or any other type of cancer based on mutation type (missense or truncating). However, the occurrence of BC may be associated with truncating mutations in certain binding domains of the ATM protein (e.g., P53/BRCA1, β-adaptin, and FAT domains; $P = 0.006$), suggesting that the risk of BC is associated with the alteration of binding domains rather than with the length of the predicted ATM protein (Cavaciuti et al. 2005). Recently Renwick et al. (2006) analysing 443 breast cancer families showed that mutations in ATM gene give to the carriers a relative risk of 2.37 to develop cancer.

Somatic *ATM* mutations have been reported in several forms of leukaemia and lymphoma, including acute lymphoblastic leukaemia (ALL), chronic lymphocytic leukaemia (CLL), T-cell prolymphocytic leukaemia (T-PLL), and mantle zone lymphoma (Stankovic et al. 1998, Stilgenbauer et al. 2000, Fang et al. 2003, Yamaguchi et al. 2003, Eclache et al. 2004). In general, the spectrum of *ATM* mutations differs for each of these; breast cancer mutations tend to be different from those seen in individuals with AT (Bernstein et al. 2003), while *ATM* mutations of T-ALL cases are similar to those seen in AT patients (Liberzon et al. 2004).

Epidemiological studies also suggest that AT carriers are also at an increased risk for heart disease (Swift 1985, Swift et al. 1991).

### Other manifestations

AT patients have been reported to show cardiac anomalies under heart ultrasound examination. In 5 out of 11 AT children Bastianon et al. (1993) reported mitral valve prolapse and aortic root dilatation, later confirmed in other AT young patients (personal observation).

More than 50% of AT patients in one series (Jabado et al. 2000) manifested glucose intolerance associated with insulin resistance and hyperglycaemia. Growth retardation is present in many of these children; by adolescence weight and height will drop below the third percentile, especially in patients with chronic sinopulmonary infections. Patients who attain puberty are likely to achieve growth within the normal range. No specific hormonal deficit is known that would account for the tendency of children with AT to grow less than normal. How-

ever, all sexes may have delayed or absent pubertal changes often associated with gonadal atrophy, and in later years associated with insulin-resistant diabetes in a significant minority of cases (Crawford 1998, Jabado et al. 2000).

Females with AT often have delayed menstruations, with equally delayed development of secondary sexual characteristics. The ovaries are sometimes absent or hypoplastic and female AT patients may be sterile. However, many male AT patients ejaculate and at least those few who have been studied produced sperm. Atm-knockout mice are however anovulatory and aspermic, respectively. Rare instances of long-surviving AT patients who conceived children are reported in the literature (Stankovic et al. 1998).

Mild-liver associated laboratory abnormalities, such as alkaline phosphatase and serum transaminase levels, are elevated in about half of children with AT. Fatty infiltration and portal round cell infiltration have been observed in some liver biopsies: however these manifestations are not diagnostic nor life-threatening and they do not require any specific treatment.

### Imaging and neurophysiology

MRI and sporadically made CT scan often show evidence of nonspecific cerebellar atrophy involving the vermis and/or the hemispheres and manifesting as decreased size of the cerebellum, increase prominence of the cerebellar folial and fissures, and enlargement of the fourth ventricle (Barkovich 2005, Cardeur et al. 1983, Edelstein et al. 2005). Atrophy of AT is panvermian and, according to Tavani et al. (2003), progresses with age (Fig. 6), starting from early childhood. In our experience, the atrophy usually does not appear at MRI before the age of 2–3 years: initially, the vermis is more markedly involved than the cerebellar hemispheres (Farina et al. 1994) but the brain stem and the cerebral cortex are involved as well (Fig. 6). More severe atrophy is associated with longer duration of disease and more severe ataxia (Barkovich 2005) (Fig. 6f, g). Occasionally, affected adolescents (Fig. 7a, b) and older AT patients (Fig. 7c) may show high T2 signal foci in the cerebral white matter, pos-

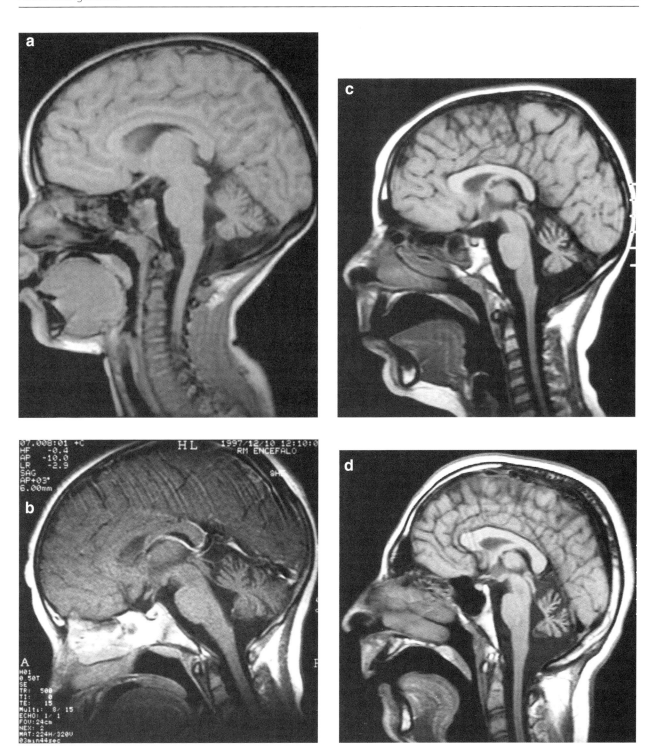

**Fig. 6.** Sagittal (**a–g**) and coronal (**h**) T1-weighted magnetic resonance images of the brain in AT individuals at different ages [8 yrs (**a**), 12 yrs (**b**), 15 yrs (**c**), 17 yrs (**d**), 25 yrs (**d**), 29 yrs (**e**), 34 yrs (**f**) and 43 yrs (**g, h**)] show the progression of cerebellar, brainstem and cortical atrophy. Note the relative preservation of the brainstem and higher segments of the cord in the initial phases (**a, b**) as compared to the late stages of disease (**l–g**) (c, e, g are courtesy of Prof. A. Federico and M. T. Dotti, Institute of Neuroscience, University of Siena, Siena, Italy).

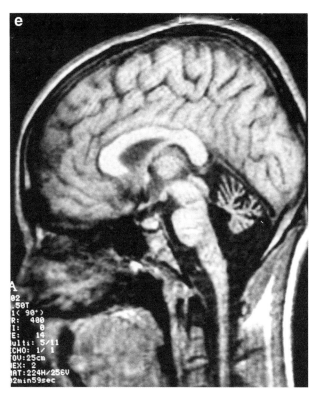

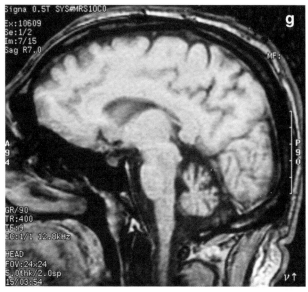

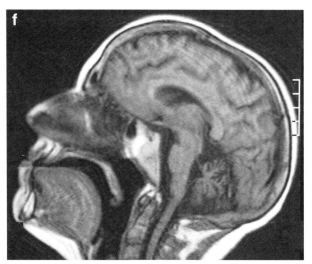

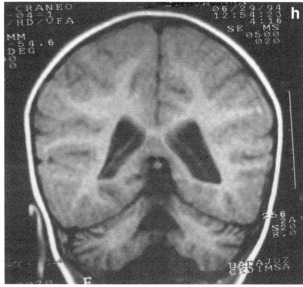

**Fig. 6.** (Continued)

sibly indicating degenerative changes of the progeroid type (Edelstein et al. 2005, Sardanelli et al. 1995). In younger AT patients cerebral white matter typically shows no focal signal intensity changes. Absence of such cerebral changes is considered to exclude macroscopic brain teleangiectasia (Sardanelli et al. 1995). Haemorrhage may occur as a result of rupture of parenchymal telangiectasias. Cerebral infarcts may result from emboli that are shunted through vascular malformations within the lungs (Barkovich 2005).

Proton MR spectroscopy features in AT closely correlate with the morphologic neuroimaging findings of posterior fossa atrophy (i.e., profound loss of all metabolites – NAA, Cr and

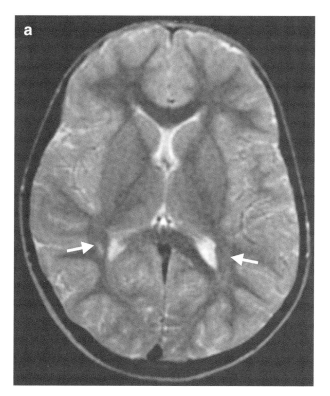

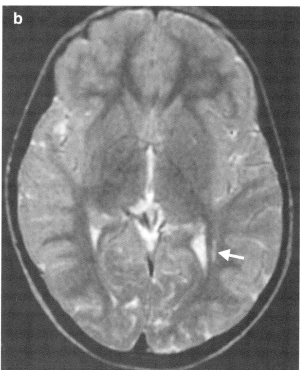

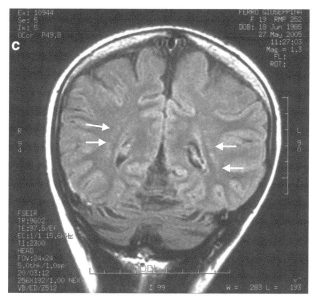

**Fig. 7.** Axial T2-weighted (**a, b**) and coronal T1-weighted (**c**) magnetic resonance images of the brain in a 18-year-old boy (**a, b**) and a 27-year-old woman (**c**) with AT showing high signal lesions in the periventricular white matter (white arrows). Note the speckled aspect of these anomalies (**c**), which reflects the likely telangiectasic nature of the lesions (c, courtesy of Prof. D. Di Bella, Pediatric Radiology Unit, Institute of Radiology and Department of Pediatrics, University of Catania, Catania, Italy).

Cho – in the cerebellar vermis) (Lin et al. 2006, Wallis et al. 2007), a trend for decreased metabolites within the cerebellar hemispheres (Lin et al. 2006) with significantly lower NAA/Cho and higher Cho/Cr ratios in adult vs. younger AT patients (Wallis et al. 2007).

Radiological findings, either on MRI and/or lateral skull radiographs, of simple mucosal thickening to decreased or absent adenoidal tissue in the nasopharynx are so typical in AT that (along with cerebellar atrophy) are of diagnostic value. Chest X-rays studies may show a small or absent thymic shadow, decreased mediastinal lymphoid tissue, and pulmonary changes similar to those seen in cystic fibrosis. Hypoplastic peripheral lymphoid tissue is such a consistent clinical finding in AT that the appearance of lymphadenopathy or even easily palpable lymph nodes has been highly suggestive of lymphoma.

Electromyogram (EMG) and nerve conduction velocities are frequently normal in young children. In the later stages of the disease, when the anterior horn cells are involved and peripheral neuropathy has occurred, the EMG shows signs of denervation and the nerve conduction velocity is reduced, especially in sensory fibres.

Electrooculography is valuable in corroborating the characteristic oculomotor abnormality of AT and differentiating AT from Friedreich ataxia.

## Pathology

The cerebellum atrophies early, being visibly smaller on MRI examination by seven or eight years of age (see above, Imaging and neurophysiology), with concomitant loss of Purkinje cells and depletion of granule cells: this is the major pathological marker of AT in the CNS. No vascular abnormalities are usually found, except late degenerative gliovascular nodules in the white matter and telangiectasic vessels in the leptomeninges (Edelstein et al. 2005). Lesions of the basal ganglia are found only occasionally. In addition there is loss of neurons in the olivary nuclei, substantia nigra and oculomotor nuclei, as well as spongy degeneration and abnormal vasculature in the cerebral cortex. Degeneration of spinal tracts (dorsal columns and dorsal ganglial cells) and anterior horn cells is often present in older cases.

Microscopic nucleomegaly also occurs in the cells of tissues throughout the body.

Biopsy specimens have shown that the typical skin changes in AT are similar to those seen in cumulative actinic damage and, thus, are suggestive of progeric changes. The predilection of both the progeric skin changes and the oculocutaneous telangiectases for sun-exposed areas further suggests increased propensity to actinic damage.

## Pathogenesis and molecular genetics

The gene mutated in Ataxia Telangiectasia patients has been mapped in 1988 (Gatti et al. 1988) on the long arm of chromosome 11 at region q22–23. In the following years, the joined efforts of an international Consortium allowed the progressive restriction of this region to a 500 kb interval (Foroud et al. 1991, Gatti et al. 1994, Lange et al. 1995) and, in 1995, the identification of the *ATM* gene by positional cloning (Savitsky et al. 1995).

The AT Mutated gene (*ATM*) extends over 150 kb of genomic DNA, includes 66 exons (62 coding), and has an open reading frame of 9168 nucleotides. The *ATM* gene product contains 3056 amino acids and is a member of the phosphatidylinositol (PI) 3-kinase family of proteins, with the kinase domain in its C-terminal region (Savitsky et al. 1995) (Fig. 8). The patients are mostly compound heterozygotes for two different mutations inherited by their parents, but the homozygotes for the same mutation are not infrequent, especially in highly inbred populations. More than 400 unique mutations, spread all over the ATM gene, have been identified in AT patients, without evidence of any mutational hot spots (Fig. 9). Most of these changes are predicted to give rise to a truncated protein that is highly unstable, effectively producing a null phenotype (~85%). However, a significant number of missense mutations has been recorded (~10%) and recent data suggest that many of these have dominant interfering effects (Scott et al. 2002, Spring et al. 2002, Concannon 2002, Concannon and Gatti 1997). Recurrent mutations are reported in Norway, the Netherlands, Costa Rica, the English Midlands, Italy, Japan, Poland, and among people of Irish English, Utah Mormon, African American, Israeli Jewish, and Amish/Mennonite descent (Gilad et al. 1996, Ejima and Sasaki 1998, Laake et al. 1998, Stankovic et al. 1998, Telatar et al. 1998). For several of these mutations the carriers share common haplotypes, indicating a founder effect. A regularly updated ATM mutation Database Web site is available (http://chromium.liacs.ml/loud).

The *ATM* gene plays a key role in several pathways involved in cell-cycle control, oxidative stress,

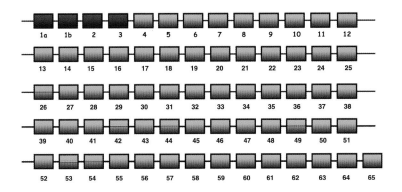

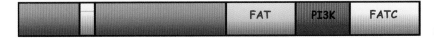

**Fig. 8.** The *ATM* gene and its protein structure.

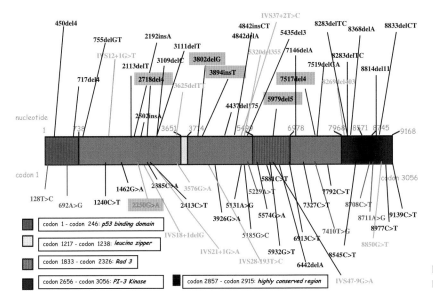

**Fig. 9.** Spectrum of *ATM* gene mutations in Italian AT patients.

and DNA repair (Lavin and Shiloh 1997, Shiloh 2003). It acts recognizing and facilitating the repair of a subcategory of double strand breaks (DSBs) or a form of damage, like oxidative stress, that is converted into a DSB in DNA (Fig. 10); this recognition would probably be the trigger for ATM to activate a number of cell cycle checkpoints. The ATM protein is present in the nucleus as an inactive dimer and is activated in response to DNA DSBs by an auto-phosphorylation on ser-1981 that causes the dissociation of the dimer to form active monomeric forms, which are capable to initiate the phosphorylation of multiple intermediates involved in DNA

repair and cell cycle control (Bakkenist and Kastan 2003). The double strand break is generally regarded as the most toxic DNA lesion. DSBs are induced by a number of different mechanisms, including exposure to ionising radiations and radiomimetic drugs, collapse of replication forks when the replication machinery encounters single-stranded breaks (SSBs) in the template DNA, and programmed cleavage by specific endonucleases during meiotic recombination and immunoglobulin gene rearrangements (for reviews, see Valerie and Povirk 2003, Petrini and Stracker 2003). SSBs are mainly generated directly by oxidative stress and, if not rapidly processed, are

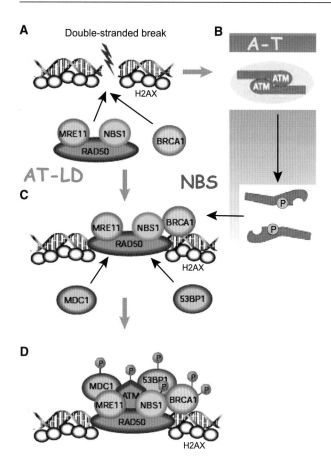

**Fig. 10.** Pathways involved in recognition and facilitation of sub-categories of double strand breaks (DSBs) in the ATM and NBS genes (see text for explanation) (modified from Bakkenist and Kastan 2003, Mckinnon 2004).

converted to DSBs (Caldecott 2003). There are two major types of DBS repair pathway, homologous recombination repair (HRR) and non-homologous end-joining (NHEJ), which are fundamentally different because of the dependence on DNA homology in HHR (Johnson and Jasin 2001). Errors in DSBs repair generate small deletions or insertions at the site of the lesion and can result in chromosome translocations and genomic instability, finally leading to cancer.

Progressive neurodegeneration, a major characteristic of AT, has been reported to be associated with cerebellar defects involving ectopic migration and loss of Purkinje cells. However, it is evident that other regions of the brain and the CNS are affected by loss of ATM (Sedgwick and Boder 1991). Given the important role for ATM in recognising and signalling DNA double strand breaks, it is understandable that post-

mitotic cells would be vulnerable in AT patients. It has been suggested that a checkpoint defect in AT post-mitotic cells would be responsible for this vulnerability (Yang and Herrup 2005); this hypothesis is supported by the evidence of a mitotic spindle defect in AT cells post-irradiation (Takagi et al. 1998).

The initiating event in the damage response is the change in the chromatin structure, that rapidly triggers the activation of ATM, as indicated by the auto-phosphorylation of ATM at serine-1981 and subsequent ATM dimer dissociation (Bakkenist and Kastan 2003). A direct role for ATM in DSBs repair has not been conclusively demonstrated except for correlative findings. ATM, by an as yet unknown mechanism, senses DSBs and phosphorylates proteins involved in HRR, such NBS1 at three sites (ser-343, ser-397 and ser-615) (Gatei et al. 2000, Lim et al. 2000), BLM at two sites (thr-99 and thr-122) (Beamish et al. 2002), BRCA1 at three sites (ser-1387, ser-1423, ser-1524) (Gatei et al. 2001), Rad51 at thr-54 and thr-315 indirectly through c-Abl (Chen et al. 1999), and SMC1 at ser-957 and ser-966 (Kim et al. 2002). Many of these proteins have been found in 'repair foci' (Celeste et al. 2002), which formation is explained by the co-localization of Mre11 with Rad50 or Rad51 at sites of DSBs. It is not clear whether these foci constitute repair-competent complexes or result from the accumulation of proteins that failed to repair the damage (Paull 2000). The earliest (1–3min) recorded event during foci formation is the phosphorylation of histone H2AX at S139 by ATM (Paull et al. 2000, Burma et al. 2001), followed by colocalisation of BRCA1, RAD54, and either RAD50 or RAD51 (Gatei et al. 2000b, Paull et al. 2000). The phosphorylation of H2AX is believed to serve as a focal point for the assembly of repair proteins at the DSB resulting in irradiation-induced foci (IRIFs), since cells that do not express H2AX show impaired recruitment of NBS1, 53BP1 and BRCA1 (Celeste et al. 2002).

## Variability within the classical AT phenotype

Within the classical phenotype of AT, some variability can be appreciated. In general, however, the older patients with fully expressed disease manifest a very homogeneous syndrome. Thus, it is the onset and progression of signs and symptoms that provide most of the variability (Chun and Gatti 2004). Variability exists in *laboratory findings* (e.g., ATM protein levels, serum AFP) and *radiosensitivity* (reviewed by Chun and Gatti 2004; see below under diagnosis) as well; variability is also seen with the *cancer phenotype*, as within the same families some patients may develop several primary cancers while other affected siblings live into later life without cancer. Rare AT patients do not develop noticeable *ataxia* until their teens or even later; partial ATM kinase activity has been hypothesized as a possible explanation for these phenotypes (Chun and Gatti 2004). We have seen two AT children (with known *ATM* mutations) and are aware of other two clinically identified (Nardocci, personal communication 2004) who had a classical AT phenotype with early onset ataxia and during their second decade switched to an intention dyskinetic syndrome with preserved gait and no other associated movements abnormalities. Notably, one of such children is able in her teens to ski and ride horses. Two other AT patients studied and molecularly confirmed by us presented until puberty a classical AT phenotype with recurrent infections, but after that age had no

more infections and reached their thirties still walking and being in a relatively good health.

Occasionally, patients presenting with few clinical features of AT, other than progressive ataxia, have been described as "AT Variants" (Chessa et al. 1992, Fiorilli et al. 1985a, Taylor et al. 1987, Ying and Decouteau 1981). Molecular analysis allowed us to classify these patients in three groups: (1) individuals with laboratory evidence of AT who have been shown to have mutations in the *ATM* gene (McConville et al. 1996, Gilad et al. 1998); (2) patients who show clinical and cellular AT phenotype without telangiectasias: some have mutations in *ATM* gene, some other in Mre11 gene, a DSB repair gene which is part of the MNR complex – this condition is referred as *AtaxiaTelangiectasia-Like Disorder* (*ATLD*) (Petrini 1999; Stewart et al. 1999, Pitts et al. 2001, Delia et al. 2004) (Fig. 11; see also table 1 in chapter 51); and (3) patients presenting with a neurologic disorder very similar to AT who lack multisystemic involvement, have normal alpha-fetoprotein and chromosomal stability and no hypersensitivity to ionising radiations: this condition is referred as *Ataxia with Oculomotor Apraxia Type 1* (*AOA1*) or *AT-like syndrome* (Date et al. 2001, Moreira et al. 2001).

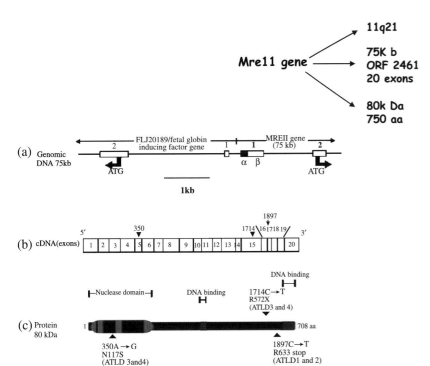

**Fig. 11.** Mre11 gene and protein (modified from Taylor et al. 2004).

## Natural history

The primary features of AT include progressive gait and truncal ataxia with onset between one and four years of age; progressively slurred speech; oculomotor apraxia; choreoathetosis (writhing movements); oculocutaneous telangiectasia, usually by six years of age; frequent infections, with accompanying evidence of serum and cellular immunodeficiencies; susceptibility to cancer, usually leukaemia or lymphoma; and hypersensitivity to ionising radiation. Other features include premature aging with greying of the hair. Endocrine abnormalities, such as insulin-resistant diabetes mellitus, have also been observed. The AT syndromic pathway varies little from family to family in its late stages (Boder 1985, Chun and Gatti 2004, Gatti 2002; Perlman et al. 2003).

**Lifespan.** Over the past twenty years, the expected lifespan of individuals with AT has increased considerably; most individuals now live beyond 25 years of age. Some have survived into their 40s and 50s (Dork et al. 2004). In older individuals pulmonary failure, with or without identifiable infections, is the major cause of failing health and death. Life-threatening lymphocytic infiltrations of the lung have been reported (Tangsinmankong et al. 2001).

## Diagnosis

Diagnosis of AT relies upon clinical findings, the disease being suspected in young children who have signs of progressive cerebellar dysfunction including gait and truncal ataxia, slurred speech, and oculomotor apraxia. The onset of cerebellar features is generally between one and four years of age. A small cerebellum is often observed on MRI examination but may not be obvious in very young individuals. The appearance of telangiectasias (between 2 and 8 years of age) and the recurrence of sinopulmonary infections confirm the clinical diagnosis.

Laboratory tests can be performed to support the diagnosis: first, the levels of serum alpha-fetoprotein, which are elevated in more than 95% of individuals with AT (Stray-Pedersen et al. 2007) and the levels of IgA, which are reduced in ~60% of the patients; both these analyses can be easily done in a routine laboratory. More specialistic analyses include

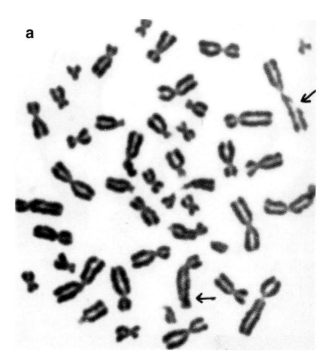

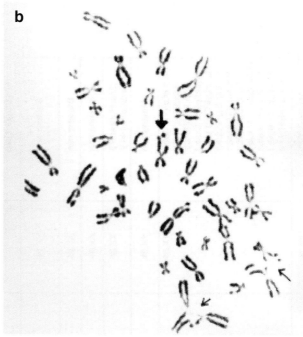

**Fig. 12.** Chromosomal and chromatid damages secondary to radiohypersensitivity in AT patients.

the routine karyotype of peripheral blood cells with the search for a 7; 14 chromosome translocation and in vitro radiosensitivity assay (rate of induced chromosomal breakage, colony surviving assay, radioresistant DNA synthesis) (Figs. 12, 13). All these tests are now overpassed by the use of Western Blot analysis which allows the determination of the amount and functionality of ATM protein in the patient' cells. Immunoblotting is considered the most definitive clinical test for establishing a diagnosis of AT, as about 90% of individuals with AT have no detectable ATM protein, approximately 10% have trace amounts, and about 1% have normal amounts of ATM-lacking protein kinase activity ("kinase-dead") (Fig. 14). A lymphoblastoid cell line established from the patient is routinely used; this procedure requires four to six weeks, thus prolonging turnaround time but permitting in the majority of cases the definition of the diagnosis. The establishment of a lymphoblastoid cell line is everywhere a useful procedure, allowing the repetition of all the diagnostic tests and providing a renewable source of RNA and DNA for subsequent identification of *ATM* mutations – the ultimate confirmation of a diagnosis of AT.

Molecular genetic testing of the *ATM* gene has always been a long-time spending analysis; the recent use of DHPLC (Denaturing High Performance Liquid Chromatography) and direct sequencing has shortened the times for a positive response (Bernstein et al. 2003). In fact, PTT (Protein Truncation Test) detects approximately 70% of *ATM* mutations (Telatar et al. 1996), while DHPLC detects more than 85% of *ATM* mutations (Bernstein et al. 2003).

In few cases in which the *ATM* mutations couldn't be identified the linkage analysis with the short-tandem repeat (STR) and single-nucleotide polymorphism (SNP) markers will permit the detection of the carriers between the family members with an accuracy approaching 100%, because at least two of the used markers are intragenic.

The identification of *ATM* gene mutations is important to understand the molecular basis of

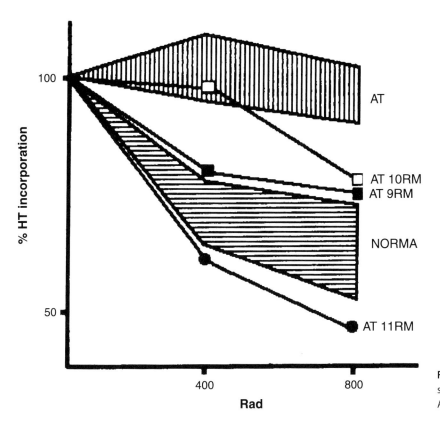

**Fig. 13.** Curve/dosage ideogram of radiosensitivity in classical AT vs. "variant" AT (AT 9RM, AT 10RM, AT 11RM) and normal subjects.

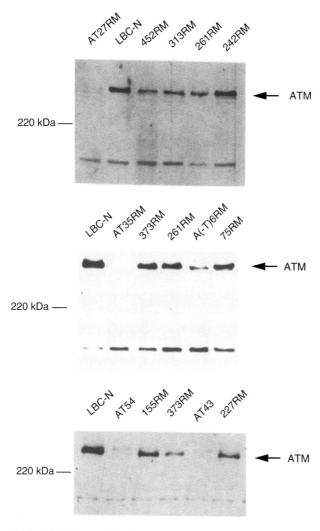

**Fig. 14.** ATM immunoblotting sequences.

## Differential diagnosis

Establishing the diagnosis of ataxia-telangiectasia is most difficult in very young children, primarily because the full syndrome is not yet apparent. The most common misdiagnosis is cerebral palsy. Diagnosis of AT is questionable when accompanied by severe mental retardation, seizures, non-progressive ataxia, or microcephaly. Not unexpectedly, mutations in genes specifying proteins in pathways controlled by or involving *ATM* leads to phenotypes overlapping with AT (Shiloh 2003). Mutations in Nbs1 and Mre11 give rise to Nijmegen Breakage Syndrome (NBS) and AT-LD respectively, both of which show considerable overlap in clinical and cellular phenotype with AT (Saar et al. 1997, Stewart et al. 1999, Delia et al. 2004). *ATM* is dependent upon Nbs1 as part of the Mre11 complex as a sensor of double strand breaks and in turn phosphorylates this protein to enhance its activity in DNA repair and as an adaptor molecule for phosphorylation of other downstream substrates of *ATM*.

Patients presenting Ataxia with Oculomotor Apraxia type 1 (AOA1) share with AT patients a common neurological phenotype but no multisystemic involvement neither elevated alpha-fetoprotein, decreased IgA levels, chromosomal instability and hypersensitivity to ionising radiations. The AOA1 patients show ataxia with onset in childhood, choreoathetosis, dystonia, severe oculomotor apraxia; the disease is slowly progressive and the prognosis is favourable due to the absence of recurrent infections and neoplasia. The gene responsible for the disease in Japanese as well in Portuguese patients was identified by two distinct groups in the two populations in 2001 and was called *APTX* (Date et al. 2001, Moreira et al. 2001). This gene encodes for a protein called aprataxin, which is a member of the HIT superfamily, involved in DNA Single Strand Breaks repair and response to genotoxic agents causing oxidative stress (Gueven et al. 2004, Mosesso et al. 2005). Ataxia with Oculomotor Apraxia type 2 (AOA2) presents with the same neurological and cellular phenotypes but elevated alphafetoprotein levels; the onset is between 10 and 22 years (Le Ber et al. 2004, Criscuolo et al. 2006). The gene defective in AOA2 was cloned in 2004 and

the disease, and is essential for pre- and post-natal diagnosis and genetic counselling. Prenatal genetic testing has been performed initially through the establishment of radiosensitivity of the foetal cells; this approach produced often false negative result (personal observation). More recently, linkage analysis has been successfully used when the mutation(s) were not known. Direct molecular prenatal diagnosis, giving 100% of accuracy, is possible whenever the familial mutation(s) are known (Chessa et al. 1999).

Preimplantation genetic diagnosis has recently been performed in at risk couples for AT (Verlinsky et al. 2007).

called SETX (Moreira et al. 2004); it encodes for a protein, the senataxin, which is also probably involved in SSBs repair (Suraweera et al. 2007). Both the AOA new syndromes could be misdiagnosed as AT, but the clinical features together with normal levels of ATM protein will help for the correct diagnosis.

## Management, follow-up and treatment

The prevention of primary manifestations of AT has been so far unsuccessful. Therapeutic supports as early and continued physical therapy minimizes contractures, which appear in almost all individuals with time and lead to other physical problems, while IVIG replacement therapy appears to reduce the number and severity of infections in patients presenting with them. A wheelchair is necessary by ten years of age in patients with the classical form of the disease. Antioxidants (e.g., vitamin E or alpha-lipoic acid) are recommended, although there has been no formal testing for their efficacy in AT individuals (Reliene and Schiestl 2007). The predisposition to malignancy suggests the need to monitor early signs with periodic medical visits. Due to the hypersensitivity to ionising radiations, the use of radiotherapy and some radiomimetic chemotherapeutic agents should be monitored carefully; conventional doses are potentially lethal and peculiar protocols must be applied. In vitro studies suggest the possibility of a successful therapy in that 15% of patients carrying single-nucleotide changes that introduce premature termination codons. The in vitro use of aminoglycoside antibiotics showed their potential to read through premature termination codons inducing full-length ATM protein and return of ATM functions (Lai et al. 2004). One caveat in this approach is the toxicity of aminoglycosides which would not allow at this moment their use in patients.

Recently, two studies have attempted pharmacological treatment of central nervous system signs/symptoms in AT. Gazulla et al. (2006, 2007) treated a 34-year-old mann with adult onset AT with a combination of pregabalin (225 mg/day) and tiagabine (7.5 mg/day). Pregabalin treatment improved the patient's gait (he was able to walk for more than 10 m without support), and the addition of tiagabine in-

creased the distance of unsupported walking to more than 20 m and facilitated execution of half turns. Such improvements were sustained for an unspecified period, after which they disappeared, and the drugs were withdrawn. In the study of Buoni et al. (2006), a 3-year-old boy with classic AT symptoms and molecular evidence of AT experienced marked reduction of neurological signs following corticosteroids therapy (bethametasone 0.05 mg/kg every 12 h). The child's parents had previously noted reduction of neurological signs and symptoms during bethametasone treatment for asthmatic bronchitis attacks. Bethametasone reduced neurological signs within the first 2–3 days: a dramatic reduction of the disturbance of stance and gait with increased control of the head, neck and skilled movements (including climbing up the stairs) was apparent after 4 weeks of treatment (see videos available to subscribers at http://www.archneurol.com). The most notable adverse effect was increased appetite and body weight, and fluid retention (moon-like face). The findings of Buoni et al. (2006) have been recently confirmed by Broccoletti et al. (2008).

## References

Assencio-Ferreira VJ, Bancovsky I, Diamant AJ, Dias Gherpelli JL, Alves Moreira F (1981) Computed tomography in ataxia-telangiectasia. J Comput Ass Tom 5: 660–661.

Athma P, Rappaport R, Swift M (1996) Molecular genotyping shows that ataxia-telangiectasia heterozygotes are predisposed to breast cancer. Cancer Genet Cytogenet 92: 130–134.

Bakkenist CJ, Kastan MB (2003) DNA damage activates ATM through intermolecular auto-phosphorylation and dimer dissociation. Nature 421: 499–506.

Barkovich AJ (2005) The phakomatoses. In: Barkovich AJ (ed.) Pediatric neuroimaging, 4th ed. Philadelphia: Lippincott Williams & Wilkins, pp. 440–505.

Bastianon V, Fiorilli M, Giglioni E, Businco L, Chessa L (1993) Cardiac anomalies in ataxia-telangiectasia. Am J Dis Child 147: 20–21.

Beighton P, Beighton G (1997) Denise Louis-Bar. In: The men behind the syndrome. London: The Parthenon Publishing Group, pp. 110–111.

Bernstein JL, Teraoka S, Haile RW, Borresen-Dale AL, Rosenstein BS, Gatti RA, Diep AT, Jansen L, Atencio DP, Olsen JH, Bernstein L, Teitelbaum SL, Thompson WD, Concannon P (2003) Designing and implementing quality control for multi-center screening of mutations in the ATM gene among women with breast cancer. Hum Mutat 21: 542–550.

Biemond A (1957) Paleocerebellar atrophy with extrapyramidal manifestations in association with bronchiectasis and telangiectasis of the conjunctiva bulbi as a familial syndrome. In: van Bogaert L, Radermecker J (eds.) Proceedings of the First International Congress of Neurological Sciences, Brussles, July 1957. London: Permagon Press, p. 206.

Boder E (1985) Ataxia telangiectasia: an overview. In: Gatti RA, Swift M (eds.) Ataxia-telangiectasia: genetics, neuropathology and immunology of a degenerative disease of childhood. New York: Alan R Liss, pp. 1–63.

Boder E (1987) Ataxia-telangiectasia. In: Gomez MR (ed.) Neurocutaneous diseases. A practical approach. Boston: Butterworths, pp. 95–117.

Boder E, Sedgwick RP (1957) Ataxia-telangiectasia: a familial syndrome of progressive cerebellar ataxia, oculocutaneous telangiectasia and frequent pulmonary infection. A preliminary report on 7 children, an autopsy, and a case history. Univ South Calif Med Bull 9: 15–28.

Boder E, Sedgwick RP (1958) Ataxia-telangiectasia. A familial syndrome of progressive cerebellar ataxia, oculocutaneous telangiectasia and frequent pulmonary infection. Pediatrics 21: 526–534.

Boder E, Sedgwick RP (1963) Ataxia-telangiectasia: a review of 101 cases. In: Walsh G (ed.) Little Club Clinics in Dev Med no. 8. London: Heinemann Medical Books, pp. 110–118.

Bott L, Lebreton J, Thumerelle C, Cuvellier J, Deschildre A, Sardet A (2007) Lung disease in ataxia-telangiectasia. Acta Paediatr May 24 [Epub ahead of print].

Bretsky P, Haiman CA, Gilad S, Yahalom J, Grossman A, Paglin S, Van Den Berg D, Kolonel LN, Skaliter R, Henderson BE (2003) The relationship between twenty missense ATM variants and breast cancer risk: the Multiethnic Cohort. Cancer Epidemiol Biomarkers Prev 12: 733–738.

Broccoletti T, Del Giudice E, Amorosi S, Russo I, Di Bonito M, Imperati F, Romano A, Pignata C (2008) Steroid-induced improvement of neurological signs in ataxia-telangiectasia patients. Eur J Neurol 15: 223–228.

Buoni S, Zannolli R, Sorrentino L, Fois A (2006) Betamethasone and improvement of neurological symptoms in ataxia-telangiectasia. Arch Neurol 63: 1479–1482.

Caldecott KW (2003) DNA single-strand break repair and spinocerebellar ataxia. Cell 112: 7–10.

Carney JP, Maser RS, Olivares H, Davis EM, Le Beau M, Yates Jr III, Hays L, Morgan WF, Petrini JH (1998) The hMre11/hRad50 protein complex and Nijmegen breakage syndrome: linkage of double-strand break repair to the cellular DNA damage response. Cell 93: 477–486.

Cavaciuti E, Laugé A, Janin N, Ossian K, Hall J, Stoppa-Lyonnet D, Andrieu N (2005) Cancer risk according to type and location of ATM mutation in ataxia-telangiectasia families. Genes Chromosomes Cancer 42: 1–9.

Centerwall WR, Miller MM (1958) Ataxia, telangiectasia, and sinopulmonary infections. A syndrome of slowly progressive deterioration in childhood. Am J Dis Child 95: 385–396.

Chenevix-Trench G, Dork T, Scott C, Hopper J (2002) Dominant negative ATM mutations in breast cancer families. J Natl Cancer Inst 94: 952.

Chessa L, Petrinelli P, Antonelli A, Fiorilli M, Elli R, Marcucci L, Federico A, Gandini E (1992) Heterogeneity in Ataxia Telengiectasia: classical phenotype associated with low cellular radiosensitivity. Am J Med Genet 42: 741–746.

Chessa L, Lisa A, Fiorani O, Zei G (1994) Ataxia Telangiectasia in Italy: genetic analysis. Int J Rad Biol 66: S31–S33

Chessa L, Piane M, Prudente S, Carducci C, Mazzilli MC, Pachì A, Negrini M, Narducci MG, Russo G, Frati L (1999) Molecular prenatal diagnosis of Ataxia Telangiectasia heterozygosity by direct mutational assays. Prenatal Diagnosis 19: 542–545.

Chun HH, Gatti RA (2004) Ataxia-telangiectasia, an evolving phenotype. DNA Repair 3: 1187–1196.

Clemins JJ, Horowitz AL (2000) Abnormal white matter signal in Ataxia Telangiectasia. Am J Neuroradiol 21: 1483–1485.

Concannon P (2002) ATM heterozygosity and cancer risk. Nat Genet 32: 89–90.

Concannon P, Gatti RA (1997) Diversity of ATM gene mutations detected in patients with ataxia-telangiectasia. Hum Mutat 10: 100–107.

Crawford TO (1998) Ataxia-telengiectasia. Semin Pediatr Neurol 5: 287–294.

Crawford TO, Mandir AS, Lefton-Greif MA, Goodman SN, Goodman BK, Sengul H, Lederman HM (2000) Quantitative neurologic assessment of ataxia-telangiectasia. Neurology 54: 1605–1509.

Criscuolo C, Chessa L, Di Giandomenico S, Mancini P, Saccà F, Grieco GS, Piane M, Barbieri F, De Michele G, Banfi S, Pierelli F, Rizzuto N, Santorelli FM, Gallosti L, Filla A, Casali C (2006) Ataxia with oculomotor apraxia type 2: a clinical, pathology and genetic study. Neurology 66: 1207–1210.

Date H, Onodera O, Tanaka H, Iwabuchi K, Uekawa K, Igarashi S, Koike R, Hiroi T, Yuasa T, Awaya Y (2001) Early-onset ataxia with ocular motor apraxia and hypoalbuminemia is caused by mutations in a new HIT superfamily gene. Nat Genet 29: 184–188.

Delia D, Mizutani S, Panigone S, Tagliabue E, Fontanella E, Asada M, Yamada T, Taya Y, Prudente S, Saviozzi S, Frati L, Pierotti MA, Chessa L (2000) ATM protein and p53-

serine phosphorylation in Ataxia-telangiectasia (AT) patients and AT heterozygotes. Brit J Cancer 82: 1938–1945.

Delia D, Fontanella E, Ferrario C, Chessa L, Mizutani S (2003) DNA damage- induced cell cycle-phase regulation of p53 and p21waf21 in normal and ATM-defective cells. Oncogene 22: 7866–7869.

Delia D, Piane M, Buscemi G, Savio C, Palmeri S, Lulli P, Carlessi L, Fontanella E, Chessa L (2004) Mre11 mutations and impaired ATM-dependent responses in an Italian family with Ataxia Telangiectasia Like Disorder (ATLD). Hum Mol Genet 13: 2155–2163.

Demaerell Ph, Kendall BE, Kingsley D (1992) Cranial CT and MRI in diseases with DNA repair defects. Neuroradiology 34: 117–121.

Dotti MT, Federico A, Guazzi G (1994) Atassia telangiectasia: aspetti neurologici e neuroradiologici. Nuova Riv Neurol 4: 113–117.

Drolet BA, Drolet B, Zvulunov A, Jacobsen R, Troy J, Esterly NB (1997) Cutaneous granulomas as a presenting sign in ataxia-telangiectasia. Dermatology 194: 273–275.

Easton DF (1994) Cancer risks in A-T heterozygotes. Int J Radiat Biol 66: S177–S182.

Eclache V, Caulet-Maugendre S, Poirel HA, Djemai M, Robert J, Lejeune F, Raphael M (2004) Cryptic deletion involving the ATM locus at 11q22.3 approximately q23.1 in B-cell chronic lymphocytic leukemia and related disorders. Cancer Genet Cytogenet 152: 72–76.

Edelstein S, Naidich TP, Newton TH (2005) The rare phakomatoses. In: Tortori-Donati P (ed.) Pediatric neuroradiology. Brain. Berlin: Springer, pp. 819–854.

Ejima Y, Sasaki MS (1998) Mutations of the ATM gene detected in Japanese ataxia-telangiectasia patients: Possible preponderance of the two founder mutations 4612del165 and 7883del5. Hum Genet 102: 403–408.

Evrard P, Beya A, Provis M (1990) Denise Louis-Bar. In: Ashwal S (ed.) The founders of child neurology. San Francisco: Norman Publishing, pp. 774–777.

Fang NY, Greiner TC, Weisenburger DD, Chan WC, Vose JM, Smith LM, Armitage JO, Mayer RA, Pike BL, Collins FS, Hacia JG (2003) Oligonucleotide microarrays demonstrate the highest frequency of ATM mutations in the mantle cell subtype of lymphoma. Proc Natl Acad Sci USA 100: 372–377.

Fiorilli M, Carbonari M, Crescenzi M, Russo G, Aiuti F (1985a) T-cell receptor genes and ataxia-telangiectasia. Nature 313: 186.

Fiorilli M, Antonelli A, Russo G, Crescenzi M, Carbonari M, Petrinelli P (1985b) Variant of ataxia-telangiectasia with low-level radiosensitivity. Hum Genet 70: 274–277.

FitzGerald MG, Bean JM, Hegde SR, Unsal H, MacDonald DJ, Harkin DP, Finkelstein DM, Isselbacher KJ, Haber DA (1987) Heterozygous ATM mutations do not contribute to early onset of breast cancer. Nat Genet 15: 307–310.

Foroud T, Wei S, Ziv Y, Sobel E, Lange E, Chao A, Goradia T, Huo Y, Tolun A, Chessa L, Charmley P, Sanal O, Salman N, Julier C, Concannon P, McConville C, Taylor M, Shiloh Y, Lange K, Gatti RA (1991) Localization of an ataxia-telangiectasia locus to a 3-cM interval on chromosome 11q23: linkage analysis of 111 families by an international consortium. Am J Hum Genet 49: 1263–1279.

Frappart PO, McKinnon PJ (2006) Ataxia-telangiectasia and related diseases. Neuromolecular Med 8: 495–512.

Gatti RA (2006) Ataxia-telangiectasia. Gene Reviews. http://www.geneclinics.org/profiles/ataxia-telangiectasia/

Gatti RA, Berkel I, Boder E, Braedt G, Charmley P, Concannon P, Ersoy F, Foroud T, Jaspers NG, Lange K, Lathrop GM, Leppert M, Nakamura Y, O'Connell P, Paterson M, Salser W, Sanal O, Silver J, Sparkes RS, Susi E, Weeks DE, Wei S, White R, Yoder F (1988) Localization of an ataxia-telangiectasia gene to chromosome 11q22-23. Nature 336: 577–580.

Gatti RA, Boder E, Vinters HV, Sparkes RS, Norman A, Lange K (1991) Ataxia-telangiectasia: an interdisciplinary approach to pathogenesis. Medicine 70: 99–117.

Gatti RA, Lange E, Rotman G, Chen X, Uhrhammer N, Liang T, Chiplunkar S, Yang L, Udar N, Dandekar S, Sheikhavandi S, Wang Z, Yang HM, Polikow J, Elashoff M, Teletar M, Sanal O, Chessa L, McConville C, Taylor M, Shiloh Y, Porras O, Borresen A-L, Wegner R-D, Curry C, Gerken S, Lange K, Concannon P (1994) Genetic haplotyping of ataxia-telangiectasia families localizes the major gene to a 850 kb region on chromosome 11q23.1. Int J Rad Biol 66: S57–S62.

Gazulla J, Benavente I, Sarasa Barrio M (2006) Adult-onset ataxia-telangiectasia. A clinical and therapeutic observation. Neurologia 21: 447–451.

Gazulla J, Benavente I, Sarasa M (2007) New therapies for ataxia-telangiectasia. Arch Neurol 64: 607–608.

Geoffroy-Perez B, Janin N, Ossian K, Lauge A, Croquette MF, Griscelli C, Debre M, Bressac-de-Paillerets B, Aurias A, Stoppa-Lyonnet D, Andrieu N (2001) Cancer risk in heterozygotes for ataxia-telangiectasia. Int J Cancer 93: 288–293.

Gilad S, Bar-Shira A, Harnik R, Shkedy D, Ziv Y, Khosravi R, Brown K, Vanagaite L, Xu G, Frydman M, Lavin MF, Hill D, Tagle DA, Shiloh Y (1996) Ataxia-telangiectasia: founder effect among north African Jews. Hum Mol Genet 5: 2033–2037.

Gilad S, Chessa L, Khosravi R, Russel P, Galanty Y, Piane M, Gatti RA, Jorgensen TJ, Shiloh Y, Bar-Shira A (1998) Genotype-phenotype relationships in ataxia-telangiectasia (A-T) and A-T variants. Am J Hum Genet 62: 551–561.

Giovanetti A, Mazzetta F, Caprini E, Aiuti A, Marziali M, Pierdominici M, Cossarizza A, Chessa L, Quinti I,

Russo G, Fiorilli M (2002) The T cell receptor Vβ repertoire is restricted in ataxia-telangiectasia by skewed usage of variable genes, decreased thymic output and peripheral T cell expansion. Blood 100: 4082–4089.

Gomez MR (1987) Neurocutaneous diseases. A practical approach. Boston: Butterworths.

Gotoff SP, Amirmokri E, Liebner EJ (1967) Ataxia-telangiectasia. Neoplasia, untoward response to x-irradiation, and tuberous sclerosis. Am J Dis Child 114: 617–625.

Gueven N, Becherel OJ, Kijas AW, Chen P, Howe O, Rudolph JH, Gatti R, Date H, Onodera O, Taucher-Scholz G, Lavin MF (2004) Aprataxin, a novel protein that protects against genotoxic stress. Hum Mol Genet 13: 1081–1093.

Jabado N, Concannon P, Gatti RA (2000) Ataxia-telangiectasia. In: Klockgether T (ed.) Handbook of Ataxia Disorders. New York: Marcel Dekker, pp. 163–190.

Jablonski S (1969) Illustrated dictionary of eponymic syndromes and diseases and their synonyms, vol 35. Philadelphia: Saunders, pp. 191.

Johnson RD, Jasin M (2001) Double-strand-break-induced homologous recombination in mammalian cells. Biochem Soc Trans 29: 196–201.

Jozwiak S, Janniger CK (2006) Ataxia-telangiectasia. E-Medicine from the web. http://www.emedicine.com/derm/topic691.htm

Khan AO, Oystreck DT, Koenig M, Salih MA (2008) Ophthalmic features of ataxia telangiectasia-like disorder. J AAPOS 12: 186–189.

Laake K, Telatar M, Geitvik GA, Hansen RO, Heiberg A, Andresen AM, Gatti RA, Borresen-Dale A-L (1998) Identical mutation in 55% of the ATM alleles in 11 Norwegian AT families: evidence for a founder effect. Eur J Hum Genet 6: 235–244.

Lai CH, Chun HH, Nahas SA, Mitui M, Gamo KM, Du L, Gatti RA (2004) Correction of ATM gene function by aminoglycoside-induced read-through of premature termination codons. Proc Natl Acad Sci USA 101: 15676–15681.

Lange E, Borresen A-L, Chen X, Chessa L, Chiplunkar S, Concannon P, Dandekar S, Gerken S, Lange K, Liang T, Mc Conville C, Polakow J, Porras O, Rotman G, Sanal O, Sheikhavandi S, Shiloh Y, Sobel E, Taylor M, Teletar M, Teraoka S, Tolun A, Udar N, Uhrhammer N, Vanagaite L, Wang Z, Wapelhorst B, Wright J, Yang H-M, Yang L, Ziv Y, Gatti RA (1995) Localization of an ataxia-telangiectasia gene to ≈(500-kb interval on chromosome 11q23.1: linkage analysis of 176 families by an international consortium. Am J Hum Genet 57: 112–119.

Lavin MF, Shiloh Y (1997) The genetic defect in ataxia-telangiectasia. Annu Rev Immunol 15: 177–202.

Lefton-Greif MA, Crawford TO, Winkelstein JA, Lougblin GM, Korner CB, Zaburak M, Lederman HM (2000) Oropharyngeal dysphagia and aspiration in patients with ataxia-telangiectasia. J Pediatr 136: 225–231.

Leuzzi V, Elli R, Antonelli A, Chessa L, Cardona F, Marcucci L, Petrinelli P (1993) Neurological and cytogenetic study in early-onset ataxia-telangiectasia patients. Eur J Pediatr 152: 609–612.

Lewis RF, Lederman HM, Crawford TO (1999) Ocular motor abnormalities in Ataxia Telangiectasia. Ann Neurol 46: 287–295.

Liberzon E, Avigad S, Stark B, Zilberstein J, Freedman L, Gorfine M, Gavriel H, Cohen IJ, Goshen Y, Yaniv I, Zaizov R (2004) Germ-line ATM gene alterations are associated with susceptibility to sporadic T-cell acute lymphoblastic leukemia in children. Genes Chromosomes Cancer 39: 161–166.

Lin DD, Crawford TO, Lederman HM, Barker PB (2006) Proton MR spectroscopic imaging in ataxia-telangiectasia. Neuropediatrics 37: 241–246.

Louis-Bar D (1941) Sur un syndrome progressif comprenant des télangiectasies capillaries cutnées et conjonctivales symetrique naevoide et de troubles cerebellaux. Confin Neurol (Basel) 4: 432–442.

Martin L (1964) Aspect choreoathetosique du syndrome d'ataxie-telangiectasie. Acta Neurol Belg 64: 802–819.

McKinnon PJ (2004) ATM and ataxia telangiectasia. EMBO Rep 5: 772–776.

Miller VS (2004) Ataxia-telangiectasia. In: Roach ES, Miller VS (eds). Neurocutaneous disorders. New York: Cambridge University Press, pp. 112–116.

Moreira MC, Barbot C, Tachi N, Kozucha N, Uchida E, -Gibson T, Mendonca P, Costa M, Barros J, Yanagisawa T, Watanabe M, Ikeda Y, Aoki M, Nagata T, Coutinho P, Sequeiros J, Koenig M (2001) The gene mutated in ataxia-ocular apraxia 1 encodes the new HIT-Zn-finger protein aprataxin. Nat Genet 29: 189–193.

Moreira MC, Klur S, Watanabe M, Németh AH, Le Ber I, Moniz J-C, Tranchant C, Aubourg P, Tazir M, Schöls L, Pandolfo M, Schulz JB, Pouget J, Calvas P, Shizuka-Ikeda M, Shoji M, Tanaka M, Izatt L, Shaw CE, M'Zahem A, Dunne E, Bomont P, Benhassine T, Bouslam N, Stevanin G, Brice A, Guimarães J, Mendonça P, Barbot C, Coutinho P, Sequeiros J, Dürr A, Warter J-M, Koenig M (2004) Senataxin, the ortholog of a yeast RNA helicase, is mutant in ataxia-ocularapraxia 2. Nat Genet 36: 225–227.

Mosesso P, Piane M, Palitti F, Pepe G, Penna S, Chessa L (2005) The novel human gene Aprataxin is involved in the DNA Single Strand Break Repair Complex. Cell Mol Life Sci 62: 485–491.

Nowak R (1995) Discovery of AT gene sparks biomedical research bonanza. Science 23: 1700–1701.

Nowak-Wegrzyn A, Crawford TO, Winkelstein JA, Carson KA, Lederan HM (2004) Immunodeficiency and infections in ataxia-telangiectasia. J Pediatr 144: 505–511.

Olsen JH, Hahnemann JM, Borresen-Dale AL, Brondum-Nielsen K, Hammarstrom L, Kleinerman R, Kaariainen H, Lonnqvist T, Sankila R, Seersholm N, Tretli S, Yuen J, Boice JD Jr, Tucker M (2001) Cancer in patients with ataxia-telangiectasia and in their relatives in the nordic countries. J Natl Cancer Inst 93: 121–127.

Paller AS, Massey RB, Curtis MA, Pelachyk JM, Dombrowski HC, Leickly FE, Swift M (1991) Cutaneous granulomatous lesions in patients with ataxia-telangiectasia. J Pediatr 119: 917–922.

Peterson RD, Kelly WD, Good RA (1964) Ataxia-telangiectasia: its association with a defective thymus, immunologic-deficiency disease, and malignancy. Lancet 1: 1189–1193.

Petrini JH, Stracker TH (2003) The cellular response to DNA double-strand breaks: defining the sensors and mediators. Trends Cell Biol 13: 458–462.

Petrini JHJ (1999) The mammalian Mre11-Rad50-Nbs1 protein complex: integration of functions in the cellular DNA-damage response. Am J Hum Genet 64: 1264–1269.

Pitts SA, Kullar HS, Stankovic T, Stewart GS, Last JIK, Bedenham T, Armstrong SJ, Piane M, Chessa L, Taylor AMR, Byrd PJ (2001) hMRE11: genomic structure and a null mutation identified in a transcript protected from nonsense-mediated mRNA decay. Hum Molec Genet 10: 1155–1162.

Rasio D, Negrini M, Croce CM (1995) Genomic organization of the ATM locus involved in ataxia-telangiectasia. Cancer Res 55: 6053–6057.

Reliene R, Schiestl RH (2007) Antioxidants suppress lymphoma and increase longevity in atm-deficient mice. J Nutr 137: 229S–232S.

Renwick A, Thompson D, Seal S, Kelly P, Chagtai T, Ahmed M, North B, Jayatilake H, Barfoot R, Spanova A, McGuffog L, Evans DG, Eccles D, Easton DF, Stratton MR, The Breast Cancer Susceptibility Collaboration (UK), Rahman N (2006) ATM mutations that cause ataxia-telangiectasia are breast cancer susceptibility alleles. Nat Genet 38: 873–875.

Roach ES, Miller VS (2004) Neurocutaneous disorders. New York: Cambridge University Press.

Sardanelli F, Parodi RC, Ottonello C, Renzetti P, Saitta S, Lignana E, Mancardi GL (1995) Cranial MRI in ataxia-telangiectasia. Neuroradiology 37: 77–82.

Savitsky K, Bar-Shira A, Gilad S, Rotman G, Ziv Y, Vanagaite L, Tagle DA, Smith S, Uziel T, Sfez S, Ashkenazi M, Pecker I, Fridman M, Harnik R, Patanjali SR, Simmons A, Clines GA, Sartiel A, Gatti RA, Chessa L, Sanal O, Lavin MF, Jaspers NGJ, Taylor AMR, Arlett CF, Miki T, Weissman SM, Lovett M, Collins FS, Shiloh Y (1995) A single Ataxia Telangiectasia gene with a product similar to PI-3 kinase. Science 268: 1749–1753.

Saxon A, Stevens RH, Golde DW (1979a) T-cell leukemia in ataxia-telangiectasia. N Engl J Med 25: 945.

Saxon A, Stevens RH, Golde DW (1979b) Helper and suppressor t-lymphocyte leukemia in ataxia-telangiectasia. N Engl J Med 29: 700–704.

Scharnetzky M, Kohlschutter AK (1980) Computerised tomographic findings in a case of ataxia-telangiectasia (Louis-Bar syndrome). Neuropediatrics 11: 384–387.

Scott SP, Bendix R, Chen P, Clark R, Dork T, Lavin MF (2002) Missense mutations but not allelic variants alter the function of ATM by dominant interference in patients with breast cancer. Proc Natl Acad Sci USA 99: 925–930.

Sedgwick RP, Boder E (1960) Progressive ataxia in childhood with particular reference to ataxia-telangiectasia. Neurology 10: 705–715.

Sedgwick RP, Boder E (1972) Ataxia-telangiectasia. In: Vinken PJ, Bruyn GW (eds.) Handbook of clinical neurology, vol 14. Amsterdam: North Holland, pp. 267–339.

Sedgwick RP, Boder RE (1991) Ataxia-telangiectasia. In: Vianney De Jong JMB (ed.) Hereditary neuropathies and spinocerebellar atrophies. Amsterdam: Elsevier, pp. 347–423.

Shiloh Y (2003) ATM and related protein kinases: safeguarding genome integrity. Nat Rev Cancer 3: 155–168.

Shiloh Y, Andegeko Y, Tsarfaty I (2004) In search of drug treatment for genetic defects in the DNA damage response; the example of ataxia-telangiectasia. Semin Canc Biol 14: 295–305.

Sommer SS, Buzin CH, Jung M, Zheng J, Liu Q, Jeong SJ, Moulds J, Nguyen VQ, Feng J, Bennett WP, Dritschilo A (2002) Elevated frequency of ATM gene missense mutations in breast cancer relative to ethnically matched controls. Cancer Genet Cytogenet 134: 25–32.

Spring K, Ahangari F, Scott SP, Waring P, Purdie DM, Chen PC, Hourigan K, Ramsay J, McKinnon PJ, Swift M, Lavin MF (2002) Mice heterozygous for mutation in Atm, the gene involved in ataxia-telangiectasia, have heightened susceptibility to cancer. Nat Genet 32: 185–190.

Stankovic T, Kidd AM, Sutcliffe A, McGuire GM, Robinson P, Weber P, Bedenham T, Bradwell AR, Easton DF, Lennox GG, Haites N, Byrd PJ, Taylor AM (1998) ATM mutations and phenotypes in ataxia-telangiectasia families in the British Isles: expression of mutant ATM and the risk of leukemia, lymphoma, and breast cancer. Am J Hum Genet 62: 334–345.

Stewart GS, Maser RS, Stankovic T, Bressan DA, Kaplan MI, Jaspers NJ, Raams A, Byrd PJ, Petrini JH, Taylor AM (1999) The DNA double-strand break repair gene *hMre11* is mutated in individuals with an ataxia-telangiectasia-like-disorder. Cell 99: 477–486.

Stilgenbauer S, Schaffner C, Winkler D, Ott G, Leupolt E, Bentz M, Moller P, Muller-Hermelink HK, James MR, Lichter P, Dohner H (2000) The ATM gene in the pathogenesis of mantle-cell lymphoma. Ann Oncol 11(Suppl 1): 127–130.

Swift M (1985) Genetics and epidemiology of ataxia-telangiectasia. In: Gatti RA, Swift M (eds.) Ataxia-telangiectasia: genetics, neuropathology, and immunology of a degenerative disease of childhood. New York: Alan R Liss, pp. 133–144.

Stray-Pedersen A, Borresen-Dale AL, Paus E, Lindman CR, Burgers T, Abrahamsen TG (2007) Alpha fetoprotein is increasing with age in ataxia-telangiectasia. Eur J Paediatr Neurol May 29 [Epub ahead of print].

Subba Rao K (2007) Mechanisms of disease: DNA repair defects and neurological disease. Nat Clin Pract Neurol 3: 162–172.

Suraweera A, Becherel OJ, Chen P, Rundle N, Woods R, Nakamura J, Criscuolo C, Filla A, Chessa L, Gueven N, Lavin MF (2007) Senataxin defective in ataxia oculomotor apraxia type 2 is involved in the defence against oxidative DNA damage. J Cell Biol 18: 969–979.

Swift M, Morrell D, Massey RB, Chase CL (1991) Incidence of cancer in 161 families affected by ataxia-telangiectasia. N Engl J Med 325: 1831–1836.

Syllaba L, Henner K (1926) Contribution `a l'indépendance de l'athètose double idiopathique et congénitale. Rev Neurol (Paris) 1: 541–562.

Takagi M, Delia D, Chessa L, Iwata S, Shigeta T, Kanke Y, Goi K, Asada M, Eguchi M, Yamada T, Kodama C, Mizutani S (1998) Defective control of apoptosis, radiosensitivity and spindle checkpoints in Ataxia Telangiectasia. Cancer Res 51: 253–266.

Tavani F, Zimmerman RA, Berry GT, Sullivan K, Gatti RA, Blingham P (2003) Neuroradiology 45: 315–319.

Taylor AM, Groom A, Byrd PJ (2004) Ataxia-telangiectasia-like disorder (ATLD)-its clinical presentation and molecular basis. DNA Repair 3: 1219–1225.

Taylor AMR, Harnden DG, Arlett CF, Harcourt SA, Lehmann AR, Stevens S, Bridges BA (1975) Ataxia-telangiectasia: a human mutation with abnormal radiation sensitivity. Nature 258: 427–429.

Taylor AMR, Flude E, Laher B, Stacey M, McKay E, Watt J, Green SH, Harding AE (1987) Variant forms of ataxia telangiectasia. J Med Genet 24: 669–677.

Telatar M, Wang Z, Udar N, Liang T, Bernatowska-Matuszkiewicz E, Lavin M, Shiloh Y, Concannon P, Good RA, Gatti RA (1996) Ataxia-telangiectasia: mutations in ATM cDNA detected by protein-truncation screening. Am J Hum Genet 59: 40–44.

Telatar M, Teraoka S, Wang Z, Chun HH, Liang T, Castellvi-Bel S, Udar N, Borresen-Dale AL, Chessa L, Bernatowska-Matuszkiewicz E, Porras O, Watanabe M, Junker A, Concannon P, Gatti RA (1998) Ataxia-telangiectasia: identification and detection of founder-effect mutations in the ATM gene in ethnic populations. Am J Hum Genet 62: 86–97.

Teraoka SN, Malone KE, Doody DR, Suter NM, Ostrander EA, Daling JR, Concannon P (2001) Increased frequency of ATM mutations in breast carcinoma patients with early onset disease and positive family history. Cancer 92: 479–487.

Terplan KL, Krauss RF (1969) Histopathologic brain changes in association with ataxia-telangiectasia. Neurology 19: 446–454.

Thieffry S, Arthuis M, Aicardi J, Lyon G (1961) L'ataxie-telangiectasie. Rev Neurol (Paris) 105: 390–405.

Thorstenson YR, Roxas A, Kroiss R, Jenkins MA, Yu KM, Bachrich T, Muhr D, Wayne TL, Chu G, Davis RW, Wagner TM, Oefner PJ (2003) Contributions of ATM mutations to familial breast and ovarian cancer. Cancer Res 63: 3325–3333.

Valerie K, Povirk LF (2003) Regulation and mechanisms of mammalian double-strand break repair. Oncogene 22: 5792–5812.

Verlinsky Y, Rechitsky S, Sharapova T, Laziuk K, Barsky I, Verlinsky O, Tur-Kaspa I, Kuliev A (2007) Preimplantation diagnosis for immunodeficiencies. Reprod Biomed Online 14: 214–223.

Wallis LI, Griffiths PD, Ritchie SJ, Romanowski CA, Darwent G, Wilkinson ID (2007) Proton spectroscopy and imaging at 3T in ataxia-telangiectasia. AJNR 28: 79–83.

Wells CE, Shy GM (1957) Progressive familial choreoathetosis with cutaneous telangiectasia. J Neurol Neurosurg Psychiatr 20: 98–104.

Who named it? (2006) The world's most comprehensive dictionary of medical eponyms. http://www.whonamedit.com

Yamaguchi M, Yamamoto K, Miki T, Mizutani S, Miura O (2003) T-cell prolymphocytic leukemia with der(11)t(1;11)(q21;q23) and ATM deficiency. Cancer Genet Cytogenet 146: 22–26.

Yang Y, Herrup K (2005) Loss of neuronal cell cycle control in ataxia-telangiectasia: a unified disease mechanism. J Neurosci 25: 2522–2529.

Ying KL, Decoteau WE (1981) Cytogenetic anomalies in a patient with ataxia, immune deficiency, and high alpha-fetoprotein in the absence of telangiectasia. Cancer Genet Cytogenet 4: 311–317.

Zhang P, Dilley C, Mattson MP (2007) DNA damage responses in neural cells: focus on the telomere. Neuroscience Jan 3; epub ahead of print.

# Chapter 50

# NIJMEGEN BREAKAGE SYNDROME

Corry Weemaes and Luciana Chessa

Department of Paediatrics, Radboud University Nijmegen Medical Centre, Nijmegen, The Netherlands (CW);
Department of Experimental Pathology and Medicine, University "La Sapienza", Rome, Italy (LC)

## Introduction

Nijmegen Breakage syndrome (NBS) is a rare autosomal recessive condition characterized by microcephaly, typical face, short stature, chromosomal instability, immunodeficiency, X-ray hypersensitivity and predisposition to malignancies (Hiel et al. 2000, Weemaes et al. 1981). It is caused by mutations in the *NBS1* gene located in chromosome 8q21 (Varon et al. 1998) and belongs to the group of chromosomal instability/DNA repair disorders, together with Bloom syndrome (BS), Fanconi anemia (FA), ataxia-telangiectasia (A-T), and ataxia-telangiectasia-like disorder (ATLD).

## Historical perspective and eponyms

The NBS syndrome was first described by Weemaes et al. (1981). Three Czech families, with Seemanová syndrome (Seemanová et al. 1985), were later identified as having NBS.

Genetic complementation studies of Jaspers et al. (1988) noted a strong similarity between NBS cells and ataxia-telangiectasia (A-T) cells; however, they also described the NBS cells as genetically distinct from A-T, grouping individuals with either Nijmegen breakage syndrome or Czech breakage syndrome into A-T variant group 1 (V1). Germans with "*Berlin breakage syndrome*" (Wegner et al. 1999) were grouped into A-T complementation group V2 (Jaspers et al. 1988). Subsequently, *NBS1* mutations were found in all individuals studied from the V1 and V2 groups, indicating that these individuals had NBS, not ataxia-telangiectasia.

## Incidence and prevalence

Since the first description in 1981 (Weemaes et al. 1981) more than 150 patients have been recognized. The disease appears to be prevalent among the eastern/central European populations, in particular among the Czech and Polish people (Chrzanovska et al. 1995, Seemanová et al. 1985) but has been detected all over the world (Hiel et al. 2000).

## Clinical manifestations

### Microcephaly

Microcephaly (an head circumference/occipitofrontal circumference – OFC below the 3rd percentile) is the most constant sign of the disorder. It has been observed in all children. Most patients are born with a head circumference below the 3rd percentile (Fig. 1A, C), the remainder developing microcephaly during the first year (Hiel et al. 2000). The range of OFC at birth varied between 26.5 and 36.0 cm. Those children who were born with normal OFC develop progressive and severe microcephaly during the first months of life. No correlation was detected between head circumference at birth and mental development (Hiel et al. 2000, Varon et al. 2000).

### Psychomotor development and behavior

In general, developmental milestones are reached at expected time during the first year of life. Nor-

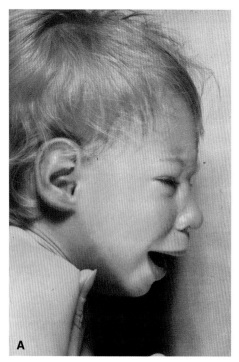

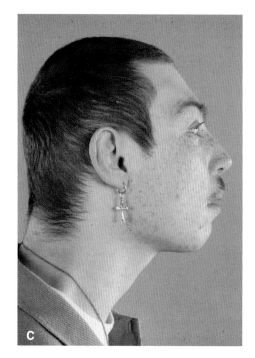

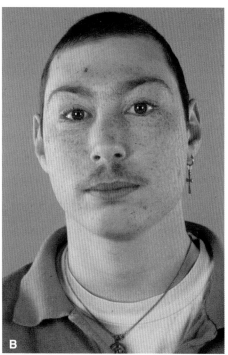

**Fig. 1.** Microcephaly in a child (**A**) and an adolescent (**B, C**) with NBS: note the typical distinctive facial appearance with the sloping forehead and receding mandible; prominent midface with a relatively long nose and long philtrum; upward slanting palpebral fissures accompanied by epicanthic folds; and the relatively large and dysplastic ears.

mal intelligence or mental retardation of various degree were both reported, but usually conclusions were made from a single evaluation. Longitudinal studies of Polish patients indicate decline of the intellectual function with age. The majority of children tested in infancy and pre-school age had IQ scores indicated a normal or borderline intelligence.

## Facial characteristics

All patients have a typical distinctive facial appearance, characterized by a sloping forehead and receding mandible, a prominent midface with a relatively long nose and long philtrum, upward slanting palpebral fissures in most, usually accompanied by epicanthic folds, and relatively large and dysplastic ears in some (Fig. 1A–C). The craniofacial characteristics become more obvious with age, probably because of progressive microcephaly (Fig. 1C). Subtle scleral telangiectasia is seen in some (Hiel et al. 2000).

## Growth retardation

After about a two-year period of distinct postnatal growth retardation, a slight improvement of growth rate (including body height and weight, but no head circumference) is usually observed. Most patients grow around the 3rd centile, some achieve 10th or even 25th percentile (Wegner et al. 2007).

## Sexual maturation

Long-term follow-up observation of a large group of Polish patients drew attention to poor development of secondary sex characteristics in NBS females, who reached pubertal age (lack of development of genital organs and breasts, primary amenorrhea). Endocrinology evaluation indicates for ovarian failure. The affected NBS females fail to reach sexual maturity due to hypergonadotropic hypogonadism. In males only a slight delay in onset of puberty may be observed. Offspring have never been reported, however, firm conclusions on fertility are hampered by the young age of the patients (Chrzanowska et al. 2000).

## Skin manifestations

Skin pigmentation abnormalities include *café-au-lait* spots (usually two to five, irregular in shape) and/or depigmented spots, which are present in about half of the patients (Fig. 2). In three Polish patients by the age of adolescence vitiligo has been observed, with progression with age (Figs. 3–4). Freckles on cheeks and nose are mentioned. Less frequently sun sensitivity of eyelids is observed, and occasionally cutaneous telangiectasia (particularly on the back) is seen. Multiple pigmented nevi and cavernous or flat hemangioma can also occur. Usually hair is thin in infants and toddlers, but later on improvement is observed. Gray hair appears by adolescence reflecting progeric changes. Cutaneous noncaseating granulomas have been recorded in NBS patients (Yoo et al. 2008).

## Recurrent infections

Most common are respiratory tract infections and sinusitis. Recurrent bronchopneumonia may result in bronchiectasis. Urinary and/or gastrointestinal tract infections are relatively frequent as well as otitis media. Opportunistic infections are very rare, just as in patients with ataxia-telangiectasia.

## Malignancies

Malignancy is the most common cause of death in patients with NBS. Based on available records an approximately 50-fold risk of early onset of cancer, and a greater than 1000-fold risk of lymphoma are estimated for patients with NBS (Wegner et al. 2007). Cancer was noted in 40% (22/55) patients (NBS registry in Nijmegen – Hiel et al. 2000). The great majority of malignancies are of lymphoid origin, and are developed before the age of 20 years (median age 9 years). Most frequent are non-Hodgkin's lymphomas (B-cell predominate over T-cell); lymphoblastic leukemia (ALL, both precursor B and T) and Hodgkin's disease have also been diagnosed (Hiel et al. 2000, Gladkowska-Dura et al. 2000). Other malignancies were glioma, meningioma, medulloblastoma, rhabdomyosarcoma, gonadoblastoma, Ewing sarcoma (Hiel et al. 2000, Van der Burgt et al. 1996, Wegner et al. 2007). Untill now, skin tumors have not been mentioned.

## Immunodeficiency

### Humoral immunity

The most frequently observed defects were combined deficit of IgG and IgA, followed by an iso-

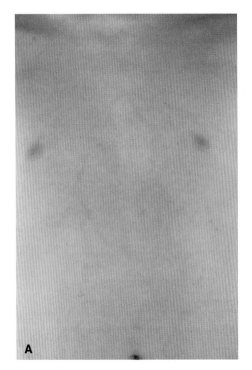

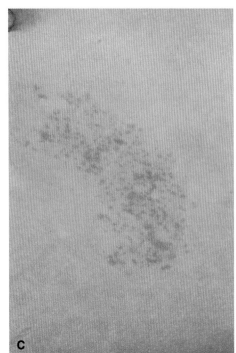

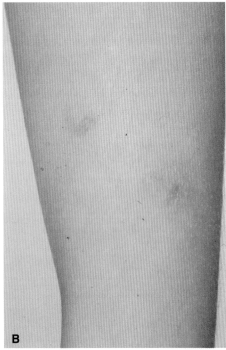

**Fig. 2.** Café-au-lait spots in the trunk (**A**) and upper limb (**B**) of a girl with NBS and vascular lesions in the abdomen (**C**) of an adolescent with NBS.

lated IgG deficiency (Hiel et al. 2000). The most characteristic feature of humoral disturbances was deficiency of one or more IgG subclasses found in all investigated Polish NBS patients. Even if total IgG levels were normal, selective deficiency of IgG4, and IgG2 were common (Gregorek et al. 2002). Levels of specific antibodies to pneumococcal polysaccharides were variable. In 9 of 17 patients hu-

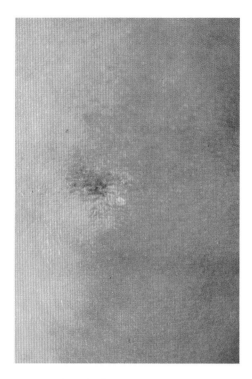

**Fig. 3.** Vitiligo-like lesions in the trunk in NBS.

moral immunodeficiency showed evident progression with time (Gregorek et al. 2002).

## Cell-mediated immunity

T-cell immunity was impaired in a great majority of NBS patients. The most commonly reported defects were mild to moderate lymphopenia, expressed as a low percentage of CD3+ T-cell population, a low proportion of CD4+ (helper) T-cell subset, and a decreased CD4+/CD8+ ratio (Hiel et al. 2000, Van der Burgt et al. 1996, Wegner et al. 1999). A deficiency of CD4/CD45RA+ ("naive") cells and an excess of CD4/CD45RO+ ("memory") cells has been observed in Polish patients (Michalkiewicz et al. 2003). A high number of NK (natural killer) cells was also noted.

## Other developmental anomalies

Minor skeletal defects as polydactyly clinodactyly of the 5th fingers and/or partial syndactyly of the 2nd/3rd toes have been encountered in about half of patients.

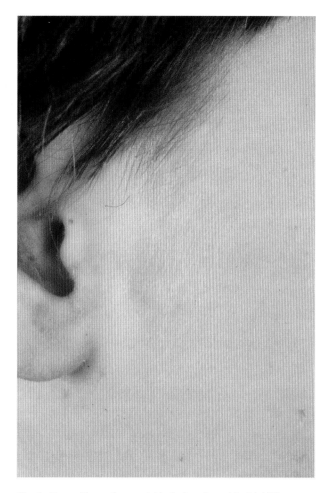

**Fig. 4.** Ear malformation and skin lesions in a girl with NBS.

Less common are anal atresia/stenosis, avarian dysgenesis, hydronephrosis and hip dysplasia (Hiel et al. 2000). Urogenital malformations (horshoe kidney, hypospadias, cryptorchismus) were noted several times. Among the other abnormalities tracheal hypoplasia, cleft lip/palate, choanal atresia, cardiovascular defect (PDA) were each reported once. Ultrasonographic examination revealed polysplenia in 20% of cases.

## Neuroimaging

Cranial MRI scan may reveal developmental abnormalities. Small brain size may be relatively frequently associated with other CNS developmental abnormalities, like corpus callosum agenesis, arachnoid

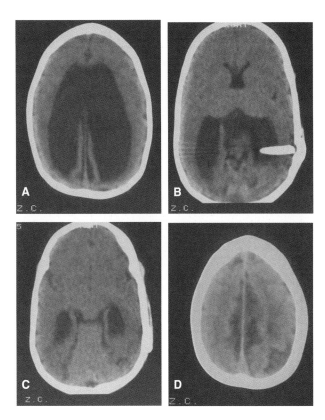

**Fig. 5.** Axial CT scan study in a child with NBS showing colpocephaly (**A**, **B**) with corpus callosum agenesis (**B**), high tentorium (**C**) and wide interhemispheric fissure (**D**).

cysts, neuronal migration disorder, and hydrocephaly. Studies of Polish NBS patients showed in all cases decreased size of the frontal lobes and narrow frontal hornes of the lateral ventricles; four of them also had partial agenesis of corpus callosum accompanied by colpocephaly and temporal horns dilatation (Bekiesinska-Figatowska et al. 2000, Chrzanowska et al. 2001). Of the four children with partial agenesis three suffered from epilepsy (Bekiesinska-Figatowska et al. 2000). Hydrocephalus, occipital cyst, schizencephaly and partial agenesis of corpus callosum were reported in other patients (Fig. 5).

## Natural history

Children with NBS generally have lower than normal birth weight and are small for gestational age. If not present from birth, microcephaly develops during the first months of life and progresses to severe microcephaly. Growth failure during the first two years of life results in height that is usually less than the third percentile by two years of age. The linear growth rate tends to be normal after two years of age, but individuals remain small for age. As microcephaly progresses, the facial features tend to become distinct, with sloping forehead, upslanting palpebral fissures, prominent midface, long nose, and small jaw. The ears may be large. Developmental milestones are attained at the usual time during the first year. Borderline delays in development and hyperactivity may be observed in early childhood. Intellectual abilities tend to decline over time and most children tested after the age of seven years have mild-to-moderate mental retardation. The children are described as having a cheerful, shy personality with good interpersonal skills. Respiratory infections are the most common. Recurrent pneumonia and bronchitis may result in pulmonary failure and early death. Chronic diarrhea and urinary tract infections may also occur.

According to Wegner et al. (2007), even more than 40% of the individuals reported to date have developed malignancies between the ages of one and 34 years. In the Polish Registry (83 patients) non-Hodgkin lymphomas were reported in 30 patients, (those of B cell origin slightly exceeded those of T cell origin), followed by lymphoblastic leukaemia/lymphoma in 8 patients (T-LBL/ALL, T-ALL, pre-B-ALL) and Hodgkin disease in 3 patients (Gladkowska-Dura et al. 2000). Several children have developed solid tumors, such as medulloblastomas, glioma, and rhabdomyosarcoma (Bakhshi et al. 2003, Distel et al. 2003, Hiel et al. 2001, Meyer et al. 2004). A second malignancy has developed in at least 7 patients.

Wegner et al. (2007) report a high incidence of premature ovarian failure in both prepubertal girls with NBS and adolescent and post-adolescent women with NBS, as evidenced by elevated serum concentration of gonadotrophins in both groups and primary amenorrhea and lack of secondary sexual development in the latter. Whether gonadal failure is part of the phenotype in males is not yet clear. Irregular skin pigmentation, manifested as hyperpigmented or hypopigmented irregular spots, is seen in most individuals. Congenital malformations, usually observed in single cases, include hydrocephalus, preaxial polydactyly, occipital cyst, choanal atresia, cleft lip and palate, tracheal hypoplasia, horseshoe kidney, hydronephrosis, hypospadias, anal stenosis/ atresia, and congenital hip dysplasia.

## Pathogenesis and molecular genetics

Cells from NBS patients were reported to display hypersensitivity to ionizing radiations and abnormal cell cycle checkpoints (Shiloh 1997). These cellular phenotypes are identical to those seen in ataxia-telangiectasia (A-T), which is caused by mutations in ATM, and in AT-like disease (AT-LD), caused by mutations in MRE11.

The mapping and positional cloning of a gene for NBS, called *NBS1*, clearly indicates that it is distinct from AT and AT-LD (Matsuura et al. 1997, Saar et al. 1997) (Fig. 6). *NBS1* is the only gene known to be associated with Nijmegen breakage syndrome. The *NBS1* gene contains 16 exons encompassing a genomic sequence of more than 48,979 bp on chromosome 8q21 (Tauchi 2000) (Fig. 6). The human *NBS1* gene is transcribed as two mRNAs of 2.6 and 4.8 kb, which differ in the lengths of their

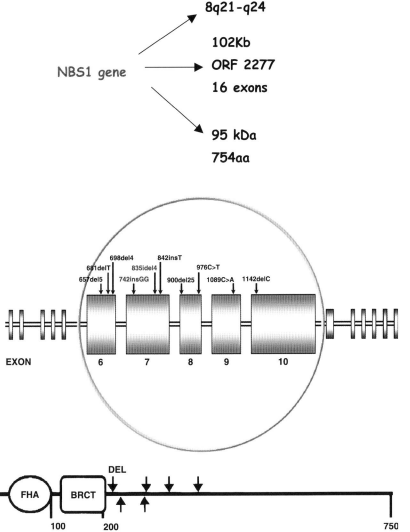

**Fig. 6.** Molecular structure of *nibrin*: the NBS protein. The protein has an FHA (fork head associated) domain, which is usually present in all transcription factors, and a BRCT (Brest Cancer Carboxyl-terminal) domain in the N-terminal position. The main function of either domain is still unclear however these domains have been observed in several protein involved in DNA repair and in the cell cycle control (modified from Varon et al. 1998 and from http://nijmegenbreakagesyndrome.net).

3′-untranslated regions. Both transcripts contain a single open reading frame coding for an ubiquitous protein, called nibrin or p95, which consists of 754 amino acids and has a predicted molecular weight of 85 kd. Nibrin shows three functional regions: the N-terminus (amino acids 1–183), a central region (amino acids 278–343) and the C-terminus (amino acids 665–693) (D'Amours and Jackson 2002, Tauchi et al. 2001). The N-terminal region includes a fork head-associated (FHA) domain and a BRCA1 C-terminus (BRCT) domain. FHA and BRCT domains are often found in eukaryotic nuclear proteins that are involved in cell-cycle checkpoints or DNA repair (Fig. 6). The C-terminal region of NBS1 binds to the MRE11/RAD50 complex.

Cells derived from NBS patients also exhibit decreased homologous recombination (Tauchi et al. 2002), accelerated shortening of telomeres (Ranganathan et al. 2001), and disruption of the G1-, G2-, and intra-S-phase checkpoints after irradiation (Buscemi et al. 2001, Shiloh 1997), phenotypes all indicating a critical role of *NBS1* in maintaining genomic stability. In fact, nibrin forms a complex with RAD50 and MRE11 (D'Amours and Jackson 2002), the so-called R/M/N complex, which is supposed to be the first sensor of DNA double strand breaks damage.

All disease-causing *NBS1* mutations identified to date are predicted to result in the truncation of the protein. The predominant mutation is the 657del5, which accounts for more than 90% of all mutant alleles in NBS and is characteristic of all the patients of Slavic origin, with a well defined founder effect (Cerosaletti et al. 1998). Each of the other mutations occurs in one or a small number of families and are clustered in the region from exon 6 to exon 10 (Fig. 6). There are no known phenotype-genotype correlations. A number of polymorphisms and rare variants in the *NBS1* gene have been described; some of them have been reported in various cancer cases and controls. Alleles at these sites are all in very strong linkage disequilibrium in the general population.

*NBS1* mRNA is always detectable in cell lines from individuals with NBS, but full-length nibrin is not detectable by Western blotting. Although some *NBS1* alleles produce residual levels of protein, this is not functional.

## Diagnosis

When a possible diagnosis of NBS is suspected, the following tests must be performed:

- *Karyotype analysis*: inversions and translocations involving chromosomes 7 and 14 are observed in PHA-stimulated lymphocytes in 10–50% of metaphases in NBS cells. The breakpoints most commonly involved are 7p13, 7q35, 14q11, and 14q32, where the loci for immunoglobulin and T cell-receptor genes are mapped.
- *Radiosensitivity*: following exposure to ionizing radiation and radiomimetics in vitro, the NBS cells show a decrease of colony-forming ability and an increase in the rate of chromosomal breakage.
- *Western blotting*: this test is used to determine if the protein is present or absent; a lymphoblastoid cell line established from the patient is routinely used.

The definitive diagnosis requires the demonstration of disease-causing mutations in the *NBS1* gene. All the patients from Poland, the Czech Republic, and the Ukraine tested to date are homozygous for the common mutation 657del5. In the other countries, about 70% of individuals tested to date are homozygous for the common mutation, 15% are homozygous for a different mutation, and 15% are compound heterozygous for 657del5 and a second mutation.

Diagnostic testing can be performed on a single sample of heparinized blood. First, the presence of the 657del5 mutation is determined; if the common mutation is not found, immunoblotting to evaluate the levels of nibrin and radiosensitivity tests are per-

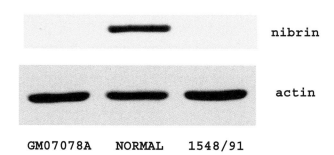

**Fig. 7.** Levels of nibrin in two NBS cellular lines.

formed. If all the three tests are normal, the diagnosis of NBS is extremely unlikely.

## Differential diagnosis

Recurrent infections, poor growth, and immunodeficiency can be observed in other inherited immunodeficiencies. Some inherited immunodeficiencies (e.g., X-linked agamma globulinemia (Bruton's agammaglobulinemia) and X-linked severe combined immunodeficiency) also demonstrate radiosensitivity (in colony survival assays).

Individuals homozygous for the 1089C > A mutation in the *NBS1* gene share features of Fanconi anemia (Gennery et al. 2004).

Occasionally individuals with the *ATM* gene mutation A-T$_{Fresno}$ have symptoms of both NBS and ataxia-telangiectasia (A-T) (Curry et al. 1989, Gilad et al. 1998).

Microcephaly, midface prominence, and mental retardation suggest syndromes such as Seckel syndrome (O'Driscoll et al. 2003) and Rubinstein-Taybi syndrome; however, cells from these individuals are not typically radiosensitive by colony survival assay (unpublished). Seeman et al. (2004) suggest that *NBS1* mutations account for a significant number of children with primary microcephaly in the Czech Republic. Other forms of autosomal recessive microcephaly have been linked chromosomes 9q, 8p, and 19q (Moynihan et al. 2000).

Individuals with ligase IV syndrome (O'Driscoll et al. 2001) may present with features of NBS, including microcephaly, short stature, midface prominence, immunodeficiency, and radiosensitivity. However, the immunodeficiency (pancytopenia) in individuals with ligase IV syndrome is typically more severe than in individuals with NBS. Ligase IV syndrome, caused by mutations in *LIG4*, is not associated with an increase in chromosomal instability or t(7; 14). The two disorders can be differentiated by molecular genetic testing of the *LIG4* and *NBS1* genes.

The early growth failure in NBS may suggest other disorders of growth, such as thyroid hormone or growth hormone deficiency, or primary disorders of bone growth (i.e., a skeletal dysplasia).

**Table 1.** Main phenotypic differences between ataxia-telangiectasia (A-T), Nijmegen breakage syndrome (NBS) and ataxia-telangiectasia like disorders (ATLD)

| Clinical phenotype | A-T | NBS | ATLD |
|---|---|---|---|
| Progressive cerebellar ataxia | + | − | |
| Oculomotor apraxia | + | − | + |
| Neurologic abnormalities | − | + | − |
| Neuron degenerations | + | − | + |
| Cancer proneness | + | + | nd |
| Immunodeficiency | + | + | − |
| Telangiectasias | + | − | − |
| Cellular phenotype | | | |
| Radiosensitivity | + | + | + |
| Chromosomal fragility | + | + | + |
| Radioresistent DNA synthesis | + | + | + |
| p53 Accumulation | − | + | + |

Because lymphoma may be the presenting finding in NBS, the diagnosis of NBS should be considered before radiotherapy is initiated in individuals with lymphoma who are younger than three years of age (Bakhshi et al. 2003, Distel et al. 2003, Meyer et al. 2004).

## Management, follow-up and treatment

Because of chromosomal instability, Vitamin E and folic acid supplementation in doses appropriate for body weight is recommended.

No treatment for NBS is known. In individuals with severe humoral immunodeficiency and frequent infections, IVIg should be considered.

- Periodic follow-up to monitor mental and physical growth and frequent infections is indicated.
- Weight loss may signal the presence of a malignancy.

## References

Bakhshi S, Cerosaletti KM, Concannon P, Bawle EV, Fontanesi J, Gatti RA, Bhambhani K (2003) Medulloblastoma with adverse reaction to radiation therapy in Nijmegen breakage syndrome. J Pediatr Hematol Oncol 25: 248–251.

Bekiesinska-Figatowska M, Chrzanowska KH, Sikorska J, Walecki J, Krajewska-Walasek M, Jóźwiak S, Kleijer WJ (2000) Cranial MRI in the Nijmegen breakage syndrome. Neuroradiology 42: 43–47.

Buscemi G, Savio C, Zannini L, Miccichè F, Masnada D, Nakanishi M, Tauchi H, Komatsu K, Mizutani S, Khanna KK, Chen P, Concannon P, Chessa L, Delia D (2001) Chk2 activation dependance on Nbs1 after DNA damage. Molec Cell Biol 21: 5214–5222.

Carney JP, Maser RS, Olivares H, Davis EM, Le Beau M, Yates JR 3rd, Hays L, Morgan WF, Petrini JH (1998) The hMre11/hRad50 protein complex and Nijmegen breakage syndrome: linkage of double-strand break repair to the cellular DNA damage response. Cell 93: 477–486.

Cerosaletti KM, Lange E, Stringham HM, Weemaes C, Smeets D, Solder B, Belohradsky BH, Taylor AM, Karnes P, Elliott A, Komatsu K, Gatti RA, Boehnke M, Concannon P (1998) Fine localization of the Nijmegen breakage syndrome gene to 8q21: evidence for a common founder haplotype. Am J Hum Genet 63: 125–134.

Chrzanowska KH, Kleijer WJ, Krajewska-Walasek M, Białecka M, Gutkowska A., Goryluk-Kozakiewicz B, Michałkiewicz J, Stachowski J, Gregorek H, Łysoń-Wojciechowska G, Janowicz W, Jóźwiak S (1995) Eleven polish patients with microcephaly, immunodeficiency, and chromosomal instability: the Nijmegen breakage syndrome. Am J Med Genet 57: 462–471.

Chrzanowska KH, Romer T, Krajewska-Walasek M, Gajtko-Metera M, Szarras-Czapnik M, Abramczuk D, Varon R, Rysiewski H, Janas R, Syczewska M (2000) Evidence for a high rate of gonadal failure in female patients with Nijmegen breakage syndrome. Eur J Hum Genet 8(Suppl 1): 73.

Chrzanowska KH, Stumm M, Bekiesińska-Figatowska M, Varon R, Białecka M, Gregorek H, Michałkiewicz J, Krajewsa-Walasek M, Jóźwiak S, Reis A (2001) Atypical clinical picture of the Nijmegen breakage syndrome associated with developmental abnormalities of brain. J Med Genet 38: e3.

Curry CJ, O'Lague P, Tsai J, Hutchison HT, Jaspers NG, Wara D, Gatti RA (1989) ATFresno: a phenotype linking ataxia-telangiectasia with the Nijmegen breakage syndrome. Am J Hum Genet 45: 270–275.

Cybulski C, Gorski B, Debniak T, Gliniewicz B, Mierzejewski M, Masojc B, Jakubowska A, Matyjasik J, Zlowocka E, Sikorski A, Narod SA, Lubinski J (2004) NBS1 is a prostate cancer susceptibility gene. Cancer Res 64: 1215–1219.

D'Amours D, Jackson SP (2002) The Mre11 complex: at the crossroad of DNA repair and checkpoint signaling. Nat Rev Mol Cell Biol 3: 317–327.

Distel L, Neubauer S, Varon R, Holter W, Grabenbauer G (2003) Fatal toxicity following radio- and chemotherapy of medulloblastoma in a child with unrecognized Nijmegen breakage syndrome. Med Pediatr Oncol 41: 44–48.

Falck J, Coates J, Jackson SP (2005) Conserved modes of recruitment of ATM, ATR and DNA-PKcs to sites of DNA damage. Nature 434: 605–611.

Gennery AR, Slatter MA, Bhattacharya A, Barge D, Haigh S, O'Driscoll M, Coleman R, Abinun M, Flood TJ, Cant AJ, Jeggo PA (2004) The clinical and biological overlap between Nijmegen breakage syndrome and Fanconi anemia. Clin Immunol 113: 214–219.

Gilad S, Chessa L, Khosravi R, Russell P, Galanty Y, Piane M, Gatti RA, Jorgensen TJ, Shiloh Y, Bar-Shira A (1998) Genotype-phenotype relationships in ataxia-telangiectasia and variants. Am J Hum Genet 62: 551–561.

Gładkowska-Dura M, Chrzanowska KH, Dura WT (2000) Malignant lymphoma in Nijmegen breakage syndrome. Ann Pediatr Pathol 4: 39–46.

Gregorek H, Chrzanovska KH, Michalkiewicz J, Syczewska M, Madalinski K (2002) Heterogeneity of humoral immune abnormalities in children with Nijmegen breakage syndrome: an 8-year follow-up study in a single centre. Clin Exp Immunol 130: 219–324.

Hiel JA, Weemaes CM, van den Heuvel LP (The International Nijmegen Breakage Syndrome Study Group) (2000) Nijmegen Breakage Syndrome. Arch Dis Child 82: 400–406.

Hiel JA, Weemaes CM, van Engelen BG, Smeets D, Ligtenberg M, van Der Burgt I, van Den Heuvel LP, Cerosaletti KM, Gabreels FJ, Concannon P (2001) Nijmegen breakage syndrome in a Dutch patient not resulting from a defect in NBS1. J Med Genet 38: E19.

Jaspers NG, Gatti RA, Baan C, Linssen PC, Bootsma D (1988) Genetic complementation analysis of ataxia telangiectasia and Nijmegen breakage syndrome: a survey of 50 patients. Cytogenet Cell Genet 49: 259–263.

Maser RS, Zinkel R, Petrini JH (2001) An alternative mode of translation permits production of a variant NBS1 protein from the common Nijmegen breakage syndrome allele. Nat Genet 27: 417–421.

Matsuura S, Weemaes C, Smeets D, Takami H, Kondo N, Sakamoto S, Yano N, Nakamura A, Tauchi H, Endo S, Oshimura M, Komatsu K (1997) Genetic mapping using microcell-mediated chromosome transfer suggests a locus for Nijmegen breakage syndrome at chromosome 8q21-24. Am J Hum Genet 60: 1487–1494.

Matsuura S, Kobayashi J, Tauchi H, Komatsu K (2004) Nijmegen breakage syndrome and DNA double strand break repair by NBS1 complex. Adv Biophys 38: 65–80.

Meyer S, Kingston H, Taylor AM, Byrd PJ, Last JI, Brennan BM, Trueman S, Kelsey A, Taylor GM, Eden OB

(2004) Rhabdomyosarcoma in Nijmegen breakage syndrome: strong association with perianal primary site. Cancer Genet Cytogenet 154: 169–174.

Michalkiewicz J, Barth C, Chrzanovska K, Gregorek H, Sysczewska M, Weemaes CMR, Madalinski K, Dzierzanowska D, Stachowski J (2003) Abnormalities in the T and NK lymphocyte phenotype in patients with Nijmegen breakage syndrome. Clin Exp Immunol 134: 482–490.

Michallet AS, Lesca G, Radford-Weiss I, Delarue R, Varet B, Buzyn A (2003) T-cell prolymphocytic leukemia with autoimmune manifestations in Nijmegen breakage syndrome. Ann Hematol 82: 515–517.

Moynihan L, Jackson AP, Roberts E, Karbani G, Lewis I, Corry P, Turner G, Mueller RF, Lench NJ, Woods CG (2000) A third novel locus for primary autosomal recessive microcephaly maps to chromosome 9q34. Am J Hum Genet 66: 724–727.

New HV, Cale CM, Tischkowitz M, Jones A, Telfer P, Veys P, D'Andrea A, Mathew CG, Hann I (2005) Nijmegen breakage syndrome diagnosed as Fanconi anaemia. Pediatr Blood Cancer 44: 494–499.

O'Driscoll M, Cerosaletti KM, Girard PM, Dai Y, Stumm M, Kysela B, Hirsch B, Gennery A, Palmer SE, Seidel J, Gatti RA, Varon R, Oettinger MA, Neitzel H, Jeggo PA, Concannon P (2001) DNA ligase IV mutations identified in patients exhibiting developmental delay and immunodeficiency. Mol Cell 8: 1175–1185.

O'Driscoll M, Ruiz-Perez VL, Woods CG, Jeggo PA, Goodship JA (2003) A splicing mutation affecting expression of ataxia-telangiectasia and Rad3-related protein (ATR) results in Seckel syndrome. Nat Genet 33: 497–501.

Ranganathan V, Heine WF, Ciccone DN, Rudolph KL, Wu X, Chang S, Hai H, Ahearn IM, Livingston DM, Resnick I, Rosen F, Seemanova E, Jarolim P, DePinho RA, Weaver DT (2001) Rescue of a telomere length defect of Nijmegen breakage syndrome cells requires NBS and telomerase catalytic subunit. Curr Biol 11: 962–966.

Saar K, Chrzanovska KH, Stumm M, Jung M, Numberg G, Wienker TF, Seemanová E, Wegner RD, Reis A, Sperling K (1997) The gene for the ataxia-telangiectasia variant, Nijmegen breakage syndrome, maps to a 1-cM interval on chromosome 8q21. Am J Hum Genet 60: 605–610.

Seeman P, Gebertova K, Paderova K, Sperling K, Seemanova E (2004) Nijmegen breakage syndrome in 13% of age-matched Czech children with primary microcephaly. Pediatr Neurol 30: 195–200.

Seemanová E, Passarge E, Beneskova D, Houstek J, Kasal P, Sevcikova M (1985) Familial microcephaly with normal intelligence, immunodeficiency, and risk for lymphoreticular malignacies: a new autosomal recessive disorder. Am J Med Genet 20: 639–648.

Shiloh Y (1997) Ataxia telangiectasia and the Nijmegen breakage syndrome: related disorders but genes apart. Annu Rev Genet 31: 635–662.

Steffen J, Varon R, Mosor M, Maneva G, Maurer M, Stumm M, Nowakowska D, Rubach M, Kosakowska E, Ruka W, Nowecki Z, Rutkowski P, Demkow T, Sadowska M, Bidzinski M, Gawrychowski K, Sperling K (2004) Increased cancer risk of heterozygotes with NBS1 germline mutations in Poland. Int J Cancer 111: 67–71.

Tauchi H (2000) Positional cloning and functional analysis of the gene for Nijmegen breakage syndrome, *NBS1*. J Radiat Res 41: 9–17.

Tauchi H, Kobayashi J, Morishima K, Matsuura S, Nakamura A, Shiraishi T, Ito E, Masnada D, Delia D, Komatsu K (2001) The Forkhead-associated domain of NBS1 is essential for nuclear foci formation after irradiation, but not essential for hRAD50/hMRE/NBS1 complex DNA repair activity. J Biol Chem 276: 12–15.

Tauchi H, Kobayashi J, Morishima K, van Gent D, Shiraishi T, Verkaik NS, van Heems D, Ito E, Nakamura A, Sonoda E, Takata M, Takeda S, Matsuura S, Komatsu K (2002) Nbs1 is essential for DNA repair by homologous recombination in higher vertebrate cells. Nature 420: 93–98.

Van der Burgt I, Chrzanowska KH, Smeets D, Weemaes C (1996) Nijmegen breakage syndrome. *Syndrome of the month*. J Med Genet 33: 153–156.

Varon R, Vissinga C, Platzer M, Cerosaletti KM, Chrzanowska KH, Saar K, Beckmann G, Seemanova E, Cooper PR, Nowak NJ, Stumm M, Weemaes CRM, Gatti RA, Wilson RK, Digweed M, Rosenthal A, Sperling K, Concannon P, Reis A (1998) Nibrin, a novel DNA double-strand break repair protein, is mutated in Nijmegen breakage syndrome. Cell 93: 467–476.

Varon R, Seemanová E, Chrzanowska KH, Hnateyko O, Piekutowska-Abramczuk D, Krajewska-Walasek M, Sykut-Cegielska J, Sperling K, Reis A (2000) Clinical ascertainment of Nijmegen breakage syndrome (NBS) and prevalence of the major mutation, 657del5, in three Slav populations. Eur J Hum Genet 8: 900–902.

Weemaes CMR, Hustinx TWJ, Scheres JMJC, van Munster PJJ, Bakkeren JAJM, Taalman RDFM (1981) A new chromosomal instability disorder: the Nijmegen breakage syndrome. Acta Paediatr Scand 70: 557–564.

Wegner R-D, German JJ, Chrzanowska K, Digweed M, Sperling K (2007) Chromosomal instability syndromes other than ataxia telangiectasia. In: Ochs HD, Smith CIE, Puck JM (eds.) Primary immunodeficiency diseases. A molecular and genetic approach, 2nd ed, New York: Oxford University Press, pp. 427–453.

Yoo J, Wolgamot G, Torgerson TR, Sidbury R (2008) Cutaneous noncaseating granulomas associated with Nijmegen breakage syndrome. Arch Dermatol 144: 418–419.

# Chapter 51

# XERODERMA PIGMENTOSUM

**Miria Stefanini and Kenneth H. Kraemer**

Institute of Molecular Genetics, National Research Council of Italy, Pavia, Italy (MS);
Basic Research Laboratory, National Cancer Institute, Bethesda, MD, USA (KHK)

## Introduction

Xeroderma pigmentosum (XP) is an autosomal recessive disease characterized by sun sensitivity, photophobia, early onset of freckling, and subsequent neoplastic changes on sun-exposed surfaces.

Approximately half of the patients with XP have a history of acute sun sensitivity from early infancy, acquiring severe sunburn with blistering or persistent erythema on minimal sun exposure. The other patients give a history of normal tanning without excessive burning. In all patients, numerous freckle-like hyperpigmented macules appear on sun-exposed skin. Repeated sun exposure results in dry and parchment-like skin with increased pigmentation, hence the name xeroderma pigmentosum ("dry pigmented skin"). If not protected from sunlight, XP patients develop skin cancer, predominantly basal and squamous cell carcinomas and melanomas. The dramatic correlation between photosensitivity and cutaneous carcinogenesis in XP is apparent from the study of Kraemer et al. (1987), who evaluated clinical abnormalities in XP by abstracting published descriptions of 830 patients in articles obtained from a survey of the medical literature from 1874 to 1982. Among XP patients under 20 years of age, the frequencies of melanoma and of basal cell carcinoma or squamous cell carcinoma of the skin appeared to be more than 1000-fold greater than those observed for the United States (US) general population. The authors estimated that the median age of onset of cutaneous symptoms in XP was between one and two years, the median age of onset of the first skin neoplasm was eight years for basal and squamous cell carcinoma, nearly 50 years earlier than that of the US general population, and 19 years for malignant melanoma. This attests to the value of DNA repair processes in protecting people against skin cancer.

Ocular abnormalities are almost as common as the cutaneous abnormalities, but they are strikingly limited to the structures of the anterior portion of the eye (lids, cornea, and conjunctiva), that is the area exposed to sunlight. Photophobia is often present and may be associated with prominent conjunctival injection. Continued sunlight exposure may result in severe keratitis, leading to corneal opacification and vascularization, and in neoplasms (epithelioma, squamous cell carcinoma, and melanoma). In XP patients there is also a greatly increased frequency of cancer of the oral cavity, particularly squamous cell carcinoma of the tip of the tongue, a presumed sun-exposed area. There is a smaller increase in internal tumors including neoplasms of the nervous system (astrocytoma of the brain or spinal cord, Schwannoma of the face).

About 20% of XP patients have neurologic manifestations, including acquired microcephaly, diminished or absent deep tendon stretch reflexes, progressive sensorineural hearing loss, and progressive cognitive impairment. The onset may be early in infancy or delayed until the second decade.

Since 1968, when Cleaver first described that cultured skin fibroblasts from XP patients were defective in the repair of DNA damage induced by ultraviolet (UV) light, our knowledge on the genetic and molecular basis of this disorder has been incredibly expanded. Now we know that most XP cases are defective in one of seven genes (called *XPA* to *XPG*) whose products are involved in nucleotide excision repair (NER), a repair system that removes UV-induced lesions and other types of damage from DNA. In about 25% of cases, the so-called XP variant form, the defect is in an eighth gene, DNA polymerase eta, whose product is required for replicating UV-damaged DNA, through a DNA damage tolerance pathway called translesion DNA synthesis (TLS) (Masutani et al. 1999, Johnson et al. 1999).

In recent years, the genes for most forms of XP have been cloned, opening up the possibility of sequencing the responsible gene in XP patients. DNA repair investigations in XP enable clinicians to establish correct and early diagnoses of new patients, which is essential for proper genetic counseling of the families involved.

## Historical perspective and terminology (eponyms, etc.)

Xeroderma pigmentosum was first described by Moriz Kaposi, born Moriz Kohn on 1837 in Kaposvár (Hungary). He died on 1902 in Vienna (Austria). Kaposi changed his name (alluding to the Kapos River in Hungary) when he moved to Vienna and married the daughter of the professor of dermatology, Ferdinand von Hebra. Hebra and Kaposi wrote the first textbook of dermatology which was translated into English in 1874 and in which Kaposi described XP.

As detailed in the review of Kraemer et al. (1987), in which most of the papers relevant for the history of XP are referenced, XP with neurologic abnormalities was first reported in 1883 by Albert Neisser, who described two sibs showing cutaneous abnormalities typical of XP in association with progressive neurologic degeneration beginning in the second decade. Neurologic involvement in XP was emphasized in 1932 by the Italian physicians Carlo De Sanctis and Aldo Cacchione, who reported a condition, which they called "xerodermic idiocy", in three brothers with XP who had mental retardation, progressive neurologic deterioration, dwarfism, and gonadal hypoplasia. Subsequently, an XP patient with any neurologic abnormality was considered affected by the De Sanctis–Cacchione syndrome. With clarification of the spectrum of XP disease, this term is now reserved for XP with progressive and severe mental deterioration, microcephaly, markedly re-

tarded growth leading to dwarfism, and immature sexual development. The complete De Sanctis–Cacchione syndrome has been recognized in very few cases, although many XP patients have one or more of its neurologic features.

In 1968, the pathophysiology of XP was elucidated by James Cleaver, who reported that cultured skin fibroblasts from three patients were unable to repair normally lesions induced in their DNA by UV radiation, as a consequence of a failure of nucleotide excision repair (NER). Soon thereafter, this excision repair defect was demonstrated *in vivo* in patients' epidermal cells (Epstein et al. 1970). These exciting findings suggested that the DNA repair defect present in XP patients might cause their clinical abnormalities, particularly their malignancies, through somatic mutations resulting from their unrepaired UV-damaged DNA.

In 1970, Jung described two XP patients with manifestations after 30 years of age, whose cells were completely normal in excision repair but had an uncharacterized deficiency in DNA synthesis after UV-irradiation. The term "pigmented xerodermoid" was coined to define this condition similar to XP but characterized by a significantly later onset, generally milder symptoms, a protracted course of the disease, and normal excision repair (Jung and Bantle 1971). One year later, Burk et al. (1971a, b) reported a patient who also was excision repair proficient but with clinically severe XP symptoms. This new class of XP patients was designated "XP variant" (XP-V). Cases of pigmented xerodermoid and of XP-V were reported for almost a decade (Cleaver 1972; Robbins and Burk 1973; Robbins et al. 1972, 1975; Kleijer et al. 1973; Hofmann et al. 1978). In 1975, Lehmann et al. described striking differences between XP-V and normal cells on examination of the size of DNA newly synthesized in UV-irradiated cells. XP-V cells failed to convert newly synthesized DNA from low to high molecular weight after UV irradiation. In particular, the time taken for the newly synthesized DNA to attain a high molecular weight similar to that in unirradiated controls was much longer than in normal cells. This conversion of low- to high-molecular weight DNA was drastically inhibited by caffeine, which had very little effect in normal cells.

The interpretation attributed to these observations was that XP-V cells were defective in postreplication repair, a pathway operating during the S phase of cell cycle, that allows progression of DNA replication in the presence of replication-blocking lesions (Lehman et al. 1975). In 1980, Cleaver et al. showed that the defects in cells of pigmented xerodermoid and XP-V patients are indistinguishable as based on an extensive analysis of repair and replication. Consequently, the term pigmented xerodermoid was announced to be redundant (Fisher et al. 1980). For a long time, it was suspected that the gene mutated in XP-V could encode a protein required for replicating UV-damaged DNA. Finally in 1999, Masutani et al. (1999) and Johnson et al. (1999) succeeded in isolating a human homologue of the yeast Rad30 protein, called DNA polymerase eta, that was able to continue replication on damaged DNA by bypassing UV-induced thymine dimers in XP-V cell extracts. These authors unequivocally demonstrated that DNA polymerase eta is the gene responsible for XP-V by showing that mutations in DNA polymerase eta gene were present in XP-V patients. Recombinant human DNA polymerase eta corrected the inability of XP-V cell extracts to carry out DNA replication by bypassing thymine dimers on damaged DNA (Masutani et al. 1999).

Coming back to the excision-repair deficient form of XP, during the 5 years following Cleaver's discovery, progress on the NER defective form of XP went relatively rapidly. DNA repair investigations performed in fibroblast strains from approximately 60 patients suggested the presence of genetic heterogeneity in the NER defective form of XP by showing different degrees in the severity of clinical symptoms and in the residual repair activity among patients. The first demonstration of genetic heterogeneity in the NER defective form of XP was attained by de Weerd-Kastelein et al. (1972), by combining somatic cell hybridization procedures with analysis of UV-induced DNA repair synthesis (UDS) at the single cell level. These authors measured the level of UDS by autoradiography following fusion of different pairs of XP fibroblast strains. Correction of DNA repair deficiency was observed in heterokaryons from some crosses, indicating that each strain used

as parental in the fusion was able to supply what the other was lacking. This implies that the strains used as parental in the fusion have different defects and, therefore, they can be assigned to different complementation groups. Genetic analysis in about fifty XP cases led to the identification of five genetically different forms of XP, that were named A to E, in order of increasing residual DNA repair synthesis (de Weerd-Kastelein et al. 1973, 1974; Paterson et al. 1974; Robbins et al. 1974; Bootsma et al. 1975; Bootsma 1978; Cleaver 1975; Kraemer et al. 1975a, b; Giannelli and Pawsey 1976). In 1979, two further complementation groups (XP-F and XP-G) were identified in the excision-repair defective form of XP (Arase et al. 1979; Keijzer et al. 1979). In this productive period, also the outlines of nucleotide excision repair in human cells were worked out (reviewed in Bootsma et al. 1991).

Following these cellular biochemistry studies, progress in understanding the role of the functions defective in XP and the related repair processes, was relatively sluggish until the late 1980s. The possibility to explore the molecular and biochemical bases of XP was opened up by the development of a cell-free system to study NER (Wood et al. 1988) and by the cloning of the genes responsible for the excision repair defective form of XP. The *XPA* gene was cloned by Tanaka and coworkers using transfection of an XP-A cell line as an initial step (Tanaka et al. 1989). Most of the other XP genes were identified taking advantage of the results obtained from characterization of UV-sensitive mutants isolated in laboratory from rodent cell lines. The human genes able to complement the repair defect of the rodent mutants were cloned by transfection of UV-sensitive rodent mutants with human DNA followed by selection for UV-resistant transfectants and recovery of the correcting gene (reviewed in Hoeijmakers 1993). These human genes were designated "excision repair cross-complementing" (ERCC) followed by a number that refers to the rodent complementation group whose defect was corrected. Reintroduction of the ERCC genes into different XP strains showed that most of the ERCC genes did correspond to the genes that were defective in the different XP complementation groups. The name of the XP genes have now superseded those of the corresponding ERCC genes, although the official Human Genome Organization (HUGO) names are still ERCC2 for XPD, ERCC3 for XPB, ERCC4 for XPF and ERCC5 for XPG.

Further consistent advances were made in recent years. The identification of other hereditary disorders defective in NER, namely Cockayne syndrome and trichothiodystrophy, provided additional tools to explore the molecular basis of NER, leading to the discovery of unexpected connections between NER and transcription. The cloning of the gene defective in the XP variant form stimulated investigations on DNA damage tolerance in human cells that is still subject of active research. Although great advances have been made in understanding the etiology of the DNA repair diseases since XP was first identified as a DNA-repair deficient human disease nearly 40 years ago, we are still far from the point of applying this knowledge to clinical trials. Therefore one of the main goals of the current research is to relate, in ways that will finally help patients, the clinical features of the NER diseases to the emerging picture of the involved molecular pathways.

Further information on the history of XP and on the exciting development of the related research field can be found in the papers of Bootsma (2001) and Cleaver (2005a), two scientists who greatly contributed with their discoveries to the clarification of the pathogenesis of XP.

# Incidence and prevalence

XP occurs with an estimated incidence of about one in a million of live births in the United States and Europe. It is more common in Japan (from 1:40.000 to 1:100.000) (Hirai et al. 2006), North Africa (Tunisia, Algeria, Morocco, Libya, and Egypt), the Middle East (Turkey, Israel, and Syria) and areas where the consanguineous marriages are common (Kraemer et al. 1987). Patients have been reported worldwide in all races including whites, blacks, Asians and Native Americans. Consistent with autosomal recessive inheritance, there is no significant difference between the sexes.

# Clinical manifestations

Patients with XP are hypersensitive to UV radiation both at the clinical and cellular level. Therefore, they show cutaneous and ocular abnormalities that are usually strikingly limited to sun-exposed areas of the body (Fig. 1A, B). If aggressive UV avoidance is not introduced early, first skin cancer may appear in early childhood. It is worth mentioning that there is great variability in the age at onset and in the severity of symptoms, depending on the mutated gene and the amount of sun exposure. Neurologic involvement has been reported in about 20–30% of XP patients. Neurological abnormalities are usually associated with mutations in the *XPA*, *XPB*, *XPD*, or *XPG* gene (Fig. 1C–E). In XP, neurologic symptoms can differ in severity and age at onset, but all share a progressive character.

## Skin abnormalities

Approximately half of the patients with XP have a history of acute sun sensitivity from early infancy, acquiring severe sunburn with blistering or persistent erythema lasting several weeks on minimal sun exposure (Fig. 1D). The other XP patients give a history of normal tanning without increased burning. In all patients, numerous freckle-like hyperpigmented macules appear on sun-exposed area of the skin (Fig. 1D). The median age of onset of first cutaneous symptoms is one to two years (Kraemer et al. 1994a). Following continued sun exposure, most XP patients develop xerosis (dry skin) poikiloderma (the constellation of hyper- and hypopigmentation, atrophy, and telangiectasia), and premalignant actinic keratoses at an early age (Fig. 1A).

If rigorous protection from UV radiation is not introduced from early life, XP patients can develop skin cancer. Neoplasms are predominantly basal cell and squamous cell carcinomas, but also include melanomas, keratoacanthomas and sarcomas (Fig. 1B). The median age of onset of the first skin neoplasm was 8 years for basal and squamous cell carcinoma, nearly 50 years earlier than that of the general population, and 19 years for malignant melanoma. In XP

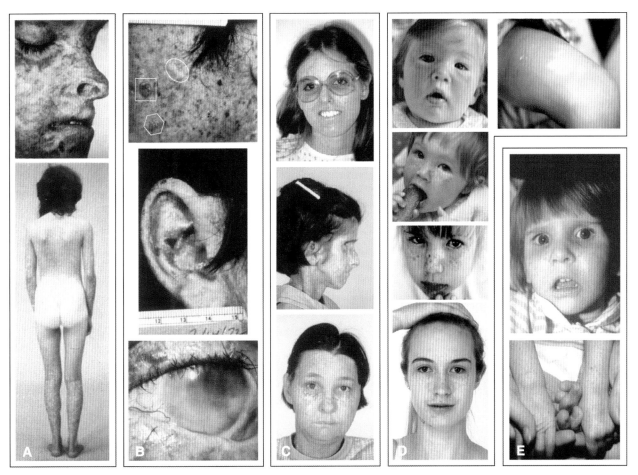

**Fig. 1.** Xeroderma pigmentosum. (**A**) The face of a 16 year old patient (top) that shows dry skin with hyperpigmentation, hypopigmentation, atrophy and cheilitis and a posterior view of the same patient (bottom) that shows the absence of pigmentary changes on areas protected from sunlight. (**B**) The face of a 14 year old patient (top) that shows freckle-like changes with different amounts of pigmentation, an actinic keratosis (in the polygon), a basal cell carcinoma (in the square) and a scar with telangiectasia (in the ellipse) at the site of the removal of another neoplasm. A pinna of a 22 year old patient (middle) that shows pigmentary abnormalities and a crusted squamous cell carcinoma. The eye of the same patient (bottom) that shows secondary telangiectasia invading the cloudy cornea, and atrophy and loss of the lashes of the lower lid. (**C**) The face of three patients with neurological abnormalities classified into XP-A (XP12BE, top), XP-B (XP11BE, middle) and XP-D (XP6BE, bottom) group, respectively. (**D**) The XP-G patient XP65BE at different ages (from top to bottom): at age 6 months (top left) she experienced severe sunburn of her face on minimal sun exposure, with erythema and swelling on the skin of forehead, cheeks, and periorbital area. At age 9 months, she developed erythema and peeling of skin of the malar area of the face following sun exposure. At age 4.5 years, she showed pigmentary changes on her nose, malar area, and other portions of the face. Furthermore, she experienced blistering sunburn on upper thigh (top left). Note spared area above the knee where sunscreen was applied. At age 14 years, she shows minimal pigmentary changes on face and sparing of neck and hand since she used measures to protect her skin from sun exposure. (**E**) The XP-G patient XP82DC at 3 years of age has deep-set eyes characteristic of CS and irregular lentiginous pigmentation on her face characteristic of XP (top) indicating the XP/CS complex. She has characteristic XP pigmented lesions on her forearms and dorsa of hands (bottom) along with thin, translucent skin with readily visible veins. The small size of her hands is apparent in comparison to the hands of her mother. Panels A, B modified from van Steeg and Kraemer (1999), and panels D, E modified from Emmert et al. (2002).

patients under 20 years of age, the frequencies for melanoma and for basal and squamous cell carcinoma were more than 1000-fold higher than in the US general population (Kraemer et al. 1987). The finding that also black patients with XP show an increased frequency of skin cancer indicates that normally functioning DNA repair systems provide greater protection against cutaneous carcinogenesis than does the natural pigmentation of black skin. If not protected from sunlight, many patients die of malignancy early in adulthood.

## Ocular abnormalities

Ocular abnormalities have been reported in 80% of XP patients. Clinical findings are strikingly limited to the anterior, UV-exposed structures (lids, cornea, and conjunctiva). The posterior portions of the eye are rarely affected, because UV-light is absorbed by anterior eye portions and only visible light (400–800 nm) reaches the retina. Photophobia is often present and may be associated with prominent conjunctival injection. Continued UV exposure of the eye may result in severe keratitis leading to corneal opacification and vascularization (Fig. 1B, bottom). The lids may develop loss of lashes and atrophy of the skin of the lids results in the lids turning out (ectropion), or in (entropion), or complete loss of the lids in severe cases. Benign conjunctival inflammatory masses or papillomas of the lids may be present. Epithelioma, squamous cell carcinoma, and melanoma of UV-exposed portions of the eye are common.

## Other neoplasias

It has been estimated that all of the sites exposed to UV radiation have about a thousand-fold increased risk of developing tumors in XP patients. Besides skin and eye cancer, a greatly increased frequency of cancer of the oral cavity, particularly squamous cell carcinoma of the tip of the tongue, a presumed sun-exposed area, has been reported (Kraemer et al. 1994b). In XP patients there is also a smaller increase in internal tumors, predominately gliomas of the brain and spinal cord and Schwannoma of the facial nerve. Two of our

patients who were cigarette smokers developed lung cancer. The carcinogens in cigarette smoke produce DNA damage that is repaired by the same nucleotide excision repair system that is defective in XP. Rarely leukemias and uterine, breast, pancreatic, gastric, renal, and testicular tumors have been reported. Overall, the literature reports suggest an approximate ten to twenty-fold increase in internal neoplasms (Kraemer et al. 1994a). The development of these tumors might be related to the persistence of DNA lesions induced by environmental carcinogens and normally repaired by NER.

## Neurologic abnormalities

Neurologic abnormalities have been reported in approximately 20% of the patients and are commonly observed in cases with mutations in either the *XPA*, *XPB*, *XPD*, or *XPG* gene (Fig. 1C–E). The onset may be early in infancy or delayed until the second decade. The neurologic abnormalities may be mild (e.g., isolated hyporeflexia) or severe, with progressive intellectual impairment, sensorineural deafness beginning with high-frequency hearing loss, spasticity, or seizures. When neurological problems do occur, however, they usually tend to worsen over time.

The most severe form, known as the De Sanctis–Cacchione syndrome, involves the cutaneous and ocular manifestations of classic XP plus additional neurologic and somatic abnormalities including microcephaly, progressive mental deterioration, low intelligence, hyporeflexia or areflexia, choreoathetosis, ataxia, spasticity, reduced nerve conduction velocity, Achilles tendon shortening with eventual quadraparesis, markedly retarded growth leading to dwarfism, and immature sexual development. Progressive sensorineural deafness, abnormal electroencephalographic findings and epilepsy can also occur. The complete De Sanctis–Cacchione syndrome has been recognized in very few patients; however, many XP patients have one or more of its neurologic features. In clinical practice, deep tendon reflex testing and routine audiometry can usually serve as a screen for the presence of XP-associated neurologic abnormalities.

The predominant neuropathologic abnormality found at autopsy in patients with neurologic symptoms was loss (or absence) of neurons, particularly in the cerebrum and cerebellum. There is evidence for a primary axonal degeneration in peripheral nerves, in some cases with secondary demyelination (Rapin et al. 2000).

## Natural history

XP is an example of accelerated photo-aging. If aggressive UV avoidance is not introduced early, accumulated sunlight-induced DNA damage is likely to result in skin cancer in the first decade of life. Some patients show exquisite acute sun sensitivity with severe burning on minimal sun exposure. However, many individuals with XP have no symptoms of increased sunburning on minimal sun exposure, but tan, freckle, and then develop skin cancers if not protected from sunlight. A dramatic increase in the frequency of all types of major skin cancers in areas exposed to sunlight is a typical feature of XP, and patients often die at an early age from the consequences of multiple cutaneous neoplasms with local invasion, metastasis, or secondary infection.

Individuals with onset in infancy have a particularly poor prognosis. However, there is evidence that early diagnosis and rigorous protection from exposure to UV radiation will reduce the frequency of skin cancers and prolong life (Slor et al. 2000). As reported by Lehmann (2003) in the UK, thanks to an excellent relationship between the XP family support group, clinicians and manufacturers of UV-resistant products, families have been able to provide effective protection in the home and school environment by covering windows with UV-resistant film. Affected individuals wear UV-opaque headgear and gloves when outside. By adhering to this level of protection, some XP children have skin which appears essentially normal. While in these circumstances the skin cancer problem appears to be under control, the XP patients have been followed for a relatively short period of time. Long-term follow-up will be needed to determine the duration of this beneficial regimen. There is no evidence that sun protection will prevent the neurological abnormalities, which are found in about 20% of affected patients.

Apart from the skin abnormalities, a proportion of XP patients have neurological abnormalities resulting from progressive neuronal death. These vary in age of onset and severity and are usually associated with mutations in the *XPA*, *XPB*, *XPD*, or *XPG* genes. This neurodegeneration has been theorized as being caused by unrepaired DNA damage in non-dividing neurons (Robbins 1988). Since UV does not reach the central nervous system, the DNA damage to neurons may be caused by oxidative damage. While most forms of oxidative damage are repaired by base excision repair, some oxidative DNA lesions, such as cyclo-adenine or cyclo-guanine are repaired by NER (Brooks et al. 2000, Brooks 2007, Kuraoka et al. 2000, D'Errico et al. 2006). It appears that persons with the most severe reductions in their DNA repair ability are the most likely to have such problems. While nothing can prevent or stop neurological problems from occurring, it is important to be aware of them. Therefore, XP patients should have a screening neurological examination including a hearing test and evaluation of deep tendon reflexes. If neurological abnormalities are detected then periodic neurological evaluations may detect disease progression. Early testing and treatment for potential neurological problems may lessen the unfortunate results of undetected abnormalities. For example, detection of hearing loss and subsequent use of a hearing aid may lessen difficulties in communication and in school.

## Pathogenesis/molecular genetics

At the cellular level, XP is characterized by varying degrees of spontaneous chromosomal instability (Lanza et al. 1997) and normal frequency of sister chromatid exchanges (SCEs). Following UV irradiation or exposure to carcinogens forming bulky adducts on DNA, XP cells typically show hypersensitivity to the killing effect of UV light, reduced extent of "host cell reactivation" (i.e., capacity to repair damaged DNA of infecting viruses), increased mu-

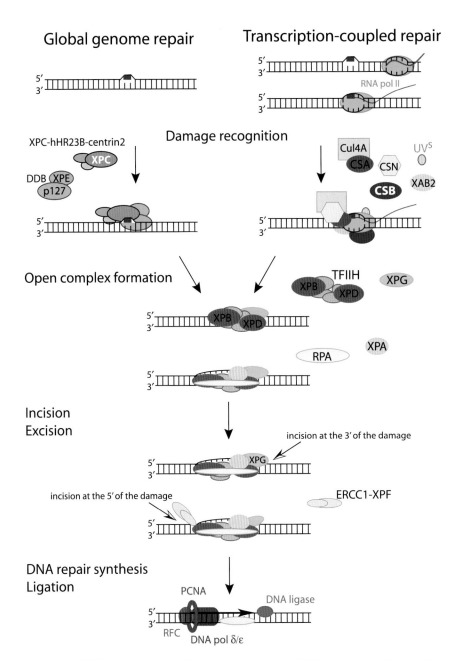

**Fig. 2.** Nucleotide excision repair (NER) and modalities of global genome repair (GGR) and transcription-coupled repair (TCR) in human cells. Damage in the non-transcribed regions of the genome is recognized by binding of XPE and XPC protein complexes through GGR. Damage in the transcribed strand of active genes is recognized by the arrest of RNA polymerase II (Pol II) that is relieved through an assembled protein complex that includes CSA and CSB proteins. The subsequent stages are identical. The XPB and XPD helicases of the multi-subunit transcription factor TFIIH open ~30 base pairs of DNA around the damage and the stability of the unwound region is guaranteed by the physical presence of XPA, RPA (replication protein A) and XPG. XPA monitors the increased DNA deformability whereas RPA stabilizes the open intermediate by binding to the undamaged strand. Once the open complex is assembled and the lesion correctly positioned, the structure-specific endonucleases XPG and ERCC1-XPF respectively cleave 3' and 5' of the borders of the opened stretch only in the damaged strand, generating a a damage-containing oligomer of 24–32 nucleotides. Precise incision locations may vary depending on the type of lesion, but the incisions are made asymmetrically around the lesion, they are independent of each other and the 3'-incision precedes the 5'-incision. The regular DNA replication machinery then completes the repair. RPA promotes the arrival of the replication factors proliferating cell nuclear antigen (PCNA) and replication factor C (RFC) to initiate DNA resynthesis. Repair synthesis is carried out by DNA polymerases $\delta/\varepsilon$ using the undamaged daughter strand as template and the repair patch is sealed by DNA ligase 1.

tability and increased frequency of chromosomal aberrations, and SCEs.

The clinical and cellular photosensitivity typical of XP results from an inability to handle damage generated in cellular DNA by the ultraviolet component of sun-light. Eight genetically distinct XP groups have been recognized that reflect mutations in distinct genes. The products of seven of these genes (named from *XPA* to *XPG*) are involved in nucleotide excision repair (NER), the sole pathway that in human cells removes the two major photoproducts generated in DNA by UV light (namely, the cyclobutane pyrimidine dimers -CPD- and the 6−4 photoproducts). An eighth gene, encoding DNA polymerase eta (polη), is responsible for the XP variant form that is defective in translesion DNA synthesis (TLS). For a comprehensive overview of cellular and molecular aspects of XP and related DNA repair processes see Friedberg et al. (2006). For recent reviews on specific topics see Andressoo and Hoeijmakers (2005), Bohr et al. (2005), Cleaver (2005b), Ford (2005), Gong et al. (2005), Reardon and Sancar (2005), Thoma (2005), Essers et al. (2006), Gillet and Scharer (2006), Laine and Egly (2006), Leibeling et al. (2006) and Park and Choi (2006).

## Pathways defective in XP

NER is a versatile repair system present in prokaryotes and eukaryotes that corrects any damage that both distorts the DNA molecule and alters its chemistry. Beside UV-induced damage, it acts on a wide variety of other bulky helix-distorting lesions caused by chemical mutagens (such as bulky chemical adducts, certain types of crosslinks and other lesions that result in large local distortion of the DNA structure). The repair of some endogenous free-radical-induced lesions, such as cyclo-adenine or cyclo-guanine, is also dependent on NER (Brooks et al. 2000, Kuraoka et al. 2000). The individual steps in the NER reaction mechanism are now understood in broad outline (Fig. 2). NER requires the co-ordinated action of more than 30 gene products and operates through two different modalities: transcription-coupled repair (TCR), which rapidly removes lesions from

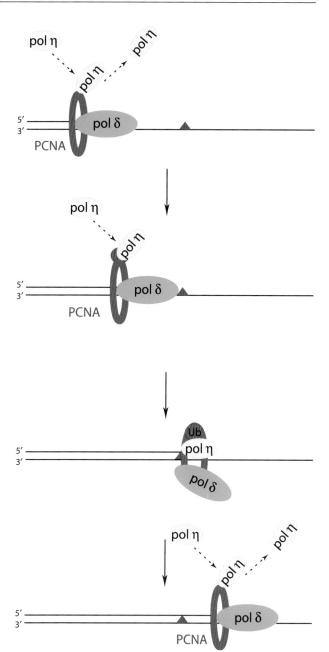

**Fig. 3.** Translesion synthesis (TLS) past a lesion with polymerase η (modified from Lehmann 2006). During DNA replication polη is only transiently associated with proliferating cell nuclear antigen (PCNA). When the replication fork is stalled at a lesion site (red triangle), PCNA becomes ubiquitinated (Ub) thereby increasing its affinity for polη and increasing its ability to displace the replicative polymerase (polδ) and carry out TLS. By this means the cell is able to replicate DNA past unrepaired damage.

transcribed strand of active genes, and global-genome repair (GGR), that slowly repairs the rest of the genome. These two sub-pathways differ in their initial damage recognition steps. The recognition events are followed by a common pathway involving unwinding of damaged DNA, dual incision in the damaged strand, removal of the damage-containing oligonucleotide, repair synthesis in the resultant gap using the undamaged complementary strand as a template and ligation of the repair patch to the contiguous parental DNA strand.

Translesion DNA synthesis (TLS) is a DNA damage tolerance pathway that utilizes multiple specialized DNA polymerases to replicate past sites of base damage (Friedberg et al. 2005, Lehmann 2006). The current model for TLS is the "DNA polymerase switch model" in which the replicative DNA polymerase blocked by DNA damage is transiently replaced by one (or several) DNA polymerases, specially designed to bypass lesions in DNA before resuming regular DNA synthesis (Fig. 3). Compared to the high-fidelity replicative DNA polymerases, these special DNA polymerases have more flexible base-pairing properties. They can bypass lesions by incorporating nucleotides opposite sites of base damage, thus taking over temporarily from the blocked replicative DNA polymerase $\delta/\epsilon$, and possibly from

pol$\alpha$. The DNA polymerase $\eta$, that is mutated in the variant form of XP, has the property of being able to synthesize across UV-induced CPD. However, this bypass has biased fidelity and may contribute to mutagenesis at UV photoproducts (McCulloch et al. 2004). There are indications that pol$\eta$ can also bypass other types of base damage (abasic sites, N-2-AAF-guanine adducts, and cis-platin DNA intrastrand cross-links).

The function and features of the genes responsible for XP are reported in Table 1.

## Clinical, cellular and molecular characteristics of the XP groups

Cells from NER-defective XP patients show a reduced ability to perform UV-induced DNA repair synthesis. This defect has been used as cellular parameter in a classical complementation test based on somatic cell hybridisation, that has led to the identification of seven distinct complementation groups in the NER-defective form of XP, designated XP-A to XP-G. In contrast, XP variant patients have been so far assigned to a single group, called XP-V.

The gene responsible for the repair defects has been defined in more than 400 XP patients and

**Table 1.** Genes responsible for xeroderma pigmentosum

| Gene name (synonyms) | Accession number | Chromosome location[a] | Size (aa) | Pathway | Function |
|---|---|---|---|---|---|
| *XPA* | NM_000380 | 9q22.33 | 273 | NER | binds damaged DNA in preincision complex and verifies the damage |
| *XPB (ERCC3)* | NM_000122 | 2q14.3 | 782 | NER | 3'–5' DNA helicase, subunit of TFIIH that catalyzes unwinding in preincision complex |
| *XPC* | NM_004628 | 3p25.1 | 940 | NER (GGR) | binds damaged DNA in complex with HR23B and centrin 2 |
| *XPD (ERCC2)* | NM_000400 | 19q13.32 | 760 | NER | 5'–3' DNA helicase, subunit of TFIIH that catalyzes unwinding in preincision complex |
| *XPE (DDB2)* | NM_000107 | 11p11.2 | 427 | NER (GGR) | binds damaged DNA, E3 ubiquitin ligase |
| *XPF (ERCC4)* | NM_005236 | 16p13.12 | 916 | NER | operates 5' incision in complex with ERCC1 |
| *XPG (ERCC5)* | NM_000123 | 13q33.1 | 1186 | NER | operates 3' incision |
| *XPV* (Pol$\eta$) | NM_006502 | 6p21.1 | 713 | TLS | bypass polymerase |

*NER* Nucleotide excision repair; *GGR* global genome repair sub-pathway; *TLS* translesion synthesis.
[a]From http://www.cgal.icnet.uk/DNA_Repair_Genes.html. See also Wood et al. (2005).

**Table 2.** Clinical and cellular features of the eight complementation groups of xeroderma pigmentosum

| Group | Patient number[a] | Clinical symptoms[b] | | Cellular response to UV[c] | | |
|---|---|---|---|---|---|---|
| | | Cancer | Neurological anomalies | UV sensitivity | UDS % normal | RRS |
| XP-A | 216 | ++ | ++/+ | +++ | <5 | − |
| XP-B | 7 | +/− | ++/+ | ++ | 10–40 | − |
| XP-C | 61 | + | − | ++ | 15–30 | + |
| XP-D | 44 | +/− | ++/− | ++ | 2–55 | − |
| XP-E | 12 | +/− | − | + | >50 | + |
| XP-F | 24 | +/− | −/++ | + | 15–30 | − |
| XP-G | 6 | +/− | ++/+/− | ++ | 2–25 | − |
| XP-V | 117 | + | − | +/+++* | 100 | + |

[a]Modified from Moriwaki and Kraemer (2001).

[b]Cases with different severity in terms of age at onset and frequency of skin tumours or neurological abnormalities (++, +); cases reported as cancer-free at the last clinical examination or without neurological involvement (−). See text for details between and within each complementation group.

[c]UV-sensitivity: survival partially (+) or drastically (+++) reduced compared with normal. In XP-V cells XP-V cells are only slightly sensitive to UV irradiation, but this sensitivity is dramatically increased by post-irradiation incubation in caffeine (*). Caffeine sensitization is specific to the XP variants and does not occur in any of the other groups.

UDS (Unscheduled DNA Synthesis) The ability to perform UV-induced DNA repair synthesis is expressed as a percentage of that in normal cells; RRS recovery of RNA synthesis rate after UV normal (+) or defective (−).

clinical and cellular features of each XP group are listed in Table 2. The different groups show different frequencies: the majority of patients belong to groups A, C and D. XP-A is more frequent in Japan, whereas XP-C is the most frequent in US and Europe. While patients with defects in each complementation group may show distinctive clinical and cellular features, there is marked phenotypic heterogeneity within each complementation group. The progression of the disease is usually faster and neurological abnormalities are usually associated with the patients showing the greatest skin photosensitivity whose cells are most sensitive to killing by UV (Andrews et al. 1978). The main features emerged from mutation analysis in patients belonging to the various XP groups are reported in Table 3.

**The XP-A group** is frequently characterized by severe clinical symptoms and a low capacity to perform UV-induced DNA repair synthesis (<5% of normal). The age of onset of cutaneous alterations and tumors is early and only few exceptional patients do not display neurological abnormalities

(Stefanini et al. 1980, Cleaver and Kraemer 1989, Chang et al. 1989). Analysis of over 100 patients led to the identification of many mutations (reviewed in States et al. 1998 and in Moriwaki and Kraemer 2001). Many are severely truncating mutations, which completely abolish NER and include one founder mutation (a G–C transversion at the 3′ splice acceptor site in intron 3, which causes abnormal splicing) identified in more than 90% of Japanese patients (Nishigori et al. 1994). A diagnostic test for this mutation based on the polymerase chain reaction (PCR) and differences in enzymatic digestion of normal and mutated products has been developed for rapid diagnosis of XP-A homozygotes and heterozygotes as well as for prenatal diagnosis (Kore-eda et al. 1992). This mutation has been estimated to be present in heterozygous form in about 1% of the Japanese population or in about 1 million people (Hirai et al. 2006). The few missense mutations that have been identified are in the zinc-finger domain of the *XPA* gene and interfere with DNA binding. These mutations result in very severe clinical features. Milder XP-A cases

**Table 3.** Mutational analysis in patients with xeroderma pigmentosum

| Gene[a] | Analyzed cases (families)[b] | Recurrent mutations | Mutated products[c] |
|---|---|---|---|
| XPA | >100 | yes | truncated products (single aa substitutions) |
| XPB | 2 (1) | yes | single aa substitution and frameshift (truncated |
| | 5 (4)* | | products in the second allele) |
| XPC | 39 (34) | no | truncated products (single aa substitutions) |
| XPD | 29 (25) | yes | single aa substitutions (deletions) |
| | 6 (6)* | | |
| XPE | 9 | no | truncated products, single aa substitutions |
| XPF | 9 | yes | truncated products, single aa substitutions |
| XPG | 4 (3) | no | single aa substitutions, truncated products |
| | 9 (9)* | | |
| XPV | 40 | no | truncated products, single aa substitutions |

[a]See XP mutation database http://xpmutations.org/ for mutations identified in these genes.
[b]The symbol * indicates the number of cases (families) with the XP/CS phenotype. See text for details.
[c]Severely truncated polypeptides because of either stop codons, frameshifts, splice abnormalities or genomic DNA deletions. Changes identified in single or rare cases are between brackets.

generally have at least one allele with a mutation outside of the DNA binding region (exons 2–5, aminoacids 98–219), such as the exon 6 mutation (arg228stop) common in Japanese and Tunisian patients. A few other mild cases have mutations close to a splice site such that alternative splicing may allow the production of a low level of normal protein (Sidwell et al. 2006).

**The XP-B group** consists of six families (Oh et al. 2006). In 4 of the families the affected patients have clinical symptoms of the XP/Cockayne syndrome (CS) complex. In one family two sisters have XP without CS with deafness as the only neurological abnormality. They both had ocular melanoma. The remaining family has two siblings with trichothiodystrophy (TTD). XPB is a subunit of TFIIH, the multiprotein complex involved in basal transcription and NER. Since the transcriptional function of TFIIH is vital for life, XPB is an essential gene, and the paucity of XP-B families suggests that the transcriptional function of the XPB gene is very intolerant of mutations.

**The XP-C group** is one of the more common forms of XP. Its pathological phenotype is rather homogeneous. The patients usually show skin and ocular symptoms, whereas mild mental retardation

has been reported for only one case (XP1MI). Differences in the severity of skin disorders depend on age, climate, and life-style (essentially the protection from the sun). XP-C cells exhibit drastically reduced UV-induced DNA repair synthesis levels (10–20% of normal), normal recovery of RNA synthesis at late times after irradiation, survival levels markedly reduced in proliferating cultures but significantly affected only at high UV doses in non-proliferating cultures. This pattern of response to UV light reflects a specific defect in GGR, the NER sub-pathway that removes damage from the non-transcribed strand of active genes and from the inactive regions of the genome. Normal TCR in XP-C cells results in normal rates of recovery of RNA synthesis. In non-dividing cells, the ability to carry out GGR is of relatively minor importance since only the actively transcribed regions of DNA are utilized, and non-dividing XP-C cells consequently have close to normal survival levels.

The mutations that have been identified in the *XPC* gene are distributed across the gene, with no indication of any hotspots or founder effects. Most of the mutations are predicted to cause premature termination of the protein as a result of frameshifts, nonsense mutations, insertions, deletions or splicing abnormalities. In the patients analyzed thus far, the lack of the *XPC* protein in some patients and the presence of a mutated protein in others both result in similar clinical phenotypes and confer the same degree of cellular sensitivity to UV light. All the XP-C patients show severe reduction in the *XPC* transcript level and undetectable levels of XPC protein (Khan et al. 2006). The only exception is represented by one patient carrying the missense mutation Trp690Ser on its paternal allele. This is the only case reported so far, in which the XPC protein is present, although at lower than normal levels (Chavanne et al. 2000). This does not result either in milder clinical features or in a less severe cellular response to UV. One family in Turkey was reported with 3 sisters having full length normal *XPC* mRNA transcripts at a level of 3–5% of normal cells. These patients had a splice lariat mutation that was associated with relatively mild skin disease (Khan et al. 2004). Parents of XP-C patients who are heterozygous for a mutation in the *XPC* gene have levels of XPC mRNA that are intermediate between the level in the patients and that in normal donors (Khan et al. 2006).

**The XP-D group** is characterized by a great heterogeneity both at clinical and cellular levels. Remarkable differences among patients concern the severity of cutaneous lesions, the presence of neurological abnormalities and the age of onset of tumors. At the cellular level, different degrees of alteration in the response to UV irradiation have been observed both in terms of survival and of UV-induced DNA repair synthesis. The complexity of the function altered in the XP-D group is stressed also by the observation that the XP-D defect has been identified in many patients with XP or with trichothiodystrophy (TTD) and in rare cases showing the clinical symptoms of Cockayne syndrome (CS) or TTD, in addition to the XP phenotype (reviewed in Lehmann 2001, 2003; Stefanini 2006). Mutation analysis in 29 XP patients indicated the XP phenotype is often associated with mutations in the helicase motifs of XPD. Most of the mutations result in a single amino acid change and 80% of mutations are localized at a single site, arg683 (Frederick et al. 1994; Takayama et al. 1995;

Taylor et al. 1997; Kobayashi et al. 1997, 2002; Viprakasit et al. 2001).

The spectrum of *XPD* mutations in XP, TTD and XP/CS patients indicates that the site of mutation generally determines the clinical phenotype. Different sites are mutated in the different pathological phenotypes with the exception of two alleles (resulting in either substitution of arg616 or a leu461val change associated with deletion of amino acid region 716–730) that were found both in XP and TTD patients. It has been suggested that some alleles are irrelevant for the pathological phenotype because they behave as null alleles (Taylor et al. 1997). Therefore the pathological phenotype in the patients who are compound heterozygotes for these "null" mutations is determined by the change on the second allele that was found always different in XP and TTD cases. Clinical symptoms of different severity have been recently reported in XP patients from two distinct families with the common R683W mutation in one allele and different mutations in the second allele. In one family the XP patient had many skin cancers and died in the fourth decade with severe neurological degeneration. The other family had two affected children. Both are now in their 20's and neither has skin cancer or any neurological abnormalities. Thus in this family the second *XPD* allele appears to play a large role in determining the clinical phenotype (Boyle et al. 2006).

**The XP-E group** is one of the least severe forms of XP, with only mild dermatological manifestations, no neurological abnormalities, late onset of tumours and a partially reduced UV response. XP-E patients are mutated in the *DDB2* gene, encoding the smaller (48kDa) subunit of the heterodimeric Damaged DNA Binding protein DDB. The identified mutations comprise both missense and truncating mutations, but all XP-E patients show a rather homogeneous mild phenotype (Nichols et al. 1996, 2000; Itoh et al. 1999; Rapic-Otrin et al. 2003). This is consistent with cellular studies, which suggest that XPE is only involved in GGR of cyclobutane pyrimidine dimers (CPDs) and not in TCR, or in GGR of 6–4 photoproducts (reviewed in Tang and Chu 2002). However, recently an XP-E family with many skin cancers including melanomas and squamous cell carcinoma of the jaw has been found (Oh et al. 2005).

**The XP-F group** comprises mildly affected patients generally without neurologic abnormalities. Most were described in Japan (reviewed in Cleaver et al. 1999). The repair synthesis level is generally reduced to less than 10% of normal whereas in several cases the survival is not drastically reduced. In the seven patients analysed by Matsumura et al. (1998), at least one allele was a missense mutation, suggesting the presence of a partially functional protein. A different mutation has been found in two European patients reported in the literature, that are respectively homozygote and compound heterozygote for a C2377T transition resulting in the Arg788Trp change (Sijbers et al. 1996, 1998). Two XP-F kindreds with severe adult onset neurodegeneration leading to death in 2 patients have been recently found (Imoto et al. 2005).

**The XP-G group** is rather rare (13 cases from 12 families), but nevertheless very heterogenous. It comprises 4 patients with XP without neurological disease (3 families), 7 patients in which XP features are associated with severe early onset CS symptoms and 2 patients with mild combined features of XP and CS. Nearly all XP-G patients have very low levels of UDS. Sequence analysis of the *XPG* gene has shown that patients with the milder symptoms have missense mutations, which retain some DNA repair activity (Emmert et al. 2002). In contrast, the mutations leading to a combined phenotype of XP and CS all result in severely truncated and/or unstable XPG proteins (reviewed in Clarkson 2003).

**The XP-V group** includes about 20% of XP cases. These patients show late onset and slow progression of clinical symptoms. They typically develop skin cancers around the age of 20–30 years and exhibit rare to no neurological abnormalities. XP-V cells are only slightly sensitive to UV irradiation, but this sensitivity is dramatically increased by post-irradiation incubation in caffeine. They are unable to recover normal levels of DNA replicative synthesis after UV. The replication fork appears to stop or to be interrupted during semiconservative replication at sites of DNA damage as a consequence of mutations

in the gene encoding DNA polymerase eta, which is required for effecting TLS past UV photoproducts. The dramatic proneness to skin cancer of XP-V individuals testifies to the importance of this DNA polymerase in cancer avoidance.

DNA polymerase eta has a dynamic cellular organization: it is mostly localized uniformly in the nucleus but is associated with replication foci during S phase. Following exposure to UV light or carcinogens, it accumulates at replication foci stalled at DNA damage. The polymerase activity of pol eta resides entirely in the first 511 amino acids of the protein. The C-terminal 70 amino acids containing a bipartite nuclear location signal (NLS), are needed for nuclear localization of pol eta. A further 50 amino acids are required for relocalization of pol eta into multiple intranuclear foci following UV irradiation. The C-terminal 120 amino acids are necessary and sufficient to target the protein into foci after DNA damage and truncated proteins lacking these domains fail to correct the defects in XP-V cells (Broughton et al. 2002).

Mutational analysis has been carried out in about 40 cases (reviewed in Gratchev et al. 2003). Mutations in the majority of the XP-V patients result in severely truncated proteins. The mutations can be divided into three categories: 1) both alleles result in a truncated protein of less than 410 amino acids (severe truncation), 2) at least one allele is a missense mutation, and 3) at least one allele results in a truncated protein of more than 520 amino acids (C-terminal truncation). Mutations found in two XP-V patients leave the polymerase motifs intact but cause loss of the C-terminal 70 amino acids, containing the localization domains. The resulting protein appears functional *in vitro*, whereas *in vivo*, it is not. This finding indicates that the XP phenotype may be caused by the protein not being correctly localized in the cell.

## Diagnosis, follow-up and management

The diagnosis of XP is made clinically based on skin, eye, and neurologic manifestations. The occurrence of consanguinuity in the family history may aid in diagnosis.

Evaluations at initial diagnosis may include:

- baseline examination of the skin (all sun exposed sites and sun shielded areas);
- baseline clinical photographs of the entire skin surface with close-ups (including a ruler) of individual lesions;
- examination of the scalp that may be facilitated by use of a hair dryer (using a cool setting) to blow the hair aside;
- examination of the lip and adjacent tip of the tongue since cancers in this area are often preceded by signs of sun damage, including actinic cheilitis and prominent telangiectasia;
- use of the Schirmer test to detect dry eyes;
- examination of the lids and anterior UV exposed portions of the globe (eversion of the lids may be necessary to detect cancers of the mucosal surface);
- measurement of occipital frontal head circumference;
- deep tendon reflex testing, and routine audiometry as a screen for the presence of XP-associated neurologic abnormalities;
- MRI of the brain and nerve conduction velocities if other neurologic problems are detected.

Specific functional assays on living cells are available to evaluate the cellular response to UV light. These assays can demonstrate UV hypersensitivity to differentiate XP from other photosensitive disorders. XP can usually be conclusively diagnosed by analysing patient's cells for the appropriate DNA repair defect. Cells from XP patients with NER defects show a reduced ability to perform UV-induced DNA repair synthesis (unscheduled DNA synthesis, UDS) and are hypersensitive to killing by UV. In contrast cells from patients with the XP variant

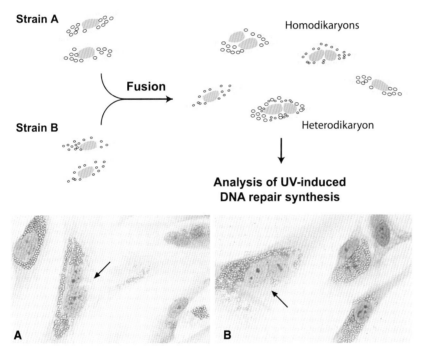

**Fig. 4.** Classical complementation assay by cell fusion for nucleotide excision repair (NER) defects and heterodikaryons showing either recovery (**A**) or persistency (**B**) of the repair defect present in the fibroblast strains used as partners in the fusion. The fibroblast strains used as partners in the fusion are grown for three days in medium containing latex beads of different sizes that are incorporated into the cytoplasm as a marker. The cells are fused and, two days later, analyzed for their ability to perform UV-induced DNA repair synthesis (UDS) by autoradiography. The two cell strains are classified in the same complementation group if the heterodikaryons (identified as binuclear cells containing beads of different sizes) fail to recover normal UDS levels. Conversely, the recovery of normal UDS levels in the heterodikaryons indicates that the cell strains used as partners in the fusion are carrier of genetically different defects.

form which is defective in TLS have normal post-UV UDS and normal post-UV survival but are sensitized to UV killing by caffeine.

The residual level of UDS in NER-defective XP is not sufficient to form the basis for gene assignment and the mutated gene can be identified by using specific assays. The classical complementation assay is carried out by fusing fibroblasts of the patient under evaluation with fibroblasts representative of the distinct XP groups (XP-A to XP-G) and by analyzing the capacity to perform UV-induced DNA repair synthesis (UDS) in heterodikaryons (Fig. 4). The restoration after fusion of normal UDS levels allows the classification of patients into different complementation groups (i.e., they are defective in different genes) whereas the maintenance of impaired UDS levels indicates that the patients are in the same complementation group (i.e., they are defective in the same gene).

In parallel to the classical complementation tests based on cell fusion, genetic analysis may be carried out also by analyzing the level of UDS in patient's cells after microinjection with different plasmids, each expressing one XP gene. An alternative assay makes use of a host-cell reactivation assay by co-transfecting a UV-treated plasmid plus plasmids expressing wild type XP cDNA of different complementation groups (Emmert et al. 2002, 2006).

Once cells from a patient are assigned to a known complementation group, the definition of the inactivating mutations may be carried out. The results of cellular and genetic analysis are fundamental for enabling clinicians to establish correct and early diagnoses of new patients, which is pivotal for proper genetic counselling of the families involved. Prenatal diagnosis is available for at risk pregnancies in families in which the repair defect in the affected member(s) has been already characterized at the cellular level. The definition of the mutated alleles offers a tool for detection of heterozygotes in the family since carriers are asymptomatic and show a normal cellular response to UV.

Knowledge of the responsible gene and underlying inactivating mutations may or may not be predictive of the future course of the clinical disease. There is marked phenotypic heterogeneity within XP com-plementation groups. Only a few severe mutations have been followed for a long period of time in a relatively large number of patients to be of predictive value. For example, the homozygous founder mutation in the *XPA* gene in Japan has been found to be associated with severe, rapid neurodegeneration (Nishigori et al. 1994). On the other hand, rare cases have been identified in which the effects of the defective XP gene are probably modified by other unidentified genes. A few families have been reported in which even affected siblings show different clinical courses despite the same mutations and style of life (Stefanini et al. 1980; Slor and Kraemer, unpubl. observations). This is an area of active research.

There is no cure for XP. The main goal of treatment is to protect oneself from UV exposure and thus prevent the damaging effects it can have on the skin. XP patients should follow general precautionary measures, such us:

– To adopt sun avoidance methods that include i) the use of protective clothing (long sleeves and pants, shirts with collars, tightly woven fabrics that don't let light through), hats (wide-brimmed) and eyewear (face shields specifically made to protect from UV light), ii) the application of sunscreens with a high sun-protective factor in all sun-exposed areas, iii) the avoidance of outdoor activities that should be kept to a minimum if at all necessary and carried out at night time if possible. Because XP shows hypersensitivity to UVA and UVB, found in sunlight, and UVC, found in some artificial light sources, it is useful to measure UV light in patient home, school, or work environment with a light meter so that high levels of environmental UV (such as halogen lamps) can be identified and eliminated if possible. While no standards exist for perfectly safe UV exposure in individuals with XP, the use of UV meters can alert individuals to unexpected sources of high levels of environmental UV.
– To undergo skin examinations by a dermatologist or other knowledgeable health professional at least every 3–6 months. Patients and their parents should be educated to look for abnormal pigmented lesions or the appearance of basal cell or squamous cell carcinoma.

- Since cells from XP patients are also hypersensitive to environmental mutagens, such as benzo(a) pyrene found in cigarette smoke, prudence dictates that individuals should be protected against these agents.
- To report immediately to the doctor any suspicious spots or growths.
- To undergo frequent eye examinations by an ophthalmologist.
- To undergo baseline testing for potential neurological problems. Routine neurologic examination is indicated because progressive neurologic abnormalities are present in a minority of individuals with XP and may not be detected in young children.
- Many XP patients have been treated with standard doses of X-radiation for inoperable skin or internal cancers. Although XP patients are not usually hypersensitive to therapeutic X-rays, cultured cells from a few XP-G patients were found to be hypersensitive to X-radiation. Clinical hypersensitivity to ionizing radiation has been recently reported in an XP-C patient due the presence of a defective radiosensitivity gene, distinct from *XPC* (Arlett et al. 2006). If X-ray therapy is necessary, for example to treat an inoperable brain or spinal cord tumor (DiGiovanna et al. 1998), the patient may be tested with a low initial dose.
- Caution should be taken in suggesting the use of photodynamic therapy (PDT) that has been described as an option for the treatment of a variety of conjunctival, skin, and other carcinomas, including in one XP patient. A recent report indicates that the use of PDT for the treatment of eye malignancies in one patient with De Sanctis-Cacchione syndrome was unsuccessful and worsened the evolution of the lesions (Procianoy et al. 2006). Therefore, it has to be taken into account that PDT may be seriously harmful in the treatment of patients with XP.

Individuals with onset in infancy have a particularly poor prognosis. However, there is evidence that early diagnosis and rigorous protection from exposure to UV radiation will reduce the frequency of skin cancers and prolong life (Slor et al. 2000). Patients with xeroderma pigmentosum and their families will face many challenges in daily living. Constant educat-ing and reminding of the need to protect oneself from sunlight is fundamental in the management of XP.

Therapy with a high dose of an oral retinoid (13 cis retinoic acid) was found to be effective in preventing new skin cancers in XP patients (Kraemer et al. 1988). However, there was considerable toxicity and when the treatment was stopped new skin cancers appeared. Subsequently, some patients were found to respond to lower doses of medication with less toxicity.

Gene therapy is the ideal goal for curing XP, but there are many hurdles to be crossed before this ideal becomes a reality. As a first stage in development of gene therapy approaches, skin from XP-C patients has been reconstructed *in vitro* (Bernerd et al. 2005). As expected, the XP skin was highly sensitive to the effects of UV-irradiation, and should provide a good model for first attempts at gene therapy.

An alternative approach has used "Enzyme therapy". A bacterial DNA repair enzyme, denV T4 endonuclease in a topical liposome-containing preparation, has been reported to reduce the frequency of new actinic keratoses and basal cell carcinomas in individuals with XP in one research study (Yarosh et al. 2001). However, this treatment has not yet been approved for general use by the US Food and Drug Administration.

Both of these approaches offer long-term hope for XP cures, but for the near future, complete protection from solar UV-irradiation is by far the best strategy for cancer avoidance. Alleviation of the neurological abnormalities associated with XP remains a major challenge for the future.

## Resources

Several XP patient support groups have been established throughout the world. Their websites are an important source of information. Their activities include summer camps with activities at night or in UV sheltered environments, providing UV meters for families, offering UV shielding for windows and providing information and support.

The booklet "Understanding Xeroderma Pigmentosum," prepared by the National Institutes of Health, is available on the Internet at www.cc.nih.

gov/ccc/patient_education/pepubs/xp5_18.pdf. This booklet provides information about XP for patients, their families, educators, students, health professionals, media inquiries, and others interested in learning more about XP.

A web site listing disease-causing mutations in XP and CS genes has been established: http://xpmutations.org/

## Patient support groups

The Xeroderma Pigmentosum Society is an educational, advocacy, and support organization for XP patients and their families: Xeroderma Pigmentosum Society Inc., Box 4759, Poughkeepsie, NY 12602-4759; Web site: http://www.xps.org; e-mail: xps@toll-free (877) XPS-CURE (877-977-2873).

Another support group is the XP Family Support Group, 8375 Folsom Blvd Suite 201, Sacramento Ca, 95826. Their website is http://www.xpfamilysupport.org/

There is an XP Support Group in the United Kingdom. Their website is http://xpsupportgroup.org.uk/

A support group in France called Enfants de la lune has a website http://www.orpha.net/nestasso/AXP/

A support group in Germany has a website http://www.xerodermapigmentosum.de/

## Acknowledgments

We apologize to our colleagues for being able to cite only a limited number of original papers and for the use of reviews, owing to space and reference limitations. We thank the members of our research groups for their contribution to the work over the years. Studies by MS mentioned in the text have been supported by grants from the Associazione Italiana per la Ricerca sul Cancro, the European Community (contracts SC1-232, CHRX-CT94-0443, QLG1-1999-00181 and MRTN-CT-2003-503618), the Italian Ministry of Education, University and Research, and the Fondazione Cariplo to MS. Research by KHK was supported by the Intramural Research Program of the NIH and the Center for Cancer Research of the National Cancer Institute.

## References

Andressoo JO, Hoeijmakers JH (2005) Transcription-coupled repair and premature ageing. Mutat Res 577: 179–194.

Andrews AD, Barrett SF, Robbins JH (1978) Xeroderma pigmentosum neurological abnormalities correlate with colony-forming ability after ultraviolet radiation. Proc Natl Acad Sci USA 75: 1984–1988.

Arase S, Kozuka T, Tanaka K, Ikenaga M, Takebe H (1979) A sixth complementation group in xeroderma pigmentosum. Mutat Res 59: 143–146.

Arlett CF, Plowman PN, Rogers PB, Parris CN, Abbaszadeh F, Green MH, McMillan TJ, Bush C, Foray N, Lehmann AR (2006) Clinical and cellular ionizing radiation sensitivity in a patient with xeroderma pigmentosum. Br J Radiol 79: 510–517.

Bernerd F, Asselineau D, Frechet M, Sarasin A, Magnaldo T (2005) Reconstruction of DNA repair-deficient xeroderma pigmentosum skin in vitro: a model to study hypersensitivity to UV light. Photochem Photobiol 81: 19–24.

Bohr VA, Sander M, Kraemer KH (2005) Rare diseases provide rare insights into DNA repair pathways, TFIIH, aging and cancer. DNA Repair 4: 293–302.

Bootsma D, De Weerd-Kastelein EA, Kleijer WJ, Keyzez W (1975) Genetic complementation analysis of xeroderma pigmentosum. Basic Life Sci 5B: 725–728.

Bootsma D (1978) Xeroderma pigmentosum. In: Hanawalt PC, Friedberg EC, Fox CF (eds.) DNA repair mechanisms. ICN-UCLA Symposium on molecular and cellular biology. New York: Academic Press, pp. 589–601.

Bootsma D, Hoeijmakers JHJ (1991) The genetic basis of xeroderma pigmentosum. Ann Genet 34: 143–150.

Bootsma D (2001) The "Dutch DNA Repair Group", in retrospect. Mutat Res 485: 37–41.

Boyle J, Ueda T, Gonzalez V, Oh KS, Imoto K, Inui H, Busch DB, Khan SG, Tamura D, DiGiovanna JJ, Kraemer KH (2006) Splice mutations in the XPD gene and absence of neurological symptoms. J Invest Dermatol 126: 79.

Brooks PJ (2007) The case for 8,5′-cyclopurine-2′-deoxynucleosides as endogenous DNA lesions that cause neurodegeneration in xeroderma pigmentosum. Neuroscience 145: 1407–1417.

Brooks PJ, Wise DS, Berry DA, Kosmoski JV, Smerdon MJ, Somers RL, Mackie H, Spoonde AY, Ackerman EJ, Coleman K, Tarone RE, Robbins JH (2000) The oxidative DNA lesion 8,5′-(S)-cyclo-2′-deoxyadenosine is repaired by the nucleotide excision repair pathway and blocks gene expression in mammalian cells. J Biol Chem 275: 22355–22362.

Broughton BC, Cordonnier A, Kleijer WJ, Jaspers NGJ, Fawcett H, Raams A, Garritsen VH, Stary A, Avrili M, Boudsocq F, Masutani C, Hanaoka F, Fuchs RP, Sarasin A, Lehmann AR (2002) Molecular analysis of mutations in DNA polymerase eta in xeroderma pigmentosum-variant patients. Proc Natl Acad Sci USA 99: 815–820.

Burk PG, Lutzner MA, Clarke DD, Robbins JH (1971a) Ultraviolet-stimulated thymidine incorporation in xeroderma pigmentosum lymphocytes. J Lab Clin Med 77: 759–767.

Burk PG, Yuspa SH, Lutzner MA (1971b) Xeroderma pigmentosum and DNA repair. Lancet 1: 601.

Chang HR, Ishizaki K, Sasaki MS, Toguchida J, Kato M, Nakamura Y, Kawamura S, Moriguchi T, Ikenaga M (1989) Somatic mosaicism for DNA repair capacity in fibroblasts derived from a group A xeroderma pigmentosum patient. J Invest Dermatol 93: 460–464.

Chavanne F, Broughton BC, Pietra D, Nardo T, Browitt A, Lehmann AR, Stefanini M (2000) Mutations in the XPC gene in families with xeroderma pigmentosum and consequences at the cell, protein, and transcript levels. Cancer Res 60: 1974–1982.

Clarkson SG (2003) The XPG story. Biochimie 85: 1113–1121.

Cleaver JE (1968) Defective repair replication of DNA in xeroderma pigmentosum. Nature 218: 652–656.

Cleaver JE (1972) Xeroderma pigmentosum: variants with normal DNA repair and normal sensitivity to ultraviolet light. J Invest Derm 58: 124–128.

Cleaver JE (1975) Xeroderma pigmentosum: biochemical and genetic characteristics. Ann Rev Genet 9: 19–38.

Cleaver JE, Arutyunyan RM, Sarkisian T, Kaufmann WK, Greene AE, Coriell L (1980) Similar defects in DNA repair and replication in the pigmented xerodermoid and the xeroderma pigmentosum variants. Carcinogenesis 1: 647–655.

Cleaver JE, Kraemer KH (1989) Xeroderma pigmentosum. In: Scriver CR, Beaudet AL, Sly WS, Valle D (eds.) The metabolic basis of inherited diseases. New York: McGraw-Hill, pp. 2949–2971.

Cleaver JE, Thompson LH, Richardson AS, States JC (1999) A summary of mutations in the UV-sensitive disorders: xeroderma pigmentosum, Cockayne syndrome, and trichothiodystrophy. Hum Mutat 14: 9–22.

Cleaver JE (2005a) Mending human genes: A job for a lifetime. DNA Repair 4: 635–638.

Cleaver JE (2005b) Cancer in xeroderma pigmentosum and related disorders of DNA repair. Nat Rev Cancer 5: 564–573.

D'Errico M, Parlanti E, Teson M, de Jesus BM, Degan P, Calcagnile A, Jaruga P, Bjoras M, Crescenzi M, Pedrini AM, Egly JM, Zambruno G, Stefanini M, Dizdaroglu M, Dogliotti E (2006) New functions of XPC in the protection of human skin cells from oxidative damage. EMBO J 25: 4305–4315.

De Sanctis C, Cacchione A (1932) L'idiozia xerodermica. Rivista Sperimentale di Freniatria e Medicina Legale delle Alienazioni Mentali 56: 269–292.

de Weerd-Kastelein EA, Keijzer W, Bootsma D (1972) Genetic heterogeneity of xeroderma pigmentosum demonstrated by somatic cell hybridization. Nature New Biol 238: 80–83.

de Weerd-Kastelein EA, Kleijer WJ, Sluyter ML, Keijzer W (1973) Repair replication in heterokaryons deprived from different repair-deficient xeroderma pigmentosum strains. Mutat Res 19: 237–243.

de Weerd-Kastelein EA, Keijzer W, Bootsma D (1974) A third complementation group in xeroderma pigmentosum. Mutat Res 22: 87–91.

DiGiovanna JJ, Patronas N, Katz D, Abangan D, Kraemer KH (1998) Xeroderma pigmentosum: spinal cord astrocytoma with 9-year survival after radiation and isotretinoin therapy. J Cutan Med Surg 2: 153–158.

Emmert S, Slor H, Busch DB, Batko S, Albert RB, Coleman D, Khan SG, Abu-Libdeh B, DiGiovanna JJ, Cunningham BB, Lee MM, Crollick J, Inui H, Ueda T, Hedayati M, Grossman L, Shahlavi T, Cleaver JE, Kraemer KH (2002) Relationship of neurologic degeneration to genotype in three xeroderma pigmentosum group G patients. J Invest Dermatol 118: 972–982.

Emmert S, Wetzig T, Imoto K, Khan SG, Oh KS, Laspe P, Zachmann K, Simon JC, Kraemer KH (2006) A novel complex insertion/deletion mutation in the XPC DNA repair gene leads to skin cancer in an Iraqi family. J Invest Dermatol 126: 2542–2544.

Epstein JH, Fukuyama K, Reed WB Epstein WL (1970) Defect in DNA synthesis in skin of patients with xeroderma pigmentosum demonstrated in vivo. Science 168: 1477–1478.

Essers J, Vermeulen W, Houtsmuller AB (2006) DNA damage repair: anytime, anywhere? Curr Opin Cell Biol 18: 240–246.

Fischer E, Jung EG, Cleaver JE (1980) Pigmented xerodermoid and XP-variants. Arch Dermatol Res 269: 329–330.

Ford JM (2005) Regulation of DNA damage recognition and nucleotide excision repair: another role for p53. Mutat Res 577: 195–202.

Frederick GD, Amirkhan RH, Schultz RA, Friedberg EC (1994) Structural and mutational analysis of the xeroderma pigmentosum group D (XPD) gene. Hum Mol Genet 3: 1783–1788.

Friedberg EC, Lehmann AR, Fuchs RP (2005) Trading places: how do DNA polymerases switch during translesion DNA synthesis? Mol Cell 18: 499–505.

Friedberg EC, Walker GC, Siede W, Wood RD, Schultz RA, Ellenberger T (2006) Xeroderma pigmentosum: a disease associated with defective nucleotide excision repair or defective translesion synthesis. In: DNA repair and mutagenesis. Washington DC: ASM Press, pp. 863–894.

Giannelli F, Pawsey SA (1976) DNA repair synthesis in human heterokaryons. III. The rapid and slow complementing varieties of xeroderma pigmentosum. J Cell Sci 20: 207–213.

Gillet LC, Scharer OD (2006) Molecular mechanisms of mammalian global genome nucleotide excision repair. Chem Rev 106: 253–276.

Gong F, Kwon Y, Smerdon MJ (2005) Nucleotide excision repair in chromatin and the right of entry. DNA Repair 4: 884–896.

Gratchev A, Strein P, Utikal J, Goerdt S (2003) Molecular genetics of Xeroderma pigmentosum variant. Exp Dermatol 12: 529–536.

Hirai Y, Kodama Y, Moriwaki S, Noda A, Cullings HM, Macphee DG, Kodama K, Mabuchi K, Kraemer KH, Land CE, Nakamura N (2006) Heterozygous individuals bearing a founder mutation in the XPA DNA repair gene comprise nearly 1% of the Japanese population. Mutat Res 601: 171–178.

Hoeijmakers JHJ (1993) Nucleotide excision repair. II: From yeast to mammals. Trends Genet 9: 173–177.

Hofmann H, Jung EG, Schnyder UW (1978) Pigmented Xerodermoid: first report of a family. Bull Cancer 65: 347–350.

Imoto K, Slor H, Orgal S, Khan SH, Oh KS, Busch DB, Nadem C, Ueda T, Gadoth N, Jaspers NG, Kraemer KH (2005) Xeroderma pigmentousm group F patients with late onset neurological disease. J Invest Dermatol 124: A78.

Itoh T, Mori T, Ohkubo H, Yamaizumi M (1999) A newly identified patient with clinical xeroderma pigmentosum phenotype has a non-sense mutation in the DDB2 gene and incomplete repair in (6−4) photoproducts. J Invest Dermatol 113: 251–257.

Johnson RE, Kondratick CM, Prakash S, Prakash L (1999) hRAD30 mutations in the variant form of xeroderma pigmentosum. Science 285: 263–265.

Jung EG (1970) New form of molecular defect in xeroderma pigmentosum. Nature 228: 361–362.

Jung EG, Bantle K (1971) Xeroderma pigmentosum and pigmented xerodermoid. Birth Defects Orig Artic Ser 7: 125–128.

Khan SG, Metin A, Gozukara E, Inui H, Shahlavi T, Muniz-Medina V, Baker CC, Ueda T, Aiken JR, Schneider TD, Kraemer KH (2004) Two essential splice lariat branchpoint sequences in one intron in a xeroderma pigmentosum DNA repair gene: mutations result in reduced XPC mRNA levels that correlate with cancer risk. Hum Mol Genet 13: 343–352.

Khan SG, Oh KS, Shahlavi T, Ueda T, Busch DB, Inui H, Emmert S, Imoto K, Muniz-Medina V, Baker CC, DiGiovanna JJ, Schmidt D, Khadavi A, Metin A, Gozukara E, Slor H, Sarasin A, Kraemer KH (2006) Reduced XPC DNA repair gene mRNA levels in clinically normal parents of xeroderma pigmentosum patients. Carcinogenesis 27: 84–94.

Keijzer W, Jaspers NG, Abrahams PJ, Taylor AM, Arlett CF, Zelle B, Takebe H, Kinmont PD, Bootsma D (1979) A seventh complementation group in excision-deficient xeroderma pigmentosum. Mutat Res 62: 183–190.

Kleijer WJ, de Weerd-Kastelein EA, Sluyter ML, Keijzer W, de Wit J, Bootsma D (1973) UV-induced DNA repair synthesis in cells of patients with different forms of xeroderma pigmentosum and of heterozygote. Mutat Res 20: 417–428.

Kobayashi T, Kuraoka I, Saijo M, Nakatsu Y, Tanaka A, Someda Y, Fukuro S, Tanaka K (1997) Mutations in the XPD gene leading to xeroderma pigmentosum symptoms. Hum Mutat 9: 322–331.

Kobayashi T, Uchiyama M, Fukuro S, Tanaka K (2002) Mutations in the XPD gene in xeroderma pigmentosum group D cell strains: confirmation of genotype-phenotype correlation. Am J Med Genet 110: 248–252.

Kore-eda S, Tanaka T, Moriwaki S, Nishigori C, Imamura S (1992) A case of xeroderma pigmentosum group A diagnosed with a polymerase chain reaction (PCR) technique. Usefulness of PCR in the detection of point mutation in a patient with a hereditary disease. Arch Dermatol 128: 971–974.

Kraemer KH, Coon HG, Petinga RA, Barrett SF, Rahe AE, Robbins JH (1975a) Genetic heterogeneity in xeroderma pigmentosum: complementation groups and their relationship to DNA repair rates. Proc Nat Acad Sci USA 72: 59–63.

Kraemer KH, De Weerd-Kastelein EA, Robbins JH, Keijzer W, Barrett SF, Petinga RA, Bootsma D (1975b) Five complementation groups in xeroderma pigmentosum. Mutat Res 33: 327–340.

Kraemer KH, Lee MM, Scotto J (1987) Xeroderma pigmentosum. Cutaneous, ocular, and neurologic abnormalities in 830 published cases. Arch Dermatol 123: 241–250.

Kraemer KH, DiGiovanna JJ, Moshell AN, Tarone RE, Peck GL (1988) Prevention of skin cancer in xeroderma pigmentosum with the use of oral isotretinoin. N Engl J Med 318: 1633–1637.

Kraemer KH, Levy DD, Parris CN, Gozukara EM, Moriwaki S, Adelberg S, Seidman MM (1994a) Xeroderma pigmentosum and related disorders: examining the linkage between defective DNA repair and cancer. J Invest Dermatol 103 (5 Suppl): 96S–101S.

Kraemer KH, Lee MM, Andrews AD, Lambert WC (1994b) The role of sunlight and DNA repair in melanoma and nonmelanoma skin cancer: The xeroderma pigmentosum paradigm. Arch Dermatol 130: 1018–1021.

Kuraoka I, Bender C, Romieu A, Cadet J, Wood RD, Lindahl T (2000) Removal of oxygen free-radical-induced 5',8-purine cyclodeoxynucleosides from DNA by the nucleotide excision-repair pathway in human cells. Proc Natl Acad Sci USA 97: 3832–3837.

Laine JP, Egly JM (2006) When transcription and repair meet: a complex system. Trends Genet 22: 430–436.

Lanza A, Lagomarsini P, Casati A, Ghetti P, Stefanini M (1997) Chromosomal fragility in the cancer-prone disease xeroderma pigmentosum preferentially involves bands relevant for cutaneous carcinogenesis. Int J Cancer 74: 654–663.

Lehmann AR, Kirk-Bell S, Arlett CF, Paterson MC, Lohman PHM, De Weerd-Kastelein EA, Bootsma D (1975) Xeroderma pigmentosum cells with normal levels of excision repair have a defect in DNA synthesis after UV-irradiation. Proc Natl Acad Sci USA 72: 219–223.

Lehmann AR (2001) The xeroderma pigmentosum group D (XPD) gene: one gene, two functions, three diseases. Genes Dev 15: 15–23.

Lehmann AR (2003) DNA repair-deficient diseases, xeroderma pigmentosum, Cockayne syndrome and trichothiodystrophy. Biochimie 85: 1101–1111.

Lehmann AR (2006) Clubbing together on clamps: The key to translesion synthesis. DNA Repair 5: 404–407.

Leibeling D, Laspe P, Emmert S (2006) Nucleotide excision repair and cancer. J Mol Histol 37: 225–238.

Masutani C, Kusumoto R, Yamada A, Dohmae N, Yokoi M, Yuasa M, Araki M, Iwai S, Takio K, Hanaoka F (1999) The XPV (xeroderma pigmentosum variant) gene encodes human DNA polymerase eta. Nature 399: 700–704.

Matsumura Y, Nishigori C, Yagi T, Imamura S, Takebe H (1998) Characterization of molecular defects in xeroderma pigmentosum group F in relation to its clinically mild symptoms. Hum Mol Genet 7: 969–974.

McCulloch SD, Kokoska RJ, Masutani C, Iwai S, Hanaoka F, Kunkel TA (2004) Preferential cis-syn thymine dimer bypass by DNA polymerase eta occurs with biased fidelity. Nature 428: 97–100.

Moriwaki S, Kraemer KH (2001) Bridging a gap between clinic and laboratory. Photodermatol Photoimmunol Photomed 17: 47–54.

Nichols AF, Ong P, Linn S (1996) Mutations specific to the xeroderma pigmentosum group E Ddb phenotype. J Biol Chem 271: 24317–24320.

Nichols AF, Itoh T, Graham JA, Liu W, Yamaizumi M, Linn S (2000) Human Damage-specific DNA-binding Protein p48. Characterization of XPE mutations and regulation following UV irradiation. J Biol Chem 275: 21422–21428.

Nishigori C, Moriwaki S, Takebe H, Tanaka T, Imamura S (1994) Gene alterations and clinical characteristics of xeroderma pigmentosum group A patients in Japan. Arch Dermatol 130: 191–197.

Oh KS, Schmidt D, Kraemer KH (2005) A new xeroderma pigmentosum group E kindred with a R273H mutation in the DDB2 gene has features mimicking XP variant cells. J Invest Dermatol 124: A81.

Oh KS, Khan SG, Jaspers NG, Raams A, Ueda T, Lehmann A, Friedmann PS, Emmert S, Gratchev A, Lachlan K, Lucassan A, Baker CC, Kraemer KH (2006) Phenotypic heterogeneity in the XPB DNA helicase gene (ERCC3): xeroderma pigmentosum without and with Cockayne syndrome. Hum Mutat 27: 1092–1103.

Park CJ, Choi BS (2006) The protein shuffle. Sequential interactions among components of the human nucleotide excision repair pathway. FEBS J 273: 1600–1608.

Paterson MC, Lohman PH, Westerveld A, Sluyter ML (1974) DNA repair monitored by an enzymatic assay in multinucleate xeroderma pigmentosum cells after fusion. Nature 248: 50–52.

Procianoy F, Cruz AA, Baccega A, Ferraz V, Chahud F (2006) Aggravation of eyelid and conjunctival malignancies following photodynamic therapy in De Sanctis-Cacchione syndrome. Ophthal Plast Reconstr Surg 22: 498–499.

Rapic-Otrin V, Navazza V, Nardo T, Botta E, McLenigan M, Bisi DC, Levine AS, Stefanini M (2003) True XP group E patients have a defective UV-damaged DNA binding protein complex and mutations in DDB2 which reveal the functional domains of its p48 product. Hum Mol Genet 12: 1507–1522.

Rapin I, Lindenbaum Y, Dickson DW, Kraemer KH, Robbins JH (2000) Cockayne syndrome and xeroderma pigmentosum. Neurology 55: 1442–1449.

Reardon JT, Sancar A (2005) Nucleotide excision repair. Prog Nucleic Acid Res Mol Biol 79: 183–235.

Robbins JH, Levis WR, Miller AE (1972) Xeroderma pigmentosum epidermal cells with normal UV-induced thymidine incorporation. J Invest Dermatol 59: 402–408.

Robbins JH, Burk PG (1973) Relationship of DNA repair to carcinogenesis in xeroderma pigmentosum. Cancer Res 33: 929–935.

Robbins JH, Kraemer KH, Lutzner MA, Festoff BW, Coon HG (1974) Xeroderma pigmentosum. An inherited diseases with sun sensitivity, multiple cutaneous neoplasms, and abnormal DNA repair. Ann Int Med 80: 221–248.

Robbins JH, Kraemer KH, Flaxman BA (1975) DNA repair in tumor cells from the variant form of xeroderma pigmentosum. J Invest Dermatol 64: 150–155.

Robbins JH (1988) Xeroderma pigmentosum. Defective DNA repair causes skin cancer and neurodegeneration. JAMA 260: 384–388.

Sidwell RU, Sandison A, Wing J, Fawcett HD, Seet JE, Fisher C, Nardo T, Stefanini M, Lehmann AR, Cream JJ (2006) A novel mutation in the XPA gene associated with unusually mild clinical features in a patient who developed a spindle cell melanoma. Br J Dermatol 155: 81–88.

Sijbers AM, de Laat WL, Ariza RR, Biggerstaff M, Wei YF, Moggs JG, Carter KC, Shell BK, Evans E, de Jong MC, Rademakers S, de Rooij J, Jaspers NG, Hoeijmakers JH, Wood RD (1996) Xeroderma pigmentosum group F caused by a defect in a structure-specific DNA repair endonuclease. Cell 86: 811–822.

Sijbers AM, van Voorst Vader PC, Snoek JW, Raams A, Jaspers NG, Kleijer WJ (1998) Homozygous R788W point mutation in the XPF gene of a patient with xeroderma pigmentosum and late-onset neurologic disease. J Invest Dermatol 110: 832–836.

Slor H, Batko S, Khan SG, Sobe T, Emmert S, Khadavi A, Frumkin A, Busch DB, Albert RB, Kraemer KH (2000) Clinical, cellular, and molecular features of an Israeli xeroderma pigmentosum family with a frameshift mutation in the XPC gene: sun protection prolongs life. J Invest Dermatol 115: 974–980.

States JC, McDuffie ER, Myrand SP, McDowell M, Cleaver JE (1998) Distribution of mutations in the human xeroderma pigmentosumgroup A gene and their relationships to the functional regions of the DNA damage recognition protein. Hum Mutat 12: 103–113.

Stefanini M, Keijzer W, Dalprà L, Elli R, Nazzaro Porro M, Nicoletti B, Nuzzo F (1980) Differences in the level of UV repair and in clinical symptoms in two sibs affected by xeroderma pigmentosum. Human Genetics 54: 177–182.

Stefanini M (2006) Trichothiodystrophy, a disorder highlighting the crosstalk between DNA repair and transcription. In: Balajee A (ed.) DNA repair and human diseases. Landes Bioscience, pp. 30–46.

Takayama K, Salazar EP, Lehmann A, Stefanini M, Thompson LH, Weber CA (1995) Defects in the DNA repair and transcription gene ERCC2 in the cancer- prone disorder xeroderma pigmentosum group D. Cancer Res 55: 5656–5663.

Tanaka K, Satokata I, Ogita Z, Uchida T, Okada Y (1989) Molecular cloning of a mouse DNA repair gene that complements the defect of group-A xeroderma pigmentosum. Proc Natl Acad Sci USA 86: 5512–5516.

Tang J, Chu G (2002) Xeroderma pigmentosum complementation group E and UV-damaged DNA-binding protein. DNA Repair 1: 601–616.

Taylor EM, Broughton BC, Botta E, Stefanini M, Sarasin A, Jaspers NG, Fawcett H, Harcourt SA, Arlett CF, Lehmann AR (1997) Xeroderma pigmentosum and trichothiodystrophy are associated with different mutations in the XPD (ERCC2) repair/transcription gene. Proc Natl Acad Sci USA 94: 8658–8663.

Thoma F (2005) Repair of UV lesions in nucleosomes – intrinsic properties and remodeling. DNA Repair 4: 855–869.

van Steeg H, Kraemer KH (1999) Xeroderma pigmentosum and the role of UV-induced DNA damage in skin cancer. Mol Med Today 5: 86–94.

Viprakasit V, Gibbons RJ, Broughton BC, Tolmie JL, Brown D, Lunt P, Winter RM, Marinoni S, Stefanini M, Brueton L, Lehmann AR, Higgs DR (2001) Mutations in the general transcription factor TFIIH result in beta-thalassaemia in individuals with trichothiodystrophy. Hum Mol Genet 10: 2797–2802.

Wood RD, Robins P, Lindahl T (1988) Complementation of the xeroderma pigmentosum DNA repair defect in cell-free extracts. Cell 53: 97–106.

Wood RD, Mitchell M, Lindahl T (2005) Human DNA repair genes. Mutat Res 577: 275–283.

Yarosh D, Klein J, O'Connor A, Hawk J, Rafal E, Wolf P (2001) Effect of topically applied T4 endonuclease V in liposomes on skin cancer in xeroderma pigmentosum: a randomised study. Xeroderma Pigmentosum Study Group. Lancet 357: 926–929.

# Chapter 52

# COCKAYNE SYNDROME

**Miria Stefanini and Martino Ruggieri**

Institute of Molecular Genetics, National Research Council of Italy, Pavia, Italy (MS);
Institute of Neurological Science, National Research Council of Italy, Catania, Italy (MR)

## Introduction

Cockayne syndrome (CS) is a rare autosomal recessive disorder characterised by pre- or post-natal growth failure, leading to a characteristic appearance of so-called cachectic dwarfism, progressive neurologic dysfunction, signs of premature ageing, gait defects, ocular and skeletal abnormalities and otherwise clinically heterogeneous features that commonly include cutaneous photosensitivity but no cancer. In 1992, Nance and Berry have suggested a classification of the disease into three clinically different subtypes: – "classical CS" or type I (CSI), in which classical CS symptoms become manifest within the first few years of life, – "severe CS" or type II (CSII), with more severe symptoms already manifest prenatally, and a mild form, characterised by late onset and slow progression of symptoms (Nance and Berry 1992).

About 50% of the patients with symptoms diagnostic for CS show an abnormal cellular response to ultraviolet (UV) light, characterised by inability to recover normal RNA and DNA synthesis levels at late times after irradiation and hypersensitivity to the killing effects of UV exposure. Genetic analysis led to the definition of two distinct complementation groups, designated CS-A and CS-B, whose corresponding genes (*CSA* and *CSB*) have been cloned. CS cells representative of both groups fail to perform preferential repair of the transcribed strand of transcriptionally active genes at the rate seen in normal cells, but they are capable of removing UV-induced damage from the non-transcribed part of the genome at the normal rate. Hypersensitivity to UV light in CS has therefore been attributed to a specific defect in functions involved in transcription-coupled repair (TCR),

the nucleotide excision repair (NER) sub-pathway that specifically removes DNA damage blocking the progression of the transcription machinery in actively transcribed regions of DNA. Recent experimental evidence suggests that CSA and CSB proteins are involved also in some aspects of transcription as well as in the repair of oxidative DNA damage. Impairments in these processes are likely to be responsible for the ageing features and the progressive neurological degeneration typically observed in CS patients.

Some of the major clinical symptoms of CS have been described in a few rare cases that show in combination the cutaneous alterations of xeroderma pigmentosum (XP). All these patients, assigned to a clinical entity designated XP/CS, have been classified into the XP-B, XP-D, and XP-G groups and are mutated in either the *XPB*, *XPD* or *XPG* gene.

In recent years our knowledge on the genetic and molecular basis of CS has been consistently expanded. Methods are available to assess the cellular response to UV, to detect the gene responsible for the pathological phenotype in the DNA repair defective patients and to identify the underlying mutation(s). However, we have still to fully understand the functions of the CSA and CSB proteins, to elucidate the mechanism of TCR at the molecular level and to identify the disease gene(s) responsible for the clinical outcome of CS in patients with a normal cellular response to UV.

## Historical perspective and eponyms

Cockayne syndrome is named after **Edward Alfred Cockayne** (1880–1956), a London specialist in paediatrics who, in 1936, described a 7-year 11 month-old girl and her 6-year 3-month-old brother who were affected with a condition characterised by cachectic dwarfism, progressive mental retardation, and an odd facial appearance where loss of subcutaneous fat resulted in a "wizened" appearance with typical "bird-headed" facies and prominent "Mickey Mouse" ears. Other features described in the initial report (Cockayne 1936) included microcephaly, enophthalmos, prominent maxillae, disproportionately long extremities in comparison with the size of the trunk (with particular enlargement of the hands and feet), erythematous scaly photosensitive dermatitis, thick cranial vault, shallow pituitary fossa, carious dentition and anorexia. Cockayne followed the development of these children and ten years later wrote a second account reporting additional findings including cataracts, extreme inanition, secondary hypomenorrhea, spasticity of the lower extremities with flexion contractures, cardiac arrhythmias, proteinuria, marked delay in pubertal development pigmentary degeneration of the retina, optic atrophy, and progressive hearing loss (Cockayne 1946). In this report, Cockayne emphasised the progressive nature of the disease. More than 60 cases have subsequently been reported (reviewed in Soffer et al. 1979, Jin et al. 1979), many of them in siblings of both sexes, suggesting an autosomal recessive inheritance.

The sensitivity of many CS patients to sunlight prompted an examination of their sensitivity to UV at the cellular level. Hypersensitivity to killing by UV light was clearly shown in a number of CS cells (Schmickel et al. 1977, Andrews et al. 1978, Hoar and Waghorne 1978, Wade and Chu 1979, Marshall et al. 1980, Lehmann and Mayne 1981). This feature was paralleled by increased mutability (reviewed in Arlett and Harcourt 1982) and by the inability to recover DNA synthesis at late time after irradiation (Lehmann et al. 1979), and to reactivate UV-irradiated adenoviruses (Rainbow and Howes 1982). These observations led to the suggestion that CS patients might be defective in some aspect of DNA repair (Lehmann and Mayne 1981). This notion was reinforced by the demonstration that CS cells were also slightly sensitive to ionising radiations and to

some chemicals generating bulky adducts in DNA, which are substrate for nucleotide excision repair (reviewed in Arlett and Lehmann 1978, Friedberg et al. 2006a).

However, the analysis of several aspects of excision repair failed to show any difference in the response of normal and CS cells to UV exposure (Mayne et al. 1982 and references therein). No defects in unscheduled DNA synthesis (UDS) or in post-replication daughter-strand repair were detected after UV irradiation, pointing to a cellular DNA-repair defective phenotype distinct from those typical of XP (for further information see Chapter 51).

In 1982, Mayne and Lehmann demonstrated that RNA synthesis in human fibroblasts is depressed following exposure to UV irradiation, presumably reflecting inhibition of transcription as a result of DNA damage. In contrast to normal cells, which recover rapidly from this inhibition, CS cells showed a significant delay in RNA synthesis recovery (Mayne and Lehmann 1982). As well as giving an additional indication of a defect in the cellular response to UV-induced DNA damage, these observations provided a cellular diagnostic test for CS. Since then, the abnormality in RNA synthesis following UV exposure has been used successfully as a diagnostic test in patients whose diagnosis was ambiguous and in prenatal diagnosis of pregnancies at risk (Lehmann et al. 1985, 1993; Cleaver et al. 1994; Kleijer et al. 2006). It has also provided a biochemical parameter for measurement of genetic complementation. Pairs of CS cell strains have been fused together and the resulting heterokaryons exposed to UV light. Restoration of normal rates of RNA (or DNA) synthesis indicates that the parental strains in the cross contain genetically different defects and are classified into different complementation groups. In contrast, the absence of correction of the defect after fusion indicates the presence of the same genetic defect, and parental strains are classified in the same group. Analysis performed on twelve patients with CS, led to the identification of two distinct complementation groups, designated CS-A (to which were assigned two cases) and CS-B (with ten cases, including two siblings) (Tanaka et al. 1981, Lehmann 1982, Miyauchi et al. 1994). Using this assay, an individual who also had XP, and was the sole known representative of XP complementation group B was classified in a third complementation group, designated CS group C (Lehmann 1982). Later on, this designation was considered confusing and it has been withdrawn (Lehmann et al. 1994).

In the mid-1980s, a fundamental tool for understanding the modalities of NER in mammalian cells and the biological roles of the function altered in CS-A and CS-B patients was provided by a group led by P. Hanawalt. Bohr and his colleagues (Bohr et al. 1985) devised an elegant experimental technique for monitoring the kinetics of removal of the major UV-induced DNA lesions (i.e., cyclobutane pyrimidine dimers, CPD) from defined genes. This technical strategy coupled the sensitivity of Southern hybridisation for examining defined regions of the genome with the substrate specificity of pyrimidine dimer-DNA glycosylase, a DNA repair enzyme that incises DNA at CPD that are formed as a consequence of exposure to UV light. Using this technique, it was shown that the rate of loss of CPD from a transcriptionally active gene was faster that in the genome overall. This phenomenon was referred to as the preferential repair of transcriptionally active gene (Bohr et al. 1985, 1987; Mellon et al. 1986). More refined analysis of the phenomenon using hybridisation probes for each of the two DNA strands revealed that in many transcriptionally active eukaryotic genes the transcribed strand is repaired more rapidly than the nontranscribed strand (Mellon et al. 1987, Hanawalt and Mellon 1993, Hanawalt 2002). The observation that in mammalian cells preferential repair and strand-specific repair of transcriptionally active genes are confined to genes that are transcribed by RNA polymerase II, has led to the view that these two repair modalities are mechanistically related and reflect the operation of a NER mode that is somehow coupled to the process of transcription elongation by RNA polymerase II at sites of base damage (Friedberg 1996a).

In 1990, Venema and colleagues demonstrated that UV-irradiated CS cells fail to repair transcriptionally active DNA with a similar rate and to the same extent as normal cells (Venema et al. 1990). Further studies provided evidence for defective exci-

sion repair of CPD in transcribed genes in CS cells and normal excision repair of other photoproducts (Barrett et al. 1991, Parris and Kraemer 1993). Analysis of the removal of UV-induced CPD using strand specific probes indicated that in CS cells the preferential repair of the transcribed strand does not take place, damage in these regions being repaired at the same (slow) rate as in the bulk of the DNA (Van Hoffen et al. 1993). Some CS cell strains were described to be also slightly deficient in the repair of UV-induced damage located on the nontranscribed strand of active genes (Van Hoffen et al. 1993). Based on these cellular studies, it was proposed that the CSA and CSB proteins might have a similar role to the transcription-repair coupling factor identified in *Escherichia coli* (Selby et al. 1991, Selby and Sancar 1993).

In the same period, Nance and Berry performed a comprehensive review of 140 CS patients to serve as a resource for physicians and other caregivers of CS patients regarding the important characteristics of the syndrome, and to identify which manifestations are of particular significance in the long term prognosis of patients (Nance and Berry 1992). This paper represents a major milestone in elucidating the clinical features of CS. The authors first proposed diagnostic criteria for CS that include 1) poor growth, 2) neurodevelopmental and later neurological dysfunction, with evidence of predominant white-matter involvement, and at least three of the following clinical features: 3) cutaneous photosensitivity, 4) progressive pigmentary retinopathy and/or cataract, optic disk atrophy, miotic pupils, or decreased lacrimation, 5) sensorineural hearing loss, 6) dental caries, and 7) a characteristic physical appearance, that of "cachectic dwarfism", with a characteristic stance in the ambulatory patients. The last four criteria are more likely to be present in the older child than in the infant or toddler. Furthermore, Nance and Berry (1992) assigned patients with CS to three clinical subtypes. Clinical subtype I corresponds to classic CS and accounted for about 85% of cases. An extremely severe phenotype was assigned to clinical subtype II and included about 20 children with onset in infancy, sometimes even prenatally, who died in the first few years of life. Subtype II had intrauterine growth failure, congenital cataracts, or other structural eye abnormalities, and infants developed the typical facies and other CS features very early. Clinical subtype III was limited to four patients who presented with mild or atypical phenotypes because of normal intelligence, linear growth, or reproductive capacity. Afterward, the wide clinical presentations in CS has been confirmed in CS patients additionally reported in the literature (Pasquier et al. 2006, Rapin et al. 2006).

The correlation between clinical symptoms and the failure of RNA synthesis to recover to normal rates after UV irradiation was explored in 1993 by Lehmann et al. (1993). These authors analysed the response to UV in 52 cases for whom a clinical diagnosis of CS was considered a possibility. Twenty-nine patients showed the defect characteristic of CS cells, and 23 had a normal response. The comparison of the clinical features of the "defective RNA synthesis" and "normal RNA synthesis" groups showed that all patients had growth and mental retardation, microcephaly, and, in most cases, abnormal facial features, these being in many cases the reasons for the initial suspicion of diagnosis of CS. Tremor and cataracts did not differ greatly between the two groups. Pigmentary retinopathy, dental caries and gait abnormalities were found much more frequently in the "defective RNA synthesis" than in the "normal RNA synthesis" group. This suggests that these features are good positive indicators for a diagnosis of CS, although their absence does not exclude it. Photosensitivity -manifested as a persistent erythema after sun exposure, accompanied in some instances by dermatitis- was the clinical feature that correlated most strongly with defective RNA synthesis. Only five patients with normal RNA synthesis were photosensitive whereas photosensitivity was absent in one case with defective RNA synthesis (Lehmann et al. 1993). The correlation between the cellular diagnosis and the clinical features required by Nance and Berry (1992) showed that three or more of the required characteristics were present in 18 out of the 29 patients with defective UV response and in 4 out of the 23 patients with normal response to UV. In conclusion, this study showed that in the absence of a specific laboratory test, a patient can be diagnosed

with confidence as having CS if growth and mental retardation, microcephaly, pigmentary retinopathy, gait defects, and dental caries are present (Lehmann et al. 1993). The status of a small number of patients who have normal RRS, but nevertheless have several of the clinical features of CS, remains obscure still at present.

The genes defective in the CS-A and CS-B complementation groups were cloned in 1995 and 1992, respectively (Troelstra et al. 1992, Henning et al. 1995). However, the limited number of patients which have been subject to complementation analysis were impeding studies aimed at determining the correlation between clinical phenotypes and molecular defects. In 1996, a complementation test - in which the fusion products were unequivocally identified using latex beads-less laborious than the previous ones was set up (Stefanini et al. 1996). In this assay, cells of two different CS donors are labelled with beads of different size, fused and analysed for their ability to recover RNA synthesis at late times after UV-irradiation. Restoration of normal RNA synthesis rate in heterodikaryons, which can be easily recognized as binuclear cells containing beads of both sizes, indicates that the partners in the fusion are in different complementation groups, whereas a failure to effect this recovery implies that they are in the same group. Seventeen out of the twenty-two CS patients analysed in this study were assigned to group B, the remaining five (of which two belong to the same family) fell into group A (Stefanini et al. 1996). Therefore, the relative frequencies of CS-A and CS-B defects in the newly characterised CS patients were similar to those found in the twelve cases described previously with CS-B being the most common group (Tanaka et al. 1981, Lehmann 1982, Miyauchi et al. 1994). Intriguingly, no "new" CS genetic defect was identified in this analysis of twenty-one families from eight different countries and representing several different ethnic groups. This indicates that if defects in any gene other than *CSA* and *CSB* can result in the CS phenotype (in the absence of XP features), they must, if they exist at all, be extremely rare.

In the last decade, many studies have supported the notion that CS-A and CS-B cells are defective in a DNA repair mode that is transcription-dependent (reviewed in Friedberg et al. 2006b). However, it is still an unresolved question whether this is the primary molecular defect responsible for the complex clinical outcome of the disorder. An attractive hypothesis is that CS cells have a defect in transcription affecting the expression of certain genes, which is compatible with embryogenesis but not with normal post-natal development. Defective transcription may impair the normal processing of DNA damage during transcription-dependent repair (Friedberg 1996b). Recent experimental evidence indicates that CSA and CSB proteins are involved also in some aspects of transcription as well as in the repair of oxidative DNA damage (reviewed in Friedberg et al. 2006b). Impairments in these processes might explain the ageing features and the progressive neurological degeneration typically observed in CS patients. A current model proposes that the severity and early onset of the developmental and neurological defects in CS patients are due to excessive cell death and progressive transcription insufficiency in tissues that undergo rapid cell proliferation, high levels of transcription, and other metabolic activities that may generate reactive oxygen species, particularly during embryonic development and early childhood (Spivak 2004).

Meanwhile, in vitro and in vivo studies have widely investigated the role of CSB and CSA in TCR of UV lesions (Fousteri et al. 2006; Lainé and Egly 2006a, b) and their functional relationships has been unravelled (Groisman et al. 2006). Additional information is emerging from the analysis of CS mouse models (Wijnhoven et al. 2007), although DNA repair pathways differ in significant ways between rodents and humans, and therefore, the use of mouse model systems for study of human DNA repair has limitations. A major challenge for the future is to clarify the pathogenesis of CS by correlating the roles played by the CSA and CSB proteins in repair and transcription with the differing clinical features of the disorder.

## Incidence

CS is an autosomal recessive disorder that is rare worldwide. About 200 cases have been described in the literature and an incidence of less than 1 case per 250,000 live births has been reported for the United States. The syndrome has been described in children from almost every ethnic background. Consistent with autosomal recessive inheritance, there is no significant difference between the sexes.

## Clinical manifestations

The cardinal clinical features of CS are pre- or post-natal growth failure, leading to a characteristic appearance of so-called cachectic dwarfism, and progressive neurological dysfunction. Associated clinical features are gait defects, progressive pigmentary retinopathy and other ocular anomalies such as cataracts and optic disc atrophy, sensorineural hearing loss, dental caries and cutaneous photosensitivity. The disease is clinically heterogeneous, with a wide range in type and severity of symptoms. A subdivision into three clinically different classes of the disease has been suggested by Nance and Berry (1992): (i) a classical form, or CS I (which includes the majority of cases), showing the first two symptoms listed above and at least three of the others; (ii) a severe CS form, or CS II, characterized by early onset and severe progression of symptoms, with low birth weight and poor or absent physical and neurological development; and (iii) a mild form, characterized by late onset and slow progression of symptoms.

*Cerebro-oculo-facial syndrome* (COFS), which is also referred to as Pena-Shokeir syndrome type II, overlaps clinically with the severe form of CS. Furthermore, the clinical hallmarks of CS have been reported in rare patients showing in combination the cutaneous alterations of XP. All these cases have been assigned to a clinical entity designated XP/CS. Clinical features of COFS and XP/CS complex phenotype are reported at the end of this section.

## Skin manifestations

Photosensitivity is a prominent feature and is usually seen in 50% of patients with CS. In the *classical form* dermatitis appears on the sun-exposed parts of the body early in life, by the second year of life, with a butterfly arrangement on the face (Fig. 1A). The forehead is spared, but the pinnae and chin are involved (Lindenbaum et al. 2001, Rapin et al. 2000). Acute sensitivity leads to erythema that desquamates leaving

post-inflammatory pigmentary changes (hyperpigmentation) and scarring in older patients (Rapin et al. 2006). As the children grow up they typically develop the appearance of "cachectic dwarfism". The freckles and dyspigmentation seen in XP are not features of

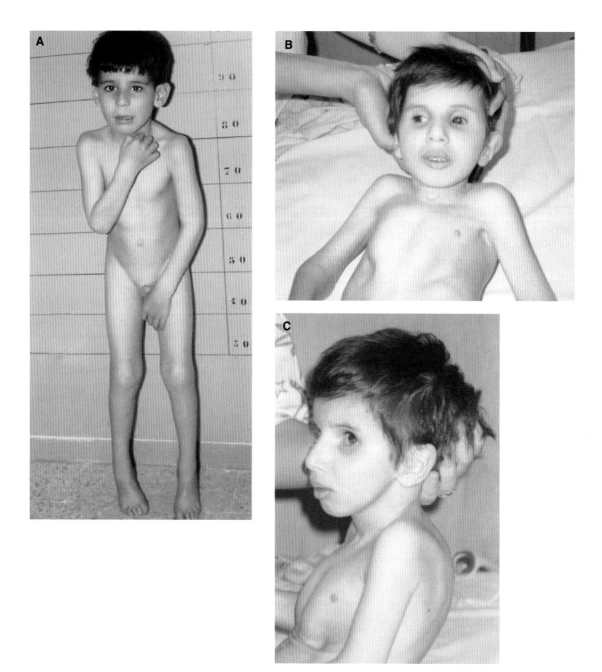

**Fig. 1.** (**A**) Phenotypic appearance of affected individuals; (**B**, **C**) typical facial appearance; (**D**) body disproportion and associated musculoskeletal abnormalities.

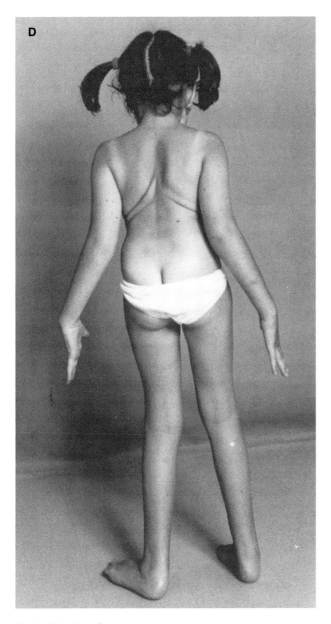

**Fig. 1.** (Continued)

this disease. Seborrheic dermatitis may also be present. The scalp hair and, sometimes, the eyebrows are diminished. Subcutaneous fat appears to be decreased throughout the body except for the suprapubic areas (the eccrine sweat glands are abnormally small for the patients' age). Remarkably, in striking contrast with XP, and with the only exception of patients who fall into the XP/CS complex phenotype, no significant increase in skin cancer is noted.

Other skin manifestations include thin, dry hair and dry, scaly skin. These findings coupled with the diminution of subcutaneous fat, contribute to the "aged" or progeric appearance of these patients.

Typical progeric, dwarf-like features are noted before the age of 2 years in the *severe form of CS*: cutaneous complications, however, are less commonly noted (Rapin et al. 2000, Wagner 2006).

## Facies

Progressive loss of subcutaneous facial fat, particularly of the cheeks, gives prominence to the facial bones. This feature, combined with microcephaly, sunken eyes, thin often beak-like nose, vermillion of the lips, and large ears, gives the patient a birdlike appearance (Fig. 1B, C). Microcephaly is radiologically apparent during the 2nd an 3rd years of life (Bensman et al. 1981, Riggs and Seibert 1972).

## Eyes

Enophthalmos is a virtually constant feature. The retina is studded with fine, speckled pigment of salt-and-pepper type, with the greater concentration in the macular area. In addition to pigmentary retinopathy, optic atrophy and arterioral narrowing are common. Congenital cataract is frequently reported in severely affected CS cases. In other patients, cataracts have developed by adolescence. A poor response to mydriasis with homatrophine or Neosynephrine (miotic pupils) has been noted. Corneal dystrophy with recurrent epithelial erosions, nystagmus, and photophobia are less frequently observed (Traboulsi et al. 1992).

## Oral manifestations

An increase in dental caries has been reported by most authors. In some cases, numerous permanent teeth were congenitally absent. Atrophy of alveolar processes, condylar hypoplasia, and short conical roots have also been observed.

## Musculoskeletal abnormalities

Proportionate dwarfism is the most prominent feature of the disorder. Growth retardation becomes evident during the second decade of life after a normal gestation, birth weight, and infancy. A low birth weight is reported in severely affected patients. Kyphosis and osteoporosis are frequent. The limbs are disproportionately long (Fig. 1D). Flexion contractures may involve the ankles, knees, and elbows. The interphalangeal joints of the hands and feet may show periarticular thickening. Overall, the progeria-like features associated to the disproportionately large hands and feet with flexion contractures of joints result in the typical "horse riding stance".

## Neurological manifestations

The earliest commonly noticed neurological abnormality is delayed psychomotor development, which usually becomes apparent at the time when sitting, walking, and speech should develop. The delay in the acquisition of functions becomes progressively greater as the patients grow older (van der Knaap and Valk 2005). In the course of the years other progressive neurological abnormalities become apparent including increasing spasticity, cerebellar signs (e.g., tremor, lack of coordination, dysarthric speech, and gait ataxia). Pyramidal signs are usually present with hypertonia and hyperreflexia. Myoclonus and involuntary choreiform and athetoid movements are rare. The gait disorder in patients who become ambulatory is striking and progressive, due to a combination of spasticity, ataxia, weakness and contractures of the hips, knees and ankles (Rapin et al. 2000, van der Knaap and Valk 2005). These manifestations are well explained by the widespread brain pathology (see below, pathology). Mental capacities vary from mildly to profoundly deficient; normal intelligence has been reported in one case (Lanning and Simila 1970). The progressive high-tone hearing loss results from gradual degeneration of all the cellular elements of the cochlea, associated with secondary degeneration of the relays of the central auditory pathway (Rapin et al. 2000). Advancing loss of vestibular function be-cause of progressive cellular death in the vestibular labyrinth, added to the cerebellar degeneration, impaired somatosensory input from the neuropathy, and increasingly poor vision contributes to the ataxia of patients with CS (Rapin et al. 2000).

In contrast to the recessive severe primary microcephalies (which occur prenatally), the typical microcephaly in CS is mainly postnatal: the brain in CS is extraordinarily small but the head circumference is normal at birth. These observations make it unlikely that the cause of the extreme microcephaly of CS is premature curtailment of neurogenesis, disordered neuronal migration, or grossly aberrant connectivity (Rapin et al. 2000). Interference with the proliferation, branching, and deployment of neuronal processes seems more plausible (indeed, lamination of the neurocortex, as well as neuronal size and configuration, are relatively preserved) (Gandolfi et al. 1984, Rapin et al. 2000). This relatively normal structural brain development, including the neocortex, may account for one of the notable features of CS (commented on by Cockayne in his original 1936 description and by Neil and Dingwall in 1950 and Brumback et al. in 1978): namely, less profoundly impaired cognition and behaviour than one might predict from the diminutive size of the brain (some 400 to 700 g), together with remarkably preserved sociality and alertness (Rapin et al. 2000).

Some patients have diminished lacrimation, decreased sweating, miotic pupils, and cool and acrocyanotic limbs. This could be due to autonomic dysfunction, but formal assessment of autonomic function has not been documented. Seizures occur late and in a minority of patients.

Overt signs of peripheral neuropathy are rare until the late stages of disease, leading to a progressive, diffuse muscular atrophy, muscle weakness, and areflexia.

## Other findings

Hypertension and renal disease are frequent complications. Elevated peripheral vein rennin and deposits of immunoglobulin and complement in the kidney vessels and glomerulus have been reported. Undescended testes, small breast, and oligomenorrhea have

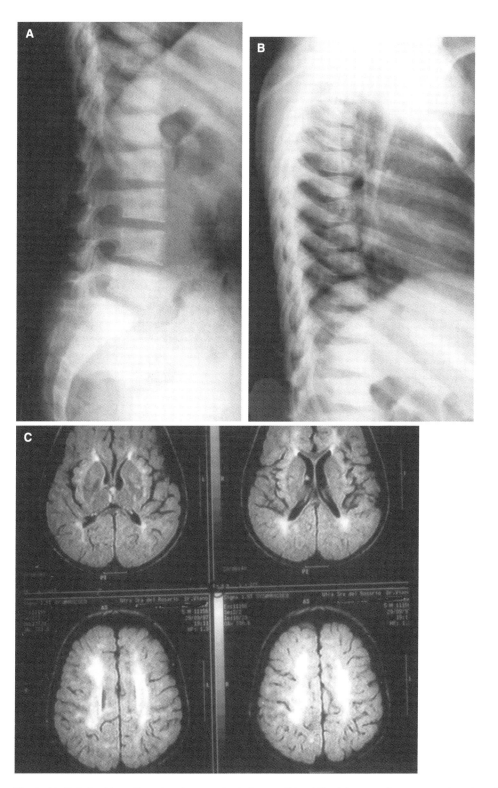

**Fig. 2.** (**A**, **B**) Spine X-ray films showing vertebral abnormalities; (**C**) axial magnetic resonance imaging of the brain in an affected child showing extensive white matter damage.

been also noted. Elevated liver function tests, enlargement of liver or spleen and emphysema have been described.

## Imaging findings

Radiographic studies show abnormalities in the skull, extremities, and spine. There is increased thickening of the bones, particularly the base and calvaria, most noticeable in the frontal and parieto-occipital regions. Microcephaly and brain atrophy are apparent on skull X-rays. Often there is associated osteoporosis. Other characteristic radiological manifestations are (reviewed in Taybi 1996) (Fig. 2A, B): (a) *spinal abnormalities* including platyspondyly with ovoid (and/or biconcave) vertebral bodies and tongue-like protrusion of the anterior aspects of the vertebral bodies (anterior notching); increase in the antero-posterior diameter of vertebral bodies; scalloping and posterior wedging of vertebral bodies; thoracic kyphosis; intervertebral calcifications; (b) *various nonspecific limb abnormalities* including hypoplasia of the iliac wings and acetabular roofs; slender long bones with narrow medullary canal; slightly bowed fibulas; large tarsal and carpal bones; asymmetric fingers; brachydactyly; marble epiphyses in the terminal phalanges of the hands; (c) osteoporosis; (d) thin elongated ribs; (e) underdevelopment and sclerosis of the mastoids; poor aeration of the paranasal sinuses; small mandible.

CT scans of the brain may demonstrate calcifications of the putamen, thalamus and cerebral and cerebellar white matter superficial to the dentate nuclei, although in some patients the calcium deposits are very subtle (Barkovich 2005, van der Knaap and Valk 2005). Cerebral, cerebellar, and brain stem atrophy with prominence of sulci and ventricular enlargement is usually seen.

Magnetic resonance imaging studies confirms the presence of variable hypoplasia and atrophy, most pronounced in brain stem and cerebellum (Fig. 2C). There is a loss of white matter volume and ventricles are mildly enlarged in most patients (Nishio et al. 1988, van der Knaap and Valk 2005). In addition, there are symmetrical white matter abnormalities. On T2-weighted images the signal intensity of the cerebral white matter is abnormally high, but usually not so high as in completely unmyelinated white matter in neonates. The white matter often seems to have a finely irregular granular aspect, probably reflecting the tigroid pattern of myelin presence. In many CS patients the moderately high signal intensity is seen throughout the hemispheric white matter, including periventricular white matter and U fibres, sometimes also the internal capsule (van der Knaap and Valk 2005). The corpus callosum has a better state of myelination. In other patients the white matter is better myelinated in the subcortical areas and the white matter hyperintensity is most marked in the periventricualr area. In the severe form (CS type II) the myelin deficiency is more profound and the cerebellum as a rule very hypoplastic.

Progressive loss of myelin (demyelination) or failure of normal myelination (dysmyelination) is characteristic of CS and is a useful criterion to differentiate CS from XP with neurological disease in which the primary histological finding is neuronal degeneration without inflammation or abnormal depositions.

## XP/CS complex phenotype

Less than two dozen patients with the XP/CS complex have been reported in the literature (reviewed in Lindenbaum et al. 2001, Rapin et al. 2000, Kraemer et al. 2007a). They combine the skin manifestations of XP with the somatic and neurological features of CS. Thus, their skin is hypersensitive to sunlight and they develop the freckling and other pigmentary changes of XP. Cutaneous manifestations may include also neoplasms on sun-exposed skin. Although XP/CS patients differ greatly in clinical severity, they all show the short stature and immature sexual development as well as the neurological and ocular abnormalities typically reported in CS (including pigmentary retinal degeneration, calcification of the basal ganglia, demyelination and cerebellar dysfunction). The disease course is one of progressive neurological degeneration. The neuropathology, like the clinical phenotype, is essentially that of CS, as pointed out by Lindenbaum et al.

(2001) who extensively reviewed the neuropathological features typically present in XP/CS cases. It is worth to recall that XP patients with neurological abnormalities (Chapter 51) may display some features of CS (such as mental retardation, spasticity, short stature, and hypogonadism) but they never show skeletal dysplasia, CNS demyelination and calcifications, and the peculiar facies of CS.

## Cerebro-oculo-facial syndrome

COFS is a rapidly progressive neurological disorder that was explicitly delineated 30 years ago, as occurring with autosomal recessive inheritance in isolated Manitoba families characterised by frequent consanguineous marriages (Pena and Shokeir 1974). Subsequent reports suggested a spectrum ranging from severe perinatal lethal forms to milder forms that allowed affected individuals to survive childhood (reviewed in Meira et al. 2000). Key features of the disorder include cerebral atrophy, hypoplasia of the corpus callosum, hypotonia, severe mental retardation, cataracts, microcornea, optic atrophy, progressive joint contractures, osteoporosis and postnatal growth deficiency. Recent observations by Helene Dolphus indicate that the eye defects in COFS are more severe but similar to those observed in CS, i.e., congenital cataract, retinal degeneration, optic atrophy and enopthalmus (reported in Kraemer et al. 2007b). As in CS, postmortem examination reveals dilated ventricles, marked myelin attenuation with a tigroid pattern of demyelination, calcific deposits, and hypoplastic cerebellum (Del Bigio et al. 1997; Sakai et al 1997).

There is no clear consensus on the criteria that differentiate COFS from CS type II. Although skeletal abnormality at birth due to foetal immobility and cataracts at birth are considered important diagnostic criteria of COFS, these two parameters may be insufficient to uniquely define this syndrome. Thus, it remains possible that COFS and CS type II are distinct syndromes with significant overlap (Bohr et al 2005). The identification of a mutation in the CSB gene in five patients related to the Manitoba Aboriginal population group within which

COFS syndrome was originally reported (Meira et al. 2000) indicates that CS and COFS syndrome share a common pathogenesis. On the basis of these findings, it was suggested that COFS syndrome no longer constitutes a distinct genetic entity but represents an allelic, clinically severe form of CS (Meira et al. 2000).

Another patient diagnosed with a severe form of COFS has been reported as having defective NER caused by mutations in the XPD gene by Graham and colleagues (2001). As a further example of the association between COFS and NER defects, these authors mention two previously characterised cases mutated in the XPG gene, who were considered as affected by XP/CS in the original reports (Hamel et al. 1996; Sigmundsson et al. 1998; Moriwaki et al. 1996).

Recently, mutations in ERCC1, another gene involved in NER, have been found in a child with symptoms compatible with a clinical diagnosis of a severe form of COFS (Jaspers et al. 2007). At birth, the patient's weight, length, and occipitofrontal circumference were <3rd percentile. The infant had microcephaly with premature closure of fontanels, bilateral microphthalmia, blepharophimosis, high nasal bridge, short filtrum, micrognathia, low-set and posteriorrotated ears, arthrogryposis with rockerbottom feet, flexion contractures of the hands, and bilateral congenital hip dislocation. On X-rays, there was no evidence for spine abnormalities. Nuclear magnetic resonance revealed cerebellar hypoplasia and a simplified gyral pattern, which was not previously described in patients with defective NER. These alterations are indicative of postmitotic neuronal migration defects and a probable cause of impaired foetal movement, which is consistent with the joint deformities of the patient at birth.

Since COFS and CS are usually considered within the same differential diagnosis and both disorders include photosensitive and non-photosensitive cases, DNA repair studies cannot be informative for the diagnosis. However, the finding of UV hypersensitivity in a patient suspected of having COFS or early onset CS would provide a cellular parameter that allows for reliable genetic counselling and management of future pregnancies (Graham et al. 2001).

## Pathology

Histopathological examination of the eyes of CS affected individuals demonstrated optic atrophy, retinal pigmentation, loss of nerve fibres and ganglion cell layers, findings consistent with those observed in demyelinating disease.

In CS there is progressive degeneration of both central and peripheral nerve tissues. Neuropathologic studies of the brain have shown microcephaly (the brain is extraordinarily small but is not grossly malformed; see also above, neurological manifestations), widespread (extra-vascular) mineralisation in the cortex, basal ganglia, and cerebellum, leptomeningeal fibrosis, patchy ependymal denudation with glial overgrowth, and patchy myelin loss, often severe, with axonal preservation in the subcortical white matter, in the basal ganglia, and, especially, in the cerebellum where exuberant proliferation of atypical dendrites of Purkinje cells and neuronal death by apoptosis have been documented. There may be very premature arteriosclerosis coupled with the calcific vasculopathy, meningeal fibrosis, excessive accumulation of lipofuscin in neurons, Alzheimer neurofibrillary tangles, and Hirano bodies (Rapin et al. 2000, Soffer et al. 1979). These features are not uniformly present and vary significantly in intensity. Brumback et al. (1978) suggested the possibility that low-pressure hydrocephalus may contribute to ventricular dilatation and clinical deterioration.

Biopsy of the sacral nerve showed the main pathologic change to be segmental demyelination with re-myelination (onion-bulb formation) and moderate decrease in the number of myelinated fibres with axonal loss.

## Natural history

### CS type I (classical form)

In the majority of CS affected individuals, prenatal growth is typically normal. Birth length, weight, and head circumference are normal. Within the first two years, however, growth and development fall below normal. By the time the disease has become fully manifest, height, weight, and head circumference are far below the 5th percentile. Progressive impairment of vision, hearing, and central and peripheral nervous system function leads to severe disability.

Additional neurological abnormalities reported in at least 10% of patients include increased tone/spasticity, hyper- or hyporeflexia, abnormal gait or inability to walk, ataxia, incontinence, tremor, abnormal or absent speech, seizures, muscle atrophy, behavioural abnormality, weak cry and poor feeding, Ophthalmologic manifestations often present are enophthalmos, pigmentary retinopathy, abnormal electroretinogram, cataracts, optic atrophy, miotic pupils, farsightedness, decreased or absent tears, strabismus, nystagmus, photophobia, narrowed retinal arterioles, and microphthalmia.

Severe dental caries occur in up to 86% of affected individuals. Absent or hypoplastic teeth, delayed eruption of deciduous teeth, and malocclusion have also been reported. Photosensitivity can be severe, but individuals are not predisposed to skin cancers. Other sporadically reported dermatological findings are anhidrosis and malar rash.

Undescended testes and/or delayed/absent sexual maturation is a common finding. No individuals with classic or severe CS forms (type I or II) have been known to reproduce. A successful (but very difficult) pregnancy has been reported in a young woman with mild CS (type III) (Lahiri and Davies 2003).

Death typically occurs in the first or second decade. The mean age of death is 12 years, but survival into the third decade has been reported.

### CS type II (severe form)

These patients have earlier onset of symptoms and are more severely affected than typical classical CS patients (Wagner 2006). They show intrauterine growth retardation, poor postnatal growth, severe and rapidly progressive neurologic impairment, and congenital cataracts or early structural eye abnormalities. Typical progeric, dwarf-like features are noted before the age of 2 years. Affected individuals have arthrogryposis or early postnatal contractures of the spine (kyphosis, scoliosis) and joints. Dental, auditory, and cutaneous complications are less commonly noted. Affected children typically die by age six to seven years.

## CS type III (mild form)

Symptoms of this CS form are typically mild and late in onset. The patients may have normal intelligence, growth and reproductive capacity (Wagner 2006). As mentioned above, the first case of successful pregnancy in a patient with mild CS has been reported in 2003 (Lahiri and Davies 2003).

## Pathogenesis/molecular genetics

About 50% of patients with symptoms diagnostic for CS have a normal response to UV. No cellular marker has been so far identified for these non photosensitive cases and nothing is known about the genes responsible for the pathological phenotype.

An altered cellular response to UV light is present in the remaining CS patients, including a few cases that do not exhibit cutaneous photosensitivity (Colella et al. 1999). Following UV irradiation cells from these CS patients cells show reduced extent of "host cell reactivation" (i.e., capacity to repair damaged DNA of infecting viruses), increased mutability, and increased frequency of chromosomal aberrations and sister chromatid exchanges. Other alterations typically observed in CS cells are: inability to recover normal RNA and DNA synthesis levels at late times after UV irradiation, substantial

sensitivity to the killing effects of UV light. The magnitude of these defects appears to be rather uniform in CS patients and does not correlate with the clinical severity of the disorder. In a few CS cases, the RNA synthesis defect appears to be intermediate between normal and bona fide CS cells (Lehmann 2003). The status of these patients remains to be determined.

The pattern of response to UV light typically present in CS cells reflects a specific defect in transcription-coupled repair (TCR), the nucleotide excision repair (NER) sub-pathway that specifically removes DNA damage blocking the progression of the transcription machinery in actively transcribed regions of DNA (see Chapter 51). In particular, CS cells are defective in the removal of CPD located on the transcribed strand of transcriptionally active genes whereas they normally repair other photoproducts and CPD located on the silent regions of the genome. Normal capability of removing damage from the non-transcribed part of the genome (called global genome repair-GGR) in CS cells results in normal level of UV-induced DNA repair synthesis (UDS).

Genetic analysis led to the definition of two distinct complementation groups, designated CS-A and CS-B, whose corresponding genes (*CSA* and *CSB*) have been cloned. The function and features of these genes are reported in Table 1.

Both CS-A and CS-B cells are proficient in checkpoint activation after UV irradiation, suggesting that a functional GGR is necessary and sufficient to activate the checkpoint response, whereas TCR may be dispensable (Marini et al. 2006).

CS cells are sensitive also to some chemicals, such as N-acetoxy-N-2-acetyl-2-aminofluorene and

**Table 1.** Genes responsible for Cockayne syndrome

| Gene name (synonyms) | Accession No. | Chromosome location[a] | Size (aa) | Function |
|---|---|---|---|---|
| CSA (CKN1, ERCC8) | NM_000082 | 5q12.1 | 396 | E3 ubiquitin ligase |
| CSB (ERCC6) | NM_000124 | 10q11.23 | 1493 | DNA-dependent ATPase and chromatin remodelling |

*ERCC8* Excision repair cross-complementing rodent complementation group 8; *ERCC6* excision repair cross-complementing rodent complementation group 6.
[a] From http://www.cgal.icnet.uk/DNA_Repair_Genes.html. See also Wood et al. (2005).

4-nitroquinoline 1-oxide, that form bulky adducts in DNA that are substrates for NER. Furthermore, they are defective in oxidative DNA damage response. This defect extends beyond the level of TCR because CS-A and CS-B cells are impaired in the repair of oxidatively induced DNA lesions that are a substrate for base excision repair (BER), a repair mechanism distinct from NER.

For a comprehensive overview of cellular and molecular aspects of CS (see Bohr et al. 2005, Cleaver 2005, Reardon and Sancar 2005, Andressoo et al. 2006, Friedberg et al. 2006a, Lainé and Egly 2006, Sarasin and Stary 2007).

## Clinical, cellular and molecular characteristics of the CS groups

More than 50 CS cases showing different degrees of severity in the pathological phenotype and coming from a wide range of ethnic backgrounds have been genetically characterised. Two thirds of the patients have been assigned to the CS-B group and the remaining one third to CS-A. CS-B is much the most prevalent group for Western CS patients, while CS-A is much more prevalent in patients of Asian origin (Lehmann and Stefanini, unpublished observations). It is worthwhile mentioning that the CS-B group includes also three cases with the severe form of CS, who showed an altered cellular response to UV even though they had no signs of clinical photosensitivity (Colella et al. 1999). The main clinical and cellular features of the two complementation groups of CS are reported in Table 2. No obvious clinical or cellular differences were observed between patients in the two groups. Patients with different clinical severity were classified in either CS-A or CS-B group, indicating that mutations in the same gene are associated with the clinical distinct forms of CS. As already mentioned, another important implication of the genetic analysis results is that, if defects in any "repair" gene other than CSA and CSB can result in the CS phenotype, they must, if they exist at all, be extremely rare.

**Table 2.** Clinical and cellular features of the two complementation groups of Cockayne syndrome

| Group | OMIM | Clinical symptoms[a] | | Cellular response to UV[b] | | |
|---|---|---|---|---|---|---|
| | | Neurological impairment | Physical impairment | UV-sensitivity | UDS, % normal | RRS |
| CS-A | 133540 | +/+++ | +/+++ | ++ | 100 | – |
| CS-B | 133540 | ++/+++ | +/+++ | ++ | 100 | – |

[a] Cases with different severity in terms of age at onset and severity of neurological and physical impairment. Mildly (+), moderately (++) or severely (+++) affected cases. See text for details.
[b] UV-sensitivity: survival consistently reduced compared with normal (3–5x) UDS (unscheduled DNA synthesis): the ability to perform UV-induced DNA repair synthesis is expressed as a percentage of that in normal cells. RRS: Recovery of RNA synthesis rate after UV is defective (5–20% of normal).

**Table 3.** Mutational analysis in patients with Cockayne syndrome CS

| Gene | Cases No. | Recurrent mutations | Mutated products[a] |
|---|---|---|---|
| CSA | 20 | yes | truncated products* (single aa substitutions) |
| CSB | 20 | yes | truncated products* (single aa substitutions) |

[a] See also XP mutation database http://xpmutations.org/for mutations identified in these genes. *Severely truncated polypeptides because of either stop codons, frameshifts, splice abnormalities or genomic DNA deletions. Changes identified in a minority of cases are between brackets.

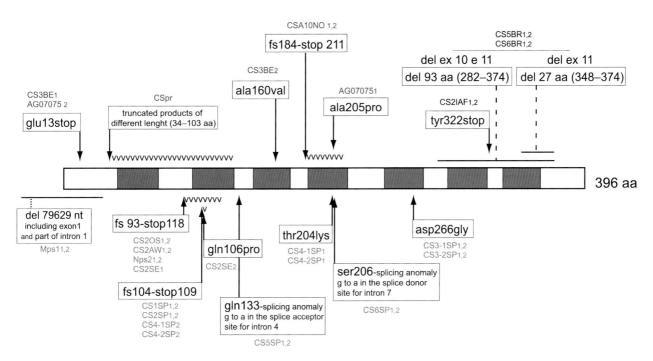

**Fig. 3.** CSA protein and inactivating aminoacid changes caused by the mutations found in 20 patients with Cockayne syndrome (CS), four of which are affected by the classical form of CS (code in blue), and three by the severe form of CS (code in black). The clinical form of CS is not reported in the remaining 13 cases (code in grey). The diagram shows the CSA protein with the seven WD repeats (red boxes). The amino acid changes are shown boxed, with the change in black on white. The numbers 1 and 2 after the patient code denote the different alleles. Patients reported by Henning et al. (1995), McDaniel et al. (1997), Ren et al. (2003), Cao et al. (2004), Komatsu et al. (2004), Ridley et al. (2005), Bertola et al. (2006), and Kleppa et al. (2006).

Causative mutations have been identified in both CS-A and CS-B patients. The main features emerged from this analysis are reported in Table 3.

Most of the mutations identified in the 20 CS-A patients reported in the literature (Fig. 3) result in severely truncated polypeptides because of either stop codons, frameshifts, splice abnormalities or genomic DNA deletions (Henning et al. 1995, McDaniel et al. 1997, Ren et al. 2003, Cao et al. 2004, Komatsu et al. 2004, Ridley et al. 2005, Bertola et al. 2006, Kleppa et al. 2006). In the majority of the patients, both alleles are affected in this way and it is highly unlikely that the corresponding mutated proteins would have any functional ability. No indications can be drawn on genotype-phenotype relationships because the clinical form is not reported for 13 cases. Stefanini and colleagues (unpublished observations) have sequenced the *CSA* gene in additional 12 CS-A patients showing differ-

ent degrees of clinical severity. Besides confirming that *CSA* is not an essential gene, mutational analysis indicated that the molecular defect does not correlate with the severity of the clinical phenotype. This observation implies that the type and severity of the clinical features in CS-A patients must be influenced by factors in the intra-uterine environment and/or genetic background.

Mutational analysis has been performed in 20 CS-B patients showing different degrees of severity in the pathological phenotype and coming from a wide range of ethnic backgrounds (Troelstra et al. 1992; Mallery et al. 1998; Colella et al. 1999, 2000; Meira et al. 2000; Horibata et al. 2004). As shown in Fig. 4, 15 of the 21 mutations resulted in severely truncated products. In 13 patients, both alleles were affected in this way, resulting in proteins that are likely to be functionally inactive. This indicates that the *CSB* gene is not essential for viability and cell

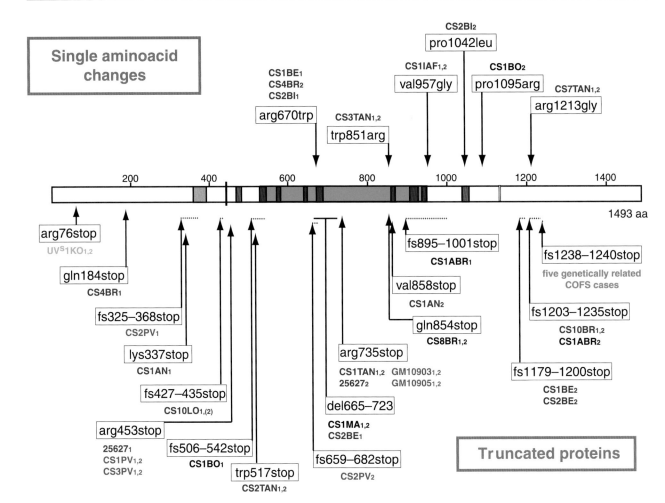

**Fig. 4.** CSB protein and inactivating aminoacid changes caused by the mutations found in 20 patients with Cockayne syndrome (CS), in 5 patients with Cerebro-Oculo-Facio-Skeletal syndrome (COFS), in two brothers with a severe form of xeroderma pigmentosum (XP), and in one case with the UV-sensitive syndrome (UVˢS). The diagram shows the CSB protein with the putative functional domains. The amino acid changes are shown boxed, with the change in black on white. The colour of the patient code refers to the disorder: CS classical form in blue, CS severe form in black, CS severe form without clinical photosensitivity in red, COFS in green, XP in violet, UVˢS in light blue. The numbers 1 and 2 after the patient code denote the different alleles. Patients reported by Troelstra et al. (1992), Mallery et al. (1998), Colella et al. (1999, 2000), Meira et al. (2000), and Horibata et al. (2004).

proliferation, an important issue to be considered in any speculation on the recently demonstrated additional function of the CSB protein in transcription. The six missense mutations are all located in the *CSB* region corresponding to aminoacids 670–1213. The mutations resulting in the changes Arg670Trp, Trp851Arg e Val957Gly lie either within or very close to the helicase domains of the protein and are likely to abolish any function associated with these domains. The location or type of mutations found in

CS-B patients does not correlate with the clinical phenotypes. Severe truncations were found in patients with either classical or early-onset forms of the disease as well as in three cases with the severe form of CS but without clinical photosensitivity (Colella et al. 1999). Conversely, both severe and moderate phenotypes are associated with truncating and missense mutations and even with the same set of mutated *CSB* alleles. The lack of clear genotype–phenotype relationships suggests that the clinical features must be influenced either by environmental factors encountered in utero or by other aspects of the genetic background. This notion has been further extended by the finding that the same inactivating mutation in the *CSB* gene (Colella et al. 2000) was associated with distinct pathological phenotypes diagnostic, respectively, for CS and for a severe form of XP (Greenhaw et al. 1992).

As reported in Fig. 4, mutations in the *CSB* gene have also been found associated with two other clinical entities. The first is COFS, an autosomal recessive disorder that, as already mentioned, shares a lot of clinical features with CS, including severe mental and physical retardation and precocious ageing. The second is a very mild disorder, designated UV-Sensitive Syndrome (UV<sup>S</sup>S), in which affected individuals have skin photosensitivity and freckling, without proneness to skin cancer or CS classical features (reviewed in Spivak 2005). The mutation detected in the *CSB* gene of two UV<sup>S</sup>S patients results in a severely truncated protein. However, no protein was detected by immunoblot analysis, suggesting that the total absence of the CSB protein may be less deleterious than the truncated or abnormal counterparts found in CS-B patients (Horibata et al. 2004).

## Functions defective in CS

CSA and CSB are the key players in TCR, a repair modality where lesion-induced stalling of the transcribing RNA polymerase II serves as a signal for recruitment of factors responsible for NER (see Chapter 51, fig. 2). By rapidly repairing damage in the transcribed strand of active genes, TCR may enable the cell to quickly resume transcription and prevent cell death. Several studies have shown that the persistence of CPD in the transcribed strand of active genes leads to apoptosis. In UV-irradiated CS-A and CS-B primary fibroblasts, the induction of p53 is not paralleled by any increase in mdm2 expression and the persistence of high levels of p53, due to the lack of its degradation by mdm2, is associated with a drastically increased apoptotic response (Conforti et al. 2000, D'Errico et al. 2005 and references therein).

The coupling between transcription and repair involves a chain of events that include chromatin remodelling, recruitment of a repair complex, recycling and/or ubiquitylation of RNA polymerase II. Both CS proteins are required for enhanced repair of actively transcribed genes and for ubiquitylation of RNA polymerase II after UV-induced damage but their precise role has still to be fully elucidated. Biochemical studies have shown that CSA and CSB reside in complexes with different activities. CSA via interaction with DDB1 is integrated in a complex with cullin 4A and Roc1 (CSA core complex), which displays E3-ubiquitin ligase activity. Following UV-irradiation, COP9/signalosome (CSN), a protein complex with ubiquitin isopeptidase activity, rapidly associates with the CSA core complex, thus silencing the CSA-associated E3-ubiquitin ligase activity (Groismann et al. 2003). CSB resides in a >700-kDa complex (van Gool et al. 1997) and interacts with RNA polymerase II, XPG, TFIIE, TFIIH and splicing factors. It has been shown that stalled RNA polymerase II at UV-damaged sites is associated with CSB, which then recruits the CSA core/CSN complex that is inactive for E3-ubiquitin ligase activity (Groismann et al. 2003). In UV-irradiated cells, CSA rapidly translocates to the nuclear matrix by a CSB-dependent mechanism, where it colocalises with hyperphosphorylated form of RNA polymerase II, engaged in transcription elongation (Kamiuchi et al. 2002). A current model proposes that CSB monitors progression of RNA polymerase II by regularly probing its elongation. When RNA polymerase II encounters DNA damage, CSB becomes more tightly recruited to participate in remodelling the DNA/RNA polymerase II interface. Depending on the type of damage, this would result in either a bypass and/or a stabilisation of RNA polymerase II to allow for the recruitment of the repair factors (Lainé and Egly 2006a). CSA and CSB display differential roles in recruitment of chromatin remodelling and repair factors to stalled RNA polymerase II *in vivo*. CSB is necessary to attract the histone acetyltransferase p300, a chromatin remodelling factor, and all the NER factors specific for TCR, including the proteins involved in the late steps of the repair process. In cooperation with CSB,

CSA is required for recruitment of the nucleosomal binding protein HMGN1, the chromatin factor XAB2, and the transcription factor TFIIS (Fousteri et al. 2006). *In vitro* studies have shown that an isolated elongating RNA polymerase II stalled at the lesion is able to sequentially recruit the repair factors and to initiate and/or mediate an ATP-dependent incision of the damaged DNA in the presence of CSB (Lainé and Egly 2006a). Therefore, it has been suggested that CSB might push the blocked RNA polymerase II forward in the vicinity of the lesion, enabling the recruitment of the repair factors in a sequential manner. Once the repair complex has assembled around the lesion, RNA polymerase II might be released, whereas CSB probably helps reposition the repair complex (Lainé and Egly 2006b). The CSA-associated ubiquitin ligase activity, silenced by CSN at the beginning of the repair process, becomes active at later stages and is responsible for the degradation of CSB. This event is required for post-repair transcription recovery (Groisman et al. 2006).

The broad range in type and severity of CS symptoms and the lack of clear genotype-phenotype relationships in CS-A and CS-B patients has led to the suggestion that CS proteins might have additional roles outside NER. This notion has been supported by several lines of evidence. CSB has been implicated in chromatin remodelling (Citterio et al. 2000) and in general transcription by RNA polymerase II (Balajee et al. 1997, Selby and Sancar 1997, van Gool et al. 1997, Tantin 1998) and RNA polymerase I (Bradsher et al. 2002). Accordingly, analysis of gene expression profile in CS-B cells has indicated a general role for CSB protein in maintenance and remodelling of chromatin structure, suggesting that CS is a disease of transcriptional deregulation caused by misexpression of growth suppressive, inflammatory, and proapoptotic pathways (Newman et al. 2003). Furthermore, CSB appeared to be involved in the repair of certain types of oxidative DNA damage (reviewed in Licht et al. 2003, Frosina 2007, Wilson and Bohr 2007). Based on the current studies, it has been proposed that CSB is an auxiliary factor in base excision repair (BER), interacting with a number of key proteins and possibly playing a general regulatory role (Wilson and Bohr 2007). A general deficiency in transcription after oxidative stress has been described in CS-B cells (Kyng et al. 2003).

Some major defects highlighted by the expression profile analysis are in the transcription of genes involved in DNA repair, signal transduction, and ribosomal functions. These findings indicate that the consequences of the CS-B defect are extensive and affect not only stress response and transcription regulation but also cell cycle checkpoints and central areas of signal transduction. Altogether these observations suggest a causal contribution of unrepaired oxidative damage to ageing and neurological degeneration (Kyng and Bohr 2005, Bohr et al. 2007). More recently, the analysis of retinopathy, that is a typical trait of CS mouse models, further supports the role of oxidative DNA lesions in CS-specific premature ageing (Gorgels et al. 2006).

Besides the inability to remove DNA damage (UV and oxidative damage) via different mechanisms (TCR/BER), an additional defect has been recently described in CS-B cells. Following UV irradiation, CSB has been shown to play a pivotal role in the transcription initiation of a certain set of protein coding genes. As a consequence, *CSB* mutations result in the disassembly of the preinitiation complex at the housekeeping promoters (Proietti-DeSantis et al. 2006). The possible link between TCR and RNA transcription following UV irradiation could rely on the role of CSB acting as a chromatin remodelling factor, which would favour the recruitment of either the transcriptional machinery at the initiation sites or the repairosome machinery at the damaged sites. The role of CSB in initiating the transcriptional program of a subset of genes after UV irradiation may explain some of the clinical symptoms exhibited by the CS patients.

Like CSB, CSA has been reported to physically interact with TFIIH (Henning et al. 1995), thus suggesting an additional role in general transcription. Recently, D'Errico and colleagues (2007) have provided the first *in vivo* evidence that also the CSA protein contributes to prevent accumulation of various oxidized DNA bases (D'Errico et al. 2007).

Furthermore, analysis of the response to UVB irradiation has shown that the CS-A defect is associated with a strong apoptotic response in fibroblasts but not in keratinocytes, which represent the target cells for skin cancer. In human keratinocytes the mechanism for elimination of heavily damaged cells relies on signalling pathways that are largely TCR/ p53-independent (D'Errico et al. 2005) and an efficient GGR might operate as a back-up system to remove transcription-blocking lesions (D'Errico et al. 2003), thus providing keratinocytes from CS patients of an efficient protection from skin cancer. The cell-type specific response to UVB detected in human (but not in mouse) cells might also account for the disparity in skin cancer rates in CS patients and CS mouse models.

## Functions defective in XP/CS and COFS patients

The XP/CS complex has been described in associations with mutations either in the *XPB*, *XPD* or *XPG* gene. Mutations in these genes are responsible for several disorders corresponding to distinct clinical entities. This puzzling heterogeneity of the clinical outcome is thought to reflect different mutation sites in the gene(s) that differentially affect the structure and/or the functionality of the corresponding protein(s).

XPB and XPD are subunits of TFIIH, a complex involved in several aspects of transcription (including RNA polymerase II transcription initiation, RNA polymerase I transcription, activated transcription) as well as in NER and cell cycle regulation. As deeply discussed in chapter 53, *XPB* and *XPD* mutations associated with the distinct disorders are located at different sites of the genes, thus differentially interfering with the stability and the conformation of the entire TFIIH complex and, consequently, with its multiple activities.

Interestingly, cells from XP/CS patients mutated in *XPD* show a peculiar breakage phenomenon by generating breaks in their DNA in response to UV damage, 8-oxoguanine and methylation damage (Berneburg et al. 2000, Theron et al. 2005). These breaks are not located at the sites of the damage but they are introduced erroneously by the NER ma-

chinery at sites of transcription initiation. It has been suggested that the presence of damage changes the conformation of TFIIH and that in normal cells the TFIIH is recruited from sites of transcription initiation to the sites of the breaks. In the XP-D/CS cells, the conformational change still occurs, but the mutated XPD component prevents the TFIIH from being recruited to the damage. The TFIIH in its "repair conformation" remains at the site of transcription initiation, and the NER nucleases cut the DNA at sites of transcription initiation (Theron et al. 2005). These DNA damage-induced breaks, which are transcription dependent, can be regarded as diagnostic for XP-D/CS. Indeed, they may provide a prognostic marker for development of later CS symptoms in XP-D patients.

The molecular pathology of XP/CS associated with XPG was less clearly understood. A recent study by K. Tanaka, J.M. Egly and colleagues (Ito et al. 2007) demonstrates that XPG forms a stable protein complex with TFIIH and is involved in maintaining the integrity of TFIIH in cooperation with XPD. The *XPG* mutations found in patients with severe XP or XP/CS phenotypes alter the architecture of TFIIH, leading to defects in nuclear receptor transactivation. As well as demonstrating that XPG plays a role in transcription in helping TFIIH to perform some of its functions, these findings support the notion that the clinical features of CS in some XP-G patients are not the consequence of defective TFIIH-dependent repair of DNA but rather result from defective transactivation of critical genes, a process that is also TFIIH dependent. These results raised the question of whether the CS patients with mutations in the *CSA* or *CSB* gene, who show the same features of CS as XP-G patients with XP/CS, have an unstable TFIIH and therefore exhibit a similar dysregulation in gene expression. By showing that CS-A and CS-B cells (as well as XP-B cells from an XP/CS patient) have an intact TFIIH, Ito and colleagues (Ito et al. 2007) demonstrated that the same features of CS could be caused by various transcriptional deficiencies.

Clinically observed similarities between COFS syndrome and CS have been followed by the discovery of a mutation in the *CSB* gene in five patients related to the Manitoba Aboriginal population group within which COFS syndrome was originally reported (Meira et al. 2000). Another patient diagnosed with a severe form of COFS has been reported as having defective NER caused by mutations in the same sites of the *XPD* gene (Graham et al. 2001) that have been found mutated also in a single XP case (asp681) or in several XP and TTD patients (arg616) in combination with other mutated *XPD* alleles. This finding might reflect the puzzling variety of pathological phenotypes that have been identified in association with defects in *XPD*. Recently, mutations in ERCC1, another gene involved in NER, have been found in a child with symptoms compatible with a clinical diagnosis of a severe form of COFS (Jaspers et al. 2007). Besides representing the first case of human ERCC1 deficiency, this unique patient reveals the importance of ERCC1-XPF during human foetal development, in particular for the CNS.

## Diagnosis, follow-up and management (including treatment)

The main diagnostic criteria of CS are low birthweight, little postnatal increase in weight and height, microcephaly, poor or absent psychomotor development, pigmentary retinopathy, sensorineural hearing loss, photosensitivity, arthrogryposis, dental caries, abnormal myelin formation, cerebellar hypoplasia, calcifications by cranial CT and reduced motor nerve conduction, characteristic radiographic findings of thickening of the calvarium, sclerotic epiphyses, vertebral and pelvic abnormalities, a characteristic physical appearance of "cachectic dwarfism" with thinning of the skin and hair, sunken eyes, and a stooped standing posture. Congenital cataracts with other structural defects of the eye (microphthalmia, microcornea, iris hypoplasia) are suggestive for the severe form of CS. The following tests have been identified as useful for diagnosis and management of CS patients: rate of growth, brain imaging, nerve conduction, auditory and vision exam, CSF protein analysis and retinal imaging. Clinicians should ensure that CS patients are examined by a neurologist (Bohr et al. 2005).

The severe form of CS can be diagnosed already at birth whereas in the classical form physical and mental retardation become manifest in childhood. Mild CS cases may have late onset and slow progression of symptoms.

About 50% of the patients with a suspected clinical diagnosis of CS show an abnormal cellular response to UV light. Laboratory testing can be useful for confirming the presence of DNA repair defects at all stages of disease progression. DNA repair investigations are suggested even in the absence of clinical photosensitivity since an altered cellular response to UV has been reported in CS patients that were not sun-sensitive and showed a normal response to both photosensitivity and UVA and UVB sensitisation tests (Colella et al. 1999).

Alterations typically observed in CS cells are inability to recover normal RNA and DNA synthesis levels at late times after irradiation, substantial sensitivity to the killing effects of UV light but normal levels of UV-induced DNA repair synthesis.

As well as representing a cellular diagnostic test for CS, the failure of RNA synthesis to recover following UV-irradiation provides a biochemical parameter for the identification of the gene responsible for the repair defect in CS patients. Genetic analysis relies on complementation assays that are usually performed by fusing fibroblasts of the patient under evaluation with fibroblasts mutated in either the *CSA* or *CSB* gene and by analysing the capacity to recover normal RNA synthesis (RRS) levels at late times after irradiation in heterodikaryons (Fig. 5). The restoration after fusion of normal RRS levels allows the classification of patients into different complementation groups (i.e., they are defective in different genes) whereas the maintenance of impaired RRS levels indicates that the patients are in the same complementation group (i.e., they are defective in the same gene). In parallel to the classical complementation tests based on cell fusion, genetic analysis may be carried out also by analysing the level of RRS in patient's cells after microinjection with plasmids expressing either the *CSA* or *CSB* gene.

Based on the available mutational data, the definition of the molecular defect is not informative for

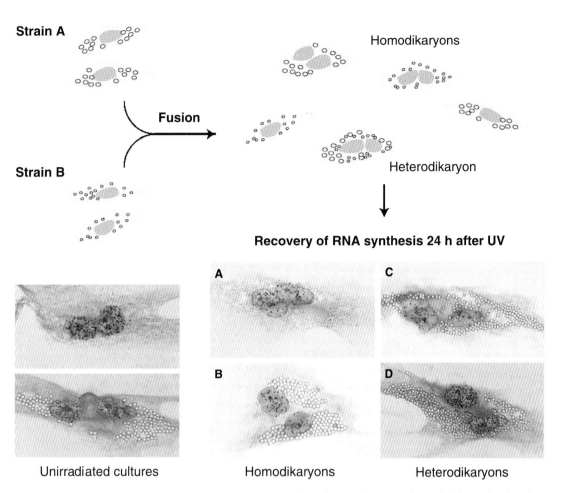

**Fig. 5.** Genetic analysis of the DNA repair defect in patients affected by Cockayne syndrome (CS) by evaluating the recovery of RNA synthesis after UV irradiation in classical complementation tests based on somatic cell hybridisation. The cell strains used as partners in the fusion (i.e., the fibroblasts of the patient under analysis and of CS patients representative of either the CS-A or CS-B complementation group) are grown for three days in medium containing latex beads of different sizes that are incorporated into the cytoplasm as a marker. The cells are fused, irradiated with UV two days later and, after further 24 h analysed for their ability to recover normal RNA synthesis rate by autoradiography. To evaluate the baseline level of RNA synthesis in the fusion partners, one sample of fused cells is treated in parallel but without UV irradiation. Since CS cells fail to recover normal rates of RNA synthesis 24 h following UV irradiation, the number of grains over the nuclei of homodikaryons (identified as binuclear cells containing beads of one size) is significantly lower in the irradiated cultures (panels **A** and **B**) than in the unirradiated cultures. The two cell strains used as partners in the fusion are classified in the same complementation group if the heterodikaryons (identified as binuclear cells containing beads of different sizes) fail to recover normal RNA synthesis levels (panel **C**). Conversely, the restoration of normal RNA synthesis levels in the heterodikaryons (panel **D**) indicates that the cell strains used as partners in the fusion are carrier of genetically different defects.

the prognosis. Lack of genotype-phenotype correlation has been found in patients mutated in the *CSB* gene and no obvious genotype-phenotype correlation is suggested by data on CS-A patients.

Management issues are: 1) comprehensive baseline evaluation at initial diagnosis to establish the

extent of disease and serial monitoring, and 2) symptomatic care.

Baseline evaluation includes measurement of growth, developmental assessment, dental and dermatologic evaluations, ophthalmologic evaluation (including electroretinogram), audiologic evaluation (including audiogram), MRI of the brain, skeletal

X-rays to document the presence of skeletal dysplasia, EMG to document the presence of a demyelinating neuropathy, Laboratory studies to assess renal and hepatic function, Testing for diabetes mellitus and disorders of calcium metabolism.

Surveillance includes yearly reassessment for known potential complications such as hypertension, renal or hepatic dysfunction, hearing loss and declining vision. Patients have to be monitored also dental caries.

Treatment for CS is generally supportive and based on symptoms. Symptomatic care includes an individualized educational program, assistive devices and assessment of safety in the home for developmental delay and gait disturbances, physical therapy to prevent contractures and maintain ambulation, feeding gastrostomy tube placement to prevent malnutrition in patients who feed poorly, and medication for spasticity. The ultimate goal of the treatment strategy for CS is to facilitate the physical and mental development and well-being of the patient, and to optimise his/her neurologic and neurosensory abilities. Hearing loss, cataracts and other ophthalmologic complications, and dental caries are treated as in the general population. Patients should avoid excessive sun exposure and use sunscreens and sunglasses liberally when outdoors.

## Resources

The Share and Care Cockayne Syndrome Network is an international network that was founded in 1981. Its website shares basic information about Cockayne syndrome.

A Web site listing disease-causing mutations in XP and CS genes has been established: http://xp-mutations.org/. Additional information is available on the of Geneskin web site http://geneskin.idi.it, that is part of an European coordination action project on rare genetic skin genetic skin diseases funded by the European Commission (LSHM-CT-2005-512117).

**Patient support group** – The Share and Care Cockayne Syndrome Network offers mutual support and networking for families with CS affected members. This includes the sharing of information between families and professionals, maintaining a registry of families, and providing referral information, a newsletter, phone support, and a pamphlet (which is available in English, Spanish, and Japanese). Share and Care has its own multilingual (English, German, Spanish, Portuguese, French and Japanese) webpage. Web site: http://www.cockayne-syndrome.org

Address: Share and Care Cockayne Syndrome Network, PO Box 282, Waterford, Virginia, 20197; e-mail: JackieClark@aol.com

## Acknowledgments

We apologize to our colleagues for being able to cite only a limited number of original papers and for the use of reviews, owing to space and reference limitations. We thank the members of our research groups for their contribution to the work over the years. Studies by MS mentioned in the text have been supported by grants from the Associazione Italiana per la Ricerca sul Cancro, the European Community (contracts SC1-232, CHRX-CT94-0443, QLG1-1999-00181 and MRTN-CT-2003-503618), the Italian Ministry of Education, University and Research, the Istituto Superiore Sanità-Programma Malattie Rare and the Fondazione Cariplo.

## References

Andressoo JO, Hoeijmakers JH, Mitchell JR (2006) Nucleotide excision repair disorders and the balance between cancer and aging. Cell Cycle 5: 2886–2888.

Andrews AD, Barrett SF, Yoder FW, Robbins JH (1978) Cockayne's syndrome fibroblasts have increased sensitivity to ultraviolet light but normal rates of unscheduled DNA synthesis. J Invest Dermatol 70: 237–239.

Arlett CF, Lehmann AR (1978) Human disorders showing increased sensitivity to the induction of genetic damage. Ann Rev Genet 12: 95–115.

Arlett CF, Harcourt SA (1982) Variation in response to mutagens amongst normal and repair-defective human cells. In: Lawrence CW (ed.) Induced mutagenesis. Molecular mechanisms and their implications for environmental protection. New York: Plenum Publishing Corp, pp. 249–266.

Balajee AS, May A, Dianov GL, Friedberg EC, Bohr VA (1997) Reduced RNA polymerase II transcription in intact and permeabilized Cockayne syndrome group B cells. Proc Natl Acad Sci USA 94: 4306–4311.

Barkovich AJ (2005) Pediatric Neuroimaging, 4<sup>th</sup> ed. Philadelphia: Lippincott Williams and Wilkinson.

Barrett SF, Robbins JH, Tarone RE, Kraemer KH (1991) Evidence for defective repair of cyclobutane pyrimidine dimers with normal repair of other DNA photoproducts in a transcriptionally active gene transfected into Cockayne syndrome cells. Mutat Res 255: 281–291.

Bensman A, Fraure C, Kaufmann HJ (1981) The spectrum of x-ray manifestations in Cockayne's syndrome. Skeletal Radiol 7: 173–177.

Berneburg M, Lowe J, Nardo T, Araujo S, Fousteri M, Green MH, Krutmann J, Wood RD, Stefanini M, Lehmann AR (2000) UV damage causes uncontrolled DNA breakage in cells from patients with combined features of XP-D and Cockayne syndrome. EMBO J 19: 1157–1166.

Bertola DR, Cao H, Albano LM, Oliveira DP, Kok F, Marques-Dias MJ, Kim CA, Hegele RA (2006) Cockayne syndrome type A: novel mutations in eight typical patients. J Hum Genet 51: 701–705.

Bohr VA, Smith CA, Okumoto DS, Hanawalt PC (1985) DNA repair in an active gene: removal of pyrimidine dimers from the DHFR gene of CHO cells is much more efficient than in the genome overall. Cell 40: 359–369.

Bohr VA, Phillips DH, Hanawalt PC (1987) Heterogeneous DNA damage and repair in the mammalian genome. Cancer Res 47: 6426–6436.

Bohr VA, Sander M, Kraemer KH (2005) Rare diseases provide rare insights into DNA repair pathways, TFIIH, aging and cancer. DNA Repair 4: 293–302.

Bohr VA, Ottersen OP, Tonjum T (2007) Genome instability and DNA repair in brain, ageing and neurological disease. Neuroscience 145: 1183–1186.

Bradsher J, Auriol J, Proietti de Santis L, Iben S, Vonesch JL, Grummt I, Egly JM (2002) CSB is a component of RNA pol I transcription. Mol Cell 10: 819–829.

Cao H, Williams C, Carter M, Hegele RA (2004) CKN1 (MIM 216400): mutations in Cockayne syndrome type A and a new common polymorphism. J Hum Genet 49: 61–63.

Citterio E, Van Den Boom V, Schnitzler G, Kanaar R, Bonte E, Kingston RE, Hoeijmakers JH, Vermeulen W (2000) ATP-dependent chromatin remodeling by the Cockayne syndrome B DNA repair-transcription-coupling factor. Mol Cell Biol 20: 7643–7653.

Cleaver JE (2005) Cancer in xeroderma pigmentosum and related disorders of DNA repair. Nat Rev Cancer 5: 564–573.

Cleaver JE, Volpe JP, Charles WC, Thomas GH (1994) Prenatal diagnosis of xeroderma pigmentosum and Cockayne syndrome. Prenat Diagn 14: 921–928.

Cockayne EA (1936) Dwarfism with retinal atrophy and deafness. Arch Dis Child 11: 1–8.

Cockayne EA (1946) Dwarfism with retinal atrophy and deafness. Arch Dis Child 21: 52–54.

Colella S, Nardo T, Mallery D, Borrone C, Ricci R, Ruffa G, Lehmann AR, Stefanini M (1999) Alterations in the CSB gene in three Italian patients with the severe form of Cockayne syndrome (CS) but without clinical photosensitivity. Hum Mol Genet 8: 935–941.

Colella S, Nardo T, Botta E, Lehmann AR, Stefanini M (2000) Identical mutations in the CSB gene associated with either Cockayne syndrome or the DeSanctis-Cacchione variant of xeroderma pigmentosum. Hum Mol Genet 9: 1171–1175.

Conforti G, Nardo T, D'Incalci M, Stefanini M (2000) Proneness to UV-induced apoptosis in human fibroblasts defective in transcription coupled repair is associated with the lack of Mdm2 transactivation. Oncogene 19: 2714–2720.

Del Bigio MR, Greenberg CR, Rorke LB, Schnur R, McDonald-McGinn DM, Zackai EH (1997) Neuropathological findings in eight children with cerebro-oculo-facio-skeletal (COFS) syndrome. J Neuropathol Exp Neurol 56: 1147–1157.

D'Errico M, Teson M, Calcagnile A, Proietti-DeSantis L, Nikaido O, Botta E, Zambruno G, Stefanini M, Dogliotti E (2003) Apoptosis and efficient repair of DNA damage protect human keratinocytes against UVB. Cell Death Differ 10: 754–756.

D'Errico M, Teson M, Calcagnile A, Nardo T, De Luca N, Lazzari C, Soddu S, Zambruno G, Stefanini M, Dogliotti E (2005) Differential role of transcription-coupled repair in UVB-induced response of human fibroblasts and keratinocytes. Cancer Res 65: 432–438.

D'Errico M, Parlanti E, Teson M, Degan P, Lemma T, Calcagnile A, Iavarone I, Jaruga P, Ropolo M, Pedrini AM, Orioli D, Frosina G, Zambruno G, Dizdaroglu M, Stefanini M, Dogliotti E (2007) The role of CSA in the response to oxidative DNA damage in human cells. Oncogene 26: 4336–4343.

Fousteri M, Vermeulen W, van Zeeland AA, Mullenders LH (2006) Cockayne syndrome A and B proteins differentially regulate recruitment of chromatin remodeling and repair factors to stalled RNA polymerase II in vivo. Mol Cell 23: 471–482.

Friedberg EC (1996a) Relationships between DNA repair and transcription. Annu Rev Biochem 65: 15–42.

Friedberg EC (1996b) Cockayne syndrome-a primary defect in DNA repair, transcription, both or neither? Bioessays 18: 731–738.

Friedberg EC, Walker GC, Siede W, Wood RD, Schultz RA, Ellenberger T (2006a) Other diseases associated with defects in nucleotide excision repair of DNA. In: DNA repair and mutagenesis. Washington, DC: ASM Press, pp. 895–918.

Friedberg EC, Walker GC, Siede W, Wood RD, Schultz RA, Ellenberger T (2006b) Heterogeneity of nucleotide excision repair in eukaryotic genomes. Washington DC: ASM Press, pp. 351–378.

Frosina G (2007) The current evidence for defective repair of oxidatively damaged DNA in Cockayne syndrome. Free Radic Biol Med 43: 165–177.

Gandolfi A, Horoupian D, Rapin I, DeTeresa R, Hyams V (1984) Deafness in Cockayne's syndrome: morphological, morphometric, and quantitative study of the auditory pathway. Ann Neurol 15: 135–143.

Gorgels TG, van der Pluijm I, Brandt RM, Garinis GA, van Steeg H, van den Aardweg G, Jansen GH, Ruijter JM, Bergen AA, van Norren D, Hoeijmakers JH, van der Horst GT (2007) Retinal degeneration and ionizing radiation hypersensitivity in a mouse model for Cockayne syndrome. Mol Cell Biol 27: 1433–1441.

Graham JM Jr, Anyane-Yeboa K, Raams A, Appeldoorn E, Kleijer WJ, Garritsen VH, Busch D, Edersheim TG, Jaspers NG (2001) Cerebro-oculo-facio-skeletal syndrome with a nucleotide excision-repair defect and a mutated XPD gene, with prenatal diagnosis in a triplet pregnancy. Am J Hum Genet 69: 291–300.

Greenhaw GA, Hebert A, Duke-Woodside ME, Butler IJ, Hecht JT, Cleaver JE, Thomas GH, Horton WA (1992) Xeroderma pigmentosum and Cockayne syndrome: overlapping clinical and biochemical phenotypes. Am J Hum Genet 50: 677–678.

Groisman R, Polanowska J, Kuraoka I, Sawada J, Saijo M, Drapkin R, Kisselev AF, Tanaka K, Nakatani Y (2003) The ubiquitin ligase activity in the DDB2 and CSA complexes is differentially regulated by the COP9 signalosome in response to DNA damage. Cell 113: 357–367.

Groisman R, Kuraoka I, Chevallier O, Gaye N, Magnaldo T, Tanaka K, Kisselev AF, Harel-Bellan A, Nakatani Y (2006) CSA-dependent degradation of CSB by the ubiquitin-proteasome pathway establishes a link between complementation factors of the Cockayne syndrome. Genes Dev 20: 1429–1434.

Hamel BC, Raams A, Schuitema-Dijkstra AR, Simons P, van der Burgt I, Jaspers NG, Kleijer WJ (1996) Xeroderma pigmentosum – Cockayne syndrome complex: a further case. J Med Genet 33: 607–610.

Hanawalt P, Mellon I (1993) Stranded in an active gene. Curr Biol 3: 67–69.

Hanawalt PC (2002) Subpathways of nucleotide excision repair and their regulation. Oncogene 21: 8949–8956.

Henning KA, Li L, Iyer N, McDaniel LD, Reagan MS, Legerski R, Schultz RA, Stefanini M, Lehmann AR, Mayne LV, Friedberg EC (1995) The Cockayne syndrome group A gene encodes a WD repeat protein that interacts with CSB protein and a subunit of RNA polymerase II TFIIH. Cell 82: 555–564.

Hoar DI, Waghorne C (1978) DNA repair in Cockayne syndrome. Am J Hum Genet 30: 590–601.

Horibata K, Iwamoto Y, Kuraoka I, Jaspers NG, Kurimasa A, Oshimura M, Ichihashi M, Tanaka K (2004) Complete absence of Cockayne syndrome group B gene product gives rise to UV-sensitive syndrome but not Cockayne syndrome. Proc Natl Acad Sci USA 101: 15410–15415.

Ito S, Kuraoka I, Chymkowitch P, Compe E, Takedachi A, Ishigami C, Coin F, Egly JM, Tanaka K (2007) XPG stabilizes TFIIH, allowing transactivation of nuclear receptors: implications for Cockayne syndrome in XP-G/CS patients. Mol Cell 26: 231–243.

Jaspers NG, Raams A, Silengo MC, Wijgers N, Niedernhofer LJ, Robinson AR, Giglia-Mari G, Hoogstraten D, Kleijer WJ, Hoeijmakers JH, Vermeulen W (2007) First reported patient with human ERCC1 deficiency has cerebro-oculo-facio-skeletal syndrome with a mild defect in nucleotide excision repair and severe developmental failure. Am J Hum Genet 80: 457–466.

Jin K, Handa T, Ishihara T, Yoshii F (1979) Cockayne syndrome: report of two siblings and review of literature in Japan. Brain Dev 1: 305–312.

Kamiuchi S, Saijo M, Citterio E, de Jager M, Hoeijmakers JH, Tanaka K (2002) Translocation of Cockayne syndrome group A protein to the nuclear matrix: possible relevance to transcription-coupled DNA repair. Proc Natl Acad Sci USA 99: 201–206.

Kleijer WJ, van der Sterre ML, Garritsen VH, Raams A, Jaspers NG (2006) Prenatal diagnosis of the Cockayne syndrome: survey of 15 years experience. Prenat Diagn 26: 980–984.

Kleppa L, Kanavin OJ, Klungland A, Stromme P (2007) A novel splice site mutation in the Cockayne syndrome group A gene in two siblings with Cockayne syndrome. Neuroscience 145: 1397–1406.

Komatsu A, Suzuki S, Inagaki T, Yamashita K, Hashizume K (2004) A kindred with Cockayne syndrome caused by multiple splicing variants of the CSA gene. Am J Med Genet A 128: 67–71.

Kraemer KH, Patronas NJ, Schiffmann R, Brooks BP, Tamura D, DiGiovanna JJA (2007a) Xeroderma pigmentosum, trichothiodystrophy and Cockayne syndrome: a complex genotype-phenotype relationship. Neuroscience 145: 1388–1396.

Kraemer KH, Sander M, Bohr VA (2007b) New areas of focus at workshop on human diseases involving DNA repair deficiency and premature aging. Mech Ageing Dev 128: 229–235.

Kyng KJ, May A, Brosh RM Jr, Cheng WH, Chen C, Becker KG, Bohr VA (2003) The transcriptional response after oxidative stress is defective in Cockayne syndrome group B cells. Oncogene 22: 1135–1149.

Kyng KJ, Bohr VA (2005) Gene expression and DNA repair in progeroid syndromes and human aging. Ageing Res Rev 4: 579–602.

Lahiri S, Davies N (2003) Cockayne's syndrome: case report of a successful pregnancy. BJOG 110: 871–872.

Lainé JP, Egly JM (2006a) Initiation of DNA repair mediated by a stalled RNA polymerase IIO. EMBO J 25: 387–397.

Lainé JP, Egly JM (2006b) When transcription and repair meet: a complex system. Trends Genet 22: 430–436.

Lanning M, Simila S (1970) Cockayne's syndrome. Report of a case with normal intelligence. Z Kinderheilkd 109: 70–75.

Lehmann AR, Kirk-Bell S, Mayne L (1979) Abnormal kinetics of DNA synthesis in ultraviolet light-irradiated cells from patients with Cockayne's syndrome. Cancer Res 39: 4237–4241.

Lehmann AR, Mayne LV (1981) The response of Cockayne's syndrome cells to UV irradiation. In: Seeberg E, Kleppe K (eds.), Chromosome damage and repair. New York: Plenum Publishing Corp, pp. 367–371.

Lehmann A (1982) Three complementation groups in Cockayne syndrome. Mutat Res 106: 347–356.

Lehmann AR, Francis AJ, Giannelli F (1985) Prenatal diagnosis of Cockayne's syndrome. Lancet 1: 486–488.

Lehmann AR, Thompson AF, Harcourt SA, Stefanini M, Norris PG (1993) Cockayne's syndrome: correlation of clinical features with cellular sensitivity of RNA synthesis to UV irradiation. J Med Genet 30: 679–682.

Lehmann AR, Bootsma D, Clarkson SG, Cleaver JE, Mc Alpine PJ, Tanaka K, Thompson LH, Wood RD (1994) Nomenclature of human DNA repair genes. Mutat Res 315: 41–42.

Licht CL, Stevnsner T, Bohr VA (2003) Cockayne syndrome group B cellular and biochemical functions. Am J Hum Genet 73: 1217–1239.

Lindenbaum Y, Dickson D, Rosenbaum P, Kraemer K, Robbins I, Rapin I (2001) Xeroderma pigmentosum/cockayne syndrome complex: first neuropathological study and review of eight other cases. Eur J Paediatr Neurol 5: 225–242. Review.

Mallery DL, Tanganelli B, Colella S, Steingrimsdottir H, van Gool AJ, Troelstra C, Stefanini M, Lehmann AR (1998) Molecular analysis of mutations in the CSB (ERCC6) gene in patients with Cockayne syndrome. Am J Hum Genet 62: 77–85.

Marini F, Nardo T, Giannattasio M, Minuzzo M, Stefanini M, Plevani P, Muzi Falconi M (2006) DNA nucleotide excision repair-dependent signaling to checkpoint activation. Proc Natl Acad Sci USA 103: 17325–17330.

Marshall RR, Arlett CF, Harcourt SA, Broughton BA (1980) Increased sensitivity of cell strains from Cockayne's syndrome to sister-chromatid-exchange induction and cell killing by UV light. Mutat Res 69: 107–112.

Mayne LV, Lehmann AR (1982) Failure of RNA synthesis to recover after UV irradiation: an early defect in cells from individuals with Cockayne's syndrome and xeroderma pigmentosum. Cancer Res 42: 1473–1478.

Mayne LV, Lehmann AR, Waters R (1982) Excision repair in Cockayne syndrome. Mutat Res 106: 179–189.

McDaniel LD, Legerski R, Lehmann AR, Friedberg EC, Schultz RA (1997) Confirmation of homozygosity for a single nucleotide substitution mutation in a Cockayne syndrome patient using monoallelic mutation analysis in somatic cell hybrids. Hum Mutat 10: 317–321.

Meira LB, Graham JM Jr, Greenberg CR, Busch DB, Doughty AT, Ziffer DW, Coleman DM, Savre-Train I, Friedberg EC (2000) Manitoba aboriginal kindred with original cerebro-oculo-facio-skeletal syndrome has a mutation in the Cockayne syndrome group B (CSB) gene. Am J Hum Genet 66: 1221–1228.

Mellon I, Bohr VA, Smith CA, Hanawalt PC (1986) Preferential DNA repair of an active gene in human cells. Proc Natl Acad Sci USA 83: 8878–8882.

Mellon I, Spivak G, Hanawalt PC (1987) Selective removal of transcription-blocking DNA damage from the transcribed strand of the mammalian DHFR gene. Cell 51: 241–249.

Miyauchi H, Horio T, Akaeda T, Asada Y, Chang HR, Ishizaki K, Ikenaga M (1994) Cockayne syndrome in two adult siblings. J Am Acad Dermatol 30: 329–335.

Moriwaki S, Stefanini M, Lehmann AR, Hoeijmakers JH, Robbins JH, Rapin I, Botta E, Tanganelli B, Vermeulen W, Broughton BC, Kraemer KH (1996) DNA repair and ultraviolet mutagenesis in cells from a new patient with xeroderma pigmentosum group G and cockayne syndrome resemble xeroderma pigmentosum cells. J Invest Dermatol 107: 647–653.

Nance MA, Berry SA (1992) Cockayne syndrome: review of 140 cases. Am J Med Genet 42: 68–84.

Neil CS, Dingwall MM (1950) A syndrome resembling progeria. A review of two cases. Arch Dis Child 25: 213–221.

Newman JC, Bailey AD, Weiner AM (2003) Cockayne syndrome group B protein (CSB) plays a general role in chromatin maintenance and remodeling. Proc Natl Acad Sci USA 103: 9613–9618.

Nishio H, Kodama S, Matsuo T, Ichihashi M, Ito H, Fujiwara Y (1988) Cockayne syndrome: magnetic resonance images of the brain in a severe form with early onset. J Inherit Metab Dis 11: 88–102.

Parris CN, Kraemer KH (1993) Ultraviolet-induced mutations in Cockayne syndrome cells are primarily caused by cyclobutane dimer photoproducts while repair of other photoproducts is normal. Proc Natl Acad Sci USA 90: 7260–7264.

Pasquier L, Laugel V, Lazaro L, Dollfus H, Journel H, Edery P, Goldenberg A, Martin D, Heron D, Le Merrer M, Rustin P, Odent S, Munnich A, Sarasin A, Cormier-Daire V (2006) Wide clinical variability among 13 new Cockayne syndrome cases confirmed by biochemical assays. Arch Dis Child 91: 178–182.

Pena SD, Shokeir MH (1974) Autosomal recessive cerebro-oculo-facio-skeletal (COFS) syndrome. Clin Genet 5: 285–293.

Proietti-De-Santis L, Drane P, Egly JM (2006) Cockayne syndrome B protein regulates the transcriptional program after UV irradiation. EMBO J 25: 1915–1923.

Rainbow AJ, Howes M (1982) A deficiency in the repair of UV and gamma-ray damaged DNA in fibroblasts from Cockayne's syndrome. Mutat Res 93: 235–247.

Rapin I, Lindenbaum Y, Dickson DW, Kraemer KH, Robbins JH (2000) Cockayne syndrome and xeroderma pigmentosum. Neurology 55: 1442–1449.

Rapin I, Weidenheim K, Lindenbaum Y, Rosenbaum P, Merchant SN, Krishna S, Dickson DW (2006) Cockayne syndrome in adults: review with clinical and pathologic study of a new case. J Child Neurol 21: 991–1006.

Reardon JT, Sancar A (2005) Nucleotide excision repair. Prog Nucleic Acid Res Mol Biol 79: 183–235.

Ren Y, Saijo M, Nakatsu Y, Nakai H, Yamaizumi M, Tanaka K (2003) Three novel mutations responsible for Cockayne syndrome group A. Genes Genet Syst 78: 93–102.

Ridley AJ, Colley J, Wynford-Thomas D, Jones CJ (2005) Characterisation of novel mutations in Cockayne syndrome type A and xeroderma pigmentosum group C subjects. J Hum Genet 50: 151–154.

Riggs W Jr, Seibert J (1972) Cockayne's syndrome. Roentgen findings. Am J Roentgenol Radium Ther Nucl Med 116: 623–633.

Sakai T, Kikuchi F, Takashima S, Matsuda H, Watanabe N (1997) Neuropathological findings in the cerebro-oculo-facio-skeletal (Pena-Shokeir II) syndrome. Brain Dev 9: 58–62.

Sarasin A, Stary A (2007) New insights for understanding the transcription-coupled repair pathway. DNA Repair 6: 265–269.

Schmickel RD, Chu EHY, Trosko JE, Chang CC (1977) Cockayne syndrome-cellular sensitivity to UV light. Pediatrics 60: 135–139.

Selby CP, Witkin EM, Sancar A (1991) Escherichia coli mfd mutant deficient in "mutation frequency decline" lacks strand-specific repair: in vitro complementation with purified coupling factor. Proc Natl Acad Sci USA 88: 11574–11578.

Selby CP, Sancar A (1993) Molecular mechanism of transcription-repair coupling. Science 260: 53–58.

Selby CP, Sancar A (1997) Human transcription-repair coupling factor CSB/ERCC6 is a DNA-stimulated AT-Pase but is not a helicase and does not disrupt the ternary transcription complex of stalled RNA polymeraseII. J Biol Chem 272: 1885–1890.

Sigmundsson J, Jaspers NGJ, Raams A, Grompe M (1998) Acase of xeroderma pigmentosum-Cockayne syndrome complex due to a mutation in the repair endonuclease XPG. Am J Hum Genet Suppl 63: A120.

Soffer D, Grotsky HW, Rapin I, Suzuki K (1979) Cockayne syndrome: unusual neuropathological findings and review of the literature. Ann Neurol 6: 340–348.

Spivak G (2004) The many faces of Cockayne syndrome. Proc Natl Acad Sci USA 101: 15273–15274.

Spivak G (2005) UV-sensitive syndrome. Mutat Res 577: 162–169.

Stefanini M, Fawcett H, Botta E, Nardo T, Lehmann AR (1996) Genetic analysis of twenty-two patients with Cockayne syndrome. Hum Genet 97: 418–423.

Tanaka K, Kawai Y, Kumahara Y, Ikenaga M, Okada Y (1981) Genetic complementation groups in Cockayne syndrome. Somat Cell Genet 7: 445–455.

Tantin D (1998) RNA polymerase II elongation complexes containing the Cockayne syndrome group B protein interact with a molecular complex containing the transcription factor IIH components xeroderma pigmentosum B and p62. J Biol Chem 273: 27794–27799.

Taybi H (1996) Cockayne syndrome. In: Tayby H, Lachman RS (eds.) Radiology of syndromes, metabolic disorders, and skeletal dysplasias, 4th ed. St. Louis: Mosby, pp. 100–101.

Troelstra C, van Gool A, de Wit J, Vermeulen W, Bootsma D, Hoeijmakers JH (1992) ERCC6, a member of a subfamily of putative helicases, is involved in Cockayne's syndrome and preferential repair of active genes. Cell 71: 939–953.

Traboulsi EI, De Becker I, Maumenee IH (1992) Ocular findings in Cockayne syndrome. Am J Ophthalmol 114: 579–583.

Theron T, Fousteri MI, Volker M, Harries LW, Botta E, Stefanini M, Fujimoto M, Andressoo J, Mitchell J, Jaspers NGJ, McDaniel LD, Mullenders L, Lehmann AR (2005) Transcription-associated breaks in xeroderma pigmentosum group D cells from patients with combined features of xeroderma pigmentosum and Cockayne Syndrome. Mol Cell Biol 25: 8368–8378.

Van der Knaap M, Valk J (2005) Cockayne syndrome. In: van der Knaap M, Valk J (eds.) Magnetic resonance of myelination and myelin disorders, 3rd ed. Berlin: Springer, pp. 259–267.

van Gool AJ, Citterio E, Rademakers S, van Os R, Vermeulen W, Constantinou A, Egly JM, Bootsma D, Hoeijmakers JH (1997) The Cockayne syndrome B protein, involved in transcription-coupled DNA repair, resides in an RNA polymerase II-containing complex. EMBO J 16: 5955–5965.

van Hoffen A, Natarajan AT, Mayne LV, van Zeeland AA, Mullenders LH, Venema J (1993) Deficient repair of the transcribed strand of active genes in Cockayne's syndrome cells. Nucleic Acids Res 21: 5890–5895.

Venema J, Mullenders LH, Natarajan AT, van Zeeland AA, Mayne LV (1990) The genetic defect in Cockayne syndrome is associated with a defect in repair of UV-induced DNA damage in transcriptionally active DNA. Proc Natl Acad Sci USA 87: 4707–4711.

Wade MH, Chu EH (1979) Effects of DNA damaging agents on cultured fibroblasts derived from patients with Cockayne syndrome. Mutat Res 59: 49–60.

Wagner AM (2006) Xeroderma pigmentosum, Cockayne's syndrome and Trichothiodystrophy. In: Harper J, Oranje A, Prose N (eds.) textbook of pediatric dermatology, 2nd ed, vol. 2, pp. 1557–1582.

Wijnhoven SW, Hoogervorst EM, de Waard H, van der Horst GT, van Steeg H (2007) Tissue specific mutagenic and carcinogenic responses in NER defective mouse models. Mutat Res 614: 77–94.

Wilson DM 3rd, Bohr VA (2007) The mechanics of base excision repair, and its relationship to aging and disease. DNA Repair 6: 544–559.

Wood RD, Mitchell M, Lindahl T (2005) Human DNA repair genes. Mutat Res 577: 275–283.

# Chapter 53

# TRICHOTHIODYSTROPHY

**Miria Stefanini and Martino Ruggieri**

Institute of Molecular Genetics, National Research Council of Italy, Pavia (MS); Institute of Neurological Science,
National Research Council of Italy, and Department of Pediatrics, University of Catania, Catania, Italy (MR)

## Introduction

Trichothiodystrophy (TTD) is a term introduced by Vera Price and coworkers in 1980 (Price et al. 1980) to describe a group of autosomal recessive neuroectodermal disorders whose defining feature is brittle hair with a cystein content less than half of normal. The designation derives from Greek: *tricho*, hair; *thio*, sulfur; *dys*, faulty; and *trophe*, nourishment.

The clinical spectrum of TTD varies widely from patients with only the brittle, fragile hair to patients with the most severe neuroectodermal symptoms. Associated clinical features include physical and mental retardation of different severity, small stature, ichthyotic skin, nail dysplasia, decreased fertility, proneness to infections, unusual facial features, cataracts, and dental caries (Itin et al. 2001, Wagner 2006). Photosensitivity is present in about 50% of patients and is associated with an altered cellular response to UV light due to a defect in nucleotide excision repair (NER), the DNA repair pathway that removes a wide spectrum of DNA lesions, including UV-induced damage. Three genes have been identified as responsible for the *photosensitive form* of TTD, namely *XPB*, *XPD* and *TTDA* (*p8* or *GTF2H5*). The discovery that these genes encode distinct subunits of the general transcription factor IIH (TFIIH), a multi-protein complex involved in both NER and transcription, has been crucial to rationalize the TTD pathological phenotype. Clinical symptoms of TTD that are difficult to explain on the basis of a repair defect, may be easily ascribed to subtle defects in transcription. Research in this field is very active and the resulting achievements demonstrate how characterization of a genetic disorder, even if extremely rare, may offer valuable tools to gain insights into fundamental cellular processes, such as DNA repair and transcription.

On 2005, the first milestone in our understanding of the genetic and molecular basis of the *non-photosensitive form* of TTD has been accomplished. *C7orf11* has been described as the first disease gene (Nakabashi et al. 2005) and the disease locus has been designated TTDN1 (TTD non-photosensitive 1). Evidence has been provided that the non-photosensitive form of TTD is genetically heterogeneous, as previously found for photosensitive TTD. Future tasks include the cloning of the other disease-genes and the identification of their functions, a fundamental step toward developing therapeutic strategies.

## Historical perspective, terminology and eponyms

TTD, variously known as Tay's syndrome (Tay 1971), Pollitt syndrome (Pollitt et al. 1968), Amish hair–brain syndrome and Sabinas syndrome, was first described as a distinct clinical entity in 1980 to characterize the condition of patients with sulfur-deficient brittle hair and other ectodermal and neuroectodermal symptoms and signs (Price et al. 1980). The first reported case of TTD appeared more than a decade before when Salfeld and Lindley described a 10-years old patients showing ichthyosis vulgaris combined with bamboo hair formation and ectodermal dysplasia (Salfeld and Lindley 1963). In 1968, Pollitt and colleagues described two patients with trichorrhexia nodosa, low sulfur content of hair and associated mental and physical retardation. Two years later, Brown and colleagues (1970) reported a case of trichoschisis with the typical pattern of sulfur-deficient hair seen on polarized light microscopy. Tay (1971) described three siblings, two brothers and a sister, offspring of first-cousin parents of Chinese extraction living in Singapore. They all had congenital ichthyosis, brittle hair, growth retardation, progeria-like facies, and mental development delay. Microscopic examination of their hair shafts showed clean transverse fractures (Tay 1971, Happle et al. 1984). As the parents were unaffected and closely related Tay (1971), concluded that the disease was inherited as an autosomal recessive trait. In the same year Allen (1971) and few years after Jackson et al. (1974) reported a similar association with brittle hair without ichthyosis later named *BIDS syndrome* (brittle hair, intellectual impairment, decreased fertility and short stature) (Baden et al. 1976).

The acronyms *BIDS* (Baden et al. 1976), *IBIDS* (Jorizzo et al. 1980) and *PIBIDS* (Crovato et al. 1983) syndrome, have been used on the basis of the presence or absence of the following signs: Brittle hair, Ichthyosis, Impaired intelligence, Decreased fertility, Short stature, and Photosensitivity. Later, Chapman (1988), described osteosclerotic anomalies in a patient affected by TTD and added the term *SIBIDS syndrome* (osteoSclerosis, Ichthyosis, Brittle hair, Impaired intelligence, Decreased fertility, Short stature). Central osteosclerosis has since been described in multiple patients (Wagner 2006).

The term *Tay's syndrome* was first introduced by Happle et al. (1984) who comprehensively reviewed the existing cases in the literature including those reported under the acronyms of IBIDS and PIBIDS syndromes and proposed to group all these entities under a "shorter designation" (i.e., Tay's syndrome) instead of using "the ambiguous term TTD or the cumbersome acronyms BIDS, IBIDS or PIBIDS". At the same time he established differential diagnostic criteria (Happle et al. 1984). Photosensitivity was described in about 20% of the cases (18 out of 81) reported in the literature from 1963 to 1988 (reviewed in Stefanini et al. 1989) but it was suggested that photosensitivity could be often overlooked, and that the association of photosensitivity could be considerably more frequent.

Still the McKusick catalogue (OMIM 2007) has multiple entries besides the photosensitive TTD

(TTDP; OMIM #601675) and non-photosensitive TTD (TTDN1 or Amish brittle hair–brain syndrome-ABHS- or hair–brain syndrome or BIDS syndrome; OMIM #234050) including *Sabinas brittle hair syndrome* (Brittle hair and mental deficit; OMIM %211390) (Arbisser et al. 1976, Howell et al. 1981) and the *Trichorrhexis nodosa syndrome* (Pollitt syndrome; OMIM %275550).

In 1986, DNA repair investigations provided the first evidence of an altered cellular response to UV into four Italian patients who showed clinical symptoms diagnostic for TTD along with acute photosensitivity (Stefanini et al. 1986). Following UV irradiation, cells from these patients showed notable reductions in the level of survival and of UV-induced DNA repair synthesis (unscheduled DNA synthesis, UDS), a failure to recover normal DNA and RNA synthesis rate, and an increased mutability. The occurrence of these abnormalities in the cellular response to UV light indicates the presence of a defect in nucleotide excision repair (NER), a DNA repair process involved in the removal of a wide spectrum of DNA lesions, including UV-induced damage. Defects in NER had previously been identified in other two hereditary disorders, namely xeroderma pigmentosum (XP) and Cockayne syndrome (CS), characterized by peculiar and differing clinical symptoms (see Chapters 51 and 52, respectively). In particular, XP displays various manifestations of cutaneous UV-genotoxicity, notably photosensitivity, pigmentation abnormalities, and a greatly increased incidence of skin cancer.

Although the respective clinical symptoms were distinct, the altered cellular response to UV observed in the four TTD patients investigated by Stefanini and colleagues (Stefanini et al. 1986) resembled that typically detected for XP. This finding prompted investigations on genetic homology between XP and TTD by a classical complementation test based on the analysis of the capacity of fusion products to perform UV-induced DNA repair synthesis (see Fig. 4, Chapter 51 on XP). TTD cells were fused with XP cells representative of the seven NER-deficient complementation groups hitherto identified (designated XP-A to XP-G), and UDS level was analyzed in the heterodikaryons. Since parental cells in each cross were labeled with latex beads of two different sizes, heterodikaryons were unambiguously identified as binuclear cells containing beads of both sizes. Restoration of normal UDS levels was observed in all cases except in the crosses between TTD and XP-D cell strains. These results indicated that the UV hypersensitivity observed in the four Italian TTD patients was due to the presence of the XP-D defect (Stefanini et al. 1986). Very soon it was shown that NER alterations were not a common feature shared by all the patients affected by TTD. A normal cellular response to UV and a normal ability to complement the defect in repair-deficient TTD cells was observed in an Italian TTD patient without signs of photosensitivity (Stefanini et al. 1987, Fois et al. 1988). Further studies in the Italian repair-deficient TTD patients and in their relatives, namely reconstruction of genealogical trees, surname analysis, typing of blood genetic markers and cytogenetic analysis, failed to identify the mechanism underlying the association of the XP-D defect with TTD (Nuzzo et al. 1988, 1990).

In the meanwhile, DNA repair investigations were extended to other 20 TTD cases from different countries (Lehmann et al. 1988; Stefanini et al. 1992, 1993a). Cellular response to UV appeared to be normal in the 5 cases whose cutaneous photosensitivity was normal, and defective in the remaining 15, who showed all the symptoms of TTD, together with photosensitivity. Genetic analysis based on complementation studies demonstrated the presence of the XP-D defect in 12 repair-deficient cases, indicating definitively that the concurrence of TTD with XP-D was not a sporadic or casual event. Unexpectedly, in the three further repair-deficient cell strains (TTD4VI and TTD6VI from two French siblings and TTD1BR from an English patient) complementation was observed with XP-D cells. Restoration of normal UDS levels were also observed after fusion of TTD1BR cells with TTD6VI cells. These observations gave the first indication that TTD was associated with repair defects behaving differently in the functional test of complementation (Stefanini et al. 1993a). Further analysis demonstrated the repair defect in TTD1BR was complemented by all known XP complementation

groups and was not corrected by several cloned human DNA repair genes. TTD1BR was therefore a representative of a new excision-repair complementation group that was called TTD-A (Stefanini et al. 1993b). The French siblings TTD4VI and TTD6VI were assigned to the XP-B complementation group (Vermeulen et al. 1994a), a very rare defect previously identified only in three patients showing clinical symptoms of XP in association with those of CS (Robbins et al. 1974, Scott et al. 1993, Vermeulen et al. 1994b). The assignment of TTD4VI and TTD6VI to the XP-B group was later on substantiated by sequence analysis of the *XPB* cDNA that enabled the identification of the primary molecular defect (Weeda et al. 1997).

Thus, in the early 1990s genetic characterization of photosensitive TTD patients led to the identification of a new excision-repair complementation group (designated TTD-A), and to the demonstration that two defects (the XP-B and XP-D defects), previously described as responsible for XP and XP/CS pathological phenotypes, were associated with TTD. The intriguing aspect of these observations was the lack of cancer proneness in TTD, despite the presence of DNA repair defects. Even in those TTD patients in whom the DNA repair defect was the same as that in XP-D, cutaneous skin abnormalities and skin cancer typical of XP have never been observed (Lehmann 1989).

The paradox that defects in a single gene could cause different disorders was rationalized by the discovery of unexpected links between DNA repair and transcription. In 1993, a group led by J.M. Egly demonstrated that the XPB and XPD proteins were subunits of TFIIH (Schaeffer et al. 1993, 1994), a multiprotein complex that, in addition to participating to NER, is also a general transcription factor. These findings suggested that different mutations in these genes involved both in NER and transcription could differentially affect the two processes, and result in XP when only repair is affected, and in TTD when transcription is also affected (Bootsma and Hoeijmakers 1993, 1994; Lehmann 1995; Hoeijmakers et al. 1996). This hypothesis requires that the mutations associated with the distinct disorders are located at different sites in the gene. This was explored by determining in many patients the sites of mutation in the *XPD* gene that had been cloned in the meanwhile (Weber et al. 1990). The results of this work demonstrated that the site of the mutation in *XPD* determines the clinical phenotype (reviewed in Lehmann 1998, 2001, 2003). Each mutated site was indeed found in either XP or TTD or XP/CS patients. There was no example in which identical changes were found in both XP and TTD patients (Broughton et al. 1994; Frederik et al. 1994; Takayama et al. 1996, 1997; Taylor et al. 1997; Botta et al. 1998; Viprakasit et al. 2001). Investigations on Italian TTD patients with different disease severity revealed also that the moderately affected cases were homozygous for a mutation resulting in the aminocid change arg112his whereas the more severely affected cases were functionally hemizygous with only one mutated *XPD* allele resulting in the arg112his change, the other *XPD* allele being completely inactive. These data suggested that the *XPD* gene dosage affects the clinical outcome in TTD individuals (Botta et al. 1998).

Further insights were gained once genetic engineering was used to produce a mouse that contained a specific mutation in the *XPD* gene (resulting in the arg722trp change) that had been found in several patients with TTD but not in any with XP. The mouse had many of the features of TTD, including the brittle hair and small size (de Boer et al. 1998, 2002). This definitely proved that the single alteration in the *XPD* gene was responsible for all the defects associated with TTD.

Through collaborative efforts of several research groups, we have been able in the last few years not only to establish genotype–phenotype relationships, but also to better understand the mechanism of transcription and NER, and to determine the role of TFIIH in both processes and its link with cell cycle regulation (reviewed in Coin and Egly 1998, 2003; Bergmann and Egly 2001; Egly 2001; Friedberg et al. 2006; Lainé et al. 2006). A fundamental contribution to this field came from work of the group led by J. M. Egly, who discovered also the involvement of TFIIH complex in RNA polymerase I transcription (Iben et al. 2002) and in regulation of gene expression (Bastein et al. 2000, Busso et al. 2000, Chen et al. 2000, Keriel et al. 2002, Drané et al. 2004).

Meanwhile, also our understanding on the pathological basis of the photosensitive form of TTD greatly improved. It was shown that all the mutations responsible for TTD cause a decrease by up to 70% in the cellular content of TFIIH (Vermeulen et al. 2000, 2001; Botta et al. 2002). Reduced levels of TFIIH were found also in some XP-D cell strains from XP and XP/CS patients. These findings led to the suggestion that the clinical outcome of *XPD* mutations is the combined result of the reduction in TFIIH content and the effects of the specific mutations on the multiple roles of TFIIH (Botta et al. 2002). So, perhaps is not so surprising the puzzling variety of pathological phenotypes that have been recently identified in association with defects in XPD (reviewed in Stefanini 2006). The picture that is now emerging is that mutations in the *XPD* gene can be associated not only with clinical features of XP and TTD but also with a spectrum of combination of features found in XP, CS and TTD. The complexity of this phenotypic picture is no doubt a reflection of the many different roles of TFIIH. During transcription, TFIIH interacts with a variety of factors, including tissue-specific transcription factors, nuclear receptors, chromatin remodeling complexes and RNA, suggesting that in some cases the genetic background may also play a role in the clinical outcome.

Further evidence supporting a transcriptional defect in TTD has been provided by *in vitro* studies with recombinant TFIIH complexes in which the XPD subunit carries amino acid changes found in patients. All the mutations found in XP-D patients, independent of the associated pathological phenotype, affect the helicase activity of XPD, thus explaining the NER defect, but only those responsible for TTD diminish the basal transcription activity of TFIIH (Dubaele et al. 2003). *In vivo* studies demonstrated that some mutations in *XPB* and *XPD* interfere with the regulatory role of TFIIH in transcription, resulting in altered gene expression (Liu et al. 2000, 2001; Keriel et al. 2002; Drané et al. 2004; Compe et al. 2005; Weber et al. 2005). Furthermore, reduced expression of several genes in terminally differentiating cells from patients and mouse model has been shown (Stefanini et al. 1986, Mariani et al. 1992, de Boer et al. 1998, Racioppi et al. 2001, Viprakasit et al. 2001, Backendorf et al. 2005, Compe et al. 2005). These findings suggest that quantitative and conformational alterations of TFIIH in TTD patients may become limiting in terminally differentiated tissues, in which the mutated TFIIH might get exhausted before the transcriptional program has been completed. This may affect the transcription of genes that are highly expressed in differentiated cells, such as those involved in hair structure or in the neuromyelination process. This model of attenuated transcription in terminally differentiating cells in TTD has received support from studies with the fruit fly *Drosophila melanogaster* (Zurita and Merino 2003).

Whereas consistent advances have been made on TTD associated with defects in either *XPB* or *XPD* gene, the identity of the gene responsible for TTD-A has remained for years an unsolved question. Because XPB and XPD were components of TFIIH, it was investigated whether TTDA could be a protein belonging to the complex. However, no causative mutation was identified in any of the TFIIH subunits or in any of the known NER genes. Nevertheless, the TFIIH content was drastically reduced in TTD-A cells. Moreover TFIIH isolated from TTD-A cells had normal enzymatic activities and transiently restored the NER defect in these cells, suggesting that TFIIH was qualitatively not or only mildly defective (Vermeulen et al. 2000). The search for the *TTDA* gene was successfully accomplished in 2004, when Ranish and colleagues (Ranish et al. 2004) identified a new small 8 kDa component of TFIIH in yeast, that they called TFB5. Deletion of TFB5 caused UV sensitivity, slow growth on a number of carbon sources, reduced basal and activated transcription, and reduced recruitment of TFIIH to promoters. By using a combination of cellular, biochemical and molecular techniques, a group led by Wim Vermeulen cloned the human homolog of TFB5 (called *GTF2H5*, *p8* or *TTDA*) and showed that it contributes to the stability and concentration of human TFIIH complex in the cell (Giglia-Mari et al. 2004). Furthermore, they identified mutations in *GTF2H5* in four TTD-A patients from three distinct families and demonstrated that the wild-type version of this gene was

able to restore a normal response to UV and normal levels of TFIIH in TTD-A cells. As well as highlighting the powerful technologies now available in eukaryote genetics, proteomics and genomics, these studies enhance the value of clinical observations and of reporting rare patients (see Kraemer 2004, Cleaver 2005). Only three families with TTD-A had been identified but they were key to establish the 8 kDa protein as a structural subunit of TFIIH and as an essential factor for NER.

In 2005, also the first disease gene for the non-photosensitive form of TTD has been identified (Nakabayashi et al. 2005). Mutations in this gene (*C7orf11*) *TTN1*, that has been designated account for less than 20% of non-photosensitive TTD patients (Nakabayashi et al. 2005, Botta et al. 2007), suggesting the involvement of other still unknown genes.

In conclusion, although it is evident that there is still much more to learn about TTD, enormous progress has been made in our understanding of the genetic and molecular bases of this disorder. Future research will have to address the cloning of the other disease-genes and the identification of their functions, a fundamental step toward developing therapeutic strategies. Further studies are needed to dissect the individual roles of the pathways specifically altered in TTD in the acceleration of the ageing process and their contemporary tumor suppressive mode of action.

## Incidence and prevalence

TTD is a rare autosomal recessive disorder whose prevalence is unknown. Less than 200 patients have been reported in the literature and the reviewing of the published cases indicates that males and females are similarly affected. Patients have been reported worldwide.

## Clinical manifestations

All TTD patients exhibit sparse, dry and easily broken hair associated with low sulfur and cysteine content (10–50% of normal). Scalp hair anomalies ex-

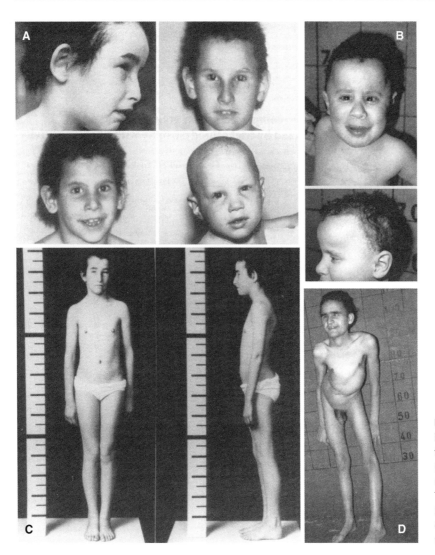

**Fig. 1.** Trichothiodystrophy. (**A**) The four Italian TTD patients firstly described as NER-defective and classified into the XP-D group (from Stefanini et al. 1986). (**B**) The face of a male patient. (**C**) A female photosensitive TTD patient aged 18 years (from Nuzzo and Stefanini 1989). (**D**) A male TTD patient with complex skeletal deformities including severe scoliosis.

tend to eyebrows and eyelashes and are associated with a wide spectrum of clinical symptoms that usually affect organs of ectodermal and neuroectodermal origin. Common features include mental and growth retardation, face characterized by receding chin, small nose, large ears and microcephaly, nail dysplasia and ichthyosis (Fig. 1). At birth, children often present with ichthyosiform erythroderma, and they may be encased in a collodion-like membrane. About 50% of the patients show an abnormal sun reaction on minimal sun exposure with blistering and persistent erythema. This photosensitivity results from inability to remove UV-induced damage but does not lead to an increased skin cancer risk.

The disorder is characterized by a wide variation in the expression and severity of the clinical features, as detailed in the comprehensive review of Itin and colleagues (Itin et al. 2001). A few mild cases have been described with hair abnormalities but without physical and mental impairment. Other patients show a pathological phenotype of moderate severity, with short stature, delayed puberty, mental development at pre-school or primary school level, axial hypotonia, reduced motor coordination and survival beyond early childhood. The most severe form is characterized by very poor mental and motor performance and speech, failure to thrive and death during early childhood. Numerous patients suffer from repeated and severe infectious illnesses, mainly of the gastrointestinal and respiratory tract. In addition, osteoporosis, hearing loss, cataracts, dental caries, and other features of premature ageing have been reported.

## Skin manifestations and annexes

*Hair abnormalities* are considered the key factors in the recognition of the disorder (Fig. 2). Scalp hair, eyebrows, and eyelashes are short, thin, brittle and dry, and show an abnormally low content of cystein and sulfur. This reflects a reduction in the content of sulfur rich hair matrix proteins that normally confer hair shaft stability. A typical tiger tail pattern of the hair of affected individuals can be seen using polarized microscopy. Quantitative and qualitative alterations of sulfur rich hair matrix proteins result in changes of the amino acid content of the hair. These anomalies provide a diagnostic test for the disorder.

*Dysplasia of nails* is frequently observed. The nails are short, broadened and may show longitudinal ridging as well as horizontal splitting. The nails have been found to be deficient in cystine (Sass et al. 2004). Thickening of the nails has been reported in two cases (Jorizzo et al. 1980, 1982; Price et al. 1980).

At birth a smooth, shiny membrane resulting in the typical appearance of a colloidon baby may cover the skin of affected individuals. *Ichthyosiform erythroderma* is often manifest during the first weeks after birth. During the first months of life, the scaling may be alligator-like but later on becomes less prominent. The ichthyosis also involves the palms and soles which may show marked thickening and deep fissures. Of note, the flexural areas of the limbs may be spared as it occurs in ichthyosis vulgaris. The ichthyosis may reduce the sweating capacity that usually turns to normal after treatment of the skin lesions. Histologically, the ichthyotic lesions reveal orthohyperkeratosis intermingled with parakeratotic strands. The granular layer appears to be reduced, and follicular plugging may be noted (Braun-Falco et al. 1981, Jorizzo et al. 1980, Salfeld and Lindley 1963, Tay 1971).

The few studies performed on the skin ultrastructural aspects have highlighted a peculiar feature of ichthyotic skin in TTD (Fois et al. 1988, Calvieri et al. 1993). Electron microscopy examination of the skin showed large membrane-bound vacuoles filled with granular-filamentous material in the cytoplasm of keratinocytes of the basal and spinous layer (Fig. 3). The tonofibril bundles were thinner and less electron dense than normal. The cytoplasm of cells of the granulous layer showed large vacuoles filled with granular material and the keratohyalin granules of the keratinocytes were small and less electron dense than normal.

*Other skin symptoms* include erythroderma, eczema, telangiectasia, hemangioma, lipoatrophy, parchment-like skin, poikiloderma, folliculitis, cheilitis, hyperpigmented eyelids, hypopigmented macules.

Approximately half of the patients with TTD exhibit cutaneous *photosensitivity* but premalignant

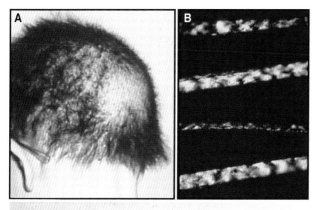

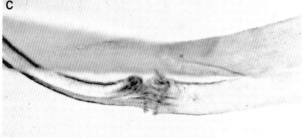

Fig. 2. Hair features in TTD. (**A**) Short, sparse and broken scalp hair. (**B**) Polarizing microscopy of hair shafts showing tiger-tail pattern (from Stefanini 2006). (**C**) Light microscopy demonstrates trichoschisis (**C**, courtesy of I. Pascual-Castroviejo, University of Madrid, Spain).

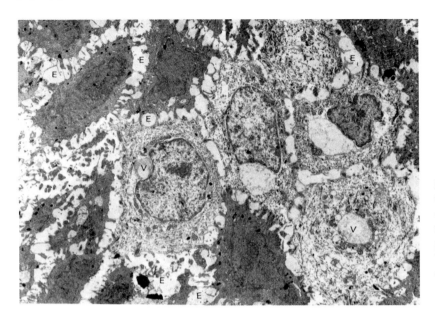

**Fig. 3.** Electron microscopy of the skin of the patient TTD5PV mutated in the *TTDN1* gene. Large membrane-bound vacuoles (*V*) filled with granulo-filamentous material are present in the cytoplasm of keratinocytes. The tonofibril bundles are thinner and less electron dense than in normal keratinocytes. Intercellular oedema (*E*) is also present (from Fois et al. 1988).

skin lesions and cutaneous tumors have never been described. Photosensitivity may be extreme in some patients, in particular photosensitivity to UVB, and impressive for UVA (Richetta et al. 2001). Only a few minutes outdoors or behind the glass pane are able to induce a severe burn with subsequent ichthyosiform erythroderma. Interestingly, photosensitivity seems to diminish with age, and it does not affect patients with congenital ichthyosis, but only those with ichthyosis that develops later in infancy (Crovato and Rebora 1985).

*Lack of subcutaneous fatty tissue* is a characteristic feature of severely affected cases (Happle et al. 1984). In women the breast tissue may be completely absent, in spite of normal development of nipples (Jorizzo et al. 1980).

## Prematurely aged facial appearance

The face has been described as progeric-like (Tay 1971) or pointed and angular (Jorizzo et al. 1980). The aged facial appearance is mainly due to sunken cheeks lacking their subcutaneous tissue. Other features include a beaked nose, receding chin and large, protruding ears (Fig. 1). Notably, all of these features are recorded in the spectrum of DNA repair disorders (see pathogenesis). Thickened epicanthal folds have been observed in some cases (Price et al. 1980, Salfeld and Lindley 1963).

## Low birth weight

Delivery is frequently preterm and birth weight is low for pregnancy age (<3000 g, ranging between 2000 and 2500 g). In some cases it was attributed to placental insufficiency and/or premature delivery (Happle et al. 1984, Ostergaard and Christensen 1996). Feeding problems have also been reported.

## Other dysmorphic features and skeletal anomalies

Typical features are growth retardation, developmental delay and microcephaly.

Skeletal deformations observed in TTD patients include (see Fig. 1D) genu valgum, coxa valga, pes valgus, cubital and tibial valgus deformity, ulnar deviation of fingers, zygodactyly, clinodactyly, scoliosis, thoracic kyphosis, lumbosacral lordosis, and metacarpal bones of the thumb reduced in size. Osteosclerosis is a rather common and characteristic finding in patients with TTD (Yoon et al. 2005 and references therein). The axial skeleton, including the skull, ribs, vertebrae, pelvis, and proximal parts of the extremities, is usually affected; peripheral osteopenia denominates "central osteosclerosis". Recently, retarded bone age has been reported in two TTD patients showing also tapered distal phalanges by hand radiographs (Wakeling et al. 2004, Yoon et al. 2005).

Dental abnormalities and caries are frequently reported.

## Neurological abnormalities

Neurological involvement in cases with TTD is frequent. A variety of neurological and developmental defects have been reported.

Mental retardation is the most common feature and impaired motor control is frequently reported. Spasticity, paralysis, ataxia, tremor, hypotonia, decreased muscle tone, seizures, and sensorineural hearing loss have all been described. Usually patients show delayed speech development, and reduced learning ability. The neurological defects present in TTD appear to be mainly related to impaired development and maturation of the nervous system (Kraemer et al. 2007a). They have decreased to absent myelin in the cerebrum. While not proven definitively, it seems that the myelin in these patients never formed properly (dysmyelination) rather than sustaining a loss of normally formed myelin (demyelination). This suggests the presence of a developmental defect as is also seen in the congenital cataracts in the eye, the problems during in utero growth, and the short stature. At

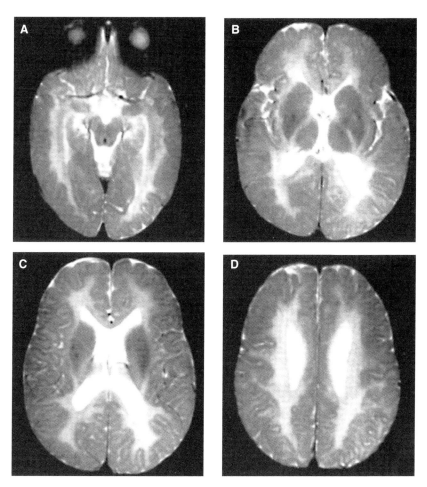

**Fig. 4.** Axial T2-weighted magnetic resonance images in a 3-year-old boy with TTD show insufficient myelination of the cerebral white matter, which has a high signal (**A–D**). Note that even the corpus callosum and internal capsule are hypomyelinated (**B**, **C**). The cerebral white matter apparently contains more myelin, but still less than normal (**A–D**) (reprinted with permission from van der Knaap and Valk 2005; fig. 33.1, page 271).

present we have no evidence of progressive neurological degeneration.

While TTD patients may have intellectual impairment, they usually are very social and have an outgoing, engaging, friendly personality. Typically, standard intelligence tests appear to underestimate their capability for social interactions (Kraemer et al. 2007a).

Other less common neuropsychiatric findings include (Itin et al. 2001) autism, paralysis, ataxia, cerebellar deficiency, intention tremor, pyramidal signs, peripheral neuropathy, hyperreflexia, absent deep tendon reflexes, hemiparesis, tetraparesis, intracranial calcifications, partial agenesis of corpus callosum, gray matter heterotopia and necrotising encephalopathy, jerky eye movements, dysarthria, irritability, lethargy, perimedullary fibrosis of spinal cord.

*Imaging.* Due to the rarity and the confusion of patients with the different syndromes with TTD, the imaging studies are sparse (Peserico et al. 1992, Battistella and Peserico 1996, Ostergaard and Christensen 1996, Porto et al. 2000). No structural abnormalities of the brain have been documented in association with TTD. Published cases in which brain magnetic resonance imaging (MRI) was performed invariably show evidence of abnormal myelination of varying degree including widespread confluent increase in signal symmetrically in all the supratentorial regions with a patchy arrangement in the cerebellar central and foliar white matter with sparing of the myelin in the brainstem (Fig. 4), indicating that central nervous system dysmyelination occurs quite commonly in TTD (van der Knaap and Valk 2005). It has been reported that the supratentorial white matter signal on both T1-weighted images and T2-weighted images resembled that of very poorly myelinated white matter, similar to that seen in both Cockayne syndrome and Pelizaeus-Merzbacher disease (van der Knaap and Valk 2005, Yoon et al. 2005). These findings were confirmed at pathology in one case recorded under the acronym PIBIDS (Tolmie et al. 1994). Cerebellar atrophy has been sporadically reported and it may be a late imaging finding in TTD. Spectroscopy studies (Porto et al. 2000) revealed increased myoinositol and decreased choline.

Recent neuroradiological studies of 6 TTD patients conducted by Patronas and colleagues using both MRI and CT scans (reported in Kraemer et al. 2007b), showed cerebral atrophy and white matter disease but no cerebellar atrophy. The MRI shows predominantly hypomyelination of the white matter of the cerebrum. Atrophy of the brain is not a major feature. Some patients may have calcification of the basal ganglia.

## Ocular abnormalities

These have been frequently reported including nystagmus, epicanthal folds, retinal dystrophy, entropion, ectropion, hypotelorism, exophthalmus/enophthalmus, esotropia, myopia, astigmatism, retrobulbar hemangioma, chorioretinal atrophy, retinal pigmentation, strabismus, reduced visual acuity, corneal dryness, myopia, hypertelorism, blepharitis, pale optic disc, and microcornea. Conjunctivitis and photophobia may also be present. Cataracts have been frequently reported in severely affected patients. As recently pointed out (Kraemer et al. 2007b), eye defects in TTD patients tend to reflect developmental defects whereas the dry eye might result from premature ageing-like phenomena or other pathological mechanisms affecting the eyes.

## Impaired sexual development

Delayed puberty and hypoplasia of female genitalia were observed in affected females whereas undescended testes and bilateral or unilateral cryptorchidism have been frequently described in male patients. Post-puberal patients have delayed and reduced development of secondary sexual characters. Fertility is reduced.

## Immune system alterations

Impaired NK cell activity and an increased susceptibility to bacterial infections localized anywhere in the body (including pneumonia, otitis, mastoiditis, sinusitis and pyelonephritis) are frequently reported.

In contrast, increased susceptibility to viral infections is not a common feature in TTD, although recent studies point at a role of XPB and XPD in a cellular defense against retroviral infection (Yoder et al. 2006).

## Hematologic alterations

The hematological features of β-thalassemia trait, and reduced level of β-globin synthesis and β-globin transcript have been reported in eleven TTD patients with characterized mutations in the *XPD* gene. These findings provide an important additional simple diagnostic tool for differential diagnosis of TTD (Viprakasit et al. 2001).

Neutropenia, anemia and hypereosinophilia have been sporadically observed.

## Other associated features

Cardiovascular alterations, including ventricular septal defect, hemangioma, telangiectasia, impairment of peripheral circulation, angioepitheliomas of the liver, and pulmonic stenosis, have been sporadically observed.

Asthma, gastrointestinal malabsorption by jejunal atrophy, multiple food intolerance and acrocheilia have also been reported.

## Natural history

Patients may have a different prognosis, depending on the type and severity of the features associated with the hair alterations. Cases that died during early infancy showed severe physical and mental retardation and frequently suffered from severe respiratory infections. Therefore, poor prognosis in TTD has been linked to severe, recurrent infectious disease with most pediatric deaths due to overwhelming bacterial infections.

The disturbed hair growth and the ichthyosis tend to improve during adolescence and adulthood. Most patients survive to adult age, although with motor and mental delay, short stature, ocular problems such as cataracts and strabismus, and prematurely aged facial appearance. Often, they are no longer prone to infections, although they suffered moderate infections during early childhood. Photosensitivity seems to diminish with age.

**Table 1.** Genes responsible for trichothiodystrophy

| Gene name (synonyms) | Accession number | Chromosome location[a] | Size (aa) | Function |
|---|---|---|---|---|
| **Photosensitive form[b]** | | | | |
| XPB (ERCC3) | NM_000122 | 2q14.3 | 782 | 3′–5′ DNA helicase essential for both transcription and NER |
| XPD (ERCC2) | NM_000400 | 19q13.32 | 760 | 5′–3′ DNA helicase necessary for NER but dispensable for *in vitro* basal transcription |
| GTF2H5 (p8, TTDA) | NM_207118 | 6p25.3 | 71 | provides stability to TFIIH, stimulates XPB ATPase activity and promotes the translocation of XPA to UV damaged sites |
| **Non-photosensitive form** | | | | |
| C7orf11 (TTDN1) | NM_138701 | 7p14.1 | 179 | transcription factor? |

*NER* nucleotide excision repair; *TFIIH* general transcription factor IIH; *GTF2H5* general transcription factor IIH, polypeptide 5. *ERCC2* excision repair cross-complementing rodent complementation group 2; *ERCC3* excision repair cross-complementing rodent complementing group 3.

[a]From http://www.cgal.icnet.uk/DNA_Repair_Genes.html. See also Wood et al. (2005).

[b]The three genes identified as responsible of the photosensitive form of TTD encode distinct subunits of TFIIH, a multiprotein complex involved in both transcription and NER.

It is worth mentioning that hair loss and other features, such as brittle hair and nails, ichthyosis and ataxia, have been reported to become more pronounced during episodes of fever in patients with a mutation in the *XPD* gene conferring thermo-instability of TFIIH (Vermeulen et al. 2001).

## Pathogenesis/molecular genetics

The remarkable progress that has been made over the last twenty years on TTD has revealed two distinct forms of the disorder characterized by the presence or absence of clinical and cellular photosensitivity. Both these forms are genetically heterogeneous and the features of the disease-genes identified so far are reported in Table 1. The molecular complexity of the pathways altered in the photosensitive form, as a consequence of quantitative and structural alterations in the transcription/repair complex TFIIH, offers a rational for the wide variation in the expression and severity of the clinical features and a clue for the role of the functions implicated in the non-photosensitive form.

### Functions defective in TTD

**All sun-sensitive TTD cases** show an altered cellular response to UV as a consequence of defects in nucleotide excision repair (NER) resulting from al-

terations in either XPB, XPD or TTDA, which are three components of TFIIH, a ten-subunit complex that is essential for various processes. Besides participating to NER, TFIIH is also engaged in RNA polymerase II transcription initiation, RNA polymerase I transcription, activated transcription, and cell cycle regulation. The multiple roles of TFIIH might explain why mutations in *XPB* and *XPD* have been found associated with a variety of hereditary disorders. As already mentioned, *XPB* has been identified as the gene responsible for rare cases with either XP, TTD or the XP/CS complex whereas *XPD* has been implicated not only in XP, TTD and XP/CS but also in other pathological phenotypes ranging from cerebro-oculo-facioskeletal syndrome to combined XP/TTD features (see also Chapters 51 and 52). This pleiotropy is likely related to different mutation sites in the *XPB* and *XPD* genes that affect in slightly different ways the stability and the conformation of TFIIH and, consequently, its functional activities.

The human transcription/repair factor IIH (TFIIH) consists of ten subunits. XPB, XPD, p62, p52, p44 and p34 form the core complex, while cdk7, MAT1, and cyclin H form the cdk-activating kinase (CAK) subcomplex. The core-TFIIH and CAK sub-complexes are bridged by the XPD subunit, which interacts with p44 on the one side and MAT1 on the other side. The recently identified 8-kDa TTDA protein connects to the core via inter-

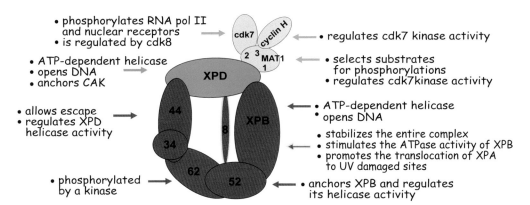

**Fig. 5.** TFIIH composition and functions of its subunits. The six subunits composing the coreTFIIH subcomplex are in red, the three subunits of the cdk-activating kinase (CAK) subcomplex are in light blue, the XPD subunit that bridge the two TFIIH subcomplexes is in green (updated from Stefanini 2006).

actions with p52 and XPD (Fig. 5). TFIIH harbors different enzymatic activities: a protein kinase displayed by the cyclin-dependent kinase cdk7, two DNA-dependent ATPases, XPB and XPD, required for the helicase function, and the ubiquitin ligase activity of p44. In the first steps of the nucleotide excision reaction, TFIIH unwinds the DNA around the lesion to allow the recruitment of the other factors of the repair machinery (see Fig. 2 in Chapter 51). In the transcription of class II genes, TFIIH participates in the initiation of RNA synthesis by opening the promoter around the start site and by phosphorylating via its cdk7 kinase the carboxy-terminal domain of the largest subunit of RNA polymerase II and some transcriptional activators including nuclear receptors. The three TFIIH subunits mutated in TTD have different roles. XPB and XPD are ATP-dependent helicases with opposite polarity and participate in the unwinding of DNA both in repair and basal transcription (Coin et al. 2007 and refer-

ence therein). The p8/TTDA subunit stabilizes the cellular concentration of TFIIH *in vivo* and stimulates NER *in vitro* (Coin et al. 2006, Giglia-Mari et al. 2006).

All the mutations found in TTD result in reduced steady-state levels of the entire TFIIH complex and modification of its architecture. As exemplified in Fig. 6, this leads to a reduced functioning of the complex in repair and transcription. Accordingly, TTD-specific mutations in the *XPD* gene have been shown to interfere with both repair and basal transcription *in vitro* (Dubaele et al. 2003). DNA repair defects, however, only marginally explain the TTD clinical outcome while a transcriptional deficiency may account for the majority of the symptoms.

Transcriptional defects in TTD are compatible with life and therefore they have to occur only under certain circumstances and/or in specific cellular compartments. Several lines of evidence support the hypothesis that quantitative and conformational al-

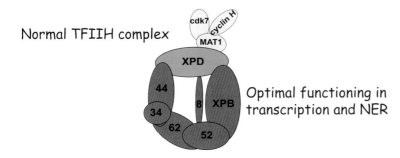

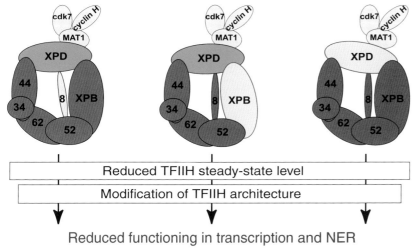

**Fig. 6.** TFIIH alterations in the photosensitive form of trichothiodystrophy. The presence of a mutated subunit results in reduced steady-state levels of the entire complex and in modifications of its conformation.

terations of TFIIH in TTD patients may become limiting in terminally differentiated tissues, in which the mutated TFIIH might be insufficient to provide adequate transcriptional activity of a diverse set of highly expressed genes. This might account for the deficiency in cysteine-rich matrix proteins in the hairshafts, for the β-globin deficiency in erythrocytes of TTD/XP-D patients showing the hematological features of β-thalassemia trait without mutations in hemoglobin genes (Viprakasit et al. 2001), and for the alterations in T cells and dendritic cells reported in few TTD patients (Stefanini et al. 1986, Racioppi et al. 2001). Accordingly, a lowered expression of differentiation markers has been described in skin and differentiating keratinocytes from the TTD mouse model (de Boer et al. 1998, Backendorf et al. 2005), and a reduced ability to terminally differentiate has been recently identified in epidermal keratinocytes from TTD patients (Botta et al. our unpublished observations). We have recently observed alterations in components of the extracellular matrix in primary skin fibroblasts from TTD patients mutated in *XPD*. Furthermore, we have provided the first evidence of a failure in the expression of the collagen type VI alpha 1 subunit (*COL6A1*) that might account for clinical symptoms that TTD share with hereditary disorders mutated in *COL6A1* (Orioli et al. submitted).

TFIIH is involved in gene expression not only by binding to core promoter elements and facilitating initiation of transcription but also by promoting specific ligand-dependent nuclear receptor-mediated transactivation of target promoters. It has been demonstrated that the TFIIH regulatory role in transcription may be hampered by the presence of a mutated subunit within the complex. Several *XPD* mutations have been showed to confer defects in the TFIIH-dependent phosphorylation of certain nuclear receptors, which fail to proper control the expression of their specific responsive genes. In particular, mutations at position arg658 (TTD), arg683t (XP), and arg722t (TTD) confer reduced transactivation by the estrogen (ERα), androgen (AR), retinoic acid (RARα and RARγ) and peroxisome proliferator-activated (PPARs) receptors (Keriel et al. 2002, Dubaele et al. 2003, Compe et al. 2005).

The finding that mutations located in the C-terminal end of *XPD*, prevent the action of nuclear receptors harboring an A/B domain regardless the associated pathological phenotype, offers a clue for understanding some developmental and neurological defects encountered in both XP and TTD patients.

The importance of the co-activator function of TFIIH in the pathogenesis of TTD has been highlighted by recent studies from J. M. Egly group (reported in Kraemer et al. 2007b) showing that the expression of myelin is dysregulated in the brain of TTD mice as a consequence of a TFIIH defect in stabilizing the thyroid receptor (TR) on the promoter region of TR-target genes. This TFIIH dysfunction appeared to have different consequences on the expression of TR-regulated genes in distinct tissues of TTD mice. Therefore, TFIIH is a tissue specific transcription factor co-activator but the tissue-specificity is conferred by the cell type-specific transcription regulatory machinery and not by TFIIH itself. As well as providing the first evidence that defects in transcriptional co-activation play a role in the neuropathology of TTD, these results have dramatic implications for understanding tissue-specific effects of mutations that alter the structure/function of TFIIH in many subtly different ways.

As far as the ageing features are concerned, it has been suggested that they might be due to unrepaired oxidative damage that compromises transcription and leads to functional inactivation of critical genes and enhanced apoptosis (de Boer et al. 2002, Wijnhoven et al. 2005, Andressoo et al. 2006a). Whereas hypersensitivity to oxidative stress has been clearly demonstrated in Cockayne syndrome (CS), a disorder that shares many features of ageing and developmental anomalies with TTD, inability to repair oxidative damage in TTD remains elusive.

The lack of skin cancer in TTD patients, despite their deficiencies in NER has been the subject of much speculation (reviewed in Lehmann 2003, Stefanini 2006). Transcriptional alterations as well as differences in immune responses, cell-cycle regulation, oxidative metabolism and apoptosis have been invoked to account for this apparent anomaly. However, we don't have yet a clear answer why XP and TTD patients defective in the same repair pathway, and even in the same gene, do show different cancer susceptibility.

Very little information is available on the defects underlying the **non-photosensitive form of TTD**. In these patients the cellular response to UV is normal, thus excluding NER deficiencies. Also the cellular amount of TFIIH is in the normal range (Botta et al. 2007). Only one disease-gene (designated *C7orf11*) has been identified so far (Nakabayashi et al. 2005). *C7orf11* is an uncharacterized open reading frame that maps to chromosome 7p14. The corresponding protein localizes to the nucleus and is expressed in fetal hair follicles, but nothing is known about its functional activity. Since non-photosensitive TTD patients share with photosensitive cases all the clinical symptoms except cutaneous photosensitivity, the genes implicated in the non-photosensitive form might encode factors involved in transcription regulation but not in DNA repair. These proteins could be transcriptional regulators of genes involved in metabolic pathways that are affected in both forms of TTD or they may be involved in conformational changes required for optimal functioning of TFIIH. We have recently obtained evidence suggesting that TFIIH alterations typically present in photosensitive TTD patients may influence the *C7orf11* expression with different tissue-specific modalities (Botta et al. our unpublished observations). This finding supports the hypothesis that *C7orf11* function might be critical for tissue-specific transcription and/or during differentiation, when a diverse set of genes must be transcribed at a very high rate.

## Clinical, cellular and molecular characteristics of the TTD groups

The genetic defects underlying the photosensitive form of TTD have been identified by using the reduced ability to perform UV-induced DNA repair synthesis typically present in patient cells, as cellular parameter in a classical complementation test based on somatic cell hybridization (illustrated in Chapter 51, Fig. 4). It is worthwhile recalling that this assay

has been set up for the NER defective form of XP and it enabled these XP patients to be classified into seven different complementation groups, designated from XP-A to XP-G (see Chapter 51). Genetic studies in TTD have demonstrated that *XPD* is the gene that accounts for the NER defect in the majority of patients whereas rare cases were found mutated in either the *XPB* or *TTDA* gene (reviewed in Lehmann 2003, Stefanini 2006). Clinical and cellular features of TTD groups and the results of patient mutation analysis are summarized in Tables 2 and 3, respectively.

**The TTD-A group** comprises four patients from three families, who exhibit similar clinical and cellular features (Stefanini et al. 1993b, Vermeulen et al. 2000, Botta et al. 2002, Giglia-Mari et al. 2004). They show a pathological phenotype of moderate severity but drastically increased cellular sensitivity to the killing effects of UV light and notable reductions in UV-induced DNA repair synthesis levels (15–25% of normal), recovery of RNA synthesis at late times after irradiation, and TFIIH cellular amounts (30–35% of normal). These findings suggest that a 3 fold reduction of TFIIH complexes with normal composition consistently reduces NER efficiency but confers subtle defects in transcription resulting in clinical features of mild/moderate severity. This implies that NER requires higher concentrations of TFIIH than does transcription.

Sequencing of the *p8/TTDA* gene revealed that the patient TTD99RO carries a homozygous C to T transition at codon 56, converting the CGA codon encoding arginine into a TGA stop codon. The English patient TTD1BR is a compound hererozygote, with one allele identical to that of TTD99RO and the other allele carrying a T to C transition at codon 21, converting the conserved leucine residue to a proline. This mutation is localized in one of the hydrophobic patches on the protein surface that are likely to mediate interactions either with TFIIH subunits or other proteins of the NER pathway (Vitorino et al. 2007). The two Italian siblings TTD13PV and TTD14PV are homozygotes for a mutation that converts the ATG start codon into an ACG codon and results in either a complete loss of protein synthesis or in the production of an N-ter-

**Table 2.** Clinical and cellular features of the four complementation groups of trichothiodystrophy

| Group | OMIM | Clinical symptoms[a] | | | Cellular response to UV[b] | | | TFIIH level[c] |
|---|---|---|---|---|---|---|---|---|
| | | Hair alterations | Neurological impairment | Physical impairment | UV-sensitivity | UDS, % of normal | RRS | |
| **Photosensitive form** | | | | | | | | |
| XP-B | 133510 | + | − | − | + | 40 | − | 43 |
| XP-D | 126340 | + | +/++ | +/++ | +/++ | 10–60 | − | 35–65 |
| TTD-A | 608780 | + | + | + | ++ | 15–25 | − | 35 |
| **Non-photosensitive form** | | | | | | | | |
| TTDN1 | 234050 | + | +/++ | +/++ | − | 100 | + | 115–120 |

[a]Neurological impairment: + moderate severity (mental development at either preschool level or primary-school level, axial hypotonia, and reduced motor coordination); ++ severe (very poor mental and motor performances and speech). Physical impairment: + moderate (survival beyond early childhood, delayed puberty, and short stature); ++ severe (death during childhood and/or failure to thrive/dystrophy).

[b]UV-sensitivity: survival partially (+) or drastically (++) reduced compared with normal. UDS (Unscheduled DNA synthesis): the ability to perform UV-induced DNA repair synthesis is expressed as a percentage of that in normal cells. RRS (Recovery of RNA synthesis): rate after UV normal (+) or defective (−).

[c]TFIIH level refers to the mean steady state of the subunits cdk7, p44, and p62 in patient cells expressed as percentage of that in normal C3PV cells analyzed in parallel (Botta et al. 2002, 2007).

**Table 3.** Mutational analysis in TTD patients

| Gene | Cases No. | Recurrent mutation | Mutated products[a] |
|---|---|---|---|
| **Photosensitive form** | | | |
| XPB | 2 (1 family) | – | single aa substitution |
| XPD | 28 (25 families) | yes | single aa substitutions (deletions frameshift in the c-terminal region) |
| TTDA | 4 (3 families) | yes | truncated products* (single aa substitutions) |
| **Non-photosensitive form** | | | |
| TTDN1 | 23 (9 kindreds) | yes | truncated products* (single aa substitution) |

[a]See also XP mutation database http://xpmutations.org/ for mutations identified in these genes. *Severely truncated polypeptides because of either stop codons, frameshifts, or genomic DNA deletions. Changes identified in single or rare cases are between brackets.

minally truncated protein (lacking the first and most conserved 15 aminoacids) when a downstream AUG at codon 16 is used. Thus, the majority of mutations identified in TTD-A patients lead either to non-functional truncated peptides or to the complete absence of the protein. This makes TTDA the first TFIIH subunit for which a complete absence is compatible with life (Giglia-Mari et al. 2004), in striking contrast with deletion mutants of each of the other TFIIH subunits, which are not viable in yeast and mammals.

**The XP-B group** consists of six families (see Chapter 51), only one of which with TTD affected members. They are two French siblings both born at term from first-cousin marriage, with a similar presentation as a collodion baby of favorable outcome. Their relatively mild symptoms (hair abnormalities without any physical and mental impairment) have led the clinician to describe them clinically as a TTD "variant" (van Neste et al. 1989). These patients were found to be homozygous for a A to C transversion resulting, at the protein level, in a threonine to proline substitution at amino acid residue 119 (Weeda et al. 1997). This mutation is associated with a partial reduction in the UDS levels (40% of normal) and in the cellular content of TFIIH (43% of normal). Interestingly, the (recombinant or immunopurified) TFIIH with the thr119pro mutated XPB subunit retains a significant fraction of wild-type basal transcription activity *in vitro* (Bergmann and Egly 2001). This finding further confirms that the XPB protein tolerates only those rare amino acid changes that only slightly interfere with its essential role in transcription.

**The XP-D group** comprises several TTD patients whose pathological phenotypes show different degrees of severity. Some cases are moderately af-

fected in terms of proneness to infections and physical and mental retardation with short stature, delayed puberty, mental development at preschool or primary school level, axial hypotonia, reduced motor coordination and survival beyond early childhood. Other cases exhibit very poor mental and motor performances and speech, marked proneness to infections, failure to thrive and death during early childhood. DNA repair investigations revealed that also NER is differentially impaired in these patients, with UDS levels ranging between 50% and less than 10% of normal. The reduced efficiency to perform UV-induced DNA repair synthesis is associated with a parallel decrease in cell survival ability after UV. No correlation was observed between the de-

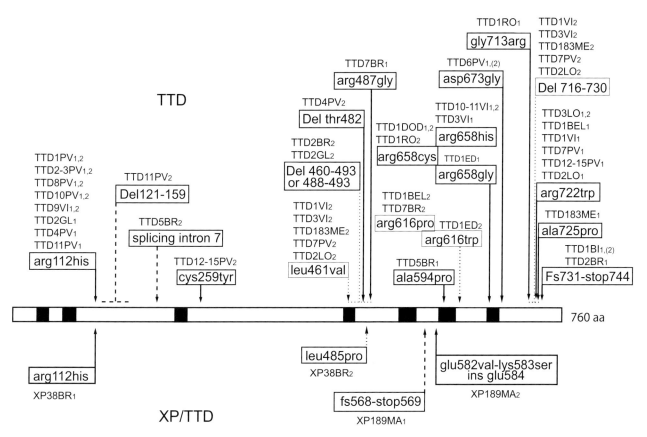

**Fig. 7.** Aminoacid changes in the XPD protein resulting from mutations described in patients with trichothiodystrophy (TTD) or combined symptoms of xeroderma pigmentosum and TTD (XP/TTD). The diagram shows the XPD protein with the helicase domains (black boxes). The amino acid changes are shown boxed. The numbers 1 and 2 after the patient code denote the different alleles. The changes responsible for the pathological phenotype, those resulting in deletions likely to affect cellular viability and mutations described as lethal (Taylor et al. 1997, Broughton et al. 2001) are indicated by solid, dashed and dotted arrows, respectively. The mutation leu461val and the deletion 716–730 have been always found associated in a single haplotype.

gree of the severity of the clinical symptoms and the repair deficiency.

The TFIIH steady-state level varies from 35% to 65% of normal, as pointed out by detailed analysis in primary fibroblasts from TTD patients representative of different types and combinations of mutated *XPD* alleles (Botta et al. 2002). The reduction in the TFIIH amount does not correlate either with the residual repair capacity or with the severity of clinical symptoms. This implies that the severity of the TTD pathological phenotype cannot be related solely to the effects of mutations on the stability of TFIIH.

As summarized in Fig. 7, mutation analysis has been so far performed in twenty eight TTD patients (Broughton et al. 1994; Takayama et al. 1996, 1997, Taylor et al. 1997; Botta et al. 1998; Viprakasit et al. 2001). Although no clear protein domains could be identified that include exclusively TTD-specific mutations, several disease-specific sites have been observed. Most of the mutations in TTD are localized at three sites and all involve a single substitution of an arginine residue (arg112, arg658, and arg722). The arg658cys mutation was shown to confer a temperature-sensitive defect in transcription and repair due to thermo-instability of TFIIH with fever-dependent reversible deterioration of TTD features (Vermeulen et al. 2001), a finding supporting the link between TFIIH instability and the hair and skin features that are the diagnostic hallmark of TTD. The arg112his change is the most common alteration in the Italian patients, of whom six were homozygotes and two were heterozygotes for this mutation. The finding that the compound heterozygotes are more severely affected at the clinical level than the arg112his homozygotes led to the suggestion that the main determinant of the severity of the clinical features might be the effective *XPD* gene dosage (Botta et al. 1998).

The mutations identified in other severely affected patients are consistent with this hypothesis. The different degrees of impairment in the cellular responses to UV in TTD appeared to be related to specific mutations. A mild UV sensitivity was found in patients with mutations resulting either in the change of arg658 or in the loss of the final portion of the XPD protein. A remarkable UV sensitivity is associated with the arg112his change whereas an intermediate UV sensitivity was associated with the arg722trp change. Two alleles, resulting in either the substitution of arg616 or the leu461val change associated with the deletion of aminoacid region 716–730, have been found in both TTD and XP individuals. These alleles are likely to be nonfunctional because they behave as null alleles in *S. pombe* (Taylor et al. 1997), they completely abolish basal transcription *in vitro* (Dubaele et al. 2003) and they have never been observed in the homozygous state, despite being relatively frequent among patients. The pathological phenotype in patients who are compound heterozygotes for one of these lethal alleles appeared to be determined by the mutation on the second allele that is always different in XP and TTD cases. Interestingly, recent evidence in TTD mouse model indicates that these null alleles can alleviate developmental delay, skin and hair features of TTD (Andressoo et al. 2006b).

Two patients have been identified with the combined clinical features of XP and TTD (Broughton et al. 2001). Although neither case had the hair brittle, hair analysis revealed a "tiger tail" appearance and partially reduced levels of sulfur-containing proteins. XP189MA, a 3-year-old girl with sun sensitivity, mental and physical developmental delay, showed an extremely reduced repair capacity and *XPD* mutations not previously reported (Fig. 7). It has been suggested that a peculiar situation in the genetic background of this patient may mitigate the effects of transcription and NER impairment, resulting in mild TTD and XP symptoms. Alternatively, the mutation present in the less severely affected allele might confer an extremely mild defect in transcription that does not completely prevent the phenotypic consequences of the repair defect, as usually found for the mutations associated with TTD. In the patient XP38BR, a 28 year-old woman with sun sensitivity, pigmentation changes and skin cancers typical of XP, a novel combination of mutated *XPD* alleles was identified (Fig. 7). One *XPD* allele had the mutation causing the arg112his substitution that has been found in several patients, all with the clinical features of TTD. The second allele contained a novel mutation resulting in the leu485pro change that was lethal in *S.*

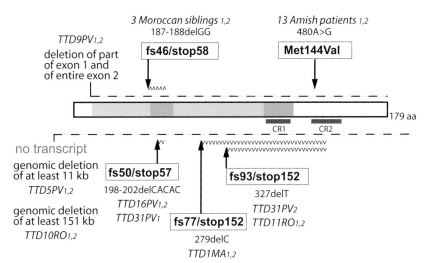

**Fig. 8.** Mutations and resulting aminoacid changes in the C7orf11 protein in non-photosensitive TTD patients. Cases described by Nakabayashi et al. (2005) (upper part) and by Botta et al. (2007) (lower part). The diagram shows the C7orf11 protein with the glycine/proline rich region in green (the low complexity regions detected by the BLASTP program are in dark green) and the two highly conserved C-terminal regions (CR1 and CR2) present among the candidate orthologs. The amino acid changes are shown boxed. Numbers 1 and 2 after the patient code denote the different alleles.

*pombe*. The level of repair of UV damage in XP38BR was substantially higher than that in other patients with the arg112his change. The peculiar clinical, cellular and molecular features of this patient might be explained by the occurrence of an as yet unidentified modifying mutation in another gene that partially suppresses the defects in transcription and repair usually associated with arg112his alteration.

**The TTDN1 group** has been recently established by Nakabayashi and coworkers (2005), who have identified *C7orf11* as the first gene responsible for non-photosensitive TTD. *C7orf11* has been sequenced in non-photosensitive TTD patients belonging to 57 families of different geographic origin (Nakabayashi et al. 2005, Botta et al. 2007). As shown in Fig. 8, mutations were found in three Moroccan siblings, an Amish kindred, and seven unrelated cases (four from Italy and one each from The Netherlands, Kuwait and Iraq). The finding that *C7orf11* is defective in a small proportion of non-photosensitive TTD cases indicates that genetic heterogeneity exists in this form of TTD, as already demonstrated for the photosensitive TTD cases.

The mutation spectrum shows that *C7orf11* is not essential for cell proliferation and viability. In three patients the gene is deleted whereas the mutations found in five cases result in frameshifts producing severely truncated proteins. A missense mutation has been reported only in the Amish kindred. Evaluation of genotype-phenotype relationships indicates

that the severity of the clinical features does not correlate with the molecular defect, suggesting that other genetic and/or environmental factors, besides the *C7orf11* mutations, are likely to be involved in determining the severity of the pathological phenotype.

## Diagnosis, follow-up and management

The main diagnostic criteria of TTD are brittle hair, mental and growth retardation, face characterized by receding chin, small nose, large ears and microcephaly, nail dysplasia and ichthyosis. The hair abnormalities are considered the key factors in the recognition of the disorder. Scalp hair, eyebrows, and eyelashes are short, thin, brittle and dry. Light microscopy reveals irregular hair surface and diameter, trichoschisis, a decreased cuticular layer with twisting, and a nodal appearance that mimics trichorrhexis nodosa. Polarization microscopy of the hair typically shows alternating light and dark bands that confer a "tiger tail" pattern. The age at which tiger tail banding is apparent, may be variable. It may not be evident until three months of age and it may not be definitive for the diagnosis of TTD in the newborn period. However, the diagnosis of TTD can be confirmed, even in the newborn period, by the amino acid analysis of the hair which shows a notably low cystine content that parallels the low total sulfur content. Also the aminoacids proline, threonine, and serine are reduced and consequently, a relative increase in methionine, phenylalanine, alanine, leucine, lysine, and aspartic acid can be found (Itin et al. 2001). Sulfur proteins are not only quantitatively but also qualitatively altered, and there is an abnormal distribution of the sulfur-rich proteins in the cortex and in hair cuticles. The fragile hair found in patients with TTD results from these alterations in hair specific cysteine-rich matrix proteins that cross-link the keratin fibers and normally confer hair shaft stability.

An inverse correlation between sulfur content and percent of hairs with shaft abnormalities (trichoschisis, trichorrhexis nodosa, or ribbon/twist) has been reported whereas no association between clinical disease severity and percent of abnormal hairs has been found (Liang et al. 2006). Hair abnormalities in TTD have been revealed also by confocal microscopy and scanning electron microscopy and it has been shown that the Raman spectral analysis of hair, nail and skin samples may provide additional diagnostic information useful for the dermatologist (Liang et al. 2006, Schlucker et al. 2006 and references therein).

A recent study confirms that in patients with clinical features suggestive of TTD, tiger tail banding seen in all hairs with polarizing microscopy, in conjunction with certain hair shaft abnormalities, provides a reliable diagnostic test (Liang et al. 2005). It must be emphasized that clinical findings of the patient should support the diagnosis of TTD. Although trichoschisis and alternating light and dark banding by polarizing microscopy are typical findings in TTD, they may occasionally occur in patients without this disorder (Itin et al. 2001).

An additional simple diagnostic tool for differential diagnosis of TTD relies on the analysis of the expression of the β-globin gene that was found reduced in all the eleven analyzed TTD patients with characterized mutations in the *XPD* gene (Viprakasit et al. 2001).

Beside hair and nails, other tissue of ectodermal and neuroectodermal origin are usually affected in TTD. As already mentioned, it is worth recalling that the clinical spectrum of associated symptoms is extensive and the disorder is characterized by a wide variation in the severity of the clinical features.

Therefore, in clinical evaluation of TTD patients a good practice would be to consider classical descriptors of the disorder as well as other clinical signs, including ocular and immunological defects, photosensitivity and pregnancy complications (Kraemer et al. 2007b).

The photosensitive form of TTD can be conclusively diagnosed by analyzing patient's cells for the appropriate DNA repair defect. Specific functional assays on *in vitro* cultured fibroblasts are available to evaluate the cellular response to UV light and to define the gene responsible for the DNA repair defect. Also the analysis of the cellular amount of TFIIH may be informative since a reduced level of the complex has been shown to be a common feature in all TTD patients mutated in *XPB*, *XPD* and *TTDA* genes (Vermeulen et al. 2000, 2001; Botta et al. 2002; Giglia-Mari et al. 2004).

Definition of the underlying molecular defect may be informative for the prognosis. The few TTD-A cases reported so far, are moderately affected. The two cases mutated in the *XPB* gene have a very mild phenotype. In TTD patients mutated in *XPD*, the severity of the pathological phenotype varies from moderate to severe and it depends on the nature of the mutated *XPD* alleles. The available mutational data suggests that the most clinically severe patients are functionally hemizygous for mutations in the *XPD* gene.

In patients with the non photosensitive form of TTD, sequencing of the *C7orf11* gene may be informative for family counseling. Mutations in this gene account for less than 20% of non photosensitive TTD patients (Botta et al. 2007) and no obvious genotype-phenotype relationships have been observed in patients with mutations in the *C7orf11* gene.

Management issues are: 1) comprehensive baseline evaluation and serial monitoring; 2) symptomatic care.

Baseline evaluation includes measurement of growth, developmental assessment, dental evaluation, dermatologic, ophthalmologic and audiologic evaluations, MRI of the brain, skeletal X-rays to document the presence of skeletal dysplasia, electromyography (EMG) and nerve conduction velocities (NCV) to document the presence of a dysmyelinating neuropathy, yearly reassessment for known potential complications such as declining vision and hearing, evaluation of hematological parameters and immune response.

Symptomatic care includes an individualized educational program, assistive devices, and assessment of safety in the home for developmental delay and gait disturbances, physical therapy to prevent contractures and maintain ambulation, feeding gastrostomy tube placement to prevent malnutrition, medication for spasticity, management of hearing loss, cataracts, and other ophthalmologic complications, dental care to minimize dental caries.

Precancerous skin alterations and tumors have never been reported in TTD. However, taking into account results showing some predisposition to cancer in the TTD mouse models, prudence dictates that TTD patients with cutaneous photosensitivity should adopt sun protective measures and undergo periodic skin examinations.

## Resources

There are not Support groups specifically intended for patients affected by trichothiodystrophy. A web site listing disease-causing mutations in TTD has been established: http://xpmutations.org/. Further Information is available on the of Geneskin web site http://geneskin.idi.it, that is part of an European coordination action project on rare genetic skin diseases funded by the European Commission (LSHM-CT-2005-512117).

## Acknowledgments

We thank the members of our research groups for their contribution to the work over the years. Studies by MS mentioned in the text have been supported by grants from the Associazione Italiana per la Ricerca sul Cancro, the European Community (contracts SC1-232, CHRX-CT94-0443, QLG1-1999-00181 and MRTN-CT-2003-503618), the Italian Ministry of Education, University and Research, and the Fondazione Cariplo.

## References

Allen R (1971) Neurocutaneous syndromes in children. Postgrad Med 50: 83–89.

Andressoo JO, Hoeijmakers JH, Mitchell JR (2006a) Nucleotide excision repair disorders and the balance between cancer and aging. Cell Cycle 5: 2886–2888.

Andressoo JO, Jans J, de Wit J, Coin F, Hoogstraten D, van de Ven M, Toussaint W, Huijmans J, Thio HB, van Leeuwen WJ, de Boer J, Egly JM, Hoeijmakers JH, van der Horst GT, Mitchell JR (2006b) Rescue of progeria in trichothiodystrophy by homozygous lethal Xpd alleles. PLoS Biol 4: e322.

Arbisser AI, Scott CI Jr, Howell RR, Ong PS, Cox HL Jr (1976) A syndrome manifested by brittle hair with morphologic and biochemical abnormalities, developmental delay and normal stature. Birth Defects Orig Artic Ser 12: 219–228.

Backendorf C, de Wit J, van Oosten M, Stout GJ, Mitchell JR, Borgstein AM, van der Horst GT, de Gruijl FR, Brouwer J, Mullenders LH, Hoeijmakers JH (2005) Repair characteristics and differentiation propensity of long-term cultures of epidermal keratinocytes derived from normal and NER-deficient mice. DNA Repair 4: 1325–1336.

Baden HP, Jackson CE, Weiss L, Jimbow K, Lee L, Kubilus J, Gold RJ (1976) The physicochemical properties of hair in the BIDS syndrome. Am J Hum Genet 28: 514–521.

Bastien J, Adam-Stitah S, Riedl T, Egly JM, Chambon P, Rochette-Egly C (2000) TFIIH interacts with the retinoic acid receptor gamma and phosphorylates its AF-1-activating domain through cdk7. J Biol Chem 275: 21896–21904.

Battistella PA, Peserico A (1996) Central nervous system dysmyelination in PIBI(D)S syndrome: a further case. Childs Nerv Syst 12: 110–113.

Bergmann E, Egly JM (2001) Trichothiodystrophy, a transcription syndrome. Trends Genet 17: 279–286.

Bootsma D, Hoeijmakers JH (1993) DNA repair. Engagement with transcription. Nature 363: 114–115.

Bootsma D, Hoeijmakers JH (1994) The molecular basis of nucleotide excision repair syndromes. Mutat Res 307: 15–23.

Botta E, Nardo T, Broughton B, Marinoni S, Lehmann AR, Stefanini M (1998) Analysis of mutations in the *XPD* gene in Italian patients with trichothiodystrophy: site of mutation correlates with repair deficiency but gene dosage appears to determine clinical severity. Am J Hum Genet 63: 1036–1048.

Botta E, Nardo T, Lehmann AR, Egly JM, Pedrini AM, Stefanini M (2002) Reduced level of the repair/transcription factor TFIIH in trichothiodystrophy. Hum Mol Genet 11: 2919–2928.

Botta E, Offman J, Nardo T, Ricotti R, Zambruno G, Sansone D, Balestri P, Raams A, Kleijer WJ, Jaspers NGJ, Sarasin A, Lehmann AR, Stefanini M (2007) Mutations in the *C7orf11* (*TTDN1*) gene in six non-photosensitive trichothiodystrophy patients: no obvious genotype-phenotype relationships. Hum Mutat 28: 92–96.

Braun-Falco O, Ring J, Butenandt O, Selzle D, Landthaler M (1981) Ichthyosis vulgaris, growth retardation, hair dysplasia, tooth abnormalities, immunologic deficiencies, psychomotor retardation and resorption disorders. Case report of 2 siblings. Hautarzt 32: 67–74.

Broughton BC, Steingrimsdottir H, Weber CA, Lehmann AR (1994) Mutations in the xeroderma pigmentosum group D DNA repair/transcription gene in patients with trichothiodystrophy. Nat Genet 7: 189–194.

Broughton BC, Berneburg M, Fawcett H, Taylor EM, Arlett CF, Nardo T, Stefanini M, Menefee E, Price VH, Sarasin A, Bohnert E, Krutmann J, Davidson R, Kraemer KH, Lehmann AR (2001) Two individuals with features of both xeroderma pigmentosum and trichothiodystrophy highlight the complexity of the clinical outcomes of mutations in the *XPD* gene. Hum Mol Genet 10: 2539–2547.

Brown AC, Belser RB, Crounse RG, Wehr RF (1970) A congenital hair defect: trichoschisis with alternating birefringence and low sulfur content. J Invest Dermatol 54: 496–509.

Busso D, Keriel A, Sandrock B, Poterszman A, Gileadi O, Egly JM (2000) Distinct regions of MAT1 regulate cdk7 kinase and TFIIH transcription activities. J Biol Chem 275: 22815–22823.

Calvieri S, Rossi A, Amorosi B, Giustini S, Innocenzi D, Micali G (1993) Trichothiodystrophy: ultrastructural studies of two patients. Pediatr Dermatol 10: 111–116.

Chapman S (1988) The trichothiodystrophy syndrome of Pollitt. Pediatr Radiol 18: 154–156.

Chen D, Riedl T, Washbrook E, Pace PE, Coombes RC, Egly JM, Ali S (2000) Activation of estrogen receptor alpha by S118 phosphorylation involves a ligand-dependent interaction with TFIIH and participation of CDK7. Mol Cell 6: 127–137.

Cleaver JE (2005) Splitting hairs – discovery of a new DNA repair and transcription factor for the human disease trichothiodystrophy. DNA Repair 4: 285–287.

Coin F, Egly JM (1998) Ten years of TFIIH. Cold Spring Harb Symp Quant Biol 63: 105–110.

Coin F, Egly JM (2003) Assay of promoter melting and extension of mRNA: role of TFIIH subunits. Methods Enzymol 370: 713–733.

Coin F, Proietti De Santis L, Nardo T, Zlobinskaya O, Stefanini M, Egly JM (2006) p8/TTD-A as a repair-specific TFIIH subunit. Molecular Cell 21: 215–226.

Coin F, Oksenych V, Egly JM (2007) Distinct roles for the XPB/p52 and XPD/p44 subcomplexes of TFIIH in damaged DNA opening during nucleotide excision repair. Mol Cell 26: 245–256.

Compe E, Drané P, Laurent C, Diderich K, Braun C, Hoeijmakers JH, Egly JM (2005) Dysregulation of the peroxisome proliferator-activated receptor target genes by XPD mutations. Mol Cell Biol 25: 6065–6076.

Crovato F, Borrone C, Rebora A (1983) Trichothiodystrophy – BIDS, IBIDS and PIBIDS? Br J Dermatol 108: 247.

Crovato F, Rebora A (1985) PIBI(D)S syndrome: a new entity with defect of the deoxyribonucleic acid excision repair system. J Am Acad Dermatol 13: 683–686.

de Boer J, de Wit J, van Steeg H, Berg RJ, Morreau H, Visser P, Lehmann AR, Duran M, Hoeijmakers JH, Weeda G (1998) A mouse model for the basal transcription/DNA repair syndrome trichothiodystrophy. Mol Cell 1: 981–990.

de Boer J, Andressoo JO, de Wit J, Huijmans J, Beems RB, van Steeg H, Weeda G, van der Horst GT, van Leeuwen W, Themmen AP, Meradji M, Hoeijmakers JH (2002) Premature aging in mice deficient in DNA repair and transcription. Science 296: 1276–1279.

Drané P, Compe E, Catez P, Chymkowitch P, Egly JM (2004) Selective regulation of vitamin D receptor-responsive genes by TFIIH. Mol Cell 16: 187–197.

Dubaele S, Proietti de Santis L, Bienstock RJ, Keriel A, Stefanini M, van Houtten B, Egly JM (2003) Basal transcription defect discriminates between xeroderma pigmentosum and trichothiodystrophy in XPD patients. Mol Cell 11: 1635–1646.

Egly JM (2001) The 14th Datta Lecture. TFIIH: from transcription to clinic. FEBS Lett 498: 124–128.

Fois A, Balestri P, Calvieri S, Zampetti M, Giustini S, Stefanini M and Lagomarsini P (1988) Trichothiodystrophy without photosensitivity: biochemical, ultrastructural and DNA repair studies. Eur J Pediatr 147: 439–441.

Frederick GD, Amirkhan RH, Schultz RA, Friedberg EC (1994) Structural and mutational analysis of the xeroderma pigmentosum group D (XPD) gene. Hum Mol Genet 3: 1783–1788.

Friedberg EC, Walker GC, Siede W, Wood RD, Schultz RA, Ellenberger T (2006) Other diseases associated with defects in nucleotide excision repair of DNA. In: DNA repair and mutagenesis. Washington, DC: ASM Press, pp. 895–918.

Giglia-Mari G, Coin F, Ranish JA, Hoogstraten D, Theil A, Wijgers N, Jaspers NG, Raams A, Argentini M, van der Spek PJ, Botta E, Stefanini M, Egly JM, Aebersold R, Hoeijmakers JH, Vermeulen W (2004) A new, tenth subunit of TFIIH is responsible for the DNA repair syndrome trichothiodystrophy group A. Nat Genet 36: 714–719.

Giglia-Mari G, Miquel C, Theil AF, Mari PO, Hoogstraten D, Ng JM, Dinant C, Hoeijmakers JH, Vermeulen W (2006) Dynamic interaction of TTDA with TFIIH is stabilized by nucleotide excision repair in living cells. PLoS Biol 4: e156. Epub 2006 May 9.

Happle R, Traupe H, Grobe H, Bonsmann G (1984) The Tay syndrome (congenital ichthyosis with trichothiodystrophy). Eur J Pediatr 141: 147–152.

Hoeijmakers JH, Egly JM, Vermeulen W (1996) TFIIH: a key component in multiple DNA transactions. Curr Opin Genet Dev 6: 26–33.

Howell RR, Arbisser AI, Parsons DS, Scott CI, Fraustadt U, Collie WR, Marshall RN, Ibarra OC (1981) The Sabinas syndrome. Am J Hum Genet 33: 957–967.

Iben S, Tschochner H, Bier M, Hoogstraten D, Hozak P, Egly JM, Grummt I (2002) TFIIH plays an essential role in RNA polymerase I transcription. Cell 109: 297–306.

Itin PH, Sarasin A, Pittelkow MR (2001) Trichothiodystrophy: update on the sulfur-deficient brittle hair syndromes. J Am Acad Dermatol 44: 891–920.

Jackson CE, Weiss L, Watson JH (1974) "Brittle" hair with short stature, intellectual impairment and decreased fertility: an autosomal recessive syndrome in an Amish kindred. Pediatrics 54: 201–207.

Jorizzo JL, Crounse RG, Wheeler CE Jr (1980) Lamellar ichthyosis, dwarfism, mental retardation, and hair shaft abnormalities. A link between the ichthyosis-associated and BIDS syndromes. J Am Acad Dermatol 2: 309–317.

Jorizzo JL, Atherton DJ, Crounse RG, Wells RS (1982) Ichthyosis, brittle hair, impaired intelligence, decreased fertility and short stature (IBIDS syndrome). Br J Dermatol 106: 705–710.

Keriel A, Stary A, Sarasin A, Rochette-Egly C, Egly JM (2002) XPD mutations prevent TFIIH-dependent transactivation by nuclear receptors and phosphorylation of RARalpha. Cell 109: 125–135.

Kraemer KH (2004) From proteomics to disease. Nat Genet 36: 677–678.

Kraemer KH, Patronas NJ, Schiffmann R, Brooks BP, Tamura D, DiGiovanna JJA (2007a) Xeroderma pigmentosum, trichothiodystrophy and Cockayne syndrome: a complex genotype–phenotype relationship. Neuroscience 145: 1388–1396.

Kraemer KH, Sander M, Bohr VA (2007b) New areas of focus at workshop on human diseases involving DNA repair deficiency and premature aging. Mech Ageing Dev 128: 229–235.

Lainé JP, Mocquet V, Egly JM (2006) TFIIH enzymatic activities in transcription and nucleotide excision repair. Methods Enzymol 408: 246–263.

Lehmann AR, Arlett CF, Broughton BC, Harcourt SA, Steingrimsdottir H, Stefanini M, Taylor AMR, Natarajan AT, Green S, King MD, McKie RM, Stephenson JBP, Tolmie JL (1988) Trichothiodystrophy: a human DNA-repair disorder with heterogeneity in the cellular response to ultraviolet light. Cancer Res 48: 6090–6096.

Lehmann AR (1989) Trichothiodystrophy and the relationship between DNA repair and cancer. Bioessays 11: 168–170.

Lehmann AR (1995) Nucleotide excision repair and the link with transcription. Trends Biochem Sci 20: 402–405.

Lehmann AR (1998) Dual functions of DNA repair genes: molecular, cellular, and clinical implications. Bioessays 20: 146–155.

Lehmann AR (2001) The xeroderma pigmentosum group D (XPD) gene: one gene, two functions, three diseases. Genes Dev 15: 15–23.

Lehmann AR (2003) DNA repair-deficient diseases, xeroderma pigmentosum, Cockayne syndrome and trichothiodystrophy. Biochimie 85: 1101–1111.

Liang C, Kraemer KH, Morris A, Schiffmann R, Price VH, Menefee E, DiGiovanna JJ (2005) Characterization of tiger-tail banding and hair shaft abnormalities in trichothiodystrophy. J Am Acad Dermatol 52: 224–232.

Liang C, Morris A, Schlucker S, Imoto K, Price VH, Menefee E, Wincovitch SM, Levin IW, Tamura D, Strehle KR, Kraemer KH, DiGiovanna JJ (2006) Structural and molecular hair abnormalities in trichothiodystrophy. J Invest Dermatol 126: 2210–2216.

Liu J, He L, Collins I, Ge H, Libutti D, Li J, Egly JM, Levens D (2000) The FBP interacting repressor targets TFIIH to inhibit activated transcription. Mol Cell 5: 331–341.

Liu J, Akoulitchev S, Weber A, Ge H, Chuikov S, Libutti D, Wang XW, Conaway JW, Harris CC, Conaway RC, Reinberg D, Levens D (2001) Defective interplay of activators and repressors with TFIH in xeroderma pigmentosum. Cell 104: 353–363.

Mariani E, Facchini A, Honorati MC, Lalli E, Berardesca E, Ghetti P, Marinoni S, Nuzzo F, Astaldi Ricotti GCB, Stefanini M (1992) Immune defects in families and patients with xeroderma pigmentosum and trichothiodystrophy. Clinical Exp Immunol 88: 376–382.

Nakabayashi K, Amann D, Ren Y, Saarialho-Kere U, Avidan N, Gentles S, MacDonald JR, Puffenberger EG, Christiano AM, Martinez-Mir A, Salas-Alanis JC, Rizzo R, Vamos E, raams A, Les C, Seboun E, Jaspers NGJ, Beckmann JS, Jackson CE, Scherer SW (2005) Identification of C7orf11 (TTDN1) gene mutations and genetic heterogeneity in nonphotosensitive trichothiodystrophy. Am J Hum Genet 76: 510–516.

Nuzzo F, Stefanini M, Rocchi M, Casati A, Colognola R, Lagomarsini P, Marinoni S, Scozzari R (1988) Chromosome and blood marker studies in families of patients affected by xeroderma pigmentosum and trichothiodystrophy. Mutat Res 208: 159–161.

Nuzzo F, Zei G, Stefanini M, Colognola R, Santachiara AS, Lagomarsini P, Marinoni S, Salvaneschi L (1990) Search for consanguinity within and among families of patients with trichothiodystrophy associated with xeroderma pigmentosum. J Med Genet 27: 21–25.

Ostergaard JR, Christensen T (1996) The central nervous system in Tay syndrome. Neuropediatrics 27: 326–330.

Peserico A, Battistella PA, Bertoli P (1992) MRI of a very rare hereditary ectodermal dysplasia: PIBI(D)S. Neuroradiology 34: 316–317.

Pollitt RJ, Jenner FA, Davies M (1968) Sibs with mental and physical retardation and trichorrhexis nodosa with abnormal amino acid composition of the hair. Arch Dis Child 43: 211–216.

Porto L, Weis R, Schulz C, Reichel P, Lanfermann H, Zanella FE (2000) Tay's syndrome: MRI. Neuroradiology 42: 849–851.

Price VH, Odom RB, Ward WH, Jones FT (1980) Trichothiodystrophy: sulfur-deficient brittle hair as a marker for a neuroectodermal symptom complex. Arch Dermatol 116: 1375–1384.

Racioppi L, Cancrini C, Romiti ML, Angelini F, Di Cesare S, Bertini E, Livadiotti S, Gambarara MG, Matarese G, Lago Paz F, Stefanini M, Rossi P (2001) Defective Dendritic Cell Maturation in a Child with DNA-excision repair deficiency and CD4 lymphopenia. Clin Exp Immunol 126: 511–518.

Ranish JA, Hahn S, Lu Y, Yi EC, Li XJ, Eng J, Aebersold R (2004) Identification of TFB5, a new component of general transcription and DNA repair factor IIH. Nat Genet 36: 707–713.

Richetta A, Giustini S, Rossi A, Calvieri S (2001) What's new in trichothiodystrophy. J Eur Acad Dermatol Venereol 15: 1–4.

Robbins JH, Kraemer KH, Lutzner MA, Festoff BW, Coon HG (1974) Xeroderma pigmentosum. An inherited diseases with sun sensitivity, multiple cutaneous neoplasms, and abnormal DNA repair. Ann Intern Med 80: 221–248.

Salfeld K, Lindley MJ (1963) On the problem of combination of symptoms in ichthyosis vulgaris with bambolo hair formation and ectodermal dysplasia. Dermatol Wochenschr 147: 118–128.

Sass JO, Skladal D, Zelger B, Romani N, Utermann B (2004) Trichothiodystrophy: quantification of cysteine in human hair and nails by application of sodium azide-dependent oxidation to cysteic acid. Arch Dermatol Res 296: 188–191.

Schaeffer L, Roy R, Humbert S, Moncollin V, Vermeulen W, Hoeijmakers JH, Chambon P, Egly JM (1993)

DNA repair helicase: a component of BTF2 (TFIIH) basic transcription factor. Science 260: 58–63.

Schaeffer L, Moncollin V, Roy R, Staub A, Mezzina M, Sarasin A, Weeda G, Hoeijmakers JH, Egly JM (1994) The ERCC2/DNA repair protein is associated with the class II BTF2/TFIIH transcription factor. EMBO J 13: 2388–2392.

Schlucker S, Liang C, Strehle KR, DiGiovanna JJ, Kraemer KH, Levin IW (2006) Conformational differences in protein disulfide linkages between normal hair and hair from subjects with trichothiodystrophy: a quantitative analysis by Raman microspectroscopy. Biopolymers 82: 615–622.

Scott RJ, Itin P, Kleijer WJ, Kolb K, Arlett C, Muller H (1993) Xeroderma pigmentosum-Cockayne syndrome complex in two patients: absence of skin tumors despite severe deficiency of DNA excision repair. J Am Acad Dermatol 29: 883–889.

Stefanini M, Lagomarsini P, Arlett CF, Marinoni S, Borrone C, Crovato F, Trevisan G, Cordone G, Nuzzo F (1986) Xeroderma pigmentosum (complementation group D) mutation is present in patients affected by trichothiodystrophy with photosensitivity. Human Genetics 74: 107–112.

Stefanini M, Lagomarsini P, Giorgi R, Nuzzo F (1987) Complementation studies in cells from patients affected by trichothiodystrophy with normal or enhanced UV photosensitivity. Mutat Res 191: 117–119.

Stefanini M, Lagomarsini P, Nuzzo F (1989) Genetic analysis in trichothiodystrophy repair deficient cells confirms the occurrence of xeroderma pigmentosum group D mutation in unrelated patients. In: Lambert MW, Laval J (eds.) DNA repair mechanisms and their biological implication in mammalian cells. New York: Plenum Press, pp. 523–533.

Stefanini M, Giliani S, Nardo T, Marinoni S, Nazzaro V, Rizzo R, Trevisan G (1992) DNA repair investigations in nine Italian patients affected by trichothiodystrophy. Mutat Res 273: 119–125.

Stefanini M, Lagomarsini P, Giliani S, Nardo T, Botta E, Peserico A, Kleijer WJ, Lehmann AR, Sarasin A (1993a) Genetic heterogeneity of the excision repair defect associated with trichothiodystrophy. Carcinogenesis 14: 1101–1105.

Stefanini M, Vermeulen W, Weeda G, Giliani S, Nardo T, Mezzina M, Sarasin A, Harper JI, Arlett CF, Hoeijmakers JHJ, Lehmann AR (1993b) A new nucleotide excision repair gene associated with the genetic disorder trichothiodystrophy. Am J Human Genet 53: 817–821.

Stefanini M (2006) Trichothiodystrophy, a disorder highlighting the crosstalk between DNA repair and transcription. In: Balajee A (ed.) DNA repair and human diseases. Landes Bioscience, pp. 30–46.

Takayama K, Salazar EP, Broughton BC, Lehmann AR, Sarasin A, Thompson LH, Weber CA (1996) Defects in the DNA repair and transcription gene ERCC2(XPD) in trichothiodystrophy. Am J Hum Genet 58: 263–270.

Takayama K, Danks DM, Salazar EP, Cleaver JE, Weber CA (1997) DNA repair characteristics and mutations in the ERCC2 DNA repair and transcription gene in a trichothiodystrophy patient. Hum Mutat 9: 519–525.

Tay CH (1971) Ichthyosiform erythroderma, hair shaft abnormalities, and mental and growth retardation. A new recessive disorder. Arch Dermatol 104: 4–13.

Taylor E, Broughton B, Botta E, Stefanini M, Sarasin A, Jaspers NGJ, Fawcett H, Harcourt SA, Arlett CF, Lehmann AR (1997) Genotype-phenotype relationships in the xeroderma pigmentosum group D (ERCC2) repair/transcription gene. Proc Natl Acad Sci USA 94: 8658–8663.

Tolmie JL, de Berker D, Dawber R, Galloway C, Gregory DW, Lehmann AR, McClure J, Pollitt RJ, Stephenson JB (1994) Syndromes associated with trichothiodystrophy. Clin Dysmorphol 3: 1–14.

Van der Knaap M, Valk J (2005) Trichothiodystrophy with photosensitivity. In: van der Knaap M, Valk J (eds.) Magnetic resonance of myelination and myelin disorders, 3rd edn. Berlin: Springer-Verlag, pp. 268–271.

Van Neste D, de Greef H, van Haute N, van Hee J, van der Maesen J, Taieb A, Maleville J, Fontan D, Bakry N, Gillespie JM, Marshall RC (1989) High sulfur protein deficient human hair: clinical aspects and biochemical study of two unreported cases of a variant type of trichothiodystrophy. In: Van Neste D (ed.) Trends in human hair and alopecia research. Dordrecht: Kluwer Academic, pp. 195–206.

Vermeulen W, van Vuuren AJ, Chipoulet M, Schaeffer L, Appeldoorn E, Weeda G, Jaspers NGJ, Priestley A, Arlett CF, Lehmann AR, Stefanini M, Mezzina M, Sarasin A, Bootsma D, Egly JM, Hoeijmakers JHJ (1994a) Three unusual repair deficiencies associated with transcription factor BTF2 (TFIIH): evidence for the existence of a transcription syndrome. Cold Spring Harb Sym 59: 317–329.

Vermeulen W, Scott RJ, Rodgers S, Muller HJ, Cole J, Arlett CF, Kleijer WJ, Bootsma D, Hoeijmakers JH, Weeda G (1994b) Clinical heterogeneity within xeroderma pigmentosum associated with mutations in the DNA repair and transcription gene ERCC3. Am J Hum Genet 54: 191–200.

Vermeulen W, Bergmann E, Auriol J, Rademakers S, Frit P, Appeldoorn E, Hoeijmakers JH, Egly JM (2000) Sublimiting concentration of TFIIH transcription/DNA

repair factor causes TTD-A trichothiodystrophy disorder. Nat Genet 26: 307–313.

Vermeulen W, Rademakers S, Jaspers NG, Appeldoorn E, Raams A, Klein B, Kleijer WJ, Hansen LK, Hoeijmakers JH (2001) A temperature-sensitive disorder in basal transcription and DNA repair in humans. Nat Genet 27: 299–303.

Viprakasit V, Gibbons RJ, Broughton BC, Tolmie JL, Brown D, Lunt P, Winter RM, Marinoni S, Stefanini M, Brueton L, Lehmann AR, Higgs DR (2001) Mutations in the general transcription factor TFIIH result in β-thalassaemia in individuals with trichothiodystrophy. Hum Mol Genet 10: 2797–2802.

Vitorino M, Coin F, Zlobinskaya O, Atkinson RA, Moras D, Egly JM, Poterszman A, Kieffer B (2007) Solution structure and self-association properties of the p8 TFIIH subunit responsible for trichothiodystrophy. J Mol Biol 368: 473–480.

Wagner AM (2006) Xeroderma pigmentosum, Cockayne's syndrome and Trichothiodystrophy. In: Harper J, Oranje A, Prose N (eds.) Textbook of pediatric dermatology, 2nd edn, Vol. 2, Oxford: Blackwell Science, pp. 1557–1582.

Wakeling EL, Cruwys M, Suri M, Brady AF, Aylett SE, Hall C (2004) Central osteosclerosis with trichothiodystrophy. Pediatr Radiol 34: 541–546.

Weber A, Liu J, Collins I, Levens D (2005) TFIIH operates through an expanded proximal promoter to fine-tune c-myc expression. Mol Cell Biol 25: 147–161.

Weber CA, Salazar EP, Stewart SA, Thompson LH (1990) ERCC2: cDNA cloning and molecular characterization of a human nucleotide excision repair gene with high homology to yeast RAD3. EMBO J 9: 1437–1447.

Weeda G, Eveno E, Donker I, Vermeulen W, Chevallier-Lagente O, Taieb A, Stary A, Hoeijmakers JH, Mezzina M, Sarasin A (1997) A mutation in the XPB/ERCC3 DNA repair transcription gene, associated with trichothiodystrophy. Am J Hum Genet 60: 320–329.

Wijnhoven SW, Beems RB, Roodbergen M, van den Berg J, Lohman PH, Diderich K, van der Horst GT, Vijg J, Hoeijmakers JH, van Steeg H (2005) Accelerated aging pathology in ad libitum fed Xpd(TTD) mice is accompanied by features suggestive of caloric restriction. DNA Repair 4: 1314–1324.

Yoder K, Sarasin A, Kraemer K, McIlhatton M, Bushman F, Fishel R (2006) The DNA repair genes XPB and XPD defend cells from retroviral infection. Proc Natl Acad Sci USA 103: 4622–4627.

Yoon HK, Sargent MA, Prendiville JS, Poskitt KJ (2005) Cerebellar and cerebral atrophy in trichothiodystrophy. Pediatr Radiol 35: 1019–1023.

Zurita M, Merino C (2003) The transcriptional complexity of the TFIIH complex. Trends Genet 19: 578–584.

# Chapter 54

# PROGERIA AND PROGEROID SYNDROMES (PREMATURE AGEING DISORDERS)

Ignacio Pascual-Castroviejo and Martino Ruggieri

Paediatric Neurology Service, University Hospital La Paz, University of Madrid, Madrid, Spain (IPC); Institute of Neurological Science, National Research Council and Department of Pediatrics, University of Caternia, Caternia, Italy (MR)

## Generalities

Progeria (from the Greek word "*gēras*" meaning "*old age*") consists on the precocious and rapid ageing and the early onset of age-related complications such as joint restriction and cerebral and myocardial infarction (Roach 2004).

Although the first recognized entity was the Hutchinson–Gilford progeria syndrome (HGPS), described by Hutchinson in 1886 and by Gilford in 1904, several additional syndromes with progeroid appearance (*premature aging disorders*) are currently recognized. Some of these syndromes give a progeroid appearance **at birth**, such as neonatal progeroid syndrome (Wiedemann-Rautenstrauch syndrome) (OMIM # 264090), Hallerman-Streiff syndrome (OMIM # 234100), Berardinelli–Seip syndrome (OMIM # 269700), Bamatter-Franceschetti syndrome (OMIM # 231070), De Barsy syndrome (OMIM # 219150), autosomal recessive cutis laxa syndrome (OMIM # 219100), and Leprechaunism (OMIM # 218040) (the latter often mistaken with Costello syndrome during the neonatal period and over the first year of life). Other ageing conditions become clinically apparent **later in life**, such as Hutchinson–Gilford syndrome (OMIM # 176670), Cockayne syndrome (OMIM # 216400), Werner syndrome (OMIM # 277700), Mandibuloacral dysplasia syndrome (OMIM # 248370), Rothmund–Thomson syndrome (OMIM # 268400), Bloon

syndrome (OMIM # 210900), and Groenblad-Strandberg syndrome (pseudoxantoma elasticum). Generalized precocious cellular aging seems a common denominator in all syndromes.

Most patients with progeria and progeroid syndromes overlap some clinical features, whilst other show differences. Currently, the natural history of the ageing process is an important clue to identify the syndrome such as occurs with Hutchinson–Gilford progeria and Werner's syndrome, typically being diagnosed in childhood and adulthood, respectively. These were considered two different entities due to LMNA mutations (seen only in patients with Hutchinson–Gilford progeria) but later the same LMNA mutation was identified in patients with Werner syndrome.

Genomic DNA analysis can help draw diagnostic lines that will clarify the cause of progreria and progeroid entities.

Little is yet known about the pathophysiology of human senescence, about the relationship between some of these syndromes and about their possible origin. In some diseases metabolic disturbances have been demonstrated (e.g., mitochondrial alterations in the Cockayne syndrome), but the primary cause, although probably of metabolic nature, remains unknown in most entities to date. Molecular genetic diagnosis of a specific progeria syndrome may have only limited clinical value at present, but future therapies might depends on having a precise molecular classification.

# HUTCHINSON–GILFORD PROGERIA SYNDROME

## Introduction

Hutchinson–Gilford progreria syndrome (HGPS) (OMIM # 176670) is an extremely rare fatal genetic disorder which is characterized by the very early and rapid aging in children, short stature, and recognizable skin and hair manifestations (Korf 2008, Toriello 2006). HGPS is caused by mutations in the lamin A gene (*LMNA*; OMIM # 150330) (Pollex and Hegele 2004) located on chromosome 1q (Eriksson et al. 2003) whose protein product is a truncated lamin A (*progerin*), lacking 50 amino acids near the C terminus (De Sandre-Giovannoli et al. 2003, Eriksson et al. 2003).

## Historical perspective and eponyms

It was first described by Hutchinson (1886) and Gilford (1904). The syndrome was given the name progreria (from the Greek, "*geras*", meaning old age) by Gilford (1904) "in recognition of the senile characters which form such a conspicuous feature of the disease from the beginning".

## Incidence and prevalence

HGPS is the best recognized progeroid entity and the reported incidence is 1 in 8 million. Since 1886, just over 100 cases of HGPS have been reported and currently there are approximately 40 known cases worldwide (Pollex and Hegele 2004).

## Clinical manifestations

Children with HGPS appear normal and healthy at birth, but distinctive clinical features appear within the first few years of life, that mainly consists of accelerated aging and severe growth retardation.

Typical facial features (Fig. 1) include micrognathia, craniofacial disproportion, alopecia, prominent eyes, nose, and scalp veins. Children have delayed growth and are short in stature and below average weight. Craniofacial abnormalities, delayed and abnormal dentition, scleroderma-like areas of skin, due to loss of subcutaneous fat, stiffness of joints, and other skeletal abnormalities including coxa valga (giving a "horse-riding" stance). Children with HGPS appear individuals who get the old age very early (De Busk 1972, Sarkar and Shinton 2001). Onset of symptoms and signs in the neonatal age has been described in a pair of monozygotic twins (Martinville et al. 1980).

Other common abnormalities are incomplete sexual maturation, atherosclerosis, a thin and high pitched voice and a pyriform thorax. As the affected people mature, the disorder causes children to age about a decade for every year of their life (Fig. 2). This means that by the age of 10, a child with HGPS would have the same respiratory, cardiovascular, and skeletal manifestations/complications as an adult, but with normal mental and emotional development (De Busk 1972).

## Imaging

Radiological abnormalities most often, consist on facial bones hypoplasia, thin and short clavicles (Fig. 3), coxa valga, accelerated bone maturation, acroosteolyses, and wormian bones of the skull.

## Natural history

Death occurs at an average age of 13 years, with al least 90% of HGPS subjects dying from progressive atherosclerosis of the coronary and cerebrovascular arteries (Baker et al. 1981, Brown 1992, Dyck et al. 1987, Matsuo et al. 1994). Survival of a few hours was described in a baby (Rodriguez et al. 1999).

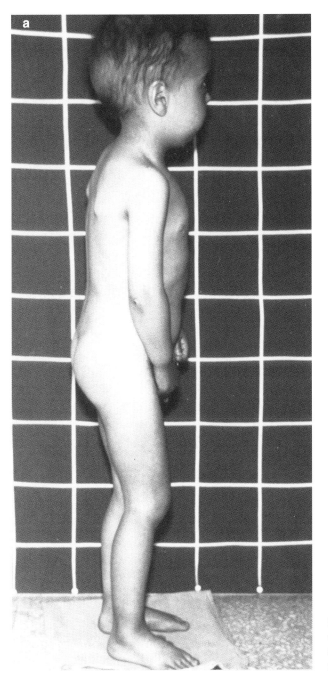

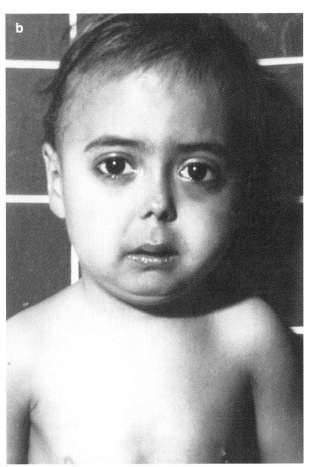

**Fig. 1.** Five-year-old child with Hutchinson–Gilford in (**a**) lateral view that shows sparse hair, contractures of elbows, knees and spine, and micrognatia; (**b**) Frontal view that shows sparse hair in the scalp, micrognatia and lack of clavicles prominence.

Death from coronary artery disease may occur before 10 years of age. Large arteries supplying the brain frequently develop atherosclerosis at an early age that cause the neurological signs and symptoms which correspond with the location of the vascular lesions (Rosman and Anslem 2001).

## Molecular genetics and pathogenesis

Recessive inheritance has been proposed, due to observations of affected individuals found in consanguineous families (Khalifa 1989, Maciel 1988, Parkash et al. 1991), or the occurrence of the syndrome in

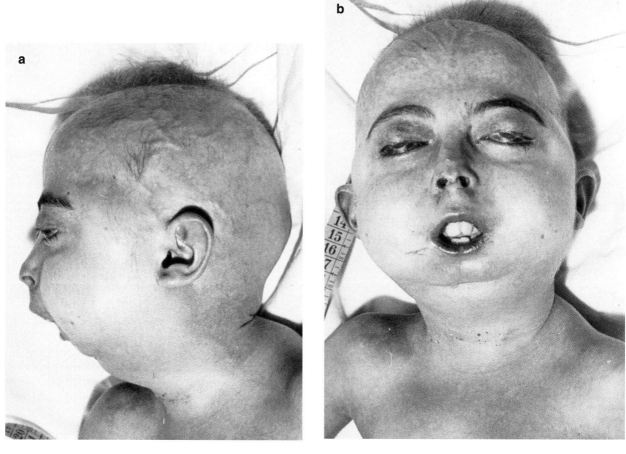

**Fig. 2.** The same patient as in Fig. 1 at 13 years of age. Severe increase of all signs of senile appearance (Courtesy of Dr. JM Santolaya).

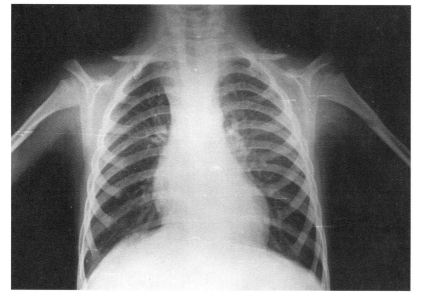

**Fig. 3.** The thoracic X-ray study shows thin and short clavicles.

pairs of affected siblings (Hadgadorn et al. 1990, Megarbane and Loiselet 1997). Progeria has been described in twins as well (Brown et al. 1992, Martinville et al. 1980, Viegas et al. 1974).

The presence of chromosomal abnormalities involving chromosome 1q23 (Brown et al. 1992, Delgado Luengo et al. 2002) were considered possible contributing factors to the disease. These cytogenetic clues proved to be critical for discovery of the HGPS gene (Pollex and Hegele 2004).

## HGPS gene

HGPS is caused by sporadic mutations in the lamin A gene (LMNA; OMIM # 150330) (Korf 2008). The HGPS gene was initially localized to chromosome 1q by observing two cases of uniparental isodisomy (i.e., the inheritance of both copies of this material from one parent) of 1q and one case with a 6-megabase paternal interstitial deletion (Eriksson et al. 2003). At least five different mutations within the LMNA gene have been found in patients with HGPS (D'Apice et al. 2004, De Sandre-Giovannoli et al. 2003, Eriksson et al. 2003, Novelli et al. 2002). Twenty five HGPS described patients harbored an identical de novo single-base substitution, a C-to-T transition at position 1824 of the coding sequence predicted to result in a silent polymorphism at codon 608 within exon 11 (G608G; OMIM # 150330.0022) (D'Apice et al. 2004). The G608G mutation causes the activation of a cryptic donor-splicing site resulting in a 150 bp deletion in the mRNA and a truncated lamin A (progerin), lacking 50 amino acids near the C terminus (De Sandre-Giovannoli et al. 2003, Eriksson et al. 2003). D'Apice et al. (2004), after studying three patients, showed G608G mutation responsible for the majority of patients with HGPS arises in the paternal germline, and they confirmed and advanced paternal age in the fathers of affected individuals.

Mutations in the lamin A gene are also responsible for mandibuloacral dysplasia, Emery-Dreifuss muscular dystrophy, Dunnigan lypodystrophy, limbgirdle muscular dystrophy 1B, Charcot-Marie-Tooth disease type 2B1 and dilated cardiomyopathy type 1A (Toriello 2006).

The discovery of the molecular basis of HGPS suggest a possible role for LMNA in aspects of the normal ageing process. Molecular diagnostic methods may provide the diagnosis during early ages before the full clinical phenotype has appeared, and may also provide reassurance by the prenatal studies (Eriksson et al. 2003).

The proteins that bind abnormally to mutant LMNA in HGPS may also play a pathogenic role in common atherosclerosis (Zastrow et al. 2004). HGPS patients develop atherosclerosis at an accelerated rate, apparently with little environmental stress, suggesting that molecular mechanisms predominate.

## Diagnosis

The increased concentration of urinary excretion of hyaluronic acid (HA) has been recognized as a biochemical marker for HGPS patients (Sweeney and Weiss 1992), although this feature is not pathognomonic of HGPS (Delgado Luengo et al. 2002). HA is an unsulfated glycosaminoglycan which plays an active role to maintain the architecture of skin, muscle, skeletal, and vascular systems (Sarkar and Shinton 2001). It has been suggested that HA acts during the morphogenesis of blood vessels in the embryo and as an antiangiogenic factor during the process of aging (Feinberg and Beebe 1983). Increase of basal growth hormone has been found in some patients (Delgado Luengo et al. 2002).

## Differential diagnosis

HGPS must be differentiated from several other conditions that develop signs of precocious senility such as Werner's syndrome; hypotrophy of adipose tissue; premature vascular occlusion and skin laxity, such as Costello syndrome, disorders with cutis laxa and fibromuscular disease. Skeletal disorder, such as mandibuloacral dysplasia exhibits some of the features of progeria, being the most frequent short stature, alopecia, hypoplasia of he clavicle and mandible, stiff joints, and persistently open cranial sutures (Hoeffel et al. 2000, Parkash et al. 1990, Parkash 1991, Toriello 1991). Despite the so characteristic appearance of patients with HGPS, that make the diagnosis very easy, differential diagnosis with several diseases may be also considered. Patients with Hallermann–Streiff, Cockayne's, and neonatal progeroid (Devos et al. 1981, Korniszewski et al. 2001, Pivnick et al. 2000) syndromes, and still less frequently others, have been mistakenly diagnosed as having progeria (Wiedemann 1987).

## Prognosis and treatment

Life span is shortened due to the involvement of almost all organic tissues and particularly of the cerebral and coronary arteries. Senile aspect appear early.

There is no therapy known for any of the complications of progeria. Patients may have a normal life during several years due to progeria usually does not effect upon the intellect during some years. Future therapies might depend on having a precise molecular classification (Hegele 2003).

## References

Baker PB, Baba N, Boesel CP (1981) Cardiovascular abnormalities in progeria. Case report and review of the literature. Arch Pathol Lab Med 105: 384–386.

Brown WT, Abdenur J, Goonewardena P, Alemzadeh R, Smith M, Friedman S (1992) Hutchinson–Gilford progeria syndrome: clinical, chromosomal and metabolic abnormalities (Abstract). Am J Hum Genet 47 (Suppl): A50.

D'Apice MR, Tenconi R, Mammi I, van den Ende J, Novelli G (2004) Paternal origin of LMNA mutations in Hutchinson–Gilford progeria. Clin Genet 65: 52–54.

De Busk FL (1972) The Hutchinson–Gilford progeria syndrome. Report of 4 cases and review of the literature. J Pediatr 80: 697–724.

Delgado Luengo W, Rojas Martinez A, Ortiz Lopez R, Martinez Basalo C, Rojas-Atencio A, Quintero M (2002) Del (1) (q23) in a patient with Hutchinson–Gilford progeria. Am J Med Genet 113: 298–301.

De Sandre-Giovannoli A, Bernard R, Cau P, Navarro C, Amiel J, Boccaccio I, Lyonnet S, Stewart CL, Munnich A, Le Merrer M, Levy N (2003) Lamin A truncation in Hutchinson–Gilford progeria. Science 300: 2055.

Devos EA, Leroy JG, Frijns JP, Van den Berghe H (1981) The Wiedemann Rautenstrauch or neonatal progeroid syndrome. Eur J Pediatr 136: 245–248.

Dyck JD, David TE, Burke B, Weebb GD, Henderson MA, Fowler RS (1987) Management of coronary disease in Hutchinson–Gilford síndrome. J Pediatr 111: 407–410.

Eriksson M, Brow WT, Gordon LB, Glynn MW, Singer J, Scott L (2003) Recurrent de novo point mutations in lamin A cause Hutchinson–Gilford progeria syndrome. Nature 423: 293–298.

Feinberg R, Beebe D (1983) Hyaluronate in vasculogenesis. Science 220: 1177–1179.

Gilford H (1904) Progeria: a form of senilism. Practitioner 73: 188–217.

Hadgadorn JL, Wilson WG, Hallen HW, Callicott JH, Beale EF (1990) Neonatal progeroid syndrome: more than one disease? Am J Med Genet 35: 91–94.

Hegele RA (2003) Drawing the line in progeria syndromes. Lancet 362: 416–417.

Hoeffel JC, Mainard L, Chastagner P, Hoeffeld CC (2000) Mandibulo-acral dysplasia. Skel Radiol 29: 668–671.

Hutchinson J (1886) Congenital absence of hair and mammary glands with atrophic condition of the skin and its appendages in a boy whose mother had been almost wholly bald from alopecia areata from the age of six. Trans Med Chir Soc (Edinburgh) 69: 473.

Khalifa MM (1989) Hutchinson–Gilford progeria syndrome: report of a Libyan family and evidence of autosomal recessive inheritance. Clin Genet 35: 125–132.

Korf B (2008) Hutchinson-Gilford progeria syndrome, aging, and the nuclear lamina. N Engl J Med 358: 552–555.

Korniszewski L, Nowak R, Okninska-Hoffmann E (2001) Wiedemann Routenstrauch (neonatal progeroid) syndrome: new case with normal telomere length in skin fibroblasts. Am J Med Genet 103: 144–148.

Maciel AT (1988) Evidence for autosomal recessive inheritance of progeria (Hutchinson Gilford). Am J Med Genet 31: 483–487.

Martinville (de) B, Sorin M, Briard ML, Fresal J (1980) Progeria de Gilford-Hutchinson à debut neonatal chez deux jumeaux monozygotes. Arch Franç Pediatr 37: 679–681.

Matsuo S, Takeuchi Y, Hayashi S, Kinagasa A, Sawada T (1994) Patient with unusual Hutchinson–Gilford syndrome (progeria). Pediatr Neurol 10: 237–240.

Megarbane A, Loiselet J (1997) Clinical manifestation of a severe neonatal progeroid syndrome. Clin Genet 51: 200–204.

Novelli G, Muchir A, Sangiuolo F, Helbling-Leclerc A, D'Apice MR, Massart C, Capon F, Sbraccia P, Federici M, Lauro R, Tudisco C, Pallotta R, Scarano G, Dallapiccola B, Merlini L, Bonne G (2002) Mandibuloacral dysplasia is caused by a mutation in LMNA-encoding lamin A/C. Am J Hum Genet 71: 426–431.

Parkash H (1991) Reply to Dr. Toriello. Am J Med Genet 41: 140.

Parkash H, Sidhu SS, Raghavan R, Deshmukh RN (1990) Hutchinson–Gilford progeria: familial occurrence. Am J Med Genet 36: 431–433.

Pivnick EK, Angle B, Kaufman RA, Hall BD, Pitukcheewanont P, Hersh JH, Fowlkes JL, Sanders LP, O'Brien JM, Carroll GS, Gunther WM, Morrow HG, Burghen GA, Ward JC (2000) Neonatal progeroid (Wiedemann-Reutenstrauch) syndrome. Am J Med Genet 90: 131–140.

Pollex RL, Hegele RA (2004) Hutchinson–Gilford progeria syndrome. Clin Genet 66: 375–381.

Reddel CJ, Weiss AS (2004) Lamin A expression levels are unperturbed at the normal and mutant alleles but display partial splice site deletion in Hutchin-son–Gilford progeria syndrome. J Med Genet 41: 715–717.

Rodriguez JL, Pérez-Alonso P, Funes R, Pérez-Rodriguez J (1999) Letal neonatal Hutchinson–Gilford progeria síndrome. Am J Med Genet 82: 242–248.

Rosman PN, Anslem I (2001) Progressive intracranial vascular disease with strokes and seizures in a boy with progeria. J Child Neurol 16: 212–215.

Sarkar PK, Shinton RA (2001) Hutchison–Gilford progeria syndrome. Postgrad Med J 77: 312–317.

Sweeney KJ, Weiss AS (1992) Hyaluronic acid in progeria and the aged phenotype? Gerontology 38: 139–152.

Toriello HV (1991) Mandibulo-acral "Dysplasia". Am J Med Genet 41: 138.

Toriello HV (2006) Premature ageing syndromes. In: Harper J, Oranje A, Prose N (eds.) Textbook of Pediatric Dermatology. 2nd ed. Oxford: Blackwell Science, pp. 1538–1556.

Viegas J, Souza LR, Salzano FM (1974) progeria in twins. J Med Genet 11: 384–386.

Wiedemann HR (1987) Progeria. In: Gomez MR (ed.) Neurocutaneos diseases. A practical approach. Stoneham: Butterworth, pp. 247–253.

Zastrow MS, Vlcek S, Wilson K (2004) Proteins that bind A-type lamins: integrating isolated clues. J Cell Sci 117: 979–987.

# NEONATAL PROGEROID SYNDROME (WIEDEMANN-RAUTENSTRAUCH SYNDROME)

## Introduction

Wiedemann-Rautenstrauch or neonatal progeroid syndrome is an autosomal recessive condition (OMIM # 264090) characterized by intrauterine growth retardation, short stature, typical facial appearance, natal teeth, lipoatrophy, and paradoxical caudal fat accumulation (Arboleda et al. 2007, Toriello 2006).

## Historical perspective and eponyms

The syndrome was described by Rautenstrauch and Snigula (1977) in two sisters with a progeria-like syndrome. Wiedemann (1979) reported two additional sibs and along with Devos et al. (1981) suggested the diagnostic term neonatal progeroid syndrome.

## Incidence and prevalence

Over twenty patients of neonatal progeroid syndrome have been described to date with similar prevalence in males and females (Korniszewski et al. 2001, Pivnick et al. 2000).

## Clinical manifestations

The neonatal progeroid syndrome is characterized by premature aging recognizable at birth. The main clinical features are intrauterine and postnatal growth failure, congenital facial appearance similar to that seen in older children with progeria, generalized lipoatrophy with specific fat accumulation in the suprabuttock region, hypotrichosis, mental retardation, macrocephaly, and natal teeth. Although the triad of intrauterine growth retardation, progeroid appearance and absence of subcutaneous fat is quite specific for this disorder, variability in the phenotype is clear and the faces of patients show different appearances. Macropenis has been reported in three patients (Pivnick et al. 2000, Wiedemann 1979), and cryptorchidism in six (Arboleda et al. 1997, Pivnick et al. 2000, Rudin et al. 1988). Psychomotor retardation is another variable manifestation of this syndrome: patients may have marked, mild or absent psychomotor delay (Pivnick et al. 2000). Feeding difficulties are common. Large hands (Fig. 4) and feet or radiological abnormalities are observed in 50% of patients (Rudin et al. 1988), and less frequently are

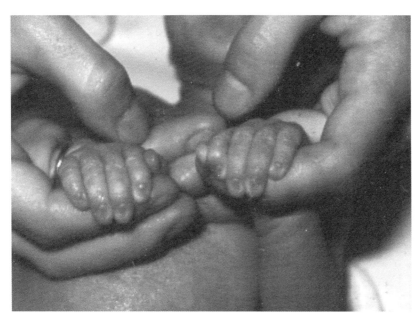

Fig. 4. Neonatal progeroid syndrome in an infant of 1 month of age who shows big fingers with small nails.

seen CNS, endocrine, and cardiovascular anomalies, vesicoureteral reflux, camptodactyly, laryngomalacia, and "sclerodermatous" skin.

## Natural history

Premature aging suggests premature cell senescence (Korniszewski et al. 2001). The life expectancy of patients with neonatal progeroid syndrome is about 7 months (Pivnick et al. 2000), although a few patients have survived the first decade (Rautenstrauch et al. 1994, Wiedemann 1979). An adolescent described by Korniszewski et al. (2001) was still alive at 16 years and 10 months. Mágarbané and Loiselet (1997) reported two sisters who survived less than 6 months.

## Pathology

Neuropathological findings in a patient who died at $5^1/_2$ years of age (Martin et al. 1984) and who had been previously reported by Devos et al. (1981), included generalized demyelination of the white matter in the central nervous system (CNS) with an accumulation of neutral fats in macrophages that are considered histological characteristics of the sudanophilic leukodystrophies type Pelizaeus-Merzbacher disease and variants. Martin et al. (1984), however, noticed significant differences between the neuropathological characteristics observed in her patient from those of previously described patients with sudanophilic leukodystrophy. Ulrich et al. (1995) noted significant demyelination of the white matter, but no sudanophilic changes. Hagadorn et al. (1990) did not find demyelination or any other anatomical or histological anomaly in a patient who died at $3^1/_2$ months of age.

## Molecular genetics and pathogenesis

Wiedemann-Rautenstrauch is an autosomal recessive condition. The pathogenesis of this disease is unknown. To date, the diagnosis is based on clinical findings. Beavan et al. (1993) described deficient decorin expression in one affected patient originally reported by Rautenstrauch and Snigula (1977): however, decorin expression returned to normal levels in adolescence in that patient.

Telomeres length have been related with other types of progeria such as Hutchinson–Gilford progeria (Allsopp 1992), but not in Werner syndrome (Matsui et al. 2000). Telomeres are specialized repetitive structures located at the ends of eukaryotic chromosomes. They play a role in the organization of the architecture of the nucleus (Blackburn 1994) and protect the chromosome ends from aberrant recombination, degradation, and fusion (Zakian 1995). The telomeric DNA is shortened every time the cells divide (Allsopp et al. 1992). The association of the progressive loss of telomeric DNA and cellular senescence is not clear despite it was found the replicative lifespan of normal cells in vitro (Bodnar et al. 1998). The only one patient with Wiedemann-Rautenstrauch in whom the length of telomere was investigated did not show shortening of fibroblasts as compared to that of normal fibroblasts (Korniszewski et al. 2001).

## Differential diagnosis

Differential diagnosis of neonatal progeroid syndrome includes other progeroid syndromes with precocious presence of the symptoms such as leprechaunism, Hallermann–Streiff syndrome, De Barsy syndrome, Berardinelli–Seip syndrome, carbohydrate deficient glycoprotein (CDG) syndrome type 1, Cockayne syndrome and Hutchinson–Gilford syndrome. Most of these entities have autosomal recessive inheritance.

Clinical features and biochemical changes that characterize some of the mentioned syndromes may facilitate the diagnosis. Cockayne syndrome is a mitochondrial disease, carbohydrate deficient glycoprotein (CDG) syndrome type 1 or Norman–Jaeken syndrome (Pascual-Castroviejo 2002) does not show aging appearance too early and have particular defined image, with severe premature cerebellar atrophy associated to primary granular cell layer of the cerebellum (Norman 1940), and characteristic biochemical findings that consist on increased serum transferrin and deficiency of phosphomannomutase (PMM) caused by a mutation in the chromosome 16p13 (Jaeken et al. 1997). De Barsy syndrome manifests clinical features at first to second year of life, with frontal losing in the young child, and later with microcephaly, short stature, narrow face with prominent nose and thin lips, corneal clouding or cataracts, abundant scalp hair, cutis laxa with atrophic skin and reduced subcutaneous fat, and most often with delay mental development. Berardinelli–Seip syndrome stars the clinical manifestations at birth or shortly after, with large hands and feet, tall stature at first, but later is normal, accelerated dentition and ossification, scalp hair abundant and curly, coarse and dry skin, and acanthosis nigricans, punctate corneal opacities, pinched face with absent bucal pad of fat, and most often mental retardation.

## Management

Treatment is symptomatic.

## References

Allsopp RC, Varizi H, Patterson C, Goldstein S, Younglai EV, Futcher AB, Greider CW, Harley CB (1992) Telomere length predicts replicative capacity of human fibroblasts. Proc Natl Acad Sci USA 89: 10114–10118.

Arboleda G, Ramírez N, Arboleda H (2007) The neonatal progeroid syndrome (Wiedemann-Rautenstrauch): a model for the study of human aging? Exp Gerontol 42: 939–943.

Arboleda H, Quintero L, Yunis E (1997) Wiedemann-Rautenstrauch neonatal progeroid syndrome: report of three new patients. J Med Genet 34: 433–437.

Beavan LA, Quentin-Hoffman E, Schonherr E, Snigula F, Leroy JG, Kresse H (1993) Deficient expression of decorin in infantile progeroid patients. J Biol Chem 268: 9856–9862.

Blackburn EH (1994) Telomeres: no end in sight. Cell 77: 621–623.

Bodnar AG, Quelletce M, Frolkis M, Holt SE, Chiu CP, Morin GB, Harley CB, Shay JW, Lichtsteiner S, Wright WE (1998) Extension of lifespan by introduction of telomerase into normal human cells. Science 279: 349–352.

Devos EA, Leroy JG, Frijns JP, Van den Berghe H (1981) The Wiedemann-Rautenstrauch or neonatal progeroid syndrome. Report of a patient with consanguineous parents. Eur J Pediatr 136: 245–248.

Hagadorn JI, Wilson WG, Hogge A, Callicott JH, Veale EF (1990) Neonatal progeroid syndrome: more than one disease? Am J Med Genet 35: 91–94.

Jaeken J, Matthijs G, Barone R, Carchon H (1997) Carbohydrate deficit glycoprotein (CDG) syndrome type 1. J Med Genet 34: 73–76.

Korniszewski L, Nowak R, Okninska-Hoffmann E, Skórka A, Gieruszczak-Bialek D, Sawadro-Rochowska M (2001) Wiedemann-Rautenstrauch (neonatal progeroid) syndrome: new case with normal telomere length in skin fibroblasts. Am J Med Genet 103: 144–148.

Mágarbané A, Loiselet J (1997) Clinical manifestation of a severe neonatal progeroid syndrome. Clin Genet 51: 200–204.

Martin JJ, Ceuterick CM, Leroy JG, Devos EA, Roelens JG (1984) The Wiedemann-Rautenstrauch or neonatal progeroid syndrome: neuropathological study of a case. Neuropediatrics 15: 43–48.

Matsui M, Misayaka J, Hamada K, Ogawa Y, Hiramoto M, Fujimori R, Aioi A (2000) Influence of aging and cell senescence on telomere activity in keratocytes. J Dermatol Sci 22: 80–87.

Norman RM (1940) Primary degeneration of the granular layer of the cerebellum: an unusual form of familial cerebellar atrophy occurring in early life. Brain 63: 365–279.

Pascual-Castroviejo I (2002) Congenital disorders of glycosylation syndromes. Dev Med Child Neurol 44: 357–358.

Pivnick EK, Angle B, Kaufman RA, Hall BD, Pitukcheewanont P, Hersh JH, Fowlkes JL, Sanders LP, O'Brien JM, Carroll GS, Gunther WM, Morrow HG, Burghen GA, Ward JC (2000) Neonatal progeroid (Wiedemann-Rautenstrauch) syndrome: report of five new cases and review. Am J Med Genet 90: 131–140.

Rautenstrauch T, Snigula F (1977) Progeria: a cell culture and clinical report of familial incidence. Eur J Pediatr 124: 101–111.

Rautenstrauch T, Snigula F, Wiedemann HR (1994) Neonatales progeroides syndrom (Wiedemann-Rautenstrauch). Eine follow-up-Studie. Klin Pediatr 206: 440–446.

Rudin C, Thommen L, Fliegel C, Steinmann B, Bühler U (1988) The neonatal pseudo-hydrocephalic progeroid syndrome (Wiedemann-Rautenstrauch): report of a new patient and review of the literature. Eur J Pediatr 147: 433–438.

Toriello HV (2006) Premature ageing syndromes. In: Harper J, Oranje A, Prose N (eds.) Textbook of Pediatric Dermatology. 2nd ed. Oxford: Blackwell Science, pp. 1538–1556.

Ulrich J, Rudin C, Bull R, Riederer BM (1995) The neonatal progeroid syndrome (Wiedemann-Rautenstrauch) and its relationship to Pelizaeus-Merzbacher's disease. Neuropathol Appl Neurobiol 21: 116–120.

Wiedemann HR (1979) An unidentified neonatal progeroid syndrome: follow-up report. Eur J Pediatr 130: 65–70.

Zakian VA (1995) Telomeres: beginning to understand the end. Science 270: 1601–1607.

# WERNER SYNDROME

## Introduction

Werner's syndrome is a rare autosomal recessively inherited disorder that is considered a segmental progeroid syndrome and is perhaps the most complete example of premature ageing syndrome. It is characterized by the combination of short stature, sclerodermatous skin, hypogonadism, proneness to diabetes, increased incidence of malignancy and early-onset graying, baldness, cataracts, atherosclerosis and osteoporosis (Toriello 2006).

## Historical perspective and eponyms

In 1904, Werner described this disease in his doctoral thesis in which he reported four siblings (brothers and sisters) who had cataract associated with scleroderma, small stature, premature ageing of the face, juvenile gray hair, and genital hypoplasia. Oppenheimer and Kugel cugned the name of "Werner's syndrome" (WS) in two reviews of this syndrome that they published in 1934 and 1941. In the paper of 1941, they also included the presence of a report of endocrine abnormalities such as osteoporosis and hyperglycemia, and a report of the first postmortem examination of a patient. A few years later Tannhauser (1945) reporting five new cases, considered the WS as the progeria of adults, and differentiated two types of progeria in adults, the Werner's and the Rothmund 'syndromes, closely related and heredofamilial, which exhibited overlapping clinical features. He provided a list of 12 major characteristics including premature senility and the possibility to occur in brothers and sisters.

## Incidence and prevalence

WS is considered a rare disorder. The incidence seems higher in Japan than in the rest of the world (about 1000 of the around 1300 patients reported worldwide are Japanese) (Yamamoto et al. 2003). However, Goto et al. (1981) reported 1 in 330.000 individuals in the Japanese population, while Piras et al. (2003) described a prevalence of 1 in 72.800 in Sardinia (Italy), explaining the high prevalence there by the consanguineous marriages, due to geographical (an island) and/or geopolitical motivations.

## Clinical manifestations

WS is regarded as a representative model disease of early senility in humans.

Symptoms rarely appear before puberty, but thereafter aging signs are evident. The most characteristics are short stature, gray hair or alopecia, cataracts, skin and subcutaneous atrophy with senile spots. Thin arms and legs, soft tissue calcification, bird-like face, refractory skin ulceration, eyelid senile retraction, or senile deformation of fingers (Fig. 5) and scleroderma-like skin changes (Fig. 6). Aging pathology diseases affect any or all organs of the body causing hypogonadism, arteriosclerotic diseases (myocardial and cerebral infarction), diabetes mellitus with hyperinsulinemia, hyperuricemia and osteoporosis from the age of 30 years, or even before. Irwing and Ward (1953) identified a total of 17 features associated with WS. Malnutrition is often seen in patients with WS (Furuhata et al. 1998)

The most severe complications of WS are malignant tumors and arteriosclerosis. The frequency of malignant tumors ranges from 5.6 to 25%, being the Japanese series which describe highest prevalence, 20.7% (85 of 411 reported patients with WS) and the highest mortality, 25 individuals (6.1%), which is considerably higher than that of the Japanese general population (0.3%) (Goto 1997, Yamamoto et al. 2003). Mesenchymal sarcoma and epithelial cancer are the most frequent tumors observed in patients with WS, with approximately the same incidence (for the general population, epithelial cancer has an

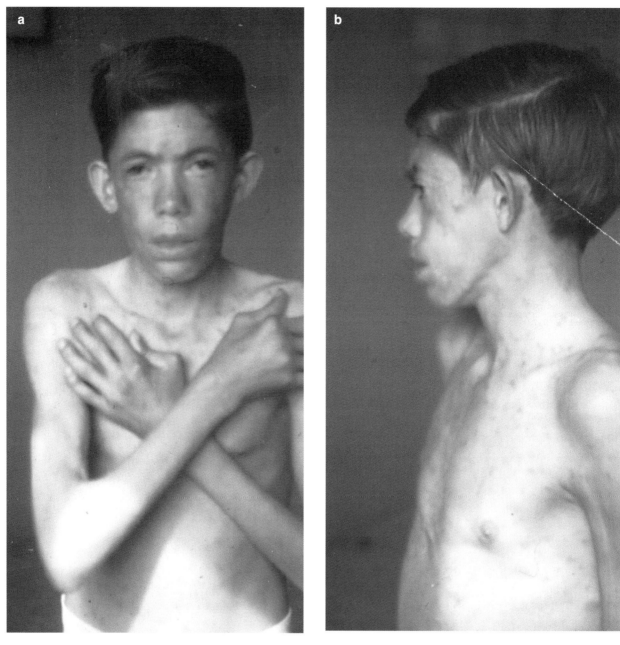

**Fig. 5.** (**a**, **b**) The frontal and lateral views of a patients of 21 years of age with Werner's syndrome who shows all signs of precocious senility manifested in skin, hands, face and eyes.

incidence rate 10 times that of mesenchymal sarcoma) (Yamamoto et al. 2003). Other tumors associated with WS are thyroid cancer, malignant melanoma, osteosarcoma, and soft tissue sarcoma. Immunological abnormalities, such as decrease in natural killer cell activities or a decrease in T-cell

subpopulations, have been associated with malignant tumor development (Goto et al. 1979), as well as DNA abnormalities (Fujiwara et al. 1977).

The second cause of dead is cardiac failure with or without myocardial infarction, but this complication occurs three times less frequent than the

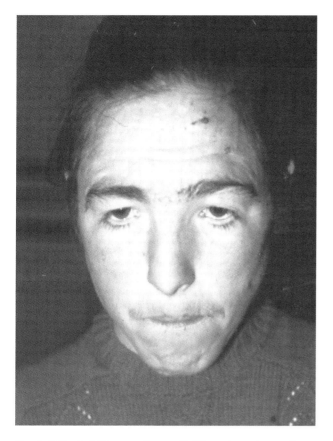

**Fig. 6.** Patient of 28 years of age with Werner's syndrome shows forehead and eyes signs of senility.

common carotid arteries, sensory and motor peripheral neuropathy, myelopathy. WS, however, may be under-recognized (Anderson and Haas 2003). Some of neurological complications are secondary to premature cerebro-vascular disease, but the pathogenesis of peripheral neuropathy and myelopathy in patients with WS is uncertain.

## Imaging

Imaging studies – conventional $T_1$ and $T_2$ -weighted MR images – do not reveal abnormalities on visual inspection. However, MR spectroscopic imaging (MRSI) and magnetization transfer (MT) may show abnormalities in these patients. They may disclose significantly lower values of normalized total brain volume and MT ratio in the white matter than age-matched normal controls. Also, proton MRSI show significantly lower values of central brain NAA/Cr in WS patients than in normal controls (De Stefano et al. 2003).

Death on average occurs at 46 years of age, due to atherosclerosis – related events or neoplasia (Goto 1987, 1997; Yamamoto et al. 2003).

malignant tumors (Yamamoto et al. 2003). Other causes are pneumonia, respiratory failure, disseminated intravascular coagulation, hepatic and renal failure, and cerebrovascular disorder. Refractory ulceration and osteomyelitis affect most frequently the extremities, with the most common site the periphery of the lower extremities. The causes of refractory ulceration may include disorders of the vasculature, such as arteriosclerotic changes in the blood vessels and decreased in local blood flow, extrinsic stimulation of the atrophic skin, and complications of generalized metabolic disorders such as diabetes mellitus.

Neurological complications are usually regarded as uncommon, but 10% of the patients manifest signs of CNS, such as epilepsy, mental retardation and schizophrenia (Goto 1997), as well as transient ischemic attacks secondary to atherosclerosis in the

## Molecular genetics and pathogenesis

WS is an autosomal recessive inherited disease. The WS locus (known as WRN) was initially located to 8p12 (Goto et al. 1992) by linkage analysis. Initial mapping placed WRN in an 8.3 centimorgan (cM) internal flanked by markers D8S137 and D8S87; D8S 339, located within this interval, was the closest marker. Subsequently, short tandem repeat polymorphism (STRP) markers at the glutathione reductase (GsR) gene and D8S 339 were shown to be in linkage disequilibrium with WS in Japanese WS patients (Yu et al. 1994), indicating that these markers are most likely close to WRN. Goddard et al. (1996) identified 18 STRP markers; probable recombinants were detected at D8S2194 (which excluded the region telomeric to this marker) and at D8S2186 (which excluded the region centromeric to this marker), making the 1.2–1.4 Mb interval from D8S2194 to D8S2186 the minimal WRN region. The predicted protein is 1432 amino acids in length and shows significant similarity to DNA helicases (Yu et al. 1996). Chen et al. (2003) reported 26 patients with wildtype WRN coding regions and were therefore categorized as cases of "atypical Werner syndrome". All of the exons of the Lamin A/C gene (LMNA) from these individuals were sequenced. The authors noted in four patients heterozygosity for novel missense mutations in LMNA, specifically A57P, R133L (in two patients) and L140R. The mutations altered relatively conserved residues within lamin A/C. Individuals with atypical Werner'syndrome with mutations in LMNA had a more severe phenotype than did those with the disorder due to mutant WRN, indicating that Werner'syndrome is molecularly by heterogeneous. LMNA mutations seem associate with various diseases and not only with WS. The specific aminoacid substitution of arginine at position 527 of lamin A/C is of particular interest, since the substitutions reported – R527P, R527H, and R 527C-result in Emery-Dreifuss muscular dystrophy (EDMD), mandibulo-acral dysplasia, and Hutchinson–Gilford progeria syndrome (HGPS), respectively (Vigouroux et al. 2003, Cao and Hegle 2003). Why mutations in LMNA result in such a wide range of apparently distinct phenotypes is unknown, However, the identification of overlapping lamin-associated disorders indicates that they represent a functional continuum of related disorders rather than separate diseases (Bonne and Levy 2003). WRN has helicase and exonuclease activities. Regulation of exonucleotic activity of WRN may be disturbed by interaction of some proteins, such as Ku 70, Ku 80 and poly (ADP-ribose) polymerase-1 (PARP-1), a 113 kDa enzyme that functions as a sensor of DNA damage (Li et al. 2004, Yu et al. 1996). WRN helicase is expressed in neurons and other cell types in the CNS. The protein participates in recombinational repair of stalled replication forms of DNA breaks, but the precise functions of this protein that prevents rapid aging is unknown. Experimentally, it has been observed in mice with enhanced telomere dysfunction, including end-to-end chromosome fusions and greater loss of telomere repeat DNA, which showed WS clinical features. These findings may indicate that telomere dysfunction may contribute to the pathogenesis of WS (Chang et al. 2004, Du et al. 2004). However, this findings need to be confirmed in humans with WS.

## Management

Tumor treatment in patients with WS is not different as in patients without WS. Surgery, chemotherapy, radiotherapy, blood transfusions may be applied in accordance with the type and the location of the tumor.

Patients with ulcer receive only conservative treatment, and those refractory receive conservative combined with surgical treatments other than amputation or with amputation in some cases, most often of one or both lower limbs. Hyperbaric oxygen therapy has been successfully applied to refractory ulceration associated with WS (Yamamoto et al. 2003). The mechanism of action of hyperbaric oxygen for ulceration involves resolution of local hypoxia due to physically elevated solubility of oxygen and promotion of the formation of fresh granulation tissue. Orthopedists must treated the patients in accordance to the particular conditions of their lesions. One common feature of WS is diabetes mellitus associated to insulin resistance, but the mechanism by which insulin resistance occurs in this syndrome is unknown. Administration of pioglitazone, a thiazolidinedione derivative, improved insulin sensitivity, glucose tolerance, lipid metabolism, and abdominal fat distribution in one patient with WS (Yokote et al. 2004).

Early detection of patients in WS families affords the opportunity for prevention of amelioration of complications, and to clarify the pathogenesis of the syndrome.

## References

Anderson NE, Haas LF (2003) Neurological complications of Werner's syndrome. J Neurol 250: 1174–1178.
Bonne G, Levy N (2003) LMNA mutations in atypical Werner's syndrome. Lancet 362: 1585–1586.

Cao H, Hegele R (2003) LMNA is mutated in Hutchinson–Gilford progeria (MIM176670) but not in Wiedemann-Rautenstrauch progeroid syndrome (MIM264090). J Hum Genet 48: 271–274.

Chang S, Multani AS, Cabrera NG, Naylor ML, Land P, Lombard D, Pathak S, Guarente L, DePinho RA (2004) Essential role of limiting telomeres in the pathogenesis of Werner syndrome. Nat Genet 36: 877–882.

Chen L, Lee L, Kudlow BA, Dos Santos HG, Sletvold O, Shafeghati Y, Botha EG, Garg A, Hanson NB, Martin GM, Mian IS, Kennedy BK, Oshima J (2003) LMNA mutations in atypical Werner's syndrome. Lancet 362: 440–445.

De Stefano N, Dotti MT, Battisti C, Sicurelli F, Stromillo ML, Mortilla M, Federico A (2003) MR evidence of structural and metabolic changes in brain of patients with Werner's syndrome. J Neurol 250: 1169–1173.

Du X, Shen J, Kugan N, Furth EE, Lombard DB, Cheung C, Pak S, Luo G, Pignolo RJ, DePinho RA, Guarente L, Johnson FB (2004) Telomere shortening exposes functions for the mouse Werner and Bloom syndrome genes. Mol Cell Biol 24: 8437–8446.

Fujiwara Y, Higashikawa T, Tatsumi M (1977) A retarded rate of DNA replication and normal level of DNA repair in Werner's syndrome fibroblasts in culture. J Cell Physiol 92: 365–374.

Furuhata T, Hirata K, Kimura Y, Yanai Y (1998) Werner's syndrome malnutrition (in Japanase). Surg Frontier 5: 71–73.

Goddard KAB, Yu CE, Oshima J, Miki T, Nakura J, Piussan C, Martin GM, Schellenberg GD, Wijsman EM (1996) Toward localization of the Werner syndrome gene by linkage disequilibrium and ancestral haplotyping: lessons learned from analysis of 35 chromosome 8p11.1-21.1 markers. Am J Hum Genet 58: 1286–1302.

Goto M, Horiuchi Y, Okumura K, Tada T, Kawata M, Ohmorit K (1979) Immunological annormalities of aging: an analysis of T Lymphocyte subpopulations of Werner's syndrome. J Clin Invest 64: 695–699.

Goto M, Tanimoto K, Horiuchi Y, Sasazuki T (1981) Family analysis of Werner's syndrome: a survey of 42 Japanese families with a review of the literature. Clin Genet 19: 8–15.

Goto M (1987) Werner's syndrome. In: Gomez MR (ed.): Neurocutaneous diseases. A practical approach. Stoneham: Butterworths, pp. 241–246.

Goto M, Rubenstein M, Weber J, Woods K, Drayna D (1992) Genetic linkage to Werner's syndrome to five markers on chromosome 8. Nature 355: 735–738.

Goto M (1997) Hierarchical deterioration of body systems in Werner's implication for normal ageing. Mech Ageing Dev 98: 239–254.

Irwing GW, Ward PB (1953) Werner's syndrome. With a report of two cases. Am J Med 15: 266–271.

Li B, Navarro S, Kasahara N, Comae L (2004) Identification and biochemical characterization of a Werner's syndrome protein complex with ku 70/80 and poly (ADP-ribose polymerase-1). J Biol Chem 279: 13659–13667.

Oppenheimer BS, Kugel VH (1934) Werner's syndrome – a heredofamilial disorder with scleroderma, bilateral cataract, precocious graying of hair, and endocrine stigmatisation. Trans Assoc Am Physicians 49: 358–370.

Oppenheimer BS, Kugel VH (1941) Werner's syndrome: report of the first necropsy and of findings in a new case. Am J Med Sci 202: 629–642.

Piras D, Cottoni F, Cerimele D (2003) Prevalence of Werner's syndrome in northern Sardinia: a new case. J Eur Acad Dermatol Venereal 17: 248–249.

Tannhauser SJ (1945) Werner's syndrome (progeria of the adult) and Rothmund síndrome: two types of closely related heredofamilial atrophia dermatoses with juvenile cataracts and endocrine features: a critical study with five new cases. Ann Intern Med 23: 559–626.

Toriello HV (2006) Premature ageing syndromes. In: Harper J, Oranje A, Prose N (eds.) Textbook of Pediatric Dermatology. 2nd ed. Oxford: Blackwell Science, pp. 1538–1556.

Vigouroux C, Caux F, Capeau J, Christin-Maitre S, Cohen A (2003) LMNA mutations in atypical Werner's syndrome. Lancet 362: 1585.

Werner CWO (1904) Über Kataract in Verbindung mit Skleroderme. Inaugural dissertation. Kiel. Schmidt und Klauning.

Yamamoto K, Imakiire A, Miyagawa N, Kasahara T (2003) A report of two cases of Werner's syndrome and review of the literature. J Orthop Surg 11: 224–233.

Yokote K, Honjo S, Kobayashi K, Fujimoto M, Kawamura H, Mori S, Saito Y (2004) Metabolic improvement and abdominal fat redistribution in Werner syndrome by pioglitazone. J Am Geriatr Soc 52: 1582–1583.

Yu CE, Oshima J, Goddard KAB, Mili T, Nakura J, Ogihara T, Poot M, Hoehn H, Fraccaro M, Piussan C, et al. (1994) Linkage disequilibrium and haplotype studies of chromosome 8p11.1-21.1 markers and Werner syndrome. Am J Hum Genet 55: 356–364.

Yu CE, Oshima J, Fu YH, Wijsman EM, Hishama F, Alisch R, Matthews S, Nakura J, Miki T, Ouais S, Martin GM, Mulligan J, Schellenberg GD (1996) Positional cloning of the Werner's syndrome gene. Science 272: 258–262.

# ROTHMUND–THOMSON SYNDROME

## Introduction

Rothmund–Thomson syndrome (RTS) (OMIM # 268400) is a rare autosomal recessive disorder whose phenotype includes early childhood onset poikiloderma, photosensitivity, with occasional occurrence of cataracts and skeletal anomalies. An increased risk of malignancy is an additional manifestation (Toriello 2006). RTS is caused by mutations in the RecQL4 gene located on chromosome 8 (Kitao et al. 1999; Lindor et al. 2000; Wang et al. 2000, 2002).

## Historical perspective and eponyms

RTS was first described in 1868 by the German ophthalmologist Auguste Rothmund in inbred family members who had a peculiar rash and bilateral juvenile cataracts (Rothmund 1868). The British dermatologist Sydney Thomson (1923) coined the term "poikiloderma congenitale" for patients with a similar rash and skeletal anomalies, but no cataracts. Taylor (1957) suggested that the two disorders were the same and proposed the combined eponym Rothmund–Thomson syndrome.

## Incidence and prevalence

RTS is a very rare entity and the prevalence is very low.

## Clinical manifestations

RTS is characterized by growth deficiency, photosensitivity with poikilodermatous skin changes, graying and hair loss, cataracts, and a predisposition to malignancy, especially osteogenic sarcoma.

The sun-sensitive rash usually starts between 3 and 6 months, but may appear soon after birth or as late as 2 years. The acute phase manifests as erythema, swelling, and blistering on the cheeks and face and spreads to the buttocks and flexure areas of limbs, sparing the abdomen, chest, and back. Over months to years, the rash gradually enters a chronic phase with reticulated pigmentation, telangiectases, and areas of punctate dermal atrophy (collectively known as poikiloderma) that persist throughout life (Fig. 7) (Wang et al. 2001). Additionally, patients with RTS may have sparse or absent hair, eyelashes, and/or eyebrows, abnormal nails and dentition, small stature of unknown etiology, absent or malformed bones, delayed bone formation, skeletal dysplasias, and osteoporosis. Patients with RTS have an increased risk of juvenile bilateral cataracts, and a prevalence of 50% has been reported (Vennos et al. 1992). Infertility has been reported in both male and female patients, but patients who had normal pregnancies have been also reported. Intelligence and immunologic function appear to be normal (Vennos and James 1995). Patients with RST show a high risk of bone cancer, specifically osteosarcoma, which has been observed in at least 20 individuals (Pujol et al. 2000). Common sites for osteosarcoma are in the tibia, femur, humerus, fibula, and radius. Tumors developed by RTS patients are mostly mesenchymal and are not associated with juvenile cataracts, which suggests that these two patients populations may be distinct. Diagnosis of osteosarcoma may be suspicious of RTS, particularly if associated with skin changes.

The most common cutaneous malignancies associated with RTS include squamous cell carcinoma, basal cell carcinoma, spindle cell carcinoma, and Bowen's disease. Skin lesion malignancies are most frequently a product of sun hypersensitivity and abnormal or reduced DNA repair capability (Shinya et al. 1993). Moreover, some cytogenetic studies provide evidence of chromosomal instability, such as acquired in vivo mosaicism (Lindor et al. 1996) and increased chromosomal radiosensitivity (Kerr et al. 1996).

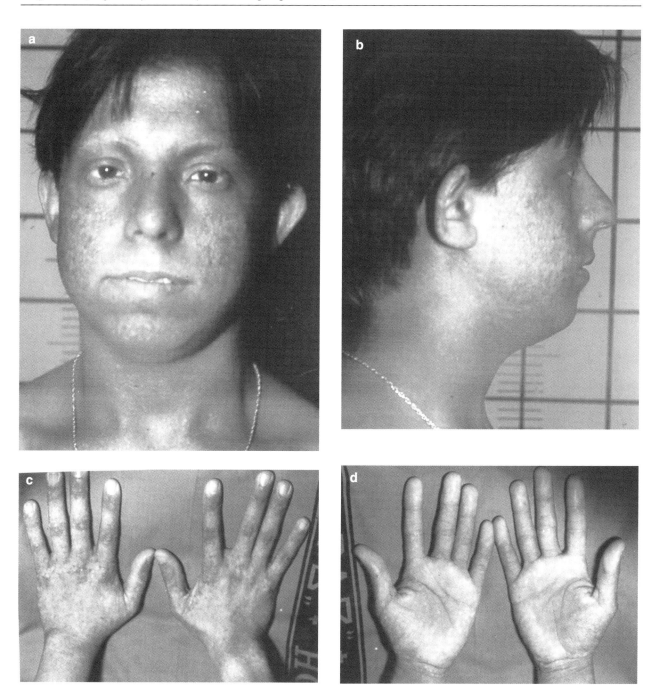

**Fig. 7.** (**a–d**) Chronic phase of the cutaneous lesions that affect face and hands in a RTS patient of 15 years of age (Courtesy of Dr. P. Lapunzina).

Linear growth is abnormal in at least two-thirds of RTS patients and when present short stature usually is moderate to severe (Lindor et al. 1996). However, most patients with the characteristic short stature of RTS have normal growth hormone levels. Provocation testing may be necessary to demonstrate growth hormone deficiency in some patients (Kaufmann et al. 1986, Lapunzina et al. 1995, Pujol et al. 2000).

## Molecular genetics and pathogenesis

RTS is an autosomal recessive disorder caused by mutations in the RecQL4 gene on chromosome 8 (Kitao et al. 1999; Lindor et al. 2000; Wang et al. 2000, 2002). The RecQL4 structure is unusual because it contains many small introns <100 bp Contraint on intron size may represent a general mutational mechanism, since human genome analysis reveals that about 15% of genes have introns, 100 bp and are therefore susceptible to size constraint. Thus, monitoring of intron size may allow detection of mutations missed by exon-by-exon approaches (Wang et al. 2002).

## Differential diagnosis

Most progeroid syndromes overlap some clinical features, although particular conditions most often permit to know the identity of the syndromes. Candidate disease to differentiate from RTS are Werner's syndrome, Bloom syndrome – both entities associated with helicase gene abnormalities as RTS – Hutchinson–Gilford progeria, Wiedemann-Rautenstrauch syndrome, Kindler syndrome (MIM 173650) or acrokeratotic poikiloderma, which is a rare genodermatosis characterized by acral bullae and photosensitivity, with additional features such as ophthalmic and skeletal abnormalities in some patients (Sharma et al. 2003), and mandibulo-acral dysplasia syndrome.

## Management

The treatment consist in avoidance of sun exposure and use of sunscreens with both UVA and UVB protection (Wang et al. 2001). Use of pulsed dye laser to treat the telangiectatic component of the rash has been reported (Potozkin and Geronemus 1991). Screening for cataracts by ophthalmologists is recommended at least annually lifelong, and surgical treatment in cataracts are discovered. Skeletal radiographs of long bones by age 5 years for all patients with RTS are recommend (Wang et al. 2001). Since patients often have underlying skeletal dysplasias. Obviously,

radiological study is necessary in patients who show clinical suspicion of pathologic features anywhere of the body. It is unclear whether RTS patients are more sensitive to the effects of chemotherapy and radiation.

Little increase in growth velocity on growth hormone replacement therapy is observed in most patients (Kaufmann et al. 1986, Lapunzina et al. 1995, Pujol et al. 2000), but good response has been seldom reported (Kerr et al. 1996).

## References

Kaufmann S, Jones M, Culler FL, Jones KL (1986) Growth hormone deficiency in the Rothmund–Thomson syndrome. Am J Med Genet 23: 861–868.

Kerr B, Ashcroft GS, Scott D, Horan MA, Ferguson MVJ, Donnai D (1996) Rothmund–Thomson syndrome: two case reports show heterogeneous cutaneous abnormalities, an association with genetically programmed aging changes, and increased chromosomal radiosensitivity. J Med Genet 33: 928–934.

Kitao S, Shimamoto A, Goto M, Miller RW, Smithson WA, Lindor NM, Furuichi Y (1999) Mutations in RECQL4 cause a subset of cases of Rothmund–Thomson syndrome. Nat Genet 22: 82–84.

Lapunzina P, Fonseca E, Gracia R, Delicado A (1995) Rothmund–Thomson syndrome and Addison disease. Pediatr Dermatol 12: 164–169.

Lindor NM, Devries EMG, Michels VV, Schad CR, Jalal SM, Donovan KM, Smithson WA, Kvols LK, Thibodeau SN, Dewald GW (1996) Rothmund–Thomson syndrome in siblings: evidence for acquired in vivo mosaicism. Clin Genet 49: 124–129.

Lindor NM, Furmichi Y, Kitao S, Shimamoto A, Arndt C, Jalal S (2000) Rothmund–Thomson syndrome due to RECQ4 helicase mutations: report and clinical and molecular comparisons with Bloom syndrome and Werner syndrome. Am J Med Genet 90: 223–228.

Potozkin JR, Geronemus RG (1991) Treatment of the poikilodermatous component of the Rothmund–Thomson syndrome with the flash lamppumped pulsed dye laser: a case report. Pediatr Dermatol 8: 162–165.

Pujol LA, Erickson RP, Heidenreich RA, Cunniff C (2000) Variable presentation of Rothmund–Thomson syndrome. Am J Med Genet 95: 204–207.

Rothmund A (1868) Ueber cataracten in vervindung mit einer eigenthemlichen hautdegeneration. Albrecht von Graefes Arch Fur Ophth 14: 159–182.

Sharma RC, Mahajan V, Sharma NL, Sharma AK (2003) Kindler syndrome. Int J Dermatol 42: 727–732.

Shinya A, Nishigori C, Miriwaki S, Takebe H, Kubota M, Ogino A, Imamura S (1993) A case of Rothmund–Thomson syndrome with reduced DNA repair capacity. Arch Dermatol 129: 332–336.

Taylor WB (1957) Rothmund's syndrome–Thomson's syndrome. Arch Dermatol 75: 236–244.

Thomson MS (1923) An hitherto undescribed familial disease. Br J Dermatol Syphilis 35: 455–462.

Toriello HV (2006) Premature ageing syndromes. In: Harper J, Oranje A, Prose N (eds.) Textbook of Pediatric Dermatology. 2nd ed. Oxford: Blackwell Science, pp. 1538–1556.

Vennos EM, Collins M, James WD (1992) Rothmund–Thomson syndrome: review of the world literature. J Am Acad Dermatol 27: 750–762.

Vennos EM, Janes WD (1995) Rothmund–Thomson syndrome. Dermatol Clin 13: 143–150.

Wang LL, Levy ML, Lewis RA, Gannavarapu A, Stockton D, Lev D (2000) Evidence for heterogeneity in Rothmund–Thomson syndrome. Am J Hum Genet 67 (Suppl 2): 376.

Wang LL, Levy ML, Lewis RA, Chintagumpala MM, Lev D, Rogers M, Rogers M, Plon SE (2001) Clinical manifestations in cohort of 41 Rothmund–Thomson syndrome patients. Am J Med Genet 102: 11–17.

Wang LL, Worley K, Gannavarapu A, Chintagumpala MM, Levy M, Plon SE (2002) Intron-size constraint as a mutational mechanism in Rothmund–Thomson syndrome. Am J Hum Genet 71: 165–167.

# BLOOM SYNDROME

## Introduction

Bloom syndrome (BS) (OMIM # 10900) is an autosomal recessive disorder characterized by growth deficiency of prenatal onset, variable degrees of immunodeficiency, and predisposition to cancers of many sites and types (German 1995). BS is caused by a mutation in the gene BLM, RECQ2 (Ellis et al. 1995). The protein encoded by BLM and lacking in BS, has DNA helicase activity (Karow et al. 1997).

## Historical perspective

The syndrome was first described in 1954 by Bloom (Bloom 1954).

## Incidence and prevalence

The Bloom's Syndrome Registry recorded from the mid-1960s to 1987 (German and Passarge 1989) 130 persons with BS.

## Clinical manifestations

Growth delay is the most characteristic clinical feature of patients with BS and most often is the first symptom of the disorder.

Other associated features, such as characteristic facies, facial telangiectasia, small testicular size, and immunodeficiency, are not present or recognizable at birth. Longitudinal growth data from 148 patients (Keller et al. 1999) showed a discrete prevalence of BS in males and confirmed that growth deficiency has a prenatal onset and persists throughout life. Growth continues by at least 1 cm per year until age 21 years for both sexes. More than half of children with BS are significantly wasted until age 8 years, but this is not related to early death or underlying malignancy (Keller et al. 1999). However, the prevalence of wasting decreases progressively after age 8 years. The mean body-mass index for adults with BS after age 25 years is low normal. Weight-for-height at the normal levels or below the 5th percentile suggests that tissue and fat mass in patients with BS are at least partially dependent on the same factors as the normal population, such as dietary intake and dehydration by illness (Keller et al. 1999). Children with BS regularly show much less interest in eating, abnormal frequent vomiting and recurrent diarrhea during infancy and early childhood than unaffected children (German 1995, Keller et al. 1999). The most serious consequences of malnutrition may be developmental delay and subsequently restricted intellectual ability, although individuals with BS have been described to have average intelligence and some have completed college or obtained higher degrees (German 1995). Decreased cellular immunity may be especially disadvantageous to children with BS as it relates to tumor surveillance.

BS predisposes to leukemias and epithelial derived tumors (adenocarcinoma of breast and gastrointestinal tract).

From the 130 individuals with BS recopilated by The Bloom's Syndrome Registry, malignant neoplasms were detected in 57 and the mean age at diagnosis was 24.8 years (German and Passarge 1989). Early-onset drusen, that represent an age – related degenerative change in normal individuals, has been recently described in a patient with BS (Aslan et al. 2004).

## Molecular genetics and pathogenesis

The BS gene (BLM), located on chromosome 15q26.1, encodes a BLM Rec Q helicase homolog intranuclear protein (Kaneko and Kondo 2004, Lindor et al. 2000). The protein has 1417 aminoacids (Ellis et al. 1995). Protein expression is in thymus, testis, brain and heart. BLM plays an important role in the maintenance of genomic stability in somatic cells (Davis et al. 2004). In budding and fission yeasts, loss of RecQ elicase function confers sensitivity to inhibitors of DNA replication, such as hydroxyurea (H$^u$), by failure to execute normal cell cycle progression following recovery from such an S-phase arrest. RecQ helicases play a conserved role in recovery from perturbations in DNA replication following S-phase arrest and hence prevent subsequent genomic instability (Davies et al. 2004). The proteins participate in recombinational repair of stalled replication forks or DNA breaks, but the precise functions of the proteins that prevent rapid aging are unknown.

Experimental observations indicate that telomere shortening exposes functions for the mouse Werner and Bloom syndromes genes, but the importance in vivo of the proteins in telomere biology has not been investigated yet (Du et al. 2004).

## Differential diagnosis

Differential diagnosis may be made with most of the progeroid syndromes, but most of these diseases show particular characteristics. The clinical similarities are especially with Rothmund–Thomson syndrome and with neonatal progeroid syndrome due to the precocious presentation of the symptoms. Werner syndrome, Hutchinson–Gilford syndrome, Cockayne syndrome and others have a later onset. These entities also have genetic differences (Lindor et al. 2000). BS is due to mutations in RecQ2 helicase (Ellis et al. 1995), while Werner syndrome is caused by mutations in RecQ3 (Yu et al. 1996), and Rothmund–Thomson syndrome is due to mutations in RecQ4 helicase (Kitao et al. 1999).

## Management

The main complication of BS is the presence of tumors, particularly leukemia. Treatment is symptomatic. Decreased cellular immunity may be related to tumor surveillance and would be at least one theoretical reason for nutritional intervention in patients with BS.

Localization of cancer susceptibility genes by genome-wide single-nucleotide polymorphism linkage-disequilibrium mapping may be applicable to the identification of novel cancer-causing genes (Mitra et al. 2004)

## References

Aslan D, Ozturk G, Kaya Z, Bideci A, Ozdogaan S, Ozdek S, Gursel T (2004) Early-onset in a girl with Bloom syndrome: probable clinical importance of an ocular manifestation. J Pediatr Hematol Oncol 26: 156–257.

Bloom D (1954) Congenital telangiectatic erythema resembling lupus erythematosus in dwarfs. Probably a syndrome entity. Am J Dis Child 88: 754–758.

Davis SL, North PS, Dart A, Lakin ND, Hickson ID (2004) Phosphorylation of the Bloom's syndrome helicase and its role in recovery from S-phase arrest. Mol Cell Biol 24: 1279–1291.

Du X, Shen J, Kugan N, Furth EE, Lombard DB, Cheung C, Pak S, Luo G, Pignolo RJ, DePinho RA, Guarente L, Johnson FB (2004) Telomere shortening exposes function for the mouse Werner and Bloom syndrome genes. Mol Cell Biol 24: 8437–8446.

Ellis NA, Groden J, Ye TZ, Straughen J, Lennon DJ, Ciocci S, Proytcheva M, German J (1995) The Bloom's syndrome gene product is homologous to RecQ elicases. Cell 83: 655–666.

German J (1995) Bloom syndrome. Dermatol Clin 13: 7–18.

German J, Passarge E (1989) Bloom's syndrome XII. Report from the Registry for 1987. Clin Genet 35: 57–60.

Kaneko H, Kondo N (2004) Clinical features of Bloom syndrome and function of the causative gene, BLM helicase. Expert Rev Mol Diagn 4: 393–401.

Karow J, Chrakraverty R, Hickson I (1997) The Bloom's syndrome gene product is 3'–5' DNA Helicase. J Biolo Chem 272: 39611–39614.

Keller C, Keller KR, Shew SB, Plon SE (1999) Growth deficiency and malnutrition in Bloom syndrome. J Pediatr 134: 472–479.

Kitao S, Shimamoto A, Goto M, Miller RW, Smithson WA, Lindor MN, Furuichi Y (1999) Mutations in RECQ4 helicase as the cause of a subset of cases of Rothmund–Thomson syndrome. Nat Genet 22: 82–84.

Lindor NM, Furnichi Y, Kitao S, Shimamoto A, Arndt C, Jalal S (2000) Rothmund–Thomson syndrome due to RECQ4 helicase mutations: report and clinical and molecular comparisons with Bloom syndrome and Werner syndrome. Am J Med Genet 90: 223–228.

Mitra M, Ye TZ, Smith A, Chuai S, Kirchohoff T, Peterlongo P, Nafa K, Phillips MS, Offit K, Ellis NA (2004) Localization of cancer susceptibility genes by genome-wide single-nucleotide polymorphism linkage-disequilibrium mapping. Cancer Res 64: 8116–8125.

Yu CE, Oshima J, Fu YM, Wijsman EM, Isama F, Alisch R, Matthews S, Nakura J, Miki T, Ouais S, Martin GM, Mulligan J, Schellenberg GD (1996) Positional cloning of Werner's syndrome gene. Science 272: 258–262.

# MANDIBULOACRAL DYSPLASIA

## Introduction

Mandibuloacral dysplasia (MAD) (OMIM # 248370) is a rare and not well-known progeroid syndrome characterized by the combination of short stature, progressive skeletal changes and skin abnormalities.

## Historical perspective and eponyms

This condition was possibly first described by Cavallazzi et al. (1960) under the term of cleidocranial dysostosis (CCD). Young et al. (1971) reported two boys whose main pathological manifestations were mandibular hypoplasia, acroosteolysis, still joints and cutaneous atrophy, naming the disorder "mandibuloacral dysplasia", which has persist to date. MAD has been diagnosed as acrogeria (Levi et al. 1970), or Werner's syndrome (Cohen et al. 1973). Most cases reported to date originate from Italy (Cavallazzi et al. 1960, Levi et al. 1970, Zina et al. 1981, Pallotta and Morgese 1984, Tenconi et al. 1986, Tudisco et al. 2000, Novelli et al. 2002).

## Incidence and prevalence

Prevalence of MAD has not been investigated, but appears to be low.

## Clinical manifestations

MAD is characterized by postnatal hypoplasia of the jaw and clavicles, short distal phalanges with acroosteolysis, broad and dysplastic nails, distal skin atrophy, later closure of the cranial fontanelles and sutures, a thin beaked nose, prominent eyes (Fig. 8), and postnatal growth retardation. Severe expression of MAD with lethal neonatal presentation has been exceptionally reported (Seftel et al. 1996). Subtotal alopecia (only in male patients), micrognathia, pre-mature loss of the teeth, dental overcrowding, hepatomegaly, acanthosis nigricans in the axillae and groin, together with mottled areas of hyperpigmentation over the lower trunk, upper thighs, and distal lower limbs, loss of subcutaneous fat in the extremities and accumulation in the trunk, face, submental region, and occiput (buffalo hump) were found in nine individuals of five consanguineous Italian families (Novelli et al. 2002).

X-ray studies usually show clavicular and mandibular hypoplasia acroosteolysis, delayed ossifi-

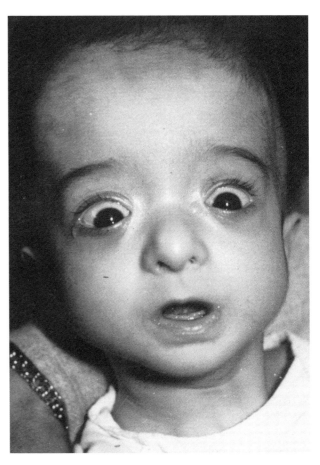

**Fig. 8.** A 3 month-old-patient with mandibuloacral dysplasia shows a thin beaked nose, enlarged forehead, prominent eyes and hypoplasia of the jaw.

cation and multiple wormian bones in the skull (as observed in cleidocranial dysplasia).

Severe insulin resistance and diabetes mellitus in MAD have been reported (Freidenberg et al. 1992, Novelli et al. 2002).

Intelligence usually is described as normal and survival also is average.

## Molecular genetic and pathogenesis

MAD is an autosomal recessive disorder and familial presentation has been often reported (Zina et al. 1981, Pallota and Morgese 1984, Tenconi et al. 1986, Novelli et al. 2002). MAD is caused by the LMNA gene, located in 1q21 (Novelli et al. 2002). This gene encodes lamins A and C (Lamin A/C). These proteins are major components of the nuclear lamina, a fibrous network underlying the inner surface of the nuclear envelope (Lin and Worman 1993). In the nine patients studied by Novelli et al. (2002), these were identified as a homozygous missense mutation (R527H) that was shared by all affected patients, and cultured skin fibroblasts showed nuclei that presented abnormal lamin A/C distribution and a dysmorphic envelope, thus demonstrating the pathogenic effect of the R527H LMNA mutation. The R527 amino acid is located in C-terminal domain common to lamin A and lamin C, and thus R527H substitution would disrupt the surface structure of the protein, altering binding fundamental sites (Novelli et al. 2002).

## Differential diagnosis

Patients with MAD have been mistakenly diagnosed as acrogeria of Gottron (Levi et al. 1970), cleidocranial dysostosis (Cavallazzi et al. 1960), Werner's syndrome (Cohen et al. 1973) or have suggested the diagnosis of Hallermann–Streiff syndrome (Shrander-Stumpel et al. 1992).

The metabolic characteristics that affect the LMNA gene may related MAD with distinct pathologies caused by other mutations in the LMNA gene, including Dunnigan-type familial partial lipodystrophy, which caused by mutations in the lamin A/C gene (LMNA{MIM150330} (Cao and Hegele 2000, Shackleton et al. 2000), and also autosomal dominant and autosomal recessive Emery-Dreifuss muscular dystrophy (Bonne et al. 1999, Raffaele di Barletta et al. 2000), limb-girdle muscular dystrophy type 1B (Muchir et al. 2000), dilated cardiomyopathy type 1A (Fatkin et al. 1999, Bécane et al. 2000), and autosomal recessive Charcot-Marie-Tooth disease type 2 (De Sandre-Giovannoli et al. 2002).

## Management

Treatment is symptomatic and affects particularly orthopedic and plastic abnormalities.

## References

Bécane HM, Bonne G, Varnous S, Muchir A, Ortega V, Hammouda EH, Urtizberea JA, Lavergne T, Fardeau M, Eymard B, Weber S, Schwartz K, Duboc D (2000) High incidence of sudden death of conduction system and myocardial disease due to lamins A/C gene mutation. Pacing Clin Electrophysiol 23: 1661–1666.

Bonne G, Raffaele di Barletta M, Varnous S, Bécane HM, Hammaouda EH, Merlini L, Muntoni F, Greenberg CR, Gary F, Urtizberea JA, Duboc D, Fardeau M, Toniolo D, Schwartz K (1999) Mutations in the gene encoding lamin A/C causes autosomal dominant Emery-Dreiffuss muscular dystrophy. Nat Genet 21: 285–288.

Cao H, Hegele RA (2000) Nuclear lamin A/C R482Q mutation in Canadian Kindreds with Dunnigan-type familial partial lipodystrophy. Hum Mol Genet 9: 109–112.

Cavallazzi C, Cremoncini R, Quadri A (1960) A case of cleidocranial dysostosis. Riv Clin Pediatr 65: 313–326.

Cohen LK, Thurmon TF, Salvaggio J (1973) Werner's syndrome. Cutis 12: 76–80.

De Sandre-Giovannoli A, Chaouch M, Kozlov S, Vallat JM, Tazir M, Kassouri M, Szepetowski P, Hammadouche T, Vandenberghe A, Stewart CL, Grid D, Levy N (2002) Homozygous defects in LMNA encoding lamin A/C nuclear envelope proteins, cause autosomal recessive axonal neuropathy in human (Charcot-Marie-Tooth disorder type 2) and mouse. Am J Hum Genet 70: 726–736.

Fatkin D, McRae C, Sasaki T, Wolff MR, Porou M, Frenneaux M, Atherton J, Vidaillet HJ Jr, Spudich S, De Girolami U, Seidman JG, Seidman C, Muntoni F, Muehle G, Johnson W, McDonough B (1999) Missense mutations in the rod domain of the lamin A/C gene as causes of dilated cardiomyopathy and conduction-system disease. N Engl J Med 431: 1715–1724.

Freidenberg GR, Cutler DL, Jones MC, Hall B, Mier RJ, Culler F, Jones KL, Lozzio C, Kaufmann S (1992) Severe insulin resistance and diabetes mellitus in mandibuloacral dysplasia. Am J Dis Child 146: 93–99.

Levi L, Bellani G, Vergani C, D'Alonso R, Fiorelli G (1970) L'acrogeria di Gottron. Descrizione di un caso. G Ital Dermatol 105: 645–651.

Lin F, Worman HJ (1993) Structural organization of the human gene encoding nuclear lamin A and nuclear lamin C. J Biol Chem 268: 16321–16326.

Muchir A, Bonne G, van der Koci AJ, van Meegen M, Baas F, Bolhuis PA (2000) Identification of mutations in the gene encoding lamins A/C in autosomal dominant limb-girdle muscular dystrophy with atrioventricular conduction disturbances (LGMD1B). Hum Mol Genet 9: 1453–1459.

Novelli G, Muchir A, Sangiuolo F, Helbling-Leclerc A, D'Apice MR, Massart C, Capon F, Sbraccia P, Federici M, Lauro R, Tudisco C, Pallotta R, Scarano G, Dallapiccola B, Merlini L, Bonne G (2002) Mandibuloacral dysplasia is caused by mutation in LMNA-encoding lamin A/C. Am J Hum Genet 71: 426–431.

Pallota R, Morgese G (1984) Mandibuloacral dysplasia: a rare progeroid syndrome. Two brothers confirm autosomal recessive inheritance. Clin Genet 26: 133–138.

Raffaele di Barletta M, Ricci E, Galluzzi G, Tonali P, Mora M, Morandi L, Romorini A, Voit T, Orstavik KH, Merlini L, Trevisan C, Biancalana V, Housmanowa-Petrusewicz I, Bione S, Ricotti R, Schwartz K, Bonne G, Toniolo D (2000) Different mutations in the LMNA gene cause autosomal dominant and autosomal recessive Emery-Dreiffuss muscular dystrophy. Am J Hum Genet 66: 1407–1412.

Seftel MD, Wright CA, Wan Po PL, de Ravel TJL (1996) Lethal neonatal mandibuloacral dysplasia. Am J Med Genet 66: 52–54.

Shackleton S, Lloyd DJ, Jackson SN, Evans R, Niermeijer MF, Singh BM, Schmidt H, Brabant G, Kumar S, Durrington PN, Gregory S, O'Rahilly S, Trembath RC (2000) LMNA, encoding lamin A/C, is mutated in partial lipodystrophy. Nat Genet 24: 153–156.

Shrander-Stumpel C, Spaepen A, Fryns JP, Dumon J (1992) A severe case of mandibuloacral dysplasia in a girl. Am J Med Genet 43: 877–881.

Tenconi R, Miotti F, Miotti A, Audino G, Ferro R, Clementi M (1986) Another Italian family with mandibuloacral dysplasia: why does it seen more frequent in Italy? Am J Med Genet 24: 357–364.

Tudisco C, Canepa G, Novelli G, Dallapiccola B (2000) Familial mandibuloacral dysplasia: report of an additional Italian patient. Am J Med Genet 94: 237–241.

Young LW, Radebaugh JF, Rubin P, Sensenbrenner JA, Fiorelli G (1971) New syndrome manifested by mandibular hypoplasia, acroosteolysis, stiff joints and cutaneous atrophy (mandibuloacral dysplasia) in two unrelated boys. Birth Defects Orig Artic Ser 7: 291–297.

Zina AM, Cravario A, Bundino S (1981) Familial mandibuloacral dysplasia. Brit J Dermatol 105: 719–723.

# BERARDINELLI–SEIP CONGENITAL LIPODYSTROPHY

## Introduction

Berardinelli–Seip congenital lipodystrophy (BSCL) syndrome (MIM 269700) is a rare, autosomal recessive disorder characterized by: (BSCL group A) generalized lipodystrophy, severe insulin resistance, hyperlipidemia, hepatomegaly, acromegaly, gigantism, acanthosis nigricans, apparent muscle hypertrophy and lack of ketoacidosis; and (BSCL group B) more severe involvement of both skeletal and nonskeletal muscle and milder endocrine involvement. Two genetic loci, BSCL1 mapping to human chromosome 9q34 (Garg et al. 1999) and BSCL 2 which maps to chromosome 11q13 (Magre et al. 2001) are responsible for the disorder.

## Historical perspective

BSCL was first described by Berardinelli in 1954, and subsequently identified by Seip (1959).

## Incidence and prevalence

The birth prevalence has been calculated as one in 50,000 live births in the Sultanate of Oman (10 cases among 500,000 live births between 1991 and 1999) (Rajab et al. 2002). However, consanguinity is very high in this country, and the true prevalence in the world population probably is much lower. Males and females are equally affected.

## Clinical manifestations

The clinical phenotype shows two groups of BSCL patients confirming its genetic heterogeneity. The first group, or group A, shows features similar to those originally described by Berardinelli (1954) and Seip (1959). This group is characterized by generalized lipodystrophy, severe insulin resistance, hyperlipidemia, hepatomegaly, acromegaly, gigantism, acanthosis nigricans, and apparent muscle hypertrophy (Fig. 9) and a lack of ketoacidosis. Patients with BSCL present with lack of body fat, delay in cognitive development, bone sclerosis, lymph nodes enlargement, and endocrine disturbances such as precocious sexual development (Rajab et al. 2002). Reduced exercise tolerance and percussion myoedema in skeletal muscle, and infantile hypertrophic pyloric stenosis, prominent veins, disturbances of cardiac rhythm, and cardiomyopathy were observed involving nonskeletal muscle (Rajab et al. 2002). The early development of acanthosis nigricans has been associated with a more severe phenotype with diabetes mellitus (Rajab et al. 2002).

The clinical phenotype in the second group, or group B, is rather different, with more severe involvement of both skeletal and nonskeletal muscle and milder endocrine involvement.

Patients with BSCL2 who were diagnosed very early showed that females developed more severe diabetes than males (Raygada and Rennert 2005). With regard to cognitive development, Raygada and Rennert (2005) reported that female patients had less impairment than male patients and performed better in school.

## Molecular genetics and pathogenesis

BSCL is a recessive disorder. Two gene loci have been identified: BSCL1 was mapped to chromosomal region 9q34 (Garg et al. 1999) and the second locus, BSCL2, was discovered on chromosome 11q13 in patients from Norway and Lebanon (Magre et al. 2001)

The BSCL2 gene encodes the seipin protein that encodes a 398-aminoacid protein, of unknown function and with little homology to known protein (Magre et al. 2001). The AGPATs gene located on chromosome 9q34 (BSCL) encodes the enzyme

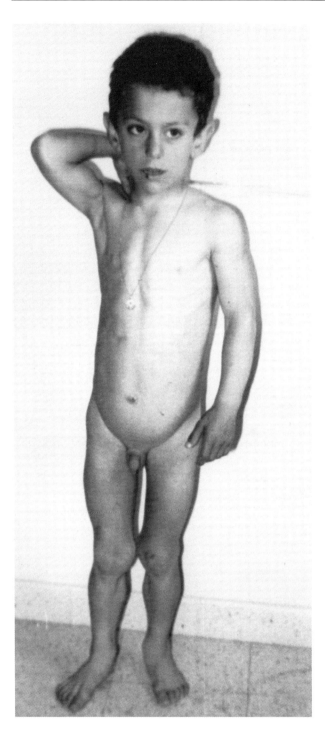

**Fig. 9.** Patient with Berardinelli–Seip shows lack of body fat and apparent muscle hypertrophy in all four extremities.

1-acyl-glycerol-3-phosphate-acyltransferase-β, which is involved in the synthesis of triglycerides (Gomes et al. 2004).

The BSCL2 protein seipin is highly expressed in brain and testis, and although the function of this gene is unknown at present, it possibly is important in the distribution of fat and insulin resistance (Rajab et al. 2002). The phenotype in BSCL2 mutations have a higher incidence of intellectual impairment and hypertrophic cardiomyopathy (Van Maldergem et al. 2002). Seipin mutations were found in patients from families originating from Europe and the Middle East. AGPAT2 mutations were found predominantly in cohorts of African ancestry.

There is also a partial late -onset form of inherited lipodystrophy referred to as Dunnigan partial lipodystrophy-, mapped to 1q21 and due to mutations in the lamin A/C gene (Shackleton et al. 2000). A novel nonsense mutation of seipin at codon 27 (R 275X) was identified in Japanase patients with BSCL (Ebihara et al. 2004).

The adipocyte hormone leptin is important in regulating energy homeostasis. Severe lipodystrophy is associated with leptin deficiency, insulin resistance, hypertriglyceridemia, and hepatic steatosis (Oral et al. 2002). Leptin has direct or indirect effects on the key organs of metabolism, including brain, liver, muscle, fat and pancreas. Leptin deficiency appears to be the main contributor to the metabolic abnormalities associated with lipodystrophy.

## Differential diagnosis

Differential diagnosis is often made with hypothalamic tumors, Thomsen congenital myotonia, and some types of muscular dystrophies.

## Management

Leptin-replacement therapy improves glycemic control and decreases triglyceride levels in patients with lipodystrophy and leptin deficiency. Leptin deficiency contributes to insulin resistance and other metabolic abnormalities associated with severe lipodystrophy (Oral et al. 2002). The optimal dose of recombinant leptin in patients with lipodystrophy remains to be determined (Oral et al. 2002).

# References

Berardinelli W (1954) Undiagnosed endocrinometabolic syndrome: report of two cases. J Clin Endocrinol 14: 193–204.

Ebihara K, Kusakabe T, Masuzaki H, Kobayashi N, Tanaka T, Chusho H, Miyanaga F, Miyazawa T, Hayashi T, Hosoda K, Ogawa Y, Nakao K (2004) Gene and phenotype analysis of congenital generalized lipodystrophy in Japanese: a novel homozygous nonsense mutation in seipin gene. J Clin Endocrinol Metab 89: 2360–2364.

Garg A, Wilson R, Barnes R, Arioglu E, Zaidi Z, Gurakan F, Kocak N, O'Rahilly S, Taylor SI, Patel SB, Bowcock AM (1999) A gene for congenital generalized lipodystrophy maps to human chromosome 9q34. J Clin Endocrinol Metab 84: 3390–3394.

Gomes KB, Fernandes AP, Ferreira ACS (2004) Mutations in the Seipin gene and AGPAT2 genes clustering in consanguineous families with Berardinelli–Seip congenital lipodystrophy from two separate geographical regions of Brazil. J Clin Endocrinol Metab 89: 357–361.

Magre J, Delepine M, Khallouf E, Gedde-Dahl T, van Maldergem L, Sobel E, Papp J, Meier M, Megarbane A, Bachy A, Verloes A, d'Abronzo FH, Seemanova E, Assan R, Baudic N, Bourut C, Czernichow P, Huet F, Grigorescu F, de Kerdanet M, Lacombe D, Labrune P, Lanza M, Loret H, Matsuda F, Navarro J, Nivelon-Chevalier A, Polak M, Robert JJ, Tric P, Tubiana-Rufi N, Vigouroux C, Weissenbach J, Savasta S, Maassen JA, Trygstad O, Bogalho P, Freitas P, Medina JL, Bonnici F, Joffe BI, Loyson G, Panz VR, Raal FJ, O'Rahilly S, Stephenson T, Kahn CR, Lathrop M, Capeau J; BSCL Working Group (2001) Identification of the gene altered in Berardinelli-Seip congenital lipodystrophy on chromosome 11q13. Nat Genet 28: 365–370.

Oral EA, Simha V, Ruiz E, Andewelt A, Premkumar A, Snell P, Wagner AJ, DePaoli AM, Reitman ML, Taylor SI, Gorden P, Garg A (2002) Leptin-replacement therapy for lipodystrophy. N Engl J Med 346: 570–578.

Rajab A, Heathcote K, Joshi S, Jeffery S, Patton M (2002) Heterogeneity for congenital generalized lipodystrophy in seventeen patients from Oman. Am J Ned Genet 110: 219–225.

Raygada M, Rennert O (2005) Congenital generalized lipodystrophy: profile of the disease and gender differences in two siblings. Clin Genet 67: 98–101.

Seip M (1959) Lipodystrophy and gigantism with associated endocrine manifestation: a new diencephalic syndrome? Acta Paediatr Scand 48: 555–574.

Shackleton S, Lloyd D, Jackson SNJ, Evans R, Niermeijer MF, Singh BM, Schmidt H, Brabant G, Kumar S, Durrington PN, Gregory S, O'Rahilly S, Trembath RC (2000) LMNA, encoding lamin A/C, is mutated in partial lipodystrophy. Nat Genet 24: 153–156.

Van Maldergem L, Magre J, Khallouf TE (2002) Genotype-phenotype correlations in Berardinelli–Seip congenital lipodystrophy. J Med Genet 39: 722–733.

# HALLERMANN–STREIFF SYNDROME

## Introduction

Hallermann–Streiff syndrome (HSS) is a rare genetic disorder characterized by head and face abnormalities including dyscephalia with abnormal head, bird-like facies and hypoplastic mandible, dental anomalies, proportionate nanism, hypotrichosis, cutaneous atrophy, microphthalmia, and congenital cataracts.

## Historical perspective and eponyms

HSS probably was first described by Aubry in 1893, who emphasized the alopecia, but did not mention other signs of this syndrome. Hallermann (1948), and Streiff (1950) distinguished the syndrome from progeria and mandibulofacial dysostosis. François (1958) reviewed 22 cases of the literature, added 2 personally studied cases, and further delineated the syndrome. The condition has also been called François syndrome, especially by French authors (Berbich et al. 1977, Barrucand et al. 1978, François 1982), and Hallermann–Streiff-François syndrome (Crevits et al. 1977). A complete review of the condition was published by Cohen (1991).

## Incidence and prevalence

Over 150 cases were reported up to 1991 (Cohen 1991) and very few patients have been reported since then. The condition is described most frequently in children, but adults are also reported (Cohen 1991, Mirshekari and Safar 2004).

## Clinical manifestations

François listed seven essential manifestations of the syndrome that included dyscephalia with abnormal head, bird-like facies and hypoplastic mandible, dental anomalies, proportionate nanism, hypotrichosis, cutaneous atrophy, microphthalmia, and con-

genital cataracts (Fig. 10). Birth weight is normal in about 64%, but prematurity and/or low birth weight occur in the other 36%. More than half of patients

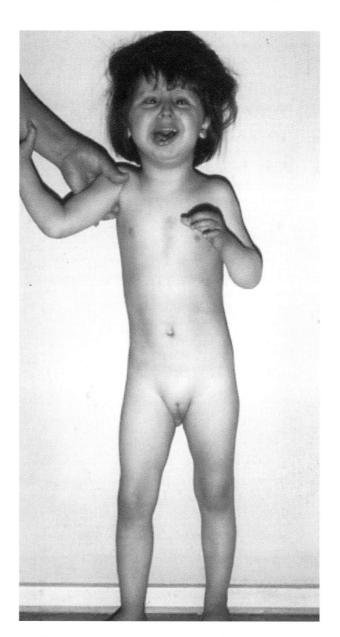

**Fig. 10.** A young patient with the typical appearance of the Hallermann–Streiff syndrome. She shows microphthalmia, bilateral cataract, and birth-like facies.

show short stature, being al least two to five standard deviations below the mean. Sexual development may be retarded and patients may show hypogenitalism with cryptorchidism, hypospadias, clitoral enlargement, breast asymmetry, and scant axillary and pubic hair (François 1982).

Mental deficiency has been noted in about 15% of patients (Cohen 1991) to 50% (Judge and Chakanovskis 1971), and hyperactivity, choreoathetosis, and generalized tonic-clonic seizures, and small cerebellum have been reported occasionally (Judge and Chakanovskis 1971, Crevits et al. 1977, Hou 2004).

The face is small with a thin, tapering, "pinched" nose, and receding chin (Sclaroff and Appley 1987) (Figs. 11 and 12). An odd-shaped, bulging skull with brachycephaly is often accompanied by frontal or parietal bossing. Some cases may present malar bone hypoplasia and microcephaly. The nose is thin, pointed, and often curved, with a tendency to septal deviation in some patients. Generalized hypotrichosis is a characteristic of HSS, being especially obvious in the scalp, brows, lashes, axillary and pubic areas. Alopecia is most prominent in the frontal and occipital areas (Fig. 13). Cutaneous atrophy is limited to the scalp and nose, showing underlying prominent veins.

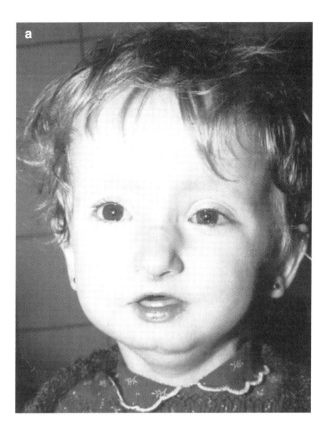

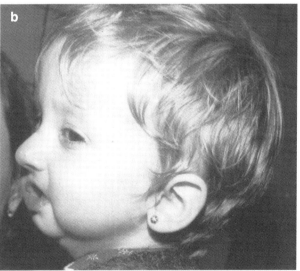

**Fig. 12.** (**a**, **b**) The same patient as in Fig. 11 at 4 years of age shows small face, microphthalmia with left eye cataract, thin nose, and micrognatia.

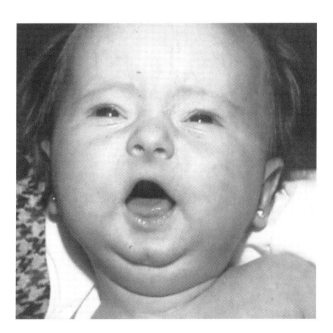

**Fig. 11.** An infant of 3 months of age shows microphthalmia and micrognatia.

Ocular abnormalities mainly consist of congenital cataracts (81–90%) and microphthalmia (78–83%), and, less frequently, nystagmus, strabismus,

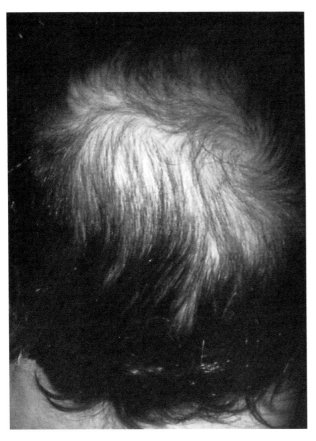

**Fig. 13.** Same patient as in Fig. 10 showing alopecia in the parieto-occipital area.

blue sclerae, sparse eyelashes and eyebrows, fundus anomalies, and others (Cohen 1991).

Dental anomalies are common (80–85%) (Cohen 1991) and may include absence of teeth, persistence of deciduous teeth, malocclusion and open bite, malformed teeth, severe and premature caries, supernumerary teeth, and natal teeth. Radiographic records have also shown malocclusion, narrowed upper arch, bilateral posterior crossbite, and anterior open bite (Defraia et al. 2003). Histopathologic study of dentoalveolar abnormalities consisted of root irregular dentin and osteodentin (Slootweg and Huber 1984).

A narrow upper airway may lead to respiratory embarrassment. Obstructive sleep apnea (OSA) has been observed in some instances. The severity of OSA in children with craniofacial anomalies ranges from mild to life-threatening. Respiratory obstruction may cause cor pulmonale (Robinow 1991).

Patients with HSS present particular anesthestic risks. Because of micrognathia, microstomia, and serious upper airway compromise, laryngoscopy and endotracheal intubation may be difficult. In some situations presurgical tracheotomy should be considered in HSS patients.

Tracheostomy is often necessary in these instances. Other anomalies or complications associated with HSS are various types of heart anomalies (Dinwiddie et al. 1978), genital anomalies, decreased GH and insulin-like growth factor-1 (Pivnick et al. 1991, Salpietro et al. 2004), pectus carinatum, and pectus excavatum, lordosis, scoliosis, and other skeletal anomalies. The most severe complication is early pulmonary infection resulting in death.

The condition is described most frequently in children, but adults are also reported (Cohen 1991, Harrod and Friedman 1991, Limeres et al. 2004, Mirshekari and Safar 2004). Familial lethal presentation, with two siblings whose autopsies showed slender long bones with a few fractures, and underossified skull has been reported (Dennis et al. 1995).

## Imaging

Radiological findings in HSS (Christian et al. 1991, Defraia et al. 2003) include large, poorly ossified skull with decreased ossification in the sutural areas, increase in the number of Wormian bones, severe mid-facial hypoplasia, prominent nasal bone, abnormally obtuse or nearly straight gonial angle, thin and gracile long bones, small vertebral bodies, aplasia of teeth, skeletal open bite, and excessive vertical dimension of the lower third of the face.

## Molecular genetics and pathogenesis

The cause of HSS in unknown to date. Virtually all cases of HSS are sporadic. The condition affects similarly both sexes. Familial patients reported have not been accepted scientifically (Cohen 1991). However, the physical appearance of several familial patients described show similar features as reported HSS patients (Harrod and Friedman 1991). A review of the literature indicates two classes of patients labeled HSS: typical and atypical. Most patients are typical who may be diagnosed at the first sigh, and few are atypical (Cohen 1991). Chromosome analyses are often normal. Increased chromosomal breakage rate, although seldom reported (Hou 2003) is suggestive of the existence of some DNA repair defects in HSS patients.

## Differential diagnosis

HSS can be distinguished from progeria and all progeroid syndromes, mandibuloacral dysplasia, mandibulofacial dysostosis, Seckel syndrome, and oculodentodigital dysplasia. However, HSS is sporadic, while progeria and progeroid syndromes most often have autosomal recessive inheritance. Seckel syndrome is characterized by severe growth deficiency, mental deficiency, microcephaly and receding forehead, but patients with this condition do not present cataracts, and malformed temporomandibular joints. Progeria differs from HSS because of premature arteriosclerosis, nail dystrophy, normal eyes, acromicria, and chronic deforming arthritis. Mandibulofacial dysostosis overlaps some signs with HSS that mainly involve malar bone, but the associated eyelid colobomas and ears anomalies, that are not present in HSS, differentiate both entities. Mandibuloacral dysplasia is characterized by delayed closure of cranial sutures, mandibular hypoplasia, dysplastic clavicles, and abbreviated terminal phalanges with acrolisthesis, overlapping only mandibular hypoplasia with HSS. Oculodentodigital dysplasia (ODDD) (Lohmann 1920) is characterized by four major manifestations: typical face with thin nose and hypoplastic nasal alae, bilateral microphthalmia with anomalies of the iris, syndactyly of fingers IV and V, and yellowish discoloration of the teeth because of enamel hypoplasia. Patients with ODDD overlap some signs with those of HSS (Spaepen et al. 1991). However, while ODDD is a dominantly inherited disorder due to mutations in the connexion 43 gene GJA1, the origin of HSS is still debated (Pizzuti et al. 2004). The facial changes of ODDD may become more obvious when growing up (Patton and Laurence 1985).

## Management

Dental extractions, scaling, restorations, and endodontics under local anesthesia, and later orthodontic rehabilitation with fixed brackets may be necessary (Limeres et al. 2004). Later, a subsequent phase of orthodontic therapy consists of dental arches for controlling the tongue thrust in the anterior open bite (Defraia et al. 2004). Surgical and prosthetic interventions are scheduled at the completion of growth to solve the skeletal discrepancy and for occlusal rehabilitation (Defraia et al. 2004). Despite numerous systemic anomalies some of these patients may undergo conventional dental procedures under local anesthesia in the dental office (Limeres et al. 2004).

Surgical treatment may include tracheotomy, mandibular advancement, mandibular and chin-hyoid advancement, palatal shortening, tonsillectomy, surgical reduction of the tongue, mandibular positioning dental appliances, and tongue retaining devices (Cohen 1991). Nonsurgical treatment may include sleep position modification, medication, continuous positive airway pressure therapy, weight loss, head and neck extension collars, etc.

Tracheostomy, although curative, is associated with major long term problems related to depression and difficulties with stoma care, and may be only performed when necessary.

Patients with HSS mostly look forward to cosmetic surgery to establish maxillomandibular harmony and to solve respiratory difficulties. Cataracts may be treated by the ophthalmologists.

## References

Aubry M (1893) Variété singulière d'alopécie congénitale: alopécie suturales. Ann Dermatol Syphil (Paris) 4: 899–900.

Barrucand D, Benradi C, Schmitt J (1978) Syndrome de François. A propos de deux cas. Rev Oto-Neuro-Ophthal 50: 305.

Berbich A, Benradi F, Sekkat A (1977) Syndrome de François. Arch Ophthalmol (Paris) 37: 723–730.

Christian CL, Lachman RS, Ayhsworth AS, Fujimoto A, Gorlin RJ, Lipson MH, Graham JM Jr (1991) Radiological findings in Hallermann–Streiff syndrome: report of five cases and a review of the literature. Am J Med Genet 41: 508–514.

Cohen MM Jr (1991) Hallermann–Streiff syndrome: a review. Am J Med Genet 41: 488–499.

Crevits L, Thiery E, Van der Eechem H (1977) Oculo-mandibular dyscephaly (Hallermann–Streiff-François syndrome) associated with epilepsy. J Neurol 215: 225–230.

Defraia E, Marinelli A, Alarashi M (2003) Case report: orofacial characteristics of Hallermann–Streiff syndrome. Eur J Pediatr Dent 4: 155–158.

Dennis NR, Fairhurst J, Moore IE (1995) Lethal syndrome of slender bones, intrauterine fractures, characteristic facial appearance, and cataracts, resembling Hallermann–Streiff syndrome in two sibs. Am J Med Genet 59: 517–520.

Dinwiddie R, Gewitz M, Taylor JFX (1978) Cardiac defects in the Hallermann–Streiff syndrome. J Pediatr 92: 77.

François MJ (1958) A new syndrome: dyscephalia with bird face and dental anomalies, nanism, hypotrichosis, cutaneous atrophy, microphthalmia and congenital cataract. Arch Ophthalmol 60: 842–862.

François MJ (1982) François dyscephalic syndrome. Birth Defects 18: 595–619.

Hallermann W (1948) Vogelgesicht und Cataracta congenital. Klin Monatsbl Augenheilkd 113: 315–318.

Harrod MJ, Friedman JM (1991) Congenital cataracts in mother, sister, and of a patient with Hallermann–Streiff syndrome: coincidence or clue? Am J Med Genet 41: 500–502.

Hou JW (2003) Hallermann–Streiff syndrome associated with small cerebellum, endocrinopathy and increased chromosomal breakage. Acta Pediatr 92: 869–871.

Judge C, Chakanovskis JE (1971) The Hallermann–Streiff syndrome. J Ment Defic Res 15: 115–120.

Limeres J, Abeleira M, Tomas I, Feijoo JF, Vilaboa C, Diz P (2004) An atypical Hallermann–Streiff syndrome. Focus on dental care and differential diagnosis. Quintessence Int 35: 49–55.

Lohmann W (1920) Beitrag zur Kenntnis des reinen Mikrophthalmus. Arch Augenheilk 86: 136–141.

Mirshekari A, Safar F (2004) Hallermann–Streiff syndrome: a case review. Clin Exp Dermatol 29: 477–479.

Patton MA, Laurence KM (1985) Three new cases of oculodentodigital (ODD) syndrome: development of the facial phenotype. J Med Genet 22: 386–389.

Pivnick EK, Burstein S, Wilroy RS, Kaufman RA, Ward JC (1991) Hallermann–Streiff-syndrome with hypopituitarism contributing to growth failure. Am J Med Genet 41: 503–507.

Pizzuti A, Flex E, Minfarelli R, Salpietro C, Zelante L, Dallapiccola B (2004) A homozygous GJA1 gene mutation causes a Hallermann–Streiff (ODDD) spectrum phenotype. Hum Mutat 23: 286.

Robinow M (1991) Respiratory obstruction and cor pulmonale in the Hallermann–Streiff syndrome. Am J Med Genet 41: 515–516.

Salpietro D, Briuglia S, Merlino V, Piraino B, Valenzise M, Dallapiccola B (2004) Hallermann–Streiff syndrome: patient with decreased GH and insulin-like growth factor-1. Am J Med Genet 125: 216–218.

Sclaroff A, Appley BL (1987) Evaluation and surgical correction of the facial skeletal deformity in Hallermann–Streiff syndrome. Int J Oral Maxilofac Surg 16: 738–744.

Slootweg PJ, Huber J (1984) Dentoalveolar abnormalities in oculomandibulo-dyscephaly (Hallermann–Streiff syndrome) J Oral Pathol 13: 147–154.

Spaepen A, Schrander-Stumpel C, Fryns JP, De Die-Smulders C, Borghgraef M, Van den Berghe H (1991) Hallermann–Streiff syndrome: clinical and psychological findings in children. Nosologic overlap with oculodentodigital dysplasia? Am J Med Genet 41: 417–420.

Streiff EB (1950) Dysmorphie mandibulo-faciale (tête d'oiseau) et alteration oculaires. Ophthalmologica 120: 79–83.

# Chapter 55

# FOCAL DERMAL HYPOPLASIA SYNDROME (GOLTZ SYNDROME)

Ignacio Pascual-Castroviejo and Martino Ruggieri

Paediatric Neurology Service, University Hospital La Paz, University of Madrid, Madrid, Spain (IPC); Institute of Neurological Science, National Research Council and Department of Pediatrics, University of Catania, Catania, Italy (MR)

## Introduction

The focal dermal hypoplasia (FDH) syndrome is a rare congenital condition (OMIM # 305600) that, as often occurs with other neurocutaneous disorders, can affect various ectodermal and mesodermal tissues besides the skin. The skin manifestations predominate and are essential for the diagnosis: these include atrophy and linear pigmentation of the skin, herniation of the fat through dermal defects and multiple papillomas of the mucous membranes or skin (Lee and Goltz 2006, Sampaio and Harper 2006). Ocular (coloboma of iris and choroid, strabismus and microphthalmia), oral (hypoplastic teeth and lip papillomas), and skeletal (syndactyly, polydactyly, camptodactyly, and absence deformities) defects as well as neurological abnormalities (mental retardation and various brain malformations) are also characteristics. The severity is variable: findings range from minimal skin manifestations to life-threatening abnormalities at birth. The multi faceted clinical presentations and multi organs involvement seen in this disorder require the knowledge and expertise of specialists from many different disciplines of medicine.

Two different forms of inheritance have been postulated: X-linked dominant with in utero lethality in males (Friedman et al. 1988, Naritomi et al. 1992) and autosomal dominant sex-limited (Burgdorf et al. 1981, Gorski et al. 1991). Various loci on the X chromosome (e.g., Xp22 region) (Friedman et al. 1988, Naritomi et al. 1992) and the long arm of chromosome 9 (Zuffardi et al. 1989) have been targeted as possible gene sites; however, no definitive sequences have been identified (Lee and Goltz 2006, OMIM 2006).

## Historical perspective and eponyms

The syndrome was first characterized by Goltz et al. (1962), who proposed the term *focal dermal hypoplasia* because of the decrease in the connective tissue of the skin (Sampaio and Harper 2006). **Robert William Goltz** is an American dermatologist, born 1923, Minnesota. He studied medicine at the University of Minnesota. In 1965 he became the first professor of dermatology at the University of Colorado, Denver. In 1970 he returned to the University of Minnesota to become head of dermatology. When he retired in 1985, he was chairman. Goltz has played an active role in his speciality and is recognised as a pioneer in dermopathology.

One year after the first report of FDH, Gorlin et al. (1963) identified in an extensive review 11 previously described patients. **Robert James Gorlin** was an American oral pathologist and geneticist, born 1923, Hudson, New York. Gorlin graduated at Columbia College, served in the US Army during World War II and then studied at the Washington University School of Dentistry, graduating in 1947. He later obtained a M.S. in Chemistry at the State University of Iowa. After a number of academic posts Gorlin in 1956 moved to the University of Minnesota School of Dentistry, where he became professor and chairman of the division of oral pathology in 1958 and regents professor in 1979. By May, 2000, he was Regents' Professor Emeritus of Oral Pathology and Genetics, department of oral sciences, University of Minnesota. Here he has served as professor of pathology, dermatology, paediatrics, obstetrics, gynaecology and otolaryngology. He died in 2006. The syndrome is known as Goltz syndrome or Goltz-Gorlin syndrome, not to be confused with Gorlin syndrome or Gorlin-Goltz syndrome (i.e., the basal cell nevus syndrome).

Jessner (1921) had described a rare disease that involved the skin, hands and feet in a 30-year-old woman consistent with FDH.

## Incidence and prevalence

Goltz estimated, in a more recent review (Goltz 1992) over 200 reported cases of FDH but minimally affected individuals may remain unrecognised. Only 10–15% of the cases are seen in males, but this incidence may be overestimated as male cases, considered a rarity, are probably reported more often (Sampaio and Harper 2006). A high incidence of miscarriages and stillbirths indicates lethality in utero, particularly in males. Persons of any race can be affected.

## Clinical manifestations

The cutaneous manifestations are emphasized in most reports; however, FDH is a generalized disease which, not only affects the skin anywhere in the body (Fig. 1), but usually shows abnormalities in other organs such as the eyes, mouth, extremities, skeletal system, renal and intestinal tracts or other internal organs, and central nervous system (CNS). This variability of expression is also observed within a family and could be explained by random inactivation of the mutant X-chromosome (see below). Generally, the findings are asymmetric, however cases of unilateral (mosaic) distribution of clinical features have been recorded (Aoyama et al. 2008). Even though most reported patients are females, more than 30 affected males have also been described (Goltz 1992).

### Skin lesions

The skin lesions can be of different types (Gellis and Feingold 1969, Rochiccioli et al. 1975):

a) Striate lesions which vary from pink, brown, pale to flesh colour and from raised to slightly depressed. They are usually asymmetric and in the distribution of Blaschko's lines, but other patterns

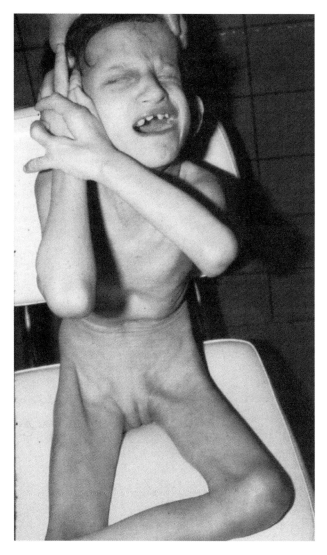

**Fig. 1.** A girl shows typical cutaneous and subcutaneous lesions distributed throughout her body.

have been observed. Occasionally there is an inflammatory phase at birth with oedematous, blistered, eroded, crusted or scaling erythematous lesions. They are usually more prominent on the limbs than on the trunk.

b) Areas of *linear dermal hypoplasia or aplasia* (appearing as atrophied skin) where the epidermis is very thin and the dermis usually is absent showing a number of different designs including striate, elliptical, round, reticulate or cribiform. The range of colours includes pink, red, brown, grey and white. Cases of total absence of skin at birth have been reported. Probably the epidermis does not develop owing to the absence of dermal substrates (these lesions are referred as congenital aplasia).

c) *Nodules of adipose tissue* which herniate through the skin, are soft and yellowish-brown in colour and appear during childhood. They can occur anywhere but are more common on the trunk and the limbs, particularly in the popliteal and cubital fossae. They can also gave a linear pattern.

d) *Angiofibromas* red-raspberry in colour which appear as verrucous papules located around the mouth, conjunctivae, vulva, and anus: these are not well demarcated and may be mistaken for warts.

e) Numerous thin and disseminated *telangiectasias* which can appear at any age and display multiple patterns which usually accompany the atrophic, striate and lipomatous lesions.

f) *Violaceous or whitish colour papillomas* usually located over the hypoplastic skin involving the mucous membranes. Deformity and disability can be associated with these lesions that sometimes achieve massive size. They are most common around the lips and eyes, on vulvar, perianal and perineal areas. They have been also reported at other sites including the oesophagus and larynx. In some instance, they are present at birth. Recurrence after excision has been observed.

g) Lesions of the scalp (*zones of alopecia*), dystrophy of the nails, and cutaneous hypohydrotic lesions.

h) Generalised skin dryness, associated with pruritus is observed in some cases as well as photosensitivity, sweat abnormalities, apocrine gland anomalies, hypoplastic dermatoglyphics on the digits and hypothenar eminence and palmar hyperkeratosis.

## Hair

The hair can be sparse and brittle. Localised areas of absence of hair in the scalp and pubic area have been reported.

## Nails

Dystrophy, atrophy, anonychia, grooving and spooning are noted in a significant number of patients.

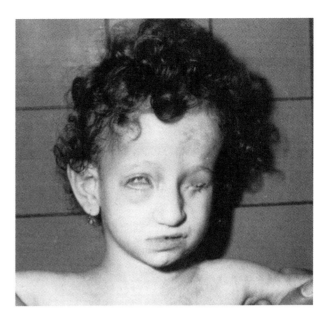

**Fig. 2.** Severe cutaneous and subcutaneous lesions in both eyes (anophthalmia), left forehead, mouth and surrounding area, and shoulders.

## Ocular anomalies

The involvement of the eys is observed in 20% of reported cases and can be a cause of handicap in these patients. Colobomas of the iris, retina or choroids are likely the most common findings. Microphthalmia or anophthalmia (Fig. 2), strabismus, and nystagmus, anomalies of the lacrimal apparatus, lacrimal duct cyst, microcornea, keratoconus, cortical and subcapsular cataracts have been also reported (Pascual-Castroviejo et al. 1982, Thomas et al. 1977, Willets 1974). In addition, papilloma of the eyelids, aniridia, heterochromia, corneal clouding, pannus, retinal non-perfusion with neovascularisation and vitreous haemorrhage, blue sclerae, irregularity of pupils, have been sporadically observed (Sampaio and Harper 2006).

## Skeletal anomalies

These abnormalities mostly involve the distal parts of the limbs. Adactyly or lack of some fingers, syndactyly (Fig. 3a) – usually of the third and fourth fingers and toes, but any combination is possible –

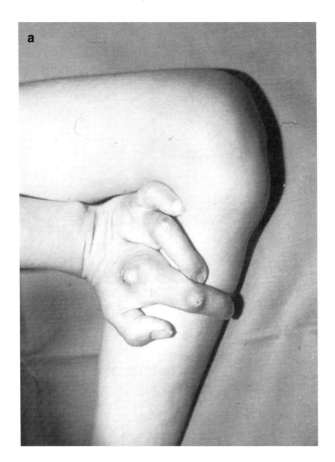

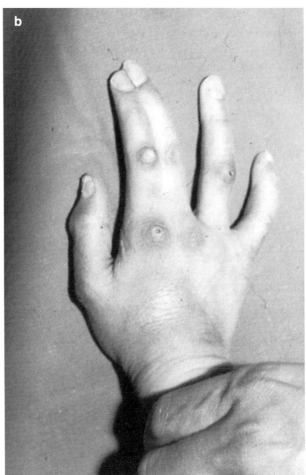

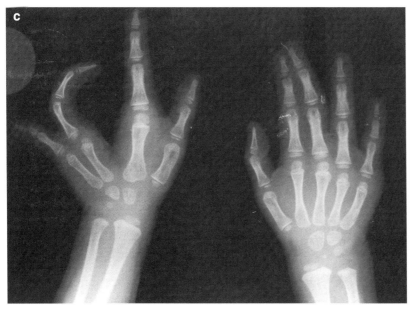

**Fig. 3.** Skeletal abnormalities. (**a**) Syndactyly of the right hand; (**b**) lobster-claw type lesion of the left hand; (**c**) X-rays of both hands show the bones and the soft tissue abnormalities in the same patient.

clinodactyly, and other more rare abnormalities. An almost unique and striking feature of FDH is the so-called *lobster-claw hand* (Fig. 3b) or *foot* with typical clinical and radiological manifestations (Fig. 3c). There are several reports of cystic lesions occurring in the maxilla, ilium, ischium, tibia, fibula, metatarsals and other bones. Most patients with FDH are of small stature. Deformities of the ribs, clavicles, asymmetry of the face, trunk, and limbs, osteopatia striata, and diffuse reduction in bone density, have also been reported in some patients (Vakilzadeh et al. 1976).

## Mouth lesions

Any external or internal region of the mouth, and respiratory tract may show some type of lesion. Dental abnormalities include congenital absent or malformed teeth and malocclusion. Tongue, gums, lips, and palate can present anomalies. Papillomas may develop anywhere in the nasal vestibule, pharynx, lanrynx, oesophagus, and mouth; these attain considerable size and their surfaces may become eroded or ulcerated, and bleeding may occur. This complication occasionally may require tracheotomy.

## Face

Typical facial features (see Figs. 1 and 2) are low-set, thin and protruding ears; pointed chin; broad nasal tip with a narrow bridge and sometimes notching of the alae nasi. Other ear deformities include asymmetric, small or deformed ears, poor development of cartilage, auricular appendages, cholesteatoma and hearing deficits. Asymmetry of the face, microcephaly, maxillary hypoplasia and facial clefts have been described.

## Soft tissue anomalies

A number of lesions affecting the soft tissues of almost any of the thoracic and abdominal organs has been reported. These include inguinal and umbilical hernia (Ginsburg et al. 1969), diaphragmatic hernia (Kunze et al. 1979), congenital heart disease such as aortic stenosis (Goltz et al. 1962), intestinal malrotation and mediastinal dextroposition (Irvine et al.

1996) and caudal appendages (Petrides et al. 2008). Reported anomalies of the urinary tract consist of absence of the kidneys, fused and horseshoe kidneys, and dilated ureters.

## Nervous system

Approximately 10–15% of patients with FDH have some degree of mental deficiency. The patients we studied showed severe mental retardation associated with severe ocular, cutaneous and skeletal abnormalities as well (Pascual-Castroviejo et al. 1982). Malformations of the CNS have been rarely reported. These included agenesis of the corpus callosum (Baughman and Worcester 1970), meningomyelocele, Arnold-Chiari malformation, hydrocephalus (Almeida et al. 1988), polymicrogyria, optic nerve tumour, partial agenesis of the corpus callosum, subependymal heterotopia optic disc anomaly (Fisher et al. 2007, Giampietro et al. 2004). Patients with less severe or even normal mental levels have also been reported. The severity of the cutaneous lesions is not correlated with central nervous system involvement: normal intelligence is noted in cases otherwise severely affected. Seizures are rare. Neurosensory and conductive hearing loss may be noted.

## Imaging

Radiography may reveal osteopathia striata which consists of longitudinal striations in the metaphyses of the bones: the lesions are usually bilateral and symmetric, manifest as linear vertical opacities that originate at an articular surface and extend into the diaphysis, where they gradually narrow and disappear paralleling the axis of the long bones, mainly involving the long bones and the sacral bone with sparing of the vertebrae and iliac bones. Prenatal ultrasonographic findings are variable ranging from non specific foetal growth delay to specific organ and/or developmental anomalies.

## Pathology

The diminution in the thickness of the dermis by defective collagen formation and fat deposits is the hallmark of the atrophic, striate and lipomatous lesions of FDH (Sampaio and Harper 2006). Ectopic fat in different patterns of distribution in the papillary dermis. mid-reticular dermis and subcutis is observed and believed to represent different degrees of the same process. In the early stages the epidermis is usually normal. Absence of epidermis and sometimes dermis is observed in the lesions of congenital aplasia. The papillomas consist of a fibrovascular stalk covered by a layer of acanthotic stratified squamous epithelium. Hyperkeratosis and pankeratosis are often present. Fat cells can be found in the mid-epidermis (Sampaio and Harper 2006). Inflammatory lesions can occur in some patients at birth and fade with time: in the acute phase there is marked oedema in the papillary dermis, perivascular lymphocytic infiltration, increased number of fibroblasts and clusters of lipocytes at the mid-dermis.

## Molecular genetics and pathogenesis

Two different forms of inheritance have been postulated: X-linked dominant (Friedman et al. 1988, Naritomi et al. 1992) and autosomal dominant sex-limited (Burgdorf et al. 1981, Gorski et al. 1991). The X-linked dominant inheritance with male lethality has been assumed to be the most likely form of inheritance. The homozygous state is incompatible with survival in affected males. In these families, miscarriage of male foetuses and stillbirths in the mothers are frequent. However, 10–15% of patients reported are male, and this represents more than 30 affected male subjects reported (Goltz 1992), some of whom survived till old age (Büchner and Itin 1992). Sporadic patients have been described in whom a new mutation might be assumed. There are few examples of father to daughter transmission (Burgdorf et al. 1981, Mahe et al. 1991): these families could represent an autosomal dominant inheritance, or the father could have been 47,XXY karyotype, or a mosaic with a gametic half-chromatid mutation or very early postzygotic mutations.

Previous studies on various loci on the X chromosome (e.g., Xp22 region) (Friedman et al. 1988, Naritomi et al. 1992) and the long arm of chromosome 9 (e.g., q932-qter) (Zuffardi et al. 1989) had been targeted as possible gene sites (Lee and Goltz 2006). Recently, Wang et al. (2007) and Grzeschik et al. (2007) have found evidence that FDH is caused by a deficiency in the gene encoding the human homolog of Drosophila Melanogaster Porcupine (PORCN) which encodes an endoplasmic reticulum transmembrane protein involved in processing of wingless proteins (e.g. WNT1). These findings have been confirmed by further studies (Leoyklang et al. 2008).

## Dysplasia of tissues

FDH manifests itself in many organs of ectodermal and mesodermal origin, but the predominant features involve structures formed by connective tissue. In the affected skin, the collagen fibres appear thin and wispy. In some areas collagen and elastin may be completely absent, and these correspond with areas of aplasia cutis congenital. These alterations suggest that fibroblastic abnormalities may lead to an alteration of collagen synthesis in FDH, especially of collagen type IV (Büchner and Itin 1992) or alteration in the growth capacity of fibroblasts, resulting in an insufficient number to produce enough collagen to form complete collagen fibres. In addition to defective collagen formation in the skin, adipose cells can appear in the dermis, especially in relation to blood vessels. This suggests that a profound dysplasia of mesodermal tissues (rather than hypoplasia) underlies the syndrome (Goltz 1992, Goltz et al. 1970).

## Differential diagnosis

FDH overlaps with several other syndromes which manifest at birth, particularly incontinentia pigmenti. Both of these neurocutaneous disorders may present with widespread skin lesions, but especially in the scalp with aplasia cutis congenital, and in the eyes, eyelids, and orbits; both also have an X-linked dominant mode of inheritance. Oculocerebro-cutaneous syndrome (OCCS) and encephalocraneocutaneous lipomatosis (ECCL) can also overlap with FDH, and the differential diagnosis may require neuroradiological studies because FDH usually does not have important cerebral or spinal anomalies, while OCCS and ECCL may show several and severe neuroanatomical alterations.

## Management

Available treatment is mainly symptomatic for most of the abnormalities found in FDH, although some of the cerebral and ocular malformations may benefit from surgery. Papillomatous lesions can be excised or treated with cautery or cryotherapy. Laser therapy is the method of choice for laryngeal papillomas. Treatment of pruriginous erythematous atrophic lesions with the vascular pulsed dye laser has been reported, with alleviation of pruritus and improvement of erythema.

## References

Almeida L, Anyane-Yeboa K, Grossman M, Rosen T (1988) Meningomyelocele, Arnold-Chiari anomaly and hydrocephalus in focal dermal hypoplasia. Am J Genet 30: 917–923.

Aoyama M, Sawada H, Shintani Y, Isomura I, Morita A (2008) Case of unilateral focal dermal hypoplasia (Goltz syndrome). J Dermatol 35: 33–35.

Baughman FA Jr, Worcester DD (1970) Agenesis of the corpus callosum in a case of focal dermal hypoplasia. Mt Sinai J Med 37: 702–709.

Büchner SA, Itin P (1992) Focal dermal hypoplasia syndrome in a male patient. Report of a case and histologic and immunohistochemical studies. Arch Dermatol 128: 1078–1082.

Burgdorf WHC, Dick GF, Soderberg MD, Goltz RW (1981) Focal dermal hypoplasia in a father and daughter. J Am Acad Dermatol 4: 273–277.

Fisher RB, Pairaudeau PW, Innes JR, Bartlett RJ, Crow YJ (2007) Focal dermal hypoplasia with subependymal heterotopia and hypoplastic corpus callosum. Clin Dysmorphol 16: 59–61.

Friedman PA, Rao KW, Teplin SW, Aylsworth AS (1988) Provisional deletion mapping of the focal dermal hypoplasia (FDH) gene to Xp22.31. Am J Hum Genet 43: A50.

Gellis SS, Feingold M (1969) Focal dermal hypoplasia (Goltz's syndrome). Picture of the month. Am J Dis Child 118: 765–766.

Giampietro PF, Babu D, Koehn MA, Jacobson DM, Mueller-Schrader KA, Moretti C, Patten SF, Shaffer LG, Gorlin RJ, Dobyns WB (2004) New syndrome: focal dermal hypoplasia, morning glory anomaly, and polymicrogyria. Am J Med Genet 124A: 202–208.

Goltz RW (1992) Focal dermal hypoplasia syndrome. An update. Arch Dermatol 128: 1108–1111.

Goltz RW, Paterson WC, Gorlin RJ, Ravits MG (1962) Focal dermal hypoplasia syndrome. Arch Dermatol 86: 708–717.

Goltz RW, Hitch JM, Ott JE (1970) Focal dermal hypoplasia syndrome. Arch Dermatol 101: 1–11.

Gorlin RJ, Meskin LM, Peterson WC Jr, Goltz RW (1963) Focal dermal hypoplasia syndrome. Acta Derm Venereol (Stockh) 43: 421–440.

Gorski JL (1991) Father-to-daughter transmission of focal dermal hypoplasia associated with nonrandom X-inactivation: support for X-linked inheritance and paternal X chromosome mosaicism. Am J Med Genet 40: 332–337.

Grzeschik KH, Bornholdt D, Oeffner F, König A, del Carmen Boente M, Enders H, Fritz B, Hertl M, Grasshoff U, Höfling K, Oji V, Paradisi M, Schuchardt C, Szalai Z, Tadini G, Traupe H, Happle R (2007) Deficiency of PORCN, a regulator of Wnt signaling, is associated with focal dermal hypoplasia. Nat Genet 39: 833–835.

Irvine AD, Stewart FJ, Binham EA, Nevin NC, Boston VE (1996) Focal dermal hypoplasia (Goltz syndrome) associated with intestinal malrotation and mediastinal dextroposition. Am J Med Genet 62: 213–215.

Jessner M (1921) Verhandlungen des Breslauer Dermatogishen Vereiningung. Arch Franc Dermatol U Syphil 133: 48.

Kunze J, Heyne K, Wiedermann HR (1979) Diaphragmatic hernia in a female newborn with focal dermal hypoplasia and marked asymmetric malformations (Goltz-Gorlin syndrome). Eur J Pediatr 13: 213–218.

Lee W, Goltz RW (2006) Focal dermal hypoplasia syndrome. e-Medicine from WebMD. http://emedicine.com/DERM/topic155.htm

Leoyklang P, Suphapeetiporn K, Wananukul S, Shotelersuk V (2008) Three novel mutations in the PORCN gene underlying focal dermal hypoplasia. Clin Genet 73: 373–379.

Mahe A, Corturier J, Mathe C, Lebras F, Bruet A, Fendler J (1991) Minimal focal dermal hypoplasia in a man: a case of father to daughter transmission. J Am Acad Dermatol 25: 879–881.

Naritomi K, Izumikawa Y, Nagataki S, Fukushima Y, Wakui K, Niikawa N, Hirayama K (1992) Combined Goltz and Aicardi syndromes in a terminal Xp deletion: are they a contiguous gene syndrome? Am J Med Genet 43: 839–843.

OMIM (2006) Ondine Mendelian Inheritance in Man. Baltimore: Johns Hopkins University. http://www.ncbi. nlm.nih.gov/omim

Pascual-Castroviejo I, Luengo dos Santos A, Baquero-Paret G (1982) Síndrome de Goltz. Presentación de dos casos. An Esp Pediatr 16: 524–526.

Petrides G, Bhat M, Holder S, Wakeling E (2008) Caudal appendage in focal dermal hypoplasia (Goltz syndrome). Clin Dysmorphol 17: 129–131.

Rochiccioli P, Dutan G, Fabre J, Marcou P, Martínez J, Abtan S (1975) Hypoplasy dermique en aire, osteopathie striée et nanisme. Pediatrie 30: 271–180.

Sampaio C, Harper J (2006) Focal dermal hypoplasia syndrome (Synonim: Goltz syndrome). In: Harper J, Oranje A, Prose N (eds.) Textbook of Pediatric Dermatology. 2nd ed. Oxford: Blackwell Science, pp. 1532–1537.

Thomas JV, Yoshizumi MO, Beyer CK, Craft JL, Albert DM (1977) Ocular manifestations of focal dermal hypoplasia syndrome. Arch Ophthalmol 95: 1997–2000.

Vakilzadeh F, Happle R, Peters P, Macher E (1976) Focal dermal hypoplasia with apocrine nevi and striation of bones. Arch Dermatol Res 256: 189–195.

Wang X, Sutton VR, Peraza-Llanes JO, Yu Z, Rosetta R, Kou YC, Eble TN, Patel A, Thaller C, Fang P, Van den Veyver IB (2007) Mutations in X-linked PORCN, a putative regulator of Wnt signaling, cause focal dermal hypoplasia. Nat Genet 39: 836–838.

Willetts GS (1974) Focal dermal hypoplasia. Br J Ophthalmol 58: 620–624.

Zuffardi O, Caiulo A, Maraschio P, Tupler R, Bianchi E, Amisano P, Beluffi G, Moratti R, Liguri G (1989) Regional assignment of the loci for adenylate kinase to 9q32 and for alpha 1-acid glycoprotein to 9q31–q32. A locus for Goltz syndrome in region 9q32-qter? Hum Genet 82: 17–19.

# Chapter 56

# EHLERS–DANLOS SYNDROMES

**Salvatore Savasta and Maurizia Valli**

Department of Paediatrics, IRCCS Hospital S. Matteo, Pavia, Italy (SS); Department of Biochemistry, Section of Medicine and Pharmacy, University of Pavia, Italy (MV)

## Introduction

Ehlers–Danlos syndrome (EDS) is an umbrella term which encompasses a heterogeneous group of connective tissue disorders with distinct inheritance patterns, biochemical defects, and prognostic implications (Byers 1997, Beighton et al. 1998, Yeowell et al. 1993). Clinically, this group of disorders is collectively characterised by fragile or hyperelastic skin, hypermobility of the large joints, vascular lesions, easy bruising and excessive scarring following an injury (Beighton 1993, Roach and Zimmermann 2004).

Continues expansion in the number of clinical entities labelled as EDS, coupled with the discovery of additional biochemical defects, led to different classification systems (Beighton et al. 1988) (Table 1) and to their revision (Beighton et al. 1998) (Table 2) with major and minor diagnostic criteria defined for each type complemented whenever possible with laboratory findings (OMIM 2006). The most recent classification, revised by Beighton et al. (1998) and designated the "Villefranche classification" (Table 2), includes six main descriptive types of EDS, according to the underlying biochemical and molecular defects, which substituted for earlier types (see Table 1) numbered with Roman numerals: classic type (EDS I and II), hypermobility type (EDS III), vascular type (EDS IV), kyphoscoliosis type (EDS VI) arthrochalasia type (EDS VIIA and VIIB) and dermatosparaxis type (EDS VIIC) (Table 2). Additional types were recognised (see Table 1) with the first four types (EDS I to EDS IV) accounting for approximately 95% of total cases. Thus, at present, at least 11 forms are recognised (Alper 1990, Beighton et al. 1998, Byers 1994, Mallory 1991, OMIM 2006) which represent clinically and genetically distinct conditions: phenotypic overlap may exist and patients may not always easily be classified in one or another subtype.

EDS related syndromes are osteogenesis imperfecta, alkaptonuria, homocystinuria, Marfan and Menkes syndrome (Hollister 1978).

## Historical perspective and eponyms

The first comprehensive description of a syndrome featuring hyperextensibility and fragility of the skin associated with hypermobility of the large joints was published by Tschernogobow (1892) in Moscow who interpreted the cause of this phenotype in a systemic defect of connective tissue. Ehler-Danlos syndrome is one of the oldest known causes of bruising and bleeding and was first described by Hippocrates in 400 BC (Parapia and Jackson 2008). The syndrome however derives its name from the reports of Edward Ehlers (1901) and Henri-Alexandre Danlos (1908), respectively, who published their observations independently and combined the pertinent features of the condition delineating the phenotype (Parapia and Jackson 2008).

**Edvard Lauritz Ehlers** (1863–1937) grew up in comfortable circumstances in Copenhagen, where his father was Mayor. After a classical education he qualified in medicine in 1891 and early in his career he developed an interest in dermatology. Thereafter he undertook postgraduate studies in Berlin, Breslau, Vienna and Paris before returning to practise in Copenhagen. In 1906 he was appointed chief of the dermatological polyclinic at the Frederiks Hospital and from 1911 until his retirement in 1932 he was director of the special service at the Kommunehos-

**Table 1.** Classification of EDS according to molecular basis (Beighton et al. 1988, OMIM 2007)

| Type | Form | Clinical features | Chromosome locus | Inheritance | Biochemical abnormality |
|------|------|-------------------|------------------|-------------|-------------------------|
| I | Gravis | Skin hyperextensibility with ecchimosis and tissue fragility; hypermobility joints; premature labour | 9q34.2–34.3; 2p31 | AD | Type V collagen (COL5A1); type V (COL5A2) |
| II | Mitis | Similar to type I and less severe | 9q34.2–34.3; 2p31 | AD | Type V collagen (COL5A1); type V (COL5A2) |
| III | Hypermobile | Marked hypermobility joints; minimal atrophic wrinkled scars | Potential allele to type IV? | AD | Probably heterogeneous |
| IV | Vascular | Thin and translucent skin; spontaneous arterial and intestinal rupture; rare hyperextensibility joints | 2q31 | AD o AR | Type III collagen |
| V | X-Linked | Similar to type II | X | XR | Unknown |
| VI | Ocular/scoliosis | Hypersensibility skin; Hypermobility joints | 1p36.3–36.2 | AR | Lysyl-hydroxylase |
| VII | Arthrochalasis multiplex congenita | General joints hyperextensibility with subluxations, fragility of skin | 17q31–22.5; 7q22.1 | AD o AR | A: collagen (COL1A1) B: collagen (COL1A2) |
| VIIC | Dermatosparaxis | Mild joints hypermobility; micrognatia and hypodontia | 5q23–q24 | AR | C: ADAMST2 |
| VIII | Periodontal | Dental and periodontal involvment with gengival resorption; variable skin laxity and joints hyperextensibility | Potential allele to type IV | AD | Unknown |
| IX | Cutis laxa, occipital horn | Occipital exostosis and typical features of types I and II | | XR | Lysyl-hydroxylase |
| X | Fibronectina | Similar to type II with petechiae and platet aggregation defect | | AR | Fibronectin deficiency |
| XI | Joint hypermobility | | | | |

pitalet (Municipal Hospital) in Copenhagen. Ehlers was an indefatigable traveller and spoke several languages. He received numerous academic honours and became president of the International Union Against Venereal Diseases. He died in 1937 at the age of 74 years after a brief but painful disease (Beighton and Beighton 1989, Who Named It? 2006). In 1899 he presented a 21-year-old law student from Bornhold Island at a clinical meeting with a history of late walking and frequent subluxations of the knees associated to formation of many haematomata on minor trauma and discoloured lesions on the elbows, knees and knuckles. In addition this young man had extensible skin and lax digits. This case was subsequently published in the dermatological literature (Ehlers 1901). Danlos presented a similar case to the Dermatological Society of Paris in 1908 (Danlos 1908).

**Henri-Alexandre Danlos** (1844–1912) spent his entire life in his native city of Paris. His father wished his son to enter a family business and his initial education was aimed in that direction, but he

**Table 2.** ≪Villefranche≫ Classification of Ehlers–Danlos syndrome (Beighton et al. 1998)

| New terminology | Old name | Inheritance | Mutated genes |
|---|---|---|---|
| Classic type | Gravis (EDS type I) | AD | *COL5A1,* |
| | Mitis (EDS type II) | | *COL5A2* |
| Hypermobility type | Hypermobile (EDS type III) | AD | *Unknown, ?* |
| | | | *TNXB?* |
| Vascular type | Arterial-ecchymosed (EDS type IV) | AD | *COL3A1* |
| Kyphoscoliosis type | Ocular-scoliotic (EDS type VI) | AR | *Lysiyl-hydroxylase* |
| Arthrochalasia type | Arthrochalasis multiplex congenital | AD | *COL1A1* |
| | (EDS type VIIA) | | *COL1A2* |
| | (EDS type VIIB) | | |
| Dermatosparaxis type | Dermatosparaxis (EDS type VIIC) | AR | *Procollagen,* |
| | | | *N-peptidase* |

himself decided he wanted to do medicine and without his parents' knowledge changed to a medical course. He qualified with distinction in 1869 and in 1874 presented his doctoral thesis that was entitled "The Relationship between Menstruation and Skin Disease" (Beighton and Beighton 1989, Who Named It? 2006). Danlos initially was most interested in laboratory work, retaining an early interest in chemistry and undertook research at the laboratory of Charles-Adolphe Wurtz (1817–1884) during the early phases of his career. In 1881, at the age of 37 years, he passed the examination for consultant status – médecin des hôpitaux – and got a well-rounded clinical training working with EFA Vulpian (1826–1887). In 1885, Danlos became chef de service at the hôpital Tenon, where he spent five years, followed by 5 years in the public service. This was an unhappy period for Danlos as he suffered a prolonged and painful illness and became withdrawn and pessimistic. In 1895, at the age of 51 years, Danlos received an appointment at the hôpital Saint Louis in Paris. He was active in general medicine and gained a reputation as a caring physician and excellent diagnostician but he was increasingly involved in the development of new therapeutic techniques in dermatology. Danlos undertook numerous meticulous studies of the use of various preparations of arsenic and mercurials in the treatment of syphilis and other skin disorders, and was a pioneer in the use of radium to treat lupus erythematosus of the skin. With Eugene Bloch he was the first to place radium in

contact with a tuberculous skin lesion. The patient illustrated by Danlos at the Paris Society of Dermatology and Syphilology in 1908 had been presented 18 months previously by his colleagues Hallopeau and Macé de Lépinay under the diagnosis of "juvenile pseudodiabetic xanthomata" (Beighton and Beighton 1989). This boy had extensibility and fragility of the skin and propensity for bruising. Danlos disagreed with the diagnosis of his colleagues and hypothesised an inherited defect of the skin, which he termed "cutis laxa" (Danlos 1908) playing his trump card against his colleagues' diagnosis by mentioning that a dermatologist from Denmark, Dr Ehlers, had reported a similar case in 1901. After three decades the eponym Ehlers–Danlos was universally accepted (Beighton and Beighton 1989).

The familial nature of this clinical association was demonstrated by Johnson (1949), and soon thereafter Jansen (1955) suggested that a genetic defect of the collagen "wicherwork" in the connective tissue probably accounted for the phenotype. McKusick (1956) included Ehlers–Danlos syndrome (EDS) in the first compilation of hereditable disorders of connective tissue. Barabas (1967), in describing a subgroup of patients with EDS who had vascular fragility, suggested the presence of genetic heterogeneity. The first molecular defect was discovered by Pinnel et al. (1972) who found lysylhydroxylase deficiency in an autosomal recessive form of EDS in which the patients were particularly prone to scoliosis and rupture of the ocular globe.

## Incidence and prevalence

The prevalence of EDS is 1 in 5000 live birth with both males and females of all racial and ethnic groups equally affected (Blereau 1996, Pyeritz 2000, Steinmann et al. 1993). All forms of the syndrome cause clinical problems, such as skin fragility, unsightly bruising and scarring, musculoskeletal discomfort and susceptibility to osteoarthritis (Byers 1997). However, with the exception of the vascular type (EDS IV), life expectancy in EDS is normal. EDS is under recognised by neurologists because many of these patients have mild clinical manifestations and do not seek medical care, or are seen by physicians in different non-neurology specialities.

## Clinical manifestations

Although much has been learned recently regarding the molecular basis of EDS, an accurate clinical diagnosis is the mainstay in distinguishing the various types of EDS (Bohm et al. 2002, De Paepe et al. 2005). All forms of EDS share the following major clinical features with variable degrees: skin hyperextensibility, joints hypermobility and excessive dislocation, easy bruising and generalized fragility of the various connective tissues (Beighton 1993, Steinmann et al. 1993, Grahame 2000) potentially affecting any part of the central nervous system (Byers 1995). The spectrum of severity ranges from almost imperceptible findings to a severe debilitating illness. The clinical and genetic heterogeneity of EDS is, in part, reflection of the underlying biochemical heterogeneity. The six major varieties of EDS so far identified are due to different abnormalities in the biogenesis of the collagens (Pope et al. 1975, Yeowell et al. 1993, Andrikopoulos et al. 1995).

## Skin abnormalities

The skin in EDS is characteristic in texture and consistency: it is soft, doughy, and velvety to the touch. When pulled, it is hyperextensible. Cutaneous fragility, manifested by splitting of the skin to

insignificant trauma, may be a prominent feature. Typically, these wounds occur over the shins, knees, elbows, forehead, and chin and often present a gaping "fish mouth" appearance owing to retraction of the adjacent skin. Upon clinical examination one can also evidence orthostatic acrocyanosis and often small, deep, palpable nodules in the subcutaneous tissue over bony prominences. Joint hypermobility is another cardinal feature, which typically involves

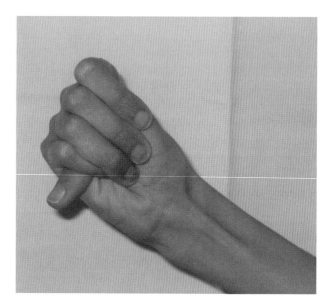

**Fig. 1.** Clinical features of Ehlers–Danlos syndrome. Hyperextensibility of the fingers.

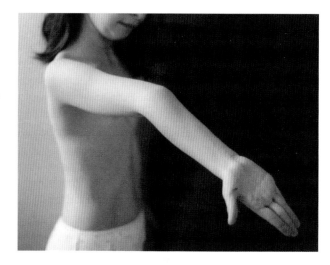

**Fig. 2.** Hyperextensibility of the elbow.

both large and small joints (Figs. 1 and 2). Congenital clubfoot is not so rare. The facies are often slightly abnormal, with epicanthial folds and ocular hypertelorism. There may be a high arched palate and frequently the patient can touch the tip of the nose with the tongue (Gorlin's sign).

## Systemic involvement

A variety of internal manifestations of connective tissue weakness may be found (Kinnane et al. 1995, Gomez-Sugranes et al. 1995, Sentongo et al. 1998, Bedda et al. 2004, Mathew et al. 2005). Intestinal diverticulas with perforation may be found from stomach to colon and repeated rectal prolapse has been seen in children below five years of age. Umbilical and inguinal hernias are common, and hiatal hernia or eventration of the diaphragm, also, may occur. Bladder diverticulas are reported and prolaps of the bladder and uterus may occur in the postpartum woman (Shukla et al. 2004). Structural abnormalities of the renal collector system and cystic malformations of the kidney may be seen. Spontaneous pneumothorax may also occur. Pregnant women often have an increased incidence of premature birth and premature rupture of foetal membranes.

Although diagnostic criteria have been promulgated for each of the different type of EDS, it is impossible to determinate the exact type of EDS in a substantial proportion of affected individuals (Beighton et al. 1986).

*EDS syndrome types I and II (classical type)* are the best recognized forms of the disorder and are characterized by moderate to severe skin extensibility, significant tissue fragility, generalized joint hypermobility and recurrent joint (sub)luxations with joint pain and early osteoarthrosis (McKusick 1986, Beighton et al. 1988, Hamel 2004) (Fig. 3). Musculoskeletal features are easily found. These features include kyphoscoliosis, hallus valgus, flat feet and genu recurvatum (Fig. 4). The facies often is characteristically "parrot like" (Fig. 5). Bruises are less common in this type than in other forms. Cardiac defects, especially mitral valvular prolapse, are sometimes present (Fig. 6). Aneurysms and dissection,

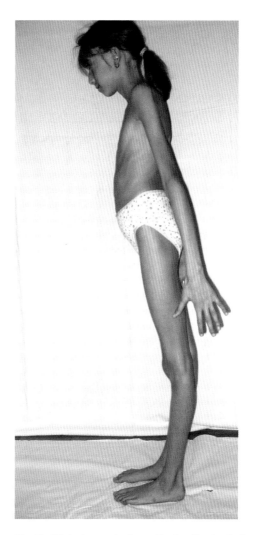

**Fig. 3.** Clinical aspect of a patient with classic form at age 12 years.

and other vascular anomalies occasionally occur with EDS types I and II (Krog et al. 1983) (Figs. 7 and 8). Hiatus hernia and anal prolapse are common. Cervix uteri insufficiency with premature labour as a result and cicatrical hernia are well-known complications (Hamel 2004). The mode of inheritance for classical type of EDS is autosomal dominant and there is a large interfamilial and intrafamilial clinical variability. The specific collagen defects for this form have been found on the collagen V (alpha-1 and -2).

Patients with *EDS type III* (Hypermobility type) show hypermobile joints, musculoskeletal complaints, luxation (especially in children), and minimal

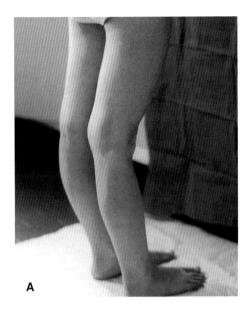

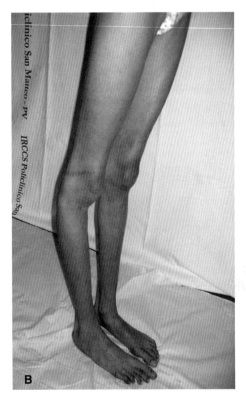

**Fig. 4.** Genu recurvatum (**A**, **B**) beyond 190°.

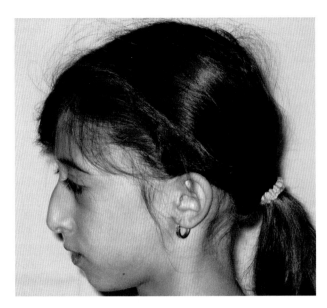

**Fig. 5.** "Parrot like" aspect of the face.

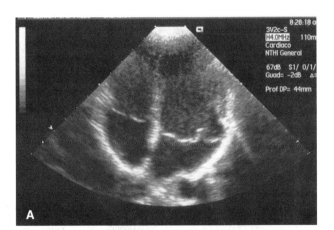

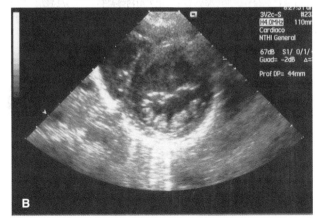

**Fig. 6.** Mitral valvular prolapse (**A**, **B**) in EDS (classic form).

atrophic wrinkled (cigarette paper or papyraceous) scars (Holzberg et al. 1987, Beighton et al. 1998). The hyperextensibility usually causes orthopaedic consequences (severe osteoarthritis) in the long term.

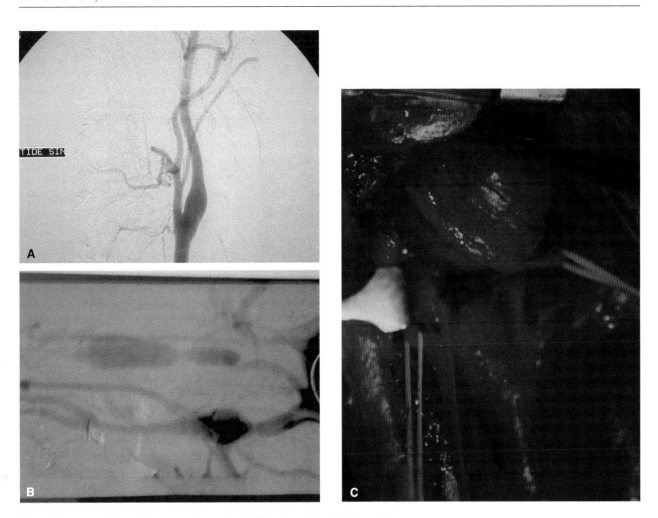

**Fig. 7.** Aneurysm of carotid artery: angiographic (**A**, **B**) and pathologic (**C**) aspects.

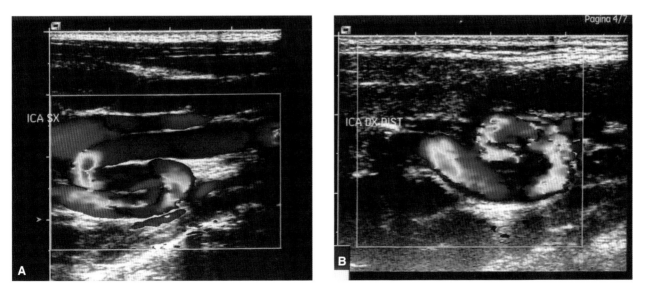

**Fig. 8.** Transcranial doppler reveals a "Kinking" image of the carotid arteries in EDS (classic form).

The disease has an incidence of 9–16% (Holzberg et al. 1987, Ciampo et al. 1997). A COL3A1 mutation (glycine substitution) was observed in a family with type III EDS, but the molecular defect that underlies this subtype is unknown (Burrows et al. 1999, Beighton et al. 1998, Narcisi et al. 1994, Iurassich et al. 2001).

*EDS type IV (vascular or arterial-ecchimotic type)* is often difficult to recognize clinically in young children, because of the paucity of clinical symptoms in childhood. This condition often comes to medical attention only after serious vascular accidents in the patients or in other affected family members. Careful clinical examination however can help to detect early symptoms of this relatively rare condition. This type of EDS is inherited as an autosomal dominant trait and it is characterised by four main clinical findings: a striking facial appearance, easy bruising, translucent skin with visible superficial veins, and spontaneous arterial, intestinal or uterine rupture (Pepin et al. 2000, Germain 2002). Severe joints hyperextensibility is rare or absent in this type: sometimes EDS-IV patients have milder laxity involving small joints or even decreased mobility with contractures. Gloviczki et al. (2005) reported a characteristic facial appearance, with thin lips, delicate, and pinched nose and prominent bones and eye in 30% of their patients and found that excessive bruising and the tendency to form haematomas was the most frequent sign (97%), while skin was not hyperextensible. Complications are uncommon during childhood, but approximately 80% of patients have already experienced at least one complication by the age of 40 (Pepin et al. 2000, Laporte-Turpin et al. 2005). Patients are typically unaware of the diagnosis until they present, often to a vascular surgeon, with spontaneous arterial rupture or dissection. This disorder is caused by type III procollagen synthesis or secretion deficiency (Pope et al. 1975). Paradoxically, although the EDS type IV has less striking clinical features, it is clearly the most malignant type and the diagnosis is often made only after a catastrophic complication or at post-mortem examination. Pepin et al. (2000) and Gloviczki et al. (2005) found that 92% of late deaths in their patients were from vascular complication.

*EDS type V (X-linked form)* is inherited as an X-linked recessive pattern. This type is similar to type II. The skin of patients with this form is highly extensible, and orthopaedic abnormalities are common. Bruising and hyperextensibility are rare.

In *EDS type VI (Kyphoscoliosis type)* patients are clinically and severely affected (Beighton et al. 1998, Heim et al. 1998, Yis et al. 2008). This disorder is a rare, autosomal-recessive form of EDS, presenting with neonatal muscular hypotonia and progressive kyphoscoliosis. The skin is extensible, bruises are common and wound healing is poor. In these patients several scars are present, some of which can be hyperpigmented. In this subgroup the ocular clinical signs are cardinal symptoms (Wenstrup et al. 1989). The ocular fragility can cause retinal haemorrhage and detachment, glaucoma, microcornea and blu sclera are described (Judisch et al. 1976) (Fig. 9). Rupture of the globe is rare but possible. In the majority of cases, the symptoms have been biochemically attributed to a deficiency of collagen lysylhydroxylase 1 (Pinnel et al. 1972, Steinmann et al. 1995). This form commonly called EDS VIA, results from different mutation in the lysylhydroxylase 1 gene. A rare subtype of EDS VI with normal lysylhydroxylase activity is designated EDS VIB. As of yet, eighteen cases of EDS type VIA and five as type VIB have been described (Gupta et al. 2000, Steinmann et al. 2002).

In *EDS type VII A–B (Artrochalasia type)* there is extreme general joint hyperextensibility with recurring subluxations. There can be congenital hip dislocation. The skin changes are less severe than those of other types; there is easy scarring because of tissue fragility, hypotonia of the muscles and kyphoscoliosis. Patients with this type are usually short in stature and microgathia, also, is present. Structural defect of pro-collagen alpha 1 and 2 was found and this form is inherited as autosomal dominant mode (Beighton et al. 1988, Giunta et al. 2008).

Patients with *EDS type VII C (Dermatosparaxis)* have mild joint hypermobility and tissue fragility. In this type, also, are present oral findings and they comprise micrognathia, hypodontia, localized microdontia or multiple tooth agenesia, opalescent tooth discoloration, root dysplasia, pulp obliteration, severe gingival hyperplasia, frontal open bite, and se-

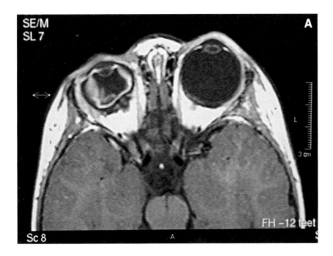

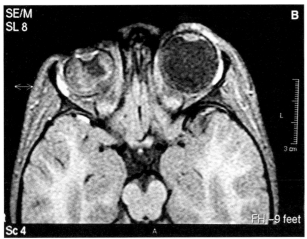

**Fig. 9.** Axial T1 weighted images of the brain at the orbital level showing retinal haemorrhage and detachment and microcornea in a patient with EDS (the scans in A and B have been taken by different TR and TE).

vere restriction of temporomandibular joints mobility (Gage et al. 1995, De Coster et al. 2003). The mode of inheritance of this form is autosomal recessive. To date, only seven cases of human dermatosparaxis have been recorded and is caused by deficient activity of procollagen-I-N-proteinase (Colige et al. 1999).

In *EDS type VIII dental* involvement with gingival periodontal inflammation are present. Skin laxity, joint hyperextensibility, and bruisability are variable. Gingival resorption and permanent loss of the teeth are common.

*Occipital horn syndrome* is an X-linked recessive form of EDS (*type IX* or *X-linked cutis laxa*) diagnosed by the presence of occipital exostosis, obstructive uropathy, and chronic diarrhoea, in additional to the typical features of EDS (Lazoff et al. 1975). Other features include bladder diverticula or rupture and bony dysplasia. This form is caused by a defect in copper metabolism, which leads to lysyl oxidase deficiency and abnormal collagen (Byers et al. 1980). Copper and ceruloplasmin are low. Other features include bladder diverticula or rupture and bony dysplasia. This type of EDS resembles a mild adult variant of Menkes' disease. In fact, the occipital horn syndrome may be the result of a point mutation in the Menkes' disease gene (Kaler et al. 1994).

*EDS type X* is an autosomal recessive form described in one family. The patients exhibited poor wound healing, petechiae, and platelet aggregation defect, which were corrected by fibronectin supplementation. Type X (fibronectina deficiency) and *type XI* (*benign hypermobile joint syndrome*) are rare forms of *EDS*. Some suggested that these types are so similar that they are better classified as one type rather than two and to remove the type XI from EDS classification.

## Nervous system abnormalities

Neurological manifestations, also, are reported in persons with EDS (Shapiro 1952, Cupo 1981) and include cerebrovascular disorders, chronic pain syndrome, peripheral neuropathy, plexopathy, heterotopic grey matter nodules in the periventricular white matter, polymicrogyria, epilepsy and spontaneous intracranial hypotension (SIH) (Pretorius et al. 1983, Herrero 1995, Thomas et al. 1997, Jacome 1999b, Gupta et al. 2000, Mathew et al. 2005).

Recurrent *headaches* may constitute the neurological presentation of EDS in the absence of structural, congenital, or acquired central nervous system lesions and are not, always, the result of the known cerebrovascular complications of EDS (Jacome 1999a). The types of headaches occurring in patients may be diverse: migraine with or without aura, tension headaches, migraine and tension headaches, blepharoclonus. The pathogenesis of headaches in EDS is uncertain. Sacheti et al. (1997) reported chronic pain in 51 patients with EDS and speculated that chronic pain in EDS may be the consequence of inherited connective tissue abnormalities; isolated tension or post-traumatic headaches in EDS perhaps could be explained on this basis. Although cortical microdysgenesis may accompany EDS, it is unknown whether this disorder of neuronal cytoarchitecture and connective tissue organisation could precipitate migraines by creating a chronic state of hyperexcitability (Chen et al. 1995, Thomas et al. 1996, Jacome 1999a, Chevassus-au-Louis et al. 1999). Holzchuch et al. (1996) reported a low arterial pulsatility index in a patient with EDS studied by transcranial doppler. These limited preliminary data of functional cerebrovascular abnormality in EDS also suggest that EDS patients may have a disorder of cerebrovascular reactivity that could explain why some of these individuals suffer migraine and are prone to stroke.

*Cerebrovascular complications* (Rubinstein et al. 1964, Hunter et al. 1982, Krog et al. 1983, Pretorius et al. 1983, Schievink et al. 1990, North 1995, Heidbreder et al. 2008) may affect patients with EDS in the form of intracranial aneurysms, subarachnoid haemorrhage, spontaneous arterial dissection, and spontaneous cavernous sinus fistula. In particular, patients with EDS type IV are at greater risk of intracranial aneurysms (Rubinstein et al. 1964, Edwards et al. 1969, Mirza et al. 1979, Pepin et al. 2000). Typically the aneurysm develops in the cavernous sinus or just at it emergence, and bilateral carotid aneurysms also have been reported (Schoolman et al. 1967, Mirza et al. 1979) (Fig. 7). Subarachnoid haemorrhage or rupture of an intracavernous carotid aneurysm to create a carotid-cavernous fistula are the most common complications. Aneurysmal rupture can occur spontaneously or during vigorous activity (North et al. 1995, Schievink et al. 1990). A fistula can develop after minor head trauma but most occur spontaneously (Krog et al. 1983, Debrun et al. 1996). Carotid-cavernous fistulae in EDS patients result from rupture of an internal carotid artery aneurysm within the cavernous sinus (Schievink et al. 1991). Bi-

lateral and recurrent carotid-cavernous fistula are rare (Halbach et al. 1990; Desal et al. 1997, 2005; Gloviczki et al. 2005). Arterial dissection has been documented in most of the intracranial and extracranial arteries and the clinical presentation depends on which artery is affected. Carotid dissection classically causes ipsilateral oculosympathetic paresis and headache (Pope et al. 1991), but more commonly leads to signs of ischemic infarction. Patients with vertebral dissection develop painful, pulsatile mass of the neck. Also, tortuosity of the carotid and intracranial arteries have been recently reported (Lees et al. 1969, Franceschini et al. 2000, Wahab et al. 2003, Zaidi et al. 2004) (Fig. 8). In patients with EDS type I aneurysms, occasionally, occur and other vascular abnormalities are rare.

Brachial and/or lumbosacral plexus *neuropathies* have been reported in EDS syndrome and attributed to pressure effects secondary to the ligament laxity (Reed 1972, De Graf 1973, Kayed et al. 1979, El-Shaker et al. 1991, Galan 1995). The exact pathogenetic mechanism of the peripheral neuropathy is unknown. Mechanical and other traumatic factors may play an important role (Kayed et al. 1979, Papapetropoulos et al. 1981). Some patients show only motor manifestation and others, motor and sensory impairment (De Graf 1973). Dislocation and subluxations due to ligament and capsular laxity are especially common in EDS type III, and may be responsible for these complications. Excessive stretching of nerves with deficient connective tissue support is probably a contributory factor. Peripheral nerve disorders in EDS tend to be chronic, are often precipitated by trauma and patients exhibit conduction block of electrical nerve impulses on electrophysiologic testing (Galan et al. 1995). Underlying hereditary neuropathy with susceptibility to pressure palsies (tomaculous neuropathy) may be present (Schady et al. 1984, Farag et al. 1989).

The role of spontaneous cerebrospinal fluid (CSF) leaks as a cause of *intracranial hypotension* is poorly understood. Schievink et al. (2003) examined the putative role of systemic connective tissue disorders in the development of this condition and reported an astonishing number of 12 of 18 patients (67%) with stigmata of either a generalized connective tissue disorder or joint hypermobility. Syndromic conditions included, also, EDS type II.

Patients with EDS syndrome and *epilepsy* have been described in the literature (Tschernogobow 1892; Herrero 1972, 1995). Jacome (1999b) studied seven patients, four of whom were referred for neurologic consultations because of their epilepsy, two because of symptoms of peripheral neuropathy, and the remaining patient because of extreme fatigue. They were diagnosed with EDS. Two cases of EDS type IX (occipital horn syndrome) and partial seizures suggestive of supplementary motor area (SMA) origin were diagnosed. Of these two, one had an area of frontal gliosis and was able to abate his seizures by hyperextending his neck; the other had a Dandy-Walker malformation and in addition pseudoseizures. The third patient of the series had complex partial seizures, pain asymbolia, and basilar artery hypoplasia. Two earlier patients with EDS and pain asymbolia were reported by Silverman et al. (1959). Other patients had complex partial seizures, focal seizures and grand mal seizures. As Jacome (1999b) in patients with EDS and epilepsy reported basilar artery hypoplasia, and Dandy-Walker malformation (including one case who was able to abate his seizures by hyperextending his neck) and as previously Thomas et al. (1996) reported one EDS patient with agenesis of the corpus callosum, one could ask whether in certain patients with EDS, prenatal insufficiency of the vertebrobasilar arterial system is present, resulting in development arrest or malformation of anatomic structures supplied by this system. In addition, a vascular disturbance of the posterior circulation could be potentially aggravated by neck hyperextension beyond physiologic limits during delivery in someone with lax connective tissue. This excessive flexibility of the neck would allow stretching or compression to already abnormal vertebral arteries due to EDS.

A disruption in the link between the extracellular matrix and cytoskeleton causes *aberrations in cellular migration* during development. This disruption may result in various congenital malformation of the vessels and brain parenchyma, including cortical dysgenesis, which at times is difficult to detect with current conventional neuroimaging techniques (Wang

et al. 1993, Sakai 1995). Any of such lesions may cause epilepsy in patient with EDS. The subjects with EDS and epilepsy may have normal interictal EEGs, as the cases of Jacome (1999b), or show nonspecific paroxysmal activity. Therefore, prolonged EEG monitoring with ictal recordings is necessary in EDS.

Thomas et al. (1996) reported a case of EDS in 24-year-old woman with complex partial and right sensory motor seizures, associated with periventricular subependymal heterotopias (PSH), agenesis of the posterior corpus callosum and aneurysms of the sinuses of Valsalva. Previously, Cupo et al. (1981) described a similar case in an EDS patient who in addition had myocardial infarction. The clinical and anatomical features reported were consistent with the classical form of EDS (types I and II). Thomas and Cupo hypothised that this form of EDS may be different from the variants previously described. Savasta et al. (2007) described PSH in a 12-year-old female with headache and EDS classic form (Fig. 10A, B and C).

Many of the clinical and neuroimaging features seen in the three cases, reported by Thomas, Cupo, and Savasta can sometimes be seen in X-linked PSH (Poussaint et al. 2000) due to FLNA mutations. A gene for PSH has been identified as filamin-1 (FLN-1; also known as FLNA) (Fox et al. 1998) an actin-cross-linking phosphoprotein expressed in nonmuscle cells originally identified from motile blood cells. It has a high level of expression in the developing cortex and is required for neuronal migration in the cerebral cortex and is subsequently downregulated in adults (Eksioglu et al. 1996).

Sheen et al. (2005) reported two familial cases and nine additional sporadic cases of EDS-variant form of PSH, characterized by nodular heterotopia, joint hypermobility, and development of aortic dilatation in early adulthood. MRI typically demonstrated bilateral nodular PSH, indistinguishable from PSH due to FLNA mutations. The female predominance of affected individuals reported by Sheen et al. (2005) and Poussant et al. (2000) suggest an X-linked inheritance pattern, although the clinical characteristics or mode of inheritance are distinct from the X-linked occipital horn syndrome (EDS type IX). Sheen et al. (2005) suggested that patients with PSH and EDS collectively do not fall into any particular EDS classification and the Ehlers–Danlos variant of PSH, in part, represents an overlapping syndrome with X-linked dominant PSH due to FLNA mutations.

*Pain* is a frequent yet poorly characterized clinical finding in EDS and significantly affect the psy-

chosocial functioning of these patients (Lumley et al. 1994). Sacheti et al. (1997) indicated that chronic, frequently debilitating pain of early onset and diverse distribution is a constant feature in most individuals affected with different types of EDS. In this study patients noted elbow pain and pain in their hands, knees and spine. Some patient had abdominal pain and others reported continuous pain in

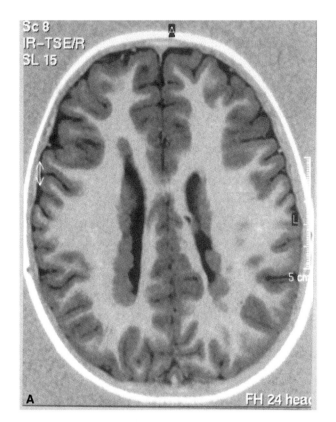

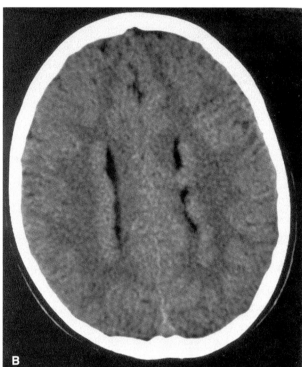

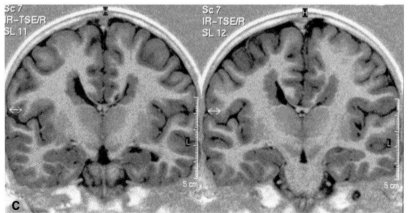

**Fig. 10.** Axial (**A**, **B**) high resolution inversion recovery T1 and T2-weighted magnetic resonance images showing multiple well-circumscribed round masses lining the lateral ventricles: characteristic bilateral subependimal heterotopia. The nodules are isointense to the cortical grey matter. (**C**) Coronal image of the same patient demonstrates grey matter nodules. (**D**) Sagittal image showing hypoplasia of the median part of corpus callosum.

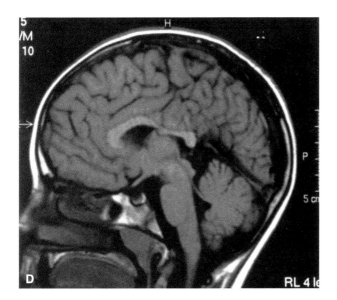

**Fig. 10.** (Continued)

their lower extremities, ankles, feet, toes, and hips. In these cases investigation is necessary to study the origin of pain and the efficacy of specific intervention in patients with EDS.

*Other neurologic manifestation* are reported in patients with EDS. One patient reported by Nagashima et al. (1981) had quadriparesis attributed to ligamentous laxity and instability of the atlanto-occipital and atlantoaxial joints. Echaniz-Laguna et al. (2000) and Ezzeddine et al. (2005) found bilateral frontal polymicrogyria in patients with EDS. Brunk et al. (2004) reported a girl with marked general joint hypermobility, thoracolumbar kyphoscoliosis and several intraspinal extramedullary lesions interpreted as spinal meningeal cysts. In this patients diagnosis of EDS was supported by the specific urinary metabolite pattern of type VI.

Mathew et al. (2005) reported *rare neurological manifestations* in four patients with EDS: bilateral optic atrophy, sensorineural deafness, demyelinating neuropathy, cerebellar ataxia, chorea, action myotonia, polymicrogyria and mirror movements.

Although not always emphasized in the medical literature, patients with EDS often report *easy fatigability* of uncertain origin, as well as *widespread muscle and joint pain*. Rowe et al. (1999) report in 12 cases a previously unappreciated association between EDS, chronic fatigue syndrome and orthostatic intolerance (Rowe et al. 1995, Stewart et al. 1999) and Vilisar et al. (2008) reported a possible association between multiple sclerosis and EDS.

## Pathology

Histologic findings in skin biopsy specimens are variable and sometimes normal (Clark et al. 1980). The abnormality is defined by thickness, array and shape of dermal collagen fibrils (Table 3) (Kobayasi 2004). Collagen fibrils show irregularities in size and orientation. Electron microscopy reveals (Fig. 11) that collagen fibres can be large or irregular in some

**Table 3.** Shape and size of collagen fibrils transversally sectioned

| Parameter | Control | EDS |
|---|---|---|
| Shape factor | 0.99 ± 0.0 | 0.88 ± 0.09 |
| Collagen fibrils diameter (nm) | 50.34 ± 0.64 | 67.21 ± 4.65 |

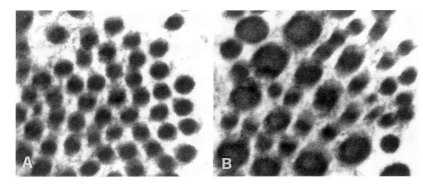

**Fig. 11.** Small (**A**) and large and irregular (**B**) collagen fibres in EDS skin biopsies seen at the electron microscope.

EDS type (types I–III) but they can be also small or various in others (Byers et al. 1979, Holbrook et al. 1981). Occasionally fibrils with a cauliflower configuration are observed (Bouma et al. 2001, Pièrard et al. 1988). Clinical variant of EDS cannot be differentiated on the basis of ultrasrucutral findings (Kobayasi et al. 1984). Age-dependent ultrasrucutral change of broad elastic fibres in skin specimen from EDS have been evaluated (Kobayasi 2005) in reticular dermis and categorized in infantile, adolescent, adult e senile pattern. A degeneration was first found in adolescent pattern by disarrayed microfibrils and degenerative matrix. Degeneration proceeded in adult pattern and ended in senile pattern. In EDS the degeneration starts earlier and it is more severe than the controls (Kobayasi 2005).

## Natural history

EDS is diagnosed and classified on the basis of medical family history, and physical examination with laboratory confirmation when possible at the protein level (collagen 1, 3 and 5 in fibroblast and tenascin-X in serum) and/or at the molecular level. Certain findings in a review of a patient's history can lead to suspicion for EDS. Reports of skin that is easily bruised, torn, or scarred are common. Poor wound healing is not rare and the use of sutures is usually a problem in patients, in whom easy dehiscence and cigarette-paper-like scars may be observed. Frequently these scars are found on the knees. The joints are hyperextensible, sometimes dramatically, but the degree of involvement is variable. In addition the patients may have frequent dislocations of the shoulders and knees but they are usually able to reduce them with no pain. Joints that the patients hyperextend may cause chronic pain. Family members with similar characteristics can contribute to a positive family history. Delayed motor development may also be present in the patient's history due to hypotonia caused by EDS. Muscle weakness is often present, and parents complain of an easy tendency to fall down and poor body control. Sometimes difficult walking is present. The mental development is normal. Seizures are associated with a poor progno-

sis. The vascular type of EDS (Type IV) is less frequent than the classic type but it is the most serious and life-threatening of all. The patients with EDS type IV, often, have a shortened lifespan and spontaneous haemorrhage, aneurysms, arterial dissection, bowel perforation and uterine rupture are major causes of morbidity and mortality. Pregnant women with the vascular type of EDS are at an increased risk for severe complications. In this type sudden death can occur after visceral perforation or after rupture of a large vessel, most commonly an abdominal or splenic vessel. The other types of EDS usually are not life-threatening, and affected patients can live healthy with a somewhat restricted life.

## Pathogenesis/molecular genetics

Patients with EDS demonstrate connective tissue abnormalities as a result of defects in the inherent strength, elasticity, integrity, and healing properties of the tissues. The specific characteristics of a particular form of EDS stem from the tissue's specific distribution of various components of the extracellular matrix. Each tissue and organ system express an array of connective proteins. The specific interactions of the various components of the matrix are tissue specific. EDS is caused by a variety of abnormalities in the synthesis and metabolism of collagen. A minimum of 29 genes contribute to the collagen protein structure, and the genes are located on 15 different chromosomes and form at least 19 identifiable forms of collagen molecules. In EDS types I and II, the classic variety, identifying the molecular structure in most affected patients is difficult. Mutations in the COL5A1 (De Paepe et al. 1997) and the COL5A2 gene encoding the a1 (V) and the a2 (V) chains, respectively of type V collagen have been shown to cause the disorder, but it is unknown what proportion of classic EDS patients carries a mutation in either gene. The COL5A1 and COL5A2 gene are located, respectively on the long arm of chromosome 2q31 and on the long arm of chromosome 9q34.2-34.3. Although one half of the mutations that cause EDS types I and II are likely to affect the COL5A1 gene, a significant portion of the mutations result in low levels of messenger RNA (mRNA) from the mutant allele as a consequence of nonsense-mediated mRNA decay (Schwarze et al. 2000).

De Paepe et al. (2005) reported in their 48 patients, a total of 17 mutations leading to a premature stop codon and five structural mutations were identified in the COL5A1 and COL5A2 genes. In three patients with a positive COL5A1 null-allele test, no causal mutation was found. Overall, in 25 out of 48 patient with classic EDS, an abnormality in type V collagen was confirmed. Variability in severity of phenotype was observed, but no significant genotype-phenotype correlations emerged form this study. The relatively low mutation detection rate suggests that other genes are involved in EDS classic form. The authors excluded the COL1A1, COL1A2, and DCN gene as major candidate genes for classic EDS, since no causal mutation in these genes was found in a number of patients who tested negative for COL5A1 and COL5A2.

All patients with confirmed type IV EDS by biochemical and molecular methods display autosomal dominant inheritance (Beighton 1993). Apparent autosomal recessive transmission may result from parental mosaicism (Beyers 1994). Patients with EDS type IV have abnormal production of type III collagen, the major collagen type in blood vessels, bowel and uterus (North et al. 1995). Many different mutations of the COL3A1 gene on chromosome 2 have been detected, including point mutations, exon skipping mutations and multi-exon deletions, all of which result in abnormal type III precollagen (Byers 1994, Pepin et al. 2000). Mutations of the COL3A1 gene are rare in aneurysm from patients without EDS IV (Hamano et al. 1998).

Autosomal recessive-type VI EDS, also known as the kyphoscoliotic type, is biochemically attributed to a deficiency in lysyl hydroxylase (LH). More than 20 mutations are identified in the LH1 gene that contributes to LH deficiency and clinical EDS type VI. Yeowell et al. (2000) identified 2 of these mutations in 5 or more unrelated patients: a large duplication of exons 10–16 and a nonsense mutation Y511X in exon 14 of the LH1 gene. Both mutations seem to originate from a single ancestral gene.

Schalkwijk et al. (2001) showed, in eight patients from five families, a new autosomal recessive type of EDS caused by mutations in the extracellular matrix protein tenascin X (TNXB) gene. This new type of EDS is similar to classic form of EDS, including hyperextensible skin, hypermobile joints and easy bruising but without delayed wound healing or atrophic scar formation (Hamel 2004). TNX deficiency is associated with abnormalities in collagen and elastic fibres (Burch et al. 1997), which are the principal components of heart valves and large vessels. Cardiac abnormalities such as mitral valve prolapse and aortic dilatation are reported to be common features of certain EDS types (Beighton et al. 1998). This new type of EDS is associated with congenital adrenal hyperplasia when it is due to a deletion encopassing the CYP21 gene (Schalkwijk et al. 2001, Burch et al. 1997).

## Management

Management of EDS includes mainly prophylactic measures, symptomatic treatment of complications and genetic counselling. It is largely supportive (e.g., physiotherapy, ergotherapy, rehabilitation) and preventive (e.g., surgical precautions, avoiding certain professions and sports, avoiding overweight); it is rarely surgical (e.g., arthrodesis). Avoidance of invasive vascular procedures such as catheterisations is particularly important for patients with EDS and vascular fragility. Monitoring patients for scoliosis is important and patients should seek regular evaluation, also, of nutrition, growth, eyes, heart, skin, and joints (Whitelaw 2004). Cardiac auscultation and evaluation are important because a murmur of mitral valve prolapse may be noted. Antibiotic prophylaxis for bacterial endocarditis is an easy but important preventive measure. Plastic re-excision of scars sometimes provides acceptable cosmetic results. Patients with EDS types IV or VI should avoid participating in dangerous contact sports. Some authors mention risks with activities that can increase intracranial pressure as a result of the Valsalva effect. An example of one such activity is playing the trumpet.

## Treatment

There is no specific treatment for EDS and individuals problems must be evaluated and cared for appropriately. Treatment of symptoms as they arise and appropriate education is valuable for patients and their families. The loose joints caused by EDS can be painful. Bracing or fusion of joint may be necessary to provide more joint stability and to reduce pain (Hagen et al. 1993). Physical therapy and occupational therapy are important additional treatments for most patients. The physical therapy can teach patients how to strengthen muscles without stressing joints and how to protect their joints. Occupational therapy is useful when devices are necessary for support or protection of joints and ligaments at risk for injury. Avoiding injury is essential and includes making homes safe to prevent falls and avoiding high-impact or collision sports. Weight lifting, stretching, and any activities that cause the joints to lock are contraindicated due to the stress on the joints. Often, children may enjoy demonstrating the hypermonility of their joints to their peers, but this should be avoided because the practice can lead to early degenerative joints disease. Skin care is significant to prevention of complications for patients with EDS because the skin is easily damaged. The patients with EDS should avoid excessive sun exposure.

Medical treatment in EDS is unsatisfactory and only one isolated report showed that patients with type VI disease benefited of 1 year of high-dose vitamin C therapy. However, high-dose vitamin C therapy is not the standard goal of care.

## Genetic counselling

Genetic counselling is part of management and recommended for parents with a family history of EDS. Affected parents should be aware of the type of EDS they have and its mode of inheritance. EDS comprises a very heterogeneous group of collagen diseases and genetic heterogeneity refers to the fact that mutations in different genes can produce the same phenotype. For example EDS type I can result from mutations in 2 collagen genes, either COL5A1 (chromosome bands 9q34.2–34.3) or COL5A2 (band 2q31) (see Tables 1 and 2).

Allelic heterogeneity may be consider in EDS. For example, mutations of type 3 collagen are suggested to be responsible for the phenotype of EDS types III, IV and VII.

Variable expression, also, is a hallmark of autosomal dominant condition. Autosomal dominant EDS exhibits both intrafamilial and interfamilial variability, which is a critical counselling issue in regard to recurrences. Important implications exist for the subtypes of EDS regarding the differences in modes of inheritance and long-term prognoses.

## Acknowledgments

We wish to thank Professor Alberto Caligaro, dean of the Faculty of Medicine and Surgery at the University of Pavia, Department of Experimental Medicine, Section of General Histology and Embryology for his skilful analysis of electron microscopy and histological specimens and collagen samples and for critical discussion of our patients; Dr. Laura Eusti, Department of Pediatrics, University of Pavia is gratefully acknowledged for her precious clinical assistance and for critically reviewing the manuscript.

## References

Alper J (1990) Genetic disorders of the skin. St. Louis: Mosby Year Book.

Andrikopoulos KL, Liu X, Keene DR, Jaenish R, Ramirez F (1995) Targeted mutation in the COL5a2 gene reveals a regulatory role for type V collagen during matrix assembly. Nat Genet 9: 31–36.

Barabas AP (1967) Heterogeneity of the Ehlers–Danlos syndrome: description of three clinical types and a hypothesis to explain the basic defect(s). BMJ 2: 612–613.

Barkovich AJ, Kjos BO (1992) Gray matter heterotopias: MR characteristics and correlation with developmental and neurologic manifestations. Radiology 182: 493–499.

Beighton P (1970) The Ehlers–Danlos syndrome. In: Heinemann W (eds.) Medical Books, London.

Beighton P (1993) The Ehlers–Danlos syndrome. In: Beighton P (eds.) Mckusic's heritable disorders of connective tissue. St. Louis: Mosby, pp. 189–257.

Beighton P, Beighton G (1989) The Man Behind the Syndrome. Berlin: Springer.

Beighton P, De Paepe A, Danks D (1988) International nosology of heritable disorders of connective tissue, Berlin,1986. Am J Med Genet 29: 581–594.

Beighton P, De Paepe A, Hal JG, Hollister DW, Pope FM, Pyeritz RE, Steinmann B, Tsipouras P (1992) Molecular nosology of heritable disorders of connective tissues. Am J Med Genet 42: 431–448.

Beighton P, de Paepe A, Steinmann B, Tsipuoras P, Wenstrup RJ (1998) Ehlers–Danlos syndrome: revised nosology. Am J Med Genet 77: 31–37.

Blereau R (1996) Three relatives with Ehlers–Danlos syndrome. Consultant 36: 2459–2460.

Bohm S, Behrens P, Martinez-Schramm A, Lohr JF (2002) Das Ehlers–Danlos syndrome. Ortopadie 31: 108–121.

Bouma P, Cabral WA, Cole WG, Marini JC (2001) COL5A1 exon 14 splice acceptor mutation causes a functional null allele, haploinsufficiency of alpha 1 (V) and abnormal heterotopic interstitial fibrils in Ehlers–Danlos syndrome II. J Biol Chem 16: 276–284.

Brunk I, Stover B, Ikonomidou C, Brinckmann J, Neumann L (2004) Ehlers–Danlos syndrome type VI with cystic malformations of the meninges in a 7-years-old girl. Eur J Pediatrics 163(4–5): 214–217.

Byers PH (1995) Disorders of collagen biosynthesis and structure. In: Beaudet Al, Sly WS, Valle D (eds.) The metabolic and molecular bases of inherited disease, 7th ed. McGraw-Hill: New York, pp. 65–71.

Byers PH (1997) Ehlers–Danlos syndrome. In: Rimoin DI, Commor JM, Pyeritz RE (eds) Energy and Rimoin's principles and practice of medical genetics, 3rd ed. New-York: Churchill Livingstone, pp. 1067–1081.

Byers PH, Holbrook KA, McGillivray B, MacLoad PM, Lowry RB (1979) Clinical and ultrastructural heterogeneity of type IV Ehlers–Danlos syndrome. Hum Genet 47: 141–150.

Byers PH, Siegel RC, Holbrook KA, Narayanan AS, Bornstein P, Hall JG (1980) X-linked cutis laxa: defective cross-link formation in collagen due to decreased lysyl oxidase activity. N Engl J Med 303: 61–65.

Chen BM, Grinnel AD (1995) Integrins and modulation of transmitter release from motor nerve terminals by stretch. Science 269: 1578–1580.

Chevassus-au-Louis N, Baraban SC, Gaiarsa JL, Ben-Ari Y (1999) Cortical malformations and epilepsy: new insight from animal models. Epilepsia 40: 811–821.

Ciampo E, Iurassich S (1997) La sindrome di Ehlers-Danlos e gli inestetismi dell'acne. Chron Dermatol 7: 343–348.

Clark JG, Kuhn C, Uitto J (1980) Lung collagen in type IV Ehlers–Danlos syndrome: ultrastructural and biochemical studies. Amer Rev Resp Dis 122: 971–978.

Colige A, Sieron AL, Li SW, Schwarze U, Petty E, Wertelecki W (1999) Human Ehlers–Danlos sindrome type VIIC and bovine dermatosparaxis are caused by mutations in the procollagen-I-N-proteinase gene. Am J Hum Genet 65: 308–317.

Cupo LN, Pyeritz RE, Olson JL (1981) Ehlers–Danlos syndrome with abnormal collagen fibrils, sinus of Valsalva aneurysms, myocardial infarction, panacinar emphisema and cerebral heterotopias. Am J Med 71: 1051–1058.

Danlos EA (1908) Un cas de cutis laxa avec tumeurs pur contusion chronique des coudes et des genous. Bull Soc Franc Dermatol Syphiligr 19: 70–72.

De Coster PJ, Malfait F, Martens LC, De Paepe A (2003) Unusual oral findings in dermatosparaxis (Ehlers-Danlos syndrome type VIIC). J Oral Pathol Med 32: 568–570.

De Graaf AS (1973) Neuralgic amyotrophy in identical twins with Ehlers–Danlos syndrome. Eur Neurol 9: 190–196.

De Paepe A, Nuytink L, Hausser I, Anton-Lamprecht I, Naeyaert JM (1997) Mutations in the COLA5A1 gene are causal in the Ehlers–Danlos syndrome I and II. Am J Hum Genet 60: 547–554.

De Paepe A, Malfait F, Coucke P, Symoens S, Loeys B, Nuytinck L (2005) The molecular basis of the classic Ehlers–Danlos syndrome: a comprehensive study of biochemical and molecular findings in 48 unrelated patients. Hum Mutat 25: 28–37.

Debrun GM, AletichVA, MillerNR, DeKeiset RJW (1996) Three cases of spontaneous direct carotid cavernous fistulas associated with Ehlers–Danlos syndrome Type IV. Surg Neurol 46: 247–252.

Desal H, Leaute F, Auffray-Calvier E, Martin S, Guillon B, Robert R, de Kersaint-Gilly A (1997) Direct carotidocavernous fistula. Clinical radiological and therapeutic studies in 49 cases. J Neuroradiol 24: 141–154.

Desal H, Toulgoat F, Raoul S, Guillon B, Bommard S, Naudou-Giron E, Auffray-Calvier E, de Kersaint-Gilly A (2005) Ehlers–Danlos syndrome type IV and recurrent carotid-cavernous fistula. Review of the literature, endovascular approach, technique and difficulties. Neuroradiology 47: 300–304.

Echaniz-laguna A, de Saint-Martin A, Lafontaine AL, Tasch E, Thomas P, Hirsh E (2000) Bilateral focal polymicrogyria in Ehlers–Danlos syndrome. Arch Neurol 57: 123–127.

Edwards A, Taylor GW (1969) Ehlers–Danlos syndrome with vertebral artery aneurysm. Proceedings of the Royal Society of Medicine 62: 734–735.

Ehlers E (1901) Danische dermatologische Gesellschaft 15. Sitzung vom 15 Dezember 1900. Dermatol Z 8: 173–175.

El-Shaker M, Watts HG (1991) Acute brachial plexus neuropathy secondary to halo-gravity traction in a patient with Ehlers–Danlos syndrome. Spine 16: 385–386.

Eksioglu Y, Scheffer IE, Cardenas P (1996) Periventricular heterotopia: an X-linked dominant epilepsy locus causing aberrant cerebral cortical development. Neuron 16: 77–87.

Ezzedine H, Sabourand P, Eschard C, El Tourjuman O, Bednarek N, Motte J (2005) Bilateral frontal polymicrogyria and Ehlers–Danlos syndrome. Arch de Pediatrie 12: 173–175.

Farag TI, Schimke RN (1989) Ehlers–Danlos syndrome: a new oculo-scoliotic type with associated polyneuropathy? Clin Genet 35: 121–124.

Franceschini P, Guala A, Licata D, Di Cara G, Franceschini D (2000) Arterial tortuosity syndrome. Am J Med Genet 91: 141–143.

Gage J, Moloney FB (1995) Collagen type in dysfunctional temporomandibular joints disks. J Prosthetdent 74: 517–520.

Galan E, Koussef BG (1995) Peripheral Neuropathy in Elhers-Danlos syndrome. Pediatr Neurol 12: 242–245.

Germain DP (2002) Clinical and genetic features of vascular Ehlers–Danlos syndrome. Ann Vasc surg 16: 391–397.

Giunta C, Chambaz C, Pedemonte M, Scapolan S, Steinmann B (2008) The arthrochalasia type of Ehlers-Danlos syndrome (EDS VIIA and VIIB): the diagnostic value of collagen fibril ultrastructure. Am J Med Genet A 146: 1341–1346.

Gloviczki P, Oderich G, Panneton JM, Thomas C, Bower TC, Noralane M, Lindor NM, Kennet JC, Cherry J, Noel AA, Kalra M, Sullivan T (2005) The spectrum, management and clinical outcome of Ehlers–Danlos syndrome type IV: a 30-year experience. J Vasc Surg 42: 98–106.

Gomez-Sugranes JR, Luengo Rodriguez de Ledesma L, Castellotte Caixal M, Ros Lopez S, Mayayo Artral E (1995) Perforation of small intestine diverticulum in Ehlers–Danlos syndrome. Rev Esp Enferm Dig 87(1): 53–55.

Grahame R (2000) Hypermobility-not a circ act. Int J Clin Pract 54(5): 314–315.

Gupta P, Gleeson AP (2000) A rare case of head injury associated with Ehlers–Danlos syndrome. Injury Int J Care Injured 31: 641–643.

Hagen K (1993) What's wrong with this patient? RN 56: 34–37.

Halbach VV, Higashida RT, Dowd CF, Barnwell SL, Hieshima GB (1990) Treatment of carotid cavernous fistulas associated with Ehlers–Danlos syndrome. Neurosurgery 26: 1021–1027.

Hamel BCJ (2004) Ehlers–Danlos syndrome. J Med 62: 141–142.

Heidbreder AE, Ringelstein EB, Dittrich R, Nabavi D, Metze D, Kuhlenbäumer G (2008) Assessment of skin extensibility and joint hypermobility in patients with spontaneous cervical artery dissection and Ehlers-Danlos syndrome. J Clin Neurosci 15: 650–653.

Heim P, Raghunath M, Meiss L, Heisse U, Myllyla R, Kohlschutter A, Steinmann B (1998) Ehlers–Danlos syndrome type VI (EDSVI): problems of diagnosis and management. Acta Paediatr 87: 708–710.

Herrero F (1995) Ehlers–Danlos syndrome and epilepsy: a case study. Epilepsia 36(3): 240.

Holbrook KA, Byers PH (1981) Ultrastrucutral characteristics of the skin in a form of the Ehlers–Danlos syndrome type IV. Lab Invest 44: 342–350.

Hollister DW (1978) Heritable disorders of connective tissues: Ehlers–Danlos syndrome. Pediatr Clin North Am 25: 575–591.

Holzberg M, Hevan-Lowe KO, Olansky AJ (1987) The Ehlers–Danlos syndrome: recognition, characterization and importance of a milder variant of the classic form. J Am Acad Dermatol 19: 656–666.

Holzschuch M, Woerrgen C, Brawanski A (1996) Transcranial Doppler sonography in a patient with Ehlers–Danlos syndrome: case report. Neurosurgery 39: 170–172.

Hunter GC, Malone JM, Moore WS, Misiarowski DL, Chvapli M (1982) Vascular manifestations in patients with Ehlers–Danlos syndrome. Arch Surg 117: 495–498.

Huttenlocher PR, Taravath S, Mojtahedi S (1994) Periventricular heterotopias and epilepsy. Neurology 44: 51–55.

Iurassich S, Rocco D, Aurilia A (2001) Type III Ehlers–Danlos syndrome. Correlations among clinical signs, ultrasound, and histologic findings in a study of 35 cases. Int J Dermatol 40: 175–178.

Jacome DE (1999a) Headache in Ehlers–Danlos syndrome. Chefalalgia 19: 791–796.

Jacome DE (1999b) Epilepsy in Ehlers–Danlos syndrome. Epilepsia 19: 467–473.

Jansen LH (1955) The structure of the connective tissue, an explanation of the symptoms of Ehlers–Danlos syndrome. Dermatologica 110: 108–120.

Johnson SAM (1949) Ehlers–Danlos syndrome: a clinical and genetic study. Arch Dermatol Syph 60: 82–105.

Judisch GF, Waziri M, Krachmer JH (1976) Ocular Ehlers–Danlos syndrome with normal lysyl hydroxylase activity. Arch Ophthalmol 94: 1489–1491.

Kaler SG, Gallo LK, Proud VK (1994) Occipital horn syndrome and a mild Menkes phenotype associated with splice site mutations at the MNK locus. Nat Genet 8: 195–202.

Kayed K, Kass B (1979) Acute multiple brachial neuropathy and Ehlers–Danlos syndrome. Neurology 29: 1620–1621.

Kinnane J, Priebe C, Caty M, Kuppermann N (1995) Perforation of the colon in an adolescent girl. Pediatr Emerg Care 11(49): 230–232.

Kobayasi T (2004) Abnormality of dermal collagen fibrils in Ehlers–Danlos syndrome. Anticipation of the abnormality for the inherited hypermobile disorders. Eur J Dermatol 14(4): 221–229.

Kobayasi T (2005) Dermal elastic fibres in the inherited hypermobile disorders. J Dermat Sci (in press).

Kobayasi T, Oguchi M, Asboe-Hansen G (1984) Dermal changes in Ehlers–Danlos sindrome. Clin Genet 25(6): 477–484.

Krog M, Almgren B, Eriksson I, Nordstrom S (1983) Vascular complications in the Ehlers–Danlos syndrome. Acta Chirurgica Scandinavica 149: 279–282.

Laporte-Turpin E, Marcoux MO, Machado G, Dulac Y, Claudet I, Grouteau E, Puget C (2005) Lethal aortic dissection in a 13-year-old boy with a vacular Ehlers–Danlos syndrome. Arch de Pediatrie 12: 1112–1115.

Lazoff SG, Rybak JJ, Parker BR, Luzzatti L (1975) Skeletal dysplasia, occipital horns, diarrhea and obstructive uropathy: a new hereditary syndrome. Birth Defects 11: 71–74.

Lees MH, Menashe VD, Sunderland CO (1969) Ehlers–Danlos syndrome associated with multiple pulmonary artery stenoses and tortuous systemic arteries. J Pediatr 75(6): 1031–1036.

Lumley MA, Jordan M, Rubinstein R, Tsipouras P, Evans MI (1994) Psychosocial functioning in the Ehelrs–Danlos syndrome. Am J Med Genet 53: 149–152.

Mallory SB, Krafchik BR (1991) What syndrome is this? Pediatr Dermatol 8(4): 348–351.

Mathew T, Sinha S, Taly AB, Arunodaya GR, Srikanth SG (2005) Neurological manifestations of Ehlers–Danlos syndrome. Neurol India 53(3): 339–341.

McKusick VA (1956) Heritable disorders of connective tissue. St Louis: Mosby.

McKusick VA (1986) Catologs of autosomal dominant autosomal recessive, and X-linked phenotypes. In: Hopkins J (ed.) Mendelian inheritance in man, 3rd ed. Baltimore: University Press.

Mirza FH, Smith PL, Lim WN (1979) Multiple aneurysms in a patient with Ehlers–Danlos syndrome: angiography without sequelae. Am J Radiol 132: 993–995.

Nagashima C, Tsuji R, Kubota M, Tajima J (1981) Atlanto-axial, atlanto-occipital dislocations, development canal stenosis in the Ehlers–Danlos syndrome. No Shinkei geka 9: 601–608.

Narcisi P, Richards AJ, Ferguson SD (1994) A family with Ehlers–Danlos syndrome type III/articular hypermobility syndrome has a glycine 637 to serine in type III collagen. Hum Mol Genet 3: 1617–1620.

North KN, White man DA, Pepin MG, Byers PH (1995) Cerebrovascular complications in Ehlers–Danlos syndrome type IV. Ann Neurol 38: 960–964.

Papapetropoulos T, Tsankanikas C (1981) Brachial neuropathy and Ehlers–Danlos syndrome. Neurology 31: 642–643.

Parapia LA, Jackson C (2008) Ehlers-Danlos syndrome-a historical review. Br J Haematol 141: 32–35.

Pepin M, Schwarze U, Superti-Fuga A, Byers PH (2000) Clinical and genetic features of Ehlers–Danlos syndrome type IV, the vascular type. N Eng J Med 342: 673–680.

Piérard GE, Lé T, Piérard-Franchimont C, Lapière CM (1988) Morphometric study of cauliflower collagen fibrils in Ehlers–Danlos syndrome type I. Collagen Rel Res 8: 453–457.

Pinnel SR, Krane SM, Kenzora JE, Glincher MJ (1972) A heritable disorder of connective tissue: hydroxylysine-deficient collagen disease. N Eng J Med 286: 1013–1020.

Pope FM, Martin GR, Lichtenstein JR (1975) Patients with Ehlers–Danlos syndrome type IV lack type III collagen. Proc Natl Acad Sci USA 72: 1314–1316.

Pope FM (1991) Molecular analysis of Ehlers–Danlos syndrome type II. Br J Rheumatol 30: 163–166.

Pouassaint TY, Fox JW, Dobyns WB, Radke R, Scheffer IE, Berkovic SF, Barnes PD, Huttenlocher PR, Walsh CA (2000) Periventricular nodular heterotopia in patients with filamin-1 gene mutations: neuroimaging findings. Pediatr Radiol 748–755.

Pretorius ME, Butler IJ (1983) Neurologic manifestation of Ehlers–Danlos syndrome. Neurology 33: 1087–1089.

Pyeritz RE (2000) Ehlers–Danlos syndrome. In: Goldmann L, Bennet JC (eds.) Cecil textbook of medicine, 21st ed. Philadelphia: Saunders, pp. 1119–1120.

Reed WB (1972) Ehlers–Danlos syndrome with neurological complications. Arch Dermatol 106: 410–411.

Rowe PC, Bou-Holaigah I, Kan JS, Calkins H (1995) Is neurally mediated hypotension an unrecognised cause of chronic fatigue? Lancet 345: 623–624.

Rowe PC, Barron DF, Calkins H, Maumenee IH, Tong PY, Geraghty MT (1999) Orthostatic intolerance and chronic fatigue syndrome associated with Ehlers–Danlos syndrome. J Pediatr 135: 494–499.

Rubinstein MK, Cohen NH (1964) Ehelrs-Danlos syndrome associated with multiple intracranial aneurysms. Neurology 14: 125–132.

Sacheti A, Szemere J, Bernstein B, Tafas T, Schechter N (1997) Chronic pain is a manifestation of the Ehlers–Danlos syndrome. J Pain Symptom Manage 14: 88–93.

Sakai LY (1995) The extracellular matrix. Sci Am 2: 58–67.

Savasta S, Crispino M, Valli M, Calligaro A, Zambelloni C, Poggiani C (2007) Subependymal periventricular heterotopias in a patient with Ehlers–Danlos syndrome: a new case. J Child Neurol 22: 317–320.

Schady W, Ochoa J (1984) Ehlers–Danlos syndrome in association with tomaculous neuropathy. Neurology 34: 1270.

Schievink WI, Limburg M, Oorthuys JW, Fleury P, Pope FM (1990) Cerebrovascular disease in Ehlers–Danlos syndrome type IV. Stroke 21: 626–632.

Schievink WI, Piepgras DG, Earnest VE, Gordon H (1991) Spontaneous carotid-cavernous fistulae in Ehlers–Danlos syndrome type IV. J Neurosurg 74: 991–998.

Schievink WI, Gordon OK, Tourje J (2003) Connective tissue disorders with spontaneous spinal cerebrospinal fluid leaks and intracranial hypotension: a prospective study. Neurosurgery 54: 65–71.

Scholman A, Kepes JJ (1967) bilateral spontaneous carotid-cavernous fistulae in Ehlers–Danlos syndrome. J Neurosurg 26: 82–86.

Schwarze U, Atkinson M, Hoffman GG, Greenspan DS, Byers PH (2000) Null alleles of the COL5A1 gene of type V collagen are a case of the classical forms of Ehlers–Danlos syndrome (type I and type II). Am J Hum Genet 66: 1757–1765.

Shapiro SK (1952) a case of Meekrin-Ehlers–Danlos syndrome with neurological manifestation. J Nerv Ment Dis 115: 64–71.

Sheen VL, Jansen A, Chen MH, Parrini E, Morgan T, Ravenscroft R, Ganesh V, Underwood T, Wiley J, Leventer R, Vaid RR, Ruiz DE, Hutchins GM, Menasha J, Willner J, Geng Y, Gripp KW, Nicholson L, Berry-Kravis E, Bodell A, Apse K, Guerrini R, Walsh CA (2005) Filamin A mutation cause periventricular heterotopia with Ehlers–Danlos syndrome. Neurology 64: 254–262.

Shukla AR, Bellah RA, Canning DA (2004) Giant bladder diverticula causing bladder obstruction. Urology 172: 1977–1979.

Silverman FN, Gilden JJ (1959) Congenital insensitivity to pain: a neurologic syndrome with bizarre skeletal lesions. Radiology 72: 176–190.

Steinmann B, Royce PM, Superti-Furga A (1993) The Ehlers–Danlos syndrome. In: Royce PM, Steinmann B (eds.) Connective tissues and its heritable disorders. Molecular, genetic, and medical aspects. New York: Wiley-Liss, pp. 351–407.

Steinmann B, Royce PM, Superti-Furga A (2002) The Ehlers–Danlos syndrome. In: Royce PM, Steinmann B (eds.) Connective tissues and its heritable disorders, 2nd ed. New York: Wiley-Liss, pp. 431–523.

Stewart JM, Gewitz MH, Weldon A, Arlievsky N, Li K, Munoz J (1999) Orthostatic intolerance in adolescent chronic fatigue syndrome. Pediatrics 103: 116–121.

Thomas P, Bossan A, Lacour JP, Chanalet S, Ortone JP, Chatel M (1996) Ehlers–Danlos syndrome with subependimal periventricular heterotopias. Neurology 46: 1165–1167.

Tschernogobow A (1892) Cutis laxa. Mhft Prakt Dermatol 14: 76.

Vilisar J, Harikrishnan S, Suri M, Constantinescu CS (2008) Ehlers-Danlos syndrome and multiple sclerosis: a possible association. Mult Scler Jan 31 [Epub ahead of print].

Wahab AA, Janahi IA, Eltohami A, Zeid A, Haque NF, Teebi AS (2003) A new type of Ehlers–Danlos syndrome associated with tortuous systemic arteries in a large kindred from Qatar. Acta Paediatr 92: 456–462.

Wang N, Butler JP, Ingber DE (1993) Mechanotransduction across the cell surface and through the cytoskeleton. Science 260: 1124–1227.

Wenstrup RJ, Murad S, Pinnel SR (1989) EDS type VI: clinical manifestation of collagen lysylhydroxylase deficiency. J Pediatr 115: 405–409.

Whitelaw SE (2004) Ehelrs-Danlos syndrome, classical type: case management. Dermatol Nurs 16(5): 433–449.

Who named it? (2006) A dictionary of medical biographies. http://www.whonamedit.com

Yeowell HN, Pinnel SR (1993) The Ehlers–Danlos syndrome. Semin Dermatol 12: 229–240.

Yiş U, Dirik E, Chambaz C, Steinmann B, Giunta C (2008) Differential diagnosis of muscular hypotonia in infants: the kyphoscoliotic type of Ehlers-Danlos syndrome (EDS VI). Neuromuscul Disord 18: 210–214.

Zaidi SHE, Peltekova V, Meyer S, Lindinger A, Paterson AD, Tsui LC, Faiyaz-UI-Haque M, Teebi AS (2004) A family exhibiting arterial tortuosity syndrome displays homozygosity for markers in the arterial tortuosity locus at chromosome 20q13. Clin Genet 67: 183–188.

# Chapter 57

# LIPOID PROTEINOSIS

**Takahiro Hamada**

Department of Dermatology, Kurume University School of Medicine, Asahimachi, Kurume, Fukuoka, Japan

## Introduction

The autosomal recessive disorder lipoid proteinosis (LiP; OMIM # 247100) is a rare genodermatosis that presents in early infancy with hoarseness, followed by pox-like and acneiform scars, along with infiltration and thickening of the skin and certain mucous membranes. The disorder is characterized by deposits of amorphous hyaline-like material in the skin and mucous membranes. Neurologic and psychiatric abnormalities such as epilepsy, sometimes in association with calcification with intracranial calcification, may also occur.

Although the etiology is still unclear, LiP was recently mapped to chromosome 1q21 and pathogenetic loss-of-function mutations were identified in the extracellular matrix protein 1 gene (*ECM1*). So far, more than 25 different pathogenic mutations in this gene have been identified. These data now may give us some implications for the pathogenesis of this disorder.

## Historical perspective and eponyms

LiP was first described in 1929 by **Erich Urbach**, an Austrian–American allergologist and dermatologist, born in 1893 in Prague and died in 1946 and **Camillo Wiethe**, an Austrian otolaryngologist born in Vienna in 1888 and died in 1949 (Urbach and Wiethe 1929, Who named it? 2006). Erich Urbach went to medical school at the University of Vienna for two years. When the 1st World War broke out he served in the Austrian army as a lieutenant and a member of the surgical group of professor Anton Freiherr von Eiselsberg (1860–1939) and was decorated for bravery. Urbach graduated doctor of medi-

cine from the University of Vienna under Wilhelm Kerl (1880–1945) in 1919. He worked in the internal departments of the Wiener allgemeines Krankenhaus under Jakob Pal (1863–1936) and Wilhelm Schlesinger (1869–1947), at the skin department under Salomon Ehrmann (1854–1926), at the Breslau skin clinic under Josef Jadassohn (1863–1936), and was an assistant at the skin department of the Rothschildspital in Vienna under Hans Königstein (1878–1954). In 1929 he was habilitated for skin and venereal diseases at his alma mater, becoming Dozent. He was subsequently assistant physician at the II skin clinic with Wilhelm Kerl. From 1936 to 1938 he was chief physician at the department of dermatology and allergy at the Merchant's hospital, Vienna, but with the advent of Hitler he migrated to the United States in 1938 and became an associate of dermatology at the University of Pennsylvania. From 1939 he was chief of the allergy department of the Jewish Hospital, Philadelphia. He was the author of many publications and published a very popular book "Allergy", with P. M. Gottlieb.

Urbach and Wiethe (1929) originally used the term '*lipoidosis cutis et mucosae*'. A decade later, Urbach changed the name to 'lipoid proteinosis cutis et mucosae', believing that the condition was associated with abnormal lipid and protein deposition in various tissues. Indeed, the condition is also sometimes referred to as Urbach-Wiethe disease. The disorder has also been referred to as 'lipoid proteinosis', 'lipoglycoproteinosis' or, due to the glass-like (hyaline) appearance of tissue sections under microscopy, 'hyalinosis cutis et mucoase' (Findlay et al. 1966, Hofer 1973). Since their report, over 300 cases of this autosomal recessive disorder have been described (Hamada 2002, Newsome 2004).

## Incidence and prevalence

LiP occurs throughout the world, although it appears to be more frequent in some countries in which consanguinity is common or a founder effect has been suspected. LiP is particularly common in the Northern Cape province of South Africa, including Namaqualand, where propagation of a mutated common ancestral allele dating back to a mid-seventeenth century settler from Germany, has been proposed (Gordon et al. 1971, Heyl 1971, Stine and Smith 1990). Recent molecular study confirmed the LiP founder effect in South Africa (Van Hougenhouck-Tulleken et al. 2004).

## Clinical manifestations

### Skin abnormalities

Skin lesions usually develop during the first few years of life or may appear later. The classic and most easily recognizable sign is the beaded eyelid papules (moniliform blepharosis) (Hamada et al. 2003), although the papular infiltration may be quite subtle in some patients (Fig. 1a). Other cutaneous changes may include waxy, yellow papules and nodules with generalized skin thickening (Fig. 1b). Hyperkeratosis may appear in regions exposed to mechanical friction, such as the hands, elbows, knees, buttocks and axillae (Fig. 1c). Sometimes the skin infiltration can appear quite verrucous. During childhood, the skin may be easily damaged by minor trauma or friction, resulting in blisters and scar formation. Pocklike or acneiform scars are particularly evident on the face and extremities (Fig. 1d). Scalp involvement may lead to loss of hair, although alopecia is not a significant finding in most cases of LiP. Histologically, LiP is characterized by deposition or accumulation of hyaline material in the dermis, which is periodic acid-Schiff (PAS)-positive, but diastase-resistant, basement membrane thickening at the dermal-epidermal junction, surrounding blood vessels and adnexal epithelia (Fig. 2a) (Muda et al. 1995). Immunofluorescence labelling with anti-type IV collagen antibody shows bright, thick bands of staining at the dermal-epidermal junction and around blood vessels consistent with basement membrane thickening (Aroni et al. 1998). Similar findings are also observed for anti-type VII collagen immunostaining (Fig. 2b) (Hamada 2002). Ultrastructural examination reveals concentric rings of excess basement membrane surrounding blood vessels and irregular reduplication of lamina densa at the dermal-epidermal junction (Fig. 2c) (Moy et al. 1987). In addition, dermal fibroblasts demonstrate characteristic cytoplasmic vacuole formation (Bauer et al. 1981, Moy et al. 1987). Abnormal lysosomes with curved tubular profiles in dermal eccrine glands and histiocytes, similar to those seen in Farber disease, have also been demonstrated in patients with LiP, which was thought to reflect an abnormality in a degradation pathway of glycolipids or sphingolipids (Navarro et al. 1999).

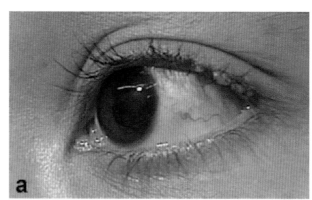
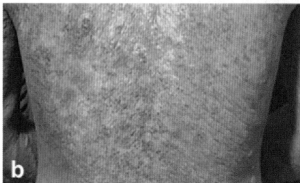

**Fig. 1.** Clinical features of LiP. (**a**) beaded papules on the upper eyelid (moniliform blepharosis); (**b**) waxy nodules and scarring on the back; (**c**) warty, infiltrated plaques on the elbow; (**d**) acneiform scars on the face.

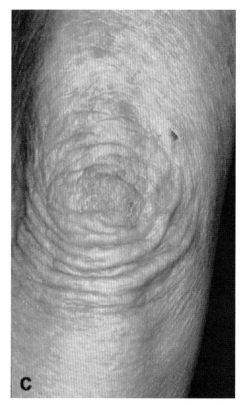

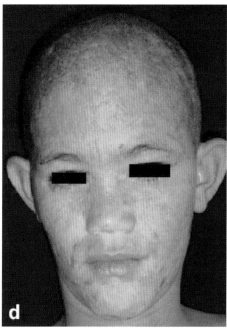

**Fig. 1.** (Continued)

## Abnormalities of other systems and organs

The first clinical sign of LiP is hoarseness, caused by infiltration of the vocal cords. In most cases this develops soon after birth or in the first year of life or, rarely, after a few years. The hoarse nature of the voice is one of the most striking clinical features in LiP (Nanda et al. 2001). The mucosa of the pharynx, tongue, soft palate, tonsils and lips are also infiltrated (Fig. 3) and this may lead to respiratory difficulty, especially in association with an upper respiratory tract infection, sometimes requiring tracheostomy (Ramsey et al. 1985). Difficulty in swallowing, symptoms of a dry mouse, recurrent episodes of inflamed parotid and submandibular glands, poor dental hygiene, and short tongue with a thickened frenulum may all occur (Hopfer 1973, Disdier et al. 1994, Aroni et al. 1998, Van Hougenhouck-Tulleken et al. 2004).

## Nervous system abnormalities

Neurologic and psychiatric abnormalities may include epilepsy and memory deficits, social and behavioral changes, paranoid symptoms, mental retardation, aggressiveness and generalized dystonia, sometimes in association with calcification in the temporal lobes or hippocampi (Friedman et al. 1984, Kleinert et al. 1987, Teive et al. 2004, Thornton et al. 2008).

The epilepsy typically manifests as complex partial seizures often with visual or olfactory hallucinations (Moy et al. 1992). Other forms of epilepsy including generalized tonic-clonic seizures, have been reported but are less frequent than partial seizures (Newsome 2004, Staut and Naidich 1998). The EEG in these patients may be abnormal without clinical epilepsy. Seizures tend to present in adulthood (Barthelemy et al. 1986, Hofer 1973, Newsome 2004).

Memory loss can occur and intelligence varies from low normal to normal. Memory impairment is often out of proportion to the overall intellectual disturbance.

Paresthesias over the skin lesions are occasionally reported and suggest peripheral nerve involvement.

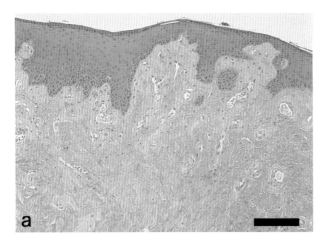

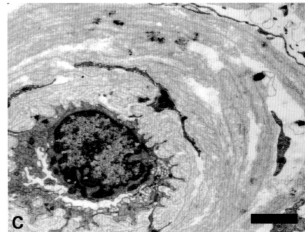

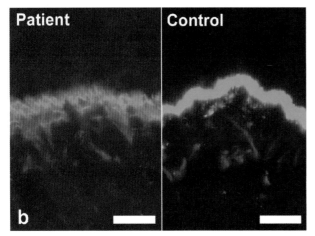

**Fig. 2.** Histological findings of LiP. (**a**) hematoxylin and eosin staining showing accumulation of hyaline material in the dermis. Bar = 0.1 mm; (**b**) immunofluorescence labelling with anti-type VII collagen antibody shows irregular, broad staining at the dermal-epidermal junction in LiP skin compared to bright, linear labelling in the control. Bar = 50 μm; (**c**) transmission electron microscopy reveals marked concentric reduplication of basement membrane around blood vessel. Bar = 2 μm.

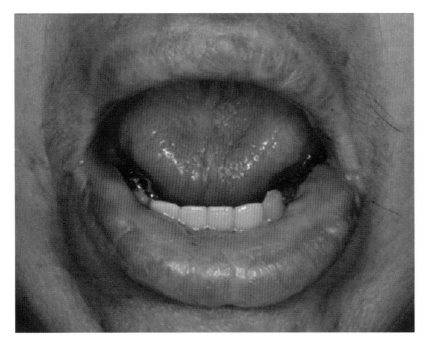

**Fig. 3.** Infiltrations on the lips and tongue.

## Imaging

Patients with LiP may develop: (a) intracranial calcifications in the medial temporal region that are located superolateral to dorsum sella projecting over the medial aspect of the orbits in the frontal view (bena-shaped; inverted commas) and in the globus pallidus, and head of the caudate. Temporal lobe calcifications occurs in 50–75% of patients, and the amygdala seems to be preferentially affected; (b) vocal cord thickening (diffuse or nodular); (c) reticular and nodular densities in the lungs (Lachman 1996).

## Natural history

Life expectancy of individuals with LiP is normal, aside from the risks of respiratory obstruction (Hofer 1973).

## Pathogenesis/molecular genetics

Increased amounts of hexuronic acid and mRNA for the alpha polypeptide of type IV collagen in cultured LiP fibroblast has been described (Bauer et al. 1981, Olsen et al. 1998), whereas decreased mRNA for type I procollagen has been demonstrated (Moy et al. 1987). Thus, collectively there appears to be an underproduction of the fibrous collagens to offset the overproduction of basement membrane collagens. Despite these and other studies, no evidence has emerged to implicate a specific skin structural protein in the primary pathogenesis of LiP.

LiP was recently shown to result from loss-of-function mutations in the extracellular matrix protein 1 gene (*ECM1*) on chromosome 1q21.2 (Hamada et al. 2002). Over 25 pathogenic mutations have been detected, most of which are specific to individual families (Fig. 4) (Hamada et al. 2002, 2003; Chan et al. 2003, 2004a, 2007; Teive et al. 2004). Mutations have been detected in all exons of *ECM1*, apart from the alternatively spliced exon 5a, but more than half of mutations occurred in exon 6 or the alternatively spliced exon 7 (Chan et al. 2004a). Another recent molecular study confirmed the LiP founder effect in the Northern Cape province of South Africa, including Namaqualand (Van Hougenhouck-Tulleken et al. 2004). A homozygous nonsense mutation in exon 7 of the *ECM1* gene, Q276X, was identified in all patients from this area. Individuals with mutations in exon 7 tended to have slightly milder phenotypes but this was not universal. No genotype-phenotype correlation was identified for presence of intracranial calcification or neuropsychiatric abnormalities. Further mutation analysis in LiP patients will be necessary to establish more robust genotype-phenotype correlation. Recently, rapid diagnosis of LiP by skin immunohistochemistry using an anti-ECM1 antibody has been reported (Chan et al. 2004b). Affected individuals showed reduced or absent skin immunostaining.

Human ECM1 encodes a glycoprotein of unknown function, the counterpart to an 85-kDa secreted protein first identified in a murine osteogenic stromal cell line, MN7 (Bhalerao et al. 1995, Johnson et al. 1997, Smits et al. 1997). Previously it has been shown that ECM1 has key roles in bone mineralization, epidermal differentiation and in aspects of

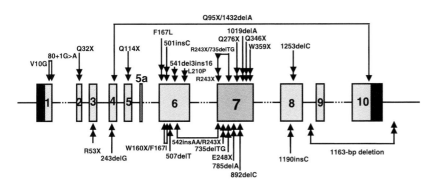

**Fig. 4.** Schematic representation of all known pathogenic mutations in the *ECM1* gene in LiP. Double arrowheads indicate homozygous mutations.

angiogenesis (Smits et al. 2000, Deckers et al. 2001, Han et al. 2001). In addition, a key interaction has recently been demonstrated between ECM1 and perlecan, a major heparan sulphate proteoglycan of basement membranes (Mongiat et al. 2003). Moreover, other recent studies have identified circulating autoantibodies against ECM1 in most patients with lichen sclerosus, a common acquired inflammatory skin disorder, that has several histopathologic features in common with LiP (Oyama et al. 2003, 2004; Chan et al. 2004c). These observations may indicate that one of the main functions of ECM1 in the dermis is to act as a form of "biological glue" maintaining dermal homeostasis, including regulation of basement membrane and interstitial collagen fibril macro-assembly as well as growth factor binding (Chan, 2004).

## Diagnosis, follow-up and management

Characteristic mucocutaneous features make the diagnosis relatively easy. Furthermore, demonstration of pathogenetic mutations in ECM1 in LiP now provides a definitive means of establishing a diagnosis through molecular gene analysis. Although there have been many therapeutic trials in LiP, including oral steroids and dimethyl sulphoxide, intralesional heparin (Hofer 1973, Wong and Lin 1988), only rarely have there been any sustained benefits, except carbon dioxide laser surgery of thickened vocal cords and infiltration around eyelids (Haneke et al. 1984, Rosenthal et al. 1997). Identification of mutations in ECM1 in LiP might provide a basis for the development of more rational forms of treatment, including trials of recombinant gene/protein for skin or respiratory mucosa.

## Differential diagnosis

Some cases of LiP had been thought to have clinico-pathological features in common with certain types of porphyria (e.g. erythropoietic protoporphyria) as well as some forms of cutaneous amyloidosis (Hofer 1973, Parker 1980, Touart and Sau

1998). Some of the ultrastructural changes seen around blood vessels may also resemble abnormalities seen in diabetic microangiopathy (Hofer 1973).

## Genetic counseling

Molecular basis of LiP could now provide feasible carrier screening, improved genetic counseling and DNA-based prenatal diagnosis, as appropriate.

## Acknowledgements

This original molecular studies referred to in this article were carried out in collaboration with the members of Genetic Skin Disease Group at St John's Institute of Dermatology for whose assistance and stimulation the author is most grateful. I am especially grateful to Prof. J. McGrath.

## References

Aroni K, Lazaris AC, Papadimitriou K, Paraskevakou H, Davaris PS (1998) Lipoid proteinosis of the oral mucosa: case report and review of the literature. Pathol Res Pract 194: 855–859.

Barthelemy H, Mauduir G, Kanitakis J, Cambazard E, Thivolet J (1986) Lipoid proteinosis with pseudomembranous conjunctivitis. J Am Acad Dermatol 14: 367–371.

Bauer EA, Santa-Cruz D, Eisen AZ (1981) Lipoid proteinosis: in vivo and in vitro evidence for a lysosomal storage disease. J Invest Dermatol 76: 119–125.

Bhalerao J, Tylzanowski P, Filie JD, Kozak CA, Merregaert J (1995) Molecular cloning, characterization and genetic mapping of the cDNA coding for a novel secretory protein of mouse. Demonstration of alternative splicing in skin and cartilage. J Biol Chem 270: 16385–16394.

Chan I (2004) The role of extracellular matrix protein 1 in human skin. Clin Exp Dermatol 29: 52–56.

Chan I, El-Zurghany A, Zendah B, Benghazil M, Oyama N, Hamada T, McGrath JA (2003) Molecular basis of lipoid proteinosis in a Libyan family. Clin Exp Dermatol 28: 545–548.

Chan I, Sethuraman G, Sharma VK, Bruning E, Hamada T, McGrath JA (2004a) Molecular basis of lipoid proteinosis in two indian siblings. J Dermatol 31: 764–766.

Chan I, Oyama N, South AP, McGrath JA, Oyama N, Bhogal BS, Black MM, Hamada T (2004b) Rapid diagnosis of lipoid proteinosis using an anti-extracellular matrix protein 1 (ECM1) antibody. J Dermatol Sci 35: 151–153.

Chan I, Oyama N, Neill SM, Wojnarowska F, Black MM, McGrath JA (2004c) Characterization of IgG autoantibodies to extracellular matrix protein 1 (ECM1) in lichen sclerosus. Clin Exp Dermatol 29: 499–504.

Chan I, Liu L, Hamada T, Sethuraman G, McGrath JA (2007) The molecular basis of lipoid proteinosis: mutations in extracellular matrix protein 1. Exp Dermatol 16: 881–890.

Deckers MM, Smits P, Karperien M, Ni J, Tylzanowski P, Feng P, Parmelee D, Zhang J, Bouffard E, Gentz R, Lowik CW, Merregaert J (2001) Recombinant human extracellular matrix protein 1 inhibits alkaline phosphatase activity and mineralization of mouse embryonic metatarsals in vitro. Bone 28: 14–20.

Disdier P, Harle JR, Andrac L, Swiader L, Weiller PJ (1994) Specific xerostomia during Urbach-Wiethe disease. Dermatology 188: 50–51.

Findlay G, Scott FP, Cripps DJ (1966) Porphyria and lipid proteinosis. Br J Dermatol 78: 69–80.

Friedman L, Mathews RD, Swanepoel PD (1984) Radiographic and computed tomographic findings in lipid proteinosis. A case report. S Afr Med J 65: 734–735.

Gordon H, Gordon W, Botha V Edelstein I (1971) Lipoid proteinosis. Birth Defects Orig Artic Ser 7: 164–177.

Hamada T (2002) Lipoid proteinosis. Clin Exp Dermatol 27: 624–629.

Hamada T, McLean WHI, Ramsay M, Ashton GHS, Nanda A, Jenkins T, Edelstein I, South AP, Bleck O, Wessagowit V, Mallipeddi R, Orchard GE, Wan H, Dopping-Hepenstal PJC, Mellerio JE, Whittock NV, Munro CS, van Steensel MAM, Steijlen PM, Ni J, Zhang L, Hashimoto T, Eady RAJ McGrath JA (2002) Lipoid proteinosis maps to 1q21 and is caused by mutations in the extracellular matrix protein 1 gene (ECM1). Hum Mol Genet 11: 833–840.

Hamada T, Wessagowit V, South AP, Ashton GH, Chan I, Oyama N, Siriwattana A, Jewhasuchin P, Charuwichitratana S, Thappa DM, Jeevankumar B, Lenane P, Krafchik B, Kulthanan K, Shimizu H, Kaya TI, Erdal ME, Paradisi M, Paller AS, Seishima M, Hashimoto T, McGrath JA (2003) Extracellular matrix protein 1 gene (ECM1) Mutations in lipoid proteinosis and genotype-phenotype correlation. J Invest Dermatol 120: 345–350.

Han Z, Ni J, Smits P, Underhill CB, Xie B, Chen Y, Liu N, Tylzanowski P, Parmelee D, Feng P, Ding I, Gao F, Gentz R, Huylebroeck D, Merregaert J, Zhang L (2001) Extracellular matrix protein 1 (ECM1) has angiogenic properties and is expressed by breast tumor cells. FASEB J 15: 988–994.

Haneke E, Hornstein OP, Meisel-Stosiek M, Steiner W (1984) Hyalinosis cutis et mucosae in siblings. Hum Genet 68: 342–345.

Heyl T (1971) Lipoid proteinosis in South Africa. Dermatologica 142: 129–132.

Hofer P (1973) Urbach-Wiethe disease (lipoglycoproteinosis; lipoid proteinosis; hyalinosis cutis et mucosae). A review. Acta Derm Suppl (Stockh) 53: 1–52.

Johnson MR, Wilkin DJ, Vos HL, Ortiz de Luna RI, Dehejia AM, Polymeropoulos MH, Francomano CA (1997) Characterization of the human extracellular matrix protein 1 gene on chromosome 1q21. Matrix Biol 16: 289–292.

Kleinert R, Cervos-Navarro J, Kleinert G, Walter GF, Steiner H (1987) Predominantly cerebral manifestation in Urbach-Wiethe's syndrome (lipoid proteinosis cutis et mucosae): a clinical and pathomorphological study. Clin Neuropathol 6: 43–45.

Lachman RS (1996) Lipoid proteinosis. In: Taybi H, Lachman RS (eds.) Radiology of syndromes, metabolic disorders, and skeletal dysplasias. 4th ed. St-Louis: Mosby, pp. 650–651.

Mongiat M, Fu J, Oldershaw R Greenhalgh R, Gown AM, Iozzo RV (2003) Perlecan protein core interacts with extracellular matrix protein 1 (ECM1), a glycoprotein involved in bone formation and angiogenesis. J Biol Chem 278: 17491–17499.

Moy LS, Moy RL, Matsuoka LY Ohta A, Uitto J (1987) Lipoid proteinosis: ultrastructural and biochemical studies. J Am Acad Dermatol 16: 1193–1201.

Muda AO, Paradisi M, Angelo C, Mostaccioli S, Atzori F, Puddu P, Faraggiana T (1995) Lipoid proteinosis: clinical, histologic, and ultrastructural investigations. Cutis 56: 220–224.

Nanda A, Alsaleh QA, Al-Sabah H, Ali AM, Anim JT (2001) Lipoid proteinosis: report of four siblings and brief review of the literature. Pediatr Dermatol 18: 21–26.

Navarro C, Fachal C, Rodriguez C, Padro L, Dominguez C (1999) Lipoid proteinosis. A biochemical and ultrastructural investigation of two new cases. Br J Dermatol 141: 326–331.

Newsome D (2004) Lipoid proteinosis. In: Roach ES, Miller VS (eds.) Neurocutaneous disorders. New York: Cambridge University Press, pp. 318–322.

Olsen DR, Chu ML, Uitto J (1998) Expression of basement membrane zone genes coding for type IV procollagen and laminin by human skin fibroblasts in vitro: elevated alpha 1 (IV) collagen mRNA levels in lipoid proteinosis. J Invest Dermatol 90: 734–738.

Oyama N, Chan I, Neill SM, Hamada T, South AP, Wessagowit V, Wojnarowska F, D'Cruz D, Hughes GJ,

Black MM, McGrath JA (2003) Autoantibodies to extracellular matrix protein 1 in lichen sclerosus. Lancet 362: 118–123.

Oyama N, Chan I, Neill SM, South AP, Wojnarowska F, Kawakami Y, D'Cruz D, Mepani K, Hughes GJ, Bhogal BS, Kaneko F, Black MM, McGrath JA (2004) Development of antigen-specific ELISA for circulating autoantibodies to extracellular matrix protein 1 in lichen sclerosus. J Clin Invest 113: 1550–1559.

Parker JM (1980) Erythropoietic protoporphyria. Cutis 26: 247–250.

Ramsey ML, Tschen JA, Wolf JE Jr (1985) Lipoid proteinosis. Int J Dermatol 24: 230–232.

Rosenthal G, Lifshits T, Monos T (1997) Carbon dioxide laser treatment for lipoid proteinosis (Urbach-Wiethe syndrome) involving the eyelids. Br J Ophthalmol 81: 252–254.

Smits P, Ni J, Feng P, Wauters J, Van Hul W, Boutaibi ME, Dillon PJ, Merregaert J (1997) The human extracellular matrix gene 1 (ECM1): genomic structure, cDNA cloning, expression pattern and chromosomal localization. Genomics 45: 487–495.

Smits P, Poumay Y, Karperien M, Tylzanowski P, Wauters J, Huylebroeck D, Ponec M, Merregaert J (2000) Differentiation-dependent alternative splicing and expression of the extracellular matrix protein 1 gene in human keratinocytes. J Invest Dermatol 114: 718–724.

Staut CCV, Naidich TP (1998) Urbach-Wiethe disease (lipoid proteinosis). Pediatr Neurosurg 28: 212–214.

Stine OC, Smith KD (1990) The estimation of selection coefficients in Afrikaaners: Huntington disease, porphyria variegata, and lipoid proteinosis. Am J Hum Genet 46: 452–458.

Teive HA, Pereira ER, Zavala JA, Lange MC, de Paola L, Raskin S, Werneck LC, Hamada T, McGrath JA (2004) Generalized dystonia and striatal calcifications with lipoid proteinosis. Neurology 63: 2168–2169.

Thornton HB, Nel D, Thornton D, van Honk J, Baker GA, Stein DJ (2008) The neuropsychiatry and neuropsychology of lipoid proteinosis. J Neuropsychiatry Clin Neurosci 20: 86–92.

Touart DM, Sau P (1998) Cutaneous deposition diseases. Part I. J Am Acad Dermatol 39: 149–171.

Urbach E, Wiethe C (1929) Lipoidosis cutis et mucosae. Virchows Arch Path Anat 273: 285–319.

Van Hougenhouck-Tulleken W, Chan I, Hamada T, Thornton H, Jenkins T, McLean WH, McGrath JA, Ramsay M (2004) Clinical and molecular characterization of lipoid proteinosis in Namaqualand, South Africa. Br J Dermatol 151: 413–423.

Who named it? (2006) A medical biography dictionary. http://www.whonamedit.com

Wong CK, Lin CS (1988) Remarkable response of lipoid proteinosis to oral dimethyl sulphoxide. Br J Dermatol 119: 541–544.

# Chapter 58

# PROGRESSIVE FACIAL HEMIATROPHY (PARRY-ROMBERG SYNDROME)

Ignacio Pascual-Castroviejo, Domenico A. Restivo, and Pietro Milone

Paediatric Neurology Service, University Hospital La Paz, University of Madrid, Madrid, Spain (IPC); Neurology Unit, Garibaldi Hospital, Catania, Italy (DAR); Institute of Radiology, University of Catania, Catania, Italy (PM)

## Introduction

Progressive facial hemiatrophy (PFH), also known as Parry-Romberg or Romberg syndrome, is a sporadic, but not so rare disease (OMIM # 141300) characterised by progressive and self-limited shrinking and deformation of one side of the face, which involves different tissues, scar-like cutaneous changes, subcutaneous connective and fatty tissue' atrophy, circumscribed osteoporosis, bone deformation accompanied usually by contralateral Jacksonian epilepsy, trigeminal neuralgia (and/or peripheral nerve dysfunction), and changes in the eyes and hair. Evidence of mendelian basis is lacking. Larner and Bennison (1993) reported discordance in a pair of monozygotic twins and Anderson et al. (2005) reported two first cousins with PFH, whose fathers were dizygotic twins and whose mothers were sisters.

## Historical perspective

Parry published the first description of hemifacial atrophy in 1825. Romberg, in 1846, detailed the clinical findings. **Caleb Hillier Parry** was a British physician, born October 21, 1755 in Cirencester, Gloucestershire and died on March 9, 1822 in Sion Place, Bath. At the age of 15 years, Parry went to Dissenter's Academy, Warrington, Lancashire, where he met his wife, and in 1773 went on to Edinburgh to study Medicine. After spending two years in London, Parry returned to Edinburgh, obtaining his medical doctorate in 1778 with a thesis on rabies. The same year he became a licentiate of the College of Physicians of London and married. The following year he commenced general practice in Bath, where he spent the rest of his life. As a physician Parry excelled as physiologist and skilled experimenter. He had life-long habit of taking detailed notes and his notes and books detail the life of a busy physician who worked long hours but still found time for research. His major contribution to medicine was the recognition of the cause of Angina. He conducted a series of experiments on sheep to investigate the circulation and the effects of impairment of the vascular supply. He was the first to suggest the correct mechanism although his explanation was ignored for more than 100 years. His "unpublished medical writings" which appeared 3 years after his death, contained the first recorded cases of congenital idiopathic dilation of the colon – Hirschprung's disease, and the PFH – as well as a detailed account of exophthalmic goitre which he first noted in 1786. Parry spent much of his spare time collecting fossils. His broad scientific contributions were recognised by his election to the Royal Society. In 1816 Parry suffered a stroke which left him with aphasia and progressive paralysis. He died in 1822.

**Ernst von Romberg** was a German physician, born on November 5, 1865, Berlin and died in 1933. He studied at Tübingen, Heidelberg, Berlin, and Leipzig, where he obtained his doctorate in 1888. He was assistant at Leipzig under Heinrich Curschmann (1846–1910) 1889–1900, and was habilitated for internal medicine in 1891, becoming professor extraordinary in 1895. In 1900, as extraordinarius, he took over the medical polyclinic in Marburg, where he was promoted to full professor (ordinarius) in 1901. In 1904 he accepted an invitation to Tübingen, moving on to Munich in 1912. Romberg was a leading researcher in the field of circulatory organs. The Ernst-von-Romberg-Strasse in Munich is named for him.

## Incidence and prevalence

The incidence of PFH is unknown. Although more than 1035 cases had been reported in the literature up to 1963, only 772 were sufficiently documented to be considered as having PFH (Rogers 1963, Tollefson and Witman 2007).

## Clinical manifestations

The onset of PFH usually is during the first two decades but it has also been reported in the fifth or sixth decade. Pensler et al. (1990) evaluated 41 patients with PFH and observed that the average age at onset of disease was 8.8 years, while a mean age at onset was 5.4 years in patients with skeletal involvement, versus 15.4 years for patients without skeletal involvement (Figs. 1 and 2).

The first sign of PFH is a progressive lowering of the skin level in unilateral areas of variable distribution, frequently preceded by hair discoloration or circumscribed alopecia. The lesion does not usually cross the midline, but may affect the cheek, nose, mouth, or ear. The subcutaneous fat seems to be responsible for most of the substantial loss (Fig. 3). The cutaneous and subcutaneous features present a slowly progressive course.

Affected persons may develop exidative neuroretinitis with retinal telangiectasias and thickening

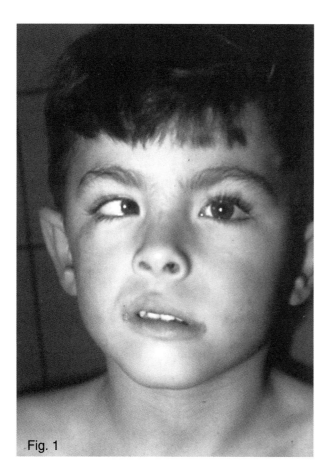
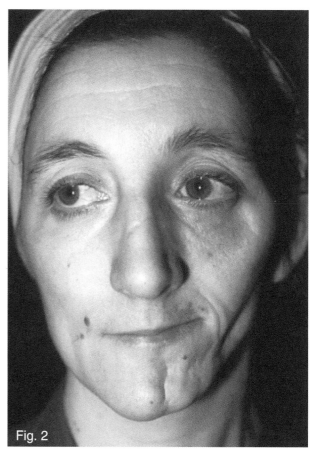

**Figs. 1 and 2.** Facial appearances of an 8-year-old boy (Fig. 1) and a 40-year-old woman (Fig. 2) showing progressive facial hemiatrophy. Cheek, nose, mouth and chin show the cutaneous and subcutaneous atrophy in the affected side.

of the vitreortinal interface (de Crecchio et al. 2008, Theodossiadis et al. 2008). Restrictive strabismus is also noted (see Fig. 1) (Khan 2007).

Epilepsy has been repeatedly reported in patients with PFH (Wolf and Verity 1974, Fry et al. 1992, Terstegge et al. 1994, Dupont et al. 1997), and most probably it is related to the CNS lesions.

## Imaging

The central nervous system (CNS) lesions usually can be demonstrated by standard imaging techniques such as CT or MRI (Moon et al. 2008) (Fig. 3). Cranial CT and MRI studies demonstrate the bony and soft tissue defects (Fig. 3D, E). Some patients also show cerebral calcifications (Fry et al. 1992). Cranial MR studies reveal areas of increased signal in the ipsilateral white matter on $T_2$-weighted images. These changes may be more common than previously believed and can be seen even in patients without neurological symptoms (Fry et al. 1992). Cerebral lesions correlate well with a prolonged clinical course. Asher and Berg (1982) reported three patients with PFH: one was observed over 43 years and showed impor-

tant facial and cerebral hemiatrophy, and two with a shorter evolution had more discrete cerebral lesion. The CNS lesion usually is homolateral to the atrophic hemifacies, but contralateral lesion has also been rarely described (Fig. 3).

## Molecular genetics and pathogenesis

Evidence of Mendelian basis is lacking. Despite that PFH has an entry in the McKusick catalogue (OMIM # 141300). Larner and Bennison (1993) reported discordance in a pair of monozygotic twins of whom only one complained of progressive wasting of the right side of his face, first noted at age 17, without imaging evidence of soft tissues, bony or cerebral abnormalities. Anderson et al. (2005) reported two first cousins with PFH, whose fathers were dizygotic twins and whose mothers were sisters.

## Pathogenesis

The specific aetiology remains unknown. A chronic inflammatory process leading to atrophy of various tis-

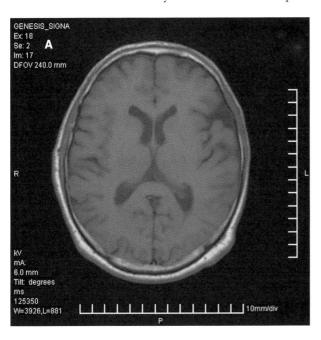
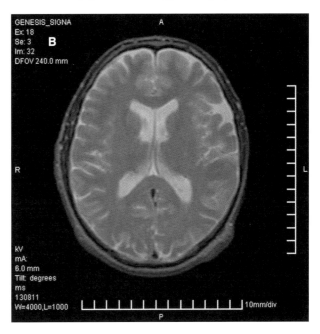

**Fig. 3.** Axial T1-weighted (**A, C, D**) and T2-weighted (**B, E**) magnetic resonance images show cortical and deep nuclei atrophy on one side contralateral to the affected facial side and loss of soft tissue (epidermis, dermis and fat tissue) on the affected side (**D, E**).

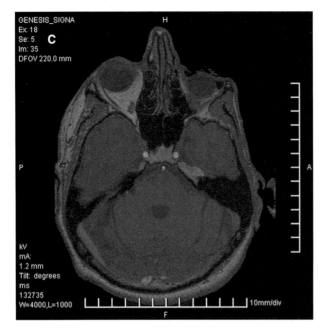

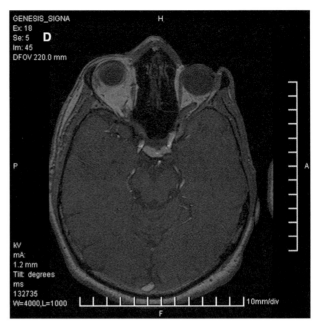

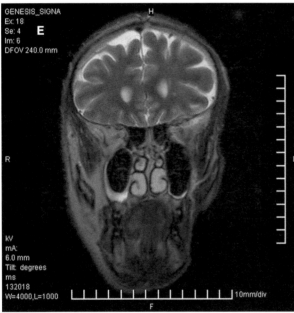

**Fig. 3.** (Continued)

sues of the face and sometimes by local invasion of parts of the brain is a highly plausible explanation for PFH (Terstegge et al. 1994). The histological findings of facial changes in PFH are unequivocal and reveal a proliferative interstitial neurovasculitis (Pensler et al. 1990). The inflammatory process is sometimes seen decades after the onset of the disease. Chronic localized meningoencephalitis with vascular involvement may be a possible underlying cause of the occasional brain involvement in PFH (Terstegge et al. 1994).

## Differential diagnosis

Differential diagnosis with circumscribed or linear scleroderma "en coup de sabre" may be necessary in some cases because of the close resemblances between both syndromes. Some authors believe that clinical differentiation of both syndromes is impossible (Ress 1976). PFH is considered the appropriate diagnosis for the two disorders because differentiation by means of laboratory and histopathological examinations apparently have not been established (Rees 1976, Pensler et al. 1990, Terstegge et al. 1994).

## Management

Management mainly consists of plastic surgery (Guerrerosantos et al. 2007, Kanchwala and Bucky 2007). Seizures need to be treated as usual in cases without PFH.

## References

Anderson PJ, Molony D, Haan E, David DJ (2005) Familial Parry-Romberg disease. Int J Pediatr Otorhonolaryngol 69: 705–708.

Asher SW, Berg BO (1982) Progressive facial hemiatrophy: report of three cases, including one observed over 43 years, and computed tomography findings. Arch Neurol 39: 44–46.

de Crecchio G, Forte R, Strianese D, Rinaldi M, D'Aponte A (2008) Clinical evolution of neuroretinitis in Parry-Romberg syndrome. J Pediatr Ophthalmol Strabismus 45: 125–126.

Dupont S, Catala M, Hasdboun D, Semah F, Baulac M (1997) Progressive facial hemiatrophy and epilepsy: a common underlying dysgenetic mechanism. Neurology 48: 1013–1018.

Fry JA, Alvarellos A, Fink CW, Blaw ME, Roach ES (1992) Intracranial findings in progressive facial hemiatrophy. J Rheumatol 19: 956–958.

Guerrerosantos J, Guerrerosantos F, Orozco J (2007) Classification and treatment of facial tissue atrophy in Parry-Romberg disease. Aesthetic Plast Surg 31: 424–434.

Kanchwala SK, Bucky LP (2007) Invited discussion: correction of hemifacial atrophy with autologous fat transplantation. Ann Plast Surg 59: 654.

Khan AO (2007) Restrictive strabismus in Parry-Romberg syndrome. J Pediatr Ophthalmol Strabismus 44: 51–52.

Larner AJ, Bennison DP (1993) Some observations on the aetiology of progressive hemifacial atrophy ("Parry-Romberg syndrome"). J Neurol Neurosurg Psychiatr 56: 1035–1039.

Moon WJ, Kim HJ, Roh HG, Oh J, Han SH (2008) Diffusion tensor imaging and fiber tractography in Parry-Romberg syndrome. Am J Neuroradiol 29: 714–715.

Parry CH (1825) Collections from the unpublished medical writings of the late Caleb Hillier Parry. London: Underwoods, pp. 478–480.

Pensler JM, Murphy GF, Mulliken JB (1990) Clinical and ultrastructural studies of Romberg' hemifacial atrophy. Plast Reconstr Surg 85: 669–674.

Rees TD (1976) Facial atrophy. Clin Plast Surg 3: 637–646.

Rogers BO (1963) Progressive facial hemiatrophy (Romberg's disease): a review of 772 cases. In: Transactions of third international congress of plastic surgery (International Congress Series No. 66) Washington: Excerpta Medica Foundation, pp. 681–689.

Romberg MH (1846) Klinishe Ergebnisse. Berlin: A Förstner, pp. 75–81.

Terstegge K, Kunath B, Felberg S, Speciali JG, Henkes H, Hosten N (1994) MR of brain involvement in progressive facial hemiatrophy (Romberg disease): reconsideration of a syndrome. Am J Neuroradiol 15: 145–150.

Theodossiadis PG, Grigoropoulos VG, Emfietzoglou I, Papaspirou A, Nikolaidis P, Vergados I, Theodossiadis GP (2008) Parry-Romberg syndrome studied by optical coherence tomography. Ophthalmic Surg Lasers Imaging 39: 78–80.

Tollefson MM, Witman PM (2007) En coup de sabre morphea and Parry-Romberg syndrome: a retrospective review of 54 patients. J Am Acad Dermatol 56: 257–263.

Wolf SM, Verity MA (1974) Neurological complications of progressive facial hemiatrophy. J Neurol Neurosurg Psychiatry 37: 997–1004.

# Chapter 59

# LINEAR SCLERODERMA (MORPHOEA) *"EN COUP DE SABRE"*

Ignacio Pascual-Castroviejo and Martino Ruggieri

Paediatric Neurology Service, University Hospital La Paz, University of Madrid, Madrid, Spain (IPC); Institute of Neurological Science, National Research Council, Catania and Department of Paediatrics, University of Catania, Catania, Italy (MR)

## Definition of localized scleroderma or morphoea

Scleroderma is a rare connective tissue disorder of unknown etiology in which increased collagen deposition occurs and results in sclerosis of the skin and subcutaneous tissue (with dermal atrophy), often affecting the underlying muscle and bone (Sampaio et al. 2006). Involvement may be diffuse (*systemic sclerosis*, which is a multisystem disease) or localized to the skin (*localized scleroderma* or *morphoea*) (Holland et al. 2006, Sampaio et al. 2006).

In childhood, localized scleroderma is more common than systemic sclerosis and shows a greater variety of clinical presentation than in adults (Sampaio et al. 2006). Morphoea may be subdivided into 6 main types: (1) *morphoea "en plaque"* or *circumscribed morphoea* (with the two variants, superficial and deep); (2) linear morphoea of the limbs and trunk; (3) *"en coup de sabre" morphoea* or *linear morphoea of the head*; (4) *generalized morphoea* (characterized by widespread sclerosis of the skin occurring with no systemic involvement); (5) *combined* (plaque and linear) *morphoea* (consisting in plaque-like lesions of the trunk with linear lesions on the leg or "en coup de sabre" lesions including the so-called forms of *morphoea and lichen sclerosus et atrophicus* and *morphoea and atrophoderma of Pasini and Pierini*); and (6) the rare and disabling *pan sclerotic morphoea* (characterized by a polymorphoea appearance of lesions with involvement of the skin, deep structures, tendons, fascia and muscles) (Holland et al. 2006, Peterson et al. 1995, reviewed in Sampaio et al. 2006). Other forms that have been described, such as *guttate morphoea* and *subcutaneous morphoea*, are to be considered variants of the above subsets and highlight the difficulty in classification and the range of overlap between the different clinical types (Sampaio et al. 2006, Uziel et al. 1994).

## LINEAR SCLERODERMA (MORPHOEA) *"EN COUP DE SABRE"*

Linear scleroderma represents a unique form of localized scleroderma that primarily affects the pediatric population, with 67% of patients diagnosed before 18 years of age (Peterson et al. 1997, Sampaio et al. 2006). Linear scleroderma frequently occurs on the limbs (linear morphoea of the limbs and trunk) but also may develop in the frontoparietal area of the forehead and scalp. When linear scleroderma occurs on the head, it is referred to as *linear scleroderma (morphoea) "en coup de sabre"* (**LScs**), given the resemblance of the skin lesions to the stroke of a sabre (see Fig. 1) (Holland et al. 2006).

Clinically, LScs is characterized by an atrophic, ban-like region of indurations involving the frontoparietal area of the forehead and scalp (Sommer et al. 2006). The cutaneous lesion most frequently is unilateral, but bilateral involvement has been described in some patients (Dilley and Perry 1968). The internal area of the eyebrow, eyelid, ala nasi and lateral zone of the nose (Fig. 1) may also be involved with progressive involution of the craniofacial bones resulting in mild to severe hemifacial atrophy similar to the Parry-Romberg syndrome (idiopathic, progressive facial hemiatrophy) (see below) (Sampaio et al. 2006, Untemberger et al. 2003).

Extracutaneous abnormalities have been described in association with LScs including ophthal-

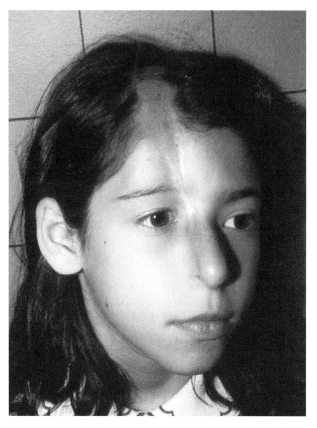

**Fig. 1.** A young adult woman shows an atrophic, band-like region involving middle-right areas of forehead, scalp, and right-lateral area of the nose.

mologic, oral and neurological changes (Holland et al. 2006). Central nervous system involvement consists in seizure disorders (mostly of the partial type), hemiparesis/muscle weakness, trigeminal neuralgia, mental deterioration, depression, decreased school performance, peripheral facial nerve palsy, oculomotor nerve palsy, migraine headache, intracranial aneurysm and subdurale hygroma (Holland et al. 2006, Unterberger et al. 2003).

## Historical perspective and eponyms

The disease was possibly first reported by Addison in 1854 who described areas of induration of the skin, called Addison's keloid (Sampaio et al. 2006). To add to the confusing nosology of scleroderma, the term "morphoea" (which is used as synonymous with the localized form of scleroderma) was first introduced by Wilson (Fox 1892) who interpreted however the disorder as leprosy (Sampaio et al. 2006). In 1868, Fagge defined Addison's keloid as morphoea. He differentiated it from Alibert's keloid (true keloid) (Fox 1892) and described the different forms of localized scleroderma, including the "en coup de sabre" variant. In 1942, Klemperer and colleagues included scleroderma in the group of collagen diseases (Sampaio et al. 2006).

## Incidence and prevalence

On the basis of a retrospective analysis of patients who developed morphoea between 1960 and 1993 in Olmsted County, Minnesota, the incidence of LScs was calculated at 0.13 cases per 100,000 population (Peterson et al. 1997). LScs is more frequent in women than in men, with a proportion of 1.5:1 to 4:1 (Falanga et al. 1986, Uziel et al. 1994).

## Clinical manifestations

### Skin manifestations

After an initial short phase of erythematous patch, a yellow-white elevated or depressed plaque develops surrounded by a blue-violet erythema (the so-called "lilac ring"). The initial stage of disease may pass unnoticed. The process develops into a more solid infiltration of the skin, resulting in atrophy with loss of hair and sebaceous glands and hyper- and hypopigmentation. In the end-phase the typical skin lesions in LScs are characterized by atrophic, ban-like region(s) of indurations, with a groove of depression in the form of "en coup de sabre" involving the frontoparietal area of the forehead and scalp. After skin and subcutis induration and atrophy, the deeper tissues become affected and the internal area of the eyebrow, eyelid, ala nasi and lateral zone of the nose (Fig. 1) may also be involved with progressive involution of the craniofacial bones resulting in mild to severe hemifacial atrophy similar to the

Parry-Romberg syndrome (idiopathic, progressive facial hemiatrophy) (Unterberger et al. 2003). The cutaneous lesion most frequently is unilateral, but bilateral involvement has been described in some patients (Dilley and Perry 1968).

## Extracutaneous involvement

Although both the systemic and localized forms of scleroderma are characterized by sclerosis of the skin and subcutaneous tissue, localized scleroderma lacks internal organ involvement. Unlike most forms of localized scleroderma (which lacks extracutaneous manifestations), the subset of linear scleroderma known as LScs has been associated with several systemic manifestations which are summarized in

**Table 1.** Extracutaneous abnormalities associated with linear scleroderma en coup de sabre [modified from Holland et al. (2006)]

**Neurological changes**
seizure disorders (mostly of the partial type)
hemiparesis/muscle weakness
trigeminal neuralgia
mental deterioration
depression
decreased school performance
peripheral facial nerve palsy
oculomotor nerve palsy
migraine headache
intracranial aneurysm
subdurale hygroma

**Ophthalmologic changes**
Ptosis
Exophthalmos
Uveitis
Motility disorders/atrophy of eye muscles
Hetrochromia of iris
Papillitis
Retrobulbar pain
Enophthalmos
Displacement of outer canthus from resorption of orbital bone
Iridocyclitis

**Oral changes**
Altered dentition
Malocclusion
Tongue atrophy

Table 1. Development of cutaneous disease typically precedes the onset of extracutaneous manifestations. Apart from the obvious changes in facial appearance, complications of LScs depend upon the extent of systemic involvement (Sampaio et al. 2006).

## Nervous system involvement

The most frequent neurologic abnormalities are seizure disorders, most commonly of the partial type (Chung et al. 1995, Dilley and Perry 1968, Ortigado Matamala et al. 1997, Ruiz-Sandoval et al. 2005).

Although the psychological changes in patients with LScs are not usually mentioned, depression, and low self-esteem are the main problems experienced, especially during adolescence and adult life. Decreased school performance of variable degrees is common in patients with LScs.

Other reported nervous system anomalies include hemiparesis/muscle weakness, trigeminal neuralgia, mental deterioration, depression, decreased school performance, peripheral facial nerve palsy, oculomotor nerve palsy, migraine headache, intracranial aneurysm cerebral vasculitis, subdurale hygroma and unilateral hippocampal atrophy (Holland et al. 2006, Korkmaz 2007, Holl-Wieden et al. 2006, Unterberger et al. 2003, Verhelst et al. 2008) (Table 1).

## Imaging

Radiographic abnormalities include skull atrophy (thinning of the skull under the skin lesion), cerebral atrophy, ventricular enlargement, parenchymal calcifications, white matter and cortical/meningeal changes (Fig. 2) (blurring of the grey-white matter interface) or multiple scattered areas of high signal intensity (on FLAIR and T2-weighted images) in the subcortical white matter. These lesions are usually subjacent to the areas of facial or scalp scleroderma (Chung et al. 1995, Ortigado-Matamala et al. 1997, Higashi et al. 2000, Grosso et al. 2003) but may also be bilateral (Holland et al. 2006). Total or partial resolution and/or recurrence or progression of radiological lesions may correlate clinically with neurological disease activity.

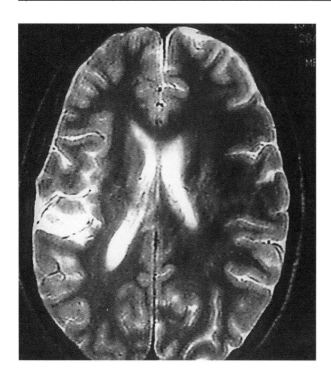

**Fig. 2.** MRI axial view shows cortical subcortical atrophy of the right cerebral hemisphere.

Abnormalities on CT and MRI studies may be seen in patients with LScs even in the absence of neurological disease (Appenzeller et al. 2004, Liu et al. 1994) and vice versa.

The lack of specificity and/or sensitive radiological findings for the associated neurological disease contributes to the difficulty in counselling these patients regarding prognosis. Certainly, the presence of radiological abnormalities warrants close clinical follow-up.

## Pathology

Histologically, the skin lesion in LScs consists of a localized area of dense collagen deposition within the dermis that may extend to involve deeper tissues including muscle, bone and even cerebral hemisphere (Chung et al. 1995, Ortigado-Matamala et al. 1997).

Histological studies of the cerebral lesion are rare and usually only done in cases with a bad response to antiepileptic drugs. Chung et al. (1995) found in a resected cerebral lesion localized band-like sclerosis of the leptomeninges and associated vessels, as well as in-

traparenchymal calcifications and anomalous, ectatic vessels. The authors suggested that LScs may represent a neurocutaneous syndrome of vascular dysplasia similar to Sturge-Weber syndrome, rather than a localized form of collagen vascular disease, as suggested by others (Falanga 1989, Pupillo et al. 1996).

Brain biopsies have been performed when concern for neoplasm arose (Holland et al. 2006). The reported histological findings have been variable: most case reported a perivascular infiltrate or vasculitis. Sclerosis, fibrosis, and gliosis involving brain parenchyma, meninges, and vasculature have also been reported (Chung et al. 1995, Obermore et al. 2003, Stone et al. 2001).

Interestingly, Stone et al. (2001) found at brain biopsy in their case an inflammatory process involving blood vessels and resulting in focal cerebral necrosis. According to these authors (Stone et al. 2001) the brain inflammation was in keeping with the intense inflammation of the dermis and subcutaneous tissue seen in the early stages of LScs supporting the hypothesis that there is an early cerebral inflammatory stage in LScs which can later progress to the end stage pathology found by Chung et al. (1995).

## Molecular genetics and pathogenesis

The pathogenesis of linear scleroderma is not completely understood. Correlations between the manifestation of the disease and trauma, endocrine changes, hormonal factors, viral and bacterial infection (the disease has been noted to start after infections such as *Borrelia burgdorferi* infection and *Epstein-Barr virus* infection), vaccination (morphoea has been described after bacille Calmette-Guerin and MMR vaccinations), the co-existence of auto-immune disease (autoantibodies have been detected in affected patients and their relatives; deposition of immunoglobulins and complement C3 have been found in skin biopsies from patients with morphoea; morphoea has presented during chronic graft-versus-host disease) and embryological maldevelopment (lesions of linear morphoea follow Blaschko's lines) have been documented (reviewed by Sampaio et al. 2006).

Most of the proposed mechanisms so far however related to systemic scleroderma: endothelial cell damage leading to increased fibroblasts activity and ischemia through luminal narrowing with subsequent modification of collagen products has been proposed as a pathogenic mechanism. The inciting event for such microvascular damage remains unknown however. As the involved areas in LScs do usually not cross the midline and may resemble innervated fields in a cranial nerve distribution, in particular the upper trigeminal dermatome, the possibility of a hyper- or hypoactivity of sympathetic nervous system or a developmental abnormality of the trigeminal nerve has been suggested (Gambichler et al. 2001). The latter hypothesis however was challenged by the findings of Stone et al. (2001) recording brain inflammation (demonstrated by brain high signal lesions and CSF oligoclonal response) in concomitance with the skin inflammatory processes.

Genetic factors also are thought to play a role, with higher incidence of connective tissue disease in family members. Morphoea has been described in siblings (Burge et al. 1969, Kass et al. 1966, Iranzo et al. 2001, Panyi 1979), in two to three generations of families (Kulin and Sybert 1966, Wadud et al. 1989) and simultaneously in a father and his daughter (Rees and Bennet 1953).

## Parry-Romberg disease and linear scleroderma "en coup de sabre"

A clear differentiation between *Parry-Romberg syndrome* and LScs is often not possible (Sampaio et al. 2006, Tollefson and Witman 2007): in Parry-Romberg facial hemiatrophy, the subcutaneous tissue, muscles and bones are affected. The overlying skin may be lax and movable without pigmentary changes (see also chapter 58). The nosological position of either disease is not yet clarified whether it is a different entity or represents one end of the spectrum of "en coup de sabre" morphoea is unclear. The latter hypothesis is more likely as these conditions share some clinical and laboratories features: central nervous system and eye involvement have been observed in both groups as well as similar autoantibod-

ies profiles (Paprocka et al. 2006, Sampaio et al. 2006, Stone et al. 2001).

## Management

Linear scleroderma is usually a self-limited disease. Regression or softening of skin lesions often occurs, but complete resolution is unusual and reactivation can occur. Adequate treatment remains elusive. Topical, intralesionale and systemic corticosteroids may reduce the inflammation of skin lesions. Systemic agents are used when more aggressive therapy is warranted and include vitamin E, vitamin D3, aminobenzoate potassium, penicillin, retinoids, diphenylhydantoine, interferon-gamma, immunosuppressive agents, and UV-A therapy (reviewed in Holland et al. 2006).

Management usually consists of plastic surgery for the craniofacial lesion (Ozturk et al. 2006, Robitschek et al. 2008) and antiepileptic pharmacological treatment. Surgical resection of the cerebral epileptogenic area may be necessary in some patient (Chung et al. 1995).

## References

Addison CH (1892) Medico-chirurgical transactions of 1854. Quoted by Fox TC: note on the history of scleroderma in England. Br J Dermatol 4: 101.

Appenzeller S, Montenegro MA, Dertkigil SS, Sampaio-Barros PD, Marques-Neto JF, Samara AM, Andermann F, Cendes F (2004) Neuroimaging findings in scleroderma en coup de sabre. Neurology 62: 1585–1589.

Burge KM, Perry HO, Stickler GB (1969) Familial scleroderma. Arch Dermatol 99: 681–687.

Chung MH, Sum JM, Morrell MJ, Houpian DS (1995) Intracerebral involvement in scleroderma en coup de sabre: report of a case with neuropathologic findings. Ann Neurol 37: 679–681.

Dilley JJ, Perry HO (1968) Bilateral lineal scleroderma en coup de sabre. Arch Dermatol 97: 688–689.

Fagge CH (1868) On keloid scleriasis, morphoea. Guy's Hosp Rep Sev 3: 255.

Falanga V, Medsger TA, Reichlin M, Rodnan GP (1986) Linear scleroderma. Clinical spectrum, prognosis, and laboratory abnormalities. Ann Int Med 104: 849–857.

Fox TC (1892) Note on the history of scleroderma in England. Br J Dermatol 4: 101.

Gambichler T, Kreuter A, Hoffmann K, Bechara FG, Altmeyer P, Jansen T (2001) Bilateral linear scleroderma "en coup de sabre" associated with facial atrophy and neurological complications. BMC Dermatol 1: 9–15.

Grosso S, Fioravanti A, Biasi G, Conversano E, Marcolongo R, Morgese G, Balestri P (2003) Linear scleroderma associated with progressive brain atrophy. Brain Dev 25: 57–861.

Higashi Y, Kanekura T, Fukumaru K, Kanzaki T (2000) Scleroderma en coup de sabre with central nervous system involvement. J Dermatol 27: 486–488.

Holland KE, Steffes B, Nocton JJ, Schwabe MJ, Jacobson RD, Drolet BA (2006) Linear scleroderma and coup de sabre with associated neurologic abnormalities. Pediatrics 117: e132–e136.

Holl-Wieden A, Klink T, Klink J, Warmuth-Metz M, Girschick HJ (2006) Linear scleroderma 'en coup de sabre' associated with cerebral and ocular vasculitis. Scand J Rheumatol 35: 402–404.

Iranzo P, Lopes I, Palou J, Herrero C, Lecha M (2001) Morphoea in three siblings. J Eur Acad Dermatol Venereol 15: 46–47.

Kass H, Hanson V, Patrick J (1966) Scleroderma in childhood. J Pediatr 68: 243–256.

Klemperer P, Pollack AD, Baehr G (1942) Diffuse collagen disease. Acute lupus erythematosus and diffuse scleroderma. J Am Med Assoc 119: 331–332.

Korkmaz C (2007) Linear scleroderma 'en coup de sabre' associated with cerebral and ocular vasculitis. Scand J Rheumatol 36: 159–160.

Kulin P, Sybert VP (1986) Hereditary hypotrichosis and localized morphoea: a new clinical entity. Pediatr Dermatol 3: 333–338.

Liu P, Uziel Y, Chuang S, Silverman E, Krafchik B, Laxer R (1994) Localized scleroderma: imaging features. Pediatr Radiol 24: 207–209.

Obermoser G, Pfausler BE, Linder DM, Sepp NT (2003) Scleroderma en coup de sabre with central nervous system and ophthalmologic involvement: treatment of ocular symptoms with interferon gamma. J Am Acad Dermatol 49: 543–546.

Ortigado-Matamala A, Martinez-Granero MA, Pascual-Castroviejo I (1997) Esclerodermia "en coup de sabre" y participación intracranial. Presentación de un caso. Neurología 12: 256–258.

Ozturk S, Acarturk TO, Yapici K, Sengezer M (2006) Treatment of "en coup de sabre" deformity with porous polyethylene implant. J Craniofac Surg 17: 696–701.

Panayi GS (1979) The immunology of connective tissue disorders. In: Medicine (series 3, no. 14). London: Medicine Education (International): 686.

Paprocka J, Jamroz E, Adamek D, Marszal E, Mandera M (2006) Difficulties in differentiation of Parry-Romberg syndrome, unilateral facial sclerodermia and Rasmussen syndrome. Childs Nerv Syst 22: 409–415.

Peterson LS, Nelson AM, Su WPD (1995) Classification of morphoea (localized scleroderma). Mayo Clin Proc 70: 1068–1076.

Peterson LS, Nelson AM, Su WPD, Mason T, O'Fallon WM, Gabriel SE (1997) The epidemiology of morphea (localized scleroderma) in Olmsted County 1960–1993. J Rheumatol 24: 73.

Pupillo G, Andermann F, Dubeau F (1996) Linear scleroderma and intractable epilepsy: neuropathologic evidence for a chronic inflammatory process. Ann Neurol 39: 277–278.

Rees RB, Bennett J (1953) Localised scleroderma in a father and daughter. Arch Dermatol 68: 360.

Robitschek J, Wang D, Hall D (2008) Treatment of linear scleroderma "en coup de sabre" with AlloDerm tissue matrix. Otolaryngol Head Neck Surg 138: 540–541.

Ruiz-Sandoval JL, Romero-Vargas S, Gutierrez-Aceves GA, Garcia-Navarro V, Bernard-Medina AG, Cerda-Camacho F, Riestra-Castaneda R, Gonzalez-Corneio S (2005) Linear scleroderma en coup de sabre: neurological symptoms, images and review. Rev Neurol 41: 534–537.

Sampaio C, Visentin MT, Howell K, Woo P, Harper J (2006) Morphoea (Synonim: localized scleroderma). In: Harper J, Oranje A, Prose N (eds.) Textbook of Pediatric Dermatology. 2nd ed., pp. 2020–2040.

Sommer A, Ganbichler T, Bacharach-Buhles M, von Rothemburg T, Altmeyer P, Kreuter A (2006) Clinical and serological characteristics of progressive facial hemiatrophy: a case series of 12 patients. J Am Acad Dermatol 54: 227–233.

Stone J, Franks AJ, Guthrie JA, Johnson MH (2001) Scleroderma "en coup de sabre": pathological evidence of intracerebral inflammation. J Neurol Neurosurg Psychiatr 70: 382–385.

Tollefson MM, Witman PM (2007) En coup de sabre morphea and Parry-Romberg syndrome: a retrospective review of 54 patients. J Am Acad Dermatol 56: 257–263.

Untemberger I, Trinko E, Engelhardt K, Muigg A, Eller P, Wagner M, Sepp N, Bauer G (2003) Linear scleroderma "en coup de sabre" coexisting with plaque-morphoea: neuroradiological manifestations and response to corticosteroids. J Neurol Neurosurg Psychiatry 74: 661–664.

Uziel Y, Krafchik BR, Silverman ED, Thorner PS, Laxer RM (1994) Localized scleroderma in childhood: a report of 30 cases. Arthritis Rheum 23: 328–340.

Verhelst HE, Beele H, Joos R, Vanneuville B, Van Coster RN (2008) Hippocampal atrophy and developmental regression as first sign of linear scleroderma "en coup de sabre". Eur J Paediatr Neurol Jan 18 [Epub ahead of print].

Wadud MA, Bose BK, Alò Nasir T (1989) Familial localized scleroderma from Bangladesh: two case reports. Bangladesh Med Res Counc Bull Ducca 15: 15–19.

# Chapter 60

# UNILATERAL SOMATIC AND INTRACRANIAL HYPOPLASIA

Ignacio Pascual-Castroviejo

Paediatric Neurology Service, University Hospital La Paz, University of Madrid, Madrid, Spain

## Introduction

Unilateral somatic and intracranial hypoplasia (USICH) does not represent a true neurocutaneous disorder, but most of its features including unilateral hypoplasia involving the upper and lower extremities, the breast and the trunk, bilateral acral abnormalities affecting especially the middle phalanges, mental retardation and partial epilepsy, overlap with the clinical and imaging findings of other neurocutaneous diseases and/or complex malformation syndromes described in this book, such as oculocerebrocutaneous/ Delleman syndrome (OCCS), encephalocraniocutaneous lipomatosis (ECCL), Proteus syndrome, Parry-Romberg syndrome, scleroderma " en coup de sabre" and Goldenhar syndrome.

## Historical perspective

This syndrome was first characterized by Pascual-Castroviejo et al. (1997).

## Incidence and prevalence

Even though no new cases have been reported since its first clinical description (Pascual-Castroviejo et al. 1997), we have seen additional patients, all women, with the same features.

## Clinical manifestations

The anomalies involve structures of ectodermal and mesodermal origin. Main clinical features are: uni-lateral hypoplasia that involve the upper and lower extremities, breast and trunk (Fig. 1), bilateral acral abnormalities affecting especially the middle phalanges (Fig. 2), mental retardation and partial epilepsy. Patients may present with hemifacial hypoplasia of the contralateral side due to the early and severe lesion of the affected cerebral hemisphere. Specific defects include several malformations ipsilateral to the hypoplastic hemibody such as unilateral cerebral brainstem (Fig. 3) and/or cerebellar hypoplasia, enlargement of the corresponding lateral ventricle with cortical polymicrogyria (Fig. 4), agenesis of the corpus callosum, microphthalmia and cataracts. All intracranial vessels on the affected side appear hypoplastic as well (Fig. 5). Despite phenotypic overlaps between USICH and some other neurocutaneous diseases described in this book (see above), the specific developmental malformation consisting of hypoplasia of the entire hemibody in women suggests that this represents a new entity.

## Molecular genetics and pathogenesis

USICH malformations correspond to different embryological periods. Hypoplasia of cerebellar hemisphere has been described in association with facial hemangioma or vascular malformation, mostly on the ipsilateral side (Pascual-Castroviejo 1978; Pascual-Castroviejo et al. 1985, 1986), and this occurs since $4^1/2$ weeks of gestational age. However, the cerebellum has the longest period of embryological development as compared to any other major structure of the brain. Congenital and acquired vascular etiologies have been suggested (De Souza et al. 1994, Granados-Alzamora et al. 2003, Pascual-Castroviejo

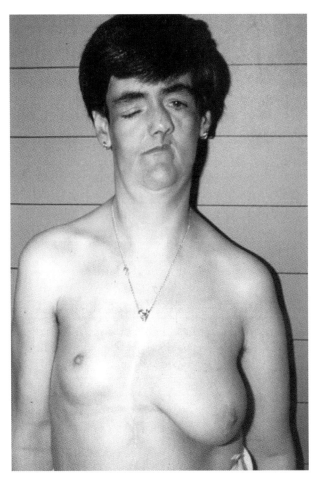

**Fig. 1.** Photograph of a patient at 30 years of age shows palpebral ptosis and breast hypoplasia on the right side and left facial atrophy.

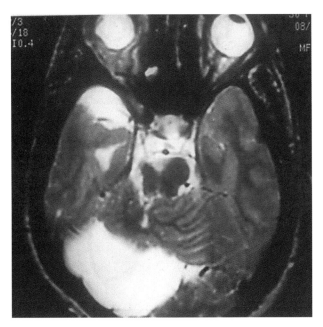

**Fig. 3.** Axial T$_2$-weighted axial MR image (400/88/2) of the upper part of the posterior fossa, the lower part of the middle fossa and the orbits shows hypoplasia of the right cerebellar hemisphere, of the right part of the mesencephalon, of the right temporal lobe and of the right eye.

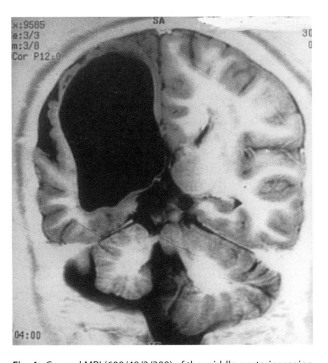

**Fig. 4.** Coronal MRI (600/48/3/300) of the middle-posterior region of the brain discloses dilatation of the right cerebral ventricle with very thin cerebral parenchymal cortical polymicrogyria, and severe hypoplasia of the right cerebellar hemisphere.

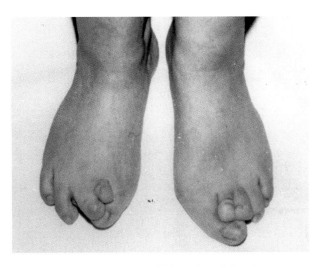

**Fig. 2.** Right foot hypoplasia and bilateral toe deformities.

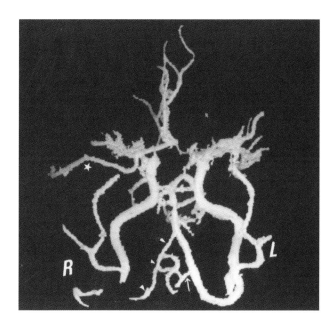

**Fig. 5.** Three-dimensional arterial phase contrast RM angiogram (48/6.9/1) in coronal view reveals the presence of only one posterior inferior cerebellar artery (PICA) which originates from the left vertebral artery of normal size (arrow), while the right vertebral artery is hypoplastic (arrowheads), and a low hypoplastic right middle cerebral artery (star).

et al. 1975, Pascual-Castroviejo 1978a). The period of cortical plate formation begins with the first wave of migrating neuroblasts from the subventricular region, at about 7–8 weeks of gestation (Sarnat 1992). The corpus callosum, however, starts to develop at 10–11 weeks and agenesis may cause changes in gyration (Muller 1990). Appearance of the middle phalanges in the hands and feet is at 12–14 weeks of gestation (Wood and Dimmick 1992). Ocular and palpebral paralysis with cataract homolateral to the remaining affected structures may be associated (likely secondary) to the cerebral hemisphere and brainstem lesions.

## Treatment

The treatment of this syndrome is symptomatic.

## References

De Souza N, Chaudhuri R, Bingham J, Cox T (1994) MRI in cerebellar hypoplasia. Neuroradiology 36: 148–151.

Granados-Alzamora V, Pascual-Pascual SI, Pascual-Castroviejo I (2003) Hipoplasia unilateral de hemisferio cerebeloso: ¿una alteración de origen vascular? Rev Neurol 36: 841–845.

Muller J (1990) Changes in cerebral sulcation in simple absence of the corpus callosum: evidence of rules controlling sulcation patterns. Can J Neurol Sci 17: 343–344.

Pascual-Castroviejo I, Tendero A, Martínez-Bermejo A, Lopez-Terradas JM, Casas C (1975) Persistence of the hypoglosal artery and partial agenesis of the cerebellum. Neuropediatrie 6: 184–189.

Pascual-Castroviejo I (1978) Vascular and nonvascular intracranial malformations associated with external capillary hemangiomas. Neuroradiology 16: 82–84.

Pascual-Castroviejo I (1978a) Vascular changes in cerebellar development defects. Neuroradiology 16: 58–60.

Pascual-Castroviejo I (1985) The association of extracranial and intracranial vascular malformations in children. Can J Neurol Sci 12: 139–148.

Pascual-Castroviejo I, Viaño J, Moreno F, Palencia R, Martínez Fernández V, Pascual-Pascual SI, Martinez-Bermejo A, Garcia-Penas JJ, Roche MC (1996) Hemangiomas of head, neck, and chest with associated vascular and brain anomalies. A complex neurocutaneous syndrome. AJNR Am J Neuroradiol 17: 461–471.

Pascual-Castroviejo I, Pascual-Pascual SI, Viaño J, Martinez V (1997) Unilateral somatic and intracranial hypoplasia. Neuropediatrics 28: 341–344.

Sarnat HB (1992) Cerebral Dysgenesis. Embryology and Clinical Expression. New York: Oxford University Press, pp. 62–71.

Wood B, Dimmick JE (1992) Skeletal system. In: Dimmick JE, Kalousek DK (eds.) Developmental Pathology of the Embryo and Fetus. Philadelphia: JB. Lippincott Company, pp. 401–423.

# Chapter 61

# OCULOCEREBROCUTANEOUS SYNDROME (DELLEMAN SYNDROME)

Ignacio Pascual-Castroviejo

Paediatric Neurology Service, University Hospital La Paz, University of Madrid, Madrid, Spain

## Introduction

Oculocerebrocutaneous syndrome (OCCS) is a rare disease (OMIM # 164180) with only around 35 patients reported so far (Hunter 2008, Tambe et al. 2003) characterized by bilateral anophthalmia and orbital cysts, typical skin lesions consisting in skin appendages, focal dermal hypoplasia/aplasia and punch-like defects, complex brain malformations (mostly of the Dandy-Walker type) associated to mental retardation and seizures, and cleft lip/palate. Happle (1987) suggested the disorder is due to an autosomal dominant lethal somatic mutation that survives by mosaicism.

## Historical perspective and eponyms

The first cases of OCCS were possibly described by ophthalmologists (Braun-Vallon et al. 1958, Dollfus et al. 1968, Ladenheim and Metrick 1956). However, these patients were studied incompletely and knowledge about the involved structures was not clarified until the report by Delleman and Oorthuys (1981) who described two unrelated children presenting with multiple congenital malformations that consisted of orbital cysts, cutaneous defects that extended anywhere in the body, skin tags, micro/anophthalmia, and malformations of the central nervous system (CNS). Despite some similarities to the Goltz (OMIM # 305600) and Goldenhar (OMIM # 164210) syndrome, a new entity was suspected. Delleman et al. (1984) added two further cases. Al-Gazali et al. (1988) reviewed 5 published cases and reported 4 new patients coining the term oculocerebrocutaneous syndrome (OCCS) or Delleman syndrome. New features were added in later reports and it is not clear that all patients described as OCCS have corresponded with the characteristics of the syndrome.

## Incidence and prevalence

McCandless and Robin (1998) suggested that the minimal diagnostic criteria for OCCS should include orbital cyst or microphthalmia, CNS cysts or hydrocephalus, and focal skin defects. However, the features of OCCS overlap with other syndromes affecting eyes, CNS and skin and a differential diagnosis must always considered. These overlapping syndromes are: encephalocraniocutaneous lipomatosis (ECCL), Goltz syndrome, nevus sebaceous of Jadassohn, Goldenhar anomaly, unilateral somatic and intracranial hypoplasia, incontinentia pigmenti, and Proteus syndrome (whose main features are described in this book). Moog et al. (1996) reported a 18-to-7 preponderance of male infants.

## Clinical manifestations

The syndrome is mainly characterized by congenital anomalies of the orbit(s), skin and CNS. OCCS is a neurocutaneous disorder with a wide spectrum of signs and symptoms that involves many organs anywhere in the body, and most often causes dysmorphologic signs. Assistance to these patients may require participation of several specialists such as pediatricians, dermatologists, pediatric neurologists, radiologists, ophthalmologists, neurosurgeons, plastic surgeons, and dysmorphologists.

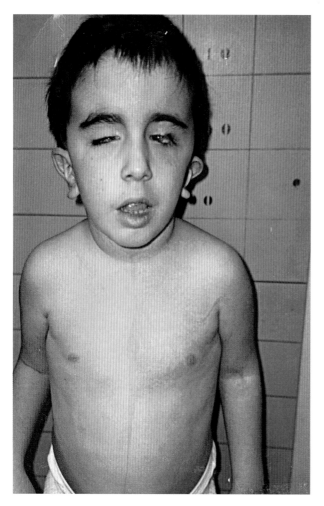

**Fig. 1.** Ocular and palpebral lesions after surgical reparation. Dysplastic left ear and cutaneous lesions on the left trunk with midline cessation of the skin changes.

## Facies

The face is asymmetric in 60% of cases. Other findings include (Fig. 1) unilateral or bilateral orbital cysts (65% with microphthalmia) and upper or lower eyelid coloboma. In the contralateral eye, persistent hyaloid artery hamartomas or opacified cornea has been reported. Cleft lip/palate has been noted in 15%.

## Skin

Almost 100% of patients have skin appendages but concentric postauricular (Fig. 1), malar, and even labial examples have been noted. Rarely, tags are pre-

sent on the trunk. Facial skin lesions have been of three types: focal hypoplasia (85%), aplasia (50%) and punch-like defects (50%). The postauricular crescent shaped hypoplastic skin lesion is pathognomonic. A few patients have involvement of the trunk. Multiple trichofolliculomas have been reported.

## Skeletal findings

These include underdeveloped orbits, zygomas, and the sphenoid part of the lateral orbital wall on the side of the involved eye (60%) as well as scoliosis and rib malformations (40%). Some patients have exhibited body asymmetry, and several have manifested hip dislocations.

## Nervous system

Most patients suffer from psychomotor retardation, seizures, dilatation of the cerebral ventricles, intracranial cysts, agenesis or hypoplasia of the corpus callosum, and cerebellar malformation, commonly consisting of Dandy-Walker malformation. Magnetic resonance imaging (MRI) reveals the presence of alterations of the neuronal migration or cortical organization, especially polymicrogyria, involving a variable part of the cerebral hemispheres and associated with deformities of the cerebral parenchyma or/and of the ventricles. Moog et al. (2005) reviewed brain imaging studies, clinical records, photographs, and pathology specimens of two new and 9 previously reported patients with OCCS. They found a consistent pattern of malformations in 8 of the 11 cases, consisting of frontal predominant polymicrogyria and periventricular nodular heterotopia, enlarged lateral ventricles or hydrocephalus, agenesis of the corpus callosum (sometimes associated with interhemispheric cysts), and a novel mid-hindbrain malformation consisting of an enlarged dysplastic tectum, absent cerebellar vermis, small cerebellar hemispheres, and a large posterior fossa fluid collection (see Fig. 2). The three remaining patients had similar but less severe forebrain abnormalities and lacked the mid-hindbrain malformation. Moog et al. (2005) suggested that the mid-hindbrain malformation is pathognomonic for OCCS and may be used to distinguish OCCS from related syndromes with comparable forebrain anomalies.

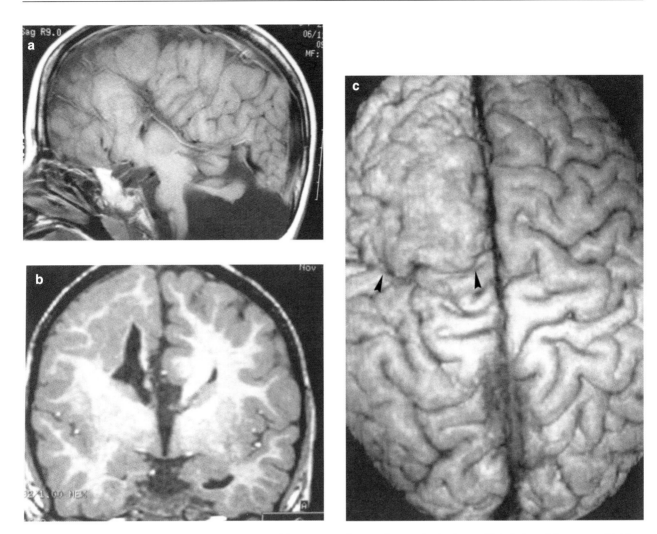

**Fig. 2.** MRI (**a**) sagittal view shows complete agenesis of the corpus callosum, abnormal sulcation and lobulation of the parasagittal face of the cerebral hemisphere, and severe cerebellar malformation. (**b**) Coronal view shows agenesis of the corpus callosum, enlarged right lateral ventricle and polymicrogyria right hemisphere. (**c**) Cortical view shows polymicrogyric right frontal lobe (arrowheads).

## Systemic involvement

Other less frequent anomalies include urogenital malformations or defects (Moog et al. 1997). Malformations usually are bilateral, but a primarily unilateral cutaneous, ocular and CNS involvement can also be observed (Hoo et al. 1991). With the description of new patients, a constellation of additional malformations, including lateral facial cleft, vertebral anomaly, ventricular septal defect, cleft lip and palate and congenital hydrocephalus became known (Leichtman et al. 1994, Angle and Hersh 1997, McCandless and Robin 1998).

## Molecular genetics and pathogenesis

Happle (1987) suggested that OCCS, like a number of other sporadically occurring disorders with an irregular distribution of skin involvement, may be the result of an autosomal dominant lethal gene that is compatible with survival only in the mosaic state. Moog et al. (1996, 1997) suggested that the pathogenic mechanism is probably disruption of the anterior neuroectodermal plate leading to neurocristopathy with primary craniofacial dysmorphogenesis. Gorlin et al. (2001) believe that the disorder has been underreported, since many examples of cystic eye represent incomplete forms. Some cases have been labeled as examples of rhabdomyomatous hamartomas.

## Differential diagnosis

These anomalies, however, overlap clinical features with other diseases described in this chapter, such as Goldenhar syndrome and others. Delineating the limits of the characteristics of every disease is very difficult or perhaps impossible till the diagnosis can be established on a genetic basis. The similarities of OCCL and ECCL consist in the overlapping of most of their clinic characteristics. These may represent different manifestations of the same disorder as has already been proposed (Loggers et al. 1992; Hunter 2006, Hennekam 1994; Moog et al. 1996, 1997, Pascual-Castroviejo et al. 2005).

## Management

The management is symptomatic and concerns many specialists, such as pediatricians for general health, pediatric neurologists for seizures, motor disease, and mental retardation, ophthalmologists for ocular anomalies, plastic surgeons for the many cutaneous lesions anywhere, etc.

## References

Al-Gazali LI, Donnai D, Berry SA, Say B, Mueller RF (1988) The oculocerebrocutaneous (Delleman) syndrome. J Med Genet 25: 773–778.

Angle B, Hersh JH (1997) Anophthalmia, intracerebral cysts, and cleft lip/palate: expansion of the phenotype in oculocerebrocutaneous syndrome. Am J Med Genet 68: 39–42.

Braun-Vallon S, Joseph R, Hezelof C, Ribierre M, Lagraulet J (1958) Un cas de teratoma de l'orbite. Bull Mem Soc Fr Ophthalmol 808–809.

Delleman JW, Oorthuys JWE (1981) Orbital cyst in addition to congenital cerebral and focal dermal malformations: a new entity? Clin Genet 19: 191–198.

Dollfus MA, Marx P, Langlois J, Clement JC, Farthomm J (1968) Congenital cyst eyeball. Am J Ophthalmol 66: 504–509.

Gorlin RJ, Cohen MM, Hennekam RCM (2001) Oculocerebrocutaneous syndrome (Dellemn syndrome). In:

Gorlin RJ, Cohen MM, Hennekam RCM (eds.) Syndromes of the Head and Neck. New York: Oxford University Press, pp. 1206–1207.

Happle R (1987) Lethal genes surviving by mosaicism: a possible explanation for sporadic birth defects involving the skin. J Am Acad Dermatol 16: 899–906.

Hennekam RC (1994) Scalp lipomas and cerebral malformations: overlap between encephalocraniocutaneous lipomatosis and oculocerebrocutaneous syndrome. Clin Dysmorphol 3: 87–89.

Hoo JJ, Kapp-Simon K, Rollnick B, Chao M (1991) Oculocerebrocutaneous (Delleman) syndrome: A pleiotropic disorder affecting ectodermal tissues with unilateral predominance. Am J Med Genet 40: 290–293.

Hunter A (2008) Oculocerebrocutaneous syndrome: an update. Am J Med Genet A 146: 674.

Hunter AG (2006) Oculocerebrocutaneous and encephalocraniocutaneous lipomatosis syndromes: blind men and an elephant or separate syndromes? Am J Med Genet A 140: 709–726.

Landenheim J, Metrick S (1956) Congenital microphthalmos with cyst formation. Am J Ophthalmol 41: 1059–1062.

Leichtman LG, Wood B, Rohn R (1994) Anophthalmia, cleft lip/palate, facial anomalies, and CNS anomalies and hypothalamic disorder in a newborn: a middle developmental field defect. Am J Med Genet 50: 39–41.

Loggers HE, Oosterwijk JC, Overweg-Plansoen WCG, van Wilsem A, Bleeker-Wagemakers EM, Bijlsma JB (1992) Encephalocraniocutaneous lipomatosis and oculocerebrocutaneous syndrome. A differential diagnostic problem. Ophthalm Paediatr Genet 13: 171–177.

McCandless SE, Robin NH (1998) Severe oculocerebrocutaneous (Delleman) syndrome: overlap with Goldenhar anomaly. Am J Med Genet 78: 282–288.

Moog U, Krüger G, Stengel B, de Die-Smulders C, Dykstra S, Bleeker-Wage-makers E (1996) Oculocerebrocutaneous syndrome: a case report, a follow-up and differential diagnostic considerations. Genet Couns 7: 257–265.

Moog U, de Die-Smulders C, Systermans JMJ, Cobben JM (1997) Oculocerebrocutaneous syndrome: report of three additional cases and etiological considerations. Clin Genet 52: 219–225.

Moog U, Jones MC, Bird LM, Dobyns WB (2005) Oculocerebrocutaneous syndrome: the brain malformation defines a core phenotype. J Med Genet 42: 913–921.

Pascual-Castroviejo I, Pascual-Pascual SJ, Velázquez-Fragua R, Lapunzina P (2005) Oculocerebrocutaneous (Delleman) syndrome: Report of two cases. Neuropediatrics 36: 50–54.

Tambe KA, Ambekar SV, Balna PN (2003) Delleman (oculocerebrocutaneous) syndrome: few variations in a classical case. Eur J Pediatr Neurol 7: 77–80.

# Chapter 62

# CEREBELLO-TRIGEMINAL DERMAL DYSPLASIA (GOMEZ-LOPEZ-HERNANDEZ SYNDROME)

Ignacio Pascual-Castroviejo and Martino Ruggieri

Paediatric Neurology Service, University Hospital La Paz, University of Madrid, Madrid, Spain (IPC); Institute of Neurological Science, National Research Council, Catania and Department of Paediatrics, University of Catania, Catania, Italy (MR)

## Introduction

Cerebello-trigeminal dermal (CTD) dysplasia (OMIM # 601853) (OMIM 2006) is an uncommon congenital disorder of the cerebellum, trigeminal nerves, cranial sutures and scalp (Muñoz et al. 2004). Clinically, CTD dysplasia is characterised by craniosynostosis, parieto-occipital scalp alopecia, trigeminal nerve anaesthesia, short stature, cerebellar abnormalities (usually of the rhombencephalosynapsis/RES type), ataxia and intellectual impairment (Brocks et al. 2000; Gomez 1979, 1987; Gomy et al. 2008; Lopez-Hernandez 1982; Munoz et al. 1997, 2004; Pascual-Castroviejo 1983; Poretti et al. 2008; Schell-Apacik et al. 2007; Tan et al. 2005).

## Historical background and eponyms

The first four cases of CTD dysplasia were reported by Gomez (1979), Lopez-Hernandez (1982) and Pascual-Castroviejo (1983). The condition is also known as *Gomez–Lopez–Hernandez syndrome*. All the first four patients had the same clinical manifestations (see below), including scarring from self-inflicted injuries, belonged to different families and only two were from the same country (Gomez 1987). Some cases in the earlier German literature could correspond to CTD dysplasia (Kayser 1921, Gross 1959, Pillat 1949). Kayser (1921) reported a boy with bilateral congenital corneal anaesthesia and difficult swallowing and chewing who was unable to stand or walk and who died of pneumonia at age 3.6 years (Gomez 1987). Pillat (1949) reported a patient with congenital trigeminal anaesthesia and symmetrical hypoplasia of the hair and part of the temporal muscles with no ap-

parent ataxia (Gomez 1987). Gross (1959) reported mental retardation, strabismus, hypertelorism and turricephaly in two patients with RES (Muñoz et al. 2004). Further cases who could have CTD dysplasia may have been reported as syndrome RES (Pavone et al. 2005, Toelle et al. 2003, Muñoz et al. 2004) because of abnormal corneal sensation (Truwit et al. 1991) or craniofacial abnormalities (Pavone et al. 2005, Toelle et al. 2003). For this and other reasons (see below) isolated RES and CTD dysplasia are currently (putatively) considered as a spectrum of disease with common aetiology (Tan et al. 2005).

## Incidence and prevalence

Twenty patients have been identified with true CTD dysplasia since 1979 (Alonso, personal communication; Bowdin et al. 2007; Brocks et al. 2000; Gomez 1979, 1987; Gomy et al. 2008; Lopez-Hernandez 1982; Muñoz et al. 1997, 2004; Pascual-Castroviejo 1983; Poretti et al. 2008; Purvis et al. 2007; Schell-Apacik et al. 2008; Tan et al. 2005; Whetsell et al. 2006). It remains unclear how many cases with RES (Pavone et al. 2005, Toelle et al. 2003) could be considered part of the CTD dysplasia spectrum (Tan et al. 2005). CTD dysplasia seems to be sporadic and all patients reported to date belong to unrelated families.

## Clinical features

The patients with CTD dysplasia show, since birth, acrocephaly with occipital flattening, moderate hypertelorism and convergent strabismus, symmetrical areas of alopecia involving the lateral skull that commonly extend to the parietal areas, but also can affect tempo-

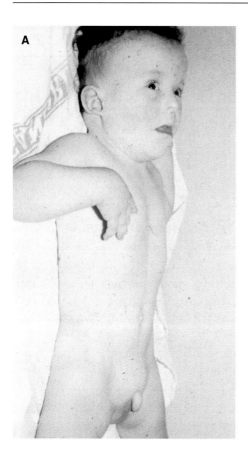

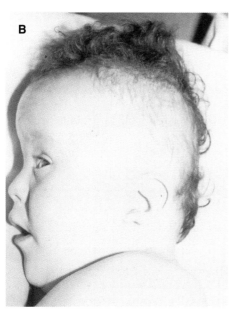

**Fig. 1.** Cerebellar trigemino dermal dysplasia. General (**A**) and lateral head and face views (**B**) show acrocephaly, open mouth, short nose, and alopecia in the parietal region of scalp.

ral and occipital regions (Fig. 1), varying degrees of bilateral trigeminal anaesthesia confirmed by EMG studies which show very prolonged latencies on R2 bilaterally and may identify an afferent lesion involving also the blink reflex (Muñoz et al. 1997, 2004).

Most patients show characteristics facial abnormalities including frontal bossing, flat occiput, hypertelorism, small nose with broad base and bulbous tip, apparently low-set and posteriorly angulated ears, thin lips and open mouth most of the time, prognatism, dental malocclusion, deciduous teeth eruption and dental abnormalities, high palate, and corneal opacities due to lack of pain sensation and to self-injuries. They all have clinodactyly of the fifth fingers and also have feeding difficulties because of masseter and temporal muscle weakness (Muñoz et al. 2004). In a male patient Brocks et al. (2000) recorded growth hormone deficiency.

Skin biopsy from areas of alopecia shows a decreased number of hair follicles (Lopez-Hernandez 1992, Muñoz et al. 1997), but preserved architecture although undeveloped head-sebaceous structures.

Postnatal motor development occurs with short stature, ataxia seizures motor and mental delay, hyperactivity and behavioural disorders. Unaided walking was obtained at age 19 months (Alonso L.G., personal communication), 2.9 years (Brocks et al. 2000), 4 years (Muñoz et al. 1997), after 5 years (Gomez 1979), and at 7 years (Lopez-hernandez 1982, Muñoz et al. 1997). In two cases there was no intellectual impairment (Alonso L.G., personal communication).

The longest follow-ups so far recorded were those of Brocks et al. (2000) in a 19 year old male followed since birth who was of short stature and showed signs of progression of his physical and psychiatric problems including hyperactivity, depression, self-injurious behaviour and bipolar disorders; and Gomy et al. (2008) in a 29-year-old patient. Mental problems and behavioural disorders in the other cases followed-up for long periods (i.e., to puberty) tended to improve with age and patients became more sociable (Muñoz et al. 1997).

## Radiographic findings

Skull X-ray studies shows brachicephaly with tower-like shape, reduced posterior fossa volume, and

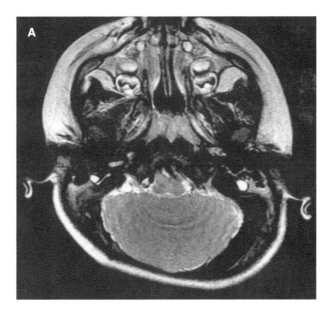

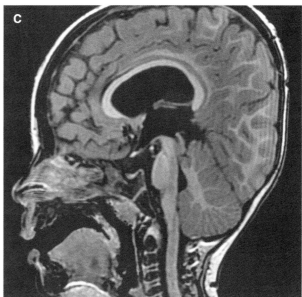

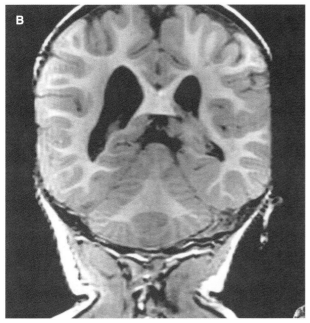

**Fig. 2.** MRI features of a young child with CTD. Axial (**A**) and coronal (**B**) images show cerebellar hemispheric fusion and absence of the vermis as well as reduced cerebellar size. (**C**) Sagittal midline image reveals markedly abnormal cerebellar lobulation and elongated fourth ventricle.

craniosynostosis with partial closure of the lambdoid sutures.

Cerebellar hypoplasia and fusion of the vermis and pons was demonstrated by Lopez-Hernandez (1982) on CT studies. MRI studies reveal RES (Brocks et al. 2000, Muñoz et al. 1997), a rare malformation that is characterized by fusion of cerebellar hemispheres and absence of the cerebellar vermis (Fig. 2). The associated central nervous system

anomalies most commonly present are fusion of the cerebellar dentate nuclei, superior cerebellar peduncles, and thalami, absence of the septum pellucidum, olivary hypoplasia, anomalies of the limbic system, hydrocephalus and azygons anterior cerebral artery (Gomy et al. 2008, Tan et al. 2005, Truwit et al. 1991, Whetsell et al. 2006). The presence of associated supratentorial lesions is a more likely cause of severe mental disease than the malformations of the

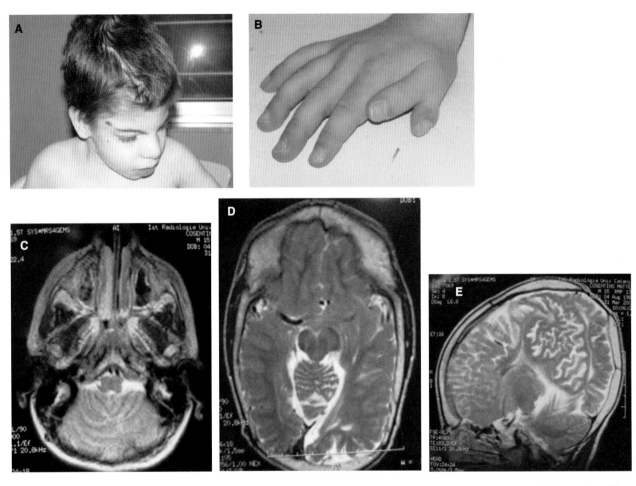

**Fig. 3.** A child with a complex malformation syndrome fitting in the group of the rhombenecephalosynapsis (RES) who have clinical features similar to CTD dysplasia: (**A**) cutis vertex rigirata with an area of alopecia in the right fronto-parietal area and a tuft of hair in the outer region of the right eyebrow; (**B**) hexadactylu with thumb duplication; and evidence of RES at axial (**C, D**) and sagittal (**E**) MRI study of the brain (reprinted with permission from Pavone et al. 2005).

posterior fossa (Muñoz et al. 1997, 2004) however the overall CNS malformation is complex and thus is almost invariably associated to neurological manifestations. Prenatal MRI of RES in a CTD dysplasia infant who had an abnormally shaped small cerebellum at antenatal ultrasound has been recently published (Tan et al. 2005).

## Pathogenesis

Pathogenesis of CTD dysplasia is not completely understood to date. The cerebellum develops late in the human embryo. The vermis is formed at

4 months of gestation, after the semilunar ganglion of the trigeminal nerve has been formed from migrating neural crest cells and thickened epidermis of each side of the head that formed placodes (Gómez 1987). In CTD dysplasia, the primordial cerebellar hemispheres, the placodes that give origin to the trigeminal nerve, and the epidermis of the occipito-parietal region that originates from the ectoderm, are affected. Failure of local epidermal development and of migration and multiplication of specific cells from a selective region in the ectoderm have been suggested as the cause of hypoplasia or dysplasia of the cerebellum, trigeminal nerves and a parieto-occipital segment of the scalp (Gomez 1987). The biology of RES is not

completely understood, but the rarity of this cerebellar malformation, which seems likely to be universally present in CTD dysplasia patients, suggests that it is one of the key features of this syndrome and that CTD dysplasia and isolated RES may have a common aetiology (Tan et al. 2005) (see also Fig. 3).

In a recent report (Schell-Apacik et al. 2008) microarrary-based comparative genomic hybridisation (array-CGH) revealed chromosomal observations including partial deletions of 1p21, 8q24.23, 10q11.2, Xq26.3 and partial duplications of 19p13.2 which, however, were classified as normal variants. Molecular analysis of the lysosomal acid phosphatase gene (ACP2) was performed by Gomy et al. (2008) with no pathogenic mutations.

## Differential diagnosis

Clinical and imaging features of CTD are very particular and differential diagnosis with other syndromes is not frequent, especially after one year of age. Differential diagnosis may be necessary to identify some patients with ataxia or severe mental retardation who show self corneal injuries. Isolated (non syndromic) RES must be carefully evaluated for the presence of associated systemic malformations suggestive of CTD dysplasia (Pavone et al. 2005, Toelle et al. 2003, Tan et al. 2005).

## Management

Treatment of CTD dysplasia is symptomatic and includes physical rehabilitation, special education, dental care, and ocular protection against self-induced corneal trauma that causes ulcers and, later, corneal opacification. Bilateral congenital trigeminal anaesthesia may require lifelong corneal protection.

The prognosis is related to the mental development, motor handicap, corneal-facial anaesthesia, and visual problems.

Follow-up of a large number of patients with CTD has not been reported in the literature and experience is limited to few cases to date.

## References

Bowdin S, Phelan E, Watson R, McCreery KM, Reardon W (2007) Rhombencephalosynapsis presenting antenatally with ventriculomegaly/hydrocephalus in a likely case of Gómez-López-Hernández syndrome. Clin Dysmorphol 16: 21–25.

Brocks D, Irons M, Sadeghi-Nadjad A, Mc Cauley R, Wheeler P (2000) Gómez-López-Hernández syndrome: expansion of the phenotype. Am J Med Genet 94: 405–408.

Gomez MR (1979) Cerebello-trigeminal and focal dermal dysplasia: a newly recognized neurocutaneous syndrome. Brain Dev 1: 253–256.

Gomez MR (1987) Cerebello-trigeminal-dermal dysplasia. In: Gomez MR (ed.) Neurocutaneous diseases. A practical approach. Stoneham: Butterworths, pp. 345–348.

Gomy I, Heck B, Santos AC, Figueiredo MS, Martinelli CE Jr, Nogueira MP, Pina-Neto JM (2008) Two new Brazilian patients with Gómez-López-Hernández syndrome: reviewing the expanded phenotype with molecular insights. Am J Med Genet A 146A: 649–657.

Gross H (1959) Die Rhombencephalosynapsis, eine systemisierte Kleinhirnfehlbildung. Arch Psychiatr Z Neurol 199: 537–552.

Kayser B (1921) Ein Fall von angeborener Trigeminuslähmung und angeborenem totalem Tränenmangel. Klin Mel Augenheilkd 66: 652–654.

Lopez-Hernandez A (1982) Craniosynostosis, ataxia, trigeminal anesthesia and parietal alopecia with pons-vermis fusion anomaly (atresia of the fourth ventricle). Report of two cases. Neuropediatrics 13: 99–102.

Muñoz MV, Santos AC, Graziadio C, Pina-Neto JM (1997) Cerebello-trigeminal-dermal dysplasia (Gómez-López-Hernández syndrome): Description of three new cases and review. Am J Med Genet 72: 34–39.

Muñoz Rojas MV, dos Santos AC, De Pina-Neto JM (2004) Cerebello-trigemino-dermal dysplasia. In: Roach ES, Miller VS (eds.) Neurocutaneous Disorders. Cambridge: Cambridge University Press, pp. 306–312.

OMIM™ (2006) Online mendelian inheritance in man. Baltimore: Johns Hopkins University. http://ncbi.nlm.nih.gov/omim

Pascual-Castroviejo I (1983) Displasia cerebelotrigeminal. Neurologia Infantil, Barcelona. Cientifico-medica: 680.

Pavone P, Incorpora G, Ruggieri M (2005) A complex brain malformation syndrome with rhombencephalosynapsis, preaxial hexadactyly plus facial and skull anomalies. Neuropediatrics 36: 279–283.

Pillat A (1949) Wiener ophthalmologische Gesellschaft. Epithelschädigung der Hornhaut bei angeborener Trigeminushypoplasie. Wien Klin Wochenschr 61: 605.

Poretti A, Bartholdi D, Gobara S, Alber FD, Boltshauser E (2008) Gómez-López-Hernández syndrome: an easily missed diagnosis. Eur J Med Genet 51: 197–208.

Purvis DJ, Ramirez A, Roberts N, Harper JI (2007) Gómez-López-Hernández syndrome: another consideration in focal congenital alopecia. Br J Dermatol 157: 196–198.

Schell-Apacik CC, Cohen M, Vojta S, Ertl-Wagner B, Klopocki E, Heinrich U, von Voss H (2008) Gomez-Lopez-Hernandez syndrome (cerebello-trigeminal-dermal dysplasia): description of an additional case and review of the literature. Eur J Pediatr 167: 23–26.

Tan TY, McGillivray G, Goergen SK, White SM (2005) Prenatal magnetic resonance imaging in Gómez-López-Hernández syndrome and review of the literature. Am J Med Genet 138A: 369–373.

Toelle SP, Valcinkaya C, Kocer N, Deonna T, Overweg-Plandsoen WCG, Bast T, Kalmanchey R, Barsi P, Schneider JFL, Capone Mori A, Boltshauser E (2003) Rhombencephalosynapsis: clinical findings and neuroimaging in 9 children. Neuropediatrics 33: 209–214.

Truwit CL, Barkovich AJ, Shanahan R, Maroldo TV (1991) MR imaging of rhombencephalosynapsis: report of three cases and review of the literature. Am J Neuroradiol 12: 957–965.

Whetsell W, Saigal G, Godinho S (2006) Gómez-López-Hernández syndrome. Pediatr Radiol 36: 552–554.

# Chapter 63

# MACRODACTYLY-LIPOFIBROMATOUS HAMARTOMA OF NERVES

Carola Duràn-Mckinster, Luz Orozco-Covarrubias, Marimar Saez-De-Ocariz, and Ramòn Ruiz-Maldonado

Department of Dermatology, National Institute of Paediatrics, Mexico City, Mexico

## Introduction

*Lipofibromatous hamartoma of nerve* (LFHN) is a very uncommon benign lipomatous tumor with specific clinicopathological characteristics which may present with or without macrodactyly. This tumor-like lesion is composed of fibrous and fatty tissues arising from the epi- and perineurium that surrounds and infiltrates the major nerves and their branches in the body (Enzinger and Weiss 1994). It is believed to be congenital and mainly affects the median nerve in the hand or more rarely the digital nerves at the peripheral level usually well before the third decade (Razzaghi and Anastakis 2005, Jung et al. 2005). An association between this condition and overgrowth of bone and macrodactyly is present in about one-third of cases (Barsky 1967).

## Historical background and eponyms

Lipofibromatous hamartoma (LFH) was first reported by Mason in 1953 and then by several other authors (Mikhail 1964, Pulvertaft 1964, Yeoman 1964). Synonyms for this condition include fatty infiltration (Yeoman 1964), intraneural lipofibroma (Houpt et al. 1989), fibrofatty proliferation (Callison et al. 1968), fibrolipomatous hamartoma, neural fibrolipoma or perineural lipoma (Razzaghi and Anastakis 2005), lipofibroma (Rowland 1977), and hamartoma (Paletta and Rybka 1972), but LFH and LFHN are the most accepted names (Johnson and Bonfiglio 1969, Razzaghi and Anastakis 2005). When accompanied by true macrodactyly, the tumor is also referred to as macrodystrophia lipomatosa (Razzaghi and Anastakis 2005).

## Incidence and prevalence

In an English language literature review of 501 articles published under the entry terms of "lipofibromatous", "hamartomas of the nerve", "macrodactyly" and "intraneural lipoma" Razzaghi and Anastakis (2005) identified some distinguishing epidemiological features including: more common prevalence among white people; sporadic occurrence across populations; increased female to male ratio when the tumor is accompanied by macrodactyly; and rare cranial nerve involvement versus the usual involvement of peripheral nerves.

## Clinical features

### General and peripheral nervous system involvement

LFHN is a tumor-like lipomatous process that involves mainly the volar aspect of the hands, wrists, and forearms and rarely occurs on the feet (Bisceglia et al. 2007). It usually manifests as a soft, slow-growing mass composed of fibrofatty tissue that surrounds and infiltrates the major nerves and their branches. Localization can be unilateral or bilateral in a asymmetrical or asymmetrical way (Bhat et al. 2005, Jung et al. 2005). The mass usually appears several years before the onset of neurological symptoms (Lowenstein et al. 2000). Subcutaneous tissues and bones may progressively enlarge. Most cases occur in the first three decades of life, although several reports have described patients who first presented past the fifth decade (Gouldesborough and Kinny 1989, Herrick et al. 1980, Kernohan et al. 1984, Marom and Helms 1999, Rusko and Larsen 1981). The affected patients have usually been aware of the presence of a mass for several years. LFHN affects peripheral nerves, the median nerve in particular, but involvement of the (proximal) ulnar nerve and the whole brachial plexus have been described (Price et al. 1995) as well as involvement of the superficial branches of the radial nerve, superficial branch of the peroneal nerve and the medial plantar nerve of the foot (reviewed in Razzaghi and Anastakis 2005). Pain, tenderness, diminished sensation, numbness, or paresthesias associated with a gradually enlarging mass are physical findings compatible with compressive neuropathy or carpal tunnel syndrome (Silverman and Enzinger 1985, Wharhold et al. 1993). Neurological deterioration ensues after some years from the mass appearance.

Meyer et al. (1998) described a case of a middle age woman who presented diverse fibrolipomatous hamartomas of the right ulnar and both median nerves, with a right-sided giant hand ("macrocheiria") due to enlarged bones and subcutaneous tissue, and an unusual late manifestation of nerve entrapment.

LFHN may infiltrate the muscle as well. Intramuscular fat deposition in biceps and tibial muscles was demonstrated by magnetic resonance (MR) imaging in three patients suffering of diverse fibrolipomatous hamartomas following the branching pattern of the nerves (De Maeseneer et al. 1997).

## Macrodactyly

The association of macrodactyly with LFHN has been largely described. Lesions presenting at birth or infancy far outnumber those recognized later in childhood or in adult life (Fig. 1). Usually, there is no history of any hereditary disorder. Macrodactyly is characterized by the increased size present since birth in one or several fingers or toes (Fig. 2). A disproportionate enlargement of digits including the nail apparatus, could be one and a half times larger than its counterparts (Fig. 3). Hands and feet are affected with almost equal frequency. Either in the

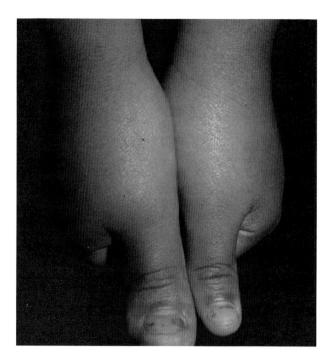

**Fig. 1.** Macrodactyly of right thumb in contrast with opposite normal finger.

hands and feet, the highest incidence of involvement is in the second and third digits, followed by the first digit; more than one digit involvement is not uncommon (Fig. 4). Enlargement of bone and subcutaneous tissue has been associated to an increase in dermal blood vessels as a nonspecific finding (Krengel et al. 2001) (Fig. 5a, b).

The natural history of the digit(s) overgrowth follows a progressive pattern and associated symptoms are variable. Some patients develop carpal tunnel syndrome later during life. Compression of the median nerve will increase and cause pain, sensory disturbance and motor weakness. The association of macrodactyly with LFHN and a vascular malformation coexisting with port-wine stains has been reported (Ban et al. 1998). In two cases of macrodactyly with nerve enlargement reported by Desai and Steiner (1990) a focal vascular proliferation within the hypertrophied lobules of adipose tissue was demonstrated. They suspected that this finding might be a part of the abnormal hamartomatous proliferation in macrodactyly. Interestingly, in large series (Razzaghi and

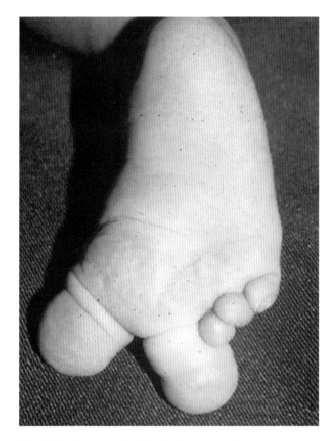

**Fig. 2.** Giant overgrowth of the first and second toes.

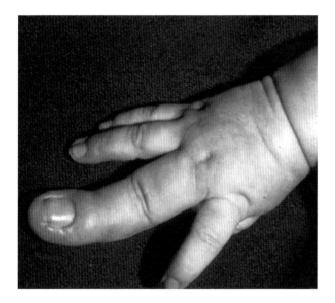

**Fig. 3.** Congenital macrodactyly of the third finger.

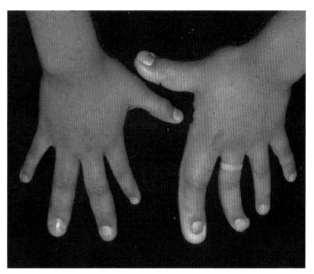

**Fig. 4.** Involvement of several fingers in both hands.

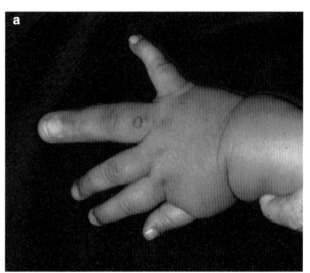

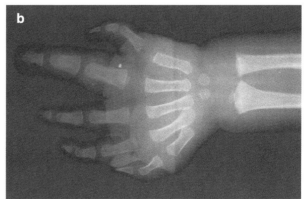

**Fig. 5.** (**a**) and (**b**) Macrodactyly of the forth digit with bone and nail enlargement.

Anastakis 2005, Syed et al. 2005) none of the affected patients had any other associated congenital anomalies.

## Imaging studies

Plain radiographs are valuable for assessing changes in the underlying skeleton when macrodactyly is present (Razzaghi and Anastakis 2005). Roentgenograms usually indicate that the bones and soft tissues of the affected digits enlarge proportionally (Roach 2004). The typical *radiological manifestations* include (Fig. 5): (1) marked proliferation of subcutaneous fat; (2) enlargement of bones (enlarged both in length and transverse diameter), marginal erosions, exostoses, joint destruction, irregular periosteal reaction, ankylosis by bands of dense bones; (3) absence of angioma or arteriovenous fistulae (Taybi 1996). Aside from the increased size and the centrifugal curvature of adjoining digits, the digits appear radiologically normal (Roach 2004). Other reported anomalies are. Early maturation of epiphyseal ossification centers in the involved area, thinning of metacarpals; thinning of metatarsals; syndactyly; polydactyly; brachydactyly; symphalangism; exostoses-like bony overgrowth along interphalangeal joints (Taybi 1996). Hypertophy and tortuosity of the digital nerve, a striking feature in macrodactyly of the hand, is notably absent in cass affecting the foot (Syed et al. 2005).

Magnetic resonance imaging (MRI) is characteristic, and allows to make the diagnosis preoperatively Jain et al. (2007). It is now being recommended in all patients suspected of having the condition. Hypertrophied nerves are characterized by fusiform nerve enlargement caused by fatty proliferation and thickening of nerve bundles. Nerve bundles appears as serpentine tubular structures, hypointense on both T1- and T2-weighted images (Sone et al. 2000). The varied amount of fatty proliferation among patients, the nerves involvement and the abnormalities in the branching pattern of nerves have been well demonstrated with MR imaging (De Maeseneer et al. 1997). Distribution of fat between fascicles is asymmetric. On coronal images the nerve has a spaghetti-like appearance that is pathognomonic for LFHN (Marom and Helms 1999, Khanna et al. 2001).

## Neurophysiologic studies

Electromyography and nerve conduction studies (EMG/NC) can show prolonged distal latency of sensory or motor innervation and fibrillations in distal muscles to confirm a compressive neuropathy (Amadio et al. 1988, Lowenstein et al. 2000, Meyer et al. 1997).

## Pathology

Histological confirmation of LFHN is not always feasible before the surgical treatment is performed.

On gross pathological examination, LFH consists of lobulated, soft, gray-yellow, sausage-shaped masses within the epineural sheath. Nerves may be markedly increased in length and diameter in the involved area: indeed, cases of fusiform median nerve enlargement of up to 17 cm in length and 30 mm in diameter have been reported (De Meseneer et al. 1997, Marom and Helms 1999). LFH can be extensive and follow nerves even up the brachial plexus. Along their course, the affected peripheral nerves do not adhere to surrounding tissue. In cases clinically associated with macrodactyly, hypertrophy of surrounding skin and soft tissue is associated with the enlargement of the bone.

In LFHN, the diffuse involvement of the nerve showing relatively bland histological changes is consistent with a hamartomatous rather than a neoplastic tumor. The lesions is described as a hamartoma because of the overgrowth of the normal connective tissue constituents: fat and fibrous tissue. Indeed, histological features are characterized by fibrofatty tissue that grows along epi- and perineurium and surrounds and infiltrates the nerve trunk. Mature fat cells have been found within the normal nerve sheath. It is thought that the proliferation of fat cells leads to enlargement of all mesenchymal components, including bone but particularly fibroadipose tissue (Silverman and Enzinger 1985). Osteocartilaginous deposits around the joints can also be found

(Nogueira et al. 1999). Neural degeneration detected by electron microscopic examination may be due to the compression of the surrounding tissue (Enzinger and Weiss 1995). The affected nerve may display other features in addition to adipose tissue, such as perineural septation of nerve fascicles and microfascicle formation.

## Pathogenesis and molecular genetics

The etiology and pathogenesis of this condition are yet unclear, but the histopathological findings support best the concept of hamartoma (Silverman and Enzinger 1985). Several potential etiologic factors have been described, including abnormal development of flexor retinaculum in children (Rowland 1977), antecedent trauma (Guthikonda et al. 1994), chronic nerve irritation (Callison et al. 1968) and nerve-mediated growth factor affecting the tissues distal to the sensory nerve tumor (Roach 2004).

Even though Barsky et al. (1967) found no report of familial occurrence megalodactyly still maintains an entry in the OMIM catalogue (OMIM # 155500) (OMIM 2006). Lacombe and Battin (1996) described 2 children diagnosed at birth as having isolated macrodactyly. Follow-up examination in these children showed development of hemihypertophy and other findings suggesting Proteus syndrome.

## Diagnosis

A carefully taken history and physical examination are the cornerstones of the correct diagnosis of LFHN (Razzaghi and Anastakis 2005). X-ray examination are valuable for assessing changes in the surrounding soft tissue and underlying bone (Taybi 1996). MRI play a major role in confirming the diagnosis (De Maeseneer et al. 1997, Khanna et al. 2001, Marom and Helms 1999) (see above "imaging studies"). EMG/NC can also provide valuable information needed to confirm the diagnosis of LFHN.

In some cases, a biopsy of the affected nerve branch must be obtained to confirm the diagnosis. When this is done, the biopsy should be studied by experienced neuropathologists so that malignant lesions such as malignant peripheral nerve sheath tumors can be ruled out.

## Differential diagnosis

Macrodactyly is not always associated to LFHN. The descriptive term of macrodactyly denotes overgrowth limited to or predominantly affecting the digits and should be distinguished from more extended malformations such as macromelia or hemihypertrophy. Clear distinction from diffuse lipomatosis with overgrowth of bone is not always possible, but diffuse lipomatosis is primarily a lesion of the subcutaneous tissue and muscle and only secondarily affects nerves.

Macrodactyly has also been described under several synonyms (see above). Enzinger and Weiss (1994) emphatically refer to them as neural fibrolipoma (lipofibromatous hamartoma of nerves) with macrodactyly.

There is a range of other, mostly congenital pathologic conditions in which localized overgrowth may mimic the clinical picture of macrodactyly. These include neurofibromatosis; primary lymphatic disorders (Milroy disease) and vascular malformations Klippel-Tranaunay and Parkes Weber syndromes as well as syndromes with hamartomatous changes (Proteus syndrome).

Diagnostic criteria to differentiate Proteus syndrome from macrodactyly due to LFHN include various localized overgrowths such as digital gigantism, hemihyperplasia with unilateral macrocephaly, epidermal nevus, and mesodermal hamartomas such as lipoma, lymphangioma, hemangioma, or fibroma. In Proteus syndrome hyperplasia of the plantar dermal tissue may results in a characteristic cerebriform appearance. Recently, hypoplastic lesions involving subcutaneous fat or muscle have been observed (Happle et al. 1997). Though Proteus syndrome comprises various other deformities, is not considered to be associated with enlarged nerves (Miura et al. 1993).

## Treatment

Treatment of LFHN associated or not to macrodactyly is usually a difficult task. Time and extent of therapeutic measures have to be considered very carefully to ensure the best functional outcome. Surgical treatments vary among patients.

Patients suffering of carpal tunnel syndrome may obtain benefit from carpal tunnel release and epineurolysis (Nogueira et al. 1999).

Another suggested approach (Roach 2004) has been to obtain serial roentgenograms of the same sex parent's hand or foot, then periodically compare the size of the child's growing digit to those of the parent at the aim of surgically obliterating the growth plate as soon as the growth size is appropriate for an adult in that family.

In principles, however, surgical excision of LFHN should not be recommended for several reasons: (1) the effects of excision are devastating in terms of motor and sensory function; (2) patients may suffer neurogenic pain after resection; (3) LFHN can involve the entire nerve all the way up to the plexus, making the resection difficult if not impossible to identify (reviewed in Razzaghi and Anastakis 2005).

In cases of LFHN without macrodactyly, most authors agree with a conservative approach that includes decompression of all compromised peripheral nerves to help alleviate pain and paresthesias to reduce the likelihood of permanent motor and sensory sequelae. If the disease is extensive consideration should be given to prophylactic decompression, even in the absence of motor and sensory symptoms.

Kotwal and Farooque (1998) reported 23 patients with macrodactyly. In eighteen patients a two-stage bulk-reducing (defatting) procedure and phalangectomy was used to shorten the digits. Good cosmetic correction was achieved in 12 patients, with satisfactory results in seven; two patients required amputation. Epiphysiodesis and epiphysectomy have been reported effective in the prevention of longitudinal overgrowth of digits. Resection of the hypertrophic nerves has been unsuccessful in preventing finger overgrowth (Ishida and Ikuta 1998).

In selected patients, other reconstructive procedures aimed at improving hand function include joint debridement, excision of osseous overgrowth and tendon transfers (i.e., opponensplasty) (Razzaghi and Anastakis 2005).

## References

Amadio PC, Reinam HM, Dobyns JH (1988) Lipofibromatous hamartoma of nerve. J Hand Surg Am 13: 65–75.

Ban M, Kamiya H, Sato M, Kitajima Y (1998) Lipofibromatous hamartoma of the median nerve associated with macrodactyly and port-wine stains. Pediatric Dermatol 15: 378–380.

Barsky AJ (1967) Macrodactyly. Bone Joint Surg 49: 1255–1266.

Bhat AK, Bhaskaranand K, Kanna R (2005) Bilateral macrodactyly of the hands and feet with post-axial involvement – a case report. J Han Surg Br 30: 618–620.

Bisceglia M, Vigilante E, Ben-Dor D (2007) Neural lipofibromatous hamartoma: a report of two cases and review of the literature. Adv Anat Pathol 14: 46–52.

Callison JR, Thoms OJ, White WL (1968) Fibrofatty proliferation of the median nerve. Plast Reconstr Surg 42: 403–413.

De Maeseneer M, Jaovisidha S, Lenchik L, Witte D, Schweitzer ME, Sartoris DJ, Resnick D (1997) Fibrolipomatous hamartoma : MR imaging findings. Skeletal Radiol 26: 155–160.

Desai P, Steiner GC (1990) Pathology of macrodactyly. Bull Hosp Jt Dis 50: 116–125.

Enzinger FM, Weiss SW (1994) Benign lipomatous tumors. In: Enzinger FM, Weiss SW (eds.) Soft tissue tumors. St. Louis: CV Mosby

Enzinger FM, Weiss SW (1995) Soft tissue tumors. 3rd ed. St Louis: CV Mosby, pp. 415–416.

Gouldesbrough DR, Kinny SJ (1989) Lipofibromatous hamartoma of the ulnar nerve at the elbow: brief report. J Bone Joint Surg Am 71: 331–332.

Guthikonda M, Renganchary SS, Balko MG, Van Loveren H (1994) Lipofibromatous hamartoma of the median nerve: case report with magnetic resonance imaging correlation. Neurosurgery 35: 127–132.

Happle R, Steijlen PM, Theile U, Karitzky D, Tinschert S, Albrecht-Nebe Helga, Küster W (1997) Patchy dermal hypoplasia as a characteristic feature of Proteus syndrome. Arch Dermatol 133: 77–78.

Herrick RT, Godsil RD Jr, Widener JH (1980) Lipofibromatous hamartoma of the radial nerve: a case report. J Hand Surg Am 5: 211–213.

Houpt P, Storm van Leeuwen JB, Van der Bergen HA (1989) Intraneural lipofibroma of the median nerve. J Hand Surg Am 14: 706–709.

Ishida O, Ikuta Y (1998) Long-term results of surgical treatment for macrodactyly of the hand. Plast Reconstr Surg 102: 1586–1590.

Jain TP, Srivastava DN, Mittal R, Gamanagatti S (2007) Fibrolipomatous hamartoma of median nerve. Australas Radiol 51 (Spec No): B98–B100.

Johnson RJ, Bonfiglio M (1969) Lipofibromatous hamartoma of the median nerve. J Bone Joint Surg Am 51: 984–999.

Jung SN, Yim Y, Kwon H (2005) Symmetric lipofibromatous hamartoma affecting digital nerves. Yonsei Med J 46: 169–172.

Kernohan J, Dakin PK, Quain JS, Helal B (1984) An "unusual" giant lipofibroma in the palm. J Hand Surg Br 9: 347–348.

Khanna G, Sundaram M, Rotman M, Janney CG (2001) Fibrolipomatous hamartoma of the nerve. Orthopedics 24: 836, 919–920.

Kotwal PP, Farooque M (1998) Macrodactyly. J Bone Joint Surg Br 80: 651–653.

Krengel S, Fustes-Morales A, Carrasco D, Vázquez M, Durán-McKinster C, Ruiz-Maldonado R (2001) Macrodactyly: report of eight cases and review of the literature. Pediatric Dermatol 17: 270–276.

Lacombe B, Battin J (1996) Isolated macrodactyly and Proteus syndrome. Clin Dysmorphol 5: 255–257.

Lowenstein J, Chandnani V, Tomaino MM (2000) Fibrolipoma of the median nerve: a case report and review of the literature. Am J Orthop 29: 797–798.

Marom EM, Helms CA (1999) Fibrolipomatous hamartoma: pathognomonic on MR imaging. Skeletal Radiol 28: 260–264.

Mason ML (1953) Presentation of a case: proceedings of the American society for surgery of the hand. J Bone Joint Surg Am 35: 273–274.

Meyer BU, Roricht S, Scmitt R (1998) Bilateral fibrolipomatous hamartoma of the median nerve with macrocheiria and late-onset nerve entrapment syndrome. Muscle Nerve 21: 656–658.

Mikhail IK (1964) Median nerve lipoma in the hand. J Bone Joint Surg Br 46: 726–730.

Miura H, Uchida Y, Ihara K, Sugioka Y (1993) Macrodactyly in Proteus syndrome. J Hand Surg 1118B: 308–309.

Nogueira A, Pena C, Martinez MJ, Sarasua JG, Madrigal B (1999) Hyperostotic macrodactyly and lipofibromatous hamartoma of the median nerve associated with carpal tunnel syndrome. Chir Main 18: 261–271.

Paletta FX, Rybka FJ (1972) Treatment of hamartoma of the median nerve. Ann Surg 176: 217–222.

Price AJ, Compson JP, Calonje E (1995) Fibrolipomatous hamartoma of the nerve arising in the brachial plexus. J Hand Surg 20: 16–18.

Pulventraft RG (1964) Unusual tumours of the median nerve. J Bone joint Surg Br 46: 731–733.

Razzaghi A, Anastakis DJ (2005) Lipofibromatous hamartoma: review of early diagnosis and treatment. J Can Chir 48: 394–399.

Roach ES (2004) Macrodactyly-nerve fibrolipoma. In: Roach ES, Van Miller S (eds.) Neurocutaneous disorders. New York: Cambridge University Press, pp. 323–325.

Rowland SA (1977) Case report: ten year follow-up of lipofibroma of the median nerve in the palm. J Hand Surg Am 2: 316–317.

Rusko RA, Larsen RD (1981) Intraneural lipoma of the median nerve: case report and literature review. J Hand Surg Am 6: 388–391.

Silverman TA, Enzinger FM (1985) Fibrolipomatous hamartoma of nerve. A clinicopathologic analysis of 26 cases. Am J Surg Pathol 9: 7–14.

Sone M, Ehara S, Tamakawa Y, Nishida J, Honjoh S (2000) Macrodystrophia lipomatosa: CT and MR findings. Radiat Med 18: 129–132.

Syed A, Sherwani R, Azam O, Haque F, Akhter K (2005) Congenital macrodactyly: a clinical study. Acta Orthop Belg 71: 399–404.

Taybi H (1996) Macrodystrophia lipomatosa. In: Taybi H, Lachman RS (eds.) Radiology of Syndromes, Metabolic Disorders and Skeletal Dysplasia, 4th ed. St. Louis: Mosby, pp. 292–293.

Warhold LG, Urban M, Bora EW, Brooks JSJ, Peters SB (1993) Lipofibromatous hamartomas of the median nerve. J Hand Surg 18A: 1032–1037.

Yeoman FM (1964) Fatty infiltration of the median nerve. J Bone Joint Surg Br 46: 737–739.

# Chapter 64

# CHIME SYNDROME (ZUNICH SYNDROME)

Janice Zunich and Nancy Esterly

Indiana University School of Medicine – Northwest, Gary, Indiana, USA (JZ); Medical College of Wisconsin, Milwaukee, Wisconsin, USA (NE)

## Introduction

CHIME syndrome is the acronym for a multisystem disorder consisting of **C**oloboma, **H**eart defects, **I**chthyosiform dermatosis, **M**ental retardation, and **E**ar anomalies with hearing loss. Characteristic features of CHIME syndrome include: (1) retinal coloboma; (2) congenital heart defects; (3) migratory ichthyosiform dermatosis at or within a few weeks of birth; (4) moderate to severe mental retardation; (5) seizure disorder exacerbated by high environmental temperatures and fever; (6) ear anomalies and mild to moderate conductive hearing loss secondary to increased desquamation in the auditory canal; (7) genitourinary abnormalities (hydronephrosis, bicornuate uterus); and (8) dysmorphic features consisting of brachycephaly, hypertelorism, broad, flat nasal root, short philtrum, full lips, anomalous dentition, low set, small nipples, brachydactyly, and broad second toes. Additional associated manifestations include feeding difficulties, recurrent respiratory infections in childhood, and large size at birth. Autosomal recessive inheritance is presumed on the basis of recurrence in a sib pair. A molecular basis for the disorder has not been determined.

## Historical perspective and eponyms

Initially described in 1983, the first report of CHIME syndrome was that of a young boy with a migratory ichthyosiform eruption, hypertelorism, bilateral retinal colobomata, conductive hearing loss, cleft palate, tooth anomalies, seizure disorder, developmental delay, and large size (Zunich and Kaye 1983). The association of an ichthyosiform dermatosis with retinal colobomata suggested a new neuroectodermal syndrome. The occurrence of congenital heart defects in two additional cases (Zunich and Kaye 1984, Zunich et al. 1988) led to the proposal of the acronym at the 1988 APS/SPR meeting. The occurrence of CHIME syndrome in the younger brother of the index case suggested autosomal recessive inheritance (Zunich et al. 1988). Subsequent case reports have established genitourinary anomalies as a cardinal feature (Shashi et al. 1995, Tinschert et al. 1996, Schnur et al. 1997, Sidbury and Paller 2001). The condition has also been reported as Zunich Neuroectodermal syndrome (Tinschert et al. 1996, OMIM # 280000).

## Incidence and prevalence

The incidence of CHIME syndrome is unknown. Only 8 cases have been reported in the literature (Zunich and Kaye 1983, 1984; Zunich et al. 1988; Ladda and Zunich 1990; Shashi et al. 1995; Tinschert et al. 1996; Schnur et al. 1997; Sidbury and Paller 2001) with another case unreported (personal communication). A possible tenth case is a male fetus terminated at 21 weeks gestation following ultrasound identification of severe hydronephrosis. Examination identified several craniofacial features consistent with those of his affected sister (personal communication). Excluding the fetus, the female: male ratio of CHIME syndrome is 1.25:1.0.

## Clinical manifestations

### Skin abnormalities

The onset of the rash is at birth or within the first 4–6 weeks. The cutaneous eruption is migratory and pruritic, characterized by scaling plaques with sharply marginated figurate borders (Fig. 1). In some

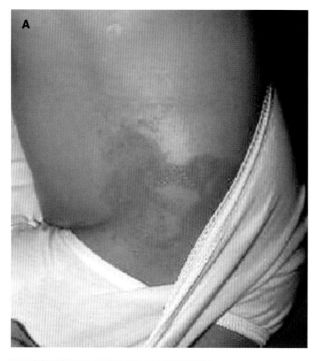

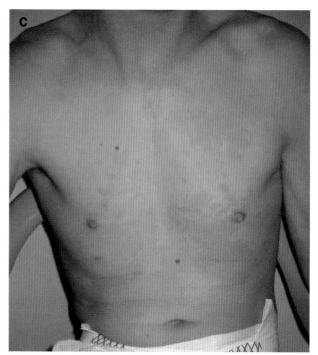

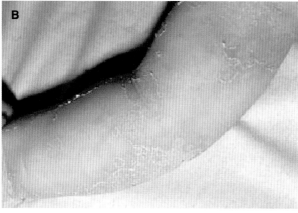

**Fig. 1.** (**A–C**) Cutaneous eruption. Note the figurate border of the plaque. (**B**) Desquamation and erythema.

patients, the rash is psoriasiform while in others it is more ichthyotic. As the rash moves elsewhere, it leaves behind normal skin. There is a lamelliform appearance to the cheeks. The palms and soles are thickened and brightly erythematous with an absence of scales.

Scalp hair, though normal in texture, is fine and somewhat sparse in younger children. Hair is poorly pigmented but seems to darken with age. Eyebrows and eyelashes are normal. Trichorrhexis nodosa has been noted in only one case. In other cases, no abnormalities of the hair shaft were identified. Additional dermatologic abnormalities reported include

lipomas (3 cases), dystrophic nails (2 cases), and recurrent skin infections (2 cases).

Histopathologic examination of biopsy specimens from patients show similar changes consisting of disordered keratinization, deep rete pegs in the dermis, and demyelination in the deep dermis.

## Nervous system abnormalities

Mild cerebral atrophy has been reported on CT scan or MRI in five cases with mildly enlarged ventricles

(Tinschert et al. 1996) and communicating hydro-cephalus (personal communication) noted in single cases. Seizure disorder has occurred in nearly all with onset usually before age 1. Grand mal, petit mal, and myoclonic seizures have all been reported. Abnormal EEG findings were identified in only one of four cases studied (Shashi et al. 1995). High environmental temperatures and fever appear to exacerbate seizures which are often difficult to control.

Moderate to severe psychomotor retardation and especially speech delay are present in nearly all cases. A single child is reported to be only mildly to moderately delayed with a nonverbal IQ of 82 at age 8 (personal communication). Three children are nonverbal and four have only limited language. Receptive language is somewhat better than expressive language skills.

Wide-based gait has been described in all cases. Hypotonia has also been noted infrequently (Ladda and Zunich 1990). Behavior problems are common and include autistic mannerisms and violent behavior towards both oneself and others. Teeth grinding, hitting, and biting have all been reported. In several cases, behaviors have worsened after puberty and seem to be correlated with the degree of discomfort resulting from the rash.

Bilateral retinal colobomata are identified in nearly all cases with choroidal colobomata noted in two individuals (Tinschert et al. 1996, Shashi et al. 1995). Additional, though less frequent, eye findings include myopia, hyperopia, ptosis, heterochromia irides, corneal clouding, esotropia, and exotropia.

All cases have mild to moderate conductive hearing loss, that apparently result from significant desquamation of the auditory canal although one case had abnormal auditory evoked responses. Myringotomy has not been successful in improving hearing.

## Craniofacial abnormalities

Characteristic craniofacial features in CHIME syndrome (Table 1) include brachycephaly, fine, sparse hair, hypertelorism, epicanthal folds, flat, broad nasal root and tip, short philtrum, and wide mouth with full lips (Fig. 2). Though head circumference is normal at birth, microcephaly is usually recognized within the

**Table 1.** Clinical characteristics of CHIME syndrome

| Clinical characteristics of CHIME syndrome | Incidence | |
|---|---|---|
| | No. | % |
| **Skin and hair** | | |
| Migratory ichthyosiform dermatosis | 9/9 | 100 |
| Sparse, fine hair as children | 7/7[*] | 100 |
| Thickened palms and soles | 5/6[*] | 83 |
| **Craniofacial** | | |
| Brachycephaly | 8/9 | 89 |
| Hypertelorism | 9/9 | 100 |
| Epicanthal folds | 8/9 | 89 |
| Flat, broad nasal root/tip | 9/9 | 100 |
| Cupped ears, rolled helices | 9/9 | 100 |
| Short philtrum | 5/9 | 55 |
| Full lips | 5/9 | 55 |
| Wide mouth | 8/9 | 89 |
| Anomalies in spacing, size, number of teeth | 7/8[†] | 88 |
| **Neurologic** | | |
| Mental retardation | 9/9 | 100 |
| Seizures | 9/9 | 100 |
| Behavior problems, autistic mannerisms | 5/8[†] | 63 |
| Wide-based gait | 6/6[†] | 100 |
| Conductive hearing loss | 9/9 | 100 |
| Microcephaly | 5/6[*] | 83 |
| **Ophthalmologic** | | |
| Retinal coloboma | 8/9 | 89 |
| Choroidal coloboma | 2/9 | 22 |
| Myopia, hyperopia | 3/9 | 33 |
| Esotropia, exotropia | 2/9 | 22 |
| Corneal clouding | 1/9 | 11 |
| **Cardiac** | | |
| Congenital heart defects | 7/9 | 78 |
| **Genitourinary** | | |
| Hydronephrosis | 5/9 | 55 |
| Renal agenesis | 1/9 | 11 |
| Bicornuate uterus | 2/5 females | 40 |
| **Gastrointestinal** | | |
| Feeding difficulties, problems chewing solids | 4/9 | 44 |
| Gastroesophageal reflux | 2/9 | 22 |

(Continued)

**Table 1.** (Continued)

| Clinical characteristics of | Incidence | |
|---|---|---|
| CHIME syndrome | No. | % |
| **Musculoskeletal** | | |
| Brachydactyly | 7/9 | 78 |
| Deviation of fingers and toes, clinodactyly | 7/9 | 78 |
| Club foot, joint contractures | 4/9 | 44 |
| **Dermatoglyphics** | | |
| High percentage of arches | 3/4* | 75 |
| **Recurrent infections in childhood** | | |
| Respiratory, sinus | 6/9 | 67 |
| Skin | 2/9 | 22 |
| **Miscellaneous** | | |
| Broad second toe | 8/9 | 89 |
| Small, low set nipples | 5/7* | 71 |
| **Growth** | | |
| Birth weight >90th percentile | 3/7* | 43 |
| Birth length >90th percentile | 4/7* | 57 |

*Not stated in all cases.
†Not able to be evaluated in some cases because of young age or early demise.

first year. The ears have rolled helices and are described in some cases as small, low set, or cupped. The teeth are small and irregularly shaped with increased spacing. Both bifid teeth and extra teeth have been described (3 cases). Infrequently, cleft palate, submucous cleft, and bifid uvula have occurred.

## Abnormalities of other systems

Cardiovascular defects have been identified in 70% and include tetralogy of Fallot, transposition, VSD (2 cases), peripheral pulmonic stenosis, subaortic stenosis, and dilated aortic root. While not initially recognized in the first 3 reported cases, genitourinary anomalies have subsequently been noted in all cases and include hydronephrosis (4 cases), unilateral renal agenesis, duplication of the collecting system with ureter entering the vagina, ectopic renal pelvis, bicornuate uterus (2 cases), and cryptorchidism. Menarche has been normal in two females and normal pubertal development has been reported in the four oldest cases (2 males and 2 females).

Though brachydactyly is the most common skeletal abnormality, clinodactyly of the 5th digits

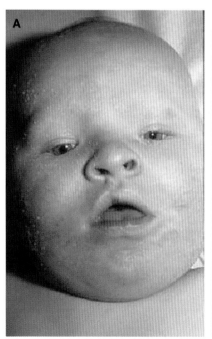 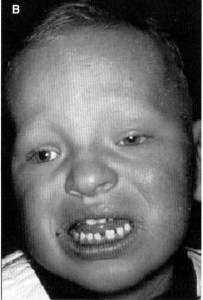 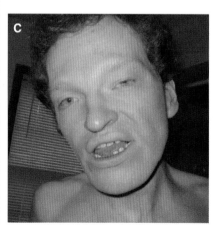

**Fig. 2. (A–C)** CHIME syndrome: index case at 1 year, 4 years, and 27 years of age. Note the hypertelorism, epicanthal folds, broad nasal root and tip, short philtrum, full lips, and increased spacing of dentition.

and deviation of the fingers and toes have frequently been present. Deviation of the toes progresses in older individuals, necessitating surgical correction (personal data). Less frequent skeletal features include scoliosis, pectus excavatum, club foot, joint contractures, subluxation of the hip, and dislocation of the radial heads. Coronal craniosynostosis requiring surgery occurred in one case (personal communication).

Feeding problems have occurred in 50% with both difficulty swallowing and chewing solids. Food often needs to be pureed for several years. Rarely, gastrointestinal anomalies have been reported and include gastroesophageal reflux (2 cases), low anal agenesis, hepatomegaly with normal liver biopsy (Schnur et al. 1997), and lymphocytic colitis.

Recurrent respiratory infections in childhood are common. One affected individual died of pneumonia at age 1 (Ladda and Zunich 1990). Recurrent sinus infections have also been noted occasionally (Zunich et al. 1985). No identifiable cause of the recurrent infections has been identified. Immunologic function studies were normal in 2 cases as was a lung biopsy in a single case. One instance of a malignancy was reported in a 4 1/2-year-old girl who developed acute lymphoblastic leukemia (Schnur et al. 1997). The significance of this is not known.

Birth weight and length greater than the 90th percentile have been noted in slightly more than one-third of cases. Bone age was normal in 3 cases. While some affected individuals have demonstrated decreased growth velocity with age (Shashi et al. 1995), others have attained normal heights.

Additional notable features include small, low set nipples and an increased percentage of arches (60–100%) on dermatoglyphics. A common but peculiar finding in 70% of cases is a broad second toe (Fig. 3). On X-ray, this appears to be the result of soft tissue enlargement and not an underlying bony abnormality.

## Pathogenesis and molecular genetics

The pathogenesis and molecular basis of CHIME syndrome remain elusive. Amino acids, organic acids,

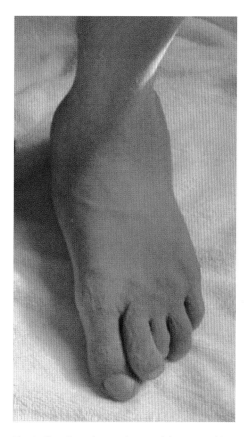

**Fig. 3.** Note broad second toe and deviation of first and second toes.

and chromosomal analysis including subtelomeres have all been normal. Although initially thought to represent a neuroectodermal syndrome, the major associated features of congenital heart defects and genitourinary anomalies suggest that the condition is truly a multisystem disorder of multiple congenital anomalies/mental retardation resulting from abnormalities of neuroectodermal, mesenchymal and mesodermal derivatives.

## Natural history

The ichthyosiform dermatosis can be present at birth or shortly thereafter. Onset of seizures has occurred between 3 weeks and 14 months. Affected individuals seem to have decreased sweating (personal data), possibly complicated by their skin condition, which may be responsible for exacerbation of seizures with high environmental temperatures and fever. Psychomotor delay is apparent on routine developmental screening in infancy. Although recurrent infections are common in childhood, general health is usually good in older individuals in spite of their associated malformations.

The first 3 reported cases are now 29 (female), 27 and 19 (both males). They require polytherapy for seizure control and management of behaviors and daily skin care. Orthopedic complications including scoliosis, deviation of toes, and hip dysplasia have recently become evident. The female lives in a group home for the developmentally disabled and the males remain with their family.

## Management and follow-up

Evaluation of the infant suspected of having CHIME syndrome should include renal ultrasound, echocardiography, and a detailed ophthalmologic examination. Auditory evoked responses to screen for conductive hearing loss is recommended. If normal, repeat hearing evaluations at 9 months and 2 years should be obtained since hearing deficits are so pervasive. Developmental testing at routine intervals beginning in infancy will determine which interventional therapies are necessary. Should seizures develop, EEG and neuroimaging studies would be recommended. In the majority of cases, however, findings on neuroimaging studies have often been nonspecific. Dermatologic evaluation can assist the family in management of the rash. Referral to other medical specialists will be determined by the associated complications of the condition.

## Differential diagnosis

The major clinical features of CHIME syndrome readily distinguish it from other ichthyosiform disorders such as KID (Keratitis-Ichthyosis-Deafness) syndrome (Nazzaro et al. 1990) and Refsum disease (Gibberd et al. 1985) in which deafness is neurosensory, not conductive, and intelligence is normal. Although both mental retardation and seizures can be associated with Sjogren-Larsson (Jagell et al. 1981),

Netherton (Julius and Keeran 1971), and Rud (Maldonado et al. 1975) syndromes, neither Sjogren-Larsson nor Netherton syndromes has hearing loss. Hearing loss reported in Rud syndrome is neurosensory and not conductive. Punctate keratitis and corneal opacities characterize Sjogren-Larsson syndrome and, rarely, retinitis pigmentosa has been seen in Rud syndrome, but retinal coloboma has not been reported.

CHARGE Association (Blake et al. 1998) and CHIME syndrome share several features: coloboma, heart defects, genitourinary anomalies, and psychomotor delay. Hearing loss is present in both, though neurosensory in CHARGE and not conductive. However, facial features are distinctly different between the two conditions and ichthyosiform skin changes have not been reported in CHARGE.

A newly reported autosomal recessive syndrome with midline brain malformation and mental retardation overlaps some features with CHIME syndrome including coloboma of the eye, heart defects, ichthyosiform dermatosis, ear defects and the nervous system defects (Al-Gazali et al. 2008). However, several features described in CHIME are not present in this newly defined syndrome (Al-Gazali et al. 2008) including deafness, seizures, digedontia, and hair abnormalities.

## Treatment

Optimal treatment measures for the eruption have yet to be determined as there is a paucity of patients studied. Caretakers advocate restricted bathing and daily hydrating agents with the use of emollients and keratolytics. Others have advocated frequent bathing. One patient showed modest improvement to isotretinoin (Accutane®). Other therapies, both developmental and medical, will be determined by the clinical extent of involvement and associated complications.

## Genetic counseling

CHIME syndrome is presumed to be an autosomal recessive disorder because of the recurrence of the condition in two brothers. Another affected sib pair is suspected (personal communication, Dr. Anne Turner). The sister was prenatally diagnosed with hydronephrosis at 15 weeks gestation and additionally has retinal colobomata, dilated aortic root, bicornuate uterus, hearing loss, moderate to severe delay, seizure disorder and characteristic dysmorphia. In a subsequent pregnancy, her mother's prenatal ultrasound identified a male fetus with extensive hydronephrosis. The fetus was suspected of being affected and the pregnancy was electively terminated at 21 weeks. Examination of the fetus identified several features consistent with his affected sister, including hypertelorism, overfolded helices, and broad, flat nasal bridge. All other cases have been isolated in families. Nevertheless, because of sibling recurrence, autosomal recessive inheritance needs to be considered a likely possibility with a maximum recurrence risk of 25% for parents of an affected child. Prenatal ultrasound to screen for cardiac or renal malformations may provide presumptive evidence of an affected fetus. In the absence of molecular testing for CHIME syndrome, confirmation of the diagnosis in a fetus would not be possible.

# References

Al-Gazali L, Hertecant J, Algawi K, El Teraifi H, Dattani M (2008) A new autosomal recessive syndrome of ocular colobomas, ichthyosis, brain malformations and endocrine abnormalities in an inbred Emirati family. Am J Med Genet A 146: 813–819.

Blake KD, Davenport SLH, Hall BD, Hefner MA, Pagon RA, Williams MS, Lin AE, Graham JM (1998) CHARGE association: An update and review for the primary pediatrician. Clin Pediatr 37: 159–174.

Gibberd FB, Billimoria JD, Goldman JM, Clemens ME, Evans R, Whitelaw MN, Retsas S, Sherrat RM (1985) Heredopathia atactica polyneuritiformis: Refsum's disease. Acta Neurol Scand 72: 1–17.

Jagell S, Gustavson K-H, Holmgren G (1981) Sjogren-Larsson syndrome in Sweden. A clinical, genetic, and epidemiological study. Clin Genet 19: 233–256.

Julius CE, Keeran M (1971) Netherton's syndrome in a male. Arch Dermatol 104: 422–424.

Ladda RL, Zunich J (1990) Ichthyosis-coloboma-heart defect-deafness-mental retardation. In: Buyse ML (ed.) Birth Defects Encyclopedia. Cambridge: Blackwell, pp. 945–946.

Maldonado RR, Tamayo L, Carnevale A (1975) Neuroichthyosis with hypogonadism (Rud's syndrome). Int J Dermatol 14: 347–352.

Nazzaro V, Blanchet-Bardon C, Lorette G, Civatte J (1990) Familial occurrence of KID (keratitis, ichthyosis, deafness) syndrome. Case reports of a mother and daughter. J Am Acad Dermatol 23: 385–388.

OMIM™ (2006) Online Mendelian Inheritance in Man. Baltimore: Johns Hopkins University. http://www.ncbi.nlm.nih.gov/omim

Schnur RE, Greenbaum BH, Hewmann WR, Christensen K, Buck AS, Reid CS (1997) Acute lymphoblastic leukemia in a child with the CHIME neuroectodermal dysplasia syndrome. Am J Med Genet 72: 24–29.

Shashi V, Zunich J, Kelly TE, Fryburg JS (1995) Neuroectodermal (CHIME) syndrome: an additional case with long term follow up of all reported cases. J Med Genet 32(6): 465–469.

Sidbury R, Paller AS (2001) What syndrome is this? Pediatr Dermatol 18(3): 252–254.

Tinschert S, Anton-Lamprecht I, Albrecht-Nebe H, Audring H (1996) Zunich neuroectodermal syndrome: migratory ichthyosiform dermatosis, colobomas, and other abnormalities. Pediatr Dermatol 13(5): 363–371.

Zunich J, Kaye CI (1983) New syndrome of congenital ichthyosis with neurologic abnormalities. Am J Med Genet 15: 331–333.

Zunich J, Kaye CI (1984) Letter to the editor: Additional case report of new neuroectodermal syndrome. Am J Med Genet 17: 707–710.

Zunich J, Esterly NB, Holbrook KA, Kaye CI (1985) Congenital migratory ichthyosiform dermatosis with neurologic and ophthalmologic abnormalities. Arch Dermatol 1212: 1149–1156.

Zunich J, Esterly NB, Kaye CI (1988) Autosomal recessive transmission of neuroectodermal syndrome. Arch Dermatol 124: 1188–1189.

# Chapter 65

# HYPOHIDROTIC ECTODERMAL DYSPLASIA (HED)

Martino Ruggieri and Ignacio Pascual-Castroviejo

Institute of Neurological Science, National Research Council, Catania and Department of Paediatrics, University of Catania, Catania, Italy (MR); Paediatric Neurology Service, University Hospital La Paz, University of Madrid, Madrid, Spain (IPC)

## Definition of the ectodermal dysplasias

The ectodermal dysplasias (EDs) represent a complex and highly diverse group of congenital heritable disorders affecting tissues of ectodermal origin. The main characteristics of the group, which encompasses more than 170 conditions (Irvine 2006, OMIM 2006), consist in developmental abnormalities of two or more ectodermal appendages/structures including skin, hair, teeth, nail and sweat glands, many of which have overlapping clinical features (Irvine 2006). Other structures derived from embryonic ectoderm include the mammary gland, thyroid gland, thymus, anterior pituitary, adrenal medulla, central nervous system, external ear, melanocytes, cornea, conjunctiva, lacrimal gland and lacrimal duct. The broader definition endeavouring all ectodermal derived structures, according to a recent review (Irvine 2006), has definite benefits in that the problems encountered by many patients and families are similar regardless of the specific subtype of ED. In addition, the wide-ranging classification is also helpful as several EDs are now known to share similar genetic mechanisms (Irvine 2006).

## History of terminology of ectodermal dysplasia

The first clinical report with features of what would be currently classified as ED is by Danz who in 1792 described two Jewish boys with congenital absence of hair and teeth (Danz 1792). The term "ectodermal dysplasia" did not appear in the literature until Weech coined it in 1929. Prior to this report isolated descriptions or small series of patients with hypotrichosis, hypodontia, onychodysplasia and anhidrosis had been described under various terms including "dystrophy of hair and nails", "imperfect development of skin, hair and teeth" and "congenital ectodermal defect". The designation coined by Weech specified some essential aspects of EDs: (1) most disturbances affected tissues of ectodermal origin; (2) these disturbances were developmental; and (3) heredity played a causative role (Irvine 2006). When Weech published his report in the late '20 (Weech 1929) he had in mind the X-linked anhydrotic form of ED (Christ-Siemens-Touraine syndrome; CST; or hypohidrotic ectodermal dysplasia, HED, OMIM # 305100) in males but noted that it had also been reported in females and occasionally could be inherited as a non-sex-linked trait (Irvine 2006): since then many clinicians have used the term ED to refer to CST syndrome and to the autosomal recessive and dominant forms of HED. As more clinical reports of patients with similar but subtly distinct patterns of abnormalities were recorded, the term "ectodermal dysplasia" became extended to include many different genetic entities. In an attempt to encapsulate this heterogeneity and the diversity of symptoms, Touraine (1936) proposed the term "ectodermal polydysplasia". Several other attempts, including hidrotic and anhidrotic forms soon followed but all failed to reflect the complexity of ectodermal appendages anomalies associated with the various forms of EDs. Currently, the most widely accepted and used definition of EDs is that reported in the paragraph below (Irvine 2006). Notably, many conditions that, by definition, lie within the broader spectrum of EDs (e.g., incontinentia pigmenti, Goltz syndrome) are often considered separately for practical reasons: these conditions are given in-depth coverage elsewhere.

## Classification of the ectodermal dysplasias

More than 170 different pathological conditions have been reported as EDs (Irvine 2006, Freire-Maia and Pinheiro 1984, OMIM 2006, Pinheiro et al. 1994, Priolo et al. 2000, 2001), and these are often associated with a broad spectrum of anomalies of ectodermal-derived organs and systems including the central nervous system (Clarke 1987, Irvine 2006). Until the end of the 20th century, classification systems for EDs were, because of lack of molecular understanding, based on clinical features. The most comprehensive accounts of clinical features and inheritance patterns of EDs are to be found in the 1984 monograph by Freire-Maia and Pinheiro and subsequent publication by Pinheiro and Freire-Maia (1994). Their classification designated conditions by groups depending on the presence of features in hair, nails, teeth or sweat glands, and assigned conditions to groups using a "1234 system" to collate conditions that had involvement of the hair (1), teeth (2) nails (3) or sweat glands (4) to groups such as 1-2 or 1-2-3. We refer the reader to the thorough review by Irvine (2006) for a comprehensive contemporaneous consideration of the breadth of ED conditions in the tradition of Freire-Maia and Pinheiro (Irvine 2006).

The last decade has watched several important insights into the molecular basis of several of the EDs which have either confirmed clinical impressions or contributed to pool or split several ED forms (Irvine 2006). Thus, new approaches to classification have endeavoured these most recent molecular insights and classified EDs under the broad categories of; (a) defects in nuclear tumour necrosis factor-like-κβ (*NF-*κβ) signalling pathways; (b) transcription factors (*TP63*-phenotypes) and homeobox genes; (c) gap junctions (*connexin* proteins: *GJA*, *GJB* and *GJC*); and (d) epithelial structural (*cytokeratins*) or adhesive (*desmosomal* components) molecules.

The X-linked, autosomal dominant and recessive hypohidrotic ectodermal dysplasias, whose phenotypic appearances are identical, are due to mutations in tumour necrosis factor-like/NF-κβ signalling pathways.

# HYPOHIDROTIC ECTODERMAL DYSPLASIA

## Introduction

Hypohidrotic ectodermal dysplasia (HED) is the most common of the EDs and is characterised by hypotrichosis, hypodontia, hypohidrosis and distinctive facial features. HED is included in both classifications of EDs, the most permissive of Freire-Maia and Pinheiro (1984) and Pinheiro and Freire-Maia (1994) and the more restrictive ones of Priolo et al. (2000), including 46 entities, and Irvine (2006) which integrate either the molecular genetic data and the corresponding clinical findings.

Three inherited types of HED are known: (1) X-linked recessive HED (XLRHED; OMIM # 305100) which is the most frequent (Irvine 2006, Reed et al. 1970); and two rarer forms: (2) autosomal dominant HED (ADHED; OMIM # 129490) and autosomal recessive HED (ARHED; OMIM # 224900) (Baala et al. 1999, Irvine 2006, Munoz et al. 1997). The phenotypic appearance of the XLRHED and autosomal types (ADHED and ARHED) are identical. The autosomal forms of HED are caused by mutations in the *Downless* (DL) gene while the X-linked form is caused by mutations in the *EDA1* gene which maps to Xq12-13.1 and encodes two isoforms of a transmembrane protein, *ectodysplasin-A* (EDA), that has homology to the TNF family (Irvine 2006).

## Historical perspective and eponyms

HED (also known as anhidrotic ectodermal dysplasia or Christ–Siemens–Touraine syndrome or Weech syndrome (Christ 1932, Siemens 1937, Weech 1929) was first reported by Thurman in 1848, but earlier descriptions may be found. Thedani (1921) determined that HED was an X-linked disorder and later reported that female carriers manifest varying signs of the conditions. Weech (1929) observed the depression of gland function and coined the term "anhidrotic ectodermal dysplasia", while Christ defined the condition as a "congenital ectodermal defect", and Siemens named the disorder as "anhidrosis hypotrichotica". Felsher (1944) pointed that the skin is rarely, if ever, completely anhidrotic and suggested the term "hypohidrotic" instead of "anhidrotic" which is most often used.

## Incidence and prevalence

HED is a rare condition.

## Clinical manifestations

Clinically, HED is characterized by: a) fine and sparse hair; b) few and often pointed teeth; c) diminished or absent eccrine function that mainly affects mucosal and sweat glands. The inability to sweat is responsible for the most dangerous consequences of the disorder with the chance of putting affected infants and children at risk for life-threatening and brain-damaging episodes of hyperthermia (Cambiaghi et al. 2000). Intolerance to heat, with severe incapacitation and hyperpyrexia may occur after only mild exertion or even following meals. In X-linked HED, the affected patients are most often hemizygous male individuals, since in heterozygous female carriers the severity of the disorder varies considerably; most females only have a mild or "partial" involvement and, most often, are not referred to a physician (Cambiaghi et al. 2000). Autosomal recessive HED is similar to the hemizygous form of X-linked HED from a clinical viewpoint except that males and females are equally affected.

Patients with HED most often show a quite characteristic phenotype and individuals from different families look enough alike as brothers.

## Craniofacial features

The facies appears as an inverted triangle, with marked frontal bossing, concave midface, different degrees of depressed nasal bridge, saddle nose and

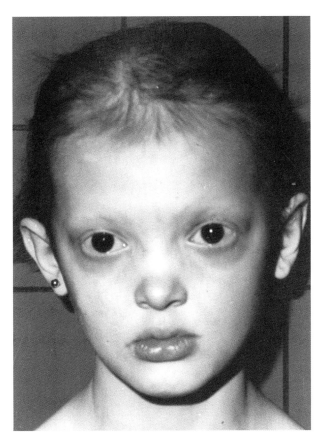

**Fig. 1.** Hypohydrotic ectodermal dysplasia in a 7-year-old girl: the facies is characterized by frontal bossing, depressed nasal bridge, thin hair, and pouting lips.

protuberant lips (Fig. 1). Fine linear wrinkles are often noted about the eyes and mouth, or evident periorbital pigmentation. A third of affected males have ears that are described as simple or satyr. The distinctive facial features may not be obvious at birth but become more noticeable with age. Carrier females may exhibit similar facial features.

## Skin

In children and adults the skin is soft, thin and dry because of the absence of sebaceous glands (Fig. 2). Eczema is not uncommon, especially during the first years of life. At birth, affected males may demonstrate marked scaling or peeling of their skin that

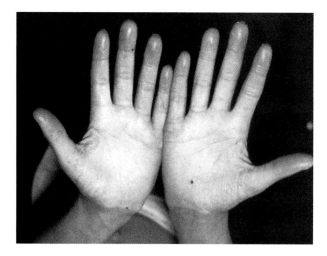

**Fig. 2.** The palms of the same patient as in Fig. 1 shows dry skin.

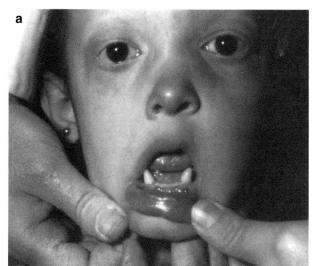

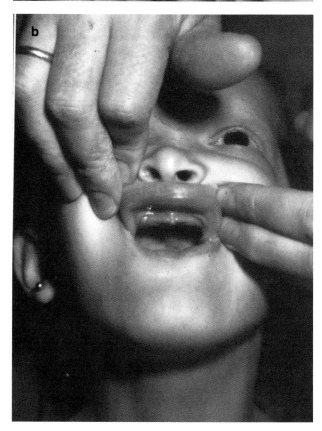

**Fig. 3.** Same patient as in Figs. 1 and 2. (**a**) Periorbital pigmentation and presence only of canines in the lower arcade; (**b**) Anodontia in the upper arcade.

may be mistaken for a colloidon membrane. Periorbital hyperpigmentation around the eyes is a characteristic features of the disorder. Small milia-like papules may be found on the face.

## Hair

Hair is scant, fine, stiff, short, and most often blond, in scalp, axillary and pubic regions, and may be completely lacking in the eyelashes, brows or in entire body. Secondary sexual hair in the beard, pubic and axillary regions is variably present. Approximately, 70% of obligate female carriers of X-linked HED describe their hair as being sparse or fine.

## Oral manifestations

Oral manifestations consist of hypodontia or, more often, anodontia reflecting complete lack of dental ectoderm. Teeth is originate from both ectodermal and mesodermal tissue, while odontoblasts from, a mesodermal component, and do not differentiate in the absence of an ectodermal layer (Glasstone 1935–1936). The few teeth that may be present are often delayed in eruption (Fig. 3), and when present, the incisors, canines and bicuspids, are often conical in crown form (Gorlin and Pindborg 1964). The shape of the crown is determined by the inner enamel or ameloblastic layer of the tooth germ. Oral, pharyngeal and nasal mucosa most often appear dry and atrophic. Dental roentgenograms show the hypodontia or anodontia and the conical form of tooth crowns (Fig. 4).

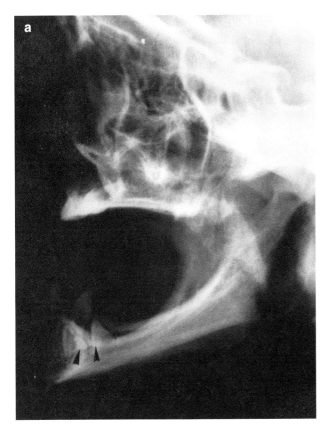
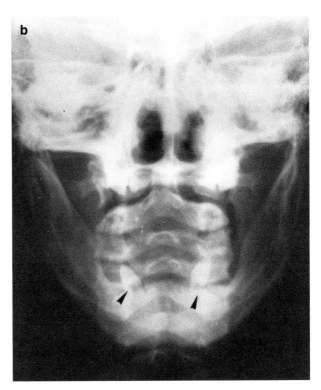

Fig. 4. Dental roentgenograms of the same patient. Sagittal and coronal views confirm the presence of two canines in the mandible (arrow heads) and anodontia of the other teeth.

## Other ectodermal structures

Aplastic or hypoplastic mammary glands, and primary hypogonadism (Mohler 1959) have been also reported. The finger and the toe nails are usually normal. Thin, brittle nail plates with longitudinal ridges have been described in some individuals.

## Eye involvement

Ocular symptoms and signs consist in alterations of the meibomian glands (95.45%) which are detected by meibomianoscopy, reduction of eyebrowns (94.4%), and lashes alterations (91.6%) (Kaercher 2004).

## Other clinical features

Diminished or absent mucous glands of the tracheal, bronchial, oesophageal, gastric and colonic mucosa cause problems with recurrent bronchitis, pneumonia, dysphagia, and gastro-oesophageal reflux and constipation. Reactive airways associated with wheezing are a common problem.

Individuals with HED most frequently show normal intelligence, and mental retardation is seldom associated with this condition.

## Molecular genetics and pathogenesis

HED most frequently manifests as X-linked recessive form or more rarely, as autosomal recessive or autosomal dominant (Baala et al. 1999, Shimomura et al. 2004, Zonana et al. 2000).

The gene responsible for X-linked HED, known as *EDA1* gene (mouse model known as *tabby*), is located at Xq12-q13.1 and affects a transmembrane protein (*ectodysplasin-A* or EDA) (Na et al. 2004) expressed by keratinocytes, hair follicles, and sweat glands, possibly having a key role in epithelial-mesenchymal signalling (Kere et al. 1996). Mutations in the domains of EDA are thought to have an effect on solubility or cleavage of ectodysplasin-A (EDA) rendering it non functional: cleavage of EDA is necessary to enable solubility and functionality of EDA. The two longest isoforms of EDA, EDA-1 and EDA-2 bind to two different receptors: EDA-1 binds to the EDAR protein and EDA-2 binds to another X-linked receptor, XEDAR.

The gene responsible for autosomal dominant/recessive HED, known as *Downless* (DL) (mouse model known as *downless*), has been mapped to chromosome 2q11-q13 (Monreal et al. 1999, Shimomura et al. 2004) and encodes a member of the tumour necrosis factor receptor (TNFR) super-family which functions as an ectodysplasin receptor (EDAR).

The EDA-EDAR pathway has been further refined when the molecular basis of a third mouse homologue has been identified: the *crinckled* mouse (*cr*) which is a spontaneous mouse mutant with an identical phenotype to *downless* and *tabby*. The causative gene of *crinckled* has been identified in an adapter protein (EDAR-associated death domain, termed *EDARADD*) for the EDA-EDAR complex (Fig. 5). Mutations in this gene have been also identified in patients with autosomal recessive HED. The EDARADD domain interacts with the intracellular domain of EDAR, linking to downstream signals leading to NF-κβ activation. In addition, EDARADD associates with TRAF (tumour necrosis factor receptor/TNFR-associated factor) 1, 2 and 3.

NF-κβ activation by the EDAR pathway is NEMO dependent: thus, loss of function mutations

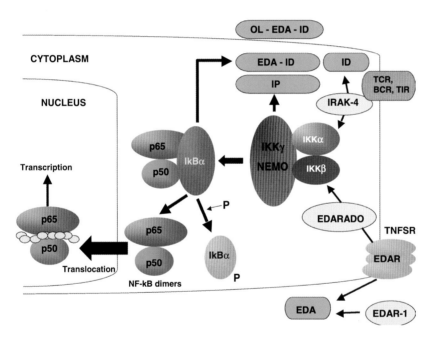

**Fig. 5.** Overview of the NF-κβ-related pathways and their role in human ectodermal dysplasias. EDA, hypohidrotic/anhidrotic ectodermal dysplasia; EDA-1, etodysplasin a; EDA-ID, anhidrotic ectodermal dysplasia with immunodeficiency; EDAR, EDA receptor; EDARADD, EDAR-associated death domain; ID, immune deficiency; κβα (aka: NFKBIA), alpha nuclear factor of kappa light chain gene enhancer in B cells inhibitor; IKKα, alpha kinase of inhibitor of kappa light polypeptide gene enhancer in B cells; IKKβ, beta kinase of inhibitor of kappa light polypeptide gene enhancer in E cells; IKKγ, gamma kinase of inhibitor of kappa light polypeptide gene enhancer in B cells; IP, incontinentia pigmenti; IRAK-4, interleukin-1-reeptor-associated kinase-4; NEMO, (aka: IKKγ) NFκB essential modulator (gamma kinase of inhibitor of kappa light polypeptide gene enhancer in B cells); NFκB essential modulator (gamma kinase of inhibitor of kappa light polypeptide gene enhancer in B cells); NFκB, nuclear factor kappa-B; OL-EDA-ID, anhidrotic ectodermal dysplasia with immunodeficiency, osteopetrosis and lymphoedema; TCR, T-cell receptor; BCR, B-cell receptor; TIR, Toll/IL-1 receptor superfamily; TNFSR, TNF superfamily (Adapted from Irvine 2006).

in the EDAR pathway are similar to those in the IKKγ gene (known as NEMO) which regulates the expression of multiple genes which functions in controlling the immune and stress response, cell adhesion, protection against apoptosis and inflammatory reactions. NF-κB factor is composed of homo- and heterodimers of 5 proteins belonging to the *Rel* family and is sequestered in the cytoplasm by inhibitory proteins of the IκB family. In response to various stimuli such as tumour necrosis factor (TNF), interleukin-1 (IL-1), and lipopolysaccharide, the inhibitory molecule is phosphorylated and then degraded, allowing NF-κB to enter the nucleus and activate transcription of targeted genes. The kinase phosphorylating IκB (IKK) is a complex of three molecules IKK1/IKKα, IKK2/IKKβ, and NEMO. IKK1 and IKK2 act as catalytic subunits, while NEMO is a structural and regulatory subunit vital to the function of the unit as a whole (Fig. 5). The absence of NEMO results in no NF-κB activity in response to stimuli (Bruckner 2004).

Several studies have shed light on how abnormalities in the NF-κB pathway produce skin and systemic lesions in HED and/or in IP (reviewed in Bruckner 2004 and Irvine 2006). The activation of NF-κB is critical in preventing apoptosis induced by TNF-α. Male NEMO knockout mice die early in utero and often demonstrate massive liver apoptosis. On the other hand, female mice heterozygous for NEMO deficiency (IKKγ$^{\pm}$) develop transitory skin changes that are phenotypically and histologically similar to those of HED and IP. The skin of these mice contains elevated levels of several cytokines and chemokines such as TNF-α (Makris et al. 2000). IP lesions of human skin strongly express eotaxin, an eosinophil-selective chemokine that is activated by NF-κb (Jean-Baptiste et al. 2002). These findings suggest that in the vesicular stage of IP and in the skin of HED, IKK-γ$^{-}$ cells undergo apoptosis, while IKK-γ$^{+}$ cells in turn upregulate the production of TNF-α, IL-1, eotaxin and other cytokines and chemokines. This further drives apoptosis of IKK-γ$^{-}$ cells and also produces an influx of eosinophils into the skin. As the population of IKK-γ$^{-}$ cells declines, inflammation subsides, heralding the end of the 1st stage of disease. Residual IKK-γ$^{-}$ cells that undergo apoptosis in response to circulating cytokines explain the recurrence of vesicular lesions with febrile illnesses (Brucker 2004). The mechanism producing subsequent skin changes, as well as other findings associated with IP and HED, are poorly understood. The skin of NEMO knockout mice over expresses cytokeratins 6 and 17 which are markers of an inflammatory response, in part explaining the hyperkeratotic lesions. The pathogenesis of the hyperpigmented lesions is unclear, as these areas often do not correspond to preceding inflammation, making purely post inflammatory hyperpigmentation unlikely. Atrophic skin changes may represent residual scarring but may also be due to developmental malformation of the affected areas.

## Hypohidrotic ectodermal dysplasia with immunodeficiency (EDA-ID)

Mutations in IKK-gamma (NEMO) have been shown to cause incontinentia pigmenti (IP) (Bloch-Sulzberger type) (Smahi et al. 2000). IKK-gamma is required for the activation of a transcription factor known as "nuclear factor Kappa B" and plays an important role in T- and B-cell function. Males with HED and immune-deficiency (ID) (HED-ID) (OMIM # 300291) from four families studied sequentially by Zonana et al. (2000) revealed 10 mutations affecting the carboxy-terminal end of IKK-gamma protein, a domain believed to connect the IKK signalsome complex to upstream activators. The findings defined this new-linked recessive immunodeficiency syndrome, distinct from other types of HED and immunodeficiency syndromes. Affected males with HED-ID have significant morbidity and mortality from recurrent infections despite therapy (Zonana et al. 2000). Even though the common IKK-gamma mutations seen in IP are lethal for males in utero, and only decrease the immunity in patients with X-linked HED-ID in the four families described by Zonana et al. (2000), it has been suggested that mutations that preserve some IKK-gamma function may be responsible for HED-ID (Zonana et al. 2000).

## Diagnosis

The value of tests in supporting the diagnosis of HED has been studied and demonstrated that non-invasive trichogram and sweat testing results can support the diagnosis of HED, but are not sensitive or highly specific; horizontally sectioned 4-mm punch biopsy specimens of the scalp or palms that lack eccrine structures are diagnostic of HED; scalp biopsy shows more sensitivity (67%), with a specificity of 100%, than palmar biopsy, and a scalp biopsy specimen with detectable eccrine structures suggests that a patient does not have HED (Rouse et al. 2004).

## Differential diagnosis

HED shows several facets in the clinical features that overlap with those observed in other neurocutaneous disorders. HED chondroectodermal dysplasia, focal dermal hypoplasia, and incontinentia pigmenti (IP) show almost identical conical teeth. Alopecia is seen in the progeria of Hutchinson-Gilford, Rothmund-Thomson syndrome, ichthyosis follicularis and sixteen additional overlapping entities (Mégarbané et al. 2004). The clinical features of HED also resemble Rapp-Hodgkin, Bowen-Amstromg and CHAND syndromes (Sahin et al. 2004), hypotrichosis and nail dysplasia syndrome (Harrison and Sinclair 2004), and the Johanson-Blizzard syndrome (1971) which is an autosomal recessive inherited disorder (Mardini et al. 1978) characterized by alae nasi hypoplasia, scalp and hair ectodermal abnormalities, absence of teeth, genito-urethro-anal anomalies, malabsorption, microcephaly, deafness and dwarfism (Schussheim et al. 1976).

## Management

The intolerance of subjects with HED to heat requires these patients to take precautions to protect them from high temperatures, sun exposure and abundant meals.

The oral rehabilitation of patients with HED is important for better social living, self esteem, and oral function (Della Valle et al. 2004).

In the current absence of any effective treatment for HED, comprehensive, accurate prenatal or postnatal genetic testing and counselling can provide valuable information.

## References

Baala L, Hadj Rabia S, Zlogotora J, Kabbaj K, Chhoul H, Munnich A, Lyonnet S, Sefiani A (1999) Both recessive and autosomal dominant forms of anhidrotic/hypohidrotic ectodermal dysplasia map to chromosome 2q11-q13. Am J Hum Genet 64: 651–653.

Bruckner AL (2004) Incontinentia pigmenti: a window to the role of NF-κB function. Semin Cut Med Surg 23: 116–124.

Cambiaghi S, Restano L, Päkkönen K, Caputo R, Kere J (2000) Clinical findings in mosaic carriers of hypohidrotic ectodermal dysplasia. Arch Dermatol 136: 217–224.

Christ J (1932) Über die Korrelationen der Kongenitalen Defekte des Ectoderms untereinander mit besonderer Berücksichtigung ihrer Beziehungen zum Auge. Zbl Haut Geschlkr 40: 1–21.

Clarke A (1987) Hypohidrotic ectodermal dysplasia. J Med Genet 24: 659–663.

Danz DFG (1792) Sechste Bemerkung. Von Menschen ohne Haare und Zähne. Stark Arch Geburtch Frauenz Neugeb Kinderkr 4: 684.

Della Valle D, Chevitarese AB, Maia LC, Farinhas JA (2004) Alternative rehabilitation treatment for a patient with ectodermal dysplasia. J Clin Pediatr Dent 28: 103–106.

Felsher Z (1944) Hereditary ectodermal dysplasia. Report of a case with experimental study. Arch Dermatol Syph 49: 410–414.

Freire-Maia N, Pinheiro M (1984) Ectodermal dysplasias: a clinical and genetic study. New York: Alan R. Liss.

Glasstone S (1935–1936) Development of tooth germs in vitro. J Anat 70: 260–266.

Gorlin RJ, Pindborg JJ (1964) Anhidrotic ectodermal dysplasia. In: Gorlin RJ, Pindborg JJ (eds.) Syndromes of the head and neck. New York: McGraw-Hill, pp. 303–311.

Harrison S, Sinclair R (2004) Hypotrichosis and nail dysplasia: a novel hidrotic ectodermal dysplasia. Australas J Dermatol 45: 103–105.

Irvine AD (2006) Ectodermal dysplasia. In: Harper J, Oranje A, Prose N (eds.) Textbook of Pediatric Dermatology. Oxford: Blackwell Science, pp. 1412–1466

Jean-Baptiste S, O'Toole EA, Chen M, Guitart J, Paller A, Chan LS (2002) Expression of eotaxin, an eosinophil-selective chemokine, parallels eosinophil accumulation in the vesiculobullous stage of incontinentia pigmenti. Clin Exp Immunol 127: 470–478.

Johanson A, Blizzard B (1971) A syndrome of congenital aplasia of the alae nasi, deafness, hypothyroidism, dwarfism, absent permanent teeth, and malabsorption. J Pediatr 79: 982–987.

Kaercher T (2004) Ocular symptoms and signs in patients with ectodermal dysplasia syndromes. Graefes Arch Clin Exp Ophthalmol 242: 495–500.

Kere J, Srivastava AK, Montonen O (1996) X-linked an-hidrotic (hypohidrotic) ectodermal dysplasia is caused by mutation in a novel transmembrane protein. Nat Genet 13: 409–416.

Makris C, Godfrey VL, Krahn-Senftleben G, Takahashi T, Roberts JL, Schwarz T, Feng L, Johnson RS, Karin M (2000) Female mice heterozygous for IKK gamma/NEMO deficiencies develop a dermatopathy similar to the human X-linked disorder incontinentia pigmenti. Mol Cell 5: 969–979.

Mardini MK, Ghandour M, Sakati NA, Nyhan VL (1978) Johanson-Blizzard syndrome in a large imbred kin-dred with three involved members. Clin Genet 14: 247–250.

Mégarbané H, Zablit C, Waked N, Lefranc G, Tomb R, Mégarbané A (2004) Ichthyosis follicularis, alopecia, and photophobia (IFAP) syndrome: report of a new family with additional features and review. Am J Med Genet 124A: 323–327.

Mohler DN (1959) Hereditary ectodermal dysplasia of the anhidrotic type associated with primary hypogonadism. Am J Med 27: 682–688.

Monreal AW, Ferguson BM, Headon DJ, Street SL, Overbeek PA, Zonana J (1999) Mutations in the human homo-logue of mouse dl cause autosomal recessive and domi-nant hypohidrotic ectodermal dysplasia. Nat Genet 22: 366–369.

Munoz F, Lestringant G, Sybert V, Frydman M, Alswaini A, Frossard PM, Jorgenson R, Zonana J (1997) De-finitive evidence for an autosomal recessive form of hypohidrotic ectodermal dysplasia clinically indistin-guishable from the more common X-linked disorder. Am J Hum Genet 61: 94–100.

Na GY, Kim do W, Lèe SJ, Chung SL, Park DJ, Kim JC, Kim MK (2004) Mutation in the ED1 gene, A la 349 Thr, in a Korean patient with X-linked hypohidrotic ec-todermal dysplasia developing de novo. Pediatr Derma-tol 21: 568–572.

OMIM (2006) ondine Mendelian Inheritance in Man. Baltimore: Johns Hopkins University Press. http://ncbi.nlm.nih.gov/omim

Pinheiro M, Freire-Maia N (1994) Ectodermal dysplasias: a clinical classification and a causal review. Am J Med Genet 53: 153–162.

Priolo M, Silengo M, Lerone M, Ravazzolo R (2000) Ecto-dermal dysplasias: not only "skin" deep. Clin Genet 58: 415–431.

Priolo M, Laganà C (2001) Ectodermal dysplasias: a new clinical-genetic classification. J Med Genet 38: 579–585.

Reed WB, Lopez DA, Landing BH (1970) Clinical spec-trum of anhidrotic ectodermal dysplasia. Arch Derma-tol 102: 134–143.

Rouse C, Siegfried E, Breer W, Nahass G (2004) Hair and sweat glands in families with hypohidrotic ectodermal dysplasia. Further characterization. Arch Dermatol 140: 850–855.

Sahin MT, Turel-Ermertcan A, Chan I, McGrath JA, Ozturkcan S (2004) Ectodermal dysplasia showing clinical overlap between AEC, Rapp-Hodgkin and CHAND syndromes. Clin Exp Dermatol 29: 486–488.

Schussheim A, Choi SJ, Silverberg M (1976) Exocrine pan-creatic insufficiency with congenital anomalies. J Pedi-atr 89: 782–784.

Shimomura Y, Sato N, Miyashita A, Hashimoto T, Ito M, Kuwano R (2004) A rare case of hypohidrotic ectodermal dysplasia caused by compound heterozygous mutations in the EDAR gene. J Invest Dermatol 123: 649–655.

Siemens HW (1937) Studien über Vererbung von Hautkrankheiten. XII. Anhidrosis hypotrichotica. Arch Dermat Syph 175: 565.

Smahi A, Courtois G, Vabres P, Yamaoka S, Hewertz S, Munnich A, Israel A, Heiss NS, Klauck SM, Kioschis P, Wiemann S, Poustka A, Esposito T, Bardaro T, Gianfrancesco F, Ciccodicola A, D'Urso M, Woffendin H, Jakins T, Donnai D, Stewart H, Kenwrick SJ, Aradhya S, Yamagata T, Levy M, Lewis RA, Nelson DL (2000) Genomic rearrangement in NEMO impairs NF-Kappa B activation and is a cause of incontinentia pigmenti: The International Incontinentia Pigmenti (IP) Consortium. Nature 405: 466–472.

Thadani KI (1921) A toothless type of man. J Hered 12: 87–88.

Thurman J (1848) Two cases in which skin, hair and teeth were very imperfectly developed. Proc Roy Med Chir Soc 31: 71–81.

Touraine A (1936) L'anidrose hereditaires avec hypotrichose et anodontie (polydysplasie ectodermique hereditaire). Presse Med 44: 145–149.

Weech AA (1929) Hereditary ectodermal dysplasia. Am J Dis Child 37: 766–790.

Zonana J, Elder ME, Schneider LC, Orlow SJ, Moss C, Golabi M, Shapira SK, Farndon PA, Wara DW, Emmal SA, Ferguson BM (2000) A novel X-linked disorder of immune deficiency and hypohidrotic ecto-dermal dysplasia is allelic to incontinentia pigmenti and due to mutations in IKK-gamma (NEMO). Am J Hum Genet 67: 1555–1562.

# Chapter 66

# COSTELLO SYNDROME AND THE RAS-EXTRACELLULAR SIGNAL REGULATED KINASE (ERK) PATHWAY

**Ignacio Pascual-Castroviejo and Martino Ruggieri**

Paediatric Neurology Service, University Hospital La Paz, University of Madrid, Madrid, Spain (IPC); Institute of Neurological Science, National Research Council, Catania and Department of Paediatrics, University of Catania, Catania, Italy (MR)

## Introduction

*Costello syndrome* is a multiple congenital malformation/mental retardation (MCA/MR) syndrome (OMIM # 218040) characterized by prenatally increased growth with subsequent (postnatal) growth retardation (usually as a result of severe postnatal feeding difficulties), distinctive coarse face (full lips, large mouth) with macrocephaly, loose skin resembling cutis laxa, diffuse hypotonia and laxity of the small joints with ulnar deviation of the wrists and fingers, tight Achilles tendons, non-progressive cardiomyopathy and/or congenital heart disease (usually valvar pulmonic stenosis), arrhythmia (usually supraventricular or paroxysmal tachycardia; most distinctively, chaotic atrial rhythm or multifocal atrial tachycardia) developmental delay and an outgoing friendly behaviour or hyperhemotionality (Galera et al. 2006; Hennekam 2003; Johnson et al. 1998; Rauen 2007a, b; Van Eeghen et al. 1999). Skin abnormalities include: (a) *cardinal manifestations* such as thick, loose skin on the dorsal aspects of the hands and feet and deep palmar and plantar creases; (b) *important manifestations* including benign tumours of ectodermal origin such as papillomas, calcified epitheliomas, dermoid cysts, mammary fibroadenosis, and syringomas appearing in the face and nasolabial regions or in other moist body surfaces; and (c) *other manifestations* such as diffuse hyperpigmentation, acanthosis nigricans and curly and sparse scalp hair (Johnson et al. 1998, Nguyen et al. 2007, Weiss et al. 2004). Patients may have a predisposition for malignancies (approximately 15% risk of malignant tumours), mainly abdominal and pelvic rhabdomyosarcoma and neuroblastoma in young children and transitional cell carcinoma of the bladder in adolescents and young adults (Gripp and Lin 2007).

Costello syndrome is inherited in an autosomal dominant manner and is caused by activating germline mutations in the HRAS proto-oncogene (OMIM # 190020) (Aoki et al. 2005; Estep et al. 2006; Gripp et al. 2006a, b; Kerr et al. 2006; Rauen 2007b). To date, most probands with Costello syndrome have the disorder as a result of a de novo mutation: parents of probands have not been proven to be affected (Gripp and Lin 2007).

Remarkable phenotypic overlaps exist between Costello syndrome and other syndromes encompassing MCA/MR and heart disease ("*neuro-cardio-faciocutaneous syndromes*") (Bentires-Alj et al. 2006), including *Noonan syndrome* (OMIM # 163950), *Cardio-facial-cutaneous (CFC) syndrome* (OMIM # 115150) (Noonan 2006, Rauen 2007), *LEOPARD syndrome* (OMIM # 151100) and *neurofibromatosis type1* (OMIM # 162200) (for reviews see also Allanson 2007, Bentires-Alj et al. 2006, Gripp and Lin 2007, Rauen 2007b). These overlaps are explained by the fact that the protein products of the causative genes of all these conditions interact in a common RAS/MAPK pathway (see below) (Rauen 2007a, Roberts et al. 2006). For these reasons the group of neuro-cardio-faciocutaneous syndrome have been tentatively renamed "*RAS/MAPK syndromes*" (Aoki et al. 2008). RAS is a critical signalling hub in the cell, which controls vital cellular functions including cell cycle progression, cell survival, motility, transcription, translation and membrane trafficking (Rauen 2007).

The pathogenesis of Costello syndrome is unclear, but there are many clues for a disturbed elastogenesis, possibly through a disturbed elastin-binding protein reuse by chondroitin sulphate-bearing proteoglycans accumulation (Hennekam 2003, Rauen 2007). It has been postulated that a chondroitin sulphate may induce shedding of EBP from Costello cells and prevent normal recycling of this reusable tropoelastin chaperone (Hinek et al. 2005). Subsequent accumulation of chondroitin 6-sulphate in cardiomyocytes contributes to the development of the hypertrophic cardiomyopathy of Costello syndrome (Hinek et al. 2005).

## Historical perspective and eponyms

In 1971, and again (in more detail) in 1977, Costello described two children with psychomotor retardation, postnatal growth failure, macrocephaly, coarse facies, short neck, sparse and curly hair, dark skin colour and nasal papillomata (Costello 1971, 1977). A similar patient was described by Der Kaloustian et al. (1991): since this report, the disorder has been recognized as a distinct entity and given the name of Costello syndrome (OMIM 2006). After recognition of the disorder as Costello syndrome, a few patients were reported as *"facio-cutaneous-skeletal syndrome"* (Borochowitz et al. 1992), but the error was corrected in subsequent papers (Borochowith et al. 1993, Der Kaloustian 1993, Martin and Jones 1993) (notably, however, still the OMIM entry shows this eponym) (OMIM 2007). Early examples of Costello syndrome were also reported as *AMICABLE syndrome* (amicable personality, mental retardation, impaired swallowing, cardiomyopathy, aortic defects, bulk, large lips and lobules, ectodermal defects) (Hall et al. 1990).

## Incidence and prevalence

About 115 patients having the clinical features of Costello syndrome have been reported until 2003, but only 103 patients were described in sufficient detail (the data on 12 patients were insufficient for complete ascertainment) (Hennekam 2003). Following this literature review, a few isolated cases

(Delrue et al. 2003) and large series (Kawame et al. 2003, Kerr et al. 2006) were described bringing the total number of reported cases to 200–300 affected individuals (Rauen 2007a). Our personal opinion is that Costello syndrome is under diagnosed, possibly because it is unknown to many paediatricians.

## Clinical manifestations

Clinical manifestations include distinct facial appearance with large head, curly hair, nasal papillomata, hyper extensible fingers (small joints), loose integument of hands and feet, hyperpigmented and hyper elastic skin, acanthosis nigricans and cognitive delay.

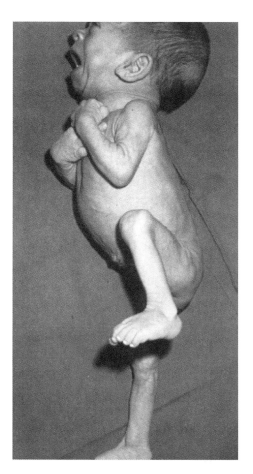

**Fig. 1.** A 4-month-old child with Costello syndrome shows generalized redundant skin and disproportion between the increased volume of the head and the thinness of the trunk and extremities.

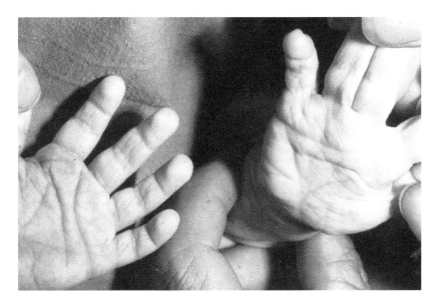

**Fig. 2.** Redundant skin, deep palmar creases and persistent fetal pads.

## Skin manifestations

Affected patients show a manifest disproportion between the excessive volume of the head and the thinness of the trunk and extremities (Fig. 1).

The most striking cutaneous sign of Costello syndrome is the redundant (loose) skin of the dorsal aspects of hands (Fig. 2) and feet (Fig. 3), face (Fig. 4) and trunk (Fig. 5), which is present since birth. This excessive skin causes deep palmar and plantar creases with or without ridges/hyperlinearity and may cause an unusual soft and velvety texture of the hands (Davies and Hughes 1994, Patton et al. 1987, Weiss et al. 2004). Nguyen et al. (2007) consider this feature a cardinal manifestation of the syndrome.

Other important skin abnormalities are tumours of ectodermal origin such as papillomas, calcified epitheliomas, dermoid cysts, mammary fibroadenosis, and syringomas (Nguyen et al. 2007). Papillomas (wart-like lesions) localized on the face, axillae, elbows, knees, vocal cords, anus, and abdomen are observed at variable ages (usually between age 2 to 6 years), and so their absence does not preclude the diagnosis of Costello syndrome: they are considered to result from friction or pressure (Siwik et al. 1998).

Acanthosis nigricans, as well as hyperkeratosis and increased skin pigmentation, are often seen

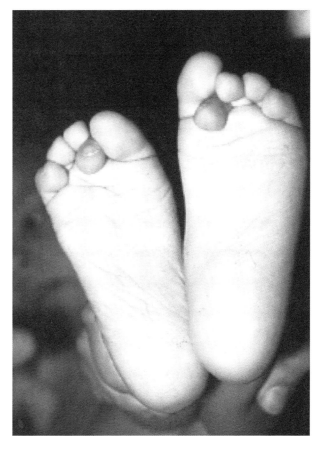

**Fig. 3.** Abundant and deep plantar creases and hyperextensibility of the second toes.

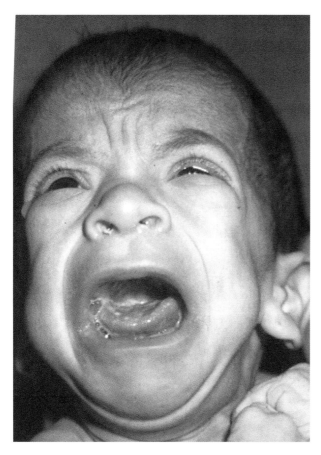

**Fig. 4.** Facial appearance of a child with Costello syndrome at age 2 months: note the redundant skin and low-set ears.

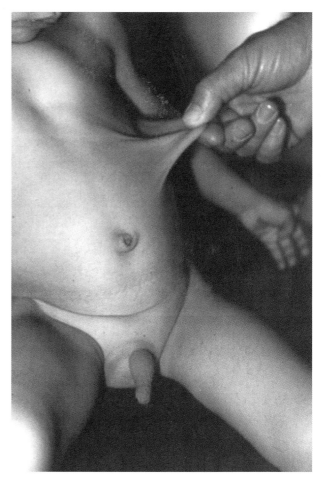

**Fig. 5.** A 2-year-old patient shows cutis laxa and pectus excavatum.

(Weiss et al. 2004). Scarce, short or thin hair is most frequently observed in Costello syndrome, but some patients show generalized hypertrichosis. Patients may show also dysplastic, thin, brittle, or deep-nails (Nguyen et al. 2007).

Other less common findings that have been reported are hyperhidrosis, multiple haemangiomas, hyperplastic nipples, supernumerary nipples, mammary fibroadenosis and unusual fat deposition (reviewed in Nguyen et al. 2007).

## Systemic features

Polyhydramnios during pregnancy is noted in about 60%, and delivery is frequently ruled by caesarean

section (Hennekam 2003). Prenatal overlap of feature of severe Noonan syndrome and Costello syndrome has been confirmed (Levaillant et al. 2006), with dysmorphologic similarities, due to oedema of foetal skin in face and extremities. Most common prenatal systemic abnormalities include increased nuchal translucency, polyhydramnios, bilateral pyelectasis and ventriculomegaly; prenatal foetal facial analysis found abnormal thickness of the skin in the prefrontal area, thick dysplastic ears, thick lips and deep-set creases in the hands and feet (Levellaint et al. 2006).

At birth, children frequently are macrosomic with increased birth weight and elevated head circumference percentiles, but they show decreased vitality with slow mobility. Poor suck is often times noted. Postnatal growth retardation is significant and persists during life. Other systemic problems, such as failure to thrive, upper airway infections, joint hyper-mobility, hoarse voice, strabismus, and psychomotor and language acquisition delay are noted very early.

A review of the main clinical features in Costello syndrome, as described in the 103 patients reported in the literature until the year 2003, was provided by Hennekam (2003). These features included: developmental delay (100%), deep palmar/plantar creases (100%), loose skin of hands and feet (99%), poor neonatal feeding (97%), coarse facies (97%), thick lips (97%), postnatal growth retardation (96%), full cheeks (92%), depressed nasal bridge (90%), birth weight >50th percentile (89%), large, fleshy ear lobes (89%), short neck (88%), hyper extensible fingers (87%), macrocephaly (84%), curly, sparse hair (82%), low-set ears (83%), epicanthal folds (82%), short bulbous nose (77%), hyperpigmentation (78%), large mouth (75%), hypertrophic cardiomyopathy (61%) and cardiac dysrhythmia (53%). Other clinical features were reported in a lower number of patients, but were confirmed in most patients, such as hyperkerato-sis, down slanting palpebral fissures, thick eyebrows, strabismus, macroglossia, apparently highly arched palate, gingival hyperplasia, teeth abnormalities, hoarse voice, broad distal phalanges, dysplastic/thin/deep-set nails, laxity of small joints, limited extension of elbow, hypotonia, increased anterior-posterior tho-rax diameter, umbilical or inguinal hernia, tight Achilles tendons, abnormal foot position, delayed bone age and outgoing personality. Endocrine abnor-malities most frequently were manifested as growth hormone deficiency and hypoglycaemia. The hypo-glycaemia is thought to be due to cortisol deficiency (Gregersen and Viljoen 2004) and patients with growth hormone deficiency have been successfully treated with biosynthetic growth hormone (Legault et al. 2001, Stein et al. 2004). It has been speculated that treatment of Costello patients with growth hor-mone may help to increase the stature and to reduce cardiac hypertrophy (Lin et al. 2002).

The anaesthesiology literature reports only mod-erate difficulties with intubations due to anatomic considerations, but no intraoperative deaths (Dearlove and Harper 1997).

## Cardiovascular abnormalities

Siwik et al. (1998) in their series of 30 patients with Costello syndrome reported cardiac disease (of any type) in 60%, structural heart disease in 30%, hyper-trophic cardiomyopathy in 20% and tachyarrhythmia in 18%. Lin et al. (2002) reviewed the incidence of hearth defects in 94 of the Costello patients in the literature and found abnormalities in 63% (including hypertrophic cardiomyopathy in 34% of patients and arrhythmias in 33%).

Many of the cardiologic abnormalities are re-lated to the elastic tissue, which is also involved in the pathogenesis of several defects in this syndrome. The main congenital defects include: ventricular or atrial septal defects (13%), pulmonary valve stenosis (13%), patent ductus arteriosus (3%), bicuspid aortic valve, aortic stenosis, mitral valve stenosis or pro-lapse, and thickening of the ventricular septum. The hypertrophic cardiomyopathy may be already pre-sent at birth, or develops in the first year of life or at later ages. Several types of dysrhythmias including supraventricular tachycardia, atrial fibrillation, atrial ectopic tachycardia, and other forms of ventricular and/or atrial origin have been reported in patients with and without overt cardiac disease, which could have some impact on the patients' longevity (Fukao et al. 1996). The most common form of arrhythmia is however the atrial tachycardia, typically supraven-tricular or paroxysmal tachycardia. Most distinctive are chaotic atrial rhythm (also known as multifocal atrial tachycardia) and ectopic atrial tachycardia (Gripp and Lin 2007). Recently, Kawame et al. (2003) described severe cardiac abnormalities in 8 of the 10 patients of their series.

Post-mortem histological, histochemical and immunohistochemical studies of the hearts of three children with Costello syndrome revealed cardio-myocyte hypertrophy, massive pericellular and intra-cellular accumulation of chondroitin sulphate-bear-ing proteoglycans and a marked reduction of elastic fibres (Hinek et al. 2005). Normal stroma was re-placed by multifocal collagenous fibrosis. Accumula-tion of chondroitin-6-sulphate was very high. In con-trast, deposition of chondroitin-4-sulphate was below the level detected in normal hearts. This finding suggests that an imbalance in sulphation of chondroitin sulphate molecules and subsequent accumulation of chondroitin-6-sulphate in cardiomyocytes contribute to the development of the hypertrophic cardiomyopathy of Costello syndrome (Hineck et al. 2005).

## Neurological abnormalities

Developmental delay and mental retardation (ranging from mild to severe) are an almost constant finding (Axelrad et al. 2004, Kawame et al. 2003). There is a characteristic nonverbal cognitive malfunctioning with variability in receptive language (Axelrad et al. 2004). Apathy and nervous personality can be present aside a pleasant, happy and outgoing behaviour (see also below). Patients may show decreased physical activity and easy fatigability, which appear to be constitutional, but one must take into consideration that congenital heart defects may be contributory. Seizures have been also reported (Kawame et al. 2003). Costello patients have been reported to have a high prevalence of obstructive sleep-related respiratory disorders including respiratory events of obstructive type during sleep, fragmented sleep structure and increased number of awakenings associated to narrowing of the upper respiratory airways (Della Marca et al. 2006).

## Behavioural and temperamental manifestations

A characteristic behaviour in infancy includes a happy and sociable personality with significant irritability, including hypersensitivity to sound and tactile stimuli, sleep disturbances (see above), and excess shyness with strangers (Axelrad et al. 2004, 2007; Kawame et al. 2003). Most affected patients have a warm and sociable personality, but they frequently are overprotected and show low frustration levels, maladaptive behaviours and poor emotional aspects (Axelrad et al. 2004). Hyperactivity with anxiety attacks and seldom self-mutilation, with an adverse reaction to psychotropic medication usually decrease or may disappear around age 2–4 years (Kawame et al. 2003).

## Neuroimaging

Ventricular dilatation is observed in more than 40% of patients who may need shunting (Pratesi et al. 1999). The presence of Chiari I malformation and syringomyelia in a patient suggested to be a possible case of Costello syndrome has been reported (Gripp et al. 2002). Brain imaging in 28 of the 38 studied patients of Costello syndrome in the literature showed some type of congenital abnormality in the cerebral ventricles, cerebral hemispheres, cerebellum, brain and corpus callosum. These abnormalities mainly consisted of mild ventricular dilatation, cerebral atrophy, Chiari malformation, tonsillar malformations, hydrocephalus, syringomyelia and isolated anomalies that involved the optic nerves, brain stem and corpus callosum (Delrue et al. 2003). In addition to the congenital brain malformations patients may have dysmielinisation of the basal ganglia and white matter (Fig. 6). Similar white matter and structural brain abnormalities are seen in CFC (Roberts et al. 2006). These abnormalities may contribute to the delay in walking and psychomotor retardation. Moyamoya vasculopathy has been also described (Shiihara et al. 2005).

## Neurophysiologic studies

Electrophysiological abnormalities have been described in nearly one third of the children of Costello syndrome, but only 20% had seizures. EEG abnormalities frequently are associated with brain imaging alterations, most often mild ventricular dilatation (Zampino et al. 1993). Different types of epilepsy have been noted such as West syndrome (Say et al. 1993), Lennox-Gastaut syndrome after a West syndrome in one patient and focalised epilepsy in another (Fujikawa et al. 2001) and tonico-clonic epilepsy (Costello 1977, Johnson et al. 1998). Patients with severe epilepsy also had brain parenchymal lesions and profound psychomotor retardation/regression (Fujikawa et al. 2001). Kawame et al. (2003) reported seizures in 50% of 10 patients with Costello syndrome without brain structural anomalies, but with behavioural and neurological features.

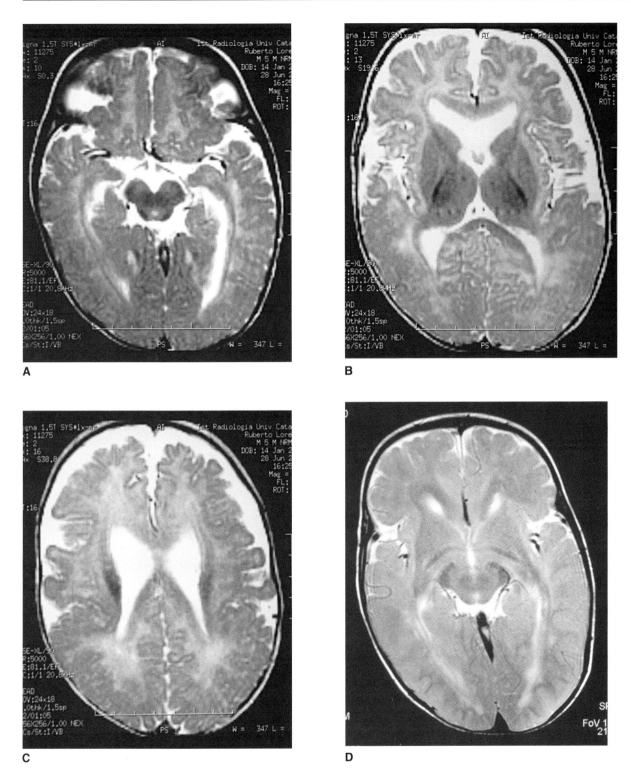

**Fig. 6.** Axial T2-weighted magnetic resonance (MR) images of the brain in a child with Costello syndrome showing at age 6 months (**A–C**) dilated ventricles and high signal lesions in the periventricular white matter and at age 2.5 years (**D–F**) partial regression of the ventricular enlargement with similar high signals in the periventricular white matter.

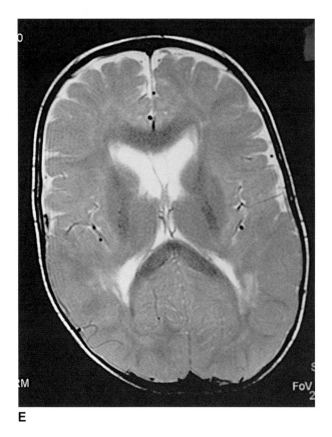

**E**

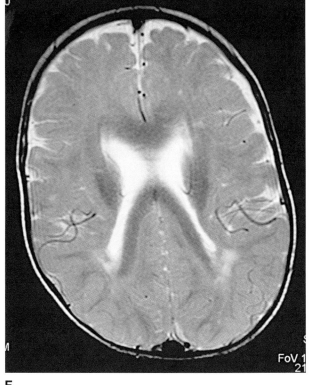

**F**

**Fig. 6.** (Continued)

## Genital abnormalities

Genital abnormalities such as undescended testes, a small penis, a hypoplastic scrotum, or large external genitalia have been observed. Libido usually is decreased.

## Tumours and malignancies

Tumour occurrence and malignancies have an estimated frequency of 17% and have been recently reviewed (Gripp et al. 2002): recommendations for screening have been proposed (Gripp et al. 2002) but also criticised (De Baum 2002). The tumours reported by Gripp et al. (2002) were ganglioneuroblastoma, bladder carcinoma (Johnson et al. 1998), vestibular schwannoma (van Eeghen et al. 1999), epithelioma (van Eeghen et al. 1999), neuroblastoma (Lurie 1994) and 10 patients with embryonal

rhabdomyosarcoma (Kerr et al. 1998, Sigaudy et al. 2000). Parameningeal rhabdomyosarcoma has been also reported (O'Neal et al. 2004). The increased incidence of tumours has been explained by the HRAS mediated RAS pathway activation (see below and also Kratz et al. 2007, Rauen 2007, Roberts et al. 2006).

The tumour screening protocol consists of abdominal and pelvic ultrasound examination every 3–6 months from birth until 8–10 years, urinary catecholamine excretion measurements every 6–12 months until 5 years, and annual screening for haematuria from 10 years on.

## Natural history

Patients with Costello syndrome maintain macrocephaly throughout their lives, but weight gain and growth are decreased and they most often show shortened height and low weight from youth to adulthood. The attained adult height has been reported to be between 116 cm and 161 cm (Hennekam 2003). Several causes have been suggested for the short height including hypothyroidism, ACTH deficiency, partial growth hormone deficiency or low response to stimulation test. A favourable response to growth hormone treatment has been reported (Gripp et al. 2006b, Legault et al. 2001).

All reported patients showed psychomotor retardation. The mean age for sitting is 23 months and for walking without help is 4 years; the first words are spoken at 4 years and 4 months, with delayed language development, and IQ test values range between 23 and 85 (mean 50) (Delrue et al. 2003). Most of these patients have a warm and sociable personality, but they frequently are overprotected and show low frustration levels, maladaptive behaviours and poor emotional aspects (Axelrad et al. 2004). Hyperactivity with anxiety attacks and seldom self-mutilation, with an adverse reaction to psychotropic medication has been reported (Van Eeghen et al. 1999). These symptoms usually decrease or may disappear around age 2–4 years (Kawame et al. 2003).

**Prenatally**, increased nuchal thickness, polyhydramnios (>90%), characteristic ulnar deviation of the wrists, and short humeri and femurs can be seen on prenatal ultrasonography. Because most features of the foetal **phenotype** are not unique and Costello syndrome is rare, the diagnosis is often not considered prenatally. Cardiac hypertrophy has not been reported, but foetal tachycardia (various forms of atrial tachycardia) has been detected in at least five foetuses subsequently diagnosed with Costello syndrome, which increases the index of suspicion of the diagnosis (Gripp and Lin 2007).

**In the neonate**, increased birth weight and head circumference (often >50th percentile) for gestational age can lead to the categorization of macrosomia. Hypoglycaemia is common. Failure to thrive and severe feeding difficulties are almost universal. Characteristic physical findings include a relatively high forehead, low nasal bridge, epicanthal folds, prominent lips and a wide mouth, ulnar deviation of wrists and fingers, loose-appearing skin with deep palmar and plantar creases, and cryptorchidism (Lo et al. 2008).

**In infancy**, severe feeding difficulties may lead to a marasmic appearance. Most infants display hypotonia, irritability, developmental delay, and nystagmus with delayed visual maturation improving with age. Cardiac abnormalities typically present in infancy or early childhood but may be recognized at any age. Approximately 75% of *HRAS* mutation-positive individuals with Costello syndrome (see below) have had some type of cardiac abnormality (Gripp et al. 2006a, b), compared to 60% of individuals with Costello syndrome diagnosed by clinical findings alone (Lin et al. 2002). In the more recent *HRAS* mutation-positive series, congenital heart defects (usually pulmonic stenosis) were noted in 25%, arrhythmia in 42%, and hypertrophic cardiomyopathy in 47%, compared to the earlier clinical series in which each of the above abnormalities was reported in about 30% of affected individuals.

**In childhood**, individuals are able to take oral feeds beginning between age two and four years. The first acceptable tastes are often strong (e.g., ketchup). The onset of speech often coincides with the willingness to feed orally. Short stature is universal, delayed bone age is common (Johnson et al. 1998), and testing may show partial or complete growth hormone deficiency. Atypically, cardiac hypertrophy detected in infancy as mild non-obstructive or non-progressive thickening may progress to severe lethal hypertrophy with "storage" (Hinek et al. 2005); most hypertrophic hearts remain stable or progress mildly. The complete natural history of cardiac hypertrophy in Costello syndrome has not been defined, but adult onset of hypertrophy has not been documented.

**Adolescents** often show delayed or disordered puberty, and may appear older than their chronologic age because of worsening kyphoscoliosis, sparse hair, and prematurely aged skin.

**Adults.** White et al. (2005) has tentatively delineated the adult phenotype in Costello syndrome reporting follow-up findings in 17 affected adults aged 16–40 years. Fourteen of these 17 adults had mild to moderate intellectual disability: 15 attained some reading and writing skills and 14 showed ongoing acquisition of new skills into adulthood. Two patients had bladder carcinoma while benign tumours included multiple ductal papillomata (n = 2) and a 4th ventricle mass (plexus papilloma? n = 1). Endocrine problems in their series were osteoporosis, central hypogonadism, and delayed puberty (White et al. 2005). Other health problems were symptomatic Chiari malformation associated to adult-onset gastro-oesophageal reflux in three cases (White et al. 2005).

**Life expectance.** Life expectance in patients with Costello syndrome is often decreased. A recent review of the literature indicates that 14 children less than 6 years of age with Costello syndrome have died of several causes, particularly of cardiac anomalies, sudden death syndrome secondary to arrhythmias or tumours, or both (Gripp et al. 2002, Hennekam 2003, Lin et al. 2000, O'Neal et al.

2004). Few patients exceed 30 years of life. We have followed a patient since the age of 11 months, who was published when he was 35 years old (Pascual-Castroviejo and Pascual-Pascual 2005): he presently is 36 years of age and is in good health (Fig. 7). The longest survival known is in a woman published by Van Eeghen et al. (1999) when she was 33 years of age and who died at 37 years because of a perforated duodenal ulcer (Hennekam 2003). Suri and Garrett (1998) reported a 32-year-old patient who died with vestibular schwannoma suggesting a possible pathogenic relationship between Costello syndrome and neurofibromatosis type 2 (see molecular genetics).

## Molecular genetics and pathogenesis

### Molecular genetics

Most of the reported patients have been isolated cases, sporadic and non familial. Consanguinity had seldom been reported (Borochowitz et al. 1992, Franceschini et al. 1999) and autosomal recessive inheritance had been postulated. Affected siblings have been published in few occasions (Berberich et al. 1999, Zampino et al. 1993, Johnson et al. 1998). Lurie (1994) reviewed 20 reported families and found that the 37 sibs of probands were all normal excluding an autosomal recessive inheritance pattern. A pair of monozygotic twins was reported by Van del Bosch et al. (2002). A single chromosomal translocation {46,XX,t (1;22) (q25;q11} associated with the condition was reported in the same patient in two distinct papers (Czeizel and Timár 1995, Maroti et al. 2002). The first to postulate autosomal dominant inheritance was van Eeghen et al. (1999) who reviewed previously reported patients and Ioan and Fryns (2002) who described Costello syndrome in a brother and sister, with minor manifestations in their mother.

Aoki et al. (2005) identified heterozygous *de novo* mutations in the *HRAS* gene (OMIM # 190020) in a cohort of 12 patients with the clinical diagnosis of Costello syndrome. Heterozygous missense mutations were found in codon 12 and codon 13 of the first coding exon, known mutation hotspots in RAS.

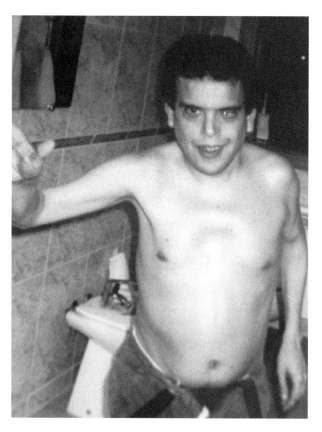

**Fig. 7.** Same patient as in Figs. 3 and 5 at age 35 years: he still shows pectus excavatum and deep palmar creases, and cataract in the left eye.

*HRAS* is a highly conserved gene located on 11p15.5 with variability of genetic sequence existing in the 3′ hypervariable region among other RAS family members (Midgley and Kerr 2002, Rauen 2007). The aminoacid substitutions in the protein product of *HRAS* caused by missense alteration found in codons 12 and 13 in Costello syndrome are well-known activating mutations in cancer (Rauen 2007).

Several studies have shown good correlation between the clinical diagnosis of Costello syndrome and the presence of heterozygous activating *HRAS* mutations (Aoki et al. 2005, Estep et al. 2006, Gripp et al. 2006b, Kerr et al. 2006, van Steensel et al. 2006, Zampino et al. 2007; reviewed in Rauen 2007a, b). The vast majority of mutations are Gly12Ser substitutions. HRAS is probably the only causal gene for Costello syndrome (Rauen 2007a). The origin of constitutional germline mutations causing Costello syndrome reflects a paternal bias (Rauen 2007a, b). Somatic mosaicism for a Gly12Ser substitution has been identified in one individual with Costello syndrome (Gripp et al. 2006a). No genotype-phenotype correlation have been noted. However, Kerr et al. (2006) suggested that the risk for malignant tumours may be higher in individuals with the G12A mutation (>55%) than in those with the G12S (<10%).

## Costello, Noonan, CFC, LEOPARD and NF1 syndromes and the RAS-extracellular signal regulated kinase (ERK) pathway

Costello syndrome shows phenotypic overlaps with other MCA/MR syndromes ("*neuro-cardofaciocutaneous syndromes*" or "*RAS/MARK syndromes*") (Aoki et al. 2008, Bentires-Alj et al. 2006) including *Noonan syndrome* (OMIM # 163950), which is caused by mutations in the protein tyrosine phosphatase SHP-2 gene *PTPN11* (>50% of cases), in the *SOS1* gene (10% of cases) and in the *KRAS* gene (<5% of cases) (OMIM # 176876) and *Cardio-facio-cutaneous (CFC) syndrome* (OMIM # 115150) caused by mutations in the BRAF gene (>75–80% of cases), mitogen-activated protein/extracellular signal-reg-

ulated kinase *MEK1* and *MEK2* genes (10–15% of cases) and in the KRAS gene (<5% of cases) (Rauen 2007b). Clinical similarities are shared also with *LEOPARD syndrome* (OMIM # 151100) and *neurofibromatosis type1* (OMIM # 162200). The clinical overlaps between all these conditions are explained by the fact that the protein products of the CFC genes, the PTPN11 Noonan gene, the NF1 gene and those of HRAS involved in the causation of Costello syndrome, all have a role in the RAS-extracellular signal regulated kinase (ERK) pathway (Fig. 8) (Allanson 2007; Gripp and Lin 2007; Rauen 2007a, b; Roberts et al. 2006). RAS genes encode guanosine triphosphate-binding proteins that serve as molecular on-off switches that activate or inhibit downstream molecules. It is a signalling pathway that is important for vital cellular functions including cell cycle progression, cell survival, motility, transcription, translation and membrane trafficking (Rauen 2007a, b; Roberts et al. 2006). Specifically, Aoki et al. (2005) hypothesised that genes mutated in Costello syndrome and in PTPN11-negative Noonan syndrome encode molecules that function upstream or downstream of SHP2 in signal pathways. In 90% of individuals with Costello syndrome they found one or another of 4 heterozygous mutations in the HRAS gene (Aoki et al. 2005): these mutations had been previously identified somatically in various tumours. These observations suggested that germ-line mutations in HRAS perturb human development and increase susceptibility to solid tumours in patients with Costello syndrome (and of haematopoietic malignancies in those with Noona syndrome) (Roberts et al. 2006). The findings of Aoki et al. (2005) were confirmed by Gripp et al. (2006b) and Estep et al. (2005). Kerr et al. (2006) identified mutations of the HRAS gene in 86% of the 37 cases analysed.

At the moment, there are more questions than answers in trying to establish why pathogenetically related syndromes display major phenotypic differences. Yet, one can firmly state that the Costello, CFC and Noonan syndrome are genetically heterogeneous. As they are all caused by mutations in genes whose protein products are part of the RAS-ERK pathway, we also understand, at least partly, why they are phenotypically similar (Roberts et al. 2006).

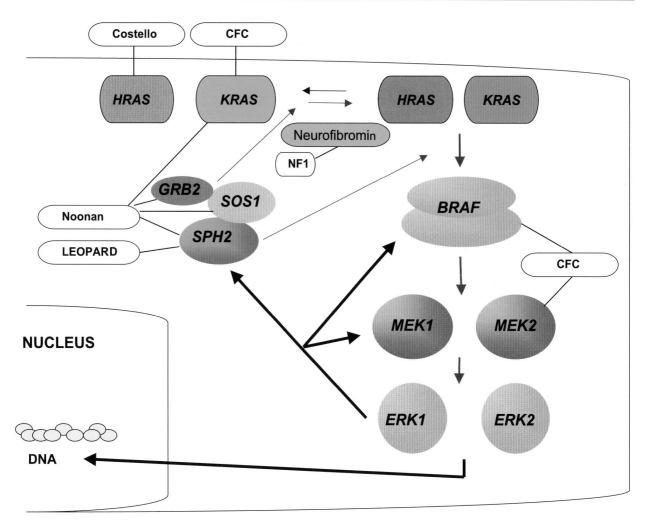

**Fig. 8.** RAS-extracellur signal-regulated kinase (ERK) signalling pathway connecting pathogenetically the Costello, Noonan, Cardiofaciocutaneous (CFC) and LEOPARD syndromes and neurofibromatosis type 1 (NF1). Inactivating HRAS and KRAS (orange and light green) are activated (dark orange and dark green) by neurofibromin (the protein product of the NF1 gene) and by SHP2, GRB2 and SOS1 (the protein products associated with the Noonan and LEOPARD genes). Red arrows and arrowhead = activation; black arrows and arrowheads = inhibition (see text for further explanation) (adapted and modified from Rauen 2007 and from Roberts et al. 2006).

## Pathogenesis

The resemblance of Costello syndrome with other disorders associated with elastic fibre degeneration such as cutis laxa, Williams-Beuren syndrome and perhaps others, may indicate a common or close origin for all these entities (Mancini et al. 2003). Histological studies showed fine, disrupted, and loosely constructed elastic fibres in the skin, tongue, pharynx, larynx, and upper oesophagus, but not in bronchi, alveoli, aorta or coronary arteries (Mori et al. 1996),

loss of anastomosing points in elastic tissue (Vila Torres et al. 1994), marked reduction of elastic fibres and replacement of normal stroma by multifocal collagen fibrosis, as well as accumulation of chondroitin-6-sulphate and decreased of chondroitin-4-sulphate (Hinek et al. 2005), all of which are in favour of a disturbed elastogenesis due to an anomaly in the elastin gene.

The human elastin gene is composed of 34 exons, and the major transcribed products are three distinct mRNAs of 3.5 Kb. These are produced by alternative exon splicing, and the distribution and function of these spliced elastins are yet not completely understood (Indik et al. 1987). Elastin is the major component of extracellular elastic fibres of skin, arteries, lungs and possibly other structures, and its normal development is an essential determinant of arterial morphogenesis (Li et al. 1998a). Elastin is composed of cross-linked tropoelastin, and formed along a scaffold of microfibrils composed off different glycoproteins. Tropoelastin is guided intracellularly by elastin – binding protein (EBP), an enzymatically inactive variant of beta-galactosidase, which is also important in elastic fibre assembly (Hinek and Rabinovitch 1994). A decreased production of tropoelastin, inadequate intracellular trafficking or release from the cell surface through inadequate functioning of EBP, or disturbed extracellular assembly either of the tropoelastin chains themselves or along the scaffold of microfibrils, may disturb elastin fibre formation (Hennekam 2003). Hinek et al. (2000) showed that cultured fibroblasts from Costello syndrome patients produce normal levels of tropoelastin and properly deposit the microfibrillar scaffold, but do not assemble elastic fibres because of a deficiency of EBP.

A production defect of tropoelastin can be found in Williams-Beuren syndrome, an abnormal microfibrillar scaffold in Marfan syndrome, and a deficient functioning of EBP Hurler syndrome. Elastin may have a role in the function of the central nervous system (CNS), since patients with Williams-Beuren syndrome, who have deletions of the elastin gene, show mental retardation. It is possible that mental retardation in Costello and Williams-Beuren syndromes arises from a defect in elastin – mediated signal transduction in the CNS (Mori et al. 1996).

## Differential diagnosis

Several diseases should be considered in the differential diagnosis of Costello syndrome (Kerr et al. 2008, Lin et al. 2008), particularly those which present cutis laxa such as leprechaunism (the diagnosis that we gave to our first patient in 1969 before Costello described his syndrome) (Davies and Hughes 1994,

Martin and Jones 1991, Patton et al. 1987, Say et al. 1993, Weis et al. 2004).

In infants and young children, Costello syndrome is difficult to distinguish from cardiofaciocutaneous (CFC) syndrome or Noonan syndrome; in older children, the distinction between Costello syndrome and Noonan syndrome is clear. Feeding problems and failure to thrive are usually more severe in infants with Costello syndrome and CFC syndrome than in infants with Noonan syndrome. The distinctive combination of *pectus carinatum* and *pectus excavatum* typifies Noonan syndrome. Costello syndrome is distinguished by ulnar deviation of the hands, marked small-joint laxity, striking excess palmar skin, the presence of papillomata, and palmar calluses.

The cardiac abnormalities in Costello syndrome, CFC syndrome, and Noonan syndrome are similar. At least one of the three following main types of cardiac abnormality was noted in about 75% of individuals with mutation-positive Costello syndrome (Gripp et al. 2006b): congenital heart defects (25%), hypertrophic cardiomyopathy (47%), and arrhythmia (mostly atrial tachycardia) (42%) (Gripp and Lin 2007). Based on two series of individuals with mutation-positive CFC syndrome (Niihori et al. 2006, Rodriguez-Viciana et al. 2006), the frequency of cardiac anomalies in general and hypertrophic cardiomyopathy in particular in Costello syndrome and CFC syndrome is similar, but congenital heart defects are more common in CFC syndrome and arrhythmia is more common in Costello syndrome. Because of the overlap between Costello syndrome and CFC syndrome, the diagnosis of individuals with a phenotype considered borderline or atypical for Costello syndrome may be clarified by molecular genetic testing.

Noonan syndrome is characterized by short stature; congenital heart defect; broad or webbed neck; unusual chest shape with superior *pectus carinatum*, inferior *pectus excavatum*, and apparently low-set nipples; developmental delay of variable degree; cryptorchidism; and characteristic facies. Varied coagulation defects and lymphatic dysplasia are frequently observed. Congenital heart defects occur in 50% and 80% of individuals (Allanson 2007). Pulmonary valve stenosis, often with dysplasia, is the most common heart defect and is found in 20–50% of individuals.

Hypertrophic cardiomyopathy, found in 20–30% of individuals, may be present at birth or appear in infancy or childhood. Other frequent structural defects include atrial and ventricular septal defects, branch pulmonary artery stenosis, and tetralogy of Fallot; less common are incomplete atrioventricular canal (premium-type atrial septal defect) and coarctation. Length at birth is usually normal. Final adult height approaches the lower limit of normal. Most school-age children perform well in a normal educational setting; 10–15% require special education. Mild mental retardation is seen in up to one-third of individuals (Van Eeghen et al. 1999). Mutations in *PTPN11* have been identified in 50% of affected individuals and *KRAS* mutations have been reported in a small number (Schubbert et al. 2006).

Some newborns or very young infants with Williams-Beuren syndrome may show similar facies to Costello syndrome, but lack the additional features that affect the skin, head circumference, increased birth weight and several other signs of the Costello syndrome, except for the frequent presentation of cardiac disease in both syndromes, will easily allow differentiation, as it occurs with I-cell, Hurler syndrome, Weaver syndrome and other related entities (Van Eeghen et al. 1999).

Cardiofaciocutaneous (CFC) syndrome resembles Costello syndrome in young children. Hypotonia, nystagmus, mild to moderate mental retardation, and postnatal growth deficiency are typical. Feeding difficulties are common but may be less severe than in Costello syndrome. The dolichocephaly, high forehead, and slightly coarse facial features may resemble Costello syndrome, but the lips are not as thick and prominent. The hair is more consistently sparse or curly, and in contrast to Costello syndrome, the eyebrows are typically sparse or absent. Skin abnormalities include severe atopic dermatitis, keratosis pilaris, ichthyosis, and hyperkeratosis; the papillomata characteristic of Costello syndrome are not seen in CFC syndrome. As in Costello syndrome, pulmonic valve stenosis is common, as is atrial septal defect. Hypertrophic cardiomyopathy has been noted in about 40% of mutation-positive individuals, similar to Costello syndrome (Niihori et al. 2006, Rodriguez-Viciana et al. 2006). Atrial

**Table 1.** Initial diagnostic work-up for Costello syndrome

Complete general and neurological examination
Plotting of growth parameters
Nutritional assessment
Cardiologic evaluation with two-dimensional and Doppler echocardiography and baseline electrocardiography
Full ophthalmology evaluation
Clinical assessment of spine and extremities, range of motion
Multidisciplinary developmental evaluation (refer to dermatologists)
Abdominal and pelvic ultrasonography
MRI study of the brain
Genetics consultation

Adapted and modified from Gripp and Lin (2007) and Rauen et al. (2008).

tachycardia had not been reported until recently; in the small number of reported cases, it has not been called chaotic atrial rhythm (Niihori et al. 2006). Malignant tumours have not been reported in CFC syndrome. The discovery of germline mutations in *BRAF*, and less commonly in *KRAS*, *MEK1*, or *MEK2*, allows for molecular confirmation of a clinical diagnosis of CFC syndrome (Gripp and Lin 2007, Niihori et al. 2006, Roberts et al. 2006, Rodriguez-Viciana et al. 2006).

## Management

The suggested work-up at the time of initial diagnosis of Costello syndrome is listed in Table 1 (see also Rauen et al. 2008).

## Treatment of Manifestations

**Growth.** Most infants require nasogastric or gastrostomy feeding. Because of gastroesophageal reflux and irritability, Nissen fundoplication is often performed. Anecdotally, **affected** children have very high caloric needs. Even after nutrition is improved through supplemental feeding, growth retardation persists.

**Cardiac.** Treatment of cardiac manifestations is generally the same as in the general population. All individuals with Costello syndrome, especially those with an identified cardiac abnormality, should be followed by a cardiologist who is aware of the spectrum of cardiac disease and its natural history (Lin et al. 2002). Ongoing studies of the natural history will be needed to define the management for older individuals. Arrhythmias have been well documented but incompletely defined from a management point of view. Malignant rhythms may require aggressive anti-arrhythmic drugs and ablation. Pharmacologic and surgical treatment (myectomy) has been used to address cardiac hypertrophy. Individuals with Costello syndrome and severe cardiac problems may choose to wear a Medic Alert® bracelet.

**Skeletal.** Ulnar deviation of the wrists and fingers responds well to early bracing and occupational and/or physical therapy. Limited extension of large joints should be addressed early through physical therapy. Surgical tendon lengthening, usually of the Achilles tendon, is often required. Kyphoscoliosis may require surgical correction.

**Central nervous system.** When seizures occur, underlying causes including hydrocephalus, hypoglycaemia, and low serum cortisone concentration need to be considered (Gregersen and Viljoen 2004).

**Cognitive.** Developmental disability should be addressed by early-intervention programs and individualized learning strategies. Speech delay and expressive language limitations should be addressed early with appropriate therapy and later with an appropriate educational plan. Alternate means of communication should be considered if expressive language is significantly limited.

**Respiratory.** A high index of suspicion should be maintained for obstructive sleep apnea as the cause for sleep disturbance.

**Dental.** Dental abnormalities should be addressed by a pediatric dentist.

**Papillomata.** Papillomata usually appear in the peri-nasal region and less commonly in the perianal region, torso, and extremities. While they are mostly of cosmetic concern, papillomata may give rise to irritation or inflammation in hard-to-clean body regions and may be removed as appropriate. Recurrent facial papillomata have been successfully managed with regular dry ice removal.

**Endocrinopathies.** Neonatal hypoglycemia has frequently been reported and a high level of suspicion should be maintained. Rarely, hypoglycemia occurs in older individuals and may present with seizures. Under these circumstances, growth hormone (GH) deficiency needs to be excluded as the underlying cause (Gripp et al. 2000). Hypoglycaemic episodes unresponsive to GH therapy responded well to cortisone replacement in another individual (Gregersen and Viljoen 2004); thus, cortisol deficiency may also be considered.

**Malignant tumours.** Treatment of malignant tumours follows standard protocols.

## Prevention of secondary complications

**Cardiac.** Certain **congenital** heart defects (notably valvar pulmonic stenosis) require antibiotic prophylaxis for subacute bacterial endocarditis (SBE), available by prescription from the cardiologist or other physician caregiver.

**Sedation.** Individuals with Costello syndrome may require relatively high doses of medication for sedation. No standardized information is available, but review of an individual's medical records documenting previously given dosages may provide guidance.

**Anesthesia** may pose a risk to individuals with some forms of unrecognised hypertrophic cardiomyopathy or those who have a predisposition to some types of atrial tachycardia.

## Surveillance

**Hypoglycemia.** Neonatal hypoglycemia has frequently been reported and a high level of suspicion should be maintained. Monitoring of blood glucose concentration should follow typical protocols for neonates at risk for hypoglycemia.

**Cardiac.** While data regarding the natural history are insufficient to determine a schedule for repeating cardiac assessments if the initial evaluation is normal, it appears that the onset of new cardiovascular abnormalities declines after adolescence. The follow-up schedule must be customized based on

**Table 2.** Follow-up cardiac evaluation for Costello syndrome

If the newborn evaluation is normal, follow-up with echocardiogram at about age six to 12 month

For those without an apparent cardiac abnormality, follow-up approximately every one to three years until about age five to ten years and less frequently if the individual remains healthy

In an **affected** adolescent with a normal baseline cardiology evaluation who maintains normal blood pressure, echocardiogram at three- to five-year intervals

For any child with a cardiac abnormality, scheduled assessment as recommended by the treating cardiologist

Because tachycardia is an important cause of death with or without underlying structural defect or cardiac hypertrophy, health professionals and caregivers should be aware of the possibility of sudden cardiovascular collapse.

Adapted and modified from Gripp and Lin (2007).

the overall clinical situation and the treating cardiologist. The cardiologist should be aware of Costello syndrome-associated heart abnormalities and schedule tests as indicated.

As more information about the natural history of cardiac abnormalities (especially hypertrophic cardiomyopathy, hypertension, and aortic dilatation) becomes available, the following recommendations may change (Table 2).

**Tumour screening** consisting of abdominal and pelvic ultrasound and urine testing for catecholamine metabolites and haematuria was proposed by Gripp et al. (2002). However, a subsequent report (Gripp et al. 2004) on elevated catecholamine metabolites in individuals with Costello syndrome without an identifiable tumour concluded that **screening** for abnormal catecholamine metabolites is not helpful.

Serial abdominal and pelvic ultrasound **screening** for rhabdomyosarcoma and neuroblastoma was proposed every three to six months until age eight to ten years. Urinalysis for haematuria was suggested annually beginning at age ten years to **screen** for bladder cancer Gripp et al. 2002.

Neither of the above **screening** approaches has yet been shown to be beneficial; however, studies are ongoing. The most important factor for early tumour

detection remains parental and physician awareness of the increased cancer risk.

**Bone density**. Osteoporosis is common in young adults with Costello syndrome (White et al. 2005), and bone density assessment is recommended as a baseline, with follow-up depending upon the initial result.

## Therapies

**Growth Hormone (GH) Treatment.** If treatment with growth hormone is contemplated, its unproven benefit and potential risks should be thoroughly discussed in view of the established risks of cardiomyopathy and malignancy in individuals with Costello syndrome and the unknown effect of growth hormone on these risks.

**Unproven benefit.** Individuals with Costello syndrome frequently have low GH levels.

True growth hormone deficiency requires GH replacement. Three individuals with GH deficiency showed increased growth velocity without adverse effects after three to seven years of replacement therapy, but two continued to have short stature (Stein et al. 2004).

It is unclear from the literature if the use of GH is beneficial in individuals with Costello syndrome with partial growth hormone deficiency. An abnormal growth hormone response on testing and a good initial growth response was reported (Legault et al. 2001).

**Cardiac hypertrophy.** Whether the anabolic actions of growth hormone accelerate pre-existing cardiac hypertrophy is not known (Lin et al. 2002). In rare cases, cardiomyopathy has progressed after initiation of growth hormone treatment; whether the relationship was causal or coincidental is unknown (Kerr et al. 2003).

**Malignancy.** The effect of growth hormone on tumour predisposition has not been determined. Two reports have raised the possibility of an association:

Bladder carcinoma occurred in a 16-year-old treated with growth hormone (Gripp et al. 2000).

A rhabdomyosarcoma was diagnosed in a 26-month-old receiving growth hormone from age 12 months (Kerr et al. 2003).

# References

Allanson JE (2007) Noona syndrome. Gene Reviews. http://www.genetests.org

Aoki Y, Niihori T, Kawame H, Kurosawa K, Ohashi H, Tanaka Y, Filocamo M, Kato K, Suzuki Y, Kure S, Matsubara Y (2005) Germline mutations in HRAS proto-oncogene cause Costello syndrome. Nature Genet 37: 1038–1040.

Aoki Y, Niihori T, Narumi Y, Kure S, Matsubara Y (2008) The RAS/MAPK syndromes: novel roles of the RAS pathway in human genetic disorders. Hum Mutat May 9 [Epub ahead of print].

Axelrad ME, Glidden R, Nicholson L, Gripp KW (2004) Adaptive skills, cognitive, and behavioral characteristics of Costello syndrome. Am J Med Genet 128A: 396–400.

Axelrad ME, Nicholson L, Stabley DL, Sol-Church K, Gripp KW (2007) Longitudinal assessment of cognitive characteristics in Costello syndrome. Am J Med Genet A 143: 3185–3193.

Bentires-Alj M, Kontaridis MI, Neel BG (2006) Stops along the RAS pathway in human genetic disease. Nat Med 12: 283–285.

Berberich MS, Carey JC, Hall BD (1999) Resolution of the perinatal and infantile failure to thrive in a new autosomal recessive syndrome with the phenotype of a storage disorder and furrowing of palmar creases. (Abstract) Proc Greenwood Genet Center 10: 78.

Bertola DR, Pereira AC, Brasil AS, Albano LM, Kim CA, Krieger JE (2007) Further evidence of genetic heterogeneity in Costello syndrome: involvement of the KRAS gene. J Hum Genet 52: 521–526.

Borochowitz Z, Pavone L, Mazor G, Rizzo R, Dar H (1992) New multiple congenital anomalies (mental retardation syndrome (MCA/1MR), with facio-cutaneous-skeletal involvement. Am J Med Genet 43: 678–685.

Borochowitz Z, Pavone L, Mazor G, Rizzo R, Dar H (1993) Facio-cutaneous-skeletal syndrome: new nosological entity or Costello syndrome? Am J Med Genet 47: 173.

Costello JM (1971) A new syndrome. NZ Med J 74: 387.

Costello JM (1977) A new syndrome: mental subnormality and nasal papillomata. Aus Pediatr J 13: 114–118.

Czeizel AE, Tímar L (1995) Hungarian case with Costello syndrome and translocation t (1; 22). Am J Med Genet 57: 501–503.

Davies SJ, Hughes HE (1994) Costello syndrome: natural history and differential diagnosis of cutis laxa. J Med Genet 31: 486–489.

Dearlove O, Harper N (1997) Costello syndrome. Paediatr Anaesth 7: 476–477.

De Baun MR (2002) Screening for cancer in children with Costello syndrome. Am J Med Genet 108: 88–90.

Della Marca G, Vasta I, Scarano E, Rigante M, De Feo E, Mariotti P, Rubino M, Vollono C, Mennuni GF, Tonali P, Zampino G (2006) Obstructive sleep apnea in Costello syndrome. Am J Med Genet A 140: 257–262.

Delrue MA, Chateil JF, Arveiler B, Lacombe D (2003) Costello syndrome and neurological abnormalities. Am J Med Genet 123A: 301–305.

Der Kaloustian VM, Moroz B, Mc Intosh N, Watters AK, Blaichman S (1991) Costello syndrome. Am J Med Genet 41: 69–73.

Der Kaloustian VM (1993) Not a new MCA/MR syndrome but probably Costello syndrome? Am J Med Genet 47: 70–71.

Estep AL, Tidyman WE, Teitell MA, Cotts PD, Rauer KA (2006) HRAS mutation in Costello syndrome: detection of constitutional activating mutations in codon 12 ans 13 and loss of wild-type allele in malignancy. Am J Med Genet 140A: 8–16.

Franceschini P, Licata D, Di Cara G, Guala A, Bianchi M, Ingrosso G, Franceschini D (1999) Bladder carcinoma in Costello syndrome: report on a patient born to consanguineous parents and review. Am J Med Genet 86: 174–179.

Fujikawa Y, Sugai K, Fukumizu M, Hanaoko S, Sasaki M, Kaga M (2001) Three cases of Costello syndrome presenting with intractable epilepsy and profound psychomotor retardation/regression. Noto Hattatsu 33: 430–435.

Fukao T, Sakai S, Shimozawa N, Kuwahara T, Kano M, Goto E, Nakashima Y, Katagiri-Kawade M, Ichihashi H, Masuno M, Orii T, Kondo N (1996) Life-threatening cardiac involvement throughout life in a case of Costello syndrome. Clin Genet 50: 244–247.

Galera C, Delcrue MA, Goizet C, Etchegovhen K, Taupiac E, Sigaudy S, Arvelier B, Philip N, Bouvard M, Lacombe D (2006) Behavioural and temperamental features of children with Costello syndrome. Am J Med Genet A 140: 968–974.

Gelb BD, Tartaglia M (2006) Noonan syndrome and related disorders: dysregulated RAS-mitogen activated protein kinase signal transduction. Hum Mol Genet 15 (Spec No 2): R220–R226.

Gregerson N, Viljoen D (2004) Costello syndrome with growth hormone deficiency, and hypoglycemia: a new report and review of the endocrine associations. Am J Med Genet 129A: 171–175.

Gripp KW, Scott CI, Nicholson L, Mc Donald-Mc Ginn DM, Ozeran JD, Jones MC, Lin AE, Zackai EH (2002) Five additional Costello syndrome patients with rhabdomyosarcoma: proposal for a tumor screening protocol. Am J Med Genet 108: 80–87.

Gripp KW, Stabley DL, Nicholson L, Hoffman JD, Sol-Church K (2006a) Somatic mosaicism for an HRAS mutation causes Costello syndrome. Am J Med Genet A 140: 2163–2169.

Gripp KW, Lin AE, Stabley DL, Nicholson L, Scott CI, Doyle D, Aoki Y, Matsubara Y, Zackai EH, Lapunzina P, Gonzalez-Meneses A, Holbrook J, Agresta CA (2006b) HRAS mutation analysis in Costello syndrome: genotype and phenotype correlation. Am J Med Genet 140A: 1–7.

Gripp KW, Lin AE (2007) Costello syndrome. Gene Reviews. http://www.genetests.org.

Hall BD, Berbereich FR, Berbereich MS (1990) AMICABLE syndrome: a new unique disorder involving facial, cardiac, ectodermal, growth and intellectual abnormalities. Proc Greenwood Genet Center 9: 103A.

Hennekam RCM (2003) Costello syndrome: an overview. Am J Med Genet Part C (Semin Med Genet) 117C: 42–48.

Hinek A, Rabinovitch M (1994) 67 Kd elastin binding protein is a protective "companion" of extracellular insoluble elastin and intracellular tropoelastin. J Cell Biol 126: 563–574.

Hinek A, Smith AC, Cutiongeo EM, Callahan JW, Gripp KW, Weksberg R (2000) Decreased elastin deposition and high proliferation of fibroblasts from Costello syndrome are related to functional deficiency in the 67-kD_elastin-binding protein. Am J Hum Genet 66: 859–872.

Hinek A, Teitell MA, Schoyer L, Allen W, Gripp KW, Hamilton R, Weksberg R, Kluppel M, Lin AE (2005) Myocardial storage of chondroitin sulfate-containing moieties in Costello syndrome patients with severe hypertrophic cardiomyopathy. Am J Med Genet 133A: 1–12.

Indik Z, Yea H, Ornstein-Goldstein N, Sheppard P, Anderson N, Rosenblood JC, Peltonen L, Rosenbloom J (1987) Alternative splicing of human elastin mRNA indicated by sequence analysis of cloned genomic and complementary DNA. Proc Natl Acad Sci USA 84: 5680–5684.

Ioan DM, Fryns JP (2002) Costello syndrome in two siblings and minor manifestations in their mother: further evidence for autosomal dominant inheritance? Genet Counsel 13: 353–356.

Johnson JP, Golabi M, Norton ME, Rosenblatt RM, Feldman GM, Yang SM, Hall BD, Fries MH, Carey JC (1998) Costello syndrome: Phenotype, natural history, differential diagnosis, and possibly cause. J Pediatr 133: 441–448.

Kawame H, Matsui M, Kurosawa K, Matsuo M, Masuno M, Ohashi H, Fueki N, Aoyama K, Miyatsuka Y, Suzuki K, Akatsuka A, Ochiai Y, Fukushima Y (2003)

Further delineation of the behavioral and neurologic features in Costello syndrome. Am J Med Genet 118A: 8–14.

Kerr B, Eden OB, Dandamudi R, Shannon N, Quarrell O, Emmerson A, Ladusans E, Gerrard M, Donnai D (1998) Costello syndrome: two cases with embryonal rhabdomyosarcoma. J Med Genet 35: 1036–1039.

Kerr B, Delrue MA, Sigaudy S, Perveen R, Marhe M, Burgelin I, Stef M, Tang B, Eden B, O'Sullivan J, De Sandre-Giovanoli A, Reardon W, Brewer C, Bennett C, Ouarell O, M'Cann E, Donnai D, Stewart F, Hennekam R, Cave H, Verloes A, Philip N, Lacombe D, Levy N, Arvelier B, Black G (2006) Genotype-phenotype correlation in Costello syndrome: HRAS mutations analysis in 43 cases. J Med Genet 43: 401–405.

Kerr B, Allanson J, Delrue MA, Gripp KW, Lacombe D, Lin AE, Rauen KA (2008) The diagnosis of Costello syndrome: nomenclature in Ras/MAPK pathway disorders. Am J Med Genet A 146: 1218–1220.

Kratz CP, Steinemann D, Niemeyer CM, Schlegelberger B, Koscielniak E, Kontny U, Zenker M (2007) Uniparental disomy at chromosome 11p15.5 followed by HRAS mutations in embryonal rhabdomyosarcoma: lessons from Costello syndrome. Hum Mol Genet 16: 374–379.

Legault L, Cagnon C, Lapointe N (2001) Growth hormone deficiency in Costello syndrome: a possible explanation for the short stature. J Pediatr 138: 151–152.

Levaillant JM, Gerard-Blanluet M, Holder-Espinasse M, Valat-Ricot AS, Devisme L, Cave H, Manouvrier-Hanu S (2006) Prenatal overlap of Costello syndrome and severe Noonan syndrome by tri-dimensional ultrasonography. Prenat Diagn 26: 340–344.

Li DY, Brooke B, Davis EC, Mechan RP, Sorensen LK, Boak BB, Eichwald E, Keating MT (1998a) Elastin is an essential determinant of arterial morphogenosis. Nature 393: 276–280.

Li DY, Faury G, Taylor DG, Davis EC, Boyle WA, Mecham RP, Stenzel P, Boak B, Keating MT (1998b) Novel arterial pathology in mice und human hemizygous for elastin. J Clin Invest 102: 1783–1787.

Lin AE, Grossfeld PD, Hamilton RM, Smoot L, Gripp KW, Proud V, Weksberg R, Wheeler P, Picker J, Irons M, Zackai E, Marino B, Scott CI Jr, Nicholson L (2002) Further delineation of cardiac abnormalities in Costello syndrome. Am J Med Genet 111: 115–129.

Lin AE, Rauen KA, Gripp KW, Carey JC (2008) Clarification of previously reported Costello syndrome patients. Am J Med Genet A 146: 940–943.

Lo IF, Brewer C, Shannon N, Shorto J, Tang B, Black G, Soo MT, Ng DK, Lam ST, Kerr B (2008) Severe neonatal manifestations of Costello syndrome. J Med Genet 45: 167–171.

Lurie IW (1994) Genetics of the Costello syndrome. Am J Med Genet 52: 358–359.

Mancini GMS, van Diggelen OP, Kleijer WJ, Di Rocco M, Farina V, Yuksel-Apak M, Kayserili H, Halley DJJ (2003) Studies on the pathogenesis of Costello syndrome. J Med Genet 40: e37.

Maroti Z, Kutsche K, Sutajova M, Gal A, Northwang HG, Czeizel AE, Tímár L, Sólyom E (2002) Refinement and delineation of the breakpoint regions of a chromosome 1;22 translocation in a patient with Costello syndrome. Am J Med Genet 109: 234–237.

Martin RA, Jones KL (1991) Delineation of the Costello syndrome. Am J Med Genet 41: 346–349.

Midgley RS, Kerr DJ (2002) Ras as a target in cancer therapy. Crit Rev Oncol Hematol 44:109–120.

Mori M, Yamagata T, Mori Y, Nokubi M, Saito K, Fukushima Y, Momoi MY (1996) Elastic fiber degeneration in Costello syndrome. Am J Med Genet 61: 304–309.

Narumi Y, Aoki Y, Niihori T, Neri G, Cave H, Verloes A, Nava C, Kavamura MI, Okamoto N, Kurosawa K, Hennekam RC, Wilson LC, Gillessen-Kaesbach G, Wieczorek D, Lapunzina P, Ohashi H, Makita Y, Kondo I, Tsuchiya S, Ito E, Sameshima K, Kato K, Kure S, Matsubara Y (2007) Molecular and clinical characterization of cardio-facio-cutaneous (CFC) syndrome: overlapping clinical manifestations with Costello syndrome. Am J Med Genet A 143: 799–807.

Nguyen V, Buka RL, Roberts BJ, Eichenfield LF (2007) Cutaneous manifestations of Costello syndrome. Int J Dermatol 46: 72–76.

Niihori T, Aoki Y, Narumi Y, Neri G, Cave H, Verloes A, Okamoto N, Hennekam RC, Gillessen-Kaesbach G, Wieczorek D, Kavamura MI, Kurosawa K, Ohashi H, Wilson L, Heron D, Bonneau D, Corona G, Kaname T, Naritomi K, Baumann C, Matsumoto N, Kato K, Kure S, Matsubara Y (2006) Germline KRAS and BRAF mutations in cardio-facio-cutaneous syndrome. Nat Genet 38: 294–296.

Noonan JA (2006) Noonan syndrome and related disorders: Alterations in growth and puberty. Rev Endocr Metab Disord 7: 251–255.

OMIM (2007) Online Mendelian Inheritance in Man. Baltimore: Johns Hopkins University Press. http://www.ncbi.nlm.nih.gov/omim.

O'Neal JP, Ramdas J, Wood WE, Pellitteri PK (2004) Parameningeal rhabdomyosarcoma in a patient with Costello syndrome.

Pascual-Castroviejo I, Pascual-Pascual SI (2005) Síndrome de Costello. Presentación de un caso con seguimiento durante 35 años. Neurología 20: 144–148.

Patton MA, Tolmie J, Ruthnum P, Bamforth S, Baraitser M, Pembrey M (1987) Congenital cutis laxa with retardation of growth and development. J Med Genet 24: 556–561.

Pratesi R, Santos M, Ferrari I (1998) Costello syndrome in two Brazilian children. J Med Genet 35: 54–57.

Rauen KA (2007) HRAS and the Costello syndrome. Clin Genet 71: 101–108.

Rauen KA (2007a) HRAS and the Costello syndrome. Clin Genet 71: 101–108.

Rauen KA (2007b) cardiofaciocutaneous syndrome. Gene Reviews. http://www.genetests.org

Rauen KA, Hefner E, Carrillo K, Taylor J, Messier L, Aoki Y, Gripp KW, Matsubara Y, Proud VK, Hammond P, Allanson JE, Delrue MA, Axelrad ME, Lin AE, Doyle DA, Kerr B, Carey JC, McCormick F, Silva AJ, Kieran MW, Hinek A, Nguyen TT, Schoyer L (2008) Molecular aspects, clinical aspects and possible treatment modalities for Costello syndrome: proceedings from the 1st International Costello Syndrome Research Symposium 2007. Am J Med Genet A 146: 1205–1217.

Roberts A, Allanson J, Jadico SK, Kavamura MI, Noonan J, Opitz JM, Young T, Neri G (2006) The cardiofaciocutaneous syndrome. J Med Genet 43: 833–842.

Rodriguez-Viciana P, Tetsu O, Tidyman WE, Estep AL, Conger BA, Cruz MS, McCormick F, Rauen KA (2006) Germline mutations in genes within the MAPK pathway cause cardio-facio-cutaneous syndrome. Science 311: 1287–1290.

Say B, Güçsavas M, Morgan H, York C (1993) The Costello syndrome. Am J Med Genet 47: 163–165.

Schubbert S, Zenker M, Rowe SL, Boll S, Klein C, Bollag G, van der Burgt I, Musante L, Kalscheuer V, Wehner LE, Nguyen H, West B, Zhang KY, Sistermans E, Rauch A, Niemeyer CM, Shannon K, Kratz CP (2006) Germline KRAS mutations cause Noonan syndrome. Nat Genet 38: 331–336.

Shiihara T, Kato M, Mitsuhashi Y, Hayakasa K (2005) Costello syndrome showing Moyamoya vasculopathy. Pediatr Neurol 32: 361–363.

Sigaudy S, Vittu G, David A, Vigneron J, Lacombe D, Moncla A, Flori E, Philip N (2000) Costello syndrome: report of six patients including one with an embryonal rhabdomyosarcoma. Eur J Pediatr 159: 139–142.

Siwik ES, Zahka KG, Wiesner GL (1998) Cardiac disease in Costello syndrome. Pediatrics 150: 706–708.

Stein RI, Legault L, Daneman D, Weksberg R, Hamilton J (2004) Growth hormone deficiency in Costello syndrome. Am J Med Genet 129A: 166–170.

Suri M, Garret C (1998) Costello syndrome with acoustic neuroma and cataract. Is the Costello locus linked to neurofibromatosis type 2 on 22q? Clin Dysmorphol 7: 149–151.

Tartaglia M, Cotter PD, Zampino G, Gelb BD, Rauen KA (2003) Exclusion of PTPN11 mutations in Costello syndrome: further evidence for distinct genetic etiologies for Noonan, cardio-facio-cutaneous and Costello syndromes. Clin Genet 63: 423–426.

Van Den Bosch T, Van Schoubroeck D, Fryuns JP, Naulaers G, Inion AM, Devriendt K (2002) Prenatal findings in a monozygotic twin pregnancy with Costello syndrome. Prenat Diagn 22: 415–417.

Van Eeghen AM, Van Gelderen I, Hennekam RCM (1999) Costello syndrome: Report and review. Am J Med Genet 82: 187–193.

van Steensel MA, Vreeburg M, Peels C, van Ravenswaaij-Arts CM, Bijlsma E, Schrander-Stumpel CT, van Geel M (2006) Recurring HRAS mutation G12S in Dutch patients with Costello syndrome. Exp Dermatol 15: 731–734.

Vila Torres J, Pineda Marfa M, Gonzalez Ensenat MA, Lloreta Trull J (1994) Pathology of the elastic tissue of the skin in Costello syndrome. An image analysis study using mathematical morphology. Anal Quant Cytol Histol 16: 421–429.

Weiss G, Confino Y, Shemor A, Trau H (2004) Cutaneous manifestation in the cardiofaciocutaneous syndrome, a variant of the classical Noonan syndrome. Report of a case and review of the literature. J Eur Acad Dermatol Venereol 18: 324–327.

White SM, Graham JM, Kerr B, Gripp K, Weksberg R, Cytrynbaum C, Reeder JL, Stewart FJ, Edwards M, Wilson M, Bankier A (2005) The adult phenotype in Costello syndrome. Am J Med Genet A 136: 128–135.

Zampino G, Mastroiacovo P, Ricci R, Zollino M, Segni G, Martini-Neri ME, Neri G (1993) Costello syndrome: Further clinical delineation, natural history, genetic definition, and nosology. Am J Med Genet 47: 176–183.

Zampino G, Pantaleoni F, Carta C, Cobellis G, Vasta I, Neri C, Pogna EA, De Feo E, Delogu A, Sarkozy A, Atzeri F, Selicorni A, Rauen KA, Cytrynbaum CS, Weksberg R, Dallapiccola B, Ballabio A, Gelb BD, Neri G, Tartaglia M (2007) Diversity, parental germline origin, and phenotypic spectrum of de novo HRAS missense changes in Costello syndrome. Hum Mutat 28: 265–272.

# Chapter 67

# ANDERSON-FABRY DISEASE

**Anna-Christine Hauser**

Department of Medicine III, Division of Nephrology and Dialysis, Medical University of Vienna, Währingergürtel 18-20, 1090 Vienna, Austria

## Introduction

Anderson-Fabry disease is a multisystemal storage disorder due to a deficiency of α-galactosidase A resulting in an accumulation of neutral glycosphingolipids. Due to its rare occurrence the disease is often misdiagnosed or the correct diagnose is delayed for many years (Weidemann et al. 2008). Dermatologists except ophthalmologists play the most important role for early diagnosis of this disorder, which can now be treated by enzyme replacement therapy. Otherwise, Anderson-Fabry disease is a lethal disorder, renal disease or stroke being the most important causes of death (Grünfeld et al. 2002, Desnick et al. 2003). Early diagnosis and treatment is essential to limit organ damage (Hauser et al. 2004b, Branton et al. 2002).

## Historical perspective and terminology

The disease was first described by Anderson and Fabry in 1898 and was called angiokeratoma corporis diffusum (Anderson 1898, Fabry 1898). In 1909, Steiner and Voerner studied the neural symptoms of the disease and, in 1925, Weicksel reported on cardiopathy, ophthalmological findings and hereditary aspects (Fabry 2002). The depositions of hitherto unknown substances in the vascular system was shown by Ruiter in 1947, which were identified by Sweely as types of glycolipids in a further step and which were localized in lysosomes by Hashimoto using electron microscopy (Fabry 2002). The disease was attributed to an enzyme defect by Brady in 1967 and Kint in 1970 (Hauser et al. 2004a). Brady performed a first trial with enzyme replacement therapy using purified ceramidetrihexosidase in 1973 (Brady et al. 1973). The most important therapeutic breakthrough was the introduction of enzyme replacement therapy with recombinant α-galactosidase A by Eng et al. and Schiffmann et al. in 2001 (Eng et al. 2001, Schiffmann et al. 2001).

## Incidence and prevalence

The disease incidence ranges from 1:40.000 to 1:117.000 live births. Anderson-Fabry disease is encountered in all racial groups with no racial or ethnic predilection (Hauser et al. 2004a, Bennett et al. 2002).

## Clinical manifestations

### Skin abnormalities

Generalized or isolated angiokeratomas are the leading dermatological findings appearing as papules of different sizes and colors, which are primarily found in the genital area, the lower abdomen and on the thighs (Larralde et al. 2004, Mohrenschlager et al. 2003), but may be present on the entire body (Fig. 1). One or more dilated blood vessels in the upper part of the dermis accompanied frequently by a dermal reaction such as acanthosis and/or hyperkeratosis can be found histologically (Schiller and Itin 1996). Larger angiokeratomas become dark red to black with a discrete verrucous overgrowth (Larralde et al. 2004). With the progression of the disease, lesions become more numerous and may eventually also affect the mucous membranes of digestive, respiratory and genitourinary tracts (Mohrenschlager et al. 2003). Such dermatological findings show a high prevalence: in a recent study, 83% of hemizygote males had widespread angiokeratomas, and 80%

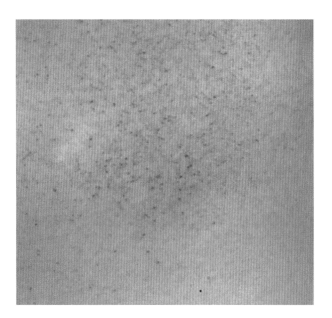

**Fig. 1.** Angiokeratomas appearing as small raised dark-red macu-lopapular discrete spots in the skin of a young male patient with Anderson-Fabry disease. They occur mainly in the area of genital and lower abdomen as well as symmetrically on the thighs. Courtesy of Department of Dermatology, Medical University Vienna, Vienna, Austria.

of heterozygote females had isolated angiokeratomas (Larralde et al. 2004). However, neither the presence nor the extent of lesions correlates with systemic morbidity (Larralde et al. 2004). In particular, they may be absent in patients with single organ manifestations such as in the cardiac and renal variants of the disease (Nakao et al. 1995, 2003). Pathogenetically, angiokeratomas seem to result from damages of the capillary wall followed by ectasia (Larralde et al. 2004).

Hypohydrosis or anhydrosis is encountered in a high percentage of male patients and seems to be less frequent in females (MacDermot et al. 2001a, b; Galanos et al. 2002). The causes are lipid accumulation in the eccrine cells as well as autonomic nervous system dysfunction (Larralde et al. 2004, Kolodny and Pastores 2002).

Lymphedema can be found in a substantial number of patients (MacDermot et al. 2001a, b). A study found fragmentation of the microlymphatic network and microlymphatic hypertension as major causes in affected patients (Amann-Vesti et al. 2003).

## Abnormalities of other systems and organs

### Eye findings

Cornea verticillata and tortuosity of conjunctival and retinal vessels are typical ocular findings (Hauser et al. 2004a). Two types of lenticular abnormalities may develop: a posterior opacity with a spoke-like appearance and a granular, anterior capsular or subcapsular wedge-shaped lipid deposit (Bennett et al. 2002). The cataracts and corneal abnormalities do not disturb the vision and are thus found only by chance (Hauser et al. 2004a, b). Eye findings can be observed in almost all affected males and in 70–90% of heterozygous women (Hauser et al. 2004a, b), and are among the first disease manifestations (Ries et al. 2003).

### Cardiac manifestations

The heart is affected in terms of left ventricular hypertrophy (LVH), mostly mild valvular affection of both mitral and aortic valves and, equally frequent in both genders, disturbance of the conduction system and anginal chest pain (Hauser et al. 2004a; Kampmann et al. 2002, 2008; Weidemann et al. 2005). Left ventricular hypertrophy is caused predominantly by an increase in contractile proteins and to less degree by Gb3 depositions, which seem to lead to a myocyte disarray. Consequently, it is associated with increased voltage electrocardiogram, while the infiltrative myocardiopathies as amyloidosis show low voltage (Kampmann et al. 2002). Affection of the conduction system leads to a wide range of arrhythmias and heart block (Hauser et al. 2004a, Kampmann et al. 2002). The frequency of cardiac rhythm disturbances increases with age (Shah and Elliot 2005).

Anginal chest pain can be found in up to 50% of Anderson-Fabry patients, often in the absence of angiographically detectable coronary artery disease. Among other factors, vasospasm due to endothelial dysfunction may be responsible for such symptoms (Kampmann et al. 2002, Hauser et al. submitted). Overall, Gb3 accumulation seems to accelerate atherosclerosis (Bodary et al. 2005).

Heart affection can be the only symptom of Anderson-Fabry disease, which is then defined as a cardiac variant (Nakao et al. 1995). In one study, about 12% of female patients with late-onset hypertrophic cardiomyopathy had Anderson-Fabry disease, with the heart being the sole organ manifestation (Chimenti et al. 2004).

**Therapy**: Non causal therapy includes routine symptomatic cardiac therapy (Kampmann et al. 2002).

## Renal manifestation

Proteinuria is an early sign of renal manifestation, often in the first decade of age in males and female patients (Warnock 2005, Mehta et al. 2004). Deterioration of renal function progresses slowly down to a glomerular filtration rate of about 60 mL/min, and is unspecific. Thereafter an accelerated decline develops to end-stage renal failure within $4\pm3$ years (mean$\pm$SD, range 1–13 years). The mean annual reduction was 12.2 ml/min in one study (Branton et al. 2002). This behavior resembles the course of diabetic nephropathy (Branton et al. 2002). The kidneys seem to be enlarged in the third decade of life followed by a decreasing renal size in the fourth and fifth decade (Stiennon and Goldberg 1980). A large ultrasonic and magnetic resonance study found abnormalities in 64.5% of males and 60% of females. Cysts, particularly parapelvic were more common and emerged earlier than in the normal population. Other findings were decreased corticomedullary differentiation and decreased cortical thickness. No renal abnormality was detected in males before 12 years of age and before 20 years of age in females (Glass et al. 2004). Renal biopsies revealed accumulation of Gb3 in the epithelial cells of Henle's loop and distal tubule as well as those of the proximal tubule. All types of glomerular cells are involved, particularly the podocytes, where in some cases Gb3 depositions were found as early as in the second trimester of fetal development (Branton et al. 2002, Sessa et al. 2001, Warnock 2005). Ultrastructural studies showed typical bodies in the cytoplasm of concentric lamellation of clear and dark layers with a periodicity of 35–50A (Sessa et al. 2001).

In the American (USRDS 2000) and the European (EDTA 1993) renal registry, the prevalence of Anderson-Fabry among chronic patients was about 0.02%. Similar to sole cardiac affection, patients with sole renal affection and end stage renal failure were identified. The residual enzyme activity was as high as in patients with full blown disease (Hauser et al. 2004a, Thadhani et al. 2002, Nakao et al. 2003).

**Therapy**: Non causal therapy should include angiotensin-converting inhibitors or angiotensin II receptor blockers for reduction of proteinuria (Warnock 2005). In the state of renal insufficiency, routine treatment for chronic renal failure should be prescribed (Ortiz et al. 2008, Warnock 2005).

## Endocrine findings

Subclinical hypothyroidism seems to be a frequent occurrence in Anderson-Fabry patients, with a prevalence of about 36% in one study. Pregnant patients should be screened for thyroid function because of an increased risk of fetal loss and abnormal neuropsychiatric development by maternal subclinical hypothyroidism (Hauser et al. 2005b). Unlike thyroid function, other endocrine functions seem undisturbed and provide a normal fertility rate in both genders (Hauser et al. 2005b).

**Therapy**: Thyroxine replacement therapy should be initiated in patients with TSH (Thyroid Stimulating Hormone) plasma levels above $10\,\mu U/ml$. In pregnant women, thyroxine therapy is indicated at lower TSH plasma levels (Hauser et al. 2005a).

## Bone affection

Anderson-Fabry disease may affect bones (Germain et al. 2005, Lien and Lai 2005). An increased risk of osteopenia and osteoporosis as well as femoral head and tibial necrosis has been described (Germain et al. 2005, Lien and Lai 2005).

**Therapy**: Given that vitamin D and calcium play a major role for the development of osteoporosis, routine antiosteoporotic therapy should be initiated (Germain et al. 2005).

## Nervous system abnormalities

### Pain

Pain is a leading symptom of Anderson-Fabry disease most often as acroparesthesias in the toes and fingers. It can be chronic and/or acute with episodic crises often triggered by changes in temperature, exercise or stress (Hauser et al. 2004a, Kolodny and Pastores 2002). The character of the pain may be described as burning, piercing, sharp, and appalling. It may be shooting in arms and legs as well as in the palms and soles. Pain emerges early in life (Mehta et al. 2004) and was present in 80% of patients at the age of 12.5 in boys and 13.2 years in girls in one study (Ramaswami et al. 2006).

Pathologically, a damage of small nerve fibers by accumulation of Gb3 in the nerve axons and dorsal root ganglia can be found. Smaller unmyelinated fibers seem to be more susceptible to Gb3 infiltration, whereas larger myelinated fibers are largely protected by myelin sheaths (Kolodny and Pastores 2002). Deposits were observed widely in the central and peripheral nervous system, most often within selected neurons of the spinal cord, brain stem, amygdale, hypothalamus and endorhinal cortex (Burlina et al. 2008, MacDermot and MacDermot 2001). Blood vessels throughout the nervous system show also widespread deposition of Gb3 (Fig. 2). The typical effect of cold exposure as pain trigger suggests the involvement of A-and C-fibers. It is assumed that pain sensation originates in abnormal ganglion cells but also from more peripheral sites, where a temperature- dependent vasoconstrictor response in stenotic small vessels could be responsible (MacDermot and MacDermot 2001). One recent study showed motor axon depolarization in Anderson-Fabry disease accompanied by normal late subexcitability, suggesting an ischemic origin of the depolarization (Tan et al. 2005).

In adults, the prevalence of pain ranges from 64 to 76% in one survey (Laaksonen et al. 2008, Mehta et al. 2004). In later life, pain may become less intense or may even disappear when the damage reaches a certain threshold (Hauser et al. 2004a, Kolodny and Pastores 2002).

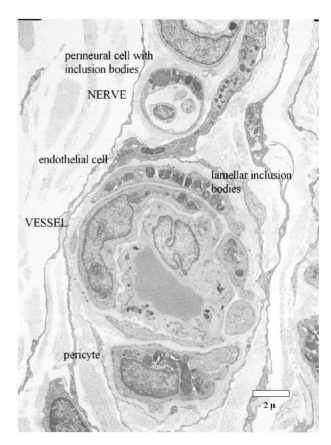

**Fig. 2.** Electron-dense cytoplasmic inclusion bodies with alternating electron dense and light regions in endothelial, perithelial and perineural cells. Findings of a young male Anderson-Fabry patient. Courtesy of Department of Dermatology, Medical University Vienna, Vienna, Austria.

### Autonomic dysfunction

Autonomic dysfunction affects tears and saliva formation, cerebrovascular reactivity, cardiac rhythm, gastrointestinal motility and pain perception. It may also be the cause of postprandial pain, nausea, and diarrhea, which can be encountered frequently in both genders (Kolodny and Pastores 2002, Mehta et al. 2004).

### Cerebrovascular complications

Ischemic but also hemorrhagic stroke and transient ischemic attack are serious manifestations of the disease predicting poor prognosis. For unknown reasons, the posterior circulation is predominantly affected (Hauser et al. 2004a, Kolodny and Pastores 2002). Deposition of glycosphingolipid in the wall of the small arteries and arterioles, dolichoectasia of intracranial arteries due to lipid involvement of the vascular smooth muscle, a prothrombotic state and probably an increased resting regional cerebral blood flow, which is reversible by enzyme replacement therapy, are major pathogenic factors (Mehta and Ginsberg 2005). In small blood vessels Gb3 depositions in endothelial and vascular smooth muscle cells cause progressive stenosis and occlusion. Conversely, in larger vessels lipid depositions may weaken the vessel wall and lead to dilatation and tortuosity. Alteration of the endothelium causes an increase in endothelial prothrombotic factors (Mehta and Ginsberg 2005). Genotypes of polymorphisms G-174C of interleukin-6, G894T of endothelial nitric oxide synthase, factor V G1691A mutation, and the A-13G and G79A of protein Z were all significantly associated with cerebral lesions in one study, suggesting that these proteins can modulate Fabry cerebral vasculopathy (Altarescu et al. 2005).

In a large study on 388 patients, 11.1% of males and 15.7% of females had suffered a stroke or transient ischemic attack (TIA) at a mean age of 35.5 and 41.4 years, respectively (Mehta et al. 2004).

In a study on patients with cryogenic stroke Fabry disease was detected among 4.9% of male and 2.4% female patients (Rolfs et al. 2005).

## Auditory symptoms

Tinnitus and hearing loss in the high tone range occur in both genders, unilaterally and bilaterally, due to lipid storage within nerve cells of the cochlea. Sudden loss of hearing could arise due to occlusion of the branch of the basilar artery to the cochlea. In contrast to vestibular deficits, the cochlear is often affected bilaterally (Kolodny and Pastores 2002, Widmer et al. 2005).

## Neuropsychiatric findings

Depression as a consequence of this very painful and disabling disease is easy to understand. A high

suicide rate and addiction to narcotics has been reported (Hauser et al. 2004a, Sadek et al. 2004).

**Therapy**: Pain can be controlled by diphenylhydantoin, carbamazepin or gabapentin. Nonsteroidal anti-inflammatory drugs are generally ineffective and may have adverse effects on kidney function. Prophylaxis with antiplatelet or anticoagulant medication should be considered for patients with a history of stroke or transient ischemia attacks. For other symptoms routine symptomatic drugs should be prescribed (Desnick et al. 2003).

## Natural history

If the disease remains untreated, the life span is reduced by about 20 years. The survival curves for male and female patients with Anderson-Fabry disease show a steep decline after the age of 35 years (MacDermot et al. 2001a, b). Renal disease or stroke are the most important causes of death (Hauser et al. 2004a, Desnick et al. 2003). In the dialysis population the mortality rates lie between diabetic and non-diabetic hemodialysis patients (Thadhani et al. 2002). At three years mean survival rate was estimated at 63% (Thadhani et al. 2002).

## Pathogenesis/molecular genetics

Anderson-Fabry disease is a lysosomal storage disorder resulting from a deficiency of the enzyme α-galactosidase A, which normally breaks globotriaosylceramide (Gb3) to galactose and lactosylceramide. In the state of enzyme deficiency, progressive systemic accumulation of neutral glycosphingolipids, primarily Gb3, occurs within lysosomes of various cell types. Endothelial and vascular muscular cells are predominantly affected, leading to vascular occlusion and clinically to ischemia with infarction of the kidney, heart and brain (Hauser et al. 2004a). Although small vessels are predominantly affected, hypertrophy of the wall of a medium sized artery was also found (Boutouyrie et al. 2002, 2001). Moreover, vascular thrombosis can occur, triggered by a prothrombotic state in Anderson-Fabry patients

(DeGraba et al. 2000). In addition to vascular cells, renal tubular cells, cardiomyocytes, valvular fibrocytes, neurones of the dorsal root ganglia and autonomic nervous systems are infiltrated (Hauser et al. 2004a).

The gene that encodes α-galactosidase A is located on the long arm of the X-chromosomes (Xq22.1) suggesting recessive X-chromosomal linked inheritance. However, due to random X-chromosome inactivation severe disease manifestation can also occur in heterozygous women (Hauser et al. 2004a). Correspondingly, discordance in female monozygotic twins has been observed (Hauser et al. 2004a). To date, over 240 gene mutations have been detected and the number of novel mutations is still rising

(Warnock 2005). It is assumed that 3–10% of patients with Anderson-Fabry disease have a newly-arising mutation. Most are present in a single family (Schaefer et al. 2005).

There is no clear relationship between a certain gene mutation and clinical signs and symptoms. Clinical involvement is variable even in patients with identical mutations or with similar levels of α-galactosidase A activity. A large number of unidentified genetic factors besides enzyme α-galactosidase A activity seem to modify the disease phenotype, creating a spectrum of disease manifestations. These manifestations range from the classic form of full blown disease (angiokeratomas, hypohydrosis, pain attacks, various cardiac, renal and neurological features

**Table 1.** Prevalence and onset of signs and symptoms among male and female adults with Anderson-Fabry disease according to several studies

| Symptoms | Prevalence (%) in adult males (n=201, mean age 35.5±13.1 years)* | Onset in males: mean years of age (95% CI)[†] | Prevalence (%) in adult females (n=165, mean age 41.4±17.1 years)* | Onset in females: mean years of age (95% CI)[†] |
|---|---|---|---|---|
| Neuropathic pain | 76 | childhood or early adolescence | 64 | childhood or early adolescence |
| Dermatological symptoms | 78 | childhood, young adults | 50 | childhood, young adults |
| Hypohydrosis or anhydrosis[†] | 56 | childhood | 32.8 | childhood |
| Lymphoedema[†] | 14 | n.a. | 8.3 | n.a |
| Dysmorphic facial features | 56 | childhood | n.a. | n.a. |
| Ophthalmologic findings | 80%[+] | childhood | 70%[+] | childhood |
| Renal symptoms | 50 | | 50 | |
| Proteinuria | 44 | childhood | 33 | childhood |
| End stage renal failure | 17 | 36.7 (32.6–40.7) | 1 | 36 (35–37) |
| Cardiac symptoms (angina, arrhythmias, and dyspoea) | 69 | young adults | 65 | young adults |
| Left ventricular hypertrophy | 46 | young adults | 28 | adults |
| Cerebrovascular events (stroke, transient ischemic attack) | 12 | 38.8 (35.2–42.9) | 27 | 52 (43.89–60.11) |
| Auditory symptoms (tinnitus, hearing loss) | 57 | adolescence | 47 | adolescence |
| Gastrointestinal symptoms | 55 | adolescence | 50 | adolescence |

Abbreviation: 95% CI, 95% confidence interval; n.a., data not available.
[†]Data from Bennett et al. (2002), MacDermot et al. (2001a, b) and Ries et al. (2003).
*Data from Mehta et al. (2004).
[+]Data from Bennett et al. (2002).
Please note that there is a large individual range of symptoms and of the onset of symptoms in Anderson-Fabry disease patients.

and associated morbidity in the absence or with very low enzyme activity) to a milder and later-onset phenotype and single organ manifestations with residual activity (Hauser et al. 2004a; MacDermot et al. 2001a, b; Warnock 2005; Schaefer et al. 2005; Branton et al. 2002). Overall, full blown disease is more often found in males than females, but single organ manifestations can be encountered in males and conversely, severe systemic organ manifestation with full blown disease can occur in females. A rough overview of the frequency of symptoms in hemizygous males and heterozygous females are shown in Table 1 (Branton et al. 2002; MacDermot et al. 2001a, b; Mehta et al. 2004; Ries et al. 2003). Ocular and dermatological findings are among the most frequent signs of the disease (Hauser et al. 2004a).

## Diagnosis, follow-up and management

### Diagnosis

Certain diagnosis can be achieved by measurement of α-galactosidase A activity in plasma or leukocytes (Hauser et al. 2004a, Warnock 2005, Branton et al. 2002). However, determination of enzyme activity is not appropriate to identify all female carriers, as 30% of carriers may have normal enzyme activities (Linthorst et al. 2005). Biopsies of the kidney or skin show lipid depositions, and in electron micrographs multilamellar myelin bodies may be found. Genetic testing can identify the mutation in GLA, the gene coding for α-galactosidase A. Prenatal diagnosis can be performed on chorionic villi or cultured amniocytes (Hauser et al. 2004a). Urinary and plasma Gb3 are not reliable markers in Anderson-Fabry disease. Plasma Gb3 can be normal in certain gene mutations (Young et al. 2005).

### Treatment

Enzyme replacement therapy, introduced in 2001, is the only causal therapy of Anderson-Fabry disease (Eng et al. 2001, Schiffmann et al. 2001). To date, two comparable α-galactosidase A drugs are available:

agalsidase alpha (Replagal TKT Europe 5SS AB, Danderyd Sweden), which is produced from genetically engineered human fibroblast cell lines, and galasidase beta (Fabrazyme Genzyme Therapeutics, Cambridge, MA, USA), which is produced from Chinese hamster ovary cell lines. Both drugs are given intravenously biweekly and are well tolerated (Hauser et al. 2004a, Breunig et al. 2003, Brenner and Grünfeld 2004). Gb3 in plasma becomes undetectable in most patients after 14 weeks of treatment (Eng et al. 2001).

Biopsy studies showed that after 6 months of therapy nearly all treated patients had a normal renal capillary endothelial histology and a normal skin endothelium (Eng et al. 2001). Normal endothelial findings of heart biopsies were observed in 75% after 6 months' therapy (Eng et al. 2001). In contrast to endothelial cells, the clearance of Gb3 was more attenuated in vascular smooth muscle cells and perineum (Thurberg et al. 2004). In the kidney, the clearance of podocytes and distal tubular cells takes longer than that of endothelial cells (Warnock 2005, Thurberg et al. 2002, Brenner and Grünfeld 2004).

The changes of pathological findings correspond largely with improvement or a stable course of clinical symptoms. A survey on 545 patients treated for more than 12 months showed stable renal function after 1 and 2 year observation period in patients with mild (GFR 60–90 mL/min/1.73 m$^2$) or moderate renal insufficiency (GFR 30–60 mL/min/1.73 m$^2$), but not in patients with advanced renal failure (Beck et al. 2004).

Moreover, a statistically significant decrease in left ventricular hypertrophy (LVH) under enzyme replacement therapy was found, particularly during the first year of treatment (Beck et al. 2004). Correspondingly, the myocardial mass may decrease (Weidemann et al. 2003, Pisani et al. 2005).

Similarly, improved pain scores were reported (Beck et al. 2004, Pisani et al. 2005). Enzyme replacement therapy significantly improved function of C-, Adelta-, and Abeta-nerve fibers and intradermal vibration receptors in Fabry neuropathy. However, a long disease history predicted a less favorable response (Hilz et al. 2004).

Despite improvement of the cerebral blood flow pattern a decline in the incidence of stroke could not be shown (Schiffmann and Ries 2005).

The individual numbers of angiokeratomas seem to remain unchanged for at least 24 months of treatment (Pisani et al. 2005). Symptoms of gastrointestinal disease subsided in patients after 6 month treatment (Banikazemi et al. 2005). All these data suggest that enzyme replacement therapy is successful, particularly if initiated early.

Co-administration of chloroquine, amiodarone, benoquin or gentamycin should be avoided because these substances could theoretically inhibit intracellular enzyme activity (Desnick et al. 2003).

Enzyme replacement therapy can be applied also in patients on maintenance hemodialysis treatment as well as in renal transplant recipients (Hauser et al. 2004a, Lorenz et al. 2003, Kosch et al. 2004, Pisani et al. 2005, Mignani et al. 2004).

Concerns arose because of the emergence of neutralizing antibodies in a high percentage of patients (Linthorst et al. 2004a). However, reports on patients receiving enzyme replacement therapy for more than 3 years and having antibodies do not suggest an attenuation of the efficacy of therapy by neutralizing antibodies (Wilcox et al. 2004).

## Differential diagnosis

Anderson-Fabry disease should be taken in the differential diagnosis of various dermatological, neurological, cardiac and renal disorders. In the case of skin findings other disorders with angiokeratomas should be considered, such as fucosidosis, sialidosis or $\alpha$- N-acetylgalactosaminidase ($\alpha$-Naga) deficiency (Kanzaki disease), GM1 and GM2 gangliosidosis and Beta-mannosidosis, which lysosomal storage disorders with autosomal inheritance are associated with generalized angiokeratomas (Linthorst et al. 2004b, Bennett et al. 2002). Angiokeratoma of Fordyce, Angiokeratoma Mibelli and Angiokeratoma circumscripta are acquired forms and appear as solitary angiokeratoma (Bennett et al. 2002, Linthorst et al. 2004b).

The character of pains may be similar to those of rheumatic fever, rheumatoid arthritis, Kanzaki disease, Raynaud's syndrome, neuropathy of many acquired (diabetic, uremic, trigeminal neuralgia) and genetic causes, such as, familial Mediterranean fever and acute intermittent porphyria. Numbness may suggest multiple sclerosis (Bennett et al. 2002). Premature stroke should take into account other causes such as systemic lupus erythemasosus, anticardiolipin antibody syndrome and many others (Hauser et al. 2004a). Cerebrovascular events within the vertebral-basilar territory may lead initially to a diagnosis of multiple sclerosis (Kolodny and Pastores 2002, Callegaro and Kaimen-Maciel 2006).

Cardiac manifestation may mimic a broad spectrum of cardiac diseases. Late onset left ventricular hypertrophy may be a striking feature of Anderson-Fabry disease (Kampmann et al. 2002; Weidemann et al. 2005). Renal affection is unspecific and may resemble various types of renal diseases (Hauser et al. 2004a; Grünfeld et al. 2002).

Corneal affection may be similar to findings after chloroquine or amiodarone therapy (Bennett et al. 2002).

## Genetic counseling

Genetic counseling should be based on medical family history, psychosocial history of probands, risk assessment and psychosocial issues (Bennett et al. 2002).

The risk assessment uses principles of X-linked recessive inheritance. However, due to random-X chromosome inactivation, heterozygous females may also show symptoms of Anderson-Fabry disease. Overall, 60–70% of carrier females show clinical expression of the disease. The percentage of females with severe full blown disease is estimated at 10% (Bennett et al. 2002). The risk of a lifelong and incurable disease is counteracted by the fact that Anderson-Fabry disease is now a treatable disorder. Enzyme replacement with recombinant $\alpha$-galactosidase A is an effective therapy to avoid and to reverse organ damage, if initiated early. Unfortunately, results of long-term therapy are currently not available. Moreover, the very high costs of this therapy may be a crucial point in some countries.

# References

Altarescu G, Moore DF, Schiffmann R (2005) Effect of genetic modifiers on cerebral lesions in Fabry disease. Neurology 64: 2148–2150.

Amann-Vesti BR, Gitzelmann G, Widmer U, Bosshard NU, Steinmann B, Koppensteiner R (2003) Severe lymphatic microangiopathy in Fabry disease. Lymphat Res Biol (3): 185–189.

Anderson W (1898) A case of angiokeratoma. Br J Dermat I: 113–117.

Banikazemi M, Ullman T, Desnick RJ (2005) Gastrointestinal manifestations of Fabry disease: Clinical response to enzyme replacement therapy. Mol Genet Metab 85(4): 255–259.

Beck M, Ricci R, Widmer U, Dehout F, de Lorenzo AG, Kampmann C, Linhart A, Sunder-Plassmann G, Houge G, Ramaswami U, Gal A, Mehta A (2004) Fabry disease: overall effects of agalsidase alfa treatment. Eur J Clin Invest 34(12): 838–844.

Bennett RL, Hart KA, O'Rourke E, Barranger JA, Johnson J, MacDermot KD, Pastores GM, Steiner RD, Thadhani R (2002) Fabry disease in genetic counseling practice: recommendations of the National Society of Genetic Counselors. J Genet Couns 11(2): 121–146.

Bodary PF, Shen Y, Vargas FB, Bi X, Ostenso KA, Gu S, Shayman JA, Eitzman DT (2005) Alpha-galactosidase A deficiency accelerates atherosclerosis in mice with apolipoprotein E deficiency. Circulation 111(5): 629–632.

Boutouyrie P, Laurent S, Laloux B, Lidove O, Grünfeld JP, Germain DP (2001) Non-invasive evaluation of arterial involvement in patients affected with Fabry disease. J Med Genet 38(9): 629–631.

Boutouyrie P, Laurent S, Laloux B, Lidove O, Grünfeld JP, Germain DP (2002) Arterial remodelling in Fabry disease. Acta Paediatr Suppl 91(439): 62–66.

Brady RO, Tallman JF, Johnson WG, Gal AE, Leahy WR, Quirk JM, Dekaban AS (1973) Replacement therapy for inherited enzyme deficiency. Use of purified ceramidetrihexosidase in Fabry's disease. N Engl J Med 289(1): 9–14.

Branton MH, Schiffmann R, Sabnis SG, Murray GJ, Quirk JM, Altarescu G, Goldfarb L, Brady RO, Balow JE, Austin Iii HA, Kopp JB (2002) Natural history of Fabry renal disease: influence of alpha-galactosidase A activity and genetic mutations on clinical course. Medicine (Baltimore) 81(2): 122–138.

Brenner BM, Grünfeld JP (2004) Renoprotection by enzyme replacement therapy. Curr Opin Nephrol Hypertens 13(2): 231–241. Review.

Breunig F, Weidemann F, Beer M, Eggert A, Krane V, Spindler M, Sandstede J, Strotmann J, Wanner C

(2003) Fabry disease: diagnosis and treatment. Kidney Int Suppl (84): S181–S185.

Burlina AP, Manara R, Caillaud C, Laissy JP, Severino M, Klein I, Burlina A, Lidove O (2008) The pulvinar sign: frequency and clinical correlations in Fabry disease. J Neurol Feb 26 [Epub ahead of print].

Callegaro D, Kaimen-Maciel DR (2006) Fabry's disease as a differential diagnosis of MS. Int MS J 13(1): 27–30.

Chimenti C, Pieroni M, Morgante E, Antuzzi D, Russo A, Russo MA, Maseri A, Frustaci A (2004) Prevalence of Fabry disease in female patients with late-onset hypertrophic cardiomyopathy. Circulation 110(9): 1047–1053. Epub 2004 Aug 16.

DeGraba T, Azhar S, Dignat-George F, Brown E, Boutiere B, Altarescu G, McCarron R, Schiffmann R (2000) Profile of endothelial and leukocyte activation in Fabry patients. Ann Neurol 47(2): 229–233.

Desnick RJ, Brady R, Barranger J, Collins AJ, Germain DP, Goldman M, Grabowski G, Packman S, Wilcox WR (2003) Fabry disease, an under-recognized multisystemic disorder: expert recommendations for diagnosis, management, and enzyme replacement therapy. Ann Intern Med 138(4): 338–346.

Eng CM, Guffon N, Wilcox WR, Germain DP, Lee P, Waldek S, Caplan L, Linthorst GE, Desnick RJ (2001) International collaborative fabry disease study group. Safety and efficacy of recombinant human alpha-galactosidase A – replacement therapy in Fabry's disease. N Engl J Med 345(1): 9–16.

Fabry H (2002) Angiokeratoma corporis diffusum-Fabry disease: historical review from the original description to the introduction of enzyme replacement therapy. Acta Paediatr Suppl 91(439): 3–5.

Fabry J (1898) Ein Beitrag zur Kenntnis der Purpura haemorrhagica nodularis. Arch Dermatol Syph 43: 187–200.

Galanos J, Nicholls K, Grigg L, Kiers L, Crawford A, Becker G (2002) Clinical features of Fabry's disease in Australian patients. Intern Med J 32(12): 575–584.

Germain DP, Benistan K, Boutouyrie P, Mutschler C (2005) Osteopenia and osteoporosis: previously unrecognized manifestations of Fabry disease. Clin Genet 68(1): 93–95.

Glass RB, Astrin KH, Norton KI, Parsons R, Eng CM, Banikazemi M, Desnick RJ (2004) Fabry disease: renal sonographic and magnetic resonance imaging findings in affected males and carrier females with the classic and cardiac variant phenotypes. J Comput Assist Tomogr 28(2): 158–168.

Grünfeld JP, Chauveau D, Levy M (2002) Anderson-Fabry disease: its place among other genetic causes of renal disease. J Am Soc Nephrol 13 [Suppl 2]: S126–S129.

Hauser AC, Lorenz M, Sunder-Plassmann G (2004a) The expanding clinical spectrum of Anderson-Fabry disease: a challenge to diagnosis in the novel era of enzyme replacement therapy. J Intern Med 255(6): 629–636.

Hauser AC, Lorenz M, Voigtländer T, Födinger M, Sunder-Plassmann G (2004b) Results of an ophthalmologic screening programme for identification of cases with Anderson-Fabry disease. Ophthalmologica 218(3): 207–209.

Hauser AC, Gessl A, Lorenz M, Voigtländer T, Födinger M, Sunder-Plassmann G (2005a) High prevalence of subclinical hypothyroidism in patients with Anderson-Fabry disease. J Inherit Metab Dis 28(5): 715–722.

Hauser AC, Gessl A, Harm F, Wiesholzer M, Kleinert J, Wallner M, Voigtländer T, Bieglmayer C, Sunder-Plassmann G (2005b) Hormonal profile and fertility in patients with Anderson-Fabry disease. Int J Clin Pract 59(9): 1025–1028.

Hauser AC, Mittermayer F, Schaller G, Harm F, Wallner M, Kleinert J, Voigtländer T, Sunder-Plassmann G (2007) Enzyme replacement therapy is associated with lower circulating ADMA levels in Anderson-Fabry patients, submitted.

Hilz MJ, Brys M, Marthol H, Stemper B, Dutsch M (2004) Enzyme replacement therapy improves function of C-, Adelta-, and Abeta-nerve fibers in Fabry neuropathy. Neurology 62(7): 1066–1072.

Kampmann C, Baehner F, Ries M, Beck M (2002) Cardiac involvement in Anderson-Fabry disease. J Am Soc Nephrol 13 [Suppl 2]: S147–S149.

Kampmann C, Wiethoff CM, Whybra C, Baehner FA, Mengel E, Beck M (2008) Cardiac manifestations of Anderson-Fabry disease in children and adolescents. Acta Paediatr 97: 463–469.

Kolodny EH, Pastores GM (2002) Anderson-Fabry disease: extrarenal, neurologic manifestations. J Am Soc Nephrol 13 [Suppl 2]: S150–S153.

Kosch M, Koch HG, Oliveira JP, Soares C, Bianco F, Breuning F, Rasmussen AK, Schaefer RM (2004) Enzyme replacement therapy administered during hemodialysis in patients with Fabry disease. Kidney Int 66(3): 1279–1282.

Laaksonen SM, Röyttä M, Jääskeläinen SK, Kantola I, Penttinen M, Falck B (2008) Neuropathic symptoms and findings in women with Fabry disease. Clin Neurophysiol 119: 1365–1372.

Larralde M, Boggio P, Amartino H, Chamoles N (2004) Fabry disease: a study of 6 hemizygous men and 5 heterozygous women with emphasis on dermatologic manifestations. Arch Dermatol 140(12): 1440–1446.

Lien YH, Lai LW (2005) Bilateral femoral head and distal tibial osteonecrosis in a patient with Fabry disease. Am J Orthop 34(4): 192–194.

Linthorst GE, Hollak CE, Donker-Koopman WE, Strijland A, Aerts JM (2004a) Enzyme therapy for Fabry disease: neutralizing antibodies toward agalsidase alpha and beta. Kidney Int 66(4): 1589–1595.

Linthorst GE, De Rie MA, Tjiam KH, Aerts JM, Dingemans KP, Hollak CE (2004b) Misdiagnosis of Fabry disease: importance of biochemical confirmation of clinical or pathological suspicion. Br J Dermatol 150(3): 575–577.

Linthorst GE, Vedder AC, Aerts JM, Hollak CE (2005) Screening for Fabry disease using whole blood spots fails to identify one-third of female carriers. Clin Chim Acta 353(1–2): 201–203.

Lorenz M, Hauser AC, Puspok-Schwarz M, Kotanko P, Arias I, Zodl H, Kramar R, Paschke E, Voigtlander T, Sunder-Plassmann G (2003) Anderson-Fabry disease in Austria. Wien Klin Wochenschr 115(7–8): 235–240.

MacDermot J, MacDermot KD (2001) Neuropathic pain in Anderson-Fabry disease: pathology and therapeutic options. Eur J Pharmacol 429(1–3): 121–125.

MacDermot KD, Holmes A, Miners AH (2001a) Anderson-Fabry disease: clinical manifestations and impact of disease in a cohort of 98 hemizygous males. J Med Genet 38(11): 750–760.

MacDermot KD, Holmes A, Miners AH (2001b) Anderson-Fabry disease: clinical manifestations and impact of disease in a cohort of 60 obligate carrier females. J Med Genet 38(11): 769–775.

Mehta A, Ricci R, Widmer U, Dehout F, Garcia de Lorenzo A, Kampmann C, Linhart A, Sunder-Plassmann G, Ries M, Beck M (2004) Fabry disease defined: baseline clinical manifestations of 366 patients in the Fabry Outcome Survey. Eur J Clin Invest 34(3): 236–242.

Mehta A, Ginsberg L, FOS Investigators (2005) Natural history of the cerebrovascular complications of Fabry disease. Acta Paediatr Suppl 94(447): 24–27.

Mignani R, Panichi V, Giudicissi A, Taccola D, Boscaro F, Feletti C, Moneti G, Cagnoli L (2004) Enzyme replacement therapy with agalsidase beta in kidney transplant patients with Fabry disease: a pilot study. Kidney Int 65(4): 1381–1385.

Mohrenschlager M, Braun-Falco M, Ring J, Abeck (2003) Fabry disease: recognition and management of cutaneous manifestations. Am J Clin Dermatol 4(3): 189–196.

Nakao S, Takenaka T, Maeda M, Kodama C, Tanaka A, Tahara M, Yoshida A, Kuriyama M, Hayashibe H, Sakuraba H (1995) An atypical variant of Fabry's disease in men with left ventricular hypertrophy. N Engl J Med 333(5): 288–293.

Nakao S, Kodama C, Takenaka T, Tanaka A, Yasumoto Y, Yoshida A, Kanzaki T, Enriquez AL, Eng CM, Tanaka H, Tei C, Desnick RJ (2003) Fabry disease: detection of undiagnosed hemodialysis patients and identification of a "renal variant" phenotype. Kidney Int 64(3): 801–807.

Ortiz A, Oliveira JP, Wanner C, Brenner BM, Waldek S, Warnock DG (2008) Recommendations and guidelines for the diagnosis and treatment of Fabry nephropathy in adults. Nat Clin Pract Nephrol Apr 22 [Epub ahead of print].

Pisani A, Spinelli L, Sabbatini M, Andreucci MV, Procaccini D, Abbaterusso C, Pasquali S, Savoldi S, Comotti C, Cianciaruso B (2005) Enzyme replacement therapy in fabry disease patients undergoing dialysis: effects on quality of life and organ involvement. Am J Kidney Dis 46(1): 120–127.

Ramaswami U, Whybra C, Parini R, Pintos-Morell G, Mehta A, Sunder-Plassmann G, Widmer U, Beck M; FOS European Investigators (2006) Clinical manifestations of Fabry disease in children: data from the Fabry Outcome Survey. Acta Paediatr 95(1): 86–92.

Ries M, Ramaswami U, Parini R, Lindblad B, Whybra C, Willers I, Gal A, Beck M (2003) The early clinical phenotype of Fabry disease: a study on 35 European children and adolescents. Eur J Pediatr 162(11): 767–772.

Rolfs A, Bottcher T, Zschiesche M, Morris P, Winchester B, Bauer P, WalterU, Mix E, Lohr M, Harzer K, Strauss U, Pahnke J, Grossmann A, Benecke R (2005) Prevalence of Fabry disease in patients with cryptogenic stroke: a prospective study. Lancet 366(9499): 1794–1796.

Sadek J, Shellhaas R, Camfield CS, Camfield PR, Burley J (2004) Psychiatric findings in four female carriers of Fabry disease. Psychiatr Genet 14(4): 199–201.

Schaefer E, Baron K, Widmer U, Deegan P, Neumann HP, Sunder-Plassmann G, Johansson JO, Whybra C, Ries M, Pastores GM, Mehta A, Beck M, Gal A (2005) Thirty-four novel mutations of the GLA gene in 121 patients with Fabry disease. Hum Mutat 25(4): 412–419.

Schiffmann R, Kopp JB, Austin HA 3rd, Sabnis S, Moore DF, Weibel T, Balow JE, Brady RO (2001) Enzyme replacement therapy in Fabry disease: a randomized controlled trial. JAMA 285(21): 2743–2749.

Schiffmann R, Ries M (2005) Fabry's disease-an important risk factor for stroke. Lancet 366(9499): 1754.

Schiller PI, Itin PH (1996) Angiokeratomas: an update. Dermatology 193(4): 275–282.

Sessa A, Meroni M, Battini G, Maglio A, Brambilla PL, Bertella M, Nebuloni M, Pallotti F, Giordano F, Bertagnolio B, Tosoni A (2001) Renal pathological changes in Fabry disease. J Inherit Metab Dis 24 [Suppl 2]: 66–70.

Shah JS, Elliott PM (2005) Fabry disease and the heart: an overview of the natural history and the effect of enzyme replacement therapy. Acta Paediatr Suppl 94(447): 11–14.

Stiennon M, Goldberg ME (1980) Renal size in Fabry's disease. Urol Radiol 2(1): 17–21.

Tan SV, Lee PJ, Walters RJ, Mehta A, Bostock H (2005) Evidence for motor axon depolarization in Fabry disease. Muscle Nerve 548–551.

Thadhani R, Wolf M, West ML, Tonelli M, Ruthazer R, Pastores GM, Obrador GT (2002) Patients with Fabry disease on dialysis in the United States. Kidney Int 61(1): 249–255.

Thurberg BL, Rennke H, Colvin RB, Dikman S, Gordon RE, Collins AB, Desnick RJ, O'Callaghan M (2002) Globotriaosylceramide accumulation in the Fabry kidney is cleared from multiple cell types after enzyme replacement therapy. Kidney Int 62(6): 1933–1946.

Thurberg BL, Randolph Byers H, Granter SR, Phelps RG, Gordon RE, O'Callaghan M (2004) Monitoring the 3-year efficacy of enzyme replacement therapy in fabry disease by repeated skin biopsies. J Invest Dermatol 122(4): 900–908.

Warnock DG (2005) Fabry disease: diagnosis and management, with emphasis on the renal manifestations. Curr Opin Nephrol Hypertens 14(2): 87–95.

Weidemann F, Breunig F, Beer M, Sandstede J, Turschner O, Voelker W, Ertl G, Knoll A, Wanner C, Strotmann JM (2003) Improvement of cardiac function during enzyme replacement therapy in patients with Fabry disease: a prospective strain rate imaging study. Circulation 108(11): 1299–1301.

Weidemann F, Breunig F, Beer M, Sandstede J, Stork S, Voelker W, Ertl G, Knoll A, Wanner C, Strotmann JM (2005) The variation of morphological and functional cardiac manifestation in Fabry disease: potential implications for the time course of the disease. Eur Heart J 26(12): 1221–1227.

Weidemann F, Strotmann JM, Breunig F, Niemann M, Maag R, Baron R, Eggert AO, Wanner C (2008) Misleading terms in Anderson-Fabry disease. Eur J Clin Invest 38: 191–196.

Widmer U, Sperling C, Romer M, Hegemann S, Straumann D, Palla A (2005) Auditory and vestibular function in Fabry Disease. Acta Paediatr Suppl 94(447): 115.

Wilcox WR, Banikazemi M, Guffon N, Waldek S, Lee P, Linthorst GE, Desnick RJ, Germain DP (2004) International Fabry Disease Study Group. Long-term safety and efficacy of enzyme replacement therapy for Fabry disease. Am J Hum Genet 75(1): 65–74.

Young E, Mills K, Morris P, Vellodi A, Lee P, Waldek S, Winchester B (2005) Is globotriaosylceramide a useful biomarker in Fabry disease? Acta Paediatr Suppl 94(447): 51–54.

# Chapter 68

# CEREBROTENDINOUS XANTHOMATOSIS

Antonio Federico, Gian Nicola Gallus, and Maria Teresa Dotti

Department of Neurological and Behavioural Science, Medical School, University of Siena, Siena, Italy

## Introduction

Cerebrotendinous xanthomatosis (CTX; OMIM # 213700) is a rare, treatable lipid storage disease characterized by abnormal deposition of cholestanol and cholesterol in multiple tissues (Bjorkhem and Boberg 1995) due to a deficiency of sterol 27-hydroxylase (EC 1.14.13.15), a member of the mitochondrial cytochrome P450 family catalyzing the initial oxidation of the side chain of sterol intermediates in hepatic bile acid synthesis (Bjorkhem and Boberg 1995, Federico et al. 1993). Together with two protein cofactors, adrenodoxin and adrenodoxin reductase, sterol 27-hydroxylase catalyses the initial steps in the oxidation of the side chain of cholesterol and also hydroxylates a spectrum of sterol substrates including vitamin $D_3$ (Bjorkhem and Boberg 1995, Russell and Setchell 1992, Dahlback and Wikvall 1988).

CTX is characterized by the association of tendon xanthomas, juvenile cataracts, and multiple progressive neurological dysfunction. Infantile-onset diarrhea (Cruysberg 2002) may be the earliest clinical manifestation. Childhood-onset cataracts are a common symptom, present in almost all patients (Verrips et al. 2000a). Tendon xanthomas are described in up to 90% of cases, low intelligence in 57%, pyramidal signs in 67% and cerebellar signs in 60% (Berginer et al. 1984, Verrips et al. 2000a). Seizures are reported in about 50% of patients (Dotti et al. 1996, Matsumuro et al. 1990). Systemic manifestations including osteoporosis (Federico et al. 1993), heart involvement and premature atherosclerosis (Berginer et al. 1993) are often found. Sterol 27-hydroxylase consists of a 33-amino acid mitochondrial signal sequence, followed by a mature protein of 498 amino acids (Cali and Russell 1991). About 50 different mutations of the *CYP27A1* gene have been identified in CTX patients drawn from various populations (Gallus et al. 2006).

## Historical perspective

CTX was first described by van Bogaert et al. in 1937, who reported two cousins with a slowly progressive neurological syndrome with cognitive and motor impairment and cataracts. Tendon xanthomas were evident only in one of the patients who underwent autopsy examination. The disease was described as a "*cholestérinose généralisée*".

Thirty years later, Menkes et al. (1968) identified the stored material as cholestanol, a metabolite of cholesterol present only in small amount in normals. Since then, increased serum cholestanol level has been a crucial diagnostic marker of the disease. More recently the human *CYP27A1* gene was localized on the long arm of chromosome 2 (Cali and Russell 1991) and the first mutations described (Cali et al. 1991). Berginer et al. in 1984 reported encouraging results of long-term chenodeoxycholic acid (CDCA) treatment on metabolic and clinical alterations.

## Incidence and prevalence

There are some ethnic subgroup with a high CTX gene frequency. The prevalence in Sephardic Jews of Moroccan extraction was estimated to be 1/108 (Berginer et al. 1981). In Jewish Moroccan, 4/100,000 CTX cases resulting from the two mutant alleles in nonconsanguineous marriages, may exist (Leitersdorf et al. 1993). The prevalence of CTX related to R362C mutation alone has been recently estimated to be approximately 1 per 50,000 among the white population

(Lorincz et al. 2005). The prevalence of CTX, reported on the website http://www.orpha.net/orphacom/cahiers/docs/GB/Prevalence_of_rare_diseases.pdf., is approximately 0.13 patients/100,000 inhabitants. Epidemiological studies are lacking.

Series of affected individuals have been reported in Israel and the USA (Berginer et al. 1984), Italy (De Stefano et al. 2001, Dotti et al. 2001), Japan (Kuriyama et al. 1991), and the Netherlands (Waterreus et al. 1987, Verrips et al. 2000a). Affected individuals have been reported in Argentina (Szlago et al. 2008), Belgium (Van Bogaert et al. 1937, Philippart and Van Bogaert 1969), Brazil (Canelas et al. 1983), Canada (Pastershank et al. 1974), France (Rogelet et al. 1992), Iran (Farpour and Mahloudji 1975), Norway (Schreiner et al. 1975), Tunisia (Ben Hamida et al. 1991), Spain (Campdelacreu et al. 2002), China (Ko and Lee 2001), and Sweden (Rystedt et al. 2002).

## Clinical manifestation

### Skin manifestations

#### Xanthomas

Tendon xanthomas, which are an hallmark of the disease, usually appear in the second or third decade of life. First estimated to be almost invariably present (Berginer et al. 1984), were recently found in less than 50% of a series of Dutch patients (Verrips et al. 2000a). In addition to the classic xanthomas of the Achilles tendon, xanthomas may also occur on the extensor tendons of the elbow and hand, the patellar tendon, and the neck tendons (Fig. 1). Xanthomas have been reported in the lung, bones and central nervous system.

### Systemic manifestations

#### Enterohepatic system

Chronic intractable diarrhea from infancy may be the earliest clinical manifestation of CTX (Cruysberg

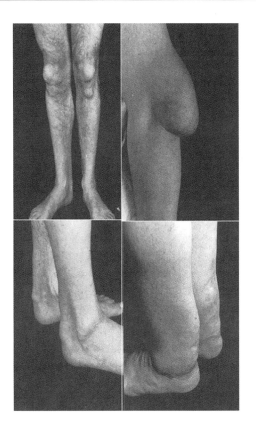

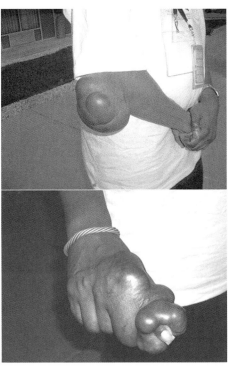

**Fig. 1.** Different localization and severity of xanthomas in CTX.

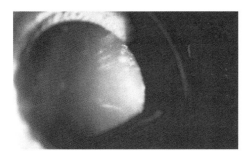

**Fig. 2.** Cataract in CTX. Infantile cataracts are one of the main early onset clinical signs.

2002, Verrips et al. 2000a). Gallstones have been reported occasionally.

## Eye

In the majority of affected individuals, cataracts are the first clinically documented finding, often appearing in the first decade of life (Verrips et al. 2000a). Cataracts (Fig. 2) may be visually significant opacities requiring lensectomy or visually insignificant cortical opacities. The appearance can include irregular cortical opacities, anterior polar cataracts, and dense posterior subcapsular cataracts (Cruysberg et al. 1995).

Other ophthalmological findings include palpebral xanthelasmas (Philippart and Van Bogaert 1969), optic nerve atrophy (Schimschock et al. 1968), and proptosis (Morgan et al. 1989). In a series of patients reported by Dotti et al. (2001) (age range 32–54 years) ocular manifestations included: cataracts in all cases, optic disk paleness in about 50% , signs of premature retinal senescence with retinal vessel sclerosis in 30%. Cholesterol-like deposits along vascular arcades and myelinated nerve fibers were present in some patients.

## Cardiovascular system

Premature atherosclerosis and coronary artery disease have been reported (Valdivielso et al. 2004, Frih-Ayed et al. 2005). Lipomatous hypertrophy of the atrial septum has been described (Dotti et al. 1998, Frih-Ayed et al. 2005).

## Skeleton

Bone involvement is characterized by granulomatous lesions in the lumbar vertebrae and femur, osteopenia with increased risk of bone fractures, and impaired adsorption of radiocalcium, which improves with chenodeoxycholic acid treatment (Berginer et al. 1993, Federico et al. 1993). Osteopenia is evident by total body densitometry in untreated individuals. Some patients may have marked thoracic kyphosis.

## Endocrine abnormalities

Hypothyroidism has occasionally been reported (Philippart and Van Bogaert 1969, Bouwes Bavinck et al. 1986, Idouji et al. 1991).

## Premature aging signs

Early-onset cataract, osteopenia with bone fractures and loss of teeth, atherosclerosis, and neurological impairment with dementia and/or parkinsonism, associated with the characteristic *facies*, suggest a generalized premature aging process (Dotti et al. 1991).

## Neurological manifestations

*Mental retardation or dementia* following slow deterioration in intellectual abilities in the second decade of life occurs in over 50% of individuals (Verrips et al. 2000a). Some individuals show mental impairment from early infancy, whereas the majority have normal or only slightly subnormal intellectual function until puberty. In the spinal form (see below), cognitive functions are almost always normal.

*Neuropsychiatric symptoms* such as behavioral changes, hallucinations, agitation, aggression, depression, and suicide attempts may be prominent.

*Pyramidal signs (i.e., spasticity) and/or cerebellar signs* are almost invariably present since 20–30 years of age. A spinal form, in which spastic paraparesis is the main clinical symptom, was described (Bartholdi et al. 2004, Verrips et al. 1999a).

*Extrapyramidal manifestations* including dystonia and atypical parkinsonism have been reported on occasional cases (Nakamura et al. 2000, Dotti et al. 2000, Grandas et al. 2002).

*Seizures* are reported in about 50% of individuals with CTX (Matsumuro et al. 1990, Clemen et al. 2005, Dotti et al. 1996).

*Peripheral neuropathy* is evident on electrophysiological studies (Arpa et al.1995, Federico et al. 1987, Ben Hamida et al. 1991), which reveal decreased nerve conduction velocities and abnormalities in somatosensory, motor, brainstem, and visual evoked potentials (Mondelli et al. 1992). Clinical manifestations related to peripheral nerve involvement are distal muscle atrophy and pes cavus. Sensory abnormalities are rarely described.

## Neuropathology

Classic CNS pathology findings in CTX include granulomatous and xanthomatous lesions in the cerebellar hemispheres, globus pallidus, and cerebellar peduncles. Demyelination and gliosis and involvement of the long tract of the spinal cord have been described (Pilo de la Fuente et al. 2008, Van Bogaert et al. 1937, Van Bogaert 1962). Nerve biopsy reveals primary axonal degeneration, demyelination, and remyelination. Mild myopathic changes with increased variability of fiber size and randomly distributed atrophic fibers have been reported (Federico et al. 1991). Ultrastructural abnormalities include mitochondrial subsarcolemmal aggregates and morphological changes of these organelles (Federico et al. 1991). Reduced respiratory chain enzyme activity has been observed (Dotti et al. 1995).

## Neuroimaging

CT and MRI of the brain typically show diffuse cerebral and cerebellar atrophy, white matter signal alterations, and bilateral focal cerebellar lesions (Berginer et al. 1981, Waterreus et al. 1987, Berginer et al. 1994, Dotti et al. 1994, De Stefano et al. 2001) (Fig. 3). Brain MRI spectroscopy shows decreased n-acetylaspartate and increased lactate level, indica-

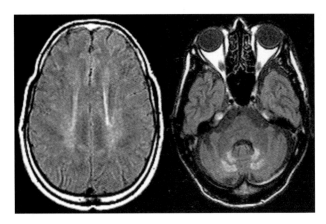

**Fig. 3.** MRI of CTX with evidence of white matter and dentate nuclei abnormalities.

tive of widespread brain mitochondrial dysfunction (De Stefano et al. 2001). The quantitative assessment of brain damage in CTX with use of magnetization transfer MR imaging has been recently described (Inglese et al. 2003).

## Natural history

CTX usually manifests in the first decade of life with diarrhea, cataract, and mild mental retardation. Adolescent-to-young-adult-onset tendon xanthomas and adult-onset progressive neurologic dysfunction are the typical manifestations. The clinical course of the disease is slowly progressive. Individual and intrafamilial variability is considerable (Dotti et al. 1996, Nagai et al. 1996, Verrips et al. 2000a, Federico and Dotti 2003, Moghadasian 2004). Early treatment with chenodeoxycholic acid (CDCA) sensibly modifies metabolic and clinical abnormalities.

## Molecular genetics

CTX is caused by a deficiency of the mitochondrial sterol 27-hydroxylase. Sterol 27-hydroxylase is a member of the cytochrome P450 family. In 1991, the cDNA for human CYP27A1 (cytochrome P450, family 27, subfamily A, polypeptide 1) was isolated by hybridizing rabbit cDNA to a liver cDNA library and its gene was localized on the long arm of chromosome 2 (Cali et al. 1991). Haplotype analysis and recombinant events allowed to map *CYP27A1* gene at the chromosome locus 2q35, between markers D2S1371 and D2S424 (Lee et al. 2001).

The structure of the human *CYP27A1* gene was explained in 1993. The promoter region is rich in guanidine and cytosine residues and contains three potential binding sites for the transcription factor SP1 and one for the liver transcription factor LF-B1 (Leitersdorf et al. 1993). *CYP27A1* gene consisting of nine exons and eight introns and spans 18.6 kb of DNA (Leitersdorf et al. 1993). The transcript is 1966 bp in size and encodes for 531 aa protein. Molecular cloning of the human sterol 27-hydroxylase cDNA has shown that the protein consists of a 498-aminoacid mature enzyme and a 33-amino acid mitochondrial signal sequence (Cali and Russell 1991).

Sterol 27-hydroxylase is expressed in many different tissues as CNS, liver, lung duodenum, and endothelial cells (Reiss 1997). The mature enzyme contains adrenodoxin-binding site (residues 351–365) and the heme-binding site (residues 435–464). These regions are the conserved part of the gene and interacts with the two protein cofactors, adrenodoxin and adrenodoxin reductase (Leitersdorf et al. 1993, Lee et al. 2001, Bjorkhem and Leitersdorf 2000). Sterol 27-hydroxylase catalyzes the initial steps in the oxidation of the side chain of cholesterol and also hydroxylates a spectrum of sterol substrates including vitamin $D_3$ (Bjorkhem and Boberg 1995, Russell and Setchell 1992, Dahlback and Wikvall 1988). Forty-nine different mutations of the *CYP27A1* gene have been reported worldwide. A review of mutations was recently reported by Gallus et al. (2006) (see Fig. 4). Many of the reported mutations involve splice sites (18%) and are predicted to affect mRNA stability or lead to the formation of abnormal mRNA with translation products that are devoid of an adrenodoxin-binding region (residues 351–356) and/or the heme-binding site (residue 453–464), important for enzyme activity. Apart from a 20% of nonsense mutations, leading to the formation of truncated peptides devoid of function, approximately 45% of mutations are missense mutations that are predicted to lead to the expression of an abnormal Cytochrome P450 27 protein. Only seven mutations are deletions and one is an insertion. About 50% of these mutations were found in the region of exons 6–8 of the *CYP27A1* gene. Overall, six mutations were found in twelve or more alleles. These muta-

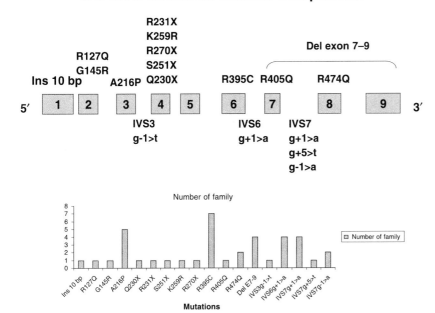

**Fig. 4.** Reports the mutations in the *CYP27A1* gene found in our population including over 30 patients.

tions occurs at aa 216, 339, 395, 474 and at a guanosine to adenosine substitution at the splice donator site of intron 6 and 7. Some of these mutations have a relatively high frequency in some ethnic groups. In the Dutch CTX patients the most frequent mutations were: the T339M (Reshef et al. 1994), the IVS7+1g>a transition in intron 7 (Garuti et al. 1996), and finally the 5–6insC in exon 1 together with the P384L missense mutation (Segev et al. 1995). The common mutations in the Japanese patients involved the same codon (R474Q and R474W). In the Italian CTX population, A216P and R395C mutations were found in 5 and 7 family, respectively.

The relationship between genotype and phenotype characteristics were extensively studied in homozygous patients by Verrips et al. (2000) and in our series of patients (unpublished data). No specific genotype-phenotype correlation has been established suggesting the presence of other factors that may modify the phenotype (Nagai et al. 1996, Dotti et al. 1996).

## Pathogenic mechanisms underling CTX

As a result of sterol 27-hydroxylase deficiency, bile acid production is decreased. The absence of the neg-

ative feedback mechanism of CDCA on 7α-hydroxylase, the rate limiting enzyme in bile acid synthesis, leads to the accumulation of intermediates as precursor for cholestanol. It has been hypothesized that the increased bile alcohols level may lead to disruption of the blood–brain barrier (Salen et al. 1987).

Cholestanol and 7-hydroxycholesterol accumulate in many tissues (Bjorkhem and Boberg 1995), including brain, leading to progressive neurological dysfunction. The storage of cholestanol in tissues other brain causes tendon xanthomas, atherosclerosis, lipomatous hypertrophy of the atrial septum and cataracts (Cali et al. 1991).

## Clinical management

Clinical improvement of individuals with CTX following chenodeoxycholic acid treatment (CDCA, a drug extensively used in the past for cholesterol gallstones) was first reported by Berginer et al. (1984). Long-term CDCA treatment (750 mg/day in adults) normalizes bile acid synthesis in serum, bile, urine, and CSF by suppressing cholestanol biosynthesis, and improves neurophysiological abnormalities (Mondelli et al. 2001) and other clinical manifestations including osteoporosis (Federico et al. 1993).

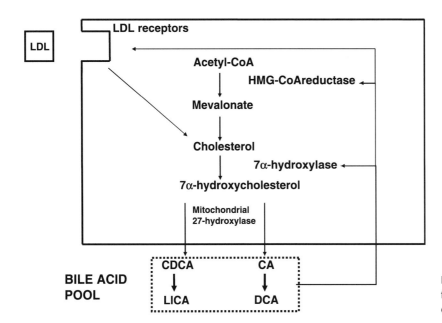

Fig. 5. Normal and abnormal steps and feedback mechanisms regulated by 27-hydroxylase activity.

Berginer et al. (1984) treated 17 patients with CDCA. All were symptomatic before treatment with evidence of Achilles tendon xanthomas (in 15 of 17), cataracts (in 12 of 17), dementia (in 13 of 17), pyramidal-tract signs (in all 17), cerebellar dysfunction (in 13 of 17), EEG changes (in 10 of 13), and abnormal cerebral CT scans (in 10 of 12). After at least 1 year of treatment, dementia cleared in 10, pyramidal and cerebellar signs disappeared in 5 and improved in 8 others, peripheral neuropathy disappeared in 6, and the EEG became normal in 5 and improved in 3 others. The CT scan improved in 7, including 1 patient in whom a cerebellar xanthoma disappeared. Mean plasma cholestanol levels declined 3-fold. The rationale of treatment with CDCA is to compensate for the pronounced deficiency of CDCA in the intrahepatic pool. The treatment produces a substantial reduction in cholestanol synthesis and lowers the cholestanol levels. Salen et al. (1987) found that treatment reduced high levels of cholesterol and cholestanol in the cerebrospinal fluid. Furthermore, untreated patients showed increased levels of apolipoprotein B and albumin. These results suggested that increased cerebrospinal fluid sterols were derived from plasma lipoproteins by means of a defective blood–brain barrier (BBB) and that treatment with CDCA reestablished selective permeability of BBB. Kuriyama et al. (1994) treated 7 CTX patients with CDCA alone, pravastatin (another inhibitor of HMG-CoA reductase), or the 2 agents in combination. CDCA treatment alone reduced serum cholestanol, but the sera of the patients on this treatment became more 'atherogenic' with an increase in total cholesterol, triglyceride, and low-density lipoprotein cholesterol, and a decrease in high-density lipoprotein cholesterol. In contrast, pravastatin made the sera markedly 'anti-atherogenic', but only modestly reduced cholestanol and sitosterol levels. However, the combination of CDCA and pravastatin resulted in improvement of serum lipoprotein metabolism, suppression of cholesterol synthesis, and reduction of cholestanol and plant sterol levels. The progression of disease was arrested in all 7 patients, but no dramatic reversal of clinical manifestations was seen.

In a long-term (11 years) treatment study with CDCA, Mondelli et al. (2001) reported that, after four months into treatment, nerve conduction velocities normalized and subsequently remained stable; motor evoked potentials (MEPs) and sensory evoked potentials (SEPs) improved slowly but continuously; clinical manifestations stabilized, but neurologic deficits did not improved. The contrast between two untreated siblings whose symptoms progressed and a third treated sibling whose symptoms stabilized suggests that treatment is beneficial (Federico, personal data).

Although CDCA is considered the best treatment for CTX (Samenuk and Koffman 2001), it has recently ceased to be available as other more effective drugs for gallstones have been utilized; its unavailability has left affected individuals without an essential drug for their disease, with the exception of affected individuals in Italy, who are closely monitored (Federico and Dotti 2001).

Inhibitors of HMG-CoA reductase alone or in combination with CDCA are also effective in decreasing cholestanol concentration and improving clinical signs (Peynet et al. 1991, Verrips et al. 1999b). However, because of clinical evidence that HMG-CoA reductase inhibitors may induce muscle damage and even rhabdomyolysis, caution is required in the use of these drugs (Federico and Dotti 1994).

Other possible treatments include low-density lipoprotein (LDL) apheresis, but the results are controversial (Mimura et al. 1993, Berginer and Salen 1994, Dotti et al. 2004).

Therapies with ursodeoxycolic acid, lovastatin, and cholestyramine have been reported to be ineffective (Batta et al. 2004, Tint et al. 1989).

Symptomatic treatments for epilepsy, spasticity, and parkinsonism have been utilized. Parkinsonism is poorly responsive to levodopa. An antihistamine drug, diphenylpyraline hydrochloride, has been reported to have an excellent effect in three individuals (Ohno et al. 2001).

Annual follow-up is recommended for clinical and laboratory investigations (neurological and neuropsychological evaluation, cholestanol level, brain MRI, echocardiography, TBD density and neurophysiological tests). Cataract extraction is typically required in at least one eye by age 50 years.

Early diagnosis of at-risk family members allows initiation of treatment that may prevent or limit disease manifestations.

## Differential diagnosis

Differential diagnosis of xanthomas include:

- *Sitosterolemia*, inherited sterol storage disease characterized by tendon xanthomas and by a strong predisposition to premature atherosclerosis. Serum concentration of plant sterols (sitosterol and campesterol) is increased. Primary neurological signs and cataracts are not present. Spastic paraparesis may occur as a result of spinal cord compression by multiple intradural, extramedullary xanthomas (Hatanaka et al. 1990).
- *Hypercholesterolemia* and *hyperlipemia* (especially type IIa), in which plasma cholestanol level is normal.

When xanthomas are not evident, the differential diagnosis includes all forms of progressive mental deterioration (Gilad et al. 1999, Verrips et al. 2000b).

## Genetic counseling

Cerebrotendinous xanthomatosis is inherited in an autosomal recessive manner.

The parents of an affected child are obligate heterozygotes and therefore carry one mutant allele. Heterozygotes (carriers) are generally asymptomatic, although an increased incidence of cardiovascular disorders and gallstones has been observed in obligate carriers.

At conception, the sibs of an affected individual have a 25% chance of being affected, a 50% chance of being asymptomatic carriers, and a 25% chance of being unaffected and not carriers.

- Once an at-risk sib is known to be unaffected, the chance of his/her being a carrier is 2/3.
- Heterozygotes (carriers) are generally asymptomatic.

The offspring of an individual with CTX are obligate heterozygotes (carriers) for a disease-causing mutation in the *CYP27A1* gene.

Sibs of the proband's parents are at 50% risk of being carriers.

## References

Arpa J, Sanchez C, Vega A, Cruz-Martinez A, Ferrer T, Lopez-Pajares R, Munoz J, Barreiro P (1995) Cerebrotendinous xanthomatosis diagnosed after traumatic subdural haematoma. Rev Neurol 23: 675–678.

Bartholdi D, Zumsteg D, Verrips A, Wevers RA, Sistermans E, Hess K, Jung HH (2004) Spinal phenotype of cerebrotendinous xanthomatosis – a pitfall in the diagnosis of multiple sclerosis. J Neurol 251: 105–107.

Batta AK, Salen G, Tint GS (2004) Hydrophilic 7 beta-hydroxy bile acids, lovastatin, and cholestyramine are ineffective in the treatment of cerebrotendinous xanthomatosis. Metabolism 53: 556–562.

Ben Hamida M, Chabbi N, Ben Hamida C, Mhiri C, Kallel R (1991) Peripheral neuropathy in a sporadic case of cerebrotendinous xanthomatosis. Rev Neurol (Paris) 147: 385–388.

Berginer VM, Salen G (1994) LDL-apheresis cannot be recommended for treatment of cerebrotendinous xanthomatosis. J Neurol Sci 121: 229–232.

Berginer VM, Berginer J, Korczyn AD, Tadmor R (1994) Magnetic resonance imaging in cerebrotendinous xanthomatosis: a prospective clinical and neuroradiological study. J Neurol Sci 122: 102–108.

Berginer VM, Berginer J, Salen G, Shefer S, Zimmerman RD (1981) Computed tomography in cerebrotendinous xanthomatosis. Neurology 31: 1463–1465.

Berginer VM, Salen G, Shefer S (1984) Long-term treatment of cerebrotendinous xanthomatosis with chenodeoxycholic acid. N Engl J Med 311: 1649–1652.

Berginer VM, Shany S, Alkalay D, Berginer J, Dekel S, Salen G, Tint GS, Gazit D (1993) Osteoporosis and increased bone fractures in cerebrotendinous xanthomatosis. Metabolism 42: 69–74.

Bjorkhem I, Boberg KM (1995) Inborn errors in bile and biosynthesis and storage of sterols other than cholesterol. In: Scriver CR, Beaudet AL, Sly WS, Valle D (eds.) The metabolic and molecular basis of inherited disease, 7th ed. New York: McGraw-Hill, pp. 2073–2099.

Bjorkhem I, Leitersdorf E (2000) Sterol 27-hydroxylase deficiency: a rare cause of xanthomas in normocholesterolemic humans. Trends Endocrinol Metab 11: 180–183.

Bouwes Bavinck JN, Vermeer BJ, Gevers Leuven JA, Koopman BJ, Wolthers BG (1986) Capillary gas chromatography of urine samples in diagnosing cerebrotendinous xanthomatosis. Arch Dermatol 122: 1269–1272.

Cali JJ, Russell DW (1991) Characterization of human sterol 27-hydroxylase. A mitochondrial cytochrome P-450 that catalyzes multiple oxidation reaction in bile acid biosynthesis. J Biol Chem 266: 7774–7778.

Cali JJ, Hsieh CL, Francke U, Russell DW (1991) Mutations in the bile acid biosynthetic enzyme sterol 27-hydroxylase underlie cerebrotendinous xanthomatosis. J Biol Chem 266: 7779–7783.

Campdelacreu J, Munoz E, Cervera A, Jauma S, Giros M, Tolosa E (2002) Cerebrotendinous xanthomatosis without tendinous xanthomas: presentation of two cases. Neurologia 17: 647–650.

Canelas HM, Quintao EC, Scaff M, Vasconcelos KS, Brotto MW (1983) Cerebrotendinous xanthomatosis: clinical and laboratory study of 2 cases. Acta Neurol Scand 67: 305–311.

Clemen CS, Spottke EA, Lutjohann D, Urbach H, von Bergmann K, Klockgether T, Dodel R (2005) Cerebrotendinous xanthomatosis: a treatable ataxia. Neurology 64: 1476.

Cruysberg JR (2002) Cerebrotendinous xanthomatosis: juvenile cataract and chronic diarrhea before the onset of neurologic disease. Arch Neurol 59: 1975.

Cruysberg JR, Wevers RA, van Engelen BG, Pinckers A, van Spreeken A, Tolboom JJ (1995) Ocular and systemic manifestations of cerebrotendinous xanthomatosis. Am J Ophthalmol 120: 597–604.

Dahlback H, Wikvall K (1988) 25-Hydroxylation of vitamin D3 by a cytochrome P-450 from rabbit liver mitochondria. Biochem J 252: 207–213.

De Stefano N, Dotti MT, Mortilla M, Federico A (2001) Magnetic resonance imaging and spectroscopic changes in brains of patients with cerebrotendinous xanthomatosis. Brain 124: 121–131.

Dotti MT, Salen G, Federico A (1991) Cerebrotendinous xanthomatosis as a multisystem disease mimicking premature ageing. Dev Neurosci 13: 371–376.

Dotti MT, Federico A, Signorini E, Caputo N, Venturi C, Filosomi G, Guazzi GC (1994) Cerebrotendinous xanthomatosis (van Bogaert-Scherer-Epstein disease): CT and MR findings. AJNR Am J Neuroradiol 15: 1721–1726.

Dotti MT, Manneschi L, Federico A (1995) Mitochondrial enzyme deficiency in cerebrotendinous xanthomatosis. J Neurol Sci 129: 106–108.

Dotti MT, Garuti R, Calandra S, Federico A (1996) Clinical and genetic variability of CTX. Eur J Neurol 3 Suppl 5: 12.

Dotti MT, Mondillo S, Plewnia K, Agricola E, Federico A (1998) Cerebrotendinous xanthomatosis: evidence of lipomatous hypertrophy of the atrial septum. J Neurol 245: 723–726.

Dotti MT, Federico A, Garuti R, Calandra S (2000) Cerebrotendinous xanthomatosis with predominant parkinsonian syndrome: further confirmation of the clinical heterogeneity. Mov Disord 15: 1017–1019.

Dotti MT, Rufa A, Federico A (2001) Cerebrotendinous xanthomatosis: heterogeneity of clinical phenotype with evidence of previously undescribed ophthalmological findings. J Inherit Metab Dis 24: 696–706.

Dotti MT, Lutjohann D, von Bergmann K, Federico A (2004) Normalisation of serum cholestanol concentration in a patient with cerebrotendinous xanthomatosis by combined treatment with chenodeoxycholic acid, simvastatin and LDL apheresis. Neurol Sci 25: 185–191.

Farpour H, Mahloudji M (1975) Familial cerebrotendinous xanthomatosis. Report of a new family and review of the literature. Arch Neurol 32: 223–225.

Federico A, Dotti MT (1994) Treatment of cerebrotendinous xanthomatosis. Neurology 44: 2218.

Federico A, Dotti MT (2001) Cerebrotendinous xanthomatosis. Neurology 57: 1743.

Federico A, Dotti MT (2003) Cerebrotendinous xanthomatosis: clinical manifestations, diagnostic criteria, pathogenesis, and therapy. J Child Neurol 18: 633–638.

Federico A, Palmeri S, Ciacci G, Rossi A, Malandrini A, Alessandrini C, Salen G, Guazzi GC (1987) Peripheral neuropathy in CTX: seven cases in two families. Neurology (suppl 1): 360.

Federico A, Dotti MT, Volpi N (1991) Muscle mitochondrial changes in cerebrotendinous xanthomatosis. Ann Neurol 30: 734–735.

Federico A, Dotti MT, Lore F, Nuti R (1993) Cerebrotendinous xanthomatosis: pathophysiological study on bone metabolism. J Neurol Sci 115: 67–70.

Frih-Ayed M, Boughammoura-Bouatay A, Ben Hamda K, Chebel S, Ben Farhat M (2005) Hypertrophy of the atrial septum in the cerebrotendinous xanthomatosis. Rev med interne 26: 992–993.

Gallus GN, Dotti MT, Federico A (2006) Clinical and molecular diagnosis of cerebrotendinous xanthomatosis with a review of the mutations in the *CYP27A1* gene. Neurol Sci 27: 143–149.

Garuti R, Lelli N, Barozzini M, Tiozzo R, Dotti MT, Federico A, Ottomano AM, Croce A, Bertolini S, Calandra S (1996) Cerebrotendinous xanthomatosis caused by two new mutations of the sterol-27-hydroxylase gene that disrupt mRNA splicing. J Lipid Res 37: 1459–1467.

Gilad R, Lampl Y, Lev D, Sadeh M (1999) Cerebrotendinous xanthomatosis without xanthomas. Clin Genet 56: 405–406.

Grandas F, Martin-Moro M, Garcia-Munozguren S, Anaya F (2002) Early-onset parkinsonism in cerebrotendinous xanthomatosis. Mov Disord 17: 1396–1397.

Hatanaka I, Yasuda H, Hidaka H, Harada N, Kobayashi M, Okabe H, Matsumoto K, Hukuda S, Shigeta Y (1990) Spinal cord compression with paraplegia in xanthomatosis due to normocholesterolemic sitosterolemia. Ann Neurol 28: 390–393.

Idouji K, Kuriyama M, Fujiyama J, Osame M, Hoshita T (1991) Hypothyroidism with increased serum levels of cholestanol and bile alcohol – analogous symptoms to cerebrotendinous xanthomatosis. Rinsho Shinkeigaku 31: 402–406.

Inglese M, DeStefano N, Pagani E, Dotti MT, Comi G, Federico A, Filippi M (2003) Quantification of brain damage in cerebrotendinous xanthomatosis with magnetization transfer MR imaging. AJNR Am J Neuroradiol 24: 495–500.

Ko KF, Lee KW (2001) Cerebrotendinous xanthomatosis in three siblings from a Chinese family. Singapore Med J 42: 30–32.

Kuriyama M, Fujiyama J, Yoshidome H, Takenaga S, Matsumuro K, Kasama T, Fukuda K, Kuramoto T, Hoshita T, Seyama Y et al. (1991) Cerebrotendinous xanthomatosis: clinical and biochemical evaluation of eight patients and review of the literature. J Neurol Sci 102: 225–232.

Kuriyama M, Tokimura Y, Fujiyama J, Utatsu Y, Osame M (1994) Treatment of cerebrotendinous xanthomatosis: effects of chenodeoxycholic acid, pravastatin, and combined use. J Neurol Sci 125: 22–28.

Lee MH, Hazard S, Carpten JD, Yi S, Cohen J, Gerhardt GT, Salen G, Patel SB (2001) Fine-mapping, mutation analyses, and structural mapping of cerebrotendinous xanthomatosis in U.S. pedigrees. J Lipid Res 42: 159–169.

Leitersdorf E, Reshef A, Meiner V, Levitzki R, Schwartz SP, Dann EJ, Berkman N, Cali JJ, Klapholz L, Berginer VM (1993) Frameshift and splice-junction mutations in the sterol 27-hydroxylase gene cause cerebrotendinous xanthomatosis in Jews or Moroccan origin. J Clin Invest 91: 2488–2496.

Lorincz MT, Rainier S, Thomas D, Fink JK (2005) Cerebrotendinous xanthomatosis: possible higher prevalence than previously recognized. Arch Neurol 62: 1459–1463.

Matsumuro K, Takahashi K, Matsumoto H, Okatsu Y, Kuriyama M (1990) A case of cerebrotendinous xanthomatosis with convulsive seizures. Rinsho Shinkeigaku 30: 207–209.

Menkes JH, Schimschock JR, Swanson PD (1968) Cerebrotendinous xanthomatosis. The storage of cholestanol within the nervous system. Arch Neurol 19: 47–53.

Mimura Y, Kuriyama M, Tokimura Y, Fujiyama J, Osame M, Takesako K, Tanaka N (1993) Treatment of cerebrotendinous xanthomatosis with low-density lipoprotein (LDL)-apheresis. J Neurol Sci 114: 227–230.

Moghadasian MH (2004) Cerebrotendinous xanthomatosis: clinical course, genotypes and metabolic backgrounds. Clin Invest Med 27: 42–50.

Mondelli M, Rossi A, Scarpini C, Dotti MT, Federico A (1992) Evoked potentials in cerebrotendinous xanthomatosis and effect induced by chenodeoxycholic acid. Arch Neurol 49: 469–475.

Mondelli M, Sicurelli F, Scarpini C, Dotti MT, Federico A (2001) Cerebrotendinous xanthomatosis: 11-year treatment with chenodeoxycholic acid in five patients. An electrophysiological study. J Neurol Sci 190: 29–33.

Morgan SJ, McKenna P, Bosanquet RC (1989) Case of cerebrotendinous xanthomatosis. I: Unusual ophthalmic features. Br J Ophthalmol 73: 1011–1014.

Nagai Y, Hirano M, Mori T, Takakura Y, Tamai S, Ueno S (1996) Japanese triplets with cerebrotendinous xanthomatosis are homozygous for a mutant gene coding for the sterol 27-hydroxylase (Arg441Trp). Neurology 46: 571–574.

Ohno T, Kobayashi S, Hayashi M, Sakurai M, Kanazawa I (2001) Diphenylpyraline-responsive parkinsonism in cerebrotendinous xanthomatosis: long-term follow up of three patients. J Neurol Sci 182: 95–97.

Pastershank SP, Yip S, Sodhi HS (1974) Cerebrotendinous xanthomatosis. J Can Assoc Radiol 25: 282–286.

Peynet J, Laurent A, De Liege P, Lecoz P, Gambert P, Legrand A, Mikol J, Warnet A (1991) Cerebrotendinous xanthomatosis: treatments with simvastatin, lovastatin, and chenodeoxycholic acid in 3 siblings. Neurology 41: 434–436.

Philippart M, Van Bogaert L (1969) Cholestanolosis (cerebrotendinous xanthomatosis). A follow-up study on the original family. Arch Neurol 21: 603–610.

Pilo de la Fuente B, Ruiz I, Lopez de Munain A, Jimenez-Escrig A (2008) Cerebrotendinous xanthomatosis: neuropathological findings. J Neurol May 6 [Epub ahead of print].

Reiss AB, Martin KO, Rojer DE, Iyer S, Grossi EA, Galloway AC, Javitt NB (1997) Sterol 27-hydroxylase: expression in human arterial endothelium. J Lipid Res 38: 1254–1260.

Reshef A, Meiner V, Berginer VM, Leitersdorf E (1994) Molecular genetics of cerebrotendinous xanthomatosis in Jews of north African origin. J Lipid Res 35: 478–483.

Rogelet P, Gerard JM, Michotte A, Masingue M, Destee A (1992) Cerebrotendinous xanthomatosis. 2 cases with magnetic resonance imaging. Rev Neurol (Paris) 148: 541–545.

Russell DW, Setchell KD (1992) Bile acid biosynthesis. Biochemistry 31: 4737–4749.

Rystedt E, Olin M, Seyama Y, Buchmann M, Berstad A, Eggertsen G, Bjorkhem I (2002) Cerebrotendinous xanthomatosis: molecular characterization of two Scandinavian sisters. J Intern Med 252: 259–264.

Salen G, Berginer V, Shore V, Horak I, Horak E, Tint GS, Shefer S (1987) Increased concentrations of cholestanol and apolipoprotein B in the cerebrospinal fluid of patients with cerebrotendinous xanthomatosis. Effect of chenodeoxycholic acid. N Engl J Med 316: 1233–1238.

Schimschock JR, Alvord EC Jr, Swanson PD (1968) Cerebrotendinous xanthomatosis. Clinical and pathological studies. Arch Neurol 18: 688–698.

Schreiner A, Hopen G, Skrede S (1975) Cerebrotendinous xanthomatosis (cholestanolosis). Investigations on two sisters and their family. Acta Neurol Scand 51: 405–416.

Segev H, Reshef A, Clavey V, Delbart C, Routier G, Leitersdorf E (1995) Premature termination codon at the sterol 27-hydroxylase gene causes cerebrotendinous xanthomatosis in a French family. Hum Genet 95: 238–240.

Szlago M, Gallus GN, Schenone A, Patiño ME, Sfaelo Z, Rufa A, Da Pozzo P, Cardaioli E, Dotti MT, Federico A (2008) The first cerebrotendinous xanthomatosis family from Argentina: a new mutation in CYP27A1 gene. Neurology 70: 402–404.

Tint GS, Ginsberg H, Salen G, Le NA, Shefer S (1989) Chenodeoxycholic acid normalizes elevated lipoprotein secretion and catabolism in cerebrotendinous xanthomatosis. J Lipid Res 30: 633–640.

Valdivielso P, Calandra S, Duran JC, Garuti R, Herrera E, Gonzalez P (2004) Coronary heart disease in a patient with cerebrotendinous xanthomatosis. J Intern Med 255: 680–683.

Van Bogaert L (1962) The framework of the xanthomatoses and their different types. 2. Secondary xanthomatoses. Rev Med Liege 17: 433–443.

Van Bogaert L, Scherer HJ, Epstein E (1937) Une forme cerebrale de la cholesterinose generalisee. Paris, Masson et Cie.

Verrips A, Nijeholt GJ, Barkhof F, Van Engelen BG, Wesseling P, Luyten JA, Wevers RA, Stam J, Wokke JH, van den Heuvel LP, Keyser A, Gabreels FJ (1999a) Spinal xanthomatosis: a variant of cerebrotendinous xanthomatosis. Brain 122 (Pt 8): 1589–1595.

Verrips A, Wevers RA, Van Engelen BG, Keyser A, Wolthers BG, Barkhof F, Stalenhoef A, De Graaf R, Janssen-Zijlstra F, Van Spreeken A, Gabreels FJ (1999b) Effect of simvastatin in addition to chenodeoxycholic acid in patients with cerebrotendinous xanthomatosis. Metabolism 48: 233–238.

Verrips A, Hoefsloot LH, Steenbergen GC, Theelen JP, Wevers RA, Gabreels FJ, van Engelen BG, van den Heuvel LP (2000a) Clinical and molecular genetic characteristics of patients with cerebrotendinous xanthomatosis. Brain 123 (Pt 5): 908–919.

Verrips A, van Engelen BG, Ter Laak H, Gabreels-Festen A, Janssen A, Zwarts M, Wevers RA, Gabreels FJ (2000b) Cerebrotendinous xanthomatosis. Controversies about nerve and muscle: observations in ten patients. Neuromuscul Disord 10: 407–414.

Waterreus RJ, Koopman BJ, Wolthers BG, Oosterhuis HJ (1987) Cerebrotendinous xanthomatosis (CTX): a clinical survey of the patient population in The Netherlands. Clin Neurol Neurosurg 89: 169–175.

# Chapter 69

# GIANT AXONAL NEUROPATHY

**Claudio Bruno and Carlo Minetti**

Muscular and Neurodegenerative Disease Unit, Department of Pediatrics, University of Genoa, Giannina Gaslini Institute, Genoa, Italy

## Introduction

Giant axonal neuropathy (GAN) (OMIM # 256850), is a rare autosomal recessive disorder characterized by a progressive motor and sensory neuropathy with early onset of cerebellar and pyramidal tract signs and mental deterioration leading to dementia (Carpenter et al. 1974, Gordon 2004, Ouvrier 1989, Yang et al. 2007). Onset occurs often before age 7, with most patients being wheelchair dependent in the first or second decade of life (Igisu et al. 1975). Death usually occurs between age 10 and 30. Most cases presented kinky hair (Treiber-Held et al. 1994).

Electrophysiological studies show signs of a severe axonal neuropathy.

The hallmark of the disease is the presence, in the peripheral nerve biopsy, of giant axonal swellings due to a massive accumulation of neurofilaments in axons (Prineas et al. 1976, Pena 1982), indicating a generalized disorganization of intermediate filaments (IF) (Herrmann and Griffin 2002).

Brain imaging findings are variable, and probably related to the stage of the disease. In some patients there are no or minimal white matter abnormalities. In other cases images reveal abnormal myelination (van der Knaap and Valk 2005).

The GAN gene, located on chromosome 16q24.1, encodes a ubiquitously expressed protein named gigaxonin, a member of the BTB/kelch superfamily proteins, with a predicted cytoskeletal role (Bomont et al. 2000). Different pathogenic mutations have been identified on different genetic backgrounds (Bomont et al. 2000, 2003; Kuhlenbaumer et al. 2002; Bruno et al. 2004; Demir et al. 2005). The genotype/phenotype correlation in this disease remains unclear.

## Historical perspective and eponyms

Berg et al. (1972) and Asbury et al. (1972) initially described the disease in a 6-year-old Caucasian girl with progressive muscle weakness, areflexia, and impairment in perceiving touch, position sense, and vibration. Electrophysiological studies were consistent with the clinical diagnosis of polyneuropathy. Sural nerve biopsy revealed enlarged axons distended by masses of tightly neurofilaments.

## Incidence and prevalence

Around 40 cases have been reported so far in the literature, without any particular ratio male/female. The prevalence of GAN is unknown.

## Clinical manifestations

### Skin appendages

Most GAN patients have hair anomalies, which usually occur before onset of neurological signs. At gross examination the hair is thick and curly, sometimes crimped and pale (Treiber-Held et al. 1994). Microscopic examination shows abnormal variation in shaft diameter and twisting *pili torti* similar to the abnormality seen in Menkes disease (Rybojad et al. 1998). At the molecular level, there is a reduction in number of bisulfur bridges, which could be the cause of the defective keratin filament alignment.

Scanning electron microscopy (SEM) showed longitudinal grooves in the hairs (Lycklama a Nijeholt et al. 1994, Treiber-Held et al. 1994).

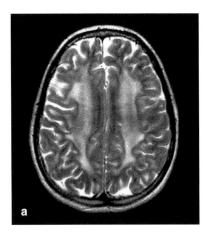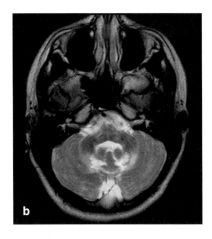

**Fig. 1.** Axial T2-weighted images of the brain in a 14-year-old girl with GAN show diffuse cerebral signal abnormalities in the centrum semiovale (sparing to some extent the U fibres) (**a**) and in the pyramidal tracts, hilus of the dentate nucleus, and cerebellar white matter (**b**). Reproduced from: van der Knaap MS, Valk J (eds.) Magnetic resonance of myelination and myelin disorders, 3rd ed. Berlin: Springer 2005, p. 439.

## Nervous system abnormalities

GAN patients show signs of central and peripheral nervous system involvement, including mental retardation, pyramidal tract signs, and cerebellar signs.

Nerve conduction studies usually show normal to moderately reduced nerve conduction velocity, reduced compound motor action potential, and absent sensory nerve action potentials EEG may present disorganized background activity with focal spikes and increased slow wave activity.

Brain magnetic resonance imaging (MRI) shows abnormal white matter signals reminiscent of leukodystrophy, and atrophy of cerebellum, brainstem, spinal cord, and corpus callosum (Fig. 1). Although imaging studies confirm CNS involvement, these abnormalities are non specific of GAN.

Magnetic resonance spectroscopy (MRS) in an 11-year old revealed normal N-acetylaspartate/creatine and increased choline/creatine and myoinositol/creatine ratios indicating significant demyelination and glial proliferation in the white matter but no neuroaxonal loss (Alkan et al. 2003). MRS of another individual revealed damage or loss of axons (reduced N-acetylaspartate and N-acetylaspartylglutamate) accompanied by acute demyelination in the white matter (elevated choline-containing compounds, myoinositol, and lactate), and generalized proliferation of glial cells in both gray and white matter (elevated choline-containing compounds and myo-inositol) (Brockmann et al. 2003).

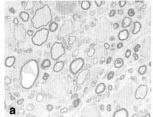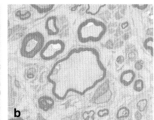

**Fig. 2.** A sural nerve biopsy in a patient with GAN reveals giant axons in transverse section (**b**, higher magnification). A decrease in the thickness of myelin layer is evident in the giant fibres as compared to normal sized fibres (**a**). Courtesy of A. Schenone, Dept. Neurology, University of Genova.

Sural nerve biopsy show the characteristic presence of giant axonal swelling, filled with neurofilaments, and reduction in numbers of myelinated fibers (Fig. 2). The giant axons are also present in the cerebral cortex, cerebellum, brainstem, and pyramidal tracts.

A generalized disorganization of intermediate filaments is also present in other cell types, such as fibroblasts and endothelial cells.

## Musculoskeletal anomalies

The patients are typically short. In addition there is scoliosis, skeletal and foot deformities with various combinations of pectus carinatum, genum-valgus, pes equino-varus, and pes planus.

## Miscellaneous findings

In some patients a peculiar facial appearance with facial diplegia, ptosis, and prominent high forehead has been reported.

An unusual and rare clinical feature is precocious puberty (Takebe et al. 1981, Demir et al. 2005).

## Natural history

GAN is an early-onset disorder usually manifesting with a delay in the acquisition of motor milestones and signs of neurological problems starting around age 6–7. Patients initially develop clumsy gait and progressive weakness of the legs.

Neurological examination shows initially signs of peripheral neuropathy, as muscular atrophy, absent reflexes, and impaired sensation. Subsequently, signs of CNS involvement such as mental retardation, cerebellar signs (ataxia, nystagmus, dysarthria), and epileptic seizures ensue. Most patients become wheelchair-dependent in the first or second decade of life and die in the second or third decade.

A subset of patients has a less severe clinical presentation, a more protracted course, and later involvement of central nervous system (CNS) indicating phenotypic variability (Malandrini et al. 1998, Bruno et al. 2004).

## Pathogenesis and molecular genetics

GAN is characterized by cytoskeletal abnormalities: the hallmark of the disease is the presence of giant axonal swelling, densely packed with aberrant neurofilaments, and abnormal microtubule network.

The GAN gene, located on chromosome 16q24.1, encodes a ubiquitously expressed protein that is composed of an amino-terminal BTB domain followed by a six kelch repeats domains. It has been shown that gigaxonin interacts with MAP1B, a microtubule (MT) associated protein involved in maintaining the integrity of cytoskeleton structure and promoting neuronal stability (Ding et al. 2002). Ablation of gigaxonin causes: (1) accumulation of

MAP1B-LC in neurons leading to cell death (Allen et al. 2005); and (2) impaired ubiquitin-proteasome system leading to a substantial accumulation of a novel microtubule-associated protein, MAP8, which in turn alters the microtubule network, traps dynein motor protein in insoluble structures and leads to neuronal death (Ding et al. 2006).

Since the first report, at least 30 GAN families of various ethnic origins and with either the *classical* or the *milder* clinical forms have been analyzed molecularly and a total of 31 different mutations have been identified (Bomont et al. 2000, 2003; Koop et al. 2007; Kuhlenbaumer 2008; Kuhlenbaumer et al. 2002; Bruno et al. 2004; Demir et al. 2005). It has been suggested that the phenotypic variability might relate to different mutations since two mild cases were associated with point mutations outside the kelch repeat domain (Kuhlenbaumer et al. 2002). However, these data were not confirmed (Bruno et al. 2004).

In addition, an Algerian family with GAN did not show linkage to chromosome 16q24.1, indicating genetic heterogeneity in GAN (Tazir et al. 2002).

## Differential diagnosis

The characteristic kinky hair changes of GAN patients might be also present in Menkes disease, which is an X-linked disease with an early severe CNS involvement (see chapter 71).

The early-onset of severe signs of peripheral neuropathy has to be put in differential diagnosis with other hereditary neuropathies of autosomal recessive inheritance.

The presence of infantile-onset signs and symptoms of both CNS and PNS involvement is characteristic also of other two neurological diseases: infantile neuroaxonal dystrophy (INAD) and metachromatic leukodystrophy (MLD). In INAD there are no hair changes and in both central and peripheral nervous system there are characteristic axonal spheroids.

MLD is a lysosomal storage disease in most cases due to arylsulfatase A deficiency.

The presence of axonal swellings in the nerve biopsy can be also caused by several toxic substances (van der Knaap and Valk 2005).

## Management and follow-up

No specific treatment is available for this disease. The treatment is exclusively symptomatic and supportive and is based mainly on physical therapy assessment.

## Genetic counseling

Giant axonal neuropathy is inherited in an autosomal recessive manner. The parents of an affected child are obligate heterozygotes and therefore carry one mutant allele. At conception, the sibs of an affected individual have a 25% chance of being affected, a 50% chance of being a carrier, and a 25% chance of being unaffected and not a carrier.

Heterozygotes (carriers) are generally asymptomatic. However, it has been proposed that certain GAN mutations might cause mild subclinical neuropathy when present at the heterozygous status.

## References

Alkan A, Kutlu R, Sigirci A, Baysal T, Yakinci C (2003) Giant axonal neuropathy. J Neuroimaging 13: 371–375.

Allen E, Ding J, Wang W, Pramanik S, Chou J, Yau V, Yang Y (2005) Gigaxonin-controlled degradation of MAP1B light chain is critical to neuronal survival. Nature 438: 224–228.

Asbury AK, Gale MK, Cox SC, Baringer JR, Berg BO (1972) Giant axonal neuropathy: a unique case with segmental neurofilamentous masses. Acta Neuropathol (Berl) 20: 237–247.

Berg BO, Rosemberg SH, Asbury AK (1972) Giant axonal neuropathy. Pediatrics 49: 894–899.

Bomont P, Cavalier L, Blondeau F, Ben Hamida C, Belal S, Tazir M, Demir E, Topaloglu H, Korinthenberg R, Tuysuz B, Landrieu P, Hentati F, Koenig M (2000) The gene encoding gigaxonin, a new member of the cytoskeletal BTB/kelch repeat family, is mutated in giant axonal neuropathy. Nat Genet 26: 370–374.

Bomont P, Ioos C, Yalcinkaya C, Korinthenberg R, Vallat JM, Assami S, Munnich A, Chabrol B, Kurlemann G, Tazir M, Koenig M (2003) Identification of seven novel mutations in the GAN gene. Hum Mutat 21: 446.

Brockmann K, Pouwels PJ, Dechent P, Elanigan KM, Frahm J, Hanefeld F (2003) Cerebral proton magnetic reso-

nance spectroscopy of a patient with giant axonal neuropathy. Brain Dev 25: 45–50.

Bruno C, Bertini E, Federico A, Tonoli E, Lispi ML, Cassandrini D, Pedemonte M, Santorelli FM, Filocamo M, Dotti MT, Schenone A, Malandrini A, Minetti C (2004) Clinical and molecular findings in patients with giant axonal neuropathy (GAN). Neurology 62: 13–16.

Carpenter S, Karpati G, Andermann F, Gold R (1974) Giant axonal neuropathy. A clinically and morphologically distinct neurological disease. Arch Neurol 31: 312–316.

Demir E, Bomont P, Erdem S, Cavalier L, Demirci M, Kose G, Muftuoglu S, Cakar AN, Tan E, Aysun S, Topcu M, Guicheney P, Koenig M, Topaloglu H (2005) Giant axonal neuropathy: clinical and genetic study in six cases. J Neurol Neurosurg Psychiatry 76: 825–832.

Ding J, Liu JJ, Kowal AS, Nardine T, Bhattacharya P, Lee A, Yang Y (2002) Microtubule-associated protein 1B: a neuronal binding partner for gigaxonin. J Cell Biol 158: 427–433.

Ding J, Allen E, Wang W, Valle A, Wu C, Nardine T, Cui B, Yi J, Taylor A, Jeon NL, Chu S, So Y, Vogel H, Tolwani R, Mobley W, Yang Y (2006) Gene targeting of GAN in mouse causes a toxic accumulation of microtubule-associated protein 8 and impaired retrograde axonal transport. Hum Mol Genet 15: 1451–1463.

Gordon N (2004) Giant axonal neuropathy. Dev Med Child Neurol 46: 717–719.

Herrmann DN, Griffin J (2002) Intermediate filaments. A common thread in neuromuscular disorders. Neurology 58: 1141–1143.

Igisu H, Ohta M, Tabira T, Hosowaka S, Goto I (1975) Giant axonal neuropathy: a clinical entity affecting the central nervous system as the peripheral nervous system. Neurology 25: 717–721.

Koop O, Schirmacher A, Nelis E, Timmerman V, De Jonghe P, Ringelstein B, Rasic VM, Evrard P, Gärtner J, Claeys KG, Appenzeller S, Rautenstrauss B, Hühne K, Ramos-Arroyo MA, Wörle H, Moilanen JS, Hammans S, Kuhlenbäumer G (2007) Genotype-phenotype analysis in patients with giant axonal neuropathy (GAN). Neuromuscul Disord 17: 624–630.

Kuhlenbäumer G (2008) Genotype-phenotype analysis in patients with giant axonal neuropathy. Neuromuscul Disord 18: 276.

Kuhlenbäumer G, Young P, Oberwittler C, Hunermund G, Schirmacher A, Domschke K, Ringelstein B, Stogbauer F (2002) Giant axonal neuropathy (GAN): case report and two novel mutations in the gigaxonin gene. Neurology 58: 1273–1276.

Lycklama a Nijeholt J, Koerten HK, de Wolff FA (1994) Giant axonal degeneration: scanning electron microscopic and biochemical study of scalp hair. Dermatology 188: 258–262.

Malandrini A, Dotti MT, Battisti C, Villanova M, Capocchi G, Federico A (1998) Giant axonal neuropathy with subclinical involvement of the central nervous system: case report. J Neurol Sci 158: 232–235.

Ouvrier RA (1989) Giant axonal neuropathy. A review. Brain Dev 11: 207–214.

Pena SD (1982) Giant axonal neuropathy: an inborn error of organization of intermediate filaments. Muscle Nerve 5: 166–172.

Prineas JW, Ouvrier RA, Wright RG, Walsh JC, McLeod JG (1976) Giant axonal neuropathy: a generalized disorder of cytoplasmic microfilament formation. J Neuropathol Exp Neurol 35: 458–470.

Rybojad M, Moraillon I, Bonafe JL, Cambon L, Evrard P (1998) Pilar dysplasia: an early marker of giant axonal neuropathy. Ann Dermatol Venereol 125: 892–83. French.

Takebe Y, Koide N, Takahashi G (1981) Giant axonal neuropathy: report of two siblings with endocrinological and histological studies. Neuropediatrics 12: 392–404.

Tazir M, Vallat JM, Bomont P, Zemmouri R, Sindou P, Assami S, Nouioua S, Hammadouche T, Grid D, Koenig M (2002) Genetic heterogeneity in giant axonal neuropathy: an Algerian family not linked to chromosome 16q24.1. Neuromuscul Disord 12: 849–852.

Treiber-Held S, Budjarjo-Welim H, Reimann D, Richter J, Kretzschmar HA, Hanefeld F (1994) Giant axonal neuropathy: a generalized disorder of intermediate filaments with longitudinal grooves in the hair. Neuropediatrics 25: 89–93.

van der Knaap MS (2005) Giant Axonal Neuropathy. In: van der Knaap MS, Valk J (eds.) Magnetic resonance of myelination and myelin disorders, 3rd ed. Berlin: Springer, pp. 436–441.

Yang Y, Allen E, Ding J, Wang W (2007) Giant axonal neuropathy. Cell Mol Life Sci 64: 601–609.

# Chapter 70

# LESCH–NYHAN SYNDROME

Ignacio Pascual-Castroviejo and Martino Ruggieri

Paediatric Neurology Service, University Hospital La Paz, University of Madrid, Madrid, Spain (IPC); Institute of Neurological Science, National Research Council and Department of Pediatrics, University of Catania, Catania, Italy (MR)

## Introduction

*Lesch–Nyhan syndrome* (**LNS**) is a rare X-linked disorder of purine metabolism associated with hyperuricemia and caused by absence or near complete absence of the enzyme *hypoxanthine-guanine phosphoriboxyl transferase* (*HGPRT*), essential for purine salvage (Nyhan 2004, Seegmiller et al. 1967, Torres and Puig 2007). The gene for HGPRT has been mapped to position Xq2.6 (OMIM # 308000). The disease phenotype includes hyperuricemia, dystonia, choreoathetosis, hypertonia, hyperreflexia, varying degrees of cognitive impairment, and the hallmark symptom of severe self-mutilation. Besides the *classical LNS* (caused by virtually 0% HGPRT activity under any conditions) several enzymatic variants (with HGPRT activities varying from 0 to 50% or near normal) have been recognised including (a) *neurological variants*; and (b) *partial variants* (Nyhan 2004).

## Historical background and eponyms

LNS was first described in the German literature by Catel and Schmidt in 1959, but the disease is better known since the report of Lesch and Nyhan in 1964, who most probably did not know the paper of Catel and Schmidt. In their original report Lesch and Nyhan (1964) described two brothers of whom the eldest was in an institution with a diagnosis of mental retardation and cerebral palsy when the younger was admitted with haematuria and found to have hyperuricemia and uricosuria and had a bizarre and compulsive, self-mutilating biting (Nyhan 2004). Both brothers exhibited involuntary choreoathetoid movements. Biochemical studies identified that the uric acid pool was enlarged and its turnover was abnormally rapid (Nyhan 1968).

In the four decades since its initial description (Lesch and Nyhan 1964) enormous clinical, biochemical and molecular genetic progresses have been made. LNS can not be classically considered a neurocutaneous disease because of the only external lesions are those caused by the self mutilation mainly of lips, fingers and hands.

## Incidence and prevalence

LNS estimated prevalence is 1 : 380000 with an unusual neurologic and behavioural phenotype (Crawhall et al. 1972).

## Clinical manifestations

### Skin manifestations and behaviour

At birth, children with LNS appear normal and gross motor milestone may be achieved appropriately until six to eight months. Choreoathetosis develops between eight and 24 months of age and a loss of early milestones is seen. Infants are hypotonic, but later they develop hypertonia and hyperreflexia. Stereotypical self-mutilation, the classic manifestation of LNS, is exhibited by four years of age or earlier (Fig. 1) in many of the affected children. Almost all children exhibit all features of LNS by eight to ten years. These features are self-mutilation (Fig. 2A) and the neurological manifestation of the disorder including spasticity, choreoathetosis

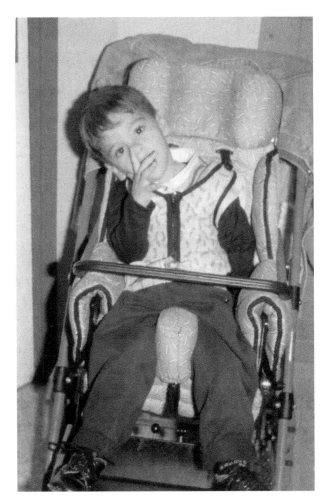

**Fig. 1.** A 3-year-old child shows dystonia and self-biting of the fingers.

Other behaviours, in order of frequency, include head banging, extension of arms when being wheelchairs, eye-poking, fingers in wheelchair spokes, and rubbing behaviours. Hierarchical cluster analysis can identify patterns of association among the types of self-mutilation (Robey et al. 2003). Some patients with LNS were reported to engage in outwardly directed behaviours that included biting, hitting, kicking, hair-pulling, spitting, and verbal insults (Anderson and Ernst 1994, Robey et al. 2003).

Special accommodations have been made in school settings, on school buses, and in group homes to limit individuals' opportunities to injury others, to spit on others and to disrupt activities with verbal aggression within the spectrum of LNS involuntary behaviours (Robey et al. 2003).

The development of communication is hampered by poor articulation due to pseudobulbar palsy and obstructed air flow. Most affected children appear to comprehend quite well. The cognitive functioning of individuals with LNS (Mattews et al. 1995) demonstrated levels that ranged from moderately mentally retarded to low average. Areas of weakness included attention, the manipulation of complex visual images, the comprehension of complex or lengthy speech, mathematical ability, and multi-reasoning. Seizures occur in approximately 50% of the patients.

## Systemic manifestations

Gouty arthritis and urate tophi, mostly located in ears, feet and hands, as well as haematuria and renal calculi are seen in the majority of LNS patients, most times as late complications. Renal failure is a severe complication that may present at any time. A megaloblastic anaemia may be common.

## Imaging

Roentgenograms have documented aspects of the self-injurious behaviour showing partial amputation of the fingers or the hands, mutilation of the face and bone fractures. The abnormal neurology is illus-

(Fig. 2B), opisthotonus, hyperreflexia and facial dystonia (Mattews et al. 1995).

The self-mutilation associated with LNS typically first appears between the age of 1 and 6 years. Fingers, hands and lips are the zones of the body more likely injured by this behaviour, but LNS patients may bite any external surface. Self-mutilation often causes the emergence of teeth. Some patients may use an external surface, such as a wheelchair component or other seating as an instrument of self-mutilation (Robey et al. 2003). The level of severity remains steady with increasing age (Anderson and Ernst 1994) and as the patient becomes older, he learns to become aggressive with speech.

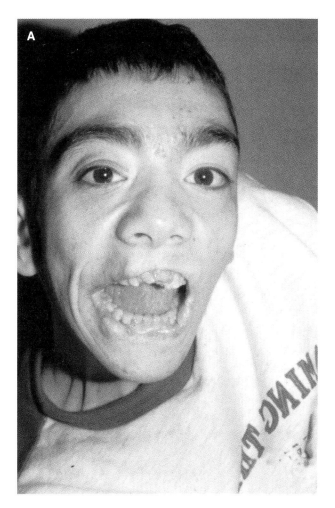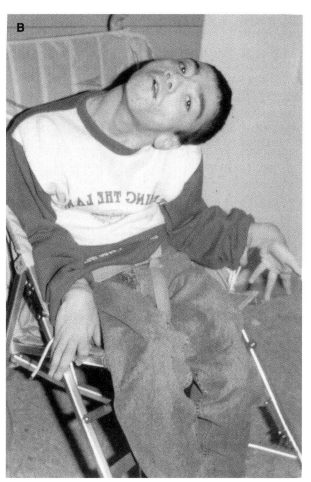

Fig. 2. (**A**) A 20-year-old patient with LNS shows facial distonia and signs of self mutilation in lips and teeth. (**B**) The same patient shows severe choreoathetosis and opisthotonos.

trated as well by conventional X-rays in the dislocated hips that are seen almost uniformly in LNS patients. The accumulation of uric acid may result in abnormal appearance on X-ray such a tophaceous gout or urinary tract calculi.

There have been very few published series that specifically focused on neuroimaging findings in LNS patients. Harris et al. (1998) provided the first MRI assessment of brain in a series of LNS patients, with emphasis on basal ganglia measurements. Volumetric studies confirmed a 34% decrease in caudate volume, a 17% decrease in total cerebral volume, and a 12% decrease in putamen volume. A PET study involving the fluorodopa F18 tracer has shown decreased dopamine storage in the putamen, caudate nucleus, frontal cortex, substantia nigra and ventral tegmentum area (Ernst et al. 1996).

## Pathology

Pathological findings for the LNS brain are nonspecific (Del Bigio and Halliday 2007). Lloyd et al. (1981), examining postmortem brains, have found that the levels of dopamine and homovanillic acid, and the activities of tyrosine hydroxylase and dopa decarboxylase in the putamen, caudate nucleus and external pallidum are all decreased in LNS. Saito et al. (1999) found decreased concentration of dopamine in the caudate nucleus of two LNS patients.

## Molecular genetics and pathogenesis

LNS is an X-linked disorder of purine metabolism caused by deficiency of hypoxanthine-guanine phosphoriboxyltransferase (HGPRT) (Melton et al. 1984). Uric acid is elevated in urine, blood and CSF. Other purines, such as xanthina and hypoxanthine are increased as well (Seegmiller 1989). Levels of uric acid in urine may be 3–4mg per mg of creatine (normal < 1mg).

The responsible gene for LNS was mapped to Xq26-q27.2. The nucleotide sequence of all nine exons has been determined (Melton et al. 1984). HGPRT gene has been localized at a position between the genes for PP-ribose-P synthetase and glucose-6-phosphate dehydrogenase (Becker et al. 1979). More than 100 mutations have been recorded to date; some 85% of these are point mutations or small deletions (Sege-Peterson and Nyhan 1997). LNS has been also described in a few females (Hara et al. 1982, Yukawa et al. 1992).

The genetic mutations cause HGPRT activity reduction to less than 0.5% of normal in several tissues including erythrocytes and fibroblast cultures. HGPRT deficiency does not permit the hypoxanthine reuse, and whatever hypoxanthine is formed is either excreted or catabolized to xanthine and uric acid. At the same time, phosphoriboxylpyrophosphate, a regulator of the purine synthesis, is increased, and this is the cause of the marked increasing of uric acid in urine, blood and CSF.

Numerous variants of the LNS have been recognized (Adler and Wrabetz 1996). Each variant have particular clinical and biochemical peculiarities that differentiate from the typical form of LNS. Table 1 summarises the spectrum of deficiency of HGPRT.

Prenatal diagnosis is possible (Zoref-Shani et al. 1989).

Uric acid itself appears not to be directly involved in producing the neurologic disorders. Increased uric acid in blood, urine and CNS, more probably is a

**Table 1.** Enzymatic variants of HGPRT and related phenotypes

| LNS variants | HGPRT activity | Clinical features |
|---|---|---|
| Classical LNS | virtually 0% under any conditions | Lesch–Nyhan syndrome |
| Neurological variant (intermediate variant) | may be virtually 0% in RBC assay unstable or altered kinetics active in whole cell assay | spasticity, choreoathetosis, good mental function, normal behaviour, hyperuricemic manifestations |
| Partial variant | 0–50% in RBC assay | gout or nephrologic complications |
| | active in whole cell assay | neurological normal |

toxic product store as a consequence of the enzymatic defect.

## Differential diagnosis

The differential diagnosis is mainly with severe mental retardation of various causes, cerebral palsy with severe dyskinesia or athetosis, disease associated with distonia, autism, some rare cases of sensory neuropathy, and congenital insensitivity to pain with anhydrosis (Barone et al. 2005).

## Management

Most of the antiobsessive substances (haloperidol, clonidine, risperidone, buspirone HCl, pimozide, clonazepam and others) have been unsuccessfully added to behavioral modification and upper limb restraints and self-abuse. Treatment with botulinum toxin injections into the bilateral masseter has lately been used and appears to represent and effective and safe treatment of severe self-mutilation in LNS without the systemic side effects and limited benefit of medication (Dabrowski et al. 2002, Zilli and Hasselmo 2008). Protection of lips, teeth and chin against self-mutilation is almost impossible, but we

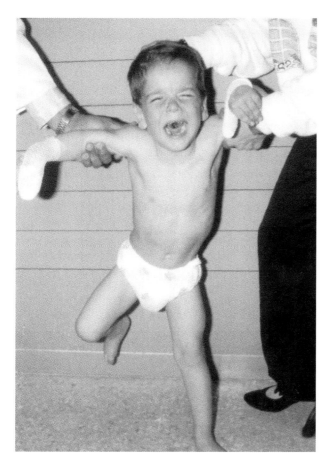

**Fig. 3.** A 4-year-old child with severe self-mutilation shows the protected hands.

must try to protect hands and fingers with bandages (Fig. 3).

The renal and arthritic manifestations of LNS are treated with allopurinol (20 mg/kg per day), a xanthine oxidase inhibitor that blocks the last steps of uric acid synthesis. Allopurinol, however, has not effect on neurological symptoms and on self-mutilation.

## References

Adler CH, Wrabetz L (1996) Lesh-Nyhan variant: distonia, ataxia, near normal intelligence, and no self-mutilation. Mov Disord 11: 583–584.

Anderson LT, Ernst M (1994) Self-injury in Lesch-Nyhan disease. J Autism Dev Disord 24: 67–81.

Barone R, Lempereur L, Anastasi M, Parano E, Pavone P (2005) Congenital insensitivity to pain with anhydrosis (NTRK1 mutation) and early onset renal disease: clinical report on three sibs with a 25-year follow-up in one of them. Neuropediatrics 36: 270–273.

Becker MA, Yen RCK, Itkin P, Gross SJ, Seegmiller JE, Bakay B (1979) Regional localization of the gene for human phosphoriboxylpyrophasphate synthetase on the X-chromosome. Science 203: 1016–1019.

Catel W, Schmidt J (1959) Über familiäre gichtische Diathese in Verbindung mit zerebralen und renalen Symptomen bei einem Kleinkind. Dtsch Med Wochenschr 84: 2145–2147.

Crawhall JC, Henderson JF, Kelley WN (1972) Diagnosis and treatmen of the Lesch–Nyhan syndrome. Pediatr Res 6: 504–513.

Dabrowski E, Leleszi JP, Smathers SA, Nigro MA (2002) Botulinum toxin as a novel treatment for self-mutilation in Lesch–Nyhan syndrome. Ann Neurol 52: S157.

Del Bigio MR, Halliday WC (2007) Multifocal atrophy of cerebellar internal granular neurons in lesch-nyhan disease: case reports and review. J Neuropathol Exp Neurol 66: 346–353.

Ernst M, Zametkin AJ, Matochik JA, Pascualvaca D, Jons PH, Hardy K, Hankerson JG, Doudet DJ, Cohen RM (1996) Presynaptic dopaminergic deficits in Lesch–Nyhan disease. N Engl J Med 334: 1568–1572.

Hara K, Kashiwamata S, Ogasawara N, Ohishi H, Natsume R, Yamanaka T, Hakamada S, Miyazaki S, Watanabe K (1982) A female case of the Leach-Nyhan syndrome. Tohoku J Exp Med 137: 275–282.

Harris JC, Lee RR, Jinnah HA, Wong DF, Yaster M, Bryan RN (1998) Craniocerebral magnetic resonance imaging measurement and findings in Lesh–Nyhan syndrome. Arch Neurol 55: 547–553.

Lesch M, Nyhan WL (1964) A familial disorder of uric acid metabolism and central nervous system function. Am J Med 36: 561–570.

Lloyd KG, Hornykiewicz O, Davidson L, Shannak K, Farley I, Goldstein M, Shibuya M, Kelley WN, Fox IH (1981) Biochemical evidence of dysfunction of brain neurotransmitters in the Lesch–Nyhan syndrome. N Engl J Med 305: 1106–1111.

Mattews WS, Solan A, Barabas G (1995) Cognitive functioning in Lesh–Nyhan syndrome. Dev Med Child Neurol 37: 715–722.

Mattews WS, Solan A, Barabas G, Robey K (1999) Cognitive functioning in Lesh–Nyhan syndrome: a 4-year follow-up study. Dev Med Child Neurol 41: 260–266.

Melton DW, Conecki DS, Brennand J, Caskey CT (1984) Structure, expression and mutation of the hypoxanthine phosphoriboxyltransferase gene. Proc Natl Acad Sci USA 81: 2147–2151.

Nyhan WZ (1968) Introduction-clinical features. In: Bland YH (ed.) Seminars on the Lesch-Nyhan syndrome. Federal Proceedings 27: 1027–1033.

Nyhan WL (2004) Lesch–Nyan syndrome. In: Roach ES, Miller VS (eds.) Neurocutaneous disorders. New York: Cambridge University Press, pp. 186–199.

Robey KL, Reck JF, Giacomini KD, Barabas G, Eddey GR (2003) Modes and patterns of self-mutilation in persons with Lesch–Nyhan disease. Dev Med Child Neurol 45: 167–171.

Saito Y, Ito M, Hanaoka S, Ohama E, Akaboshi S, Takashima S (1999) Dopamine receptor upregulation in Lesh–Nyhan syndrome: a postmortem study Neuropediatrics 30: 66–71.

Seegmiller JE, Rosenbloom FM, Kelly WN (1967) Enzyme defect associated with sex-linked human neurological disorder and excessive purine synthesis. Science 155: 1682–1684.

Seegmiller JE (1989) Contributions of Lesh–Nyhan syndrome to the understanding of purine metabolism. J Inhert Metab Dis 12: 184–196.

Sege-Peterson M, Nyhan WL (1997) Lesch-Nyhan disease and hypoxanthine-guanine phosphoriboxyltransferase deficiency. In: Rosenberg RN et al. (eds.). The molecular and genetic basis of neurological disease, 2nd ed. Boston: Butter Worth-Heinemann, pp. 1233–1252.

Torres RJ, Puig JG (2007) Hypoxanthine-guanine phosophoribosyltransferase (HPRT) deficiency: Lesch-Nyhan syndrome. Orphanet J Rare Dis 2: 48.

Yukawa T, Akazawa H, Miyake Y, Takahashi Y, Nagao H, Takeda E (1992) A female patient with Lesh–Nyhan syndrome. Dev Med Child Neurol 34: 543–546.

Zilli EA, Hasselmo ME (2008) A model of behavioral treatments for self-mutilation behavior in Lesch-Nyhan syndrome. Neuroreport 19: 459–462.

Zoref-Shani E, Bromberg Y, Goldman B, Shalli R, Barkai G, Legum C, Sperling O (1989) Prenatal diagnosis of Lesch–Nyhan syndrome: experience with three fetuses at risk. Prenat Diagn 9: 657–662.

# Chapter 71

# THE SKIN AS A CLUE FOR THE DIAGNOSIS OF INHERITED METABOLIC DISORDERS

**Enrico Bertini, May El Hachem, and Carlo Dionisi-Vici**

Unit of Molecular Medicine, Division of Dermatology and Division of Metabolic Disorders,
Bambino Gesù Children's Research Hospital, Rome, Italy

## Introduction

Dermatology may be considered as the science of skin biology, skin disease, and treatment, but it is particularly a special art of visual perception to detect clues for phenotype categorization.

The knowledge of cutaneous symptoms of inherited metabolic disorders helps to understand and diagnose inherited metabolic disorders. Sometimes the cutaneous sign is like a bookmark for the metabolic disorder; in other cases, the skin reflects complications of the diseases or adverse side effects of treatment.

Skin lesions of several types occur in inborn errors of metabolism and the principal group of lesions can be grouped in 4 main groups: 1) Vescicolobullus lesions (Table 1); 2) Photosensitivity, skin rashes and discolorations (Table 2); 3) Hyperkeratosis and ichthyosis (Table 3); 4) Skin ulceration, skin nodules, and hyperlaxity (Table 7). For simplicity we have made tables containing the list of disorders that frequently cluster for each skin lesion.

However in the text we will classify the description of skin lesions using a systematic criteria related to the subcellular organelle where the defective protein is located (mitochondrial or peroxisomal disorder) or based on the main metabolic agent that is involved by the genetic defect (porphyria, aminoacidopathy, metal toxicity disorders, etc).

## Mitochondrial disorders

Mitochondria have their own distinct DNA. Each mitochondrion contains several circular double-stranded DNA copies that are normally 16,569 base pairs in length. Each copy contains 37 genes that code for several respiratory chain structural proteins and for mitochondrial DNA transcription and translation (22 tRNAs) factors.

Mitochondrial DNA abnormalities were first linked to human disease in 1988. In that year, Leber's hereditary optic neuropathy and several progressive muscle disorders were found to be caused by mutations in mitochondrial DNA (Wallace et al. 1988, Holt et al. 1988). Aerobic metabolism depends on the hundreds of mitochondria that every cell in the body contains. Cellular dysfunction results when the proportion of mutated mitochondrial DNA strands exceeds a threshold level.

Because sperm does not contribute with mitochondria to the zygote, mutations in mitochondrial DNA are classically inherited only from the mother (maternal inheritance). Mitochondria have their own distinct DNA. The proportion of mutated mitochondria can differ widely from oocyte to oocyte. Consequently, siblings can have widely varying symptoms and severity of disease. Similarly, the proportion of mutant mitochondrial DNA differs from cell to cell in an embryo, so different daughter cell lines can have widely varying levels of cell dysfunction.

Slightly later it became evident that also defects in chromosomal DNA can also cause mitochondrial disease, because chromosomal DNA supplies most of the proteins necessary for mitochondrial DNA replication and expression. These conditions were inherited by Mendelian inheritance in a autosomal dominant or autosomal recessive fashion (Moraes et al. 1991, Tritschler et al. 1992, Zeviani et al. 1989).

**Table 1.** Vescicolobullous lesions. The numbers preceded by # or by +are referred to the data base of U.S. National Library of Medicine (http://www.ncbi.nlm.nih.gov.ezp1.harvard.edu/entrez/query.fcgi?holding=hulib). Abbreviations: *abs* abnormalities; *chr.* chromosome

| Disorders | Age at onset | Type of lesions | Other associated symptoms |
|---|---|---|---|
| Acrodermatitis enteropatica Zinc deficiency #201100 Intestinal zinc-specific transporter SLC39A4, chr. 8q24.3 | 2–4 weeks or after weaning | Skin rash Symmetric Circumorifice Retroauricular Acral Frequent secondary infection | Watery stools Failure to thrive Mucosal lesions Total alopecia Conjunctivitis |
| Methylmalonic acidemia #251000 methylmalonyl-CoA mutase deficiency; chr. 6p21 Propionic acidemia #606054 propionyl-CoA carboxylase deficiency; PPCA (13q32), PPCB (3q21-q22) | Infancy | Eczematous eruptions Circumorifice Diaper and acral areas Cutaneous detachement Desquamation | Ketoacidosis Falure to thrive Hypotonia Pancytopenia Hyperammonemia Acute decompensation |
| Holocarboxylase synthetase deficiency #253270, chr. 21q22.1 Biotinidase deficiency #253260, chr. 3p25 | Neonatal to infancy | Scaly skin rash Over whole body Prominent on diaper and intertriginous areas Patchtìy, erythmatous exudative circumorifice | Seborrheic dermatitis Keratoconjiuntivitis Alopecia Biotin-responsiveness Hypotonia Ketoacidotic coma Hyperlactacidemia Developmental delay |

**Table 2.** Photosensitivity, skin rashes and discolorations

| Disorders | Age at onset | Type of lesions | Other associated symptoms |
|---|---|---|---|
| Congenital erythropoietic porphyria see text | Neonatal and late onset | Cutaneous fragility, bullous lesions, hypertichosis dyspigmentation | |
| Erythropoietic porphyria see text | First months | | Major cutaneous signs, hemolitic anemia, splenomegaly, dark urines |
| Porphyria variegata see text | Adult | | Abdominal and neurological crisis |
| Hereditary coproporphyria see text | Adult | | Abdominal and neurological crisis, hemolitic anemia |
| Porphyria cutanea tarda see text | Adult | | Hepatic siderosis |
| Erythropoietic protoporphyria see text | <5 years | Photosensitivity Pain and edema in limbs | Hepatic failure Gallstones |
| Xeroderma pigmentosum Principal complementation groups: XPD; ERCC2; #278730; chr. 19q13.2 | 1–2 years | Freckling Hopopigmentation and hyperpigmentation of sun- | Tumors Basal carcinomas Malignant melanomas |

(Continued)

**Table 2.** (Continued)

| Disorders | Age at onset | Type of lesions | Other associated symptoms |
|---|---|---|---|
| XPA, ERCC1, +278700; chr. 9q22.3<br>XPB; ERCC3, +133510, chr. 2q21<br>XPC-HHR23B, +278720, chr. 3p25<br>XPG; ERCC5, +133530; chr. 13q33<br>XPE; DDB2, #278740, chr. 11p12<br>XPF, ERCC4, #278760, chr. 16p13.3 | | exposed skin<br>Atrophy<br>Teleangectasias<br>Tumors | Ocular signs<br>A neuronal progressive variant |
| Cockayne syndrome A;<br>#216400, ERCC8, chr. 5q11,<br>#133540, Cockayne syndrome B;<br>ERCC6, chr. 10q11, | 1–2 years | Cutaneous photosensitivity,<br>thin, dry hair | Failure to thrive, abnormal and slow growth development, progressive pigmentary retinopathy, sensorineural hearing loss, dental caries |
| Bloom syndrome<br>#210900, DNA helicase RecQ<br>protein-like-3; chr. 15q26.1 | | Facial telangiectasia in butterfly midface distribution (exacerbated by sun), spotty hypo-pigmentation spotty hyper-pigmentation, cafe-au-lait spots, hypertrichosis, photosensitivity | Prenatal onset growth retardation<br>Growth failure<br>Syndactyly<br>Polydactyly<br>Fifth finger clinodactyly |
| Hartnup disease<br>#234500, SLC6A19, chr. 5p15 | | Light-sensitive dermatitis | Intermittent cerebellar, ataxia, seizures, hypertonia delayed cognitive development, emotional instability, psychosis |
| Mitochondrial Respiratory chain abs | See text | See text | See text |
| EPEMA syndrome (etilmalonic aciduria)<br>#602473, ETHE1, chr. 19q13.32 | Early infancy | Recurring petecchiae<br>Distal acrocianosis | Congenital encephalopathy, vasculopathy, mucoid diarrhea<br>Attacs of lactic acidodsis |
| Adrenoleukodystrophy<br>#300100, ABCD1 gene, chr. Xq28 | Childhood<br>Juvenile<br>Adult | Hyperpigmentation | Progressive neurologic disorder, spastic paraplegia, peripheral neuropathy, sphincter disturbances, limb and truncal ataxia, primary adrenal insufficiency, hypogonadism |
| Wilson disease<br>#277900, ATP7B, chr. 13q14.3-q21.1 | | Reticulated brownish hyperpigmentation of the lower legs, blue lunulae | Prolonged hepatitis, hepatic cirrhosis and coma, hepatomegaly, liver failure, high liver copper, tremor, dysarthria, dysphagia, personality changes, dementia, poor motor coordination, dystonia, low serum ceruloplasmin |
| Nieman Pick A (acute infantile form) and B (chronic visceral form)<br>#257200, sphingomyelin phosphodiesterase-1, 11p15.4-p15.1 | | Brownish-yellow skin discoloration | Extreme liver and spleen enlargement, severe mental retardation and dystonia (only type A) |

Reviewing the literature of skin disorders associated with mitochondrial encephalomyopathies the most recurring sign are lipomas. Symmetric cervical lipomas are a presenting feature of Ekbom's syndrome of cervical lipomas associated with myoclonic epilepsy and ragged red muscle fibers (MERRF) and mutations in the mtDNA tRNA LysUUR 8344A-G (Ekbom 1975, Calabresi et al. 1994, Flynn et al. 1998).

**Table 3.** Hyperkeratosis and Ichthyosis (see Figs. 6, 7, and 9)

| Disorders | Age at onset | Type of lesions | Other symptoms |
|---|---|---|---|
| Tyrosinemia type II +276600, tyrosine aminotransferase deficiency, chr. 16q22.1-q22.3 | Infancy to early childhood | Painful blisters or erosions in palms and soles leading to hyperkeratosis | Keratitis, lacrimation Photophobia (conjunctivitis), hypertyrosinemia dramatically responsive to low-tyrosine diet |
| Sjogren-Larsson syndrome #270200, fatty aldehyde dehydrogenase deficiency, chr. 17p11.2 | Neonatal to infancy | Neonatal ichthiosiform erithrodermia, Collodion baby | Spastic paraplegia Mental retardation Cataract Retinitis |
| Neutral lipid storage disorder, Chanarin Dorfman disease #275630, CGI58, chr. 3p21 | Neonatal to infancy | Neonatal ichthiosiform erithrodermia Collodion baby | Hepatomegaly Slight myopathy Neuropathy Steathorrea |
| Steroid sulphatase deficiency X-linked Ichtiosis +308100, Xp22.32 | <4 months | Neonatal ichthiosiform erithrodermia | Corneal opacities Hypogonadism Short stature Chondrodysplasia punctata |
| Congenital defect of glycosilation (CDG1f) #609180, MPDU1 gene, 17p13.1-p12 | Early in infancy | Scaly, itching skin disease | Psychomotor retardation Feeding problems Growth retardation Partial growth hormone deficiency |
| Classical Refsum disease #266500, phytanoyl-CoA hydroxylase def., chr. 10pter-p11.2 | Late childhood to adulthod | Ichthiosis | Retinitis pigmentosa Ataxia Peripheral neuropathy Deafness |
| Austin disease #272200, sulfatase-modifying factor-1 gene, chr. 3p26 | 1–2 years | Ichthiosis | Coarse face Leukodystrophy Failure to thrive Hepatosplenomegaly Bone changes Mental regression Quadriplegia Vacuolated lymphocytes |
| Conradi Huntermann syndrome #302960, Sterol Δ8 isomerase deficiency, chr. Xp11.23-p11.22 Deletion of terminal short arm of X chromosome | Childhood to adulthood<br><br>Childhood | Ichthiosis "en bande" | Chondrodysplasia punctata X-linked dominant inheritance Asymmetric body |
| Trichotiodystrophy #126340, ERCC2/XPD #133510, ERCC3/XPB, #608780, TTD-A, TFB5, chr. 6p25.3 see Table X | Infancy | Ichthiosis Brittle hair Trichotiodystrophy | Short stature Mental retardation Dysmorphism Leukodystrophy Immunodeficiency |

**Table 4.** Coarse facies

| Disorders | Age at onset when first visible | Other relevant associated symptoms |
|---|---|---|
| Generalized GM1 disease +230500, beta-galactosidase deficiency, chr. 3p21.33 | Neonatal | Hydrops fetalis, Ascitis Edema Failure to thrive |
| Sialidosis type II #256550, neuraminidase, chr. 6p21.3 | Neonatal | Hypotonia, joint stiffness, osteoporosis Hirsutism |
| Galactosialidosis (early infancy) + 256540, beta-galactosidase + neuraminidase deficiency=cathepsin A, chr. 20q13.1 see Table 6 | Neonatal | |
| Sly syndrome, MPS VII + 253220, beta-glucuronidase deficiency, chr. 7q21.11. | Neonatal | |
| I-cell disease or mucolipidosis II #252500, GNPTA, chr. 12q23.3 | Neonatal | |
| Fucosidosis type I +230000, alpha-fucosidase def., chr. 1p34 | Early infancy (3–12 months) | Seizures, myoclonus, spasticity, mental retardation, leukodystrophy |
| Salla disease or Sialuria Finnish type #604369, SLC17A5, 6q14-q15 | Early infancy (3–12 months) | |
| Hurler syndrome (MPS type IH) #607014, alpha-L-iduronidase, 4p16.3 | Early infancy (3–12 months) | Inguinal hernias, ear, nose and throat infections, Hirsutism |
| Austin disease | 1–2 years | See Table 3 |
| Mannosidosis #248500, alpha-mannosidosis, 19cen-q12  #248510, beta-mannosidosis, 4q22-q25 | 1–2 years | Hypertrichosis , low anterior hairline Anterior hair whorl, heavy eyebrows macrocephaly, flat occiput, deafness Angiokeratoma, mental retardation |
| Maroteaux–Lamy (MPS VI) +253200, arylsulfatase B, chr. 5q11-q13 | 1–2 years | Normal intelligence, macrocephaly, hearing loss, glaucoma, corneal clouding, mild hirsutism |
| Hunter syndrome (MPS II) +309900, iduronate sulfatase deficiency, Xq28 | 2–6 years | Developmental delay, mental regression Scaphocephaly, macrocephaly, hearing loss, recurrent otitis media |
| Aspartylglucosaminuria (see Table 6) | 2–6 years | Developmental delay, mental regression |
| Pseduo-Hurler polyodystrophy or mucolipidosis IIIA #252600, alpha/beta-subunits precursor of GLcNAc-phosphotransferase, 12q23.3 | 2–6 years | Developmental delay, mental regression, short stature, corneal clouding, mild retinopathy |
| Sanfilippo syndrome A (MPS IIIA) #252900, N-sulfoglucosamine sulfohydrolase, chr. 17q25.3 Sanfilippo syndrome B (MPS IIIB) #252920, N-alpha-acetylglucosaminidase, chr. 17q21 | 2–6 years | Slight coarse face, abnormal behaviour, hearing loss, mild hepatomegaly, synophrys hirsutism, coarse hair |

Excluding lipomas, skin findings have been reported in several other patients as discoloration, hirsutism, and anhidrosis (Mori et al. 1991). Pigment alterations consistent with poikiloderma have been reported in some (Rötig et al. 1990, 1995; Haferkamp et al. 1994; Niaudet et al. 1994), acrocyanosis (Zupanc

**Table 5.** Alopecia and brittle hair

| Disease | Age at onset | Type of cutaneous lesion | Neurological and other symptoms |
|---|---|---|---|
| Menkes syndrome #309400, Cu(2+)-transporting ATPase, chr. Xq12-q13 | First 6 months | Brittle and fragile hair sagging cheeks, pili torti | Arrested development, hypothermia, seizures, loss of skills, mental retardation |
| Trichothiodystrophy see Table 3 | Infancy | Photosensitivity Ichthyosiform erythroderma | |
| Biotin responsive multiple carboxylase defects Holocarboxylase synthetase Biotinidase see Table 1 | Neonatal to infancy | Dermatitis, Keratocongiuntivitis, | Recurrent attacs of coma, hypotonia, ataxia, failure to thrive, ketoacidosis, hyperlactacidemia |
| Argininosuccinic aciduria #207900, argininosuccinate lyase, chr. 7 cen q 11.1 | Infancy | Trichorrhexis nodosa Dry brittle hair | Failure to thrive, severe vomiting, protein avoidance, vomiting, |
| Citrullinemia Type I #215700, argininosuccinate synthetase chr. 9q34 Type II, #603471, SLC25A13 Chr. 7q 21.3 | Infancy<br><br>Adult and neonatal onset | Dry brittle hair | hyperammonemia, hepatic fibrosis, Ataxia, coma, seizures, cerebral edema, developmental delay, mental retardation |
| Methylmalonic and propionic aciduria see Table 1 Acrodermatitis enteropatica see Table 1 | Neonatal to infancy | Periorifice bullous lesions | Chronic diarrhea Failure to thrive, hypotonia |
| Myotonic dystrophy #160900, protein kinase (DMPK), chr. 19q13.2-q13.3 | Neonatal Adulthood | Alopecia | Myopathy, cardiomyopathy |
| Ehlers-Danlos type IV (vascular type) Autosomal dominant #130050, type III collagen (COL3A1), chr. 2q31 | First year | Skin fragility, acrogeria, thin skin, easy bruisability, cigarette-paper scars, atrophic skin over ears, prominent venous markings, absent-mild skin hyperextensibility, skin changes worse in areas of lower skin temperature, molluscoid pseudotumors | Pneumothorax, gut perforation, arterial bleeding, periodontal disease, early loss of teeth thin lips |

et al. 1991, Rötig et al. 1992, Burlina et al. 1994) and vitiligo (Holt et al. 1988, McShane et al. 1991, Tulinius et al. 1995). Acrocyanosis has been reported together with Pearson syndrome (Rötig et al. 1992), and the presence of episodic acrocyanosis is part of the syndromic association of the ethylmalonic encephalopathy [EE] (Burlina et al. 1994), a devastating infantile metabolic disorder affecting the brain, gastrointestinal tract, and peripheral vessels. The gene responsible of the EE is ETHE1[#608451] (Tiranti et al. 2004) and the principal signs of the syndrome are recurrent petechiae, orthostatic acrocyanosis (Fig. 1A), and chronic diarrhea.

Other discolorations of the skin have been reported as periorbital darkening (Nørby et al. 1994); generalized hyperpigmentation associated with adrenal insufficiency (Ohno et al. 1996), cutis marmorata (Garcia-Silva et al. 1997) and jaundice in patients with

**Table 6.** Angiokeratoma

| Disorders | Age at onset | Major signs |
|---|---|---|
| Fabry disease; +301500, alpha-galactosidase A, chr. Xq22 | Childhood (male hemizygote)<br><br>Adolescent (female heterozygote) | Abdominal pain, acroparasthesias, renal failure, strokes, seizures, whorl-like corneal dystrophy, isolated angiokeratomas, corneal dystrophy |
| Fucosidosis see Table 4 | Infancy | Bone changes, coarse facies, hepatosplenomegaly, vacuolated lymphocytes |
| Galactosialidosis PPCA +256540, Protective protein/cathepsin A, ch. 20q13.1 Sialidosis types I and II; ch. 6p21.3 | Juvenile form (5–20 years)<br><br>Infantile and Juvenile forms | Bone changes, cherry red spot, corneal opacities, neurological deterioration, perinuclear cataracts, hepatosplenomegaly |
| Aspartylglucosaminuria +208400 , N-aspartyl-beta-glucosaminidase ch. 4q32-q33 | 1–5 years | Coarse face, joint laxity, lens opacities, mental regression, vacuolated lymphocytes, short stature, brachycephaly , microcephaly, acne, macroglossia, wide mouth, thick lips |
| Beta-mannosidosis See Table 4 | Adults | Nerve deafness, mental retardation, speech impairment , hypotonia aggressive behaviour, lymphedema, recurrent infections, tortuosity of conjunctival vessels |

**Table 7.** Skin ulceration, nodules, laxity, dysmorphic scaring, easy bruising

| Disease | Age at onset | Type of cutaneous lesion | Neurological and other symptoms |
|---|---|---|---|
| Prolidase deficiency +170100, peptidase A, 19cen-q13.11 | Childhood | Diffuse telangiectases, crusting erythematous dermatitis, severe progressive ulceration of lower extremities | Ptosis, ocular proptosis increased frequency of infections, systemic lupus erythematosus, developmental delay |
| Farber disease +228000, acid ceramidase, 8p22-p21.3 | Early Childhood | Lipogranulomatosis Periarticular subcutaneous nodules | Irritability, motor retardation, mental retardation, hoarse cry painful swollen joints, hepatomegaly, splenomegaly |
| Congenital defects of glycosylation 1a #212065, phospho-mannomutase-2, 16p13.3 | Birth to early childhood | Abnormal subcutaneous fat tissue distribution, fat pads 'Orange peel' skin, inverted nipples | Strabismus, retinitis pigmentosa, nystagmus, pericardial effusion, cardiomyopathy, hepatomegaly, liver fibrosis hypotonia, psychomotor retardation, ataxia, hyporeflexia, stroke-like episodes, seizures, olivopontocerebellar hypoplasia, prolonged prothrombin time, factor XI deficiency, antithrombin III deficiency, thrombocytosis |

(Continued)

**Table 7.** (Continued)

| Disease | Age at onset | Type of cutaneous lesion | Neurological and other symptoms |
|---|---|---|---|
| Ehlers Danlos syndromes (EDS) see Table 5<br>AR, EDS VI, #225400, Lysyl hydroxylase deficiency, 1p36.3-p36.2<br>%229200, EDS VIB, + macrocephaly, gene unknown<br>#130000, EDSI, 130010 EDSII (mild), collagen<br>alpha-1(V) gene<br>*120215, COL5A1, 9q34.2<br>*120190, COL5A2, 2q31<br>*120150, COL1A1, 17q21.31<br>#130020, EDSIII (benign)<br>*120180, COL3A1, 2q31<br>*600985, tenascin-XB, TNXB, 6p21.3 | Childhood<br><br>Adulhood | Joint laxity, soft skin, hyperextensible skin, moderate scarring, easy bruisability, molluscoid pseudotumors, excessive wrinkled skin (palms and soles) | Marfanoid habitus, Keratoconus, Microcornea, myopia, retinal detachment, ocular rupture, blue sclerae, epicanthal folds, glaucoma, blindness |
| EDS VII, #225410, ADAMTS2, 5q23<br>Autosomal recessive | Infancy | Skin fragility, easy bruisability soft, doughy skin, sagging, redundant skin, normal wound healing. | Blue sclerae, puffy eyelids |
| #130060, EDSVII, Autosomal dominant<br>*120150, COL1A1, 17q21.31<br>*120160, COL1A2, 7q22.1 | Childhood | Thin, velvety skin, hyperextensible skin, poor wound healing, atrophic scars easy bruisability | |
| %130080 EDS VIII (periodontosis type), AD gene unknown | Childhood | | Periodontal disease, early tooth loss |
| Occipital horn syndrome (mild variant of Menkes disease), #304150<br>see Menkes disease (see Table 5) | Early childhood | Joint laxity, soft skin, mildly extensible skin, loose, redundant skin, easy bruisability, coarse hair | Persistent, open anterior fontanel, Occipital horn exostoses, high-arched palate, hooked nose |
| Cutis laxa, #219100 Type I<br>Autosomal recessive<br>*604580, FBLN5, 14q32.1<br>*604633, FBLN4, 5q23.3 | Early infancy | Hip dislocation, lax joints, Cutis laxa | Cor pulmonale, tortuous arteries, arterial aneurysms, fibromuscular renal artery dysplasia, multiple pulmonary artery stenoses, hernias |
| Cutis laxa type II, %219200<br>Autosomal recessive<br>Gene unknown | Early infancy | Loose, redundant folds, facial skin unaffected, slow return on stretching | Widely persistent fonta-nelles, slight oxycephaly, dental caries, frontal bossing, reversed-V eyebrows, downward slanted palpebral fissures, intrauterine growth retardation, inguinal hernia |
| Pyrroline-5-carboxylate synthetase +138250, P5CS, 10q24.3 | Childhood | Familial joint hyperlaxity, skin hyperelasticity, | Cataract, mental retardation, hyperammonemia, low citrulline, ornithine and proline |
| Ullrich myopathy, #254090 collagen type VI<br>*120220, COL6A1, 21q22.3<br>*120240, COL6A2, 21q22.3<br>*120250, COL6A3, 2q37 | Birth to early infancy | Hypermobility of distal interphalangeal joints, cheloid scars, follicular keratosis | Muscle weakness, respira-tory failure, failure to thrive slender build, high-arched palate, torticollis |

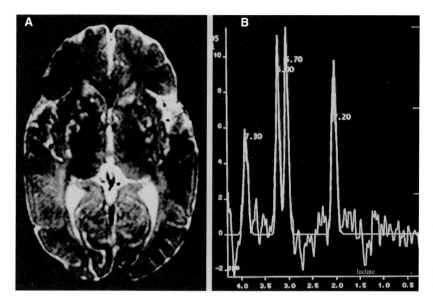

Fig. 1. Neuroradiological examination in a 1-year-old child with EPEMA syndrome. (**A**) The T2 weighted MR axial image of the brain shows iperintense areas of the basal ganglia. (**B**) Corresponds to a single voxel MR spectroscopy showing a typical lactate peak in the brain tissue (right putamen).

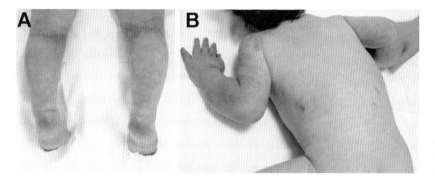

Fig. 2. Clinical dermatological appearance of the same 1-year-old child of Fig. 1 showing acrocianosis in his feet (**A**), arms and hands (**B**).

the hepatocerebral form of mitochondrial DNA depletion syndrome (MDDS) due to mutations in the nuclear-encoded mitochondrial deoxyguanosine kinase gene DGUOK; [#601465] (Mandel et al. 2001) or in the MPV17 gene [#137960] (Spinazzola et al. 2006).

Another characteristic finding of mitochondrial encephalomyopathies is hirsutism or hypertrichosis that has been reported in patients with Pearson syndrome and quite frequently in the severe Leigh syndrome with encephalomyopathy, cytochrome-c-oxidase deficiency and mutations in the SURF-1 [#185620] gene.

## Peroxisomal disorders

Peroxisomes are small, ubiquitous, cellular organelles that have an important role in oxygen, lipid, and glu-cose metabolism. More than 50 biochemical pathways have been characterized within peroxisomes. Some of the major peroxisomal functions are peroxisomal oxidation and respiration, the regulation of adipose cell number, the transport and cellular uptake of lipids, intracellular balance between free and bound fatty acids, conversion of fatty acids to their activated CoA form, penetration of fatty acids into membrane-delineated organelles, microsomal ω-oxidation, β-oxidation and ketogenesis, and the formation of glycerol for triglyceride synthesis, cholesterol synthesis, as well as sex steroid metabolism, plasmalogen biosynthesis, insulin sensitivity, catabolism of purines and D-amino acids, L-α-hydroxy acids, and urates, and metabolism of a diverse group of xenobiotics (Masters 1998, Wanders and Tager 1998, Titorenko and Mullen 2006, Wanders and Waterham 2006).

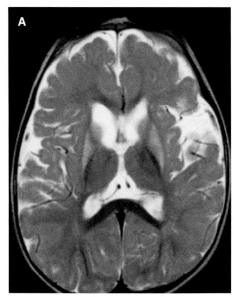

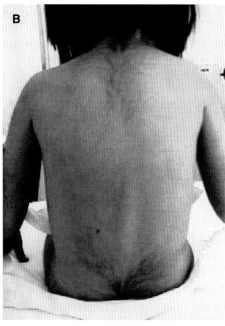

Fig. 3. (**A**) Shows the typical pattern of a Leigh syndrome in a child with citochomo c oxidase with a Surf-1 mutation: the T2 weighed MRI image shows abnormal hyperintensity of both putamen nuclei. (**B**) Shows marked hisutism in the dorsal skin ares of the same child.

There are at least 24 disorders identified that are caused by inherited peroxisomal defects (Haikoop et al. 1990, Emami et al. 1992, Hamaguchi et al. 1995, Sato et al. 1996, Baumgartner et al. 1998, Moser

and Raymond 1998, Kelley et al. 1999, DiPreta et al. 2000, Moser 1999).

Until recently peroxisomal disorders were listed under three main clinical syndromes: Zellweger syndrome (ZS), neonatal adrenoleukodystrophy (NALD), and infantile Refsum disease (IRD). Polymalformations occur in classic ZS, as well as in rhizomelic (autosomal recessive) chondrodysplasia punctata (RCDP), X-linked dominant or recessive CDP [XCDP2 (Conradi–Hunermann–Happle syndrome], autosomal recessive CDP, and congenital hemidysplasia with ichthyosiform erythroderma and limb defects (CHILD) syndrome (Emami et al. 1992, Haikoop et al. 1990, Hamaguchi et al. 1995, Sato et al. 1996, Baumgartner et al. 1998, Moser and Raymond 1998, Kelley et al. 1999). Neurologic manifestations predominate in NALD, and hepatodigestive manifestations in IRD (Baumgartner et al. 1998). However, with expansion in the understanding of the biochemical phenotypes within the spectrum of peroxisomal disorders, it has become obvious that there is little or no relationship between the clinical and biochemical phenotypes (Baumgartner et al. 1998) (see Table 9).

RCDP, XCDP2, autosomal recessive CDP, and CHILD syndrome are the syndromes most commonly associated with significant cutaneous manifestations (Table 9), and each syndrome is associated with one or more of a number of peroxisomal-related biochemical abnormalities (Table 8) or morphologic abnormalities listed in Table 9. Conversely, the same biochemical defect(s), or even the same genetic complementation group, can be associated with different clinical phenotypes, i.e., classic ZS and IRD and a form of X-linked dominant CDP (XCDP2) and CHILD syndrome (Moser 1999). Thus, a newer classification of peroxisomal disorders has been proposed based on the extent of peroxisomal dysfunction (Table 9). However, this biochemical classification is not helpful for evaluation of the clinical symptoms. Peroxisomal disorders are classified genetically as those in which the organelle is not formed normally [disorders of peroxisome biogenesis (PBD)] and those that involve a single peroxisomal enzyme (Moser 1999). Twelve PBD disorders have been defined, and molecular defects have been identified in 10 of them, all involving defects in pro-

**Table 8.** Biochemical assays for the diagnosis of peroxisomal disorders

| Biological material | Assay |
|---|---|
| Plasma | VLCFAs; phytanic and pristanic acids; THCA and DHCA; pipecolic acid, plasmalogens, and PUFAs including DHA, and 8-dehydrocholesterol and cholest-8(9)-en-3b-ol |
| Urines | Organic acids and pipecolic acid |
| Red blood cells | Plasmalogens and PUFAs including DHA |
| Fibroblasts | Plasmalogen biosynthesis, DHAPAT, and alkyl-DHAP synthase particle-bound catalase; VLCFAs, b-oxidation, and phytanic acid oxidation; immunoblotting b-oxidation proteins |
| Liver | Cytochemical localization of peroxisomal proteins, trilamellar inclusions, and insoluble lipid |

*VLCFAs* Very-long chain fatty acids; *THCA* trihydroxycholestanoic acid; *DHCA* dihydroxycholestanoic acid; *CA* cholic acid; *CDCA* chenodeoxycholic acid; *DHAPAT* dihydroxyacetone phosphate acyltransferase; *DHAP* dihydroxyacetone phosphate; *PUFAs* polyunsaturated fatty acids; *DHA* docosahexaenoic acid.

tein import mechanisms (Moser 1999). Cytoplasmic polyribosomes synthesize peroxisomal matrix proteins, which are imported posttranslationally. Factors required for this import of peroxisomal proteins are called peroxins (PEX) (Moser 1999).

CDP is a pattern of abnormal punctate calcification of dystrophic epiphyseal cartilage and certain other cartilaginous structures. Peroxisomal disorders are the most common associations. However, CDP is seen with other genetic conditions, e.g., gangliosidosis, mucolipidosis II, trisomy 21, and can be acquired *in utero* secondary to warfarin embryopathy, phenacetin, fetal alcohol, and hydantoin (Lawrence et al. 1989).

CDP is a consistent finding in a group of peroxisomal disorders, especially those with characteristic but variable cutaneous manifestations (Moser 1999). Qualitative and quantitative peroxisomal dysregulation is demonstrated in most cases of RCDP, XCDP2, autosomal dominant CDP, and CHILD syndrome, and specific genetic defects have been identified in RCDP and in some patients with XCDP2 and CHILD syndrome (Moser 1999).

The phenotypic expression of the known PEX disorders and enzymatic defects appear to vary with the nature of the mutation. In general, the severe forms manifest as classical Zellweger syndrome, while milder phenotypes manifest as NALD and infantile Refsum disease, and are associated with mutations that do not abolish function completely or are associated with mosaicism. Thus, with the

continued identification of a specific molecular defects, hopefully there will not only be better genetic counseling and better estimates of prognoses, as well as improved understanding of the divergent and overlapping spectrum of clinical findings in these diseases.

Other associated clinical findings vary but include cataracts, short stature, dysmorphic facies, a variety of skeletal malformations, and an ichthyosiform erythroderma in the neonatal period. The cutaneous manifestations range from a ichthyosiform erythroderma with adherent scales to psoriasiform hyperplasia, and are often arranged in a linear or whorled pattern on the trunk and limbs, especially in patients with X-linked dominant inheritance.

The random X chromosome inactivation (lyonization in the blastocyst) leads to the linear and whorled pattern of the cutaneous manifestations following Blashko's lines (Prendiville et al. 1991). Cutaneous manifestations often improve and may resolve in 3–6 months, especially in patients with XCDP2. However, the cutaneous lesions are commonly followed by a permanent, patterned, follicular atrophoderma in the earlier areas of hyperkeratosis.

A patchy cicatricial alopecia as well as coarse, lusterless hair can also be seen. XCDP2 has a relatively good prognosis and frequently shows asymmetrical bone defects, cataracts, and skin lesions, while RCDP is more severe as a bilateral and diffuse disease and patients usually die within the first year of life.

**Table 9.** Summary of peroxisomal disorders

| Disorder | Skin lesions | Morphology of peroxisomes | Molecular disorder |
|---|---|---|---|
| Peroxiome biogenesis disorder withloss of multiple peroxisomal functions | | Absent/ mosaicism | Caused by mutations in any of several different genes involved in peroxisome biogenesis: peroxin-1 (PEX1; 602136), peroxin-2 (PEX2; 170993), peroxin-3 (PEX3; 603164), peroxin-5 (PEX5; 600414), peroxin-6 (PEX6; 601498), peroxin-12 (PEX12; 601758), peroxin-14 (PEX14; 601791), and peroxin-26 (PEX26; 608666) |
| • Classical ZS | Facial dysmorphia | | |
| • NALD | Facial dysmorphia | | |
| • Infantile Refsum disease | Facial dysmorphia | | |
| Peroxisome biogenesis disorder with loss of at least 2 peroxisomal functions | | | PEX7 gene (601757), which encodes the peroxisomal type 2 targeting signal (PTS2) receptor |
| • RCDP (classic and atypical phenotype | Icythosiform # Limb defects | Enlarged | Deficiency of plasmalogens in phospholipids from red cells and deficient activity of the enzyme DHAPAT |
| • Unclassified peroxisomal biogenesis disorder | | Present or absent | |
| Loss of a single peroxisomal function | | | |
| • RCDP | Icythosiform # Limb defects Alopecia | Normal | Isolated DHAPAT or alkyl-DHAP XCDP2; XCDP1 synthase |
| • XCDP2 CHILD* | Icythosiform # Follicular atrophoderma Limb defects | Normal | Abnormal sterol metabolism with increased 8-dehydrocholesterol and cholest-8(9)en- 3β-ol deficiency 3β-hydroxysteroid-Δ8, Δ7-isomerase |
| • CHILD* | Icythosiform # | Decreased | DHAPAT and catalase decreased |
| • X-linked adrenoleukodystrophy | Hyperpigmentation | Present | ALD protein |
| • Peudo-NALD | | Enlarged | Acyl-CoA oxidase |
| • Bifuntional enzyme deficiency | Facial dysmorphia | Abnormal | Bi(tri)functional enzyme deficiency. |
| • Pseudo-Zellweger sindrome | Facial dysmorphia | Enlarged | Peroxisomal 3-oxoacyl-CoA thiolase |
| • Mevalonic aciduria | Morbilliform rash Edema | NA | Mevalonate kinase |
| • Trihydroxycholestanoic acidemia | Facial dysmorphia | NA | Branched chain acyl-CoA oxidase |
| • Classic Refsum disease | Icythosiform # | NA | Phytanoxyl-CoA hydroxylase |
| • Glutaric aciduria type III | | Normal | Peroxisomal glutaryl-CoA oxidase |
| • Hyperoxaluria type I | Livedo racemosa like erythema of the limbs | Smaller | Alanine glyoxylate aminotransferase |
| • Acatasemia | Ulcers/gangrene | Normal | Catalase |

*DHAPAT* Dihydroxyacetone phosphate acyltransferase; *CDP* chondrodysplasia punctata; *X* X chromosome; *X1* X-linked recessive; *X2* X-linked dominant; *CHILD* congenital hemidysplasia with ichthyosiform erythroderma and limb defects; *DHAP* dihydroxyacetone phophate; *ALD* adrenoleukodystrophy; *NALD* neonatal adrenoleukodystrophy; *CoA* coenzyme A; *NA* information not available. *ZS* Zellweger syndrome; *NALD* neonatal adrenoleukodystrophy; *RCDP* rhizomelic chondrodysplasia punctata; *XCDP2* X-linked dominant chondrodysplasia punctata. #With X-linked dominant inheritance as in XCDP2 and CHILD syndrome the icythosiform eruption follows Blaskho's line because of random inactivation of one X chromosome. *Often with a more psoriasiform with an associated inflammatory component.

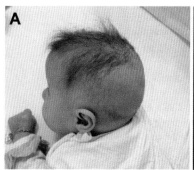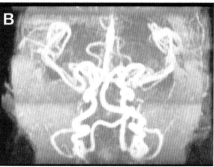

**Fig. 4.** Clinical representation of a 1 and a half year old child with a Menkes disease. (**A**) Year-old-child shows the classical aspect of the brittle and fragile hair. (**B**) Shows kinky deformation of the brain vessels.

CHILD syndrome is characterized by unilateral ichthyosiform erythroderma which, unlike XCDP2, is often inflammatory with psoriasiform hyperplasia, even though most cases show a similar X-linked dominant inheritance following Blashko's lines (Emami et al. 1992). Additional clinical findings in patients with CHILD syndrome include ipsilateral limb-reduction defects and, in some cases, ipsilateral internal organ defects. Partial resolution of the cutaneous manifestations may occur in CHILD syndrome, but it is not as characteristic as in XCDP2, and internal organ involvement is not characteristic of XCDP2.

Characteristic and very useful to suspect the diagnosis is skin discoloration in Addison disease and leukodystrophy – Adrenoleukodystrophy (ALD) or the spastic paraplegia variant called Adrenomyeloneuropathy, a X-linked disorder combining due to the deficiency of the ALD protein (see Tables 2 and 9). ALD affects approximately 1 in 20,000 to 1 in 50,000 individuals from all races. It results in the accumulation of long chain fatty acids in the nervous system, adrenal gland, and testes, which disrupts normal activity. There are seven recognized clinical forms of the disease. The childhood cerebral form appears in mid-childhood (at 4–8 years), and the other forms appear during adolescence or adulthood as Cerebral forms or Adrenomyeloneuropathy. About two-thirds of affected people develop neurological symptoms, and more than half develop abnormal adrenal function. In the childhood form, early symptoms include hyperactivity, difficulty at school, difficulty understanding spoken material, deterioration of handwriting, crossed eyes (strabismus), and

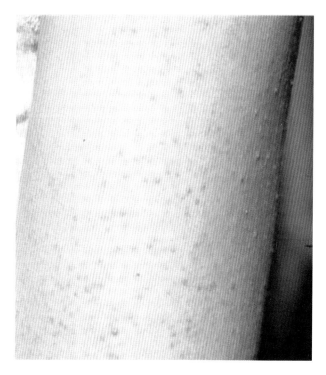

**Fig. 5.** Hyperkeratosis follicolaris: follicular papular erithematous and white lesions in a 10-years-old child affected by Ullrich congenital muscular dystrophy.

possibly seizures. As the disease progresses, particularly the severe childhood form, further signs of damage to the white matter of the brain appear; changes in muscle tone occur, stiffness and contracture deformities, swallowing difficulties, and coma. The other major component of adrenoleukodystrophy is the development of impaired adrenal gland function (similar to Addison disease). There is a deficiency of steroid hormones. This is a very signifi-

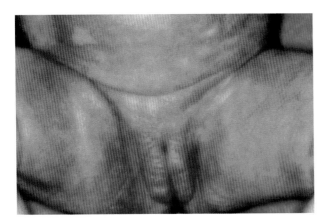

**Fig. 6.** Infiltrated erytroderma in an infant affected by early diagnosis of Chanarin-Dorfan disease.

cant development but one that can be adequately treated with corticosteroids.

In other peroxisomal diseases, there may be no cutaneous manifestations, although facial dysmorphism and/or cataracts occur in a large percentage of patients with ZS, and NALD. Patients with RD are unable to α-oxidize phytanic acid and often present with a noninflammatory ichythosiform eruption (Baumgartner et al. 1998). Although the underlying mechanism is different, an inability to α-oxidize phytanic acid also occurs in RCDP. In patients with acatalasemia, there is a catalase deficiency and an increased incidence of oral ulcerations or gangrene (Baumgartner et al. 1998).

## Aminoacidopathies

Usually, genetic disorders of aminoacid metabolism may be accompanied by distinguishing cutaneous manifestations that can be summarized as following:

1. Hypopigmentation, photosensitivity, dry skin, scleroderma-like skin lesions in phenylketonuria. (Hartmann et al. 2004) (Tables 2 and 5).
2. Painful palmoplantar hyperkeratosis in tyrosinemia type II (Saijo et al. 1991) (Table 3).
3. Black-bluish dyschromia of sun-exposed skin such as helices, nose, and sclera in alkaptonuria (ochronosis, caused by mutation in the homogentisate 1,2 dioxygenase, an enzyme involved in the

catabolism of phenylalanine and tyrosine) (Phornphutkul et al. 2002).
4. Dry, brittle hair, periorificial erythema, acrodermatitis enteropathica (maple syrup disease, homocystinuria, arginine amber acid syndrome, glutaric aciduria type I, holocarboxylase synthetase enzyme deficiency, biotinidase deficiency) (Perafan-Riveros et al. 2002) (Table 1).
5. Photosensitivity, stomatitis, glossitis, diarrhea, cerebellar ataxia, emotional instability, and amino aciduria in Hartnup syndrome due to mutations in the SLC6A19 gene, a system B(0) transporter that mediates epithelial resorption of neutral amino acids across the apical membrane in the kidney and intestine (Kleta et al. 2004) (Table 2).
6. Renal failure, pulmonary alveolar proteinosis, and skin lesions of lupus-like autoimmune symptoms (Lysinuric protein intolerance, a disorder of dibasic amino acid transport secondary to mutation of the SLC7A7 gene characterized by usually increased plasma citrulline) (Mannucci et al. 2005).

## Lysosomal diseases

Lysosomal storage disorders (LSDs)1 are a group of over 50 inherited diseases, which have a combined incidence of 1:7700 to 1:8275 live births (Meikle et al. 1999, Dionisi-Vici et al. 2002). Each disorder is caused by the dysfunction of either a lysosomal enzyme or a lysosome associated protein involved in enzyme activation, enzyme targeting, or lysosomal biogenesis. These defects lead to the accumulation of substrate that would normally be degraded in the endosome–lysosome system. In severely affected patients, this ultimately leads to the chronic and progressive deterioration of affected cells, tissues, and organs. Most LSDs display a broad spectrum of clinical manifestations, which have been previously identified as clinical subtypes [such as the Hurler/Scheie definition of mucopolysaccharidosis (MPS) I and the infantile-, juvenile-, and adult-onset forms of Pompe disease]. Some of the clinical symptoms that are observed in multiple LSDs (e.g., most of the MPSs) include bone abnormalities, organomegaly, coarse hair/facies, and central nervous system (CNS) dysfunction (Meunzer and Neufeld 2001). At the severe end of the clinical spectrum, the onset of pathology tends to be rapid and progressive, whereas at the attenuated end, disease each with a broad spectrum of clinical presentation that ranges from attenuated to severe. With the advent of molecular biology/genetics and the characterization of many of the genes associated with LSDs, it has now recognized that the range of clinical severity may in part be ascribed to different mutations within the same gene. However, genotype–phenotype correlations are not always informative.

Coarse facies is a recurrent symptom in many LSDs (Table 4). A pecular skin lesion is angiokeratoma corporis diffusum characteristic of Fabry disease, is an X chromosomal recessive α-galactosidase deficiency with deposition of ceramide trihexoside in various internal organs including kidney and heart. Typical cutaneous manifestations are erythematous-teleangiectatic papules on the periumbilical area, lower abdomen, and buttocks (angiokeratomas). (Levin 2006). Gaucher disease (acid-beta glucosidase deficiency), Niemann-Pick disease (acid sphingomyelinase deficiency) and Farber disease (acid ceramidase deficiency) may lead to the development of hyperpigmentations of the face and periarticular brown papules (Zappatini-Tommasi et al. 1992, Raddadi and Twaim 2000, Sidransky 2004).

## Porphyrias

### Porphyrin metabolism: porphyrias

The mostly genetically caused disturbances of porphyrinogens and of heme are responsible for 8 differ-

ent metabolic disorders (Table 2). Porphyrias may be either acute or nonacute. Most forms of genetic porphyria are dominantly inherited: a) #21300 Acute porphyria due to coproporphyrinogen oxidase deficiency; b) #176000 Acute intermittent porphyria, caused by mutation in the gene encoding hydroxymethylbilane synthase (HMBS; 609806), characterized by light-sensitive dermatitis and associated with the excretion of large amounts of uroporphyrin in urine also referred to as porphobilinogen deaminase (PBGD); c) #176100 Porphyria cutanea tarda is an autosomal dominant caused by Uroporphyrinogen decarboxylase; d) #176200 Porphyria variegata disorder is caused by mutations in the gene for protoporphyrinogen oxidase. Acute hepatic porphyria is ap-

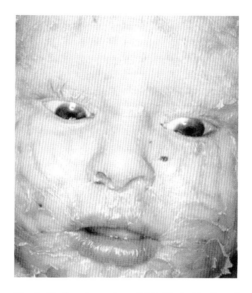

**Fig. 7.** Erythroderma in a child affected by lamellar icthyosis. Notice the large desquamation, ectropion at the level of the lower left eyelid, and mild eclabion.

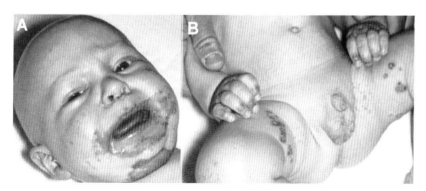

**Fig. 8.** A 6 months old male infant affected achrodermatitis enteropathica. Notice the alopecia and very rare eyelashes and eyebrows. Periorificial erosions are evident in (**A**). Bullous lesions are also seen in (**B**) localized on the perianal and perineal regions, on hand fingers. All the cutaneous manifestations appeared when the child stopped breast feeding.

parently recessive (#125270) caused by deficiency of delta-aminolevulinate dehydratase deficiency and congenital erythropoietic porphyria is caused by dominant mutations in the uroporphyrinogen III synthase gene.

Clinically porphyrias can be differentiated into erythropoietic and hepatic types (Lecha et al. 2003, Norman 2005).

## Nonacute erythropoietic porphyrias

The congenital erythropoietic porphyria is an autosomal recessive condition generally caused by mutation in the uroporphyrinogen III synthase gene (UROS; 606938) and is characterized by a severe photosensitivity, sunburns within the first summer of life, and bullae formation. The newborns show a reddish-brown urine. They experience pain and pruritus during sun exposure. Later and more chronically, symptoms include bullae formation, scars, pigment changes, mutilations, hypertrichosis, and erythrodontia in UV-A light.

The erythropoietic protoporphyria shows redness and swelling of sun-exposed skin and rarely hemorrhages.

Severe pruritus develops with delay after sun exposure. Orange-like skin may develop on the nose and the hands. In 5% of cases, liver cirrhosis develops, which more common is a protoporphyrin cholelithiasis.

## Nonacute/chronic hepatic porphyria

Porphyria cutanea tarda is a common acquired (type I) or hereditary autosomal-dominant (type II) metabolic disease with increased skin fragility of sun-exposed skin (hands, head), grayish discoloration of the face, periorbicular hypertrichosis (in women, also on the limbs), chronic conjunctivitis (ca 50% of cases), elastosis, milia, and pruritus.

Rare cutaneous manifestations include pseudoscleroderma, alopecia porphyria, centrofacial papular lymphangiectasia, purpura, lichenoid plaques of the hands, chronic erosive cheilitis, onycholysis, and recoloring of gray hair.

Porphyria cutanea tarda is associated with diabetes mellitus in 17%, with 20% of patients developing Dupuytren fibromatosis. Approximately 1% of the patients have lupus erythematosus, and 60% show homozygote or heterozygote HFE mutations. Hepatitis C infection is found more often than and independent from the hepatitis C frequency in the general population.

The extremely rare (only 40 case reports in the literature) homozygote hepatoerythropoietic porphyria shows cutaneous symptoms like those of congenital erythropoietic porphyria.

## Acute hepatic porphyrias

Acute hepatic porphyria can be caused by recessive mutations in the gene coding for delta-aminolevulinate dehydratase deficiency or dominant mutations in the gene coding for coproporphyrinogen oxidase (#121300) and may show cutaneous symptoms such as porphyria cutanea tarda.

## Metal toxicity disorders

### Iron metabolism: hemochromatosis

The most common single-gene metabolic disorder in Europe is hemochromatosis (HFE) with a prevalence of 1:400. At least 7 iron-overload disorders labeled hemochromatosis have been identified on the basis of clinical, biochemical, and genetic characteristics. a) Classic hemochromatosis is autosomal recessive (AR) #235200 caused by mutation in a gene designated HFE on chromosome 6p21.3; it has also been found to be caused by mutations in the gene encoding hemojuvelin (HJV; #608374), which maps to 1q21. b) Juvenile AR hemochromatosis or hemochromatosis type 2 is also AR, #602390. One form, designated HFE2A, is caused by mutation in the HJV gene. A second form, designated HFE2B, is caused by mutation in the gene encoding hepcidin antimicrobial peptide (HAMP; #606464), which maps to 19q13. c) Hemochromatosis type 3 (HFE3; 604250), an autosomal recessive disorder, is caused by mutation in the gene

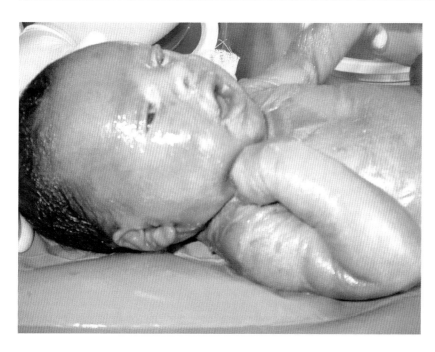

**Fig. 9.** A 10 months old child affected by trichothiodystrophy. Notice the follicular hyperkeratosis at the chins, and rare and brittle hair. Icthyosis is evident at the scalp.

encoding transferrin receptor-2 (TFR2; 604720), which maps to 7q22. d) Hemochromatosis type 4 (HFE4; #606069), an autosomal dominant disorder, is caused by mutation in the SLC40A1 gene (#604653), which encodes ferroportin and maps to 2q32.

The underlying disturbance is a defect in intestinal iron absorption (Beutler et al. 2003, Pietrangelo 2006). An early diagnosis is possible because of HFE gene analysis. The treatment of choice is blood letting.

Recently, an association with porphyria cutanea tarda could be demonstrated (Stolzel et al. 2003).

Bluish-gray hyperpigmentations are seen on the light exposed sebostatic scaling skin areas. Bronze diabetes with liver cirrhosis, hypogonadism, and loss of libido are found in more advanced cases. Hyperpigmentation of mucous membranes and conjunctival membranes occur in 15–20% of patients. There can be a loss of axillary and pubic hairs because of hepatotesticular insufficiency.

## Zinc metabolism: acrodermatitis enteropathica

Acrodermatitis enteropathica (#201100) is a rare autosomal recessive metabolic disorder caused by mutation in the intestinal zinc-specific transporter SLC39A4 (#607059).

The clinical presentation manifests in newborns. In later life, zinc deficiency can develop because of chronic alcoholism, parenteral nutrition, and chronic intestinal disease.

Characteristically, there are periorificial and acral erythemas with vesiculation mimicking acute atopic dermatitis (Fig. 8) or exudative psoriasis. Typically, one can see chronic paronychia, dystrophic nail plates, and diffuse alopecia that can develop into alopecia totalis. Chronic mucositis can develop in the oral cavity, including glossitis, on the conjunctiva, outer ear canal, and anogenital mucous membranes.

## Copper metabolism: Menkes syndrome and Wilson disease

The most common copper pathway disturbances are Menkes disease in childhood and Wilson disease in adolescence and adulthood.

Menkes disease (#309400) is a rare X-chromosomal disease due to the mutation in the gene encoding Cu(2+)-transporting ATPase, alpha polypeptide (300011) ATP7A (Shim and Harris

2003). It is manifested by cutaneous discoloration, kinky and brittle hair and central nervous symptoms with anticonvulsive resistant epilepsy and mental retardation. MRI brain angiography shows a kinky deformation of the brain vessels (Fig. 4B).

Wilson disease (#277900) is caused by mutation in the ATPase, CU(2+)-transporting, beta polypeptide (606882) ATP7B, a membrane copper-transport protein (Kitzberger et al. 2005). Clinically, patients suffer of a progressive severe dystonia, and skin manifestations are characterized by reticulated brownish hyperpigmentation of the lower legs, blue lunulae, and corneal pigmentation known as Kayser-Fleischer ring. There is additionally a premature graying of the hair and development of liver cirrhosis.

## References

Baumgartner MR, Poll-The BT, Verhoeven NM, Jakobs C, Espeel M, Roels F, Rabier D, Levade T, Rolland MO, Martinez M, Wanders RJ, Saudubray JM (1998) Clinical approach to inherited peroxisomal disorders: a series of 27 patients. Ann Neurol 44: 720–730.

Beutler E, Hoffbrand AV, Cook JD (2003) Iron deficiency and overload. Hematology Am Soc Hematol Educ Program Book, pp. 40–61.

Bieri F (1993) Peroxisome proliferators and cellular signaling pathways: a review. Biol Cell 77: 43–44.

Burlina AB, Dionisi-Vici C, Bennett MJ, Gibson KM, Servidei S, Bertini E, Hale DE, Schmidt-Sommerfeld E, Sabetta G, Zacchello F, Rinaldo P (1994) A new syndrome with ethylmalonic aciduria and normal fatty acid oxidation in fibroblasts. J Pediatr 124: 79–86.

Calabresi PA, Silvestri G, DiMauro S, Griggs RC (1994) Ekbom's syndrome: lipomas, ataxia, and neuropathy with MERRF. Muscle Nerve 17: 943–945.

Dionisi-Vici C, Rizzo C, Burlina AB, Caruso U, Sabetta G, Uziel G, Abeni D (2002) Inborn errors of metabolism in the Italian pediatric population: a national retrospective survey. J Pediatr 140: 321–327.

DiPreta EA, Smith KJ, Skelton H (2000) Cholesterol metabolsim defect associated with Conradi-Hunerman-Happle syndrome. Int J Dermatol 39: 846–850.

Ekbom K (1975) Hereditary ataxia, photomyoclonus, skeletal deformities, and lipoma. Acta Neurol Scand 51: 393–404.

Emami S, Rizzo WB, Hanley KP, Taylor JM, Goldyne ME, Williams ML (1992) Peroxisomal abnormality in fibroblasts from involved skin of CHILD syndrome. Arch Dermatol 128: 1213–1222.

Flynn MK, Wee SA, Lane AT (1998) Skin manifestations of mitochondrial DNA syndromes: case report and review. J Am Acad Dermatol 39: 819–823.

Garcia-Silva M, Ribes A, Campos Y, Garavaglia B, Arenas J (1997) Syndrome of encephalopathy, petechiae, and ethylmalonic aciduria. Ped Neurol 17: 165–170.

Haferkamp O, Scheuerle A, Schlenk R, Melzner I, Pavenstadt-Grupp I, Rodel G (1994) Mitochondrial complex I and III mutations and neutral-lipid storage in activated mononuclear macrophages and neutrophils: a case presenting with necrotizing myopathy, poikiloderma atrophicans vasculare, and xanthogranulomatous bursitis. Hum Pathology 25: 419–423.

Hamaguchi T, Bondar G, Siegfried E, Penneys NS (1995) Cutaneous histopathology of Conradi–Hunermann syndrome. J Cutan Pathol 22: 38–41.

Hartmann A, Brocker EB, Becker JC (2004) Hypopigmentary skin disorders: current treatment options and future directions. Drugs 64: 89–81.

Heikoop JC, van Roermund CW, Just WW, Ofman R, Schutgens RB, Heymans HS, Wanders RJ, Tager JM (1990) Rhizomelic chondrodysplasia punctata: deficiency of 3-oxoacyl-coenzyme A thiolase in peroxisomes and impaired processing of the enzyme. J Clin Invest 86: 126–130.

Holt IJ, Harding AE, Morgan-Hughes JA (1988) Deletions of muscle mitochondrial DNA in patients with mitochondrial myopathies. Nature 331: 717–719.

Kelley RI, Wilcox WG, Smith M, Kratz LE, Moser A, Rimoin DS (1999) Abnormal sterol metabolism in patients with Conradi-Hunermann-Happle syndrome and sporadic lethal chondrodysplasia punctata. Am J Med Genet 83: 213–219.

Kitzberger R, Madl C, Ferenci P (2005) Wilson disease. Metab Brain Dis Dec 20(4): 295–302. Review.

Kleta R, Romeo E, Ristic Z, Ohura T, Stuart C, Arcos-Burgos M, Dave MH, Wagner CA, Camargo SR, Inoue S, Matsuura N, Helip-Wooley A, Bockenhauer D, Warth R, Bernardini I, Visser G, Eggermann T, Lee P, Chairoungdua A, Jutabha P, Babu E, Nilwarangkoon S, Anzai N, Kanai Y, Verrey F, Gahl WA, Koizumi A (2004) Mutations in SLC6A19, encoding B0AT1, cause Hartnup disorder. Nat Genet 36: 999–1002.

Lawrence JJ, Schlesinger AE, Kozlowski K, Poznanski AK, Bacha L, Dreyer GL, Barylak A, Sillence DO, Rager K (1989) Unusual radiographic manifestations of chondrodysplasia punctata. Skeletal Radiol 18: 15–19.

Lecha M, Herrero C, Ozalla D (2003) Diagnosis and treatment of the hepatic porphyrias. Dermatol Ther 16: 65–72.

Levin M (2006) Fabry disease. Drugs Today (Barc) 42: 65–70.

Mandel H, Szargel R, Labay V, Elpeleg O, Saada A, Shalata A, Anbinder Y, Berkowitz D, Hartman C, Barak M, Eriksson S, Cohen N (2001) The deoxyguanosine kinase gene is mutated in individuals with depleted hepatocerebral mitochondrial DNA. Nature Genet 29: 337–341.

Mannucci L, Emma F, Markert M, Bachmann C, Boulat O, Carrozzo R, Rizzoni G, Dionisi-Vici C (2005) Increased NO production in lysinuric protein intolerance. J Inherit Metab Dis 28: 123–129.

Masters CJ (1998) On the role of the peroxisome in the metabolism of drugs and xenobiotics. Biochem Pharmacol 56: 667–673.

Meikle PJ, Hopwood JJ, Clague AE, Carey WF (1999) Prevalence of lysosomal storage disorders. JAMA 281: 249–254.

Meunzer J, Neufeld EF (2001) The mucopolysaccharidoses. In: Scriver CR, Beaudet AL, Sly WS, Vaile D (eds.) The Metabolic and Molecular Basis of Inherited Disease, 8th edn. New York: McGraw-Hill, pp. 3421–3452.

McShane M, Hammans S, Sweeney M, Holt I, Beattie T, Brett E, Harding AE (1991) Pearson syndrome and mitochondrial encephalomyopathy in a patient with a deletion of mtDNA. Am J Hum Genet 48: 39–42.

Moraes CT, Shanske S, Tritschler H-J, Aprille JR, Andreetta F, Bonilla E (1991) MtDNA depletion with variable tissue expression: a novel genetic abnormality in mitochondrial diseases. Am J Hum Genet 48: 492–501.

Mori K, Narahara K, Ninomiya S, Goto Y, Nonaka I (1991) Renal and skin involvement in a patient with complete Kearns-Sayre syndrome. Am J Hum Genet 38: 583–587.

Moser HW, Raymond GV (1998) Genetic peroxisomal disorder: why, when, and how to test. Am Neurol Assoc 44: 713–715.

Moser HW (1999) Genotype–phenotype correlations in disorders of peroxisome biogenesis. Mol Genet Metab 68: 316–327.

Niaudet P, Heidet L, Munnich A, Schmitz J, Bouissou F, Gubler MC, Rotig A (1994) Deletion of the mitochondrial DNA in a case of de Toni-Debré-Fanconi syndrome and Pearson syndrome. Ped Nephrol 8: 164–168.

Nørby S, Lestienne P, Nelson I, Nielsen I, Schmalbruch H, Sjo O, Warburg M (1994) Juvenile Kearns-Sayre syndrome initially misdiagnosed as a psychosomatic disorder. J Med Genet 31: 45–50.

Norman RA (2005) Past and future: porphyria and porphyrins. Skinmed 4: 287–292.

Ohno K, Yamamoto M, Engel AG, Harper CM, Roberts LR, Tan GH, Fatourechi V (1996) MELAS- and Kearns-Sayre-type comutation with myopathy and autoimmune polyendocrinopathy. Ann Neurol 39: 761–766.

Ostergaard E, Bradinova I, Ravn SH, Hansen FJ, Simeonov E, Christensen E, Wibrand F, Schwartz M (2005) Hy-

pertrichosis in patients with SURF1 mutations. Am J Med Genet A 138: 384–388.

Perafan-Riveros C, Franca LF, Alves AC, Sanches JA Jr (2002) Acrodermatitis enteropathica: case report and review of the literature. Pediatr Dermatol 19: 426–431.

Phornphutkul C, Introne WJ, Perry MB, Bernardini I, Murphey MD, Fitzpatrick DL, Anderson PD, Huizing M, Anikster Y, Gerber LH, Gahl WA (2002) Natural history of alkaptonuria. N Engl J Med 347: 2111–2121.

Pietrangelo A (2006) Hereditary hemochromatosis. Annu Rev Nutr 26: 251–270.

Prendiville JS, Zaparackas ZG, Esterly NB (1991) Normal peroxisomal function and absent skeletal manifestations in Conradi-Hunermann syndrome. Arch Dermatol 127: 539–542.

Raddadi AA, Twaim AA (2000) Type A Niemann-Pick disease. J Eur Acad Dermatol Venereol 14: 301–303.

Rötig A, Cormier V, Blanche S, Bonnefont J-P, Ledeist F, Romero N, Schmitz J, Rustin P, Fischer A, Saudubray JM, Munnich A (1990) Pearson's marrow-pancreas syndrome: a multisystem mitochondrial disorder in infancy. J Clin Invest 86: 1601–1608.

Rötig A, Bessis J-L, Romero N, Cormier V, Saudubray JM, Narcy P, Lenoir G, Rustin P, Munnich A (1992) Maternally inherited duplication of the mitochondrial genome in a syndrome of proximal tubulopathy, diabetes mellitus, and cerebellar ataxia. Am J Hum Genet 50: 364–370.

Rötig A, Lehnert A, Rustin P, Chretien D, Bourgeron T, Niaudet P, Munnich A (1995) Kidney involvement in mitochondrial disorders. Adv Nephrol 24: 367–378.

Saijo S, Kudoh K, Kuramoto Y, Horii I, Tagami H (1991) Tyrosinemia II: report of an incomplete case and studies on the hyperkeratotic stratum corneum. Dermatologica 182: 168–171.

Sato M, Ishikawa X, Miyachi X (1996) X-linked dominant chondrodysplasia punctata with decreased dihydroxyacetone phosphate acyltransferase activity. Dermatology 192: 23–27.

Shim H, Harris ZL (2003) Genetic defects in copper metabolism. J Nutr 133 (5 Suppl 1): 1527S–15231S. Review.

Sidransky E (2004) Gaucher disease: complexity in a "simple" disorder. Mol Genet Metab 83: 6–15.

Simonsz H, Barlocher K, Rotig A (1992) Kearns-Sayre's syndrome developing in a boy who survived Pearson's syndrome caused by mitochondrial DNA deletion. Doc Ophthalmol 82: 73–79.

Spinazzola A, Viscomi C, Fernandez-Vizarra E, Carrara F, D'Adamo P, Calvo S, Marsano RM, Donnini C, Weiher H, Strisciuglio P, Parini R, Sarzi E, Chan A, DiMauro S, Rotig A, Gasparini P, Ferrero I, Mootha VK, Tiranti

V, Zeviani M (2006) MPV17 encodes an inner mito-chondrial membrane protein and is mutated in infan-tile hepatic mitochondrial DNA depletion. Nature Genet 38: 570–575.

Stolzel U, Kostler E, Schuppan D, Richter M, Wollina U, Doss MO, Wittekind C, Tannapfel A (2003) He-mochromatosis (HFE) gene mutations and response to chloroquine in porphyria cutanea tarda. Arch Dermatol 139: 309–313.

Tiranti V, D'Adamo P, Briem E, Ferrari G, Mineri R, Lamantea E, Mandel H, Balestri P, Garcia-Silva MT, Vollmer B, Rinaldo P, Hahn SH, Leonard J, Rahman S, Dionisi-Vici C, Garavaglia B, Gasparini P, Zeviani M (2004) Ethylmalonic encephalopathy is caused by mutations in ETHE1, a gene encoding a mitochondrial matrix protein. Am J Hum Genet 74: 239–252.

Titorenko VI, Mullen RT (2006) Peroxisome biogenesis: the peroxisomal endomembrane system and the role of the ER. J Cell Biol 174: 11–17.

Tritschler H-J, Andreetta F, Moraes CT, Bonilla E, Arnaudo E, Danon MJ (1992) Mitochondrial myopathy of childhood associated with depletion of mitochondrial DNA. Neurology 42: 209–217.

Tulinius M, Oldfors A, Holme E, Larsson N, Houshmand M, Fahleson P, Sigstrom L, Kristiansson B (1995) Atypical presentation of multisystem disorders in two girls with mitochondrial DNA deletions. Eur J Ped 154: 35–42.

Wallace DC, Singh G, Lott MT, Hodge JA, Schurr TG, Lezza AM, Elsas LJ, Nikoskelainen EK (1988) Mito-chondrial DNA mutation associated with Leber's hereditary optic neuropathy. Science 242: 1427–1430.

Wanders RJ, Tager JM (1998) Lipid metabolism in peroxi-somes in relation to human disease. Mol Aspects Med 19: 69–154.

Wanders RJ, Waterham HR (2006) Biochemistry of Mam-malian peroxisomes revisited. Annu Rev Biochem 75: 295–332.

Zappatini-Tommasi L, Dumontel C, Guibaud P, Girod C (1992) Farber disease: an ultrastructural study. Report of a case and review of the literature. Virchows Arch A Pathol Anat Histopathol 420: 281–290.

Zeviani M, Servidei S, Gellera C, Bertini E, DiMauro S, DiDonato S (1989) An autosomal dominant disorder with multiple deletions of mitochondrial DNA starting at the Dloop region. Nature 339: 309–311.

Zupanc ML, Moraes CT, Shanske S, Langman CB, Ciafaloni E, DiMauro S (1991) Deletion of mitochon-drial DNA suppression in patients with combined fea-tures of Kearns-Sayre and MELAS syndromes. Ann Neurol 29: 680–683.

# Chapter 72

# SKIN INVOLVEMENT AS A CLINICAL MARKER OF NEUROMUSCULAR DISORDERS

**Raffaele Falsaperla**

Unit of Pediatrics, University Hospital "Vittorio Emanuele", Catania, Italy

The skin and the muscular skeletal tissues, despite their different embryological origin (from ectoderm the skin and from mesoderm the muscle), can be affected at the same time in some neuromuscular disorders (NMDs). In particular, skin involvement may manifest at any stage of certain NMD: some NMDs with onset during the pediatric age could present with a selective and mild skin involvement such as occurs in Bethlem myopathy or more extensively and devastatingly such as in the form of Epidermolysis Bullosa simplex associated to muscular dystrophy.

This chapter will focus only on the forms of congenital and inherited NMDs with skin involvement without mentioning the acquired NMDs such as for example Dermatomyositys or Sjogren Syndrome. In many of such forms the skin abnormalities (coupled with the underlying neuromuscular anomalies) could represent a clue for suspecting or establishing a diagnosis.

The NMDs with skin involvement can be divided into two types depending on the primary anatomic localization of the neuromuscular involvement:

Type 1 – skin involvement in NMDs affecting primarily the *muscles*;
Type 2 – skin involvement in NMDs affecting primarily the *peripheral nervous system*.

## Type 1 – Skin involvement in NMDs affecting primarily the muscles

Muscular disorders (MD) usually share a clinical picture characterized by generalized hypotonia, weakness and hypo/areflexia in the four limbs (Fig. 1).

Here below I am considering those MD, which manifest at any stage of the muscular disease a concomitant skin involvement and I will focus on the molecular basis determining the co-occurrence of muscular and skin involvement.

## Congenital muscular dystrophies

The Congenital muscular dystrophies (CMDs) are an heterogeneous group of MD with onset in the first 6 months of life and a suggestive clinical pattern characterized by generalized hypotonia, weakness (Fig. 2) and joint contractures (Fig. 3). In the past, in order to make the diagnosis of CMD the histological pattern (at muscle biopsy) had to be either dystrophic (Fig. 4) or dystrophic-like; more recently, the dystrophic pattern at muscle biopsy is no longer considered an inclusive criteria because of the newly characterized forms of CMD with myopathic patterns (Fig. 5).

Several authors of review articles have proposed classifications for the CMDs. In 2004, Muntoni and Voit suggested the following scheme (Lopate 2007):

1) *Extra cellular matrix protein defects:*
   Laminin-alpha2-deficient CMD (MDC1A) (OMIM # 607855)
   Ullrich/Bethlem CMD (UCMD 1, 2, and 3) (OMIM # 254090)
2) *Integrin-alpha7 deficiency (ITGA7) congenital myopathy (OMIM # 600536)*
3) *Glycosyltransferase (abnormal O-glucosylation [O-linked mannose pathway-OMT] of alpha-dystroglycan)*
   Walker-Warburg syndrome (WWS) (or HARD ± disease; Hydrocephalus, Agyrya, Retinal Dyspla-

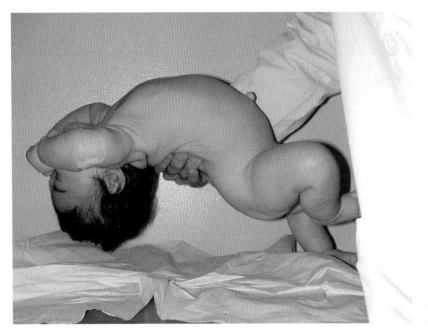

**Fig. 1.** A 3-month-old infant showing severe generalized hypotonia.

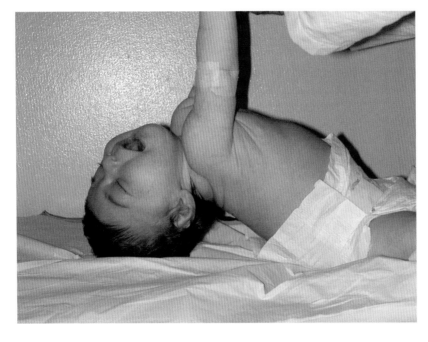

**Fig. 2.** A 3-month-old infant showing severe proximal weakness.

sia ± encephalocele) (OMIM # 236670) caused by mutations in the POMT1 (OMIM # 607423) and POMT2 (OMIM # 607439) genes; MEB (Muscle-Eye-Brain) disease (OMIM # 253380) caused by mutations in the POMGMT1 (OMIM # 606822) and in the FKRP (one patient so far; OMIM # 606596) genes (Taniguchi et al. 2003); Fukuyama CMD (FCMD) (MDC progressive with mental retardation) (OMIM # 253800) caused by mutation in the fukutin (FCMD) (OMIM # 607440) gene;

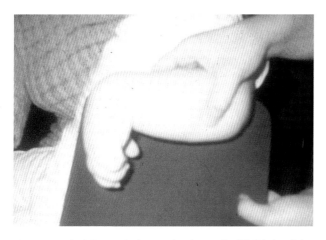

Fig. 3. A typical Congenital muscular dystrophy (CMD) sign: joint contractures.

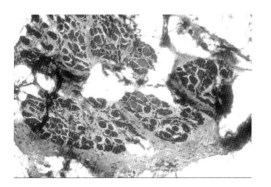

Fig. 4. Muscle biopsy: dystrophic pattern characterized by muscle-skeletal destruction with signs of necrosis and marked presence of connective tissue.

CMD plus secondary laminin deficiency 1 (MDC1B) (OMIM # 604801) with gene mapping on locus 1q42;

CMD plus secondary laminin deficiency 2 (MDC1C) (OMIM # 606612) caused by mutations in the fukitin-related protein (FKRP) gene (OMIM # 606596)

CMD with mental retardation and pachygyria syndrome (MDC1D) (OMIM # 608840) with mutations in the LARGE (OMIM # 603590) gene;

4) *Protein of the endoplasmic reticulum – Rigid-spine syndrome (RSMD1) (MCD merosin-positive with early spine rigidity)* (OMIM # 602771) with mutations in the SEPN1 gene (OMIM # 606210).

Initially, it was thought that in the CMDs there was an exclusive muscular involvement without Central Nervous System (CNS) involvement. Based on the data obtained from the most recent imaging and immunohistochemical studies (e.g., monoclonal antibodies staining: see Fig. 6) the CMDs have been subdivided into:

(a) Pure forms without gross CNS involvement;

(b) Forms with CNS involvement.

Among the *pure forms of CMD* is classified the **Ullrich congenital muscular dystrophy** (UCMD 1, 2, and 3) (OMIM # 254090). The UCMD is an au-

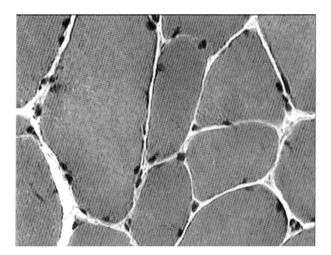

Fig. 5. Muscle biopsy: evidence of myogenic pattern with fibers variability.

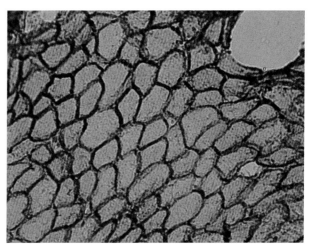

Fig. 6. Immunohistochemistry reveals a regular distribution of monoclonal antibody versus dystrophin staining.

tosomal recessive CMD caused by mutations in any of the three-collagen VI (COLVI or COL6) genes: COLVI A1 (OMIM # 120220) and COLVIA2 (OMIM # 120240) localized on chromosome 21q22.3 and COLVIA3 (OMIM # 120250) on chromosome 2q37. The onset of UCMD is extremely variable with clinical phenotypes ranging from congenital and severe hypotonia associated with kyphosis of the spine, torticollis, proximal limb contractures, hip dislocation and hyper extensibility of the distal joints to less severe clinical involvement allowing some patients to walk autonomously for a short time. Intelligence and brain magnetic resonance imaging (MRI) studies are normal as is the cardiac function. Unfortunately, respiratory involvement is common around the first-second decade of life, which impairs the quality of life leading to an unfavorable outcome. A common clinical sign, irrespective of the severity of disease, is skin involvement manifesting as rough skin consistent with follicular hyperkeratosis (Fig. 7). Additional signs of skin involvement are the formation of keloids and atrophic scars (one of the eponyms of UCMD is "Ullrich scleroatonic muscular dystrophy") (Kirschner et al. 2005). Recently, the milder (autosomal dominant) forms of UCMD have been classified as **Bethlem myopathy** (BM or be-

nign congenital BM) (OMIM # 158810) suggesting that UCMD and BM can be allelic variants of the same disease. From a pathogenic viewpoint, we know that the collagen VI microfilaments interact with the basal lamina by binding to transmembrane proteins such as integrins and NG2 proteoglycans and interacting with perlecan and decorin: in this extra-membrane network (*extra-cellular matrix*) the collagen VI micro fibrils are expressed either in muscular and cutaneous tissues. The UCMD/BM diagnosis is confirmed by low or absent signal using monoclonal antibodies directed against COLVIA1 on muscle or skin biopsy (Hicks et al. 2008). Some cases have been reported with normal COLVI expression on both tissues biopsy: this prompts the need for gene analysis in the three COLVI genes (Jimenez-Mallebrera et al. 2006). Some reports underline the need to utilize muscle MRIs for the differential diagnosis: patients with UCMD have a typical MRI pattern consistent of a diffuse involvement of the tight muscles sparing the sartorius, gracilis and adductor longus muscles (Mercuri et al. 2005). In contrast, the BM patients have a typical rectus femoris muscular involvement characterized by a central area of abnormal signal inside the muscles called "central shadow".

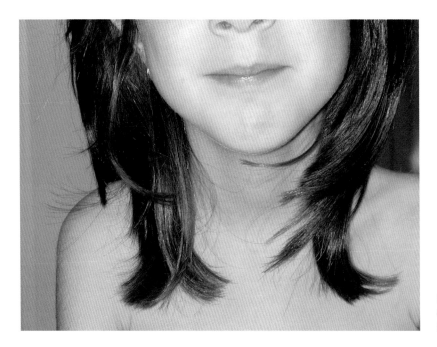

**Fig. 7.** A 7-year-old girl with Bethlem myopathy and rough skin secondary to follicular hyperkeratosis.

# Epidermolysis bullosa with muscular dystrophy (EB-MD)

**Epidermolysis Bullosa** (EB) covers a heterogeneous group of inherited (mechano-bullous) and acquired (autoimmune) disorders with one unifying diagnostic feature: fragility of skin with blister formation, following mechanical stress or trauma. The severity of skin involvement and association of extracutaneous findings produces a broad spectrum of clinical manifestations. The clinical complexity, compounded with a plethora of eponyms, has resulted in the identification of an enormous amount of different subtypes classified according to the initial site of blister formation (and the subsequent presence or lack of sequelae), and the structures and molecules involved primarily or secondarily. One of the most recently proposed classification system subdivided EB into three major groups: (1) intraepidermal (non-scarring) blistering EB; (2) sub-epidermal (junctional and dermolytic) EB; and (3) dystrophic (dermolytic, scarring) EB (Atherton et al. 2006). The major *non-scarring intraepidermal* types, EB simplex, EB herpetiformis, and epidermolytic hyperkeratosis, are caused by mutations in the keratins building up the keratinocyte cytoskeleton. The major *scarring or dermolytic* types, EB dystrophica, are caused by mutations in type VII collagen, the major protein of the anchoring fibrils, or by autoantibodies to these. The major *junctional types* (JEB), with blisters forming between the basal keratinocyte plasma membrane and the basal lamina, are caused by mutations in proteins specific for hemidesmosomes and lamina rara. Further proteins, their genes and mutations contribute to intraepidermal and JEB types (the reader is referred to a comprehensive review article by Atherton et al. 2006). In the inherited forms, the level of expression of the mutated genes along the basement membrane zone and extracutaneous tissues, the types and combinations of mutations, their positions along the mutated genes, and theirs consequences at the RNA and protein levels, when superimposed on individuals' genetic background, explain the enormous phenotype variability in this group of diseases.

Among the intraepidermal (non-scarring) blistering forms of EB there is a condition caused by anomalies of a large non-keratin phospho-protein,

**Table 1.** Myopathies with skin involvement

| Disease | Gene | Product | Inheritance | Phenotype | Skin involvement |
|---|---|---|---|---|---|
| UCMD/BM | 2q27 21q22.3 | COLVI | AD/AR | Congenital hypotonia Limb contractures Hyper extensibility of the distal joints | Keloid formation Atrophic scars Follicular hyperkeratosis |
| EB-MD | 8q24 | PLEC1 | AR | Congenital hypotonia Generalized weakness | Blistering of the skin Mild palmoplantar hyperkeratosis |
| POGL | 1q21-22 | LMNA | AD | Progeroid Syndrome | Scleroderma-like skin |
| HGPS | 1q21-22 | LMNA | AD/AR | Progeroid Syndrome | Thinning of skin |
| ASTC | 1q21-22 | LMNA | AR | Arthropathy Progeroid facies Micrognathia | Atrophic skin Chronic skin ulcers |
| MAD | 1q21-22 | LMNA | AR | Postnatal growth retardation Mandibular hypoplasia Osteolysis of clavicles Partial lipodystrophy | Acanthosis nigricans Mottled hyperpigmentation |

called *plectin* (from Greek: πλεχτιν, web or network) which belongs to the plakin protein family and shares sequence similarities with both desmoplakin and BPAG1. Plectin maps to chromosome 8q24 (human plectin gene PLEC1) and is expressed in a wide variety of tissues including stratified and non-stratified epithelia, muscle and central nervous system and turns out to be the most versatile cytoskeletal cross-linking protein. It interacts with intermediate filaments such as keratins, vimentin, desmin, or neurofilaments, with actin microfibrils, and with microtubules, linking them to each other as well as to plaque proteins of desmosomes and hemidesmosomes. In the epidermal basal keratinocytes of the skin plectin is predominantly localized to the inner plaque of hemidesmosomes and it is associated with the cytokeratin filaments of the plasma membrane (Takahashi et al. 2005). In the skeletal muscle co-localizes with the intermediate filaments such as the desmin in the Z-line structure. Plectin deficiency causes **EB simplex with Muscular Dystrophy** (MD) (EB-MD, MD-EBS or MDEBS; OMIM # 226670, formerly EBR4) also known as EB simplex and limb-girdle muscular dystrophy, a rare autosomal recessive disease characterized by generalized blistering of the skin with late-onset muscular dystrophy (Charlesworth et al. 2003). Blistering is localized on fingers and feet especially following physical trauma and is first noted at birth or early in the neonatal period, with gradual improvement but development of nail dystrophies, dental abnormalities, mild atrophy of the extremities and atrophic alopecia at adult age that are reminiscent of non-lethal JEB rather than EB simplex. At some stage of the disease there may mucous membranes (oropharyngeal, laryngeal and urethral) involvement. The muscular disease develops early in childhood or in the first years of life and mostly manifests not later than age 9 years, but sometimes only in adolescence or adulthood. Severely affected patients are finally wheel chair dependent (Koss-Harnes et al. 2004). Expressions of skin symptoms and of muscular dystrophy vary from mild to very severe, including early infant death. Immunohistochemical analysis shows a negative reaction versus plectin antibodies on skin and muscle, which is diagnostic for the disease.

## Laminopathies

The laminopathies are a heterogeneous group of genetic disorders caused by abnormalities in *lamins*, which are structural protein components (a class of intermediate filaments) of the nuclear lamina, a protein network underlying the inner nuclear membrane that determines nuclear shape and size (Jakob and Gark 2006). Three types of lamins, A, B, and C have been described in mammalian cells (OMIM 2007). Skin fibroblasts cells from many patients with laminopathies show a range of abnormal nuclear morphology including bleb formation, honeycombing, and presence of multi-lobulated nuclei (Jakob and Gark 2006). The laminopathies can manifest varied clinical features affecting many organs including cutaneous tissue, skeletal and cardiac muscle, adipose tissue, nervous system and bone (Capell and Collins 2006, Jacob and Gark 2006, Rankin and Ellard 2006). Mutations in the gene encoding lamins A and C (Lamin A/C or LMNA gene; OMIM # 150330) on chromosome 1q21.2 cause **primary laminopathies** (see below). The so-called **secondary laminopathies** are caused by mutations in the zinc metalloproteinase (ZMPSTE24) gene involved in post-translational processing of prelamin A into mature lamin A. The most recent classification distinguishes *autosomal dominant (AD)* and *autosomal recessive (AR) forms of* primary laminopathies.

The **AD forms** include Familial partial lipodystrophy of Dunnigan variety (FPLD), Puberty-onset generalized lipodystrophy, Hutchinson Gilford progeria syndrome (HGPS), Emery-Dreifuss muscular dystrophy (EDMD), limb-girdle muscular dystrophy (LGMD), dilated cardiomyopathy (DCM) type A and restrictive dermopathy.

The **AR forms** include EDMD, mandibuloacral dysplasia (MAD), Charcot-Marie-Tooth (CMT2B) and progeria-associated arthropathy.

### Autosomal dominant (AD) laminopathies due to abnormal type A lamins (LMNA)

**Dunnigan-type familial partial lipodystrophy** (FPLD). This rare disorder also known as **partial lipodystrophy type 2** (FPLD2) or familial lipodystrophy of limbs and lower trunk (OMIM # 151660), is characterized by atrophy of adipose tissue in the extremities with an excess fat accumulation on the face and neck. Affected individuals are born with normal fat distribution, but after puberty experience regional and progressive adipocyte disappearance from the upper and lower extremities and the gluteal and truncal regions, resulting in a muscular appearance with prominent superficial veins. Simultaneously, adipose tissue accumulates on the face and neck, causing a double chin, fat neck, or cushingoid appearance. Adipose tissue may also accumulate in the axillae, back, labia major, and intra-abdominal region. Acanthosis nigricans, hirsutism and menstrual abnormalities occur infrequently. Affected patients often may present profound insulin-resistant diabetes, hypertriglyceridemia and reduced level of high-density lipoprotein cholesterol (HDL). The neuromuscular and cardiac phenotype consist of incapacitating progressive limb-girdle muscular dystrophy, with calf hypertrophy, perihumeral muscular atrophy, and a rolling gait due to proximal lower limb weakness. In addition FLPD patients may have atrioventricular blocks.

**Pubertal-onset generalized lipodystrophy** (POGL). Currently there are only five reported cases in the literature with generalized lipodystrophy associated to LMNA mutations. In some cases features of an atypical progeroid syndrome including short stature, scleroderma-like skin, early graying of hair and severe insulin resistance diabetes has been reported.

**Hutchinson Gilford progeria syndrome** (HGPS). This severe progeria syndrome (OMIM # 176670), which is treated in details elsewhere in this book (see chapter 54, page 848), is characterized by precocious senility of a striking degree associated with short stature, early thinning of skin, loss of subcutaneous fat, alopecia and atherosclerosis. Affected patients usually die within the first decade of life often from coronary heart disease. A phenotype combining early-onset (prior to age 1 year) myopathy consisting in marked axial weakness and progeroid features is also caused by mutations in the LMNA gene: these individuals develop later growth failure, sclerodermatous skin changes, and osteolytic lesions.

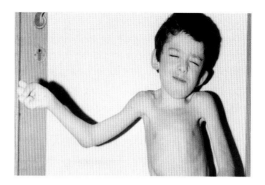

**Fig. 8.** An 8-year-old child with scapular hypotrophy and thorax asymmetry.

**Autosomal Dominant Emery-Dreifuss muscular dystrophy** (EDMD2). This is a rare AD form of MD (OMIM # 181350) with similar clinical features to the X-linked form of EDMD due to mutations in the emerin gene. In EDMD2 muscular involvement presents from 3 to 8 years and consists in early contractures of the Achilles tendons, elbows and post-cervical muscle with slowly progressive muscle wasting and weakness that involves the humero-peroneal distribution (see Fig. 8) and cardiac defects. Serum creatine kinase (CK) is not helpful in the diagnosis. For the majority of EDMD patients there is a high risk of ventricular arrhythmia. Few cases have been reported with isolated cardiac involvement.

**Limb-girdle muscular dystrophy** (LGMD). LGMD is characterized by weakness and wasting of shoulder and pelvic muscles due to necrosis and regeneration of muscle fibers. The LGMD caused by mutations in the LMNA gene mutation is called type 1B (LGMD1B; OMIM 159001). This form is a slowly progressive LGMD whose age of onset varies between 4 and 38 years old: affected patients have progressive symmetrical proximal weakness in the lower limbs and age-related cardiac involvement characterized by atrioventricular (AV) cardiac conduction disturbances. These cases benefit of pacemaker implantation.

**Dilated cardiomyopathy and cardiac conduction system defects**. Dilated cardiomyopathies (DCM) are characterized by a progressive ventricular dilatation with a marked ejection fraction (EF) reduction. The causes may be polygenic, viral and idiopathic but about half documented cases are familial. Mutations in several genes have been found to cause the familial forms of DCM (see OMIM # 115200): around 8% of these forms are due to mutations in the LMNA gene and may present with varying degrees and combinations of muscular dystrophy, partial lipodystrophy, and cardiomyopathy with conduction defects (conduction block and sinus block) (cardiomyopathy, dilated, with conduction defect 1 or CDCD1; OMIM # 115200). These patients are at high risk of sudden death and benefit of implantation of cardioverter-defibrillators (ICDs) rather than pacemakers.

**Restrictive dermopathy** (RD). Restrictive dermopathy also known as tight skin contracture syndrome (OMIM # 275210) is a lethal neonatal disorder in which tautness of the skin causes fetal akinesia or hypokinesia deformation sequence. The typical skin findings consist of shiny, rigid skin with multiple lacerations in the neck, limbs and trunk regions. It can be also caused by mutations in the ZMPSTE24 gene. Some patients with peculiar mutations show microretrognathia, sclerotic skin and joint contractures. There can be also associated hypoplastic clavicles and acro-osteolysis of terminal phalanges. Death usually occurs because of pulmonary hypoplasia and respiratory failure.

### Autosomal recessive (AR) laminopathies due to abnormal type A lamins (LMNA)

**Charcot-Marie-Tooth disease type 2B** (CMT2B). Charcot-Marie-Tooth (CMT) disease constitutes a clinically and genetically heterogeneous group of hereditary motor and sensory neuropathies, which is the most common cause of peroneal muscle atrophy. On the basis of electrophysiological criteria, CMT is divided into 2 major types: type 1 (CMT1), the *demyelinating form*, characterized by a motor median nerve conduction velocity less than 38 m/s; and type 2 (CMT2), the *axonal form*, with a normal or slightly reduced nerve conduction velocity. The AR

axonal CMT (CMT2B2) is caused by mutations in the lamin A/C gene. Onset is usually in the second decade with weakness and wasting of the distal lower limb muscles and lower limb areflexia. Motor nerve conduction velocities are normal or slightly reduced.

**Mandibuloacral dysplasia type A with partial lipodystrophy** (MADA). Mandibuloacral dysplasia (MAD) type A (MADA; OMIM # 248370) also known as craniomandibular dermatodysostosis is an uncommon disorders characterized by postnatal growth retardation, delayed cranial sutures closure, mandibular hypoplasia, osteolysis of clavicles (sometimes of the terminal phalanges too), joint stiffness and partial lipodystrophy type A. These patients have a crowing of teeth and peculiar skin abnormalities consisting in Acanthosis nigricans, mottled hypo- and hyper-pigmentation and loss of fat with secondary atrophy of the skin over hands and feet. A premature loss of teeth occurs in some patients as well as insulin resistance.

**Autosomal recessive Emery-Dreifuss muscular dystrophy**. Emery-Dreifuss muscular dystrophy (EDMD) is a relatively benign form of dystrophy, with onset in early childhood and usually only slowly progressive. The rare recessive form (OMIM # 604929), clinically, is characterized by myopathic changes in certain skeletal muscles: the patients have a motor delay due to early, severe contractures in the neck, elbows and Achilles tendons; slowly progressive muscle wasting and weakness with a humero-peroneal distribution; and a cardiomyopathy usually presenting as cardiac conduction defects (Chaouch et al. 2003). There is no skin involvement and cardiac involvement usually becomes evident as muscle weakness progresses but may exceptionally occur before there is any significant weakness (Emery 2002).

**Arthropathy syndrome with tendineous calcification** (ASTC). This peculiar and rare syndrome has a late onset (around 30 years of age) with cataract associated to arthropathy, chronic skin ulcers, progeroid facies and micrognathia. Usually these patients have generalized lipodystrophy with atrophic skin and tendineous calcifications.

## Type 2 – skin involvement in NMDs affecting primarily the peripheral nervous system

In this section I will discuss the motor and sensory neuropathies involving the axon or the myelin and the reflex sympathetic dystrophies with associated skin findings.

## Hereditary motor and sensory neuropathy (HMSN)

The neuropathies are for the majority extremely heterogeneous genetic diseases called hereditary motor and sensory neuropathies (HMSN). The oldest neuropathy discovered has been **Charcot-Marie-Tooth** (CMT), which determines a peculiar clinical sign consisting in early and selective peroneal muscular atrophy. On the basis of electrophysiological criteria, CMT is divided into 2 major types (see also above): type 1 (CMT1), the *demyelinating form*, characterized by a motor median nerve conduction velocity

**Table 2.** Neuropathies with skin involvement

| Disease | Gene | Locus | Inheritance | Phenotype | Skin involvement |
|---|---|---|---|---|---|
| CMT1 | GBJ3 | 1p35.1 | AD/AR | Distal muscular hypotrophy Deafness | Erythematous patches Hyperkeratosis of the skin |
| CMT2B | RAB7 | 3q21.3 | AD | Adult onset Muscle weakness Severe sensory lost | Recurrent foot ulcerations |
| HSAN1 | SPTLC1 | 9q22.2 | AD | Adult onset Sensory lost in distal parts Minimal autonomic involvement Deafness | Rarely |
| HSAN2 | HSN2 | 12p13.3 | AR | Childhood onset Severe sensory lost Motor symptoms | Trophic abnormalities leading amputations |
| HSAN3 | IKBKAP | 9q31 | AR | Congenital onset Severe autonomic dysfunction Loss of pain and temperature Mild motor deficit | Rarely |
| HSAN4 | NTRK | 1q21-22 | AR | Congenital onset Anhidrosis Mental retardation | Self-mutilating behavior |
| HSAN5 | NGFB | 1p13.1 | AR | Childhood onset Loss of temperature Deep pain perceptions | Trophic dysfunctions |
| POEMS Syndrome | ? | ? | ? | Sensory and motor neuropathy | Hyperpigmention Hypertrichosis Scleroderma |
| Sympathetic skin dystrophy (SSR) | ? | ? | ? | Severe pain Autonomic vasomotor dysfunction Mobility loss of the affected extremity | Trophic dysfunctions |

less than 38 m/s; and type 2 (CMT2), the *axonal form*, with a normal or slightly reduced nerve conduction velocity.

Here below I will focus only on the forms with concurrent skin involvement. One of these forms is the so-called **connexin 31 deficiency** (CMT-CX31) (Di Wei-Li et al. 2002), which is characterized by the association of neurosensorial hearing impairment and erythrokeratodermia variabilis (EKV) (Hohl 2000). The gene, known as GJB3 and its protein products (connexins) are expressed not only in the cochlea and in the auditory and sciatic nerves but also in the human epidermis (Lopez-Bigas et al. 2001). The EKV manifests as thickening of the palmo-plantar epidermis, symmetrical distributed fixed hyperkeratotic plaques and transient erythematous areas. The skin hyperactivity is triggered by trauma or changes in temperature.

Another form is the autosomal dominant for of CMT type 2B (**CMT2B**; OMIM # 600802) with onset in the second or third decades of life. In this form affected individuals experience weakness and wasting associated to severe distal sensory abnormalities (similar to those seen in common disorders such as diabetes mellitus or toxic exposures): subsequently, they may present recurrent foot ulcerations which may never heal leading to digits or limb amputations. Spontaneous shooting or lancinating pain is rarely observed. The CMT2B gene, known as RAB7, is localized on chromosome 3q21.3 and belongs to the RAB family proteins involved in vesicular transport between late endosomes and lysosomes.

## Hereditary sensory and autonomic neuropathies (HSAN)

The hereditary sensory and autonomic neuropathies (**HSAN**) are a genetically and clinically heterogeneous group of neuropathies characterized by loss of pain sensation and autonomic abnormalities. All HSAN present an exclusive involvement of the small diameter C and A delta fibers, which transmit pain sensation. The HSAN despite involving different genes have a common clinical pattern consisting in painless burns

and finger and toe mutilation presenting at different ages. The HSAN are currently subdivided into 5 types numbered by Roman numbers (I–V).

The **HSAN type I** (**HSANI**) (OMIM # 162400) is an AD form with onset within the second or third decade. The sensory abnormalities (involving sense of pain, touch, heat and cold) are predominantly distributed in distal localizations ("burning feet") with severe crises of shooting pain similar to the lightning pains of tabes dorsalis. Skin involvement consists in foot ulcers complicated in some cases by osteomyelitis. Motor involvement is variable but commonly there is distal muscle wasting and weakness. Bilateral deafness progressing to total deafness over several years is also observed. Sweating is the most frequent autonomic disturbance. At autopsy the brain is small with marked loss of ganglion cells in the sacral and lumbar dorsal root ganglia. The HSAN1 locus has been mapped to chromosome 9q22.1–q22.3: its protein product is a serine palmitoyltransferase (SPTLC1) an enzyme that catalyzes the first step in the biosynthesis of sphingolipids. A form of HSAN has been described (**HSAN1B**) without skin involvement and high frequency of cough phenomena secondary to severe gastroesophageal reflux.

The **HSAN type II** (**HSANII**) (OMIM # 201300), inherited in an AR pattern, presents during infancy or early childhood. In this type of neuropathy sensory abnormalities (e.g., numbness aggravated by cold; reduced or lost sensation to touch, pain, and temperature, with touch most severely affected) are predominant (and usually localized distally from the elbows to the fingertips and from above the knees down to the toes with a "glove and stocking" distribution) as compared to motor and autonomic disturbances. Ulcerations and infections cause spontaneous amputation of digits and surgical amputation (the condition is also known as neurogenic acro-osteolysis). The gene is localized to chromosome 12p.13.3 and the protein product is called HSN2.

**HSAN type III** (**HSAN III**) (OMIM # 223900) is an AR neuropathy peculiar for its congenital onset: it is also called familial dysautonomia (FD) or Riley-Day Syndrome, for the preponderant autonomic disturbances including alacrimia, vasomotor instability, episodic hypertension, hyperhidrosis, cyclic vomiting, skin blotching and relative indifference to pain and temperature. Notably, affected patients have associated feeding difficulties and a higher frequency of elevated body temperature. Typically there is absence of fungiform papillae on the tongue, dysmorphic signs and skeletal abnormalities. Motor deficits are mild and are typically associated to hyporeflexia in the four limbs. More than half patients die before age 30 years. Histologically, there is severe loss of unmyelinated fibers and total absence of large diameter myelinated fibers. Autopsy findings show demyelination in the medulla, pontine reticular formation, and dorsolongitudinal tracts and degeneration, pigmentation, and loss of cells in autonomic ganglia. The gene has been mapped on chromosome 9q31 and its protein product is the inhibitor of kappa light polypeptide enhancer in B-cells, kinase complex associated protein (IKBKAP). Interestingly, almost all affected patients (>99.5%) harbor the same splice site mutations caused by skipping of exon 20, which produces a truncated protein.

The **HSAN type IV (HSAN IV)** (OMIM # 256800) is a rare AR neuropathy called also congenital insensitivity to pain with anhidrosis (**CIPA**). The gene is localized on chromosome 1q21-22 and the protein product is a neurotrophic tyrosine kinase (NTRK1), which is crucial (along with NGF) in the development and function of the nociceptive reception system, as well as establishment of thermal regulation via sweating in humans. Mental retardation and self-mutilating behavior are also associated (Karkashan et al. 2002). Generalized anhidrosis can lead to febrile episodes caused by heat intolerance. Pain insensitivity usually manifest as biting of the tongue and hands with inability to sweat. Skin biopsy shows absence of epidermal and dermal innervations to the skin appendages such as for example the sweat glands.

There are two different **HSAN type V (HSAN V)** (OMIM # 608654) both inherited as AR diseases: (1) one caused by mutations in the nerve grow factor beta (NGFB) localized on chromosome 1p13.1 with childhood-onset (also known as congenital insensitivity to pain); and (2) a congenital onset form caused by mutations in the NTRK1 gene localized on chromosome 1q21-22. In contrast to

HSAN IV, HSAN V caused by abnormalities in the NGFB gene has less prominent anhidrosis with no mental retardation.

## Miscellaneous conditions

In this group are considered the syndromes not fitting into the two previous groups, which associate a neuropathy with skin changes.

One of these is the **POEMS Syndrome** characterized by polyneuropathy, organomegaly, endocrinopathy, monoclonal gammopathy and skin abnormalities (Eidner et al. 2001). This Syndrome is

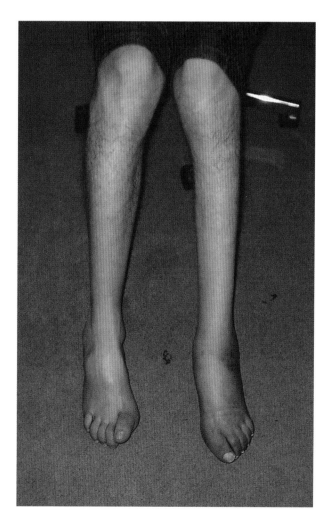

**Fig. 9.** A 30-year-old patient with Sympathetic skin dystrophy (SSD) and atrophic skin abnormalities localized to lower limbs.

a very rare, particularly outside the Japan, plasma cell disease with multi-organ involvement. It has different eponyms such as Crow-Fukase syndrome or Takatsuki syndrome. The syndrome can present as a connective tissue disease with scleroderma-like skin thickening. The skin involvement is characterized by hyperpigmentation, hypertrichosis and scleroderma. The involvement of the peripheral nervous system is consistent with a sensorial and motor neuropathy. The neuropathy was named by Vital et al. (2003) "axonal degeneration and primary degeneration". In a minority of POEMS patients have been observed on nerve biopsies uncompacted myelin lamellae (UMLs). The UMLs are located in the outer or inner part of the myelin sheath or more rarely in its middle part.

The **Sympathetic skin dystrophy** (SSD) is a complex phenomenon characterized by severe pain, autonomic vasomotor dysfunction and mobility loss in the affected extremity. The pathogenesis is not fully understood and several hypotheses have been raised. Certainly the abnormality is localized to the autonomic nervous system and it is related to hyperactivity (Bolel et al. 2006). Different methods have been used for the diagnosis including pletismography, sweating test, laser Doppler flow meter, thermography and the sympathetic skin response. In particular the latter technique is not easy as evaluates the amplitude and the latency differences with control patients. The disease can be divided into three phases: (1) the acute stage (Stage I); (2) the dystrophic phase (Stage II); and (3) the atrophic stage (Stage III). The typical abnormalities of their atrophic skin are localized to the lower limbs (see Fig. 9).

# References

Atherton DJ, Mellerio JE, Denyer JE (2006) Epidermolysis bullosa. In: Harper J, Oranje A, Prose N (eds.) Textbook of Pediatric dermatologo, 2nd ed. Oxford: Blackwell Science, pp. 1271–1303.

Bolel K, Hizmetli S, Akyuz A (2006) Sympathetic skin responses in reflex sympathetic dystrophy. Rheumatol Int 26: 788–791.

Capell BC, Collins FS (2006) Human laminopathies: nuclei gone genetically awry. Nat Rev Genet 7: 940–952.

Chaouch M, Allal Y, De Sandre-Giovannoli A, Vallat JM, Amer-el-Khedoud A, Kassouri N, Chaouch A, Sindou P, Hammadouche T, Tazir M, Levy N, Grid D (2003) The phenotypic manifestations of autosomal recessive axonal Charcot-Marie-Tooth due to a mutation in Lamin A/C gene. Neuromuscul Disord 13: 60–67

Charlesworth A, Gagnoux-Palacios L, Bonduelle M, Ortonne JP, De Raeve L, Meneguzzi G (2003) Identification of a lethal form of epidermolysis bullosa simplex associated with a homozygous genetic mutations in plectin. J Invest Dermatol 121: 1344–1348.

Di Wei-Li, Monypenny J, Common J, Kennedy C, Holland K, Leigh I, Rugg E, Zicha D, Keisell D (2002) Defective trafficking and cell death is characteristic of skin disease-associated connexion 31 mutations. Human Mol Genet 11: 2005–2014.

Eidner T, Oelzner P, Ebhardt H, Kosmehl H, Stein G, Hein G (2001) Clinical manifestation of POEMS Syndrome with features of connective tissue disease. Clin Theumatol 20: 70–72.

Hicks D, Lampe AK, Barresi R, Charlton R, Fiorillo C, Bonnemann CG, Hudson J, Sutton R, Lochmüller H, Straub V, Bushby K (2008) A refined diagnostic algorithm for Bethlem myopathy. Neurology 70: 1192–1199.

Hohl D (2000) Towards a better classification of erythrokeratodermias. Br J Dermatol 143: 1133–1137.

Jacob K, Garg A (2006) Laminopathies: multisystem dystrophy syndromes. Mol Genet Metab 87: 289–302.

Jimenez-Mallebrera C, Maioli MA, Kim J, Brown SC, Feng L, Lampe AK, Bushby K, Hicks D, Flanigan KM, Bonnemann C, Sewry CA, Muntoni F (2006) A comparative analysis of collagen VI production in muscle, skin and fibroblast from 14 Ullrich congenital muscular dystrophy patients with dominant and recessive COL6A mutations. Neuromuscul Disord 16: 571–582.

Karkashan E, Joharji HS, Al-Harbi NN (2002) Congenital Insensitivity to pain in four related Saudi families. Pediatr Dermatol 19: 333–335.

Kirschner J, Hausser I, Zou Y, Schreiber G, Christen HJ, Brown SC, Anton-Lamprecht I, Muntoni F, Hanefeld F, Bönnemann CG (2005) Ullrich congenital muscular dystrophy: connective tissue abnormalities in the skin support overlap with Ehlers-Danlos syndromes. Am J Med Genet A 132: 296–301.

Koss-Harnes D, Høyheim B, Jonkman MF, de Groot WP, de Weerdt CJ, Nikolic B, Wiche G, Gedde-Dahl T Jr (2004) Life-long course and molecular characterization of the original Dutch family with epidermolysis bullosa simplex with muscular dystrophy due to a homozygous novel plectin point mutation. Acta Derm Venereol 84: 124–131.

Lopate G (2006) Congenital muscular dystrophy. E-medicine from the WebMD. http://www.emedicine.com/neuro/topic549.htm

Lopez-Bigas N, Olive M, Rabionet R, Ben-David O, Martinez-Matos JA, Bravo O, Banchs I, Volpini V, Gasparini P, Avraham KB, Ferrer I, Arbones ML, Estivill X (2001) Connexin 31 (GBJ3) is expressed in the peripheral and auditory nerves and causes neuropathy and hearing impairment. Hum Mol Genet 10: 947–952.

Mercuri E, Lampe A, Allsop J, Knight R, Pane M, Kinali M, Bonnemann C, Flanigan K, Lapini I, Bushby K, Pepe G, Muntoni F (2005) Muscle MRI in Ullrich congenital muscular dystrophy and Bethlem myopathy. Neuromusc Disord 15: 303–310.

Muntoni F, Voit T (2004) The congenital muscular dystrophies in 2004: a century of exciting progress. Neuromuscul Disord 14: 635–649.

OMIM™ (2007) Online mendelian inheritance in man. Johns Hopkins University. http://ncbi.nlm.nih.gov/omim

Rankin J, Ellard S (2006) The laminopathies: a clinical review. Clin Genet 70: 261–274.

Taniguchi K, Kobayashi K, Saito K, Yamanouchi H, Ohnuma A, Hayashi YK, Manya H, Jin DK, Lee M, Parano E, Falsaperla R, Pavone P, Van Coster R, Talim B, Steinbrecher A, Straub V, Nishino I, Topaloglu H, Voit T, Endo T, Toda T (2003) Worldwide distribution and broader clinical spectrum of muscle-eye-brain disease. Hum Mol Genet 12: 527–534.

Takahashi Y, Rouan F, Uitto J, Ishida-Yamamoto A, Iizuka H, Owaribe K, Tanigawa M, Ishii N, Yasumoto S, Hashimoto T (2005) Plectin deficient epidermolysis bullosa simplex with 27-year-history of muscular dystrophy. J Dermatol Sci 37(2): 87–93.

Verpoorten N, De Jonghe P, Timmerman V (2006) Disease mechanism in hereditary sensory and autonomic neuropathies. Neurobiol Dis 21: 247–255.

Vital C, Vital A, Ferrer X, Viallard J, Pellegrin J, Bouillot S, Larrieu J, Lequen L, Larrieu J, Brechenmacher C, Petry K, Lagueny A (2003) Crow-Fukase (POEMS) syndrome: a study of peripheral nerve biopsy in five new cases. J Per Nerv Syst 8: 136–144.

# SUBJECT INDEX

Page numbers in **bold** denote main discussions: these may include, definition, history, incidence, clinical features, diagnosis, pathology, molecular genetics, prognosis, etc.
Numbers in *italics* refers to *tables* and *figures.*
*vs* denotes differential diagnosis

# Q

# R